AF352399

Neuroimaging of Sleep and Sleep Disorders

Neuroimaging of Sleep and Sleep Disorders

Edited by

Eric Nofzinger
The founder, Chief Medical Officer and founding CEO of Cerêve, Pittsburgh PA, USA

Pierre Maquet
Cyclotron Research Centre, University of Liège, Liège, Belgium

Michael J. Thorpy
Director, Sleep–Wake Disorders Center, Montefiore Medical Center, and Professor of Clinical Neurology, Albert Einstein College of Medicine, Bronx, NY, USA

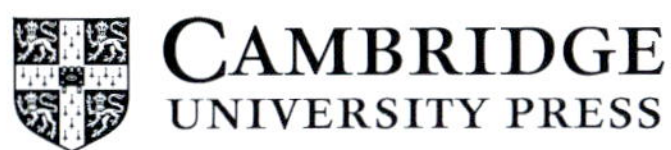

CAMBRIDGE
UNIVERSITY PRESS

CAMBRIDGE UNIVERSITY PRESS
Cambridge, New York, Melbourne, Madrid, Cape Town,
Singapore, São Paulo, Delhi, Mexico City

Cambridge University Press
The Edinburgh Building, Cambridge CB2 8RU, UK

Published in the United States of America by Cambridge University
Press, New York

www.cambridge.org
Information on this title: www.cambridge.org/9781107018631

© Cambridge University Press 2013

First published 2013

Printed and bound in the United Kingdom by the MPG Books Group

A catalog record for this publication is available from the British Library

ISBN 978-1-107-01863-1 Hardback

Contents

Section 4 Sleep and memory

Section 5 Neuroimaging of sleep disorders

Contributors

Mark S. Aloia PhD
Department of Medicine, National Jewish Health, Denver, CO;
Office of Medical & Health Affairs, Philips Healthcare, Andover,
MA, USA

Ellemarije Altena PhD
Department of Sleep & Cognition, Netherlands Institute for
Neuroscience, Amsterdam, the Netherlands; Department of
Clinical Neurosciences, University of Cambridge,
Cambridge, UK

Peter Anderer PhD
Department of Psychiatry & Psychotherapy, Medical University
of Vienna, Vienna, Austria

Christopher L. Asplund PhD
Neuroscience & Behavioral Disorders Program, Duke-NUS
Graduate Medical School, Singapore

Nitin Bangera PhD
The Mind Research Network, Albuquerque, NM, USA

Jeroen S. Benjamins PhD
Department of Sleep & Cognition, Netherlands Institute for
Neuroscience, Amsterdam, the Netherlands

Daniela Berg MD
Department of Neurodegeneration, Hertie Institute for Clinical
Brain Research and German Center for Neurodegenerative
Disorders (DZNE), University of Tübingen, Tübingen,
Germany

Bohdan Bybel MD FRCPS
Section of Nuclear Medicine, Health Sciences Centre,
University of Manitoba, Winnipeg, Manitoba, Canada

Vincenza Castronovo PhD
Sleep Disorders Center, University Vita-Salute San Raffaele and
San Raffaele Scientific Institute, Milan, Italy

Suk-tak Chan MSc PhD
Athinoula A. Martinos Center for Biomedical Imaging,
Department of Radiology, Massachusetts General Hospital,
Charlestown, MA, USA

Michael W. L. Chee MBBS FRCPEd
Neuroscience & Behavioral Disorders Program, Duke-NUS
Graduate Medical School, Singapore

Pietro Cortelli MD PhD
Department of Neurology, University of Bologna;
IRCSS Istituto delle Scienze Neurologiche di Bologna,
Bologna, Italy

Michael Czisch PhD
Max Planck Institute of Psychiatry, Munich, Germany

Joseph T. Daley MD PhD
Division of Sleep Medicine, Department of Medicine,
University of Pennsylvania, Philadelphia, PA, USA

Thien Thanh Dang-Vu MD PhD
Cyclotron Research Centre, University of Liège, Liège, Belgium;
Center for Advanced Studies in Sleep Medicine, Hôpital du
Sacré-Coeur de Montréal and University of Montreal,
Montréal, Québec, Canada

Yazmín de la Garza-Neme MD
Servicios Clínicos, Instituto Nacional de Psiquiatría Ramón de
la Fuente Muñiz, Tlalpan, México

Lourdes DelRosso MD
Division of Sleep Medicine, Department of Neurology, Louisiana
State University School of Medicine, Shreveport, LA, USA

Derk-Jan Dijk PhD
Surrey Sleep Research Centre, University of Surrey,
Guildford, UK

Maria Engström PhD
Center for Medical Image Science & Visualization,
Department of Radiology, Linköping University,
Linköping, Sweden

Thorleif Etgen MD
Department of Neurology, Kliniken Südostbayern – Klinikum
Traunstein, Traunstein, Germany; Department of Psychiatry &
Psychotherapy, Technische Universität München, Munich,
Germany

Bruce J. Fisch MD
Comprehensive Epilepsy Center and Neurodiagnostic Laboratories, Department of Neurology, University of New Mexico Health Sciences Center, Albuquerque, NM, USA

Ariane Foret MSc
Cyclotron Research Centre, University of Liège, Liège, Belgium

Patrice Fort PhD
INSERM, U1028; CNRS, UMR5292; Physiopathology of the neuronal networks responsible for the sleep-waking cycle, Lyon Neuroscience Research Center, University Lyon 1, Lyon, France

Steffen Gais PhD
Emmy Noether-Group "Memory Consolidation," General & Experimental Psychology, Ludwig Maximilians University Munich, Munich, Germany

Anne Germain PhD
Department of Psychiatry & Psychology, University of Pittsburgh School of Medicine, Pittsburgh, PA, USA

Jana Godau MD
Department of Neurodegeneration, Hertie Institute for Clinical Brain Research and German Center for Neurodegenerative Disorders (DZNE), University of Tübingen, Tübingen, Germany

Andrew L. Goertzen PhD MCCPM
Section of Nuclear Medicine, Health Sciences Centre and Department of Radiology, University of Manitoba, Winnipeg, Manitoba, Canada

William A. Gomes MD PhD
Department of Radiology, Albert Einstein College of Medicine and Montefiore Medical Center, Bronx, NY, USA

Ronald M. Harper PhD
Department of Neurobiology, David Geffen School of Medicine at UCLA, Los Angeles, CA, USA

Seung Bong Hong MD PhD
Department of Neurology, Epilepsy & Sleep Center, Samsung Medical Center, Sungkyunkwan University School of Medicine, Seoul, Korea

Romy Hoque MD
Division of Sleep Medicine, Department of Neurology Louisiana State University School of Medicine, Shreveport, LA, USA

Scott A. Huettel PhD
Center for Interdisciplinary Decision Science, Department of Psychology & Neuroscience, Duke University, Durham, NC, USA

Yuichi Inoue MD PhD
Department of Somnology, Tokyo Medical University, Tokyo, Japan

Alex Iranzo MD PhD
Neurology Service, Hospital Clínic, Institut d'Investigació Biomèdiques August Pi i Sunyer (IDIBAPS) & Centro de Investigación Biomédica en Red sobre Enfermedades Neurodegenerativas (CIBERNED), Barcelona, Spain

Mathieu Jaspar MPsych
Cyclotron Research Centre, University of Liège, Liège, Belgium

Zayd Jedidi MD
Cyclotron Research Centre, University of Liège, Liège, Belgium

Alejandro Jiménez-Genchi MD
Servicios Clínicos, Instituto Nacional de Psiquiatría Ramón de la Fuente Muñiz, Tlalpan, México

Eun Yeon Joo MD PhD
Department of Neurology, Epilepsy & Sleep Center, Samsung Medical Center, Sungkyunkwan University School of Medicine, Seoul, Korea

Gerhard Klösch MSc
Department of Neurology, Medical University of Vienna, Vienna, Austria

Karsten Krakow MD PhD
Asklepios Neurological Hospital Falkenstein, Königstein/Taunus, Germany

Rajesh Kumar PhD
Department of Neurobiology, David Geffen School of Medicine at UCLA, Los Angeles, CA, USA

Caroline Kussé MSc
Cyclotron Research Centre, University of Liège, Liège, Belgium

Hans-Peter Landolt PhD
Institute of Pharmacology & Toxicology, University of Zürich; Zürich Center for Integrative Human Physiology (ZIHP), University of Zürich; Neuroscience Center Zürich (ZNZ), University of Zurich and ETH Zürich, Zürich, Switzerland

Helmut Laufs MD
Department of Neurology and Brain Imaging Center, Goethe University, Frankfurt am Main; Department of Neurology, Universitätsklinikum Schleswig-Holstein, Kiel, Germany

Jeffrey David Lewine PhD
The Mind Research Network and Department of Neurology, University of New Mexico Health Sciences Center, Albuquerque, NM, USA

Camilo Libedinsky PhD
Neuroscience & Behavioral Disorders Program, Duke-NUS Graduate Medical School, Singapore

Michael L. Lipton MD PhD
Gruss Magnetic Resonance Research Center; Departments of Radiology, Psychiatry & Behavioral Sciences and Neuroscience, Montefiore Medical Center, Albert Einstein College of Medicine, Bronx, NY, USA

Mordechai Lorberboym MD
Department of Nuclear Medicine, Edith Wolfson Medical Center, Holon, Israel

Cheng Luo PhD
Key Laboratory for NeuroInformation of Ministry of Education, School of Life Science and Technology, University of Electronic Science and Technology of China, Chengdu, China

Pierre-Hervé Luppi PhD
INSERM, U1028; CNRS, UMR5292; Physiopathology of the neuronal networks responsible for the sleep-waking cycle, Lyon Neuroscience Research Center, University Lyon 1, Lyon, France

Paul M. Macey PhD
School of Nursing; Brain Research Institute, University of California, Los Angeles, Los Angeles, CA, USA

Pierre Maquet MD PhD
Cyclotron Research Centre, University of Liège, Liège, Belgium

Laura Mascetti MSc
Cyclotron Research Centre, University of Liège, Liège, Belgium

Christelle Meyer MSc
Cyclotron Research Centre, University of Liège, Liège, Belgium

Sarah Moens MSc
Department of Sleep & Cognition, Netherlands Institute for Neuroscience, Royal Netherlands Academy of Arts and Sciences, Amsterdam, the Netherlands

Vincenzo Muto MPsych
Cyclotron Research Centre, University of Liège, Liège, Belgium

Shadreck Mzengeza PhD
Winnipeg Cyclotron & PET Radiochemistry Facility, Department of Radiology, University of Manitoba, Winnipeg, Manitoba, Canada

Eric Nofzinger MD
Cerêve Inc., Allison Park, PA, USA

Takashi Nomura MD PhD
Division of Neurology, Department of Brain and Neurosciences, Faculty of Medicine, Tottori University, Yonago, Japan

Daniela Perani MD
Vita-Salute San Raffaele University; Department of Nuclear Medicine & Division of Neuroscience, San Raffaele Scientific Institute, Milan, Italy

Jennifer R. Ramautar PhD
Department of Sleep & Cognition, Netherlands Institute for Neuroscience, Royal Netherlands Academy of Arts and Sciences, Amsterdam, the Netherlands

Bernd Saletu MD
Department of Psychiatry & Psychotherapy, Medical University of Vienna, Vienna, Austria

Michael T. Saletu MD
Departments of Neurology; Department of Psychiatry & Psychotherapy, Medical University of Vienna, Vienna, Austria

Gerda Saletu-Zyhlarz MD
Department of Psychiatry & Psychotherapy, Medical University of Vienna, Vienna, Austria

Christina Schmidt PhD
Cyclotron Research Centre, University of Liège, Liège, Belgium; Centre for Chronobiology, Psychiatric University Clinics Basel, Basel, Switzerland

Monika Schönauer
Emmy Noether-Group "Memory Consolidation," General & Experimental Psychology, Ludwig Maximilians University Munich, Munich, Germany

Richard J. Schwab MD
Division of Sleep Medicine, Department of Medicine, University of Pennsylvania, Philadelphia, PA, USA

Sophie Schwartz PhD
Department of Neuroscience, University of Geneva, Geneva, Switzerland

Keivan Shifteh MD
Division of Neuroradiology, Montefiore Medical Center, Albert Einstein College of Medicine, Bronx, NY, USA

Sanjib Sinha MD DM
Department of Neurology, National Institute of Mental Health and NeuroSciences (NIMHANS), Bangalore, India

Victor I. Spoormaker PhD
Max Planck Institute of Psychiatry, Munich, Germany

Ryan P. J. Stocker MA
Department of Counseling Psychology, Chatham University, Pittsburgh, PA, USA

A. Jon Stoessl CM MD FRCPC FAANFCAHS
Pacific Parkinson's Research Center, University of British Columbia & Vancouver Coastal Health, Vancouver, BC, Canada

Diederick Stoffers PhD
Department of Sleep & Cognition, Netherlands Institute for Neuroscience, Royal Netherlands Academy of Arts and Sciences, Amsterdam, the Netherlands

A. B. Taly MD DM
Department of Neurology, National Institute of Mental Health and NeuroSciences (NIMHANS), Bangalore, India

Robert Joseph Thomas MD MMSc
Medicine-Division of Pulmonary, Critical Care & Sleep, Beth Israel Deaconess Medical Center, Boston, MA, USA

Michael J. Thorpy MD
Sleep-Wake Disorders Center, Montefiore Medical Center; Albert Einstein College of Medicine, Bronx, NY, USA

Emily Urry MSc
Institute of Pharmacology & Toxicology, University of Zürich; Zürich Center for Integrative Human Physiology (ZIHP), University of Zürich, Zürich, Switzerland

Jason Valerio MD MSc
Department of Medicine (Neurology), University of British Columbia, Vancouver, BC, Canada

Ysbrand D. Van Der Werf PhD
Department of Sleep & Cognition, Netherlands Institute for Neuroscience, Royal Netherlands Academy of Arts and Sciences, Department of Anatomy & Neurosciences, VU University Medical Center, Amsterdam, Amsterdam, the Netherlands

Gilles Vandewalle PhD
Cyclotron Research Centre, University of Liège, Liège, Belgium

Hans P. A. Van Dongen PhD
Sleep & Performance Research Center, Washington State University, Spokane, WA, USA

Eus J. W. Van Someren PhD
Department of Sleep & Cognition, Netherlands Institute for Neuroscience, Royal Netherlands Academy of Arts and Sciences, Department of Integrative Neurophysiology, VU University and Medical Center, Neuroscience Campus, Amsterdam, Amsterdam, the Netherlands

Vinod Venkatraman PhD
Department of Marketing, Fox School of Business, Temple University, Philadelphia, PA, USA

Frederic von Wegner MD
Clinic of Neurology and Brain Imaging Center, Goethe University, Frankfurt am Main, Germany

Thomas C. Wetter MD MA
Sleep Medicine Center, Department of Psychiatry & Psychotherapy, Medical University of Regensburg, Regensburg, Germany

Dezhong Yao PhD
Key Laboratory for NeuroInformation of Ministry of Education, School of Life Science and Technology, University of Electronic Science and Technology of China, Chengdu, China

Foreword

The daily cycle of wake and sleep is a fundamental adaptation of vertebrates to their environment. Wake and sleep are each composed of two components. Wake is made up of active waking with an ongoing stimulus-response interaction, and quiet waking with reduced environmental interaction and activation of a set of specific cortical structures, often designated the default mode network. Sleep, long a biological mystery, became amenable to experimental investigation with the development of EEG. This was followed by a long and productive period in which REM sleep was characterized, demonstrating for the first time that sleep is an active process and that all components of sleep are more complex than had even vaguely been surmised. This left two important questions to be resolved. The first is the function of sleep. It was generally accepted that sleep was important, even essential, but how? The sledgehammer approach to the question was prolonged sleep deprivation over time, resulting in death of experimental animals and, in the human, a similar fate in fatal familial insomnia. In each instance, the events leading to death are similar and attributable to prolonged stress, not an informative result. Although these studies proved a point, the question, particularly for humans with our complex behavior dominated by language and verbal memory with the capacity for time binding, is not approachable by invasive experimental methods that can be used in animals. Equally important, how does the brain generate the complex states of sleep; how does this further inform us about adaptive waking behavior; and how are the brain mechanisms of wake and sleep affected in sleep disorders and other disease states?

Until relatively recently in this long saga, the answers to these questions were not approachable with the methodology available. There is an appropriate nineteenth-century German saying, *teknik ist alles* (technology is everything). Most major problems in neuroscience have been formulated long before answers are reached. In this case, solutions to the problem of understanding brain mechanisms of wake and sleep have become approachable using functional imaging methods that have evolved over the last 20 years. Advanced EEG methodology has provided functional maps, but a downside of this is that EEG analysis is restricted to surface cortex, a serious limitation. Other early techniques methods were Single Photon Emission Computerized Tomography (SPECT) and Positron Emission Tomography (PET). These have the shortcomings of limited spatial and temporal resolution. At the same time, structural and functional magnetic resonance imaging (MRI, fMRI) were developed, with an ongoing refinement of the technology. Another method with great potential, not yet fully realized, is Magnetoencephalography (MEG). The importance of these methods, particularly fMRI with its high spatial and temporal resolution, cannot be overemphasized. In another context, fMRI has become the essential methodology of cognitive neuroscience.

In this book, *Neuroimaging of Sleep and Sleep Disorders*, a detailed review is presented with a third alloted to methodology and data from normal individuals, and two-thirds to data from disease states. Three well-known authorities in the field are editors, and the authors also are well recognized for their work. No other publication is available that covers this topic and the topics covered are extremely broad. It might be argued that the field is so new, and growing so rapidly that this is not the time for such a book, but its very size rebuts that view. My judgment is that *Neuroimaging of Sleep and Sleep Disorders* is an invaluable compendium marking the status of the field as of 2013, and will be in every medical library and on the desk, near at hand, of every worker in the field.

Robert Y Moore, MD, PhD, MD (Hon)
Love Family Professor Emeritus
Department of Neurology
University of Pittsburgh

Preface

Sleep is still largely a mysterious state that is not well understood in terms of its function and purpose. New studies indicate that it is important not only for the brain, but also for the whole body, particularly as it regulates circadian gene activity that influences most body systems. In order to understand the physiology and pathophysiology of sleep, new techniques are being developed that include new imaging methods to tell us not only about the physical structure of brain regions that are activated or deactivated by sleep and alertness, but also to help us understand the neurotransmitter mechanisms involved. This book, *Neuroimaging of Sleep and Sleep Disorders* details the important advances in the imaging of sleep disorders that holds promise to help us understand the underlying physiology and pathophysiology of sleep that will also aid in the diagnosis of sleep disorders.

The chapters presented here represent the cumulative integrated knowledge to date from several key developments in science over the past six decades. First, since the 1950s, fuelled by seminal findings in the explorations of the nature of sleep, basic science research has led to a rich understanding of the neural underpinnings of the global states of consciousness defined largely by the EEG, including waking, NREM, and REM sleep. As a result of this research, sleep is no longer impervious to scientific study, but now is understood to be a rich tapestry and integration of discrete behavioral states, each with well-defined interactions in neural circuitry. Second, at the human level, sleep has been shown to play a fundamental role in human behavior, involving interactions between homeostatic, circadian, and cognitive functions. Third, a clinical field of sleep medicine has evolved that has defined how sleep is disrupted in humans, leading to significant detrimental impacts on function, resulting in human suffering. Much of this pathology and its manifestations involves how the brain functions either normally or abnormally in clinically recognized sleep disorders, such as the insomnias, sleep apnea, narcolepsy, and the parasomnias. Fourth, a field of cognitive neuroscience has flourished in which the brain is now understood, at its highest level of organization, to have regional brain specificity for particular behaviors and cognitive processes, such as motor behavior,

sensory processing, thought, and emotion. Much of this new knowledge has come from brain imaging studies performed during waking. Fifth, there have been enormous technical developments in ways to "image" the human brain, at both the structural and functional levels, such as MR imaging, PET, and fMRI, making possible the testing of hypotheses at a regional brain level in relation to human behavior, health, and pathology. This book represents the first major overview of the wisdom generated from these cumulative scientific developments toward the study of sleep and sleep disorders.

No previous book has been published that focuses solely on neuroimaging of sleep and its disorders. This book accumulates the most recently available information on neuroimaging and is written by top specialists in the field: radiologists, sleep disorders physicians, and sleep researchers, from the USA, Europe, Canada, and Japan. The chapters are arranged in five major sections: an introduction; neuroimaging of sleep and wakefulness; neuroimaging of sleep loss and circadian misalignment; sleep and memory; and neuroimaging of the sleep disorders. The introductory section comprises chapters on the neurophysiology and the role of neuroimaging of sleep, with chapters on the fundamentals and methodology of imaging techniques. The second section specifically presents the neuroimaging of the sleep wake states, including NREM, REM, and wakefulness. Sections 3 and 4 discuss the role of neuroimaging in the understanding of sleep deprivation, and assessment of the functional responses to sleep deprivation, and how sleep is affected by circadian processes, as well as the assessment of memory by neuroimaging techniques. Section 5 presents the available information on neuroimaging of the sleep disorders, including insomnia, hypersomnias, narcolepsy, sleep-related breathing disorders, and parasomnias that includes several case presentations and the neuroimaging of alerting and sedative medications.

This volume is intended primarily for sleep disorder specialists, sleep researchers, and radiologists; however, it is suitable for neurologists, psychiatrists, and any professionals and researchers interested in the interdisciplinary field of sleep medicine. It will be of use to neurology, psychiatry and radiology residents and fellows, clinical psychologists, advanced graduate medical students, neuropsychologists, house officers, and other mental health and social workers who want to get an understanding the physiology of sleep and pathophysiological and diagnostic features of sleep disorders.

We are greatly indebted to all the authors who have contributed to this book and are appreciative of the help from the staff of the University of Cambridge Press in getting this book in print so quickly, so that the contents are up to date and current. As findings in this area are rapidly advancing, it is anticipated that future editions of this volume, *Neuroimaging of Sleep and Sleep Disorders*, will take these developments into account.

Eric, Pierre, and Michael

The role of neuroimaging in sleep and sleep disorders

1

Eric Nofzinger

Introduction

This book, entitled *Neuroimaging of Sleep and Sleep Disorders*, is a timely collection describing state-of-the-art research related to imaging the brain, both structurally and functionally, in relation to the broad topic of sleep and its disorders. The work described represents the cumulative integrated knowledge to date from several key developments in science over the past six decades. First, since the 1950s, fueled by seminal findings in the explorations of the nature of sleep, basic science research has led to an incredibly rich understanding of the neural under-pinnings of the global states of consciousness defined largely by the electroencephalogram (EEG), including waking, non-rapid eye movement (NREM) and rapid eye movement (REM) sleep. As a result of this research, sleep is no longer a mysterious state of being, impervious to scientific study, but now is understood to be a rich tapestry and integration of discrete behavioral states, each with well-defined interactions in neural circuitry. Second, at the human level, sleep has been shown to play a fundamental role in human behavior, involving interactions between homeostatic, circadian, and cognitive functions. Third, a clinical field of sleep medicine has evolved that has defined how sleep is disrupted in humans, leading to significant detrimental impacts on function, resulting in human suffering. Much of this pathology and its manifestations involves how the brain functions either normally or abnormally in clinically recognized sleep disorders such as the insomnias, sleep apnea, narcolepsy, and the parasomnias. Fourth, a field of cognitive neuroscience has flourished in which the brain is now under-stood, at it's highest level of organization, to have regional brain specificity for particular behaviors and cognitive processes, such as motor behavior, sensory processing, thought, and emo-tion. Much of this new knowledge has come from brain imag-ing studies performed during waking. Fifth, there have been enormous technical developments in ways to "image" the human brain, at both the structural and functional levels, such as magnetic resonance imaging (MRI), positron emission tomography (PET) and functional MRI (fMRI), making possi-ble the testing of hypotheses at a regional brain level in relation to human behavior, health, and pathology. This book repre-sents the first major overview of the wisdom generated from these cumulative scientific developments towards the study of sleep and sleep disorders.

Basic sleep mechanisms and neuroimaging technology

Sleep is perhaps in a unique position for study via neuroimaging. Sleep is now understood to be a manifestation of the brain, and more specifically, the result of interactions in discrete neural networks that result in the global states of consciousness we recognize at the EEG level, those of waking, NREM, and REM sleep. Importantly, the study of sleep has brought to the forefront our understanding that brain function at a global level is not a static process, but rather evolves, in a rhythmical and highly regular manner across a 24-h cycle. In no other area of neuro-imaging research has the temporal domain of brain function taken on such heightened significance. It is now understood that it is not only important to know "what" is being imaged, but "when," and that the object of study from a neuroimaging stand-point changes dramatically based on this temporal variable. Imaging brain function in waking will produce dramatically different results than imaging during sleep. Within sleep, brain activity will be globally and regionally different if studying NREM or REM sleep, or even within these larger states, if one is focusing on some discrete aspect of NREM sleep or REM sleep, such as slow waves or rapid eye movements. Even within waking, we now understand that brain function changes significantly across a normal day, from morning to evening, or with varying degrees of alertness or sleep deprivation.

The field of neuroimaging has had significant advances in the past four decades. The advent of computed tomography, or CT, allowed visualization of brain structure in a living human. CT scans provided clarity on bony structures primarily but had less ability to define internal brain structures. Limitations of CT scanning included exposure of an individual to ionizing radia-tion and limited ability to detect brain tissue differences. The development of MRI, or MR scanning, allowed for the detection of more subtle changes in brain tissues and did not involve exposure of the subject to radiation. Applications of structural imaging to sleep and sleep disorders, primarily using MR methods have defined brain structural changes that are related to pathophysiology or consequences of suffering from a specific sleep disorder.

Greater insights into the mechanisms and consequences of sleep and sleep disorders have been achieved through advances

Neuroimaging of Sleep and Sleep Disorders, ed. Eric Nofzinger, Pierre Maquet, and Michael J. Thorpy. Published by Cambridge University Press. © Cambridge University Press 2013.

Table 1.1. Functional neuroimaging tools for sleep. This table outlines various functional neuroimaging modalities and their benefits/limitations for the study of brain processes during sleep.

	MEG tomography	fMRI	H$_2$^{15}O PET	^{18}F-FDG PET	^{99m}Tc-ECD SPECT	Receptor imaging
Measure	Electrical events	Blood flow	Blood flow	Metabolism	Flow/ Metabolism	5-HT, DA, ACh, GABA
Spatial resolution	10 mm	< cm	cm	cm	cm	cm
Temporal resolution	Milliseconds	Seconds	Min	10–20 min	Min	20–90 min
Sleep in scanner?	Yes	Yes	Yes	No	No	Waking
Other	Difficult in sleep Availability, expense	Noise, technically difficult in sleep	Repeated measures possible	Long half-life limits repeated measures	Repeatable in single night	Expensive, labor intensive

FDG = fluorodeoxyglucose; ECD = ethyl cysteine dimer; 5-HT = 5-hydroxytryptamine (serotonin); DA = dopamine; ACh = acetylcholine; GABA = gamma-aminobutyric acid.

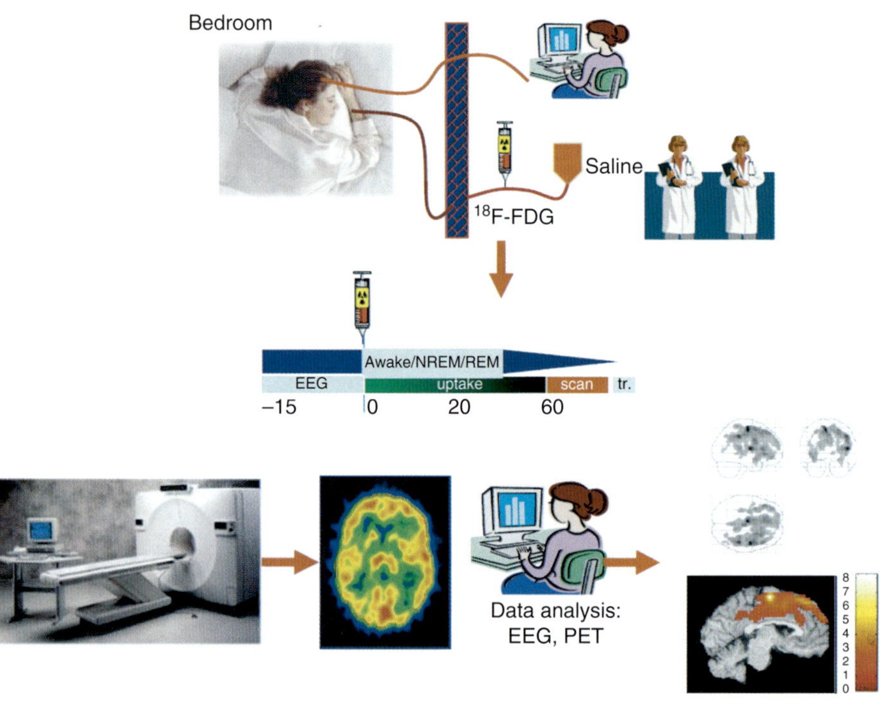

Figure 1.1 This figure depicts the application of the ^{18}F-FDG PET method for studying regional brain function during sleep. In this method (top of figure), the subject sleeps in a bedroom environment while recording equipment and technical staff for monitoring sleep and making radioisotope injections remain outside the sleeping environment in an adjacent room. The middle of the panel outlines the timing of injection and radioisotope uptake timing in relation to the temporal sequence of distinct behavioral states of waking, NREM or REM sleep. The bottom panel shows the PET scanning environment and data and image management that provide visualization of regional brain function during sleep.

in brain imaging methods that describe various aspects of neural "function." These are collectively referred to as functional neuroimaging. These include techniques such as PET, fMRI, single-photon emission computed tomography (SPECT), transcranial sonography, magnetoencephalography (MEG), low-resolution brain electromagnetic tomography (LORETA), and combined methods such as combined EEG and fMRI (Table 1.1, Figure 1.1). In each of these methods, there are assumptions between what the brain is doing (e.g., neuronal activity) and the measured process (e.g., changes in blood flow or metabolism). In most cases, these tools have been developed for the study of waking brain function and the assumptions underlying the measurements apply to waking brain activity. It is generally assumed, though probably not as rigorously validated as one

might like, that the assumptions between what the brain is doing and the measurement are similar across brain states of waking, NREM, and REM sleep. Additional research is needed in this area. Still, the applications of these methods for the study of sleep and its disorders, make up the bulk of the information related to neuroimaging of sleep and sleep disorders that we now know.

Neuroimaging of wakefulness and sleep

The earliest applications of neuroimaging to the study of sleep and its disorders were those of functional neuroimaging methods to study the global brain states of waking, NREM, and REM sleep (Figure 1.2). Prior to the application of these methods, knowledge of these gross behavioral states and their mechanisms

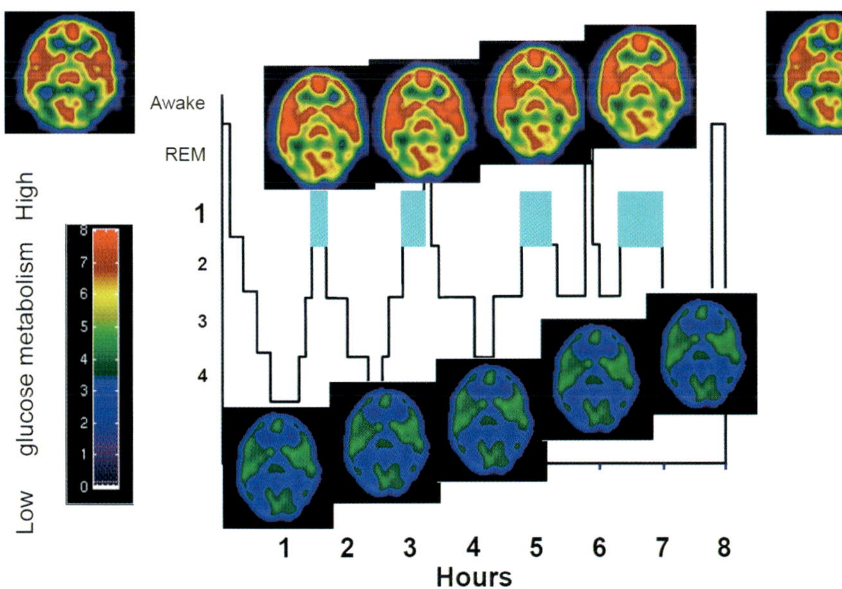

Figure 1.2 This figure depicts global changes in brain activity across the sleep/wake cycle. Global brain activity is highest in waking before and after sleep. Global brain activity is lowest in a 24-h cycle early in the night during slow wave sleep. In REM sleep, global brain activity, in connection with cortical activation at the EEG level, approximates, but does not reach, that of wakefulness. As viewed here, global brain function maintains dramatic cyclical variations in a regular manner across the sleep/wake cycle.

came largely from preclinical work. Basic science methods utilized existing neuroscience tools for assessing electrophysiology and the cellular and molecular mechanisms of sleep. The general understanding was that sleep/wake function could be defined by discrete global electrophysiological signals that differentiated various states of neural processing such as waking, NREM and REM sleep. Early brain imaging work during sleep, therefore, was somewhat exploratory and descriptive, defining large-scale changes in regional brain activity across these states of consciousness. As this had never been done before, the novelty of these early findings revolutionized our general understanding of human sleep in terms of the coordinated neural networks involved. While preclinical work had largely focused on the switches defining the regulation of sleep at a brainstem and hypothalamic level, the human sleep neuroimaging findings drew attention to the involvement or participation of higher levels of the central nervous system that likely play fundamental roles in the overall function of sleep. More recent analyses have focused on higher resolution temporal events such as phasic and non-phasic aspects of each individual state and validating neural changes in the brain as predicted from the preclinical sciences.

Neuroimaging and sleep loss and circadian misalignment

Aside from knowledge of the neural underpinnings of sleep derived from the preclinical basic science literature, there existed a long line of behavioral human sleep research that had defined the relationships between human sleep loss and performance. Extensive evidence defined both homeostatic and circadian influences on sleep and disruptions in either of these domains even in an otherwise healthy individual lead to predictable changes in alertness, cognition, and performance.

Extensive scientific progress in the area of chronobiology has also been made over the past quarter century, spawning a large academic and clinical discipline. The scientific investigation and understanding of these rhythms dramatically accelerated with the discovery of the suprachiasmatic nuclei (SCN) as the site of the biological clock [1, 2]. Extensive preclinical work has advanced our understanding of the molecular and genetic basis of circadian rhythms [3–10]. Although both photic and non-photic stimuli have been known to influence circadian rhythmicity in animals and man, light is considered to be the dominant synchronizing input [11].

Extensive applications of brain imaging have been made, largely functional neuroimaging, to help clarify the changes in regional brain function that result from perturbations in either homeostatic or circadian processes, and also have clarified the relationship between these brain changes and the behavioral consequences of these disruptions.

Sleep and memory

While disruptions in sleep were well recognized to result in changes in human behavior during waking function as measured by various performance and alertness measures, an extensive line of research was beginning to look at a potential role for sleep in terms of brain plasticity, or the capacity of the nervous system to change its structure, and its function, over a lifetime, in reaction to environmental diversity. Brain plasticity could include concepts such as synaptic plasticity, neurogenesis, and functional compensatory plasticity, concepts that had been evolving in the basic and cognitive neurosciences but previously had not been applied to the study of sleep. This area of research developed some of the most exciting hypotheses that sleep contributes importantly to processes of memory and brain plasticity. Over the past few decades, a large body of work, spanning most of the neurosciences, has provided a substantive body of evidence supporting this role of sleep in what is now known as sleep-dependent memory processing. This includes memory encoding, memory consolidation, brain plasticity, and memory reconsolidation. Extensive evidence from functional brain imaging studies support this emerging model of one of the critical functions of sleep.

Neuroimaging of sleep disorders

While disruptions in sleep are not new to humanity, significant attention to these disturbances as a public health concern worthy of medical attention and treatment has only emerged in the past four to five decades. Sleep medicine has only recently been recognized as a specialty of medicine. Its development is based on an increasing amount of knowledge concerning the physiology of sleep, circadian biology, and the pathophysiology of sleep disorders. Scientific progress combined with an increasing recognition that disorders of sleep are highly prevalent in society has led physicians to acquire knowledge necessary for the diagnosis and treatment of disorders of sleep. Centers focused on the evaluation and management of sleep disorders have developed only within the past quarter-century.

Sleep neuroimaging of sleep disorders has paralleled the development of this evolving field of medicine. Within the field of sleep disorders medicine, the polysomnographic evaluation of sleep has been the mainstay of the evaluation of sleep disruption and the effects of interventions. This is largely related to early work identifying discrete sleep stages and the evolution of sleep across a night based on electrophysiological markers of the global brain states of waking, NREM and REM sleep. Brain imaging methods can provide a needed additional breadth of knowledge in a new domain to the understanding of the neurobiology of discrete sleep disorders. Indeed, in some cases, such as primary insomnia, brain imaging studies have been shown to be more sensitive to defining pathology than traditional sleep EEG. The field of sleep neuroimaging holds promise for future use in clinical sleep medicine not only as a research tool to understand pathophysiology, but clinically in terms of diagnosis and prediction and monitoring of treatment effects. Future clinical applications will depend on advances in our understanding of individual disorders as well as technical refinements in imaging methods that should make them cost-effective and widely available for future use in sleep medicine.

Insomnia and circadian rhythm disorders

Insomnia is the most prevalent of all sleep problems. Insomnia is the subjective complaint of difficulty falling asleep, difficulty staying asleep, poor quality sleep, or inadequate sleep duration despite having an adequate opportunity for sleep. Importantly, EEG sleep alterations in insomnia are not always found in individuals with subjective complaints of insomnia. The leading neurobiological model of insomnia is that of hyperarousal. For instance, individuals with insomnia have been shown to have elevated temperature and muscle tone at sleep onset, elevated heart rate and elevated sympathovagal tone in heart rate variability, and positive correlations between wake time after sleep onset and urinary norepinephrine and dopamine metabolites [12–15]. Studies of whole-body metabolic rate, assessed by oxygen consumption, show elevated rates for individuals with insomnia compared to healthy controls, a difference that persists 24 h per day [16]. The hyperarousal of insomnia is supported by higher rates of self-reported ruminations and intrusive thoughts among insomniacs.

Perhaps among all the sleep disorders, brain imaging studies have been most helpful in elucidating the neural substrates of hyperarousal. An emerging body of evidence exists where there has been identification of regional brain alterations despite the relative absence of EEG sleep signs of the disorder. These findings hold promise that the use of brain imaging in this disorder can considerably advance our understanding of the disorder and lead to new mechanisms for treatment in a manner previously unattainable through traditional EEG sleep assessments.

Neuroimaging of central nervous system hypersomnias

Narcolepsy consists clinically of excessive daytime sleepiness in combination with cataplexy, a loss of muscle tone in response to laughter and other emotional stimuli. Some patients also experience paralysis or hallucinations at sleep onset and on awakening. A major breakthrough in our understanding of the neurobiology of this disorder occurred in the past several decades. In 1998, two peptides were identified in the hypothalamus and named hypocretin (Hcrt)-1 and Hcrt-2 [17], names reflecting their hypothalamic origin and homology to secretin. Almost simultaneously, another group of investigators independently identified the same peptides, which they named orexin-A and orexin-B, based on their appetite-stimulating effect [18]. These molecules arise from a precursor, preprohypocretin, synthesized by a small number of cells in the posterior and lateral hypothalamus, especially the perifornical area. They project to a diverse set of targets in the brain and spinal cord, especially the monoaminergic and cholinergic fields of the brainstem tegmentum comprising the ascending reticular activating system (ARAS) [19, 20].

Following preclinical findings regarding the role of the Hcrt system in narcolepsy, studies of narcoleptic patients revealed low or undetectable Hcrt-1 in the cerebrospinal fluid (CSF) of most (87%) patients with cataplexy and in some patients without cataplexy (14%) [21]. Clinical manifestations of the disease, such as cataplexy, appear to reflect a lack of Hcrt-mediated synaptic excitation of serotonergic and noradrenergic pathways normally responsible for REM sleep inhibition. The sleepiness of narcolepsy more likely reflects lack of Hcrt's excitatory influences upon histaminergic, dopaminergic, and cholinergic components of the ARAS, which normally function to promote thalamocortical arousal.

Brain imaging studies have been utilized in narcolepsy and the hypersomnias. Importantly, both structural and functional neuroimaging methods have been applied to the study of this disorder. While results to date have not been as clear as some of the preclinical genetic work in this disorder, this area remains fertile ground for future studies in understanding the neurobiology and behavioral manifestations of the disorder.

Neuroimaging of sleep-related breathing disorders

In 1965, Gastaut *et al.* documented repetitive episodes of upper-airway obstruction terminated by brief arousals that in turn fragmented nocturnal sleep in patients who subsequently would be referred to as having obstructive sleep apnea (OSA) [22]. It was postulated that sleep fragmentation was responsible for the excessive daytime somnolence observed in these patients. Subsequently, it has been determined that reductions in tidal volume (hypopneas) as well as increases in upper-airways resistance also produce sleep fragmentation and daytime sleepiness.

This major new concept in medical science stimulated considerable research in the area of sleep and breathing. An early discovery by Remmers *et al.* documented the relationship between intraluminal airway pressure and electromyogram (EMG) activity of the genioglossus muscle in the pathophysiology of upper-airway collapse in the pharyngeal segment of the airway, and tracheostomy was recognized as an effective treatment [23]. Later, Sullivan *et al.* demonstrated that the application of continuous positive airway pressure (CPAP) via the nose would prevent upper-airway collapse, normalize nocturnal sleep, and alleviate daytime hypersomnolence [24]. This latter discovery revolutionized the treatment of OSA and has resulted in the use of nasal CPAP as the most commonly used treatment of this condition.

This high prevalence in the population combined with evidence suggesting adverse cardiovascular consequences led to studies investigating these important relationships. Resulting publications established a clear association between sleep-disordered breathing and the development of hypertension, along with an increased prevalence of coronary heart disease, heart failure, and stroke at levels of an apnea-hypopnea index equal to or greater than five per hour [25–27]. Much of the growth of the field of sleep medicine can subsequently be attributed to the need for diagnostic and treatment centers to address the large population of individuals suffering from this disorder.

Brain imaging studies have rapidly evolved in the area of OSA syndrome. Brain MR studies have been performed to describe volumetric changes in discrete regions of the brain that may play a role in the pathogenesis of the disorder or as a manifestation of having OSA. MR studies have also been used extensively to define the anatomical abnormalities in the upper airways of patients with these disorders that contribute to the obstructed breathing. Functional brain imaging studies have demonstrated mechanisms related to ventilatory control in the central nervous system, the adverse consequences of sleep apnea on neural function, as well as their reversal with treatment with CPAP.

Neuroimaging of parasomnias

Parasomnias collectively refer to disorders of abnormal behavior during sleep. One of the most striking parasomnias is REM sleep behavior disorder (RBD), in which skeletal muscle remains active during dreaming, resulting in vocalization and sometimes violent activity of the arms and legs. The physiology underlying normal REM sleep atonia has been elucidated at the preclinical level and involves alterations in a descending motor inhibitory pathway from cells of the pedunculopontine nuclei that lie in close proximity to the primary REM sleep generator in the dorsal pons [28].

In humans, much interest has been generated because of the relationship between RBD and certain specific neurodegenerative disorders [29–35]. At least 50% of patients in large studies carry diagnoses of Parkinson's disease, multiple system atrophy, or dementia. There is also retrospective and prospective evidence that RBD may sometimes be the first manifestation of one of these neurological disorders, and thus at least some patients with apparently idiopathic RBD may with time evolve to develop a neurodegenerative disease. Most of the brain imaging studies in the area of parasomnias have explored these types of relationships through both structural and functional neuroimaging studies as well as in informative case studies.

Neuroimaging of other sleep-related neurological disorders

Much brain imaging work has been conducted in the area of restless legs syndrome (RLS) and periodic limb movements of sleep (PLMS). RLS may be one of the most common sleep-related disorders, with a prevalence as high as 10% [36]. Patients complain of severe discomfort in their legs while sitting or lying in bed, associated with an uncontrollable desire to move to obtain relief. Almost 90% of patients experience regular jerks of their legs while asleep, known as PLMS.

A range of studies using different methodologies has produced striking insights into the pathogenesis of the disorder. Pharmacological studies have indicated that levodopa and dopamine-receptor agonists are effective therapies for RLS, indicating that the disorder is associated with a decrease in dopaminergic function in the brain. Brain imaging studies in these disorders, then, have focused on the dopaminergic system via PET ligands in the dopamine system and functional brain imaging studies have focused on regions of the brain involved in motor behavior [37–39].

Another interesting development in understanding the pathogenesis of RLS is related to iron metabolism. Studies have revealed that RLS severity correlates with serum ferritin concentrations below 45 to 50 mg/l, values usually considered in the normal range [40, 41]. Low ferritin concentration in the CSF has been demonstrated in RLS patients with normal serum ferritin concentrations compared to controls, suggesting that low iron stores in the brain may be associated with RLS [42]. Functional imaging studies have therefore focused on assessing brain iron in regions of the brain related to motor behavior.

Neuroimaging of medication effects

Management of several sleep disorders is improved with pharmacological interventions. Examples include periodic limb movement disorders, narcolepsy, and the insomnias. Functional neuroimaging studies may provide important information regarding pharmacotherapy in several realms: drug development, assessment of mechanism of action of therapeutic compounds and assessment of treatment response/non-response to pharmacological agents.

A variety of compounds have been discovered with mechanisms of actions that may affect sleep/wake regulation. Testing in preclinical models suggest that these compounds may have novel mechanisms of action; however, the degree to which these mechanisms will translate into a clinical application are often unknown. Functional neuroimaging studies may identify the degree to which these compounds have beneficial mechanisms of action on brain structures that are known to regulate behavioral states in humans. One way of achieving this goal is to administer the compound to human subjects, then assess a functional neuroanatomical response to the compound within sleep in humans, such as a regional blood flow or metabolism. Further, these studies may help to determine the optimum dose of the compound in humans that maximizes beneficial effects of the compound, yet does not lead to adverse effects. The use of receptor ligands may clarify whether one compound has a unique mechanism of action on a specific receptor subtype that may not be shared by other compounds in its class and may therefore hold a therapeutic advantage over other agents. Finally, once a compound has been identified and shown to have effects in the central nervous system in humans, functional neuroimaging studies can then be used to determine the degree to which the compound reverses distinct alterations in neural function in a clinical population.

Future directions

The field of brain imaging in relation to sleep and its disorders has demonstrated significant promise in elucidating the basic mechanisms and functions of sleep and its disorders. As this knowledge base has evolved from multiple trends and disciplines in science and clinical sleep medicine, it is anticipated that new advances in each of these areas will lead to subsequent advances in brain imaging and sleep. It is anticipated that as technology for brain imaging evolves, these methods may eventually be utilized to generate new information regarding treatment mechanisms and will lead to the identification and prediction of treatment response and non-response in clinical sleep medicine. As increasing sample sizes evolve, results from these studies are anticipated to increase our ability to subtype individuals within a disorder based on regional brain function as opposed to an EEG criteria. It is anticipated that future brain imaging studies of sleep will evolve into a more dynamic understanding of brain function across the night. It will be possible not only to describe a person's sleep by means of EEG sleep staging but to categorize an individual's sleep on the basis of the evolution of regional brain function across the night in a type of 3-dimensional moving cerebrohypnogram, a visual movie showing how different regions of the brain are interacting across a night of sleep. Availability of this tool in future research and clinical applications is anticipated to revolutionize our understanding of sleep and its significance in all of human behavior.

Despite advances made to date, significant consideration should also be given to the development of a "Sleep Atlas" imaging resource to facilitate temporal and spatial comparisons of normal waking and sleep, and to assess the effect of factors such as age and cortical thickness across the entire lifespan. The resource would also facilitate functional imaging studies of those with sleep disorders and identifying the most important biological differences. This would be a significant improvement over existing neuroimaging atlases, which consider population variation but not sleep/wake differences in function.

References

1. Moore RY, Eichler VB. Loss of a circadian adrenal corticosterone rhythm following suprachiasmatic lesions in the rat. *Brain Res.* 1972;**42**(1):201–6.

2. Stephan FK, Zucker I. Circadian rhythms in drinking behavior and locomotor activity of rats are eliminated by hypothalamic lesions. *Proc Natl Acad Sci U S A.* 1972;**69**(6):1583–6.

3. Konopka RJ, Benzer S. Clock mutants of *Drosophila melanogaster. Proc Natl Acad Sci U S A.* 1971;**68**(9):2112–16.

4. Hardin PE, Hall JC, Rosbash M. Feedback of the *Drosophila* period gene product on circadian cycling of its messenger RNA levels. *Nature.* 1990;**343**(6258):536–40.

5. Hardin PE, Hall JC, Rosbash M. Circadian oscillations in period gene mRNA levels are transcriptionally regulated. *Proc Natl Acad Sci U S A.* 1992;**89**(24):11711–15.

6. Sehgal A, Rothenfluh-Hilfiker A, Hunter-Ensor M, *et al.* Rhythmic expression of timeless: a basis for promoting circadian cycles in period gene autoregulation. *Science.*1995;**270**(5237):808–10.

7. Darlington TK, Wager-Smith K, Ceriani MF, *et al.* Closing the circadian loop: CLOCK-induced transcription of its own inhibitors per and tim. *Science.* 1998;**280**(5369):1599–603.

8. Gekakis N, Staknis D, Nguyen HB, *et al.* Role of the CLOCK protein in the mammalian circadian mechanism. *Science.* 1998;**280**(5369):1564–9.

9. Sangoram AM, Saez L, Antoch MP, *et al.* Mammalian circadian autoregulatory loop: a timeless ortholog and mPer1 interact and negatively regulate CLOCK-BMAL1-induced transcription. *Neuron.* 1998;**21**(5):1101–13.

10. Kramer A, Yang FC, Snodgrass P, *et al.* Regulation of daily locomotor activity and sleep by hypothalamic EGF receptor signaling. *Science.* 2001;**294**(5551):2511–15.

11. Czeisler CA, Khalso SBS. The human circadian timing system and sleep/wake regulation. In: Kryger MH, Roth T, Dement W, eds. *Principles and Practice of Sleep Medicine*, 3rd edn. Philadelphia, W. B. Saunders Co. 2000; 353–75.

12. Freedman RR, Sattler HL. Physiological and psychological factors in sleep-onset insomnia. *J Abnorm Psychol.* 1982;**91**(5):380–9.

13. Monroe LJ. Psychological and physiological differences between good and poor sleepers. *J Abnorm Psychol.* 1967;**72**(3):255–64.

14. Bonnet MH, Arand DL. Heart rate variability: sleep stage, time of night, and arousal influences. *Electroencephalogr Clin Neurophysiol.*1997;**102**(5):390–6.

15. Vgontzas AN, Tsigos C, Bixler EO, *et al.* Chronic insomnia and activity of the stress system: a preliminary study. *J Psychosom Res.* 1998;**45**(1):21–31.

16. Bonnet MH, Arand DL. 24-Hour metabolic rate in insomniacs and matched normal sleepers. *Sleep.* 1995;**18**(7):581–8.

17. de Lecea L, Kilduff TS, Peyron C, *et al.* The hypocretins: hypothalamus-specific peptides with neuroexcitatory activity. *Proc Natl Acad Sci U S A.* 1998;**95**(1):322–7.

18. Sakurai T, Amemiya A, Ishii M, *et al.* Orexins and orexin receptors: a family of hypothalamic neuropeptides and G protein-coupled receptors that regulate feeding behavior. *Cell.* 1998;**92**(4):573–85.

19. Marcus JN, Aschkenasi CJ, Lee CE, *et al.* Differential expression of orexin receptors 1 and 2 in the rat brain. *J Comp Neurol.* 2001;**435**(1):6–25.

20. Kilduff TS, Peyron C. The hypocretin/ orexin ligand-receptor system: implications for sleep and sleep disorders. *Trends Neurosci.* 2000;**23**(8):359–65.

21. Nishino S, Ripley B, Overeem S, Lammers GJ, Mignot E. Hypocretin (orexin) deficiency in human narcolepsy. *Lancet.* 2000;**355**(9197):39–40.

22. Gastaut H, Roger J, Soulayrol R, *et al.* [Infantile myoclonic encephalopathy with hypsarrhythmia (West's syndrome) and Bourneville's tuberous sclerosis]. *J Neurol Sci.* 1965;**2**(2):140–60.

23. Remmers JE, deGroot WJ, Sauerland EK, Anch AM. Pathogenesis of upper airway occlusion during sleep. *J Appl Physiol.* 1978;**44**(6):931–8.

24. Sullivan CE, Issa FG, Berthon-Jones M, Eves L. Reversal of obstructive sleep apnoea by continuous positive airway pressure applied through the nares. *Lancet.* 1981;**1**(8225):862 5.

25. Peppard PE, Young T, Palta M, Skatrud J. Prospective study of the association between sleep-disordered breathing and hypertension. *N Engl J Med.* 2000;**342**(19):1378–84.

26. Nieto FJ, Young TB, Lind BK, *et al.* Association of sleep disordered breathing, sleep apnea, and hypertension in a large community-based study. Sleep Heart Health Study. *JAMA.* 2000;**283**(14):1829–36.

27. Shahar E, Whitney CW, Redline S, *et al.* Sleep-disordered breathing and cardiovascular disease: cross-sectional results of the Sleep Heart Health Study. *Am J Respir Crit Care Med.* 2001;**163**(1):19–25.

28. Hendricks JC, Morrison AR, Mann GL. Different behaviors during paradoxical sleep without atonia depend on pontine lesion site. *Brain Res.* 1982;**239**(1):81–105.

29. Olson EJ, Boeve BF, Silber MH. Rapid eye movement sleep behaviour disorder: demographic, clinical and laboratory findings in 93 cases. *Brain.* 2000;**123**(Pt 2):331–9.

30. Boeve BF, Silber MH, Ferman TJ, *et al.* REM sleep behavior disorder and degenerative dementia: an association likely reflecting Lewy body disease. *Neurology.* 1998;**51**(2):363–70.

31. Ferman TJ, Boeve BF, Smith GE, *et al.* REM sleep behavior disorder and dementia: cognitive differences when compared with AD. *Neurology.* 1999;**52**(5):951–7.

32. Boeve BF, Silber MH, Ferman TJ, Lucas JA, Parisi JE. Association of REM sleep behavior disorder and neurodegenerative disease may reflect an underlying synucleinopathy. *Mov Disord.* 2001;**16**(4):622–30.

33. Schenck CH, Bundlie SR, Mahowald MW. Delayed emergence of a parkinsonian disorder in 38% of 29 older men initially diagnosed with idiopathic rapid eye movement sleep behaviour disorder. *Neurology* 1996;**46**(2):388–93.

34. Eisensehr I, Linke R, Noachtar S, *et al.* Reduced striatal dopamine transporters in idiopathic rapid eye movement sleep behaviour disorder. Comparison with Parkinson's disease and controls. *Brain.* 2000;**123**(Pt 6):1155–60.

35. Albin RL, Koeppe RA, Chervin RD, *et al.* Decreased striatal dopaminergic innervation in REM sleep behavior disorder. *Neurology.* 2000;**55**(9):1410–12.

36. Phillips B, Young T, Finn L, *et al.* Epidemiology of restless legs symptoms in adults. *Arch Intern Med.* 2000;**160**(14):2137–41.

37. Ruottinen HM, Partinen M, Hublin C, *et al.* An FDOPA PET study in patients with periodic limb movement disorder and restless legs syndrome. *Neurology.* 2000;**54**(2):502–4.

38. Turjanski N, Lees AJ, Brooks DJ. Striatal dopaminergic function in restless legs syndrome: 18F-dopa and 11C-raclopride PET studies. *Neurology.* 1999;**52**(5):932–7.

39. Trenkwalder C, Walters AS, Hening WA, *et al.* Positron emission tomographic studies in restless legs syndrome. *Mov Disord.* 1999;**14**(1):141–5.

40. O'Keeffe ST, Gavin K, Lavan JN. Iron status and restless legs syndrome in the elderly. *Age Ageing.* 1994;**23**(3):200–3.

41. Sun ER, Chen CA, Ho G, Earley CJ, Allen RP. Iron and the restless legs syndrome. *Sleep.* 1998;**21**(4):371–7.

42. Earley CJ, Connor JR, Beard JL, *et al.* Abnormalities in CSF concentrations of ferritin and transferrin in restless legs syndrome. *Neurology.* 2000;**54**(8):1698–700.

Neuroanatomy and physiology of sleep and wakefulness

Pierre-Hervé Luppi and Patrice Fort

Introduction

In most mammals, there are three vigilance states, which are characterized by clear differences in electroencephalogram (EEG), electromyogram (EMG), and electro-oculogram (EOG) recordings. The waking state is characterized by high-frequency, low-amplitude activity on the EEG, sustained EMG activity, and ocular movement; non-rapid eye movement (NREM) or slow-wave (SWS) sleep, is characterized by low-frequency, high-amplitude delta oscillations on the EEG, low muscular activity on the EMG, and no ocular movement; and rapid eye movement (REM), or paradoxical sleep (PS) is characterized by an activated low-amplitude EEG similar to the waking EEG, but with complete disappearance of muscle tone and ocular movements.

Despite a wealth of neuropathological evidence dating back to the nineteenth century indicating that altered states of vigilance can be induced by focal brain lesions and that different neurochemical mechanisms are responsible for the succession of the three vigilance states across 24 h [1], the mechanisms underlying the switch of cortical activity from an activated (desynchronized) state during waking to a synchronized state during deep NREM and then to the activated state of PS have not yet been precisely described.

This chapter examines possible neuronal networks and mechanisms responsible for the switch from waking to NREM and REM sleep.

Mechanisms involved in waking

The activated cortical state during waking is induced by the activity of multiple waking neurochemical systems. Some of these belong to the ascending reticular activating system [2]. These include the serotonergic neurons which are mainly localized in the dorsal raphe nucleus, noradrenergic neurons in the locus coeruleus, and cholinergic neurons in the brainstem, while others are located more rostrally in the forebrain. These correspond to the cholinergic neurons in the basal forebrain, the histaminergic neurons localized in the tuberomammillary nucleus, and the orexin (hypocretin) systems in the tuberal hypothalamus [1].

Altogether, these systems control arousal characterized by high-frequency, low-amplitude cortical activation [3] and

widely project to the thalamus and/or the neocortex. When these waking systems are removed, the thalamocortical network oscillates in the delta range (i.e, the slow-wave mode of activity typical of NREM sleep) [1].

During sleep, it is believed that these waking systems are all inhibited by gamma-aminobutyric acid (GABA), the main inhibitory neurotransmitter in the brain. Indeed, it has been shown that the serotonergic neurons of the dorsal raphe nucleus and the noradrenergic neurons of the locus coeruleus are inhibited by GABA during SWS and paradoxical sleep [4, 5]. However, this is yet to be demonstrated for the other waking systems.

Gervasoni and colleagues [5] demonstrated that the unit activity of a single serotonergic neuron shows activity during waking, decreases its activity until it is nearly silent during NREM sleep, and is completely silent during REM sleep. Furthermore, by the localized application of bicuculline, a competitive antagonist of $GABA_A$ receptors, they demonstrated that these neurons ceased or decreased firing during sleep because they are tonically inhibited by GABA. Indeed, application of bicuculline during SWS and PS restored the waking activity of the neurons. Similar results had previously been obtained in noradrenergic neurons in the locus coeruleus [4].

Mechanisms involved in NREM (slow-wave sleep, SWS)

In contrast to the complex and extensive neurochemical network involved in waking, the neurons inducing SWS are localized in the lateral preoptic area and the adjacent basal forebrain. A cluster of these neurons is localized in a small nucleus called the ventrolateral preoptic nucleus (VLPO), which is situated above the optic chiasm. It has been demonstrated in rats that lesions including the VLPO induce insomnia for up to several weeks, with the reduction in the number of sleep-positive cells in the VLPO cluster linearly correlated with the reduction in the quantity of SWS and delta power [6].

GABAergic neurons projecting to the waking systems are localized in the VLPO as well as two brainstem structures, the ventrolateral periaqueductal gray and the dorsal paragigantocellular reticular nucleus [1]. The GABAergic neurons of the VLPO are active specifically during SWS [7, 8]. Sherin and

Neuroimaging of Sleep and Sleep Disorders, ed. Eric Nofzinger, Pierre Maquet, and Michael J. Thorpy. Published by Cambridge University Press. © Cambridge University Press 2013.

colleagues [9] identified a population of neurons in the VLPO that showed expression of the proto-oncogene c-Fos, a marker of neuronal activation [10], in previously sleep-deprived rats following recovery sleep. The greatest density of c-Fos-immunoreactive neurons after SWS increase were localized in the VLPO and the number of c-Fos-immunoreactive cells was directly proportional to the number of minutes of sleep during the hour before the animal was killed. This was confirmed in studies using unit recordings which demonstrated that most of the neurons in this area were specifically activated during sleep compared with the waking state [8]. Neuronal discharge, examined using a chronic microwire technique in rats, demonstrated that VLPO neurons displayed significantly elevated mean discharge rates during NREM sleep compared with waking and that discharge rates progressively increased from light to deep NREM sleep [8].

Switching from waking to NREM sleep

Figure 2.1 compares the neuronal networks responsible for waking, SWS, and paradoxical (REM) sleep. It is thought that the switch from waking to NREM sleep results from the inhibition of the waking systems by the VLPO sleep-active GABAergic neurons. Intracellular recordings in rat brain slices revealed that the VLPO comprises two cell types [11]. Two-thirds of the neurons within the VLPO were homogeneous multipolar triangular-shaped cells that showed a potent low-threshold spike. Moreover, single-cell RT-PCR showed that these cells contain mRNA for glutamic acid decarboxylase (GAD) 65 and 67, the enzymes necessary for the synthesis of GABA, proving that these neurons are of GABAergic type [11].

Based on all data available, a reciprocal interaction of wake-promoting and sleep-promoting neurons across the sleep/waking cycle has been suggested. This theory is supported by in vitro pharmacological studies in rat brain slices which revealed that VLPO neurons are indeed inhibited by most of the waking transmitters [11]. Indeed, extracellular infrared videomicroscopy demonstrated that all of the triangular multipolar neurons of the VLPO are postsynaptically inhibited by norepinephrine and acetylcholine [11]. However, serotonin postsynaptically inhibited only 50% of the neurons previously shown to be inhibited by norepinephrine and acetylcholine and excited the remaining half, suggesting the presence of two distinct subpopulations of cells (types 1 and 2). Histamine and hypocretin had neither inhibitory nor excitatory effects.

Further in vitro pharmacological investigations revealed that VLPO neurons are excited by adenosine A_{2A} agonists [12]. This study examined the hypothesis that adenosine can activate VLPO neurons via adenosine A_{2A} receptors in rat brain slices. Interestingly, the results showed that only the type-2 subpopulation of VLPO neurons that were previously shown to be excited by serotonin were excited by adenosine via postsynaptic activation of the adenosine A_{2A} receptors. Since both adenosine and serotonin progressively accumulate during waking, the authors of the study proposed that the type-2 VLPO neurons, which appear to respond to circadian and homeostatic

signals by increasing their firing, may be involved in sleep induction, whilst the type-1 neurons are most likely to play a role in the consolidation of sleep.

To summarize, in the waking rat the hypocretin neurons, for example, may be the first to start firing during waking, exciting all the other waking systems (the basal forebrain cholinergic system; the histaminergic neurons; the monoaminergic, serotonergic, and cholinergic neurons). In turn, these waking systems activate the thalamus and/or the cortex, leading to cortical activation and also, importantly, inhibit the GABAergic sleep-active neurons in the VLPO (Figure 2.1A).

At the onset of sleep, the GABAergic sleep neurons of the VLPO are activated by the circadian clock, localized in the suprachiasmatic nucleus, and the hypnogenic factor adenosine, which progressively accumulates in the brain during waking. It is the effect of this accumulation of adenosine that is the target for one of the most commonly used psychoactive drugs, caffeine [13], which acts via antagonism of the adenosine receptor. In turn these sleep-active neurons begin to inhibit the wake-active neurons in the multiple arousal centers via the neurotransmitter GABA, leading to synchronization of the thalamocortical network (Figure 2.1B). The decreases in sensory inputs is also necessary to let sleep occur since waking systems are excited by them.

Mechanisms involved in paradoxical (REM) sleep

It was first shown that PS persists following decortication, cerebellar ablation, or brainstem transections rostral to the pons. In contrast, transection at the posterior limit of the pons suppressed PS [14]. It was then demonstrated that a state resembling PS is still visible in the "pontine cat," a preparation in which all the structures rostral to the pons have been removed [14]. These results indicated that brainstem structures are necessary and sufficient to trigger and maintain the state of PS, a concept still valid today. By using electrolytic and chemical lesions, it was then evidenced that the dorsal part of the pontis oralis (PnO) and caudalis (PnC) nuclei contains the neurons responsible for PS onset [14]. Furthermore, bilateral injections of a cholinergic agonist, carbachol, into the dorsal area of the PnO and PnC, also named peri-locus coeruleus α (peri-LCα), the pontine inhibitory area (PIA), and the subcoeruleus nucleus (SubC) in cats, and more recently the sublaterodorsal tegmental nucleus (SLD) in rats, dramatically increases PS quantities [15, 16]. It was then shown by unit recordings in freely moving cats that many SLD neurons show a tonic firing selective to PS (called "PS-on" neurons) [17, 18]. It was thought that SLD PS-on neurons are cholinergic until we recently showed that they are glutamatergic.

First, in contrast to cats, carbachol iontophoresis into the rat SLD, the equivalent of the cat peri-LCα, induces waking (W) with increased muscle activity [19]. Further, only occasional cholinergic neurons were stained for c-Fos in the laterodorsal tegmental nucleus (LDT), pedunculopontine tegmental nucleus (PPT) and SLD after PS hypersomnia [20]. Finally, in rats,

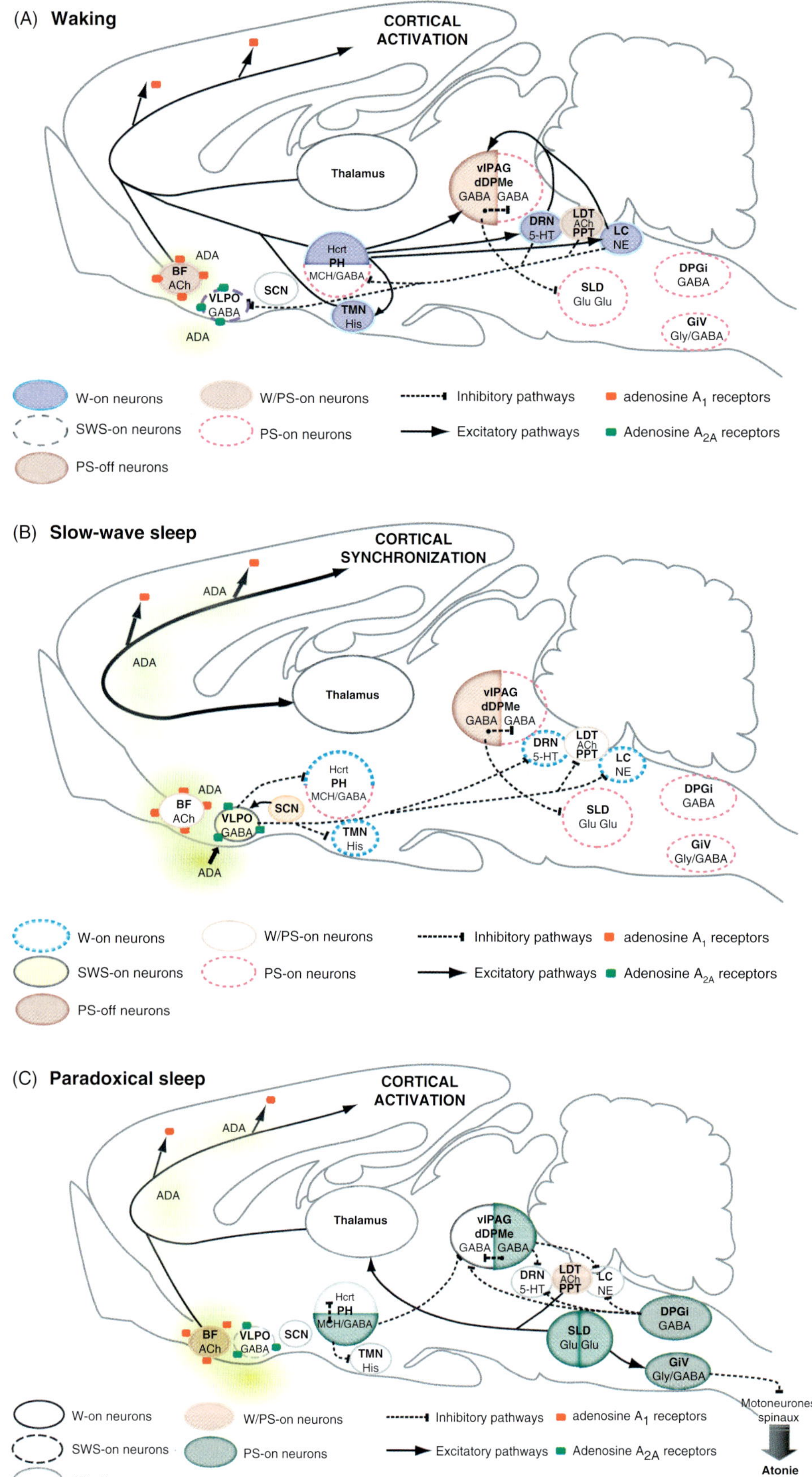

Figure 2.1 Neuronal networks responsible for waking, slow-wave (non-rapid eye movement [NREM]) sleep and paradoxical (REM) sleep (adapted from Fort *et al.* [1]). Abbreviations: 5-HT = 5-hydroxytryptamine (serotonin), ACh = acetylcholine; ADA = adenosine; BF = basal forebrain; DPGi = dorsal paragigantocellular reticular nucleus; dDPMe = deep mesencephalic reticular nucleus; DRN = dorsal raphe nucleus; GABA = gamma-aminobutyric acid; GiV = ventral gigantocellular reticular nucleus; Glu = glutamate Gly = glycine; Hcrt = hypocretin (orexin)-containing neurons; His = histamine; LC = locus coeruleus; LDT = laterodorsal tegmental nucleus; MCH = melanin concentrating hormone-containing neurons; NE = norepinephrine; PH = posterior hypothalamus; PPT pedunculopontine tegmental nucleus; PS = paradoxical sleep; SCN = suprachiasmatic nucleus; SLD = sublaterodorsal nucleus; SWS = slow-wave sleep; TMN = tuberomamillary nucleus; vlPAG = ventrolateral periaqueductal gray; VLPO = ventrolateral preoptic nucleus; W = waking.

neurochemical lesions of both the LDT and PPT induced no effect on PS and cortical activation [21]. We recently further demonstrated that most of the Fos-labeled neurons localized in the SLD after PS recovery express a specific marker of glutamatergic neurons, the vesicular glutamate transporter 2 (vGlut2) [22]. Altogether, these results indicate that the PS-on SLD neurons triggering PS are glutamatergic.

Combining Fos staining, anterograde labeling from the SLD, and glycine immunostaining in rats showing PS hypersomnia after bicuculline injection in the SLD, we also showed that the SLD sends direct efferent projections to glycinergic neurons from the alpha and ventral gigantocellular nuclei (GiA and GiV, corresponding to the cat magnocellular reticular nucleus, Mc) [19]. Further, GiA and GiV glycinergic neurons express Fos after induction of PS by bicuculline injection in the SLD [19]. In addition, glutamate release in the GiV and GiA increases specifically during PS [23] and injection of non-NMDA glutamate agonists into the GiA and GiV suppresses muscle tone while an increased tonus is induced during PS in cats with a GiA and GiV cytotoxic lesion [24, 25]. It is likely that these neurons are also GABAergic since nearly all Fos-labeled neurons localized in these two nuclei after 3 h of PS recovery following 72 h of PS deprivation express GAD67 mRNA [26].

Altogether, these results indicate that the GiV premotoneurons responsible for muscle atonia of PS co-release on motoneurons GABA and glycine that act on glycine, $GABA_A$ and $GABA_B$ receptors to hyperpolarize them.

Mechanisms of activation of SLD PS-on neurons during PS

In cats and rats, the microdialysis administration of kainic acid, a glutamate agonist, in the peri-LCα induces a PS-like state [19, 27]. A long-lasting PS-like hypersomnia can also be pharmacologically induced with a short latency in head-restrained unanesthetized rats by iontophoretic applications of bicuculline or gabazine, two $GABA_A$ receptor antagonists, into the SLD [19]. Further, application of kynurenate, a glutamate antagonist, reversed the PS-like state induced by bicuculline [19]. In the head-restrained rat, we also recorded neurons within the SLD specifically active during PS and excited following bicuculline or gabazine iontophoresis [28]. Taken together, these data indicate that the activation of SLD PS-on neurons is mainly due to the removal during PS of a tonic GABAergic tone present during W and SWS and the continuous presence of a glutamatergic input. Combining retrograde tracing with cholera toxin b subunit (CTb) injected into the SLD and GAD immunohistochemistry and Fos immunohistochemistry with GAD67 mRNA "*in situ*" hybridization after 72 h of PS deprivation, we recently demonstrated that the ventrolateral part of the periaqueductal gray (vlPAG) and the adjacent deep mesencephalic reticular nucleus (dDPMe) are the only pontomedullary structures containing a large number of GABAergic neurons activated during PS deprivation [26] projecting to the SLD. Further, injection of muscimol into the vlPAG and/or the dDPMe induces strong increases in PS quantities in cats [29] and rats [26]. Finally, neurochemical lesion of

these two structures induces profound increases in PS quantities [21]. These congruent experimental data led us to propose that PS-off GABAergic neurons within the vlPAG and the dDpMe are gating PS by tonically inhibiting PS-on neurons from the SLD during W and SWS. Our results indicate that these GABAergic neurons are crucial to gate PS although they do not rule out a secondary role for monoaminergic neurons since an increase in monoaminergic transmission either by reuptake blockers or an agonist is well known to inhibit PS. One possibility is that the monoaminergic neurons are exciting the GABAergic PS-off neurons during waking to preclude PS onset. As reported above, bicuculline application to monoaminergic neurons during SWS or PS induces a tonic firing in both types of neurons [4, 5, 30]. These results strongly suggest that an increased GABA release is responsible for the PS-selective inactivation of monoaminergic neurons. This hypothesis is well supported by microdialysis experiments in cats measuring a significant increase in GABA release in the dorsal raphe nucleus (DRN) and locus coeruleus (LC) during PS as compared to W and SWS but no detectable changes in glycine concentration [31, 32]. It seems therefore that monoaminergic cells are under a tonic GABAergic inhibition gradually increasing from W to PS.

By combining retrograde tracing with CTb and GAD immunohistochemistry in rats, we found that the vlPAG and the dorsal paragigantocellular nucleus (DPGi) [5, 33] contained numerous GABAergic neurons projecting both to the DRN and LC. They are therefore the best candidates for mediating the inhibition of monoaminergic neurons during PS. We then demonstrated by combining c-Fos and retrograde labeling that both nuclei contain numerous LC-projecting neurons selectively activated during PS rebound following PS deprivation [34, 35]. Since the possible involvement of the DPGi in PS control has not been previously investigated, we studied the firing activity of its neurons across the sleep/wake cycle in head-restrained rats [36]. In full agreement with our functional data using c-Fos, we found that the DPGi contains numerous PS-on neurons that are silent during W and SWS and fire tonically during PS. These PS-on neurons start discharging approximately 15 s before PS onset and become silent around 10 s before EEG signs of arousal. Taken together, these data highly suggest that the DPGi contains the neurons responsible for the inactivation of LC noradrenergic neurons during PS [36]. A contribution from the vlPAG in the inhibition during PS of LC noradrenergic and dorsal raphe serotonergic neurons is also likely. Indeed, an increase in c-Fos/GAD-immunoreactive neurons has been reported in the vlPAG after a PS rebound following deprivation in rats [26, 37]. In summary, a large body of data indicates that GABAergic PS-on neurons localized in the vlPAG and the DPGi hyperpolarize the monoaminergic neurons during PS. We propose that these neurons at the same time inhibit the dDPMe/vlPAG PS-off GABAergic neurons and by this mean induces a disinhibition of SLD PS-on glutamatergic neurons leading to the induction of PS. Reciprocally, PS-off GABAergic neurons could also inhibit the intermingled PS-on GABAergic neurons during W and SWS to prevent the entrance into PS. The entrance into PS would be due to the activation of PS-on GABAergic neurons by still unknown mechanisms. One possibility is that the depolarization of these neurons at the onset and during PS is due to the activation of endogenous cellular or molecular clock-like means.

The cessation of activity of these neurons at the end of PS episodes is certainly due to a completely different mechanism. Indeed, animals are entering PS slowly from SWS while in contrast they exit from it abruptly by a microarousal [38]. It indicates that the end of PS is induced by the activation of the W systems like the monoaminergic, hypocretin, or histaminergic neurons. The mechanisms responsible for their activation remain to be identified.

Role of the posterior hypothalamus, in particular MCH neurons, in PS control

To localize all brain areas activated during PS, we compared the distribution of c-Fos+ neurons in control rats, rats selectively deprived of PS for 72 h and rats allowed to recover from such deprivation [35, 39]. Surprisingly, we observed a very large number of c-Fos+ cells in the posterior hypothalamus (PH), including the zona incerta (ZI), the perifornical area (PeF), and the lateral hypothalamic area (LHA). Indeed, only a few experimental results already support the notion that the PH contributes to PS regulation. Bilateral injections of muscimol in the cat mammillary and tuberal hypothalamus induced a drastic inhibition of PS [40]. Further, neurons specifically active during PS were recorded in the PH of cats [41–43] or head-restrained rats [44]. By using double-immunostaining, we further showed that around 75% of PH cells labeled for c-Fos after PS rebound expressed GAD67 mRNA and are therefore GABAergic [45]. One-third of these GABAergic neurons were also immunoreactive for the neuropeptide melanin concentrating hormone (MCH). Almost 60% of all the MCH-immunoreactive neurons counted in PeF, ZI, and LHA were c-Fos+ [39, 46]. In support of our Fos data, it has recently been shown in head-restrained rats that hypothalamic neurons, identified ex vivo as containing MCH, fire quite exclusively during PS [47]. Importantly, MCH neurons start to fire at the onset of PS and not before and cannot therefore be responsible for the induction of the state. Nevertheless, rats receiving ICV administration of MCH showed a strong dose-dependent increase in PS and, to a minor extent, SWS quantities, due to an increased number of PS bouts [39]. Further, subcutaneous injection of an MCH antagonist decreases SWS and PS quantities [48] and mice with genetically inactivated MCH signaling exhibit altered vigilance state

architecture and sleep homeostasis [49, 50]. Thus, growing evidence indicates that MCH/GABAergic neurons play a key role in PS regulation/homeostasis. MCH and more generally GABAergic PS-on neurons in the PH might promote PS by inhibiting W active neurons like the vlPAG/dDPMe GABAergic, the monoaminergic PS-off neurons, and the hypocretinergic neurons. PS increases induced by MCH could also be due to a direct inhibition of the GABAergic dDPMe and vlPAG neurons gating PS onset while hypocretin inputs to these neurons would be excitatory to prevent PS [19, 51, 52].

A network model for PS onset and maintenance (Figure 2.1C)

PS onset would be due to the activation of glutamatergic PS-on neurons from the SLD. During W and SWS, these PS-on neurons would be inhibited by a tonic inhibitory GABAergic tone originating from PS-off neurons localized in the vlPAG and the dDpMe. These neurons would be activated during W by the hypocretin neurons and the monoaminergic neurons. The onset of PS would be due to the activation by intrinsic mechanisms of PS-on GABAergic neurons localized in the PH, DPGi, and vlPAG. These neurons would also inactivate the PS-off monoaminergic neurons during PS. The disinhibited ascending SLD PS-on neurons would in turn induce cortical activation via their projections to intralaminar thalamic relay neurons in collaboration with W/PS-on cholinergic and glutamatergic neurons from the LDT and PPT, mesencephalic and pontine reticular nuclei, and the basal forebrain. Descending PS-on SLD neurons would induce muscle atonia and sensory inhibition via their excitatory projections to glycinergic premotoneurons localized in the GiA and GiV. The exit from PS would be due to the activation of waking systems since PS episodes are almost always terminated by an arousal. The waking systems would inhibit the GABAergic PS-on neurons localized in the DPGi and vlPAG. Since the duration of PS is negatively coupled with the metabolic rate, we propose that the activity of the waking systems is triggered to end PS to restore competing physiological parameters like thermoregulation.

Acknowledgements

This work was supported by Center National de la Recherche Scientifique, Université de Lyon and Université Lyon 1. The authors have no conflicts of interest to declare.

References

1. Fort P, Bassetti CL, Luppi PH. Alternating vigilance states: new insights regarding neuronal networks and mechanisms. *Eur J Neurosci.* 2009;**29**(9):1741–53. Epub 2009/05/29.

2. Moruzzi G, Magoun HW. Brainstem reticular formation and activation of the EEG.1949. *J Neuropsychiatry Clin Neurosci.* 1995;7(2):251–67.

3. Jones BE. Basic mechanisms of sleep-wake states. In: Kryger MH, Roth T, Dement WC, eds. *Principles and Practice of Sleep Medicine.* Philadelphia, W. B. Saunders Co. 1994; 145–62.

4. Gervasoni D, Darracq L, Fort P, *et al.* Electrophysiological evidence that noradrenergic neurons of the rat locus coeruleus are tonically inhibited by GABA during sleep. *Eur J Neurosci.* 1998;**10**(3):964–70.

5. Gervasoni D, Peyron C, Rampon C, *et al.* Role and origin of the

GABAergic innervation of dorsal raphe serotonergic neurons. *J Neurosci.* 2000;**20**(11):4217–25.

6. Lu J, Greco MA, Shiromani P, Saper CB. Effect of lesions of the ventrolateral preoptic nucleus on NREM and REM sleep. *J Neurosci.* 2000;**20**(10):3830–42.

7. Sherin JE, Elmquist JK, Torrealba F, Saper CB. Innervation of histaminergic tuberomammillary neurons by GABAergic and galaninergic neurons in the ventrolateral preoptic nucleus of the rat. *J Neurosci.* 1998;**18**(12):4705–21.

8. Szymusiak R, Alam N, Steininger TL, McGinty D. Sleep-waking discharge patterns of ventrolateral preoptic/ anterior hypothalamic neurons in rats. *Brain Res.* 1998;**803**(1–2):178–88.

9. Sherin JE, Shiromani PJ, McCarley RW, Saper CB. Activation of ventrolateral preoptic neurons during sleep. *Science.* 1996;**271**(5246):216–19.

10. Morgan JI, Curran T. Stimulus-transcription coupling in the nervous system: involvement of the inducible proto-oncogenes fos and jun. *Annu Rev Neurosci.* 1991;**14**:421–51.

11. Gallopin T, Fort P, Eggermann E, *et al.* Identification of sleep-promoting neurons in vitro. *Nature.* 2000;**404**(6781):992–5.

12. Gallopin T, Luppi PH, Cauli B, *et al.* The endogenous somnogen adenosine excites a subset of sleep-promoting neurons via A2A receptors in the ventrolateral preoptic nucleus. *Neuroscience.* 2005;**134**(4):1377–90.

13. Fredholm BB, Chen JF, Masino SA, Vaugeois JM. Actions of adenosine at its receptors in the CNS: insights from knockouts and drugs. *Annu Rev Pharmacol Toxicol.* 2005;**45**:385–412. Epub 2005/04/12.

14. Jouvet M. Recherches sur les structures nerveuses et les mécanismes responsables des différentes phases du sommeil physiologique. *Arch Ital Biol.* 1962;**100**:125–206.

15. George R, Haslett WL, Jenden DJ. A cholinergic mechanism in the brainstem reticular formation: induction of paradoxical sleep. *Int J Neuropharmacol.* 1964;**3**:541–52.

16. Vanni-Mercier G, Sakai K, Lin JS, Jouvet M. Mapping of cholinoceptive brainstem structures responsible for the generation of paradoxical sleep in the cat. *Arch Ital Biol.* 1989;**127**(3):133–64.

17. Sakai K. Neurons responsible for paradoxical sleep. In: Wauquier A, Janssen Research Foundation, eds. *Sleep: Neurotransmitters and Neuromodulators.* New York, Raven Press. 1985; 29–42.

18. Sakai K, Koyama Y. Are there cholinergic and non-cholinergic paradoxical sleep-on neurones in the pons? *Neuroreport.* 1996;**7**(15–17):2449–53.

19. Boissard R, Gervasoni D, Schmidt MH, *et al.* The rat ponto-medullary network responsible for paradoxical sleep onset and maintenance: a combined microinjection and functional neuroanatomical study. *Eur J Neurosci.* 2002;**16**(10):1959–73.

20. Verret L, Leger L, Fort P, Luppi PH. Cholinergic and noncholinergic brainstem neurons expressing Fos after paradoxical (REM) sleep deprivation and recovery. *Eur J Neurosci.* 2005;**21**(9):2488–504. Epub 2005/06/04.

21. Lu J, Sherman D, Devor M, Saper CB. A putative flip-flop switch for control of REM sleep. *Nature.* 2006;**441** (7093):589–94.

22. Clement O, Sapin E, Berod A, Fort P, Luppi PH. Evidence that neurons of the sublaterodorsal tegmental nucleus triggering paradoxical (REM) sleep are glutamatergic. *Sleep.* 2011;**34**(4):419–23. Epub 2011/04/05.

23. Kodama T, Lai YY, Siegel JM. Enhanced glutamate release during REM sleep in the rostromedial medulla as measured by in vivo microdialysis. *Brain Res.* 1998;**780**(1):178–81.

24. Holmes CJ, Jones BE. Importance of cholinergic, GABAergic, serotonergic and other neurons in the medial medullary reticular formation for sleep-wake states studied by cytotoxic lesions in the cat. *Neuroscience.* 1994;**62** (4):1179–200.

25. Lai YY, Siegel JM. Pontomedullary glutamate receptors mediating locomotion and muscle tone suppression. *J Neurosci.* 1991;**11**(9):2931–7.

26. Sapin E, Lapray D, Berod A, *et al.* Localization of the brainstem GABAergic neurons controlling paradoxical (REM) sleep. *PLoS One.* 2009;**4**(1):e4272. Epub 2009/01/27.

27. Onoe H, Sakai K. Kainate receptors: a novel mechanism in paradoxical (REM) sleep generation. *Neuroreport.* 1995;**6**(2):353–6.

28. Boissard R, Gervasoni D, Fort P, *et al.* Neuronal networks responsible for paradoxical sleep onset and maintenance in rats: a new hypothesis. *Sleep.* 2000;**23**(Suppl):107.

29. Sastre JP, Buda C, Kitahama K, Jouvet M. Importance of the ventrolateral region of the periaqueductal gray and adjacent tegmentum in the control of paradoxical sleep as studied by muscimol microinjections in the cat. *Neuroscience.* 1996;**74**(2):415–26.

30. Darracq L, Gervasoni D, Souliere F, *et al.* Effect of strychnine on rat locus coeruleus neurones during sleep and wakefulness. *Neuroreport.* 1996;**8** (1):351–5.

31. Nitz D, Siegel J. GABA release in the dorsal raphe nucleus: role in the control of REM sleep. *Am J Physiol.* 1997;**273**(1 Pt 2):R451–5.

32. Nitz D, Siegel JM. GABA release in the locus coeruleus as a function of sleep/wake state. *Neuroscience.* 1997;**78**(3):795–801.

33. Luppi PH, Peyron C, Rampon C, *et al.* Inhibitory mechanisms in the dorsal raphe nucleus and locus coeruleus during sleep. In: Lydic R, Baghdoyan HA, eds. *Handbook of Behavioral State Control.* New York, CRC Press. 1999; 195–211.

34. Verret L, Fort P, Luppi PH. Localization of the neurons responsible for the inhibition of locus coeruleus noradrenergic neurons during paradoxical sleep in the rat. *Sleep.* 2003;**26**:69.

35. Verret L, Fort P, Gervasoni D, Leger L, Luppi PH. Localization of the neurons active during paradoxical (REM) sleep and projecting to the locus coeruleus noradrenergic neurons in the rat. *J Comp Neurol.* 2006;**495**(5):573–86. Epub 2006/02/25.

36. Goutagny R, Luppi PH, Salvert D, *et al.* Role of the dorsal paragigantocellular reticular nucleus in paradoxical (rapid eye movement) sleep generation: a combined electrophysiological and anatomical study in the rat. *Neuroscience.* 2008;**152**(3):849–57. Epub 2008/03/01.

37. Maloney KJ, Mainville L, Jones BE. Differential c-Fos expression in cholinergic, monoaminergic, and GABAergic cell groups of

the pontomesencephalic tegmentum after paradoxical sleep deprivation and recovery. *J Neurosci.* 1999;**19**(8):3057–72.

38. Gervasoni D, Lin SC, Ribeiro S, *et al.* Global forebrain dynamics predict rat behavioral states and their transitions. *J Neurosci.* 2004;**24**(49):11137–11147.

39. Verret L, Goutagny R, Fort P, *et al.* A role of melanin-concentrating hormone producing neurons in the central regulation of paradoxical sleep. *BMC Neurosci.* 2003;**4**(1):19.

40. Lin JS, Sakai K, Vanni-Mercier G, Jouvet M. A critical role of the posterior hypothalamus in the mechanisms of wakefulness determined by microinjection of muscimol in freely moving cats. *Brain Res.* 1989;**479**(2):225–40.

41. Alam MN, Gong H, Alam T, *et al.* Sleep-waking discharge patterns of neurons recorded in the rat perifornical lateral hypothalamic area. *J Physiol.* 2002;**538**(Pt 2):619–31.

42. Koyama Y, Takahashi K, Kodama T, Kayama Y. State-dependent activity of neurons in the perifornical hypothalamic area during sleep and waking. *Neuroscience.* 2003;**119**(4):1209–19. Epub 2003/07/02.

43. Steininger TL, Alam MN, Gong H, Szymusiak R, McGinty D. Sleep-waking discharge of neurons in the posterior lateral hypothalamus of the albino rat. *Brain Res.* 1999;**840**(1–2):138–47.

44. Goutagny R, Luppi PH, Salvert D, Gervasoni D, Fort P. GABAergic control of hypothalamic melanin-concentrating hormone-containing neurons across the sleep-waking cycle. *Neuroreport.* 2005;**16**(10):1069–73. Epub 2005/06/24.

45. Sapin E, Berod A, Leger L, *et al.* A very large number of GABAergic neurons are activated in the tuberal hypothalamus during paradoxical (REM) sleep hypersomnia. *PLoS One.* 2010; **5**(7): e11766. Epub 2010/07/30.

46. Hanriot L, Camargo N, Courau AC, *et al.* Characterization of the melanin-concentrating hormone neurons activated during paradoxical sleep hypersomnia in rats. *J Comp Neurol.* 2007;**505**(2):147–57. Epub 2007/09/14.

47. Hassani OK, Lee MG, Jones BE. Melanin-concentrating hormone neurons discharge in a reciprocal manner to orexin neurons across the sleep-wake cycle. *Proc Natl Acad Sci U S A.* 2009;**106**(7):2418–22. Epub 2009/02/04.

48. Ahnaou A, Drinkenburg WH, Bouwknecht JA, *et al.* Blocking melanin-concentrating hormone MCH1 receptor affects rat sleep-wake architecture. *Eur J Pharmacol.* 2008;**579**(1–3):177–88. Epub 2007/12/08.

49. Adamantidis A, Salvert D, Goutagny R, *et al.* Sleep architecture of the melanin-concentrating hormone receptor 1-knockout mice. *Eur J Neurosci.* 2008;**27**(7):1793–1800. Epub 2008/04/03.

50. Willie JT, Sinton CM, Maratos-Flier E, Yanagisawa M. Abnormal response of melanin-concentrating hormone deficient mice to fasting: hyperactivity and rapid eye movement sleep suppression. *Neuroscience.* 2008;**156**(4):819–29. Epub 2008/09/24.

51. Luppi PH, Boissard R, Gervasoni D, *et al.* The network responsible for paradoxical sleep onset and maintenance: a new theory based on the head-restrained rat model. In: Luppi PH, ed. *Sleep: Circuits and Function.* Boca Raton, CRC Press. 2004; 272.

52. Luppi PH, Gervasoni D, Verret L, *et al.* Paradoxical (REM) sleep genesis: The switch from an aminergic-cholinergic to a GABAergic-glutamatergic hypothesis. *J Physiol Paris.* 2006;**100**(5–6):271–83. Epub 2007/08/11.

Fundamentals of structural MR imaging

Keivan Shifteh and Michael L. Lipton

What is MRI, and how does MR work?

Magnetic resonance imaging (MRI) provides exquisitely detailed images of internal body structures and is especially useful for brain imaging. This chapter will provide an overview of the fundamental elements of MRI. Chapter 4 will introduce MRI techniques which permit assessment of brain physiology, function, and metabolism. State-of-the-art MRI machines employ large, tube-shaped superconducting magnets to produce a strong and homogeneous static magnetic field. Magnetic field strengths are measured in units of tesla (T), with typical human MRI scanners ranging from 0.3 to 3.0 T. One tesla is equal to 10 000 gauss. The Earth's magnetic field is about 0.5 gauss. Using the magnetic field, along with additional, but much weaker time-varying magnetic fields (radio frequency (RF) fields and pulsed gradient magnetic fields), computers reconstruct images from signals emitted by proton nuclei. Nuclear magnetic resonance (NMR) is the foundation on which MRI is built, although commercial interest in human applications of NMR led to the discarding of the term "nuclear" because of its negative perception. NMR is a physical phenomenon that occurs when certain elements (nuclei with an odd number of protons and/or neutrons) interact with a magnetic field. NMR is the process by which the signal detected in MRI is generated. In human tissue, which is composed largely of hydrogen-containing water (H_2O), hydrogen is the most abundant of all the NMR-capable nuclei. For this reason, human MRI is focused almost exclusively on hydrogen. Since the hydrogen nucleus contains only a single proton and nothing more, hydrogen nuclei are also referred to merely as protons. The protons within the nucleus of any atom contain electric charge and generate a magnetic field, termed a dipole, and we use a single vector to describe the magnetic field of the dipole. The orientation of this vector indicates the orientation of the dipole and the length of the vector indicates its strength. In the absence of any magnetic field external to the nucleus, orientation of the dipoles of a group of nuclei will be random. In the presence of an externally applied magnetic field, however, the dipoles will align with the externally applied magnetic field.

MRI versus CT

Computed tomography (CT) scans are more widely available, and are faster than MRI. CT is less expensive and less likely to require the patient to be sedated due to motion or claustrophobia. However, CT uses X-rays to acquire images, while MRI uses non-ionizing RF energy to generate images. MRI, unlike CT, does not expose the patient to the hazards of ionizing radiation. Contrast in CT images is generated solely by differences in the X-ray attenuation coefficient of tissues, but in MRI different nuclear properties are used to generate contrast. Both CT and MR may use intravenous contrast agents to enhance images. Contrast agents for CT are based on iodine, while contrast agents for MRI have paramagnetic properties. Both CT and MRI are able to generate 2-dimensional (2D) cross-sectional images and 3-dimensional (3D) reconstructions. MRI is generally superior to CT regarding distinguishing pathological tissue from normal tissue and identifying, mapping, and detecting tumors. CT and MRI are able to produce data that can be reconstructed in any plane. While CT and MRI provide good spatial resolution (the ability to distinguish two separate structures an arbitrarily small distance from each other), MRI provides better contrast resolution (the ability to distinguish the differences between two tissues). The strong magnetic fields of MRI can affect metal implants, including cochlear implants and cardiac pacemakers, so patients with such implants are not eligible for MRI.

Diamagnetism, paramagnetism, superparamagnetism, ferromagnetism

Four terms describe the magnetic properties of materials, such as contrast agents, used in MRI. These terms are diamagnetism, paramagnetism, superparamagnetism, and ferromagnetism.

Diamagnetic materials have no intrinsic atomic magnetic moment, but when placed in a magnetic field weakly repel the field, resulting in a small negative magnetic susceptibility. Materials like water, copper, nitrogen, barium sulfate, and most tissues are diamagnetic. The weak negative magnetic susceptibility contributes to the loss of signal seen in bowel on MRI after administration of barium sulfate suspensions.

Paramagnetic materials include oxygen and ions of various metals like iron, magnesium, and gadolinium. These ions have unpaired electrons, resulting in a positive magnetic susceptibility. Thus, paramagnetic substances generate local magnetic fields when exposed to an externally applied field. The magnitude of this susceptibility is less than 0.1% that of ferromagnetic

Neuroimaging of Sleep and Sleep Disorders, ed. Eric Nofzinger, Pierre Maquet, and Michael J. Thorpy. Published by Cambridge University Press. © Cambridge University Press 2013.

materials. The proximity of paramagnetic substances shortens the T1 and T2* relaxation rates for water protons. Gadolinium is a paramagnetic ion commonly used as an MR contrast agent. At the proper concentration, Gd contrast agents cause preferential T1 relaxation enhancement, seen as an increase in signal on T1-weighted images.

Superparamagnetic materials consist of individual domains of elements that have ferromagnetic properties in bulk. Their magnetic susceptibility is between that of ferromagnetic and paramagnetic materials. Examples of superparamagnetic materials include iron containing contrast agents for bowel, liver, and lymph node imaging.

Ferromagnetic materials generally contain iron, nickel, or cobalt. These materials include magnets, and may include objects one might find in a patient, such as some aneurysm clips, shrapnel, etc. The persistence of magnetization when the external magnetic field is removed distinguishes ferromagnetic materials from paramagnetic materials. On MR images, these materials cause susceptibility artifacts characterized by loss of signal and spatial distortion.

Spin angular momentum, precession, static magnetic field (B_0), net magnetization vector (NMV)

To be useful for MRI, the proton must have spin angular momentum, in addition to the nuclear magnetism described above. The following analogy best conveys the concept of spin angular momentum. When a figure skater enters a high-velocity spin, he or she will experience a centrifugal force that pushes him or her away from their vertical alignment. The physical phenomenon that produces this centrifugal force is called angular momentum. When nuclei are placed in a magnetic field, they will interact with the field in much the same way due to spin angular momentum; the nuclei will not remain in stationary alignment with the applied magnetic field, but will precess around the externally applied magnetic field, taking a trajectory which describes a cone whose long access is parallel to the applied field (Figure 3.1).

The rate, or frequency (ω_0), of precession is a function of the nature of the nucleus (characterized by the constant

gyromagnetic ratio, γ) and the magnetic field strength B_0. This relationship is termed the Larmor equation, $\omega_0 = \gamma \times B_0$. At any moment in time, two component vectors, one parallel to B_0 (called M_Z) and one perpendicular to it (called M_T), can describe the nuclear magnetism. If we observe a large number of protons within a magnetic field, two similar vectors can represent the nuclear magnetism of each. Because the dipoles are precessing about B_0, M_T for each dipole is rotating about B_0. However, the phase of precession of each dipole will be unique. That is, each M_T will have a unique orientation in the plane perpendicular to B_0 at any point in time. Because M_T of the numerous protons in our patient are thus randomly oriented, the vector sum of M_T for our patient will be 0. On the other hand, as described previously, M_Z will sum to some potentially measureable quantity. The vector sum of all nuclear magnetization in our patient can thus be represented by a single vector perpendicular to B_0, termed the net magnetization vector (NMV), also called M_0, with no transverse component because all of the individual spins that contribute to the NMV have random phase and as a result, their transverse components cancel each other out. While it may seem that M_0 can simply be measured to generate signals from different tissues that form an image, the fact that M_0 is so small in comparison to B_0 means that it would be impractical, if not impossible, to directly measure M_0.

In order to measure an MRI signal, we must disturb this resting state (M_0) and create a scenario where the NMV has a net transverse component. The mechanism of this process, called excitation, is beyond the scope of this chapter, but the end result of excitation is essential nonetheless. By adding energy to the patient, using an RF magnetic field, the tissue dipoles are shifted to a higher energy state, where net M_Z of our patient is lower than at rest and net M_T is present. The degree to which we observe these phenomena (decreasing M_Z and increasing M_T) depends on the amount of RF energy we apply and thereby the extent to which we shift the dipoles in our patient to a higher energy state. As M_Z declines and M_T increases, the vector sum reflecting the net magnetization of our patient changes orientation, or rotates, to form an angle with B_0. If enough energy is deposited, the NMV will rotate to a 90° angle with respect to B_0, and if more energy is deposited, the orientation with respect to B_0 will exceed 90°. This degree of rotation is called the flip angle.

Generation of net M_T is essential because net M_T is what we detect as the MRI signal. M_T precesses about B_0, thus it is a moving magnetic field. When we place a looped conducter near the patient (we call this a receiver coil), M_T will induce a voltage in the coil. The MR signal intensity is the magnitude of M_T, measured as the voltage induced in the receiver coil by the precessing M_T. Receiver coils come in many shapes, sizes, and designs, which are well beyond the scope of this chapter. Specific coils dedicated to brain or head and neck imaging will be constructed to maximize proximity of the coil to the patient in order to maximize sensitivity.

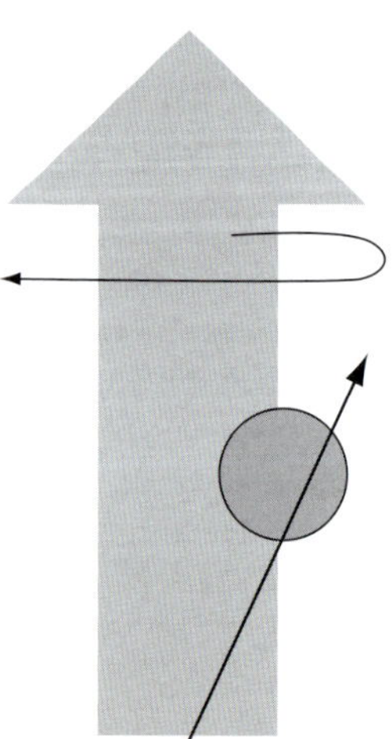

Figure 3.1 Precession. Interaction of the magnetic field of the proton with an applied magnetic field leads to precession. The vector describing the proton's magnetic field circles that describing the static magnetic field. Its path traces the surface of a cone.

Relaxation

After the NMV has been rotated with respect to B_0, when we add energy to the system, we say that the spins are "excited" by

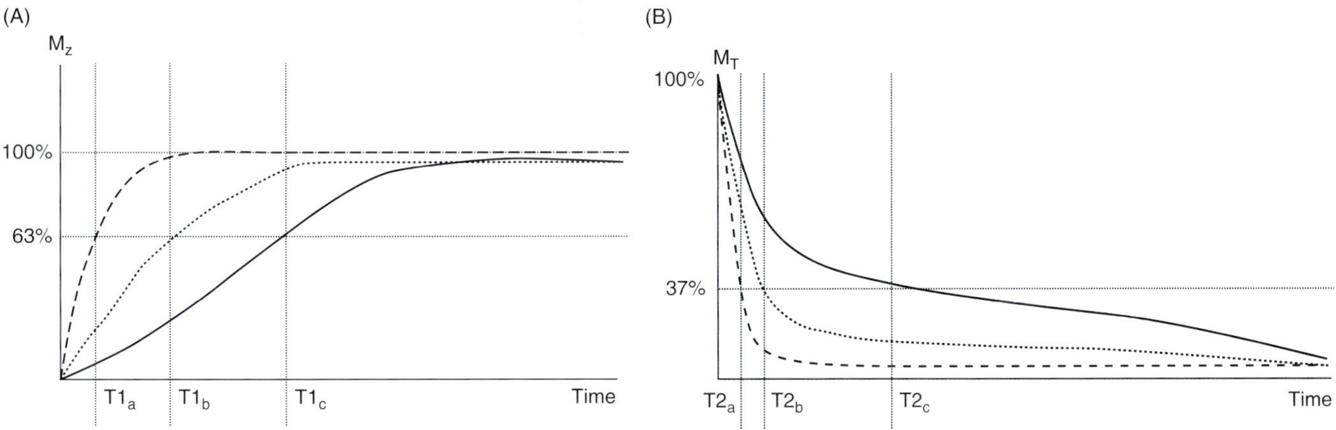

Figure 3.2 (A) Longitudinal relaxation (T1). At t = 0, a 90° RF pulse has just been delivered, and all magnetization is in the transverse plane. T1, the time at which 63% of M_Z has recovered, describes the rate of recovery. In this example, each line represents a different tissue: the dashed line represents fat, which has a short T1 ($T1_a$); the solid line represents cerebrospinal fluid (CSF), which has a long T1 ($T1_c$); and the dotted line represents brain, which has an intermediate T1 ($T1_b$). (B) Transverse relaxation (T2). At t = 0, a 90° RF pulse has just been delivered, and all magnetization is in the transverse plane. T2, the time at which 63% of M_T has dissipated and 37% remains, describes the exponential rate of signal loss. In this example, each line represents a different tissue, as described in Fig. 3.2A. Note that the tissues with long T1 also have long T2 and vice versa.

the input of RF energy. When the energy source (RF) is shut off, the system will return to a lower-energy configuration with the emission of energy equal to the amount of energy added by the RF during excitation. This return to the resting state is called relaxation. During the course of relaxation, M_T dissipates because the individual dipoles regain random phase of precession and M_Z "grows back" to reach M_0, its magnitude prior to the RF. Since dipoles in different tissues return to their resting state at different rates, we can sample the signal at varying times during relaxation to generate different signal from different tissues, which we call MRI contrast (Figures 3.2A and 3.2B).

T1, T2

The MRI examination consists of multiple types of images, each of which are chosen to provide a particular type of information about the subject tissues. These image types are often called "pulse sequences" because a unique timing and pattern of pulses of the various MRI hardware components (RF and gradient magnetic fields) is required to generate a signal suitable for transformation into an MR image.

Longitudinal and transverse relaxation must occur simultaneously, but proceed at very different rates, with transverse relaxation much more rapid than longitudinal relaxation. This phenomenon is reflected in the physical requirement that T2 be shorter than T1. The rate of recovery of longitudinal magnetization is defined by the time constant T1. The time T1 is the time required, after excitation and the resultant flip angle, to recover 63% of the remaining M_Z. Net M_T is lost as spins assume increasingly random phase such that the vector sum of the net transverse component of magnetization approaches zero. The process of transverse relaxation is by an exponential decay, governed by the time constant T2. T2 is the time required for 63% of the remaining net M_T to be lost following excitation.

The above discussion of relaxation assumes that the spatial variation of B_0 is zero. The consequence of having spatial variation in B_0 is that adjacent spins will not experience the same field strength and, consequently, will not precess at the same frequency. Following excitation spins precessing at different frequencies will lose phase coherence more rapidly than would be expected due to T2 relaxation, accelerating the loss of signal (i.e., M_T). This second process accelerates the exponential decay of the MRI signal after excitation. The additional relaxation is governed by the time constant, T2'. The time constant that describes the net rate of signal loss due to T2 and T2' is termed T2* (pronounced "T 2 star").

The spin echo

The spin echo is a method for "recovering" M_T lost due to T2' relaxation, where the phase of precessing spins becomes increasingly random as the spins precess at different ω. By applying RF, which rotates the spins 180°, the phase of the spins becomes reordered so that those precessing at lower frequencies are moved "behind" those precessing at higher frequencies. Over time, the spins "catch up" to each other, restoring phase coherence and compensating the T2' relaxation effect. If we consider adjacent spins precessing at different rates, one will be accelerating ahead of the other. If we can instantaneously invert the phase of the spins so that the one precessing faster is now "behind" the one precessing slower, the spins will come back into phase as the faster spin "catches up" with the slower one and there will be a continuous gain of phase coherence. To achieve maximal recovery of lost phase coherence due to T2' effects, we must invert the phase of the spins exactly midway between the initial RF excitation and TE (time to echo), the time at which we sample the signal. An RF pulse that flips the magnetization 180° accomplishes inversion of phase of the spins. The RF pulse must deposit twice the amount of energy as the 90° pulse in order to achieve a flip of exactly 180°.

TE (echo time) and TR (repetition time) are basic parameters of image acquisition. TE indicates the time following excitation (usually from several to just over 100 ms) when the MR signal is recorded. Sampling the signal later after excitation means that more T2 (or T2*) relaxation has occurred and the signal will thus reflect differences in T2 or T2* between tissues. This signal is thus "T2-weighted." TR describes the time between successive excitations (usually from several 10 s to several 1000 ms) and thus determines how much T1 relaxation will occur before the next excitation. If TR is very long, all tissue will be fully relaxed at the subsequent excitation and the signal then generated will not reflect differences in the T1 relaxation rate between tissues. Although TR only determines the amount of M_Z recovered before each excitation and therefore does not directly impact signal, shorter TR will yield more difference between tissue M_Z due to differences in T1, which are reflected in the subsequently generated signal. This signal will thus be "T1-weighted."

T1-weighted scans use short TE to minimize T2 contrast, and short TR, to maximize T1 contrast. Due to the short TR this scan can be run very fast, allowing the collection of high-resolution 3D data sets. Shortening of T1 by gadolinium contrast agents is best detected with a T1-weighted image, commonly collected before and after administration of the contrast agent to assess uptake of the agent. On a T1-weighted image, water and fluid-containing tissues are relatively hypointense and fat-containing tissues as well as tissue affected by paramagnetic substances which shorten T1 (e.g., methemoglobin) are relatively hyperintense. Pathologic tissues typically appear relatively hypointense on T1-weighted images (Table 3.1; Figures 3.3A and 3.3B).

T2-weighted scans use long TE to maximize T2 contrast and long TR to minimize T1 contrast. Due to the long TR, T2-weighted imaging may be time-intensive. For this reason, fast imaging techniques such as fast spin echo are almost always used to generate T2-weighted images. On a truly T2-weighted image, water- and fluid-containing tissues are hyperintense and fat-containing tissues are hypointense. A common effect of the fast imaging techniques used for T2-weighted imaging, however, is that fat-containing tissue appears very hyperintense. T2-weighted images are particularly well suited to imaging pathological tissues such as edema, which have long T2 relaxation times and appear hyperintense on T2-weighted images.

Tissue contrast is also a function of differences in the density of water protons between tissues. This spin density, also called proton density, also impacts image contrast, but its effect on the MR signal cannot be minimized or enhanced. Rather, proton density-weighted scans are created using a short TE and long TR to minimize contrast due to both T1 and T2, leaving proton density contrast dominant.

Additional contrast

Applying a 180° RF pulse *before* the RF pulse used for excitation will invert the NMV with respect to B_0. During the interval, TI, between this 180° RF pulse and the excitation RF pulse, the inverted longitudinal magnetization recovers at a rate determined by the T1 of the tissue. This approach is called inversion recovery. Tissues with different T1 will thus have different M_Z at the time of excitation and will consequently exhibit different signal. This T1 contrast is in addition to that conferred by TR. Certain choices of TI may result in M_Z from a specific population of dipoles to be zero at the time excitation occurs. As a result, this tissue will exhibit no signal at TE; it is said to be nulled and the TI is said to represent the null point for that tissue (Figure 3.4A–C).

Relatively short TI can be used to generate a STIR image, which suppresses signal from fat, which has a short T1. Long TI can be employed to suppress signal from fluids like CSF, yielding a FLAIR image. Note that inversion recovery can be used primarily to suppress signal from certain tissues, but also to

Table 3.1. Contrast modulation by TE and TR

Dominant contrast	TE	TR
T1	Short	Short
T2	Long	Long
Proton density	Short	Long

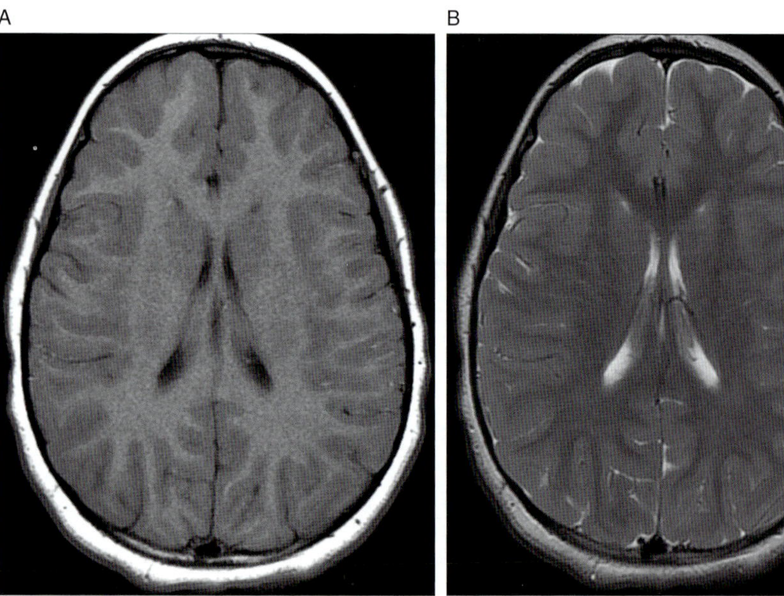

A   B

Figure 3.3 (A) Axial T1-weighted image. (B) Axial T2-weighted image.

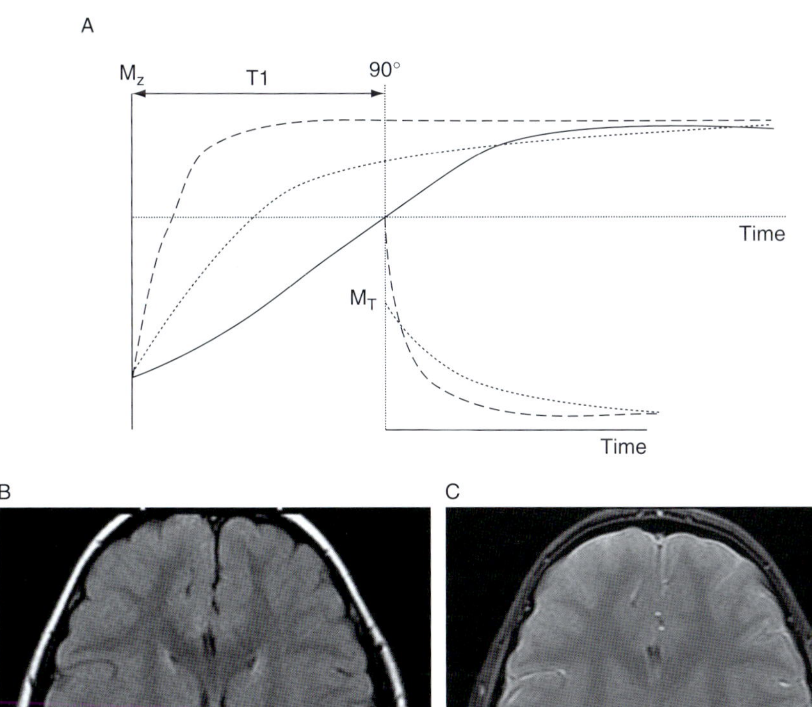

Figure 3.4 (A) Null point. The curves representing recovery of M_Z cross the X axis. At the moment the curve crossed, the tissue has no net M_Z (and also no net M_T). This point in time is termed the null point for the tissue. (B) Axial, FLAIR. (C) Axial, gradient echo.

add additional T1 contrast to an image. This latter mechanism is used commonly to generate the high contrast T1-weighted 3D gradient echo images (e.g., MP-RAGE) used in volumetric and functional MRI.

Image contrast: T1, T2, T2*

An MRI examination will be composed of several different image types, each with a unique contrast. This adds significant diagnostic power to the MRI exam when compared with CT, for example, where only one type of image contrast can be obtained. Employing multiple different contrasts also helps ensure that we avoid a potential pitfall. MRI generates image contrast by exploiting differences between tissues in their behavior within the magnetic field. Specifically, differences in T1, T2, T2*, and proton density which can be enhanced or minimized by our choice of the parameters (TE and TR) used in generating and sampling the signal. For example two different tissues whose transverse relaxation are different will lose net M_T at different rates. The tissue with the shorter T2 (or T2*) will lose M_T faster. If we set TE to occur immediately after the RF is turned off, we will detect very little difference in the M_T (read signal intensity) from the two tissues. As a result we will be unable to distinguish the tissues in our image. A longer TE, however, will reveal a large difference in signal from these tissues. To put this simply: maximal T2 contrast: long TE; minimal T2 contrast: short TE; maximal T1 contrast: short TR; minimal T1 contrast: long TR.

Contrast agents: gadolinium (Gd)

The addition of contrast agents in many cases improves sensitivity and/or specificity of the exam. Gadolinium-based contrast agents are highly paramagnetic, each gadolinium ion having nine unpaired electrons. Interaction of proton nuclei with these electrons accelerates T1 relaxation when the proton and electron are within a distance of 3 Å. Shortening of T1 decreases the time required for longitudinal relaxation to occur, thereby enhancing signal amplitude on T1-weighted images. This effect brings out differences in tissues due to differential shortening of T1; only tissues that take up the paramagnetic substance will "benefit" from this effect.

What is noise?

Noise is simply signal that does not interest us. To keep the terminology simple, we will refer to the signal arising from the subject of our image (e.g., the patient) as the signal of interest and will refer to noise as signal of no interest.

Signal-to-noise ratio: measuring image quality

We define the goal of MRI as differentiating adjacent tissues based on differences in their MR signal. If the variations in signal due to noise exceed the variations in signal we are trying to detect, such as between brain and background, we will have trouble detecting those variations in signal. The signal-to-noise ratio (SNR) is measured by obtaining measures of signal intensity from two region of interest: one placed in the image (signal of interest) and one placed in the background (signal of no interest). The more noise present in an image, the grainier it will appear. An image with very high SNR will appear to have no signal at all in the background and will look very "smooth," without graininess due to noise. Improvement in the magnitude of the MR signal can improve SNR. This can be accomplished by using different approaches. Increasing the strength of B_0, will lead to larger M_Z and, consequently, larger M_T (signal). SNR is proportional to the volume of the voxel and acquisition time. Increasing the field of view (FOV), decreasing the matrix size, and increasing the slice thickness will also improve the SNR.

Spatial resolution

The MR image, similar to CT, ultrasound, and PET, represents a slice of tissue; MRI is a tomographic or cross-sectional imaging method. In MRI, the use of gradient magnetic fields provides a spatially encoded NMR signal, which is transformed into an image using Fourier transform methods, the details of which are beyond the scope of this chapter. To be useful for diagnosis or research, any image must be physically capable of resolving signal from two locations of interest in the tissue, referred to as spatial resolution. When viewed on a computer display, the image is shown as a 2D grid of squares called pixels, but the slice of tissue that the image represents is 3D, and has a real thickness. Each pixel actually represents a prism-shaped chunk of tissue that we refer to as a voxel. The depth of the voxel is determined by the slice thickness. Spatial resolution, is a function of the number of voxels that are employed to create the image and the size of the imaging voxels. The size of the voxel depends on the number of pixels arrayed along each dimension of the image (matrix size, the dimensions of the FOV, and the slice thickness). Dividing the FOV by the matrix size gives you the voxel size; hence, increasing the FOV increases the size of the voxels and decreases the resolution. Decreasing the FOV improves the resolution. Spatial resolution defines how sharp the image appears. Low-resolution images have poor edge definition or sharpness.

Multislice versus volumetric imaging (2D vs. 3D)

In 2-dimensional (2D) imaging we acquire a set of separate images, each representing a slice of tissue. If we set up the scan so that the slices are adjacent to each other, we will represent the volume of interest as a set of contiguous slices. However, it is important to recognize that these slices are in fact independently acquired images. Furthermore, due to limitations of the MR hardware, it is not possible to generate truly contiguous slices and, for this reason, an interslice gap is commonly a feature of such scans. 3-dimensional imaging, however, offers the opportunity to image the entire volume of tissue once. This volume is then divived into a series of truly contiguous slices for purposes of display. 3-dimensional imaging is advantageous because it affords significant advantages in spatial resolution (slice thickness) and inherently higher SNR relative to 2D imaging. The major downside to 3D imaging is its cost in terms of time, which increases as a factor of the number of slices, regardless of imaging parameters. This restricts the use of 3D techniques to applications that employ very short TR, most commonly gradient echo techniques.

Magnetic resonance angiography (MRA), time-of-flight MRA (TOF-MRA)

Magnetic resonance angiography (MRA) uses the same MRI system and methods we have discussed to make images of blood vessels. Though the MRA images are cross-sectional images just like all other MR images, 3D rendering is commonly used in MRA. The most common MRA technique is based on the time-of-flight (TOF) effect, where blood protons flowing into the slice during the acquisition yield very high signal, but signal from stationary protons is suppressed. TOF thus requires no exogenous contrast agent and provides high-resolution vascular imaging that is entirely non-invasive. MRA images are simply MRI images designed to maximize contrast between the inflowing blood signal and stationary tissue signal. As a result, whereas MRA images are excellent for detection of motion (flow), they otherwise have very poor contrast for stationary tissues. The name of the game in MRA is to maximize the difference in signal intensity between flowing spins and stationary spins. To do so, signal from flow is maximized and signal from stationary tissue is suppressed. If flow is depicted as a vector, this vector describes both the direction (vector orientation) and speed (vector length) of flow. The fluid whose motion is being demonstrated with MRA is composed of particles (e.g., red blood cells). A vector will represent each individual particle, describing its direction and speed of flow. If a volume of arterial blood is then observed, the net flow detected within that volume would be determined by the individual flow vector of all particles within the volume of interest. In MRA, signal depends on the net flow vector present within a voxel of flowing blood. Key parameters for MRA include: gradient echo acquisition, short TE, and very short TR. Therefore MRA images are "T1-weighted."

How is it that MRA or MRV (MR venography) are selective for arterial or venous flow? In order to make an artery-only or vein-only image, spatial presaturation pulses must be employed. To image the carotid arteries, an RF saturation pulse selective for the region cranial to the slice of interest is applied immediately before the MRA pulse sequence begins. As a result spins flowing in the head-to-foot direction are saturated before they enter the imaging slice and, when they flow into the MRA slice, have no M_Z to be turned into signal. Thus, venous flow is suppressed, yielding an arterial image. In order to image venous flow, needs to be placed the saturation band caudal to the slice of interest. As a result, spins flowing in the foot-to-head direction are saturated and, when they flow into the MRV slice, have no M_Z to be turned into signal and therefore no arterial flow will be seen.

Conclusion

MRI provides exquisitely detailed images of internal body structures and is especially useful for brain imaging. Variation of the MR parameters yields images of multiple unique contrasts, which can be optimized to achieve superior representation of anatomy, pathology, and, as discussed in Chapter 4, function and metabolism. Further details regarding structural MRI can be found in [1–4].

Declaration of interest

The authors have nothing to disclose.

References

1. Lipton ML. *Totally Accessible MRI, a User Guide to Principles, Technology, and Applications.* New York, Springer, 2008.

2. Bushberg JT, Seibert JA, Leidholdt EM, Boone TM. *The Essential Physics of Medical Imaging,* 2nd edn. Philadelphia, Lippincott, Williams & Watkins, 2002.

3. Curry TS, III, Dowdey JE, Murray RE. *Christensen's Physics of Diagnostic Radiology,* 4th edn. Philadelphia, Lea & Febiger, 1990.

4. Stark DD, Bradley WG. *Magnetic Resonance Imaging,* 2nd edn. St. Louis, Mosby Incorporated, 1992.

Fundamentals of MRI for assessing brain function and metabolism

William A. Gomes and Michael L. Lipton

Introduction

Modern neuroimaging has revolutionized the study of brain structure and function. In particular, advanced magnetic resonance imaging (MRI) techniques allow the non-invasive collection of functional and metabolic data in human subjects that were previously restricted to invasive animal model systems. In this chapter, we review three of the most important and topical advanced MRI techniques. We first consider functional MRI (fMRI), which permits dynamic evaluation of neural activity in specific brain regions. Numerous applications for fMRI exist in sleep-related research, including examination of the neural correlates of sleep states and the consequences of sleep disturbance for waking neural function [1]. We then discuss diffusion tensor imaging (DTI), which illuminates the structure of cerebral white matter, and demonstrates the white matter connections between gray matter structures. DTI may thereby allow the identification of subtle white matter abnormalities which contribute to sleep-related disorders [2, 3]. We conclude with an introduction to magnetic resonance spectroscopy (MRS), a non-invasive method for the evaluation of brain chemistry. MRS may permit the demonstration of subtle metabolic deficits that accompany sleep disturbance [4, 5].

Functional MRI

To understand how the brain functions in the waking and sleeping states, non-invasive techniques for the evaluation of neuronal activity are required. Several such techniques are currently available, including fMRI, electroencephalography (EEG), and magnetoencephalography (MEG). Among these, fMRI is distinguished by its high spatial resolution, capacity for precise anatomical localization, and the wide availability of appropriate hardware. Funtional MRI has therefore become the predominant method for non-invasive functional brain mapping in clinical practice and basic neuroscience research. Relative limitations of fMRI include a relatively long temporal resolution, although this may be of little consequence in the study of processes with a relatively long time course, including sleep.

The goal of fMRI is to demonstrate the timing and spatial distribution of neuronal activity. In principle, this goal can be accomplished through direct measurement of the small magnetic field fluctuations associated with neuronal activity [6]. Direct demonstration of neuronal activity with MRI equipment remains difficult in practice, however. Therefore, the vast majority of contemporary fMRI experiments measure neuronal activity indirectly, through monitoring of homeostatic changes in regional blood oxygenation that accompany regional activation [7]. Increased neuronal activity results in increased metabolism, which implies increased demand for oxygen. This demand is met through increased blood flow to the activated region, a response called neurovascular coupling [8]. The regional increase in blood flow, and oxygen delivery, is larger than that required to accommodate increased neuronal metabolism. As a consequence, the neurovascular coupling response leads to a slight increase in net blood oxygenation in functionally activated regions [8]. This activity-dependent increase in blood oxygenation progresses asymptotically, reaching a plateau 4–6 s after the onset of event-related neuronal activation.

In fMRI, the slight activity-related increase in blood oxygenation level is detected through blood oxygen level-dependent (BOLD) variations of $T2^*$ in the region of neuronal activation, which are detectable as an increase in the MRI signal intensity on $T2^*$-sensitive (usually echo-planar) MRI sequences [9]. These variations in signal intensity reflect a shift in the predominant state of the hemoglobin population from deoxyhemoglobin, which is paramagnetic, to oxyhemoglobin, which is diamagnetic. The result is a slight increase in MRI signal intensity with increased brain activation. This increase follows the same time course as the underlying increase in blood oxygenation, with an initial period of asymptotic rise over 4–6 s followed by stabilization at the new, higher level.

To detect regional brain activation by fMRI, it is necessary to compare regional signal intensity during an experimental condition to a carefully selected control condition [8, 10]. This comparison is necessary because many factors, in addition to neuronal activation, influence regional signal intensity on $T2^*$-weighted images. These include static regional differences in brain oxygenation unrelated to neuronal activity, differences in tissue signal intensity unrelated to oxygenation, and MRI artifacts. Through comparison of the experimental condition to a control condition, activation-related signal changes can be separated from these confounding factors. As an example, if the goal is to demonstrate activation related to motor function, the subject might be asked to perform a motor task (e.g., finger

Neuroimaging of Sleep and Sleep Disorders, ed. Eric Nofzinger, Pierre Maquet, and Michael J. Thorpy. Published by Cambridge University Press. © Cambridge University Press 2013.

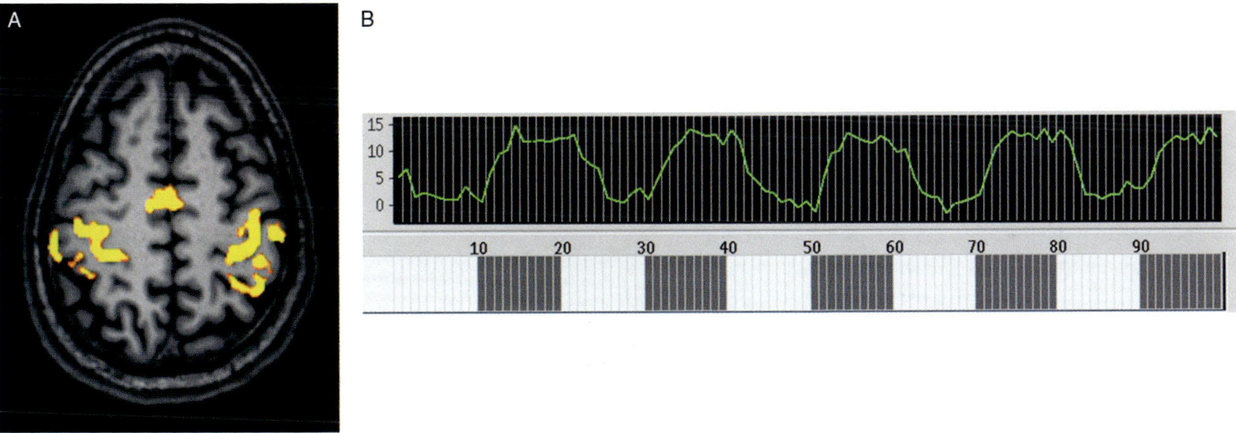

Figure 4.1 Functional MRI of a motor task. (A) Finger tapping elicits BOLD activation, displayed in yellow, in the primary motor cortex and supplemental motor area. (B) Block design of an fMRI experiment is depicted, with the resulting task-related BOLD response presented.

tapping). Images obtained during this task are compared to images obtained while the fingers were motionless, resulting in increase in the T2*-weighted MRI signal due to activation in the primary and supplemental motor areas (Figure 4.1A). Because the magnitude of the activity-related increase in T2*-sensitive MRI signal is small (≈2–4%) relative to various sources of non-activation-related signal fluctuation, it is not detectable by visual inspection of the images. Averaging of signals acquired over multiple repetitions of a task or activity is required. This can be accomplished through a "block design," in which two or more experimental conditions alternate, typically with a period of 5–10 s (Figure 4.1B) [10, 11]. T2*-weighted MRI images of the brain are obtained repeatedly throughout this process, typically at intervals of approximately 2 s. The result is a very large collection of T2*-weighted brain images obtained during the experiment, in which the desired activation data are encoded.

Extraction of the task-related BOLD activation signal from the fMRI data set requires extensive post-processing [11, 12]. First, the effects of minor head motion and various technical artifacts must be accounted for. The time-dependent signal variation in each brain voxel is then compared to the pattern expected if that portion of brain were differentially activated during the test condition. The result is a statistical map of the brain, in which each voxel is assigned a probability of covariance with the expected response pattern. Voxels that demonstrate time-dependent signal variation similar to that expected for activated brain are considered to demonstrate task-related activation. Typically, fMRI results are presented as false-colored maps, in which voxels that display statistical correlation beyond a chosen threshold are indicated (Figure 4.1).

Details of the statistical models used to create fMRI activation maps are beyond the scope of this chapter. However, it is important to note that the standard approach utilizes the General Linear Model, a statistical framework which implements linear regression techniques in the context of multiple variables [13]. Fundamental to this approach is the choice of a model for the expected time course of BOLD signal change in activated brain regions. The appropriate model is difficult to determine empirically, however, and an inappropriate choice may lead to

rejection of pertinent voxels that do not fit the chosen model with sufficient precision, a type II statistical error. Alternative statistical approaches are available, including the use of independent component analysis techniques, which do not depend on the choice of an a-priori activation model [14].

Functional MRI typically relies on the presentation of stimuli, or cues, that define the test conditions. These stimuli may be visual, auditory, or tactile. Specialized MR-compatible audio-visual systems are available that facilitate stimulus presentation and coordination of the stimuli with the MRI acquisition. Processing of fMRI data also requires specialized software. Numerous fMRI data analysis packages are available, including both commercial and open source solutions. FSL [15] and AFNI [16] are currently popular, freely available software packages that include fMRI analysis functions. Pertinent considerations for the choice of post-processing software include compatibility with the chosen activation paradigm and inclusion of the desired statistical model.

The range of potential fMRI paradigms is very large, encompassing a broad range of conscious or unconscious states. In theory, any two mental states that can be temporally defined can also be compared in an fMRI experiment. Careful paradigm design is essential to successful fMRI, however. Simple paradigms may include motor (e.g., finger tapping) or language (e.g., sentence completion) tasks. These paradigms reliably demonstrate activation of the relevant primary cortical regions. More sophisticated tasks are also available or can be created to assess memory, attention, and other higher cognitive functions [17].

Several design options are available in the construction of an fMRI paradigm [10]. The simplest is the block design, in which two or more states alternate according to a predetermined pattern (Figure 4.1). Block design has the advantage of simplicity in both implementation and post-processing, and is sufficient for many purposes. In some cases, however, a predetermined pattern of cues may be inadequate to capture the cognitive process of interest. In these cases, an event-related paradigm could be considered, in which the pertinent state occurs at irregular intervals, and may be determined retrospectively based on data obtained later in the experiment [10, 11].

Several fundamental limitations of BOLD fMRI must be acknowledged. First, the demonstration of brain activity through fMRI is necessarily indirect, in that it relies on both activity-related increase in blood flow and the consequent increase in blood oxygenation to complete a chain of inference between the neuronal activity to be measured and the fMRI statistical map that is ultimately produced. This chain of inference can be challenged at each step. It is not clear, for example, that the degree and temporal properties of neurovascular coupling remain constant across brain regions and differing experimental conditions [8, 18]. The temporal resolution of conventional fMRI is also relatively poor (approximately 2 s) relative to the time-scale of some neural processes. To address this limitation, considerable effort is currently being devoted toward the implementation of ultra-fast fMRI methods [19]. Finally, fMRI demonstrates the activation of specific brain regions in the context of a particular paradigm. From this, we can infer the involvement of that brain region in some element of the neural processes pertinent to the task. Functional MRI cannot, however, demonstrate what role that region plays, or whether that role is essential to the brain processes of interest [20].

Standard fMRI involves the comparison of brain activation, assessed through the BOLD effect, between two or more experimental conditions. As previously described, this technique depends on the association of a particular functional state with activation of corresponding brain regions. It has also been observed, however, that regional brain activity (and oxygenation) varies spontaneously in resting subjects. Furthermore, coherent temporal variation of the BOLD signal may occur across multiple brain regions in the resting state. This implies some form of functional connection among the brain areas, which are said to form a network. This observation has led to the description of a resting state, or default mode, network of functionally connected brain regions (Figure 4.2) [21]. The resting state network includes the medial temporal lobe, posterior cingulate gyrus, prefrontal cortex, and perhaps other brain regions. The precise role and significance of the default mode network remain unclear, and its significance has been questioned [22]. Nevertheless, the default mode network is perturbed in a variety of disease states [23–25]. There is currently great interest in refining our understanding of the resting state network and its role in normal brain function and in pathological states.

Diffusion tensor imaging

Neuronal axons, bundles of which form white matter tracts, are the structural substrate of functional connections between brain regions. These axonal connections vary between individuals and demonstrate plasticity in both physiological and pathological settings [26, 27]. Therefore, to understand normal and pathological brain function, we must understand the structural arrangement of white matter tracts, and how this arrangement varies between individuals. This goal can be approached in living subjects with DTI, a variant of diffusion-weighted imaging (DWI), which permits the non-invasive evaluation of regional white matter structure.

The diffusion properties of water in a simple solution (e.g., cerebrospinal fluid) are isotropic (the same in all directions). In

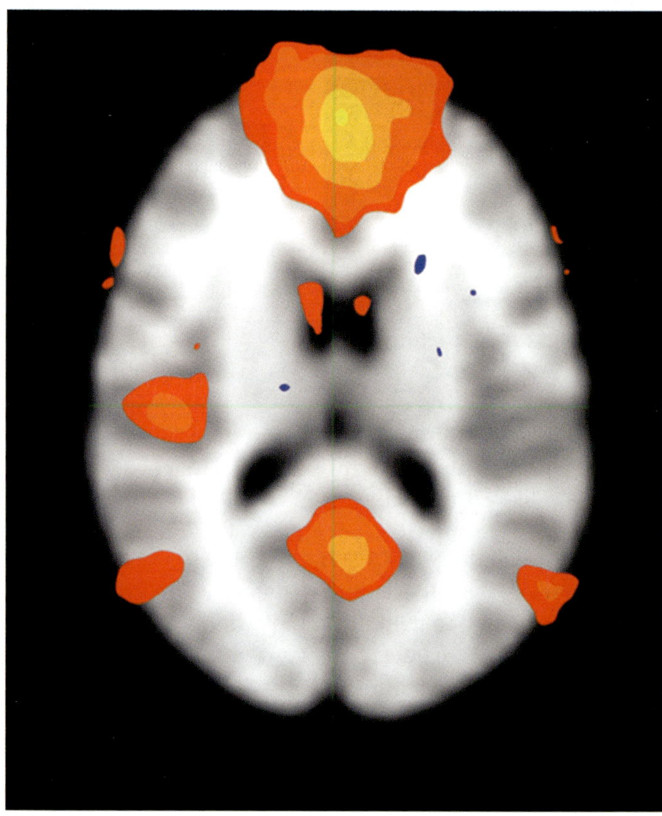

Figure 4.2 Resting state fMRI. Composite results of resting state fMRI analysis in 27 adult subjects. Synchronized activation in the default mode network is demonstrated, including cingulate, parietal, and temporal regions.

myelinated white matter, by contrast, the diffusion of water is constrained by the presence of axons and their myelin sheaths. Diffusion is therefore anisotropic (direction dependent) with relatively free diffusion along the length of axonal bundles, but slow diffusion across them. In DTI, a model of the region-specific directional diffusion properties of water is created. From this model, the regional structure of white matter is inferred.

DTI depends on the addition of diffusion sensitization gradients to standard MRI pulse sequences. With the addition of a diffusion sensitization gradient, the MRI signal intensity becomes dependent on the coefficient of diffusion along the gradient. To calculate a 3-dimensional model of diffusion, images are acquired repeatedly with systematic variation in the direction of the diffusion sensitization gradient. This collection of images, obtained with varying directional diffusion sensitization, is then processed to generate a mathematical model of the 3-dimensional distribution of diffusion coefficients for each voxel.

Three-dimensional diffusion data are represented by the diffusion tensor, a 3-dimensional ellipsoid that relates spatial direction to scalar diffusion magnitude (Figure 4.3). The tensor for a given voxel is characterized by three principal vectors (eigenvectors). The orientation of the major eigenvector (i.e., the "long axis" of the tensor) represents the predominant direction of diffusion in that voxel. In compact white matter, in which diffusion is anisotropic, the major eigenvector is substantially larger than the orthogonal medium and minor eigenvectors, corresponding to an elongated, "cigar-shaped" diffusion tensor

(Figure 4.4). In gray matter, by contrast, diffusion is relatively isotropic, and the diffusion tensor approximates a sphere.

DTI data can be assessed in several ways. First, the shape of the tensor can be assessed through comparison of the magnitude of the major eigenvector to the magnitudes of the medium and minor eigenvectors. This relationship is typically represented by the scalar value fractional anisotropy (FA), which varies from zero (isotropic diffusion) to one (unidirectional diffusion). Typical FA values in adult cerebral white matter range from approximately 0.4 to 0.7 [28]. FA maps allow depiction of the regional variation in white matter structure (Figure 4.5), with higher (brighter) values in the compact central white matter. Voxel-based comparison of FA maps between individuals or groups allows a quantitative comparison of white matter structure. Several other numerical measures derived from the diffusion tensor also prove useful in certain circumstances, including the relative anisotropy (RA) and radial diffusivity (RD). Note that FA, RA, and RD are scalar measures of the shape of the diffusion tensor, which do not account for variations in the predominant direction of diffusion. This directional information can be depicted using false color maps (Figure 4.5).

It is also of interest to distinguish between individual white matter tracts, and to characterize the structural parameters of these tracts. This can be accomplished through diffusion tractography (DT), a post-processing technique that is applied to DTI data. In DT, the directional information encoded in DTI data is used to construct an estimate of the position, course, and size of specific white matter tracts [29]. The corticospinal tracts, for example, can be demonstrated passing from the precentral gyri to the spinal cord (Figure 4.6). Numerous other white matter tracts can also be demonstrated reliably, including the superior longitudinal fasciculi, inferior longitudinal fasciculi, uncinate fasciculus, and cingulum bundle [30].

DT essentially allows the parcellation of white matter voxels into anatomically defined tracts. The tracts can then be analyzed according to their estimated size, which varies among individuals, and diffusion properties. The diffusion indices described above can be assessed in a particular tract; for example the average FA of the corticospinal tract can be measured. This approach can, theoretically, compensate for inter-individual variation in the size of white matter tracts, which might otherwise confound voxel-based DTI analysis.

A variety of DT algorithms are currently in use, which vary in their ease of implementation, reproducibility, and ability to demonstrate certain white matter tracts. The fiber assignment by continuous tracking (FACT) is most commonly used, and is

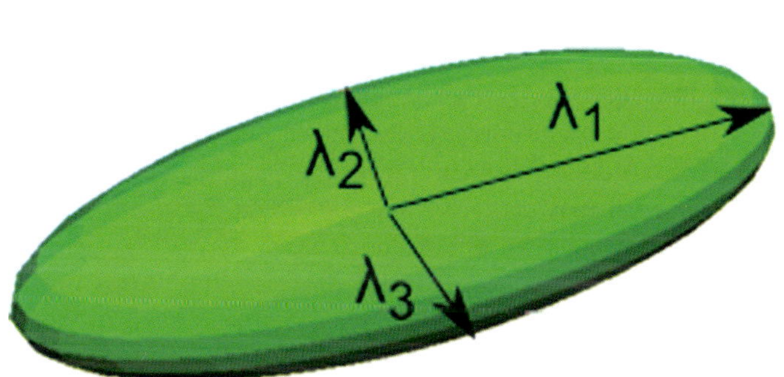

Figure 4.3 Schematic depiction of a diffusion tensor. The major (λ_1) and medium (λ_2) and minor (λ_3) eigenvectors are indicated.

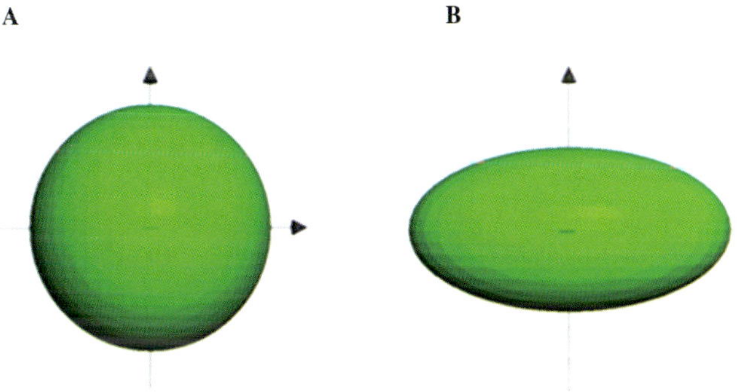

Figure 4.4 Regional variation in the diffusion tensor. Schematic depictions of diffusion tensors from gray matter (A) and white matter (B), demonstrating anisotropic diffusion in white matter.

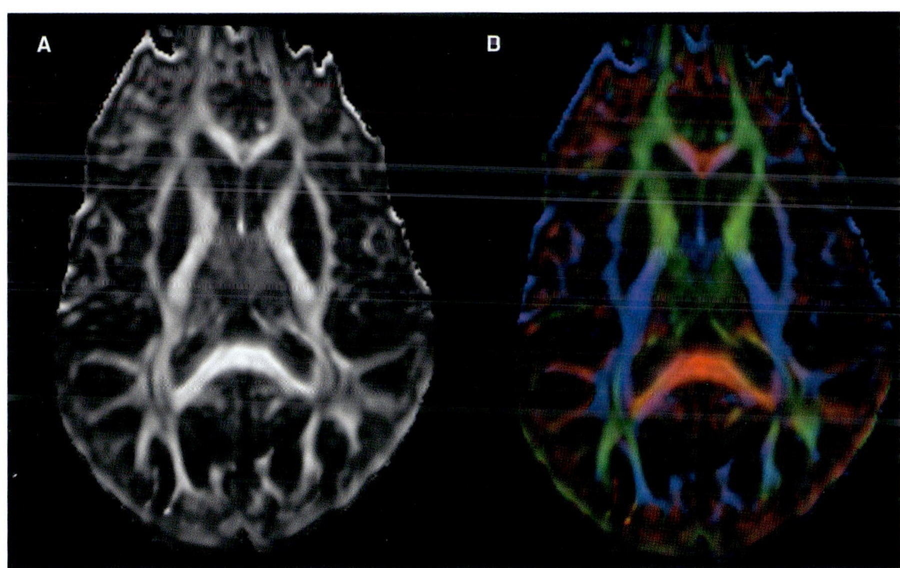

Figure 4.5 Visual representation of DTI data. (A) Anatomic map of fractional anisotropy (FA), demonstrating high FA in the central white matter. (B) Colorized fractional anisotropy map. Red indicates predominantly right–left diffusion, blue superior–inferior and green antero-posterior.

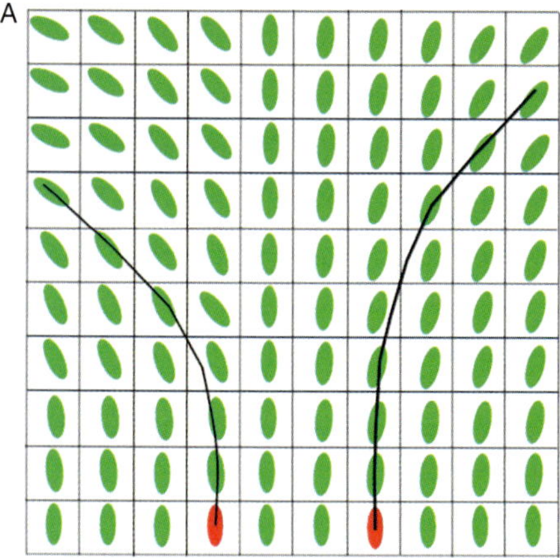
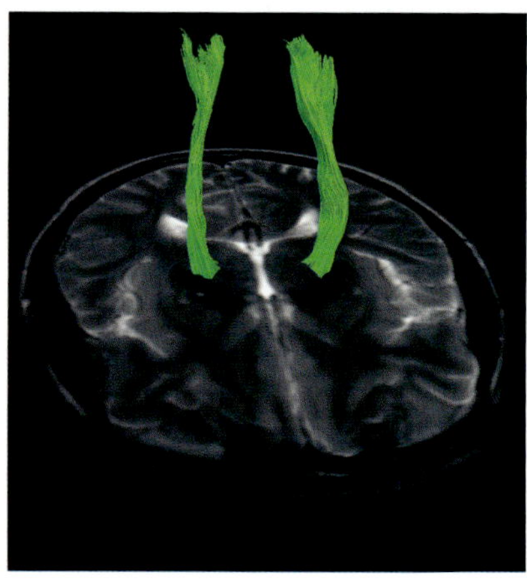

Figure 4.6 Diffusion tractography. (A) Schematic depiction of the FACT tractography algorithm, with seed voxels indicated in red. (B) Diffusion tractography of the corticospinal tracts, 3-dimensional rendering.

sufficient for many purposes [29]. In this algorithm, tracts that extend through a region of interest, or "seed," are constructed through linear, stepwise extension of tracts along the major eigenvectors of diffusion tensor data. For each voxel in the seed volume, the direction of the major eigenvector is determined. A step is then taken to the next voxel in that direction (Figure 4.6). The process is then repeated iteratively, until a termination criterion is met, to construct an estimated tract.

The FACT algorithm is remarkably successful in demonstrating major white matter tracts. There are several substantial limitations of the FACT method, however. In particular, this method can account for only one estimated fiber orientation in any one voxel. Unfortunately, this assumption does not conform to the anatomical reality that white matter tracts intermingle on a microstructural scale. This intermingling is below the resolution of standard DTI acquisitions (about 2 mm^3). In consequence, FACT-based methods underestimate the spatial extent of some tracts (e.g., portions of the corticospinal tracts) and are unable to reliably demonstrate others (e.g., the optic radiations) [30]. Several more sophisticated tractography methods are available, which attempt to address these limitations. Promising approaches include creation of a more precise model of local diffusion properties, either through a more precise diffusion-weighted acquisition, or through alternative processing schemes that do not rely on a low-order tensor model [15, 31].

Magnetic resonance spectroscopy

Standard anatomical MRI depicts the structural features of the brain, while fMRI demonstrates regional brain activity. MRS, in contrast, allows non-invasive examination of the chemical composition of the brain. MRS thereby allows for the investigation of brain metabolic processes in living subjects [32].

MRI depends on the detection of microwave-band radio-frequency (RF) signals related to the electromagnetic resonance of hydrogen (and certain other) nuclei. These signals vary slightly in frequency, depending on the chemical environment of the hydrogen nuclei. MRS exploits this slight difference in RF frequency to distinguish between metabolites.

This discussion will focus on MRS of hydrogen nuclei (^{1}H-MRS), which is the most common form of MRS in neuroscience research and clinical practice. This popularity reflects the relative ease of ^{1}H-MRS, owing to its high signal-to-noise ratio, ability to detect numerous pertinent metabolites, and availability on standard MRI equipment. Other naturally occurring isotopes are also amenable to MRS, however, including phosphorus (^{31}P), oxygen (^{17}O), and carbon (^{13}C). MRS of nuclei other than hydrogen requires specialized techniques and equipment, but can provide additional information not available through ^{1}H-MRS. In particular, ^{31}P-MRS allows examination of high-energy phosphate metabolism [5].

In ^{1}H-MRS, RF signal is elicited from a localized volume of interest (VOI) using specialized MR pulse sequences. The resulting signal is recorded and, after Fourier transformation, an RF intensity spectrum is obtained (Figure 4.7). Peaks in the RF spectrum correspond to hydrogen nuclei with differing resonant frequency. Depending on the structure of the molecule in which it is contained, an individual hydrogen moiety may be represented by one or more peaks (termed singlet and multiplet resonances, respectively).

The absolute resonant frequency depends on field strength, which varies among MRI scanners. To facilitate comparison between scanners of differing field strength, the RF spectrum is normalized to a parts-per-million (PPM) scale. For convenience, the origin of this scale (0 PPM) is assigned to the resonant frequency of a reference standard, tetramethylsilane. The distance of a peak from this origin is termed chemical shift. Signal representing a specific metabolite can then be distinguished on the basis of its characteristic chemical shift and peak structure. For historical reasons, the PPM scale is plotted such that chemical shift increases from right to left; the origin is plotted on the right.

The spatial localization techniques used in MRS differ substantially from those used in standard anatomical MRI. These differences are necessitated, in part, by the need to avoid the use of frequency encoding for spatial localization. In the simplest, single voxel, MRS techniques, a single, spatially defined VOI is stimulated, and a spectrum representing the entire VOI is obtained. Signal-to-noise considerations effectively limit single-voxel techniques to a relatively large volume – approximately 3 cm^3 using standard techniques. Therefore, while they are straightforward from the technical perspective, single-voxel techniques are limited in both resolution and anatomical coverage.

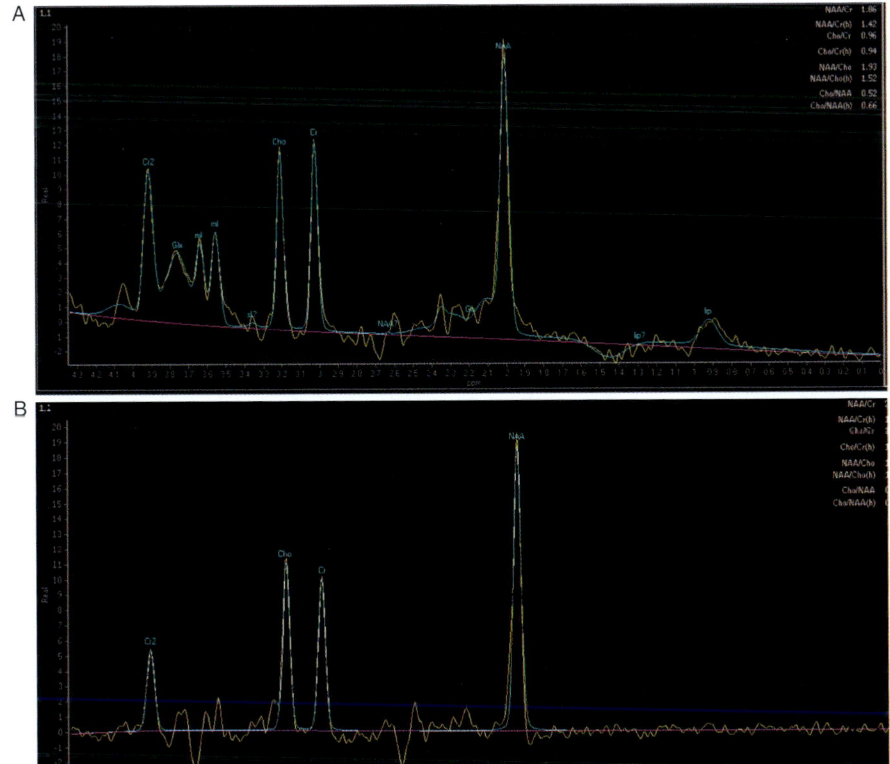

Figure 4.7 Typical short (A, TE = 30 ms) and long (B, TE = 144 ms) echo-time brain spectra obtained from cerebral white matter of a healthy adult subject.

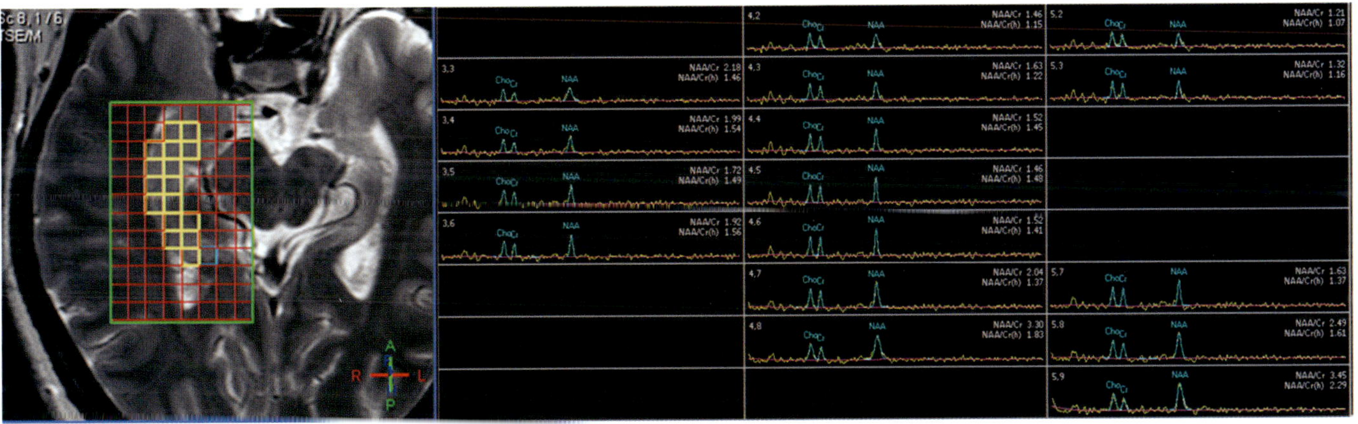

Figure 4.8 Multivoxel MRS of the hippocampus. The spectroscopic volume of interest is denoted in green, with individual voxels in red. Voxels falling within the hippocampus are highlighted (yellow), and the corresponding spectra are displayed.

These limitations of single-voxel MRS can be addressed through the use of multi voxel MRS techniques (Figure 4.8). In multivoxel MRS, a relatively large VOI is stimulated. Phase encoding techniques are then employed to obtain spatial information within the stimulated VOI. 2 dimensional phase encoding is common, although 3-dimensional techniques are increasingly employed [33]. Advantages of multivoxel techniques include improved breadth of anatomical coverage in a single MRS acquisition and the potential for smaller voxel sizes (approximately 1.0 cm^3 with typical clinical equipment). Disadvantages of multivoxel MRS include longer acquisition time, increased potential for artifact, and the requirement for highly tuned (in particular, precisely shimmed) MRI equipment.

In an unselected brain ^{1}H-MRS spectrum, the RF signal from water vastly exceeds that from any other metabolite, and the metabolite peaks of interest are therefore obscured by a large water peak. Therefore, it is typically necessary to suppress the water signal. This suppression is accomplished through specialized pulse sequences, most commonly chemically selective saturation (CHESS) [34]. In addition, large lipid resonances are present in the skull and scalp, which may also obscure metabolites of interest. It is therefore desirable to exclude the skull from the MRS excitation volume. In some cases lipid suppression techniques are required [35].

MRS yields a spectrum in which the area under a given metabolite peak is determined in part by the volume concentration of the metabolite. Many confounding biophysical and technical parameters also contribute to the observed peak area on the MRS spectrum, however. These factors are difficult to predict a priori, and analysis of an MR spectrum therefore does not provide a quantitative measure of underlying metabolite concentrations. To achieve absolute quantization of metabolite concentrations, the magnitude of MRS resonant peaks can be compared to those obtained from a standard solution of known concentration [36]. The concentration standard might be positioned beside the patient within the MR scanner, or might be scanned separately using a similar MRS protocol. Absolute quantitation is far more demanding than one might expect, however, owing to various technical considerations, including dependence of the measured MRS signal on physical properties (size, shape, mass, conductivity, position in the MRI scanner) of the sample.

Absolute quantitation of metabolite concentrations is therefore possible and desirable, but often technically difficult to achieve. One commonly used alternative is the analysis of metabolite ratios. Thus, the *N*-acetylaspartate (NAA) peak might be normalized to creatine peak area, and the ratio NAA/creatine used as an experimental measure. Creatine is frequently taken as the denominator since its levels are relatively (although not absolutely) stable across pathological conditions [32]. While absolute quantitation is clearly preferable from the theoretical perspective, analysis of metabolite ratios is simple, straightforward, and the standard in clinical MRS.

Several technical parameters influence the appearance of the ^{1}H-MRS spectrum, including which metabolites are identified and the relative size of metabolite peaks. Foremost among these parameters is the echo time (TE). The T2-decay time of MRI signal differs substantially between brain metabolites. Spectra collected at short TE (generally, 40 ms or shorter) demonstrate metabolites with both long and short decay times (Figure 4.7). In spectra obtained at long TE (typically, 144–288 ms), in contrast, signal from metabolites with shorter decay time is diminished or absent. The result is a simpler spectrum composed of only the most abundant, long decay-time metabolites. The choice of appropriate echo time depends in part on the needs of the experiment. If identification of metabolites with short decay time is required, short echo-time spectra are preferred.

A large number of metabolites are present in the normal brain. In practice, only a limited subset of these can be routinely identified with MRS. Several factors determine the visibility of metabolites by MRS, including bulk concentration, resonance structure (singlet or multiplet), and the T2-decay time. Advanced techniques are available to improve the detection of certain low abundance metabolites, including gamma-aminobutyric acid (GABA), as discussed below. The major metabolites typically demonstrated in normal brain are reviewed below, along with the chemical shift and structure of commonly used resonant peaks. For a comprehensive list of ^{1}H-MRS-visible brain metabolites, the reader is referred to Govindaraju *et al.* [37]. Further details regarding the composition and biochemical significance of MRS-visible metabolites can be found in De Graaf [32].

N-Acetylaspartate (*NAA*): singlet resonance, 2.0 PPM. NAA is a product of neuronal mitochondria, and its concentration reflects the number and metabolic integrity of neurons. NAA is present at high concentration in the normal brain, and is the predominant peak in the normal brain spectrum. The function of NAA is unknown, although roles in osmotic regulation and as a metabolic intermediate are proposed. The observed 2.0 PPM peak represents a superposition of NAA and the less-abundant metabolite, *N*-acetyl aspartyl glutamate (NAAG).

Choline: singlet resonance, 3.2 PPM. Choline-containing compounds are common constituents of cellular membranes, with a variety of biochemical functions. Increased cell proliferation, whether physiological or pathological, is associated with increased magnitude of the MRS-visible choline resonance. Increased choline on MRS is therefore a biomarker for increased cell proliferation, and correlates with histological measures such as the mitotic index. The observed peak reflects both free choline and several choline-containing metabolites.

Creatine: singlet resonance, 3.0 PPM. An intermediate in high-energy phosphate metabolism, creatine is predominantly associated with astroglia. The observed resonance actually represents a superimposition of peaks representing creatine and phosphocreatine. Compared to NAA and choline, creatine levels are relatively constant across physiological and pathological conditions.

Glutamate: complex multiplet resonances, 2.04–2.75 and 3.75 PPM. Glutamate is the primary excitatory neurotransmitter of the brain, and therefore of great interest to neuroscientists. It is also fairly difficult to quantitate, however, owing to its moderate abundance, multiplet resonance, and relatively short T2-decay time. Glutamate is best demonstrated on short echo-time spectra. The observed glutamate peaks overlap with those of glutamine, and differentiation of these compounds is difficult, especially at lower magnetic field strength.

Gamma-aminobutyric acid (GABA): multiple resonances, 1.89–3.01 PPM. GABA, the primary inhibitory neurotransmitter of the brain, is also of great interest to neuroscientists. Identification of GABA on MRS is complicated, however, by low abundance and overlap of the GABA resonances with other metabolites. Specialized spectral-editing techniques, and long acquisition times, are generally required for accurate quantitation [38].

Conclusion

The advanced neuroimaging techniques described in this chapter allow non-invasive evaluation of the intact brain at biochemical, network, and functional levels. These techniques thereby provide the foundation for an emerging body of knowledge concerning the metabolic and functional underpinnings of normal and disordered sleep. Functional neuroimaging techniques will continue to improve in coming years, opening additional opportunities for novel sleep-related investigation. In addition, it is hoped that the ubiquitous availability of MRI scanners in the modern clinical environment will allow translation of these studies into the routine clinical practice of sleep medicine.

Fundamentals of PET scanning

Bohdan Bybel, Andrew L. Goertzen, and Shadreck Mzengeza

Introduction

Positron emission tomography (PET) imaging is a proven diagnostic tomographic scintigraphic technique in which a computer-generated image of radiolabeled tracer distribution in tissues is produced through the detection of annihilation photons that are emitted when radionuclides introduced into the body decay and release positrons [1]. It has many applications in oncology, cardiology, and neurology [2]. More recently PET has been combined with computed tomography (CT), and in the near future will be combined with magnetic resonance imaging (MRI), on a single scanner to incorporate anatomical data in combination with the physiological imaging of PET to add an incremental clinical benefit for these hybrid studies [3].

PET imaging has been available for many decades in a research setting but has exploded in clinical use since the late 1990s [4]. Neurological applications are not as frequently utilized in clinical practice as oncological and, to a lesser degree, cardiac ones. In neurology, the main indications have been for localization of epileptic foci, evaluating PET ^{18}F fluorodeoxyglucose (^{18}F-FDG) patterns of cognitive impairment, and differentiating malignant recurrence of brain tumor from radiation necrosis post radiotherapy.

Extensive research in neuroimaging has enabled non-invasive measurement of biological function and evaluation of brain function associated with many physiological and pathological states. Sleep medicine literature of functional neuroimaging is still limited [5] but has many potential uses [6]. Early PET studies utilized regional cerebral blood flow (rCBF) using ^{15}O-water PET, cerebral oxygen metabolism rate (CMRO$_2$), and regional cerebral glucose metabolism (CMRglu) most often with ^{18}F-FDG [7]. Multiple PET tracers in development or early clinical use are used to look at cellular processes such as neurotransmitter synthesis and release or specific protein molecules which may have relevance for the neurological or psychiatric research questions. Serotonin and dopamine systems are probably the most studied and a new amyloid plaque agent has been developed for dementia imaging.

Measurement of rCBF has also been performed but mainly in a research setting. The most commonly used tracer for PET measurement of rCBF is ^{15}O-water. The very short half-life allows for multiple assessments (from 4 to 12 injections) of an individual at one session but also means the examination has to be performed in the immediate vicinity

of a cyclotron. Inhalation of $C^{15}O_2$ has also been described. Measurements can be made quickly in about 40 sec to 2 min and repeated every 8–10 min. The basic principle of utilizing this type of tracer is the brain possesses a mechanism by which its vascular supply can be varied in concurrence with local variations of functional activity. However, it should be noted that there is a transient uncoupling between oxygen metabolism and rCBF.

Most clinical work currently is limited to use of the glucose analog ^{18}F-FDG, which is commercially available. The principle behind this tracer is that energy metabolism of the human brain depends on the oxidation of glucose. Brain uptake is mediated via GLUT1 and GLUT3 and supported by low levels of glucose-6-phosphatase [8].

A change in the early 2000s to utilizing dual modality cameras combining PET with CT has greatly enhanced the technique. The near simultaneous imaging of molecular and anatomical information has lead to more precise localization of abnormalities and better characterization of structural changes. In addition, the imaging time has shortened, which produces more efficient instrument utilization.

Radiopharmaceuticals

The manufacture of PET radiotracers for imaging molecular processes in the human brain begins with the production of the PET radioisotope using a cyclotron. The most commonly produced radioisotopes are fluorine-18 (^{18}F), carbon-11 (^{11}C), nitrogen-13 (^{13}N), and oxygen-15 (^{15}O) (Table 5.1). Of the four common radioisotopes only ^{18}F has a radioactive half-life long enough to allow it to be shipped a significant distance, otherwise the PET radiopharmacy has to be in close proximity to the PET scanning facility. Essentially all cyclotrons used in the production of PET radioisotopes are negative ion cyclotrons which are either proton only or proton/deuteron particle cyclotrons. The low energy commercial cyclotrons have proton energy of 10–11 MeV and are usually self-shielded, for example the 11 MeV Siemens Eclipse-RD cyclotron (Figure 5.1A).

The main components of the cyclotron are: an ion source at the center of the cyclotron, a strong magnet, a pair of hollow copper electrodes, called dees because of their D-shape, to which a radiofrequency oscillator is connected, a beam extraction system and a high vacuum system. The radiofrequency oscillator is

Neuroimaging of Sleep and Sleep Disorders, ed. Eric Nofzinger, Pierre Maquet, and Michael J. Thorpy. Published by Cambridge University Press. © Cambridge University Press 2013.

Table 5.1. Cyclotron production of common PET radioisotopes

Radionuclide	Half-life (min)	Target material	Nuclear reaction	Final product
Fluorine-18	109.7	$H_2{}^{18}O$	$^{18}O(p,n)^{18}F$	$^{18}F^-$ in $H_2{}^{18}O$
Carbon-11	20.4	$^{14}N_2 + {}^{16}O_2$ (1%)	$^{14}N(p,\alpha)^{11}C$	$[^{11}C]CO_2$
Nitrogen-13	9.96	$H_2{}^{16}O$-Ethanol	$^{16}O(p,\alpha)^{13}N$	$[^{13}N]NH_3$
Oxygen-15	2.07	$^{15}N_2 + {}^{16}O_2$ (0.1–4%)	$^{15}N(p,n)^{15}O$	$[^{15}O]O_2$
		$^{15}N_2 + {}^{1}H_2$ (0.1–4%)	$^{15}N(p,n)^{15}O$	$[^{15}O]H_2O$
		$^{14}N_2 + {}^{16}O_2$ (0.1–4%)	$^{14}N(d,n)^{15}O$	$[^{15}O]O_2$
		$^{14}N_2 + CO_2$ (0.1–2%)	$^{14}(d,n)^{15}O$	$[^{15}O]CO_2$

connected to the dees such that the electrical potential on the dees is alternately positive and negative. The negatively charged particle (usually hydrogen ion) is thus accelerated in a spiral manner from the centre of the cyclotron because the dees experience a strong magnetic field and the ion particle encounters a repulsive force from the edge of one dee followed by an attractive force on the edge of the opposite dee. Once the stream of ions (proton beam) reaches the periphery it is intercepted by a carbon foil which strips electrons from the negatively charged particle to form a positively charged particle that is then directed into a beam line towards the target system containing the target material [9, 10]. Thus the target material is bombarded with a proton beam to produce a PET radioisotope. A nuclear reaction takes place in the target between the particle and the atom of the target material (Table 5.1) that gives rise to the PET radioisotope.

The radioisotope is then sent to the radiopharmacy where it is used in the preparation of a radiopharmaceutical. The preparation of the radiopharmaceutical is achieved using a computer-controlled automated synthesis module/unit housed in a shielded enclosure. The synthesis module ensures that the radioisotope is converted into a radiopharmaceutical through a series of chemical steps, as well as a formulation and dispensing process.

Radiotracers for imaging of molecular processes in the brain have to fulfill certain requirements such as (a) they should be able to cross the blood–brain barrier either passively or through an active transport, (b) they should have high affinity for the target region or receptor, (c) they should have low non-specific binding, and (d) they should not have an active efflux mechanism. Although a number of PET radiotracers have been developed for imaging molecular processes in the brain [11] only a small number have been used in neuroimaging in sleep disorder studies [12, 13]. These studies have mostly used either ^{18}F-FDG or ^{15}O-water as the radiotracer.

The ^{18}F-fluoride used in the synthesis of ^{18}F-FDG is mostly produced via the $^{18}O(p,n)^{18}F$ nuclear reaction using ^{18}O-enriched water. The ^{18}F-fluoride, dissolved in ^{18}O-water, is sent to the automated synthesis unit (ASU) such as the Bioscan Coincidence in Figure 5.1B where an anion-exchange cartridge is used to trap the ^{18}F-fluoride. The ^{18}F-fluoride is dried in a reaction vessel in the ASU and then reacted with the precursor compound (1,3,4,6-tetra-O-acetyl-2-O-trifluoromethanesulfonyl-β-D-mannopyranose commonly referred to as mannose triflate) to form the tetraacetylated ^{18}F-FDG. The two types of commercial ^{18}F-FDG ASUs differ in the way they deacetylate the tetraacetylated ^{18}F-FDG to form the injectable ^{18}F-FDG. One type such as the Coincidence (Figure 5.1B) uses the Hamacher method [14] in which the deacetylation is carried out by a base (sodium hydroxide) on a cartridge. The second method uses acid (hydrochloric acid) to deacetylate tetraacetylated ^{18}F-FDG [15].

The production of ^{15}O-water depends largely on the type of cyclotron and the nuclear reaction used to produce ^{15}O-oxygen (Table 5.1). For cyclotrons that are capable of accelerating either protons or deuterons, the preferred method for producing ^{15}O-oxygen is the bombardment of nitrogen gas mixed with a little oxygen (0.1–4%) with a deuteron beam via the $^{14}N(d,n)$ ^{15}O nuclear reaction (Table 5.1) [16, 17]. This is the cheapest and most widely used method. The small volume of ^{16}O-oxygen (usually kept as low as possible) in the target gas is needed in order to release the ^{15}O-oxygen from the target. The ^{15}O-oxygen gas is sent to a commercial ^{15}O-water synthesis box where the ^{15}O-oxygen gas is mixed with hydrogen gas and then passed over heated palladium on alumina catalytic pellets to form ^{15}O-water vapor. The ^{15}O-water vapor is then bubbled into sterile injectable saline solution. Some manufacturers have designed shielded ^{15}O-water synthesis boxes that can be located beside the PET camera. Because most CBF studies using ^{15}O-water involve several successive injections, the production process is designed such that batches of ^{15}O-oxygen are continuous produced by the cyclotron [18].

For low energy cyclotrons that are designed to accelerate protons only, ^{15}O is produced via the $^{15}N(p,n)^{15}O$ nuclear reaction in which the target material is isotopically enriched ^{15}N-N_2 gas [19]. Again a small volume of ^{16}O-oxygen is added. This method is costly because of the price of ^{15}N-N_2 gas. To reduce costs, the ^{15}O-water is separated from the ^{15}N-N_2 gas by freeze trapping ^{15}O-water at −40 °C [20]. The ^{15}N-N_2 gas is recycled and the ^{15}O-water is thawed and sent to the dispensing cell in a stream of inert gas.

A small number of ^{11}C-labeled radiotracers have been used in sleep disorder studies [12]. These include ^{11}C-dihydrotetrabenazine (C-DTBZ) [21] and ^{11}C-N-methyl-4-piperidyl benzilate (^{11}C-NMPB) [22], which have been used to assess the muscarinic cholinergic receptors, and $[^{11}C]$raclopride for D_2 receptor binding in human narcolepsy [23]. These tracers are manufactured from cyclotron produced ^{11}C-carbon dioxide which is converted into ^{11}C-methyl iodide. ^{11}C methylation of the appropriate precursor molecule gives rise to the radiotracer. High specific activity is desired for these radiotracers, which means care is taken to avoid diluting ^{11}C-carbon dioxide with atmospheric carbon dioxide.

Basic science/instrumentation

The image formation process in PET begins with the radioactive decay of a nucleus through the emission of a positron. The emitted

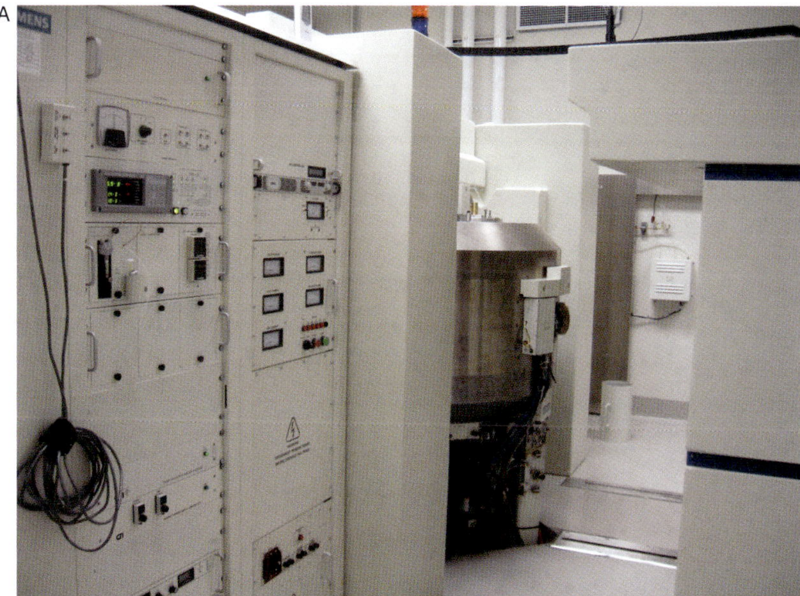

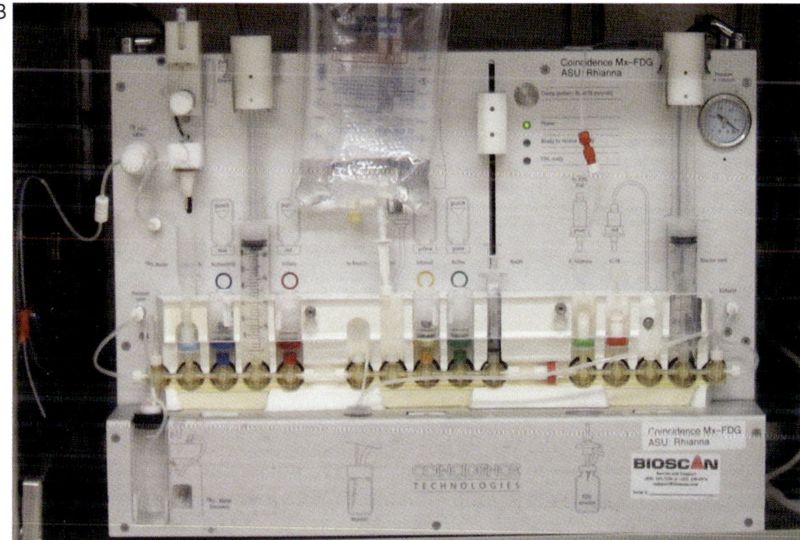

Figure 5.1 (A) Siemens Eclipse RD 11 MeV self-shielded. (B) Bioscan Coincidence ^{18}F-FDG synthesis unit loaded with cassette and reagents.

Figure 5.2 Schematic diagram of the positron emission and annihilation process.

1. Unstable, proton rich nucleus

$^{18}_{0}$F

$^{18}_{8}$O

2. Positron emitted with kinetic energy E β^- β^+

3. Positron collides with electrons until energy E is dissipated

4. Positron combines with electron to form positronium

Positronium

511 keV

180°   511 keV

5. Positron annihilates with electron

6. Mass of positron and electron converted into EM radiation. In order to conserve momentum and energy, two antiparallel annihilation photons of 511 keV are created

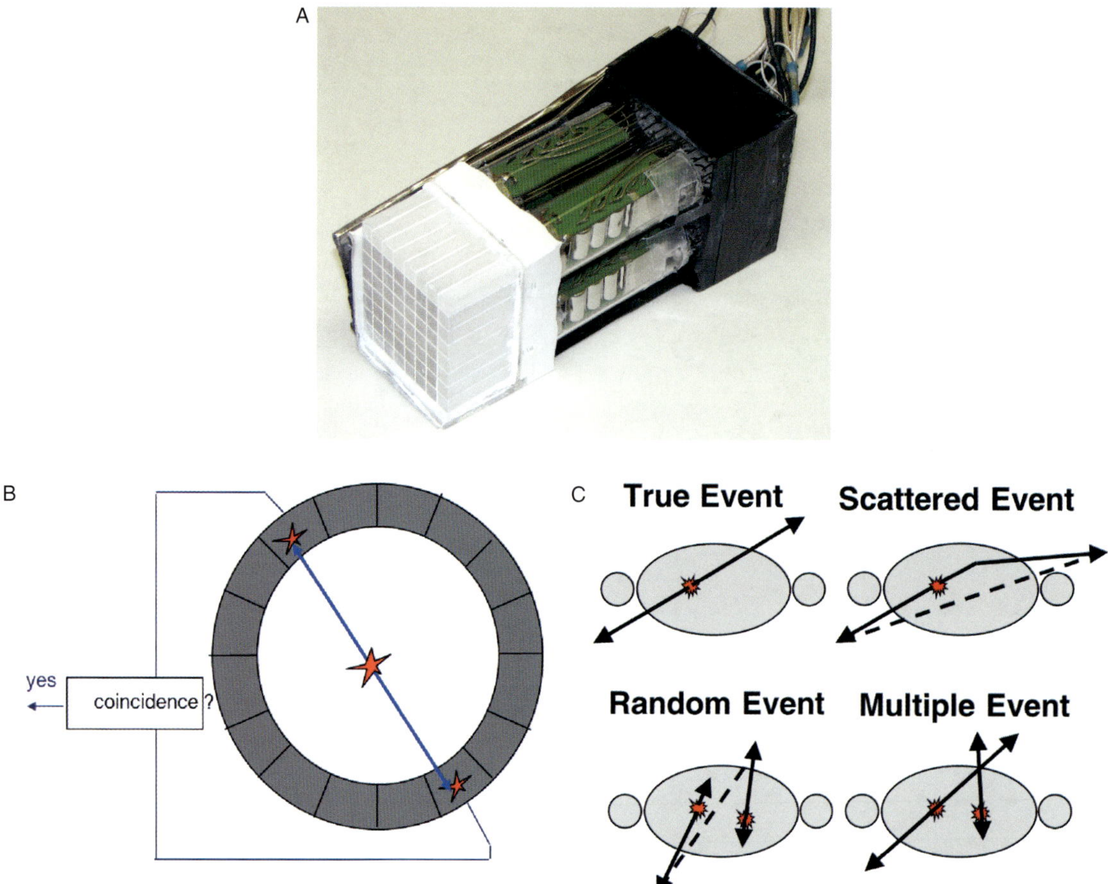

Figure 5.3 (A) Block detector from a Siemens/CTI ECAT 953B showing the 8 × 8 scintillator array coupled to the 2 × 2 PMT array. (B) Schematic of PET detector ring showing detection of coincident event. (C) Schematic showing the different types of coincidence events that are detected in PET.

positron scatters in the surrounding material, losing its kinetic energy in the process, and then annihilates with an electron. This annihilation process requires the conservation of energy and momentum, resulting in the creation of two 511 keV annihilation photons traveling antiparallel to each other. This process is shown in Figure 5.2. The 511 keV photons travel out of the subject and must be detected as a pair arriving within a narrow time window by the detectors of the PET imaging system. The position of the detectors that detect the two 511 keV photons defines the line of response (LOR) along which the positron annihilation event occurred. Through the detection of a large number of these events a distribution map of the radioactive tracer can be determined.

Detectors for PET imaging must have the following basic attributes: (1) high efficiency for stopping the 511 keV photons in order to maximize the overall detection efficiency of the PET system [24]; (2) good timing resolution in order to allow the use of a narrow coincidence timing window and thus reduce the number of accidental coincidences caused by detecting 511 keV photons originating from separate positron emission events [25]; and (3) good energy resolution in order to discriminate against lower energy events that have been scattered in the subject prior to detection [26]. The detector that currently best fits these design criteria and forms the basis for all clinical PET systems sold today is the scintillation detector.

In a scintillation detector, the 511 keV photon interacts in the scintillator material, depositing energy, and resulting in the creation of scintillation light. This light is collected and converted into an electrical signal by the photodetectors, typically an array of photomultiplier tubes (PMTs).

Figure 5.3A shows a typical scintillation detector for PET of the block detector design [27], in which a 2-dimensional scintillator crystal array is read out by a 2 × 2 array of PMTs. This design allows for only four electronics channels to be used to decode many crystal elements, for example a 13 × 13 array of $4 \times 4 \times 20$ mm^3 LSO crystals in the Siemens Biograph 16 system [28]. These detectors are arranged in a ring geometry, as shown in Figure 5.3B, with each detector operating in coincidence with each other detector in the PET system. As shown in Figure 5.3C, coincidence events can either be: (1) "true" events, in which the 511 keV photons emerge without scattering and are detected by the system; (2) "scattered" events, in which one or both of the 511 keV photons undergo Compton scattering in the subject and are subsequently detected along an LOR that is different from the true LOR if no scattering had occurred; (3) "random" events, also called accidental coincidences, in which the two 511 keV photons detected did not originate from the same positron annihilation event; and (4) "multiple" events, in which more than two 511 keV photons are detected within the coincidence window. Only true

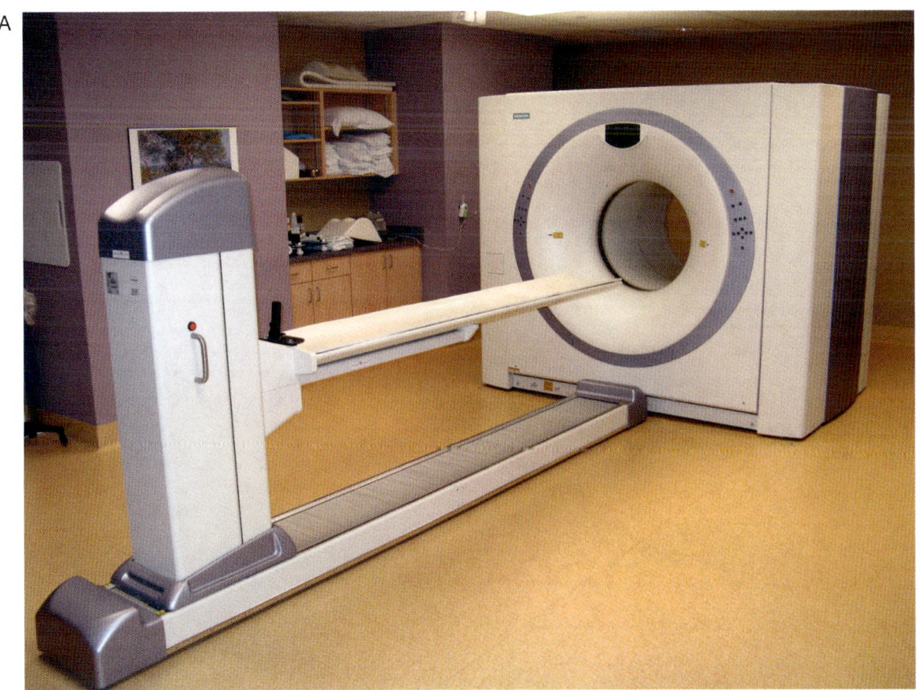

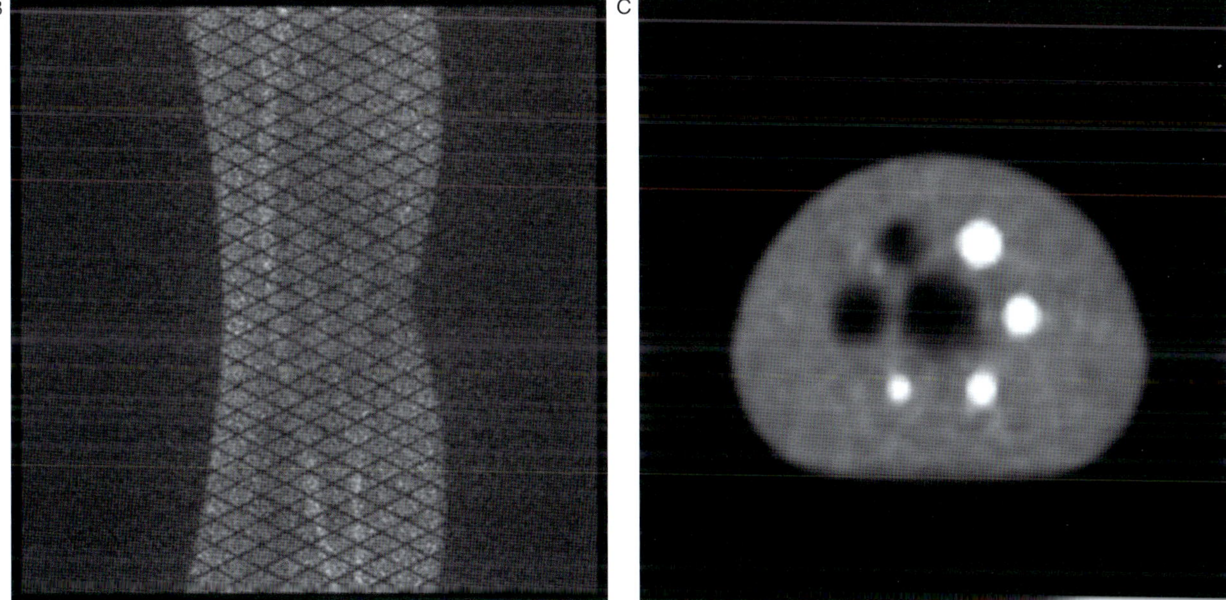

Figure 5.4 (A) Photo of a clinical PET/CT system, the Siemens Biograph 16. (B) Uncorrected sinogram data of an image quality phantom. (C) Reconstructed image generated from the data in (B) showing four "hot" regions of high radioactivity concentration and three "cold" regions that contain no radioactivity within a torso-shaped container.

events represent data that will give an accurate measure of the radiotracer distribution. The other types of coincidence events introduce bias into the image that if left uncorrected will lead to an incorrect measure of the radioactivity distribution.

The data collected in a combined PET/CT system (Figure 5.4A) are organized into a sinogram, as shown in Figure 5.4B, in which the rows represent varying angles of view and the columns represent radial offset. PET data can either be collected in static mode, in which a single time point acquisition is acquired, or in dynamic mode, in which multiple time frames are acquired. Dynamic imaging is commonly required for neuroreceptor imaging studies in which the

distribution of the tracer is changing rapidly over time and the kinetics of the tracer give information about receptor binding [29]. Images are reconstructed from sinograms using either analytical techniques such as filtered back-projection (FBP) [30] or more commonly iterative techniques such as ordered subsets expectation maximization (OSEM) [31, 32], with an example of an OSEM reconstruction seen in Figure 5.4C. A key benefit of PET is that it is quantitatively accurate, so that absolute measures of radiotracer concentration can be measured. However, to achieve this quantitative accuracy it is necessary to apply corrections for image degrading effects at either the data acquisition process or the image

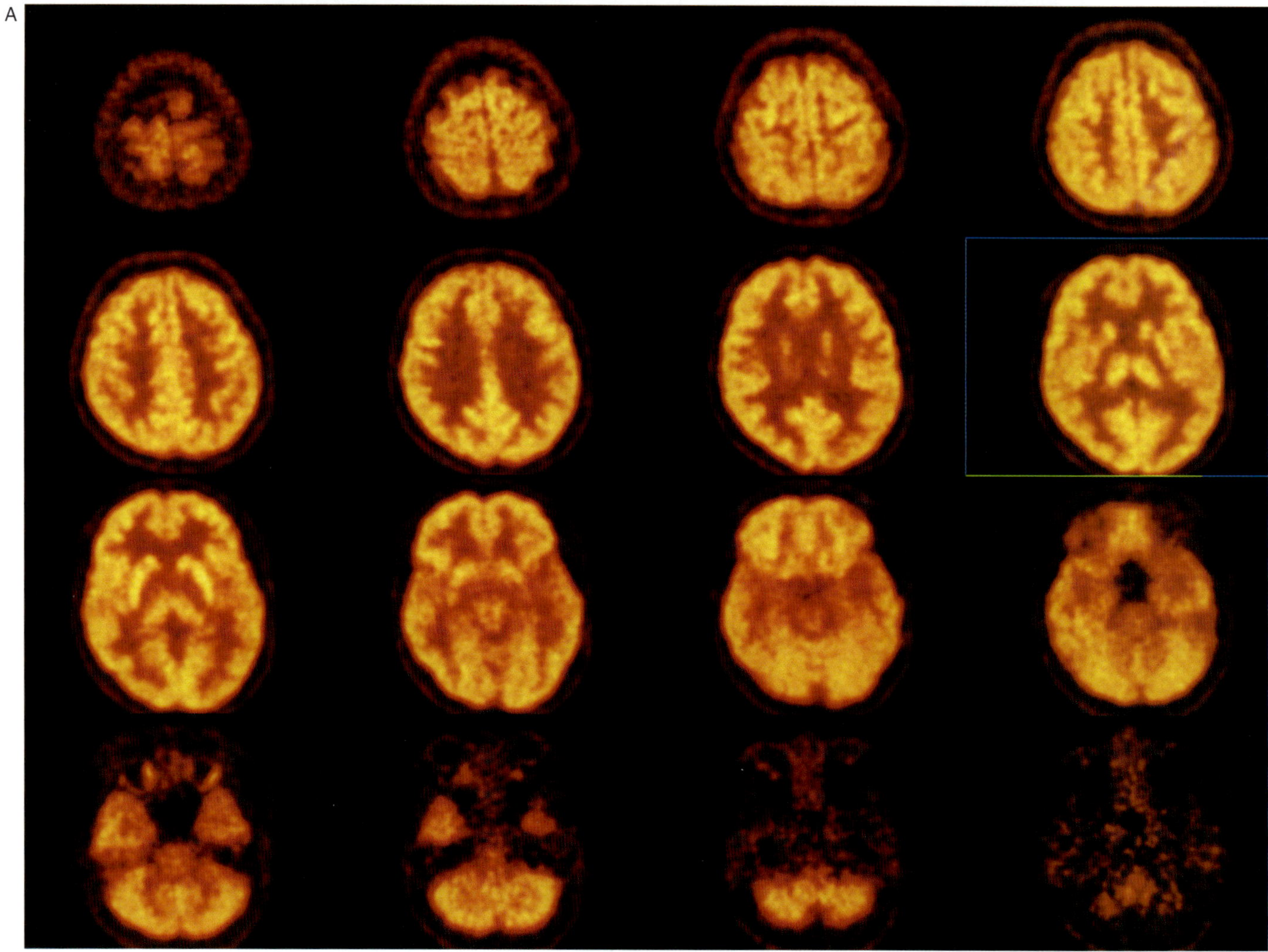

Figure 5.5 (A) Transaxial images of cerebral metabolism using ^{18}F-FDG imaging of a normal subject.

reconstruction process. These corrections must include: (1) randoms subtraction, in which either a measured or calculated estimate of the randoms event distribution is subtracted from the sinogram; (2) deadtime correction, in which the effect of count loss at high events rates is corrected for; (3) detector normalization, in which the effect of non-uniform detector response is corrected; (4) scatter correction, in which correction for the contamination of the sinogram with scattered events is applied; and (5) attenuation correction, in which the data are corrected for the effects of the attenuation of the 511 keV photons in the subject. In the case of clinical imaging, attenuation correction typically represents the single largest magnitude correction, with correction factors that often exceed a factor of 100 for LORs that pass through the body [33]. These large values of attenuation are due to the fact that the attenuation depends on the total distance traveled by both of the 511 keV photons. The problem of attenuation is less severe for neuroimaging applications of PET; however, if uncorrected for the result will be reductions in the measured

activity at the centre of the brain and apparent increase at the edge of the brain [33].

Combining PET with the anatomical imaging method of X-ray CT [34] has several key advantages for performing and interpreting PET studies. From a PET image quantitation perspective, the CT data provide a low-noise measure of the attenuation map, the acquisition of which is essential to applying an accurate attenuation correction to the data. Prior to combined PET/CT, attenuation correction was performed using a radioisotope transmission source, which was a much slower image acquisition process than a CT scan. Knowledge of the attenuation map can also aid in scatter correction and can be used in iterative reconstruction techniques. From the perspective of the clinician, combined PET and CT is essential for determining the anatomical location of regions of tracer uptake in the image, especially for radiotracers that give little, if any, anatomical information [35]. A clear sign of the benefits of combined PET and CT is that virtually all clinical PET systems sold today are of the combined PET/CT type [36].

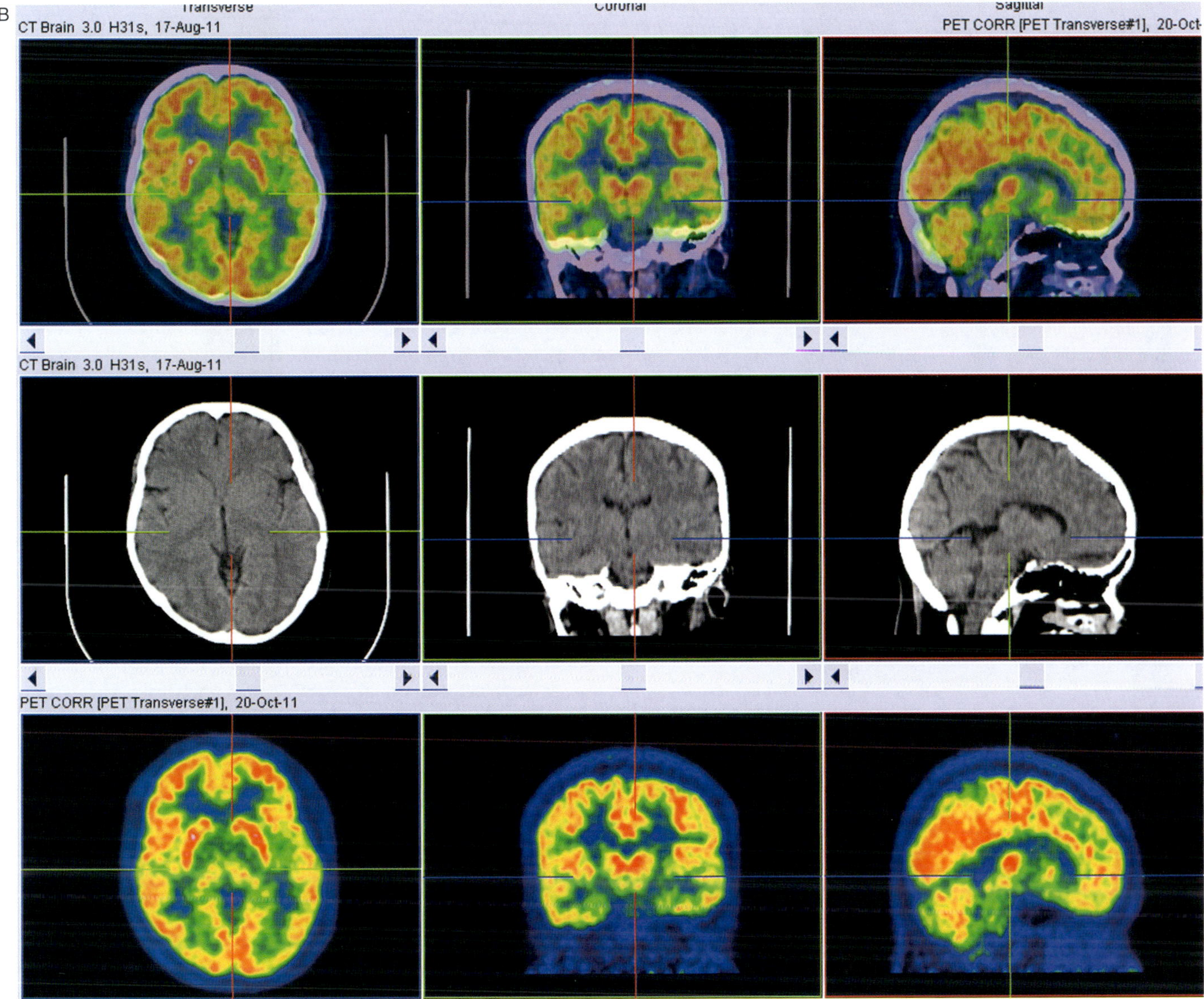

Figure 5.5 (B) CT, ^{18}F-FDG PET and fused axial, coronal, and sagittal images of the brain.

Clinical principles

Different patient protocols for PET imaging with ^{18}F FDG are present for oncological and cardiac indications [1]. The optimal technique is still evolving. Neurological studies typically follow the oncological preparation. If patient instructions are not properly followed, the potential for a non-diagnostic scan because of change in tracer distribution is increased.

Before arrival, patients should be instructed to fast and not consume beverages, except for water, for at least 4–6 h before the administration of ^{18}F-FDG to decrease physiological glucose levels and to reduce serum insulin levels to near basal levels. Oral hydration with water is encouraged. Intravenous fluids containing dextrose or parenteral feedings also should be withheld for 4–6 h.

Before injection, for brain imaging, many departments advocate the patient should be in a quiet and dimly lit room for ^{18}F-FDG administration and the subsequent uptake phase. The blood glucose level should be checked before ^{18}F-FDG administration, at least in diabetic patients. Most institutions consider rescheduling the patient if the blood glucose level is greater than 150–200 mg/dl. Administering insulin just prior to ^{18}F-FDG is not indicated since this will also cause a change in tracer distribution.

For optimal imaging of the head and neck, the arms should be positioned down along the side of the body. The dedicated scan of the brain should take a few seconds for the CT component and less than 10–15 min for the ^{18}F-FDG PET component. It should start approximately 45 min after injection of ^{18}F-FDG because of the extended uptake period for ^{18}F-FDG.

Patient preparation for other tracers is less well defined. Standardization of protocols particularly between baseline examination and post activation is essential for useful clinical information to be obtained. Imaging protocols are dependent on the tracer being utilized. A short half-life tracer like ^{15}O will need immediate imaging and a rapid acquisition, which has an advantage of identifying more transient phenomena.

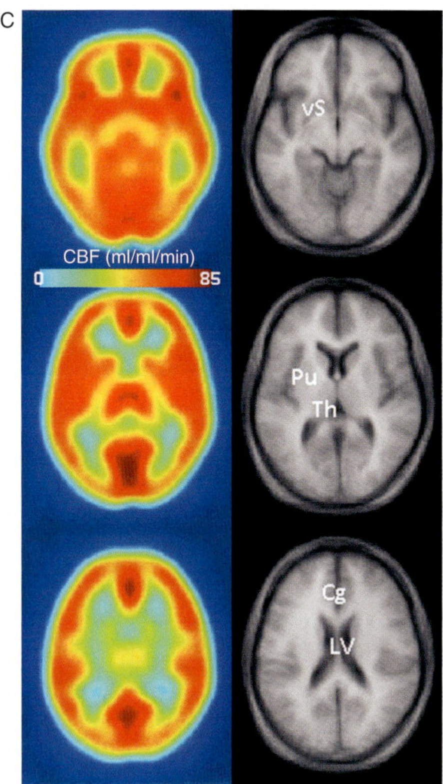

Figure 5.5 (C) Transaxial images of cerebral blood flow measured with PET ^{15}O-water with matching MRI averaged across 12 healthy subjects following spatial normalization. Three levels included ventral striatum (vS), putamen (Pu), thalamus (Th), cingulated cortex (Cg), and lateral ventricles (LV). Image courtesy of Hiroto Kuwabara MD PhD at Department of Radiology, Johns Hopkins Medical Institutes, Johns Hopkins University, Baltimore.

Although there are no absolute contraindications to PET/CT, a pregnant patient would need a very important clinical reason to go forward with a PET study; those patients who breastfeed would need to stop breastfeeding for various relatively short periods of time depending on the radiotracer administered. A history of severe claustrophobia or an inability to lie still for the duration of the scan acquisition would not allow for a diagnostic study to be completed.

As with other nuclear medicine tests, there is a relatively low but significant radiation dose to the patient with the various PET studies performed. Estimates for brain imaging radiation doses have been calculated and dose equivalents of 0.043 rem (total body) and 0.070 rem (effective dose) per mCi for ^{18}F-FDG [8] and similar rates for ^{15}O-water [8, 37] are common. As part of the exam, there is also a dose from the CT component of the exam which can range greatly depending on the protocol used.

Display/imaging

With an integrated PET/CT system, software packages provided by the vendor will register/align the CT and PET images and produce fusion images in the axial, coronal, and sagittal planes (Figure 5.5) as well as maximum-intensity-projection (MIP) images which can be reviewed in a 3-dimensional cine mode.

PET images with and without attenuation correction should be available for review.

The resolution of PET images has improved significantly with advances in technology but remains below that of MRI. Partial volume effects will make smaller defects more difficult to detect. Although one expects symmetry in brain uptake, there is some heterogeneity in normal subjects in part because of variations anatomically but also because of differences in functional status. Usually one requires a finding to be evident on more than one slice to be considered significant. Mildly increased activity is seen also in some structures such as the visual cortex and basal ganglia compared to the rest of the cerebral cortex. White matter on PET FDG imaging is reduced when compared to gray matter. There is also a change in the distribution of tracer based on the age of a patient, with infants showing a markedly different pattern to teenagers/adults. Activation of certain areas of the brain (e.g., visual cortex – when looking, motor cortex – if moving) will lead to differences in appearance when compared to the resting state. Some drugs such as barbiturates, neuroleptic drugs, antiepilepsy medications, and sedatives will also affect tracer distribution. Obviously, patients with pathological conditions such as stroke, tumor or dementia will have an altered tracer pattern.

PET rCBF imaging with ^{15}O-water can be quantified using a mathematical model using a diffusible tracer technique method [7]. However, full quantitation requires arterial catheterization and blood sampling during the scan and subsequent counting of acquired samples, cross-calibration of the scanner and counting equipment. This will allow for precise comparisons across conditions and between subjects. An alternative is to use statistical analysis based on counts obtained from imaging. There is a substantial intersubject variation so relative rCBF values can be obtained by normalizing to a reference brain region.

Software has been developed to assess imaging more quantitatively with comparison to normal subjects (most commonly in current clinical practice for ^{18}F-FDG). After the brain scan images have been aligned and normalized to a standard, the counts obtained in each designated area can be compared to a normal database. Unfortunately there can be issues with differences in individual anatomy to ensure a fit with the software program parameters. Once there is a proper registration the software will analyze each voxel to compare to the expected value and provide a statistical map that reflects the probability of change of rCBF or other parameters.

Conclusion

PET and more recently PET/CT has been utilized as a measure of functional imaging for many decades. Most studies have used ^{15}O-water and ^{18}F-FDG. Sleep disorder processes are complex and PET/CT imaging has had some success and will have a future role in investigation of this area of medicine. The quality of research continues to improve in part because of the improvements in technology and image processing and also because of development of novel tracers.

References

1. Society of Nuclear Medicine Procedure Guideline for Tumor Imaging with 18F-FDG PET/CT 1.0. 2006. http://interactive.snm.org/docs/jnm30551_online.pdf. (Accessed October 1, 2011.

2. Bybel B, Brunken RC, Shah SN, *et al.* PET and PET/CT imaging: what clinicians need to know. *Cleve Clin J Med.* 2006;**73**(12):1075–87.

3. Mitra E, Quon A. Positron emission tomography/computed tomography: the current technology and applications. *Radiol Clin North Am.* 2009;**47**:147–60.

4. Basu S, Kwee TC, Surti S *et al.* Fundamentals of PET and PET/CT Imaging. *Ann N Y Acad Sci.* 2011;**1228**:1–18.

5. Otte A, Nofzinger EA, Audenaert K *et al.* Nuclear medicine asleep in sleep research? *Eur J Nucl Med Mol Imaging.* 2002;**29**:1417–20.

6. Desseilles M, Dang-Vu T, Schwartz S *et al.* Functional neuroimaging of sleep and sleep disorders. In: Chockroverty S, ed. *Sleep Disorders Medicine.* Philadelphia, Saunders Elsevier. 2009;198–217.

7. Maquet P. Functional neuroimaging of normal human sleep by positron emission tomography. *J Sleep Res.* 2000;**9**:207–31.

8. VanHeertum RL, Tikofsky R, Ichise M. *Functional Cerebral SPECT and PET Imaging.* Philadelphia, Lippincott, Williams & Wilkins. 2010.

9. Satyamurthy N. Electronic generators. In: Phelps ME, ed. *PET Molecular Imaging and its Biological Applications.* Secaucus, Springer Science. 2004;217–69.

10. Ruth TJ. Accelerators available for isotope production. In: Welch MJ, Redvanly CS, eds. *Handbook of Radiopharmaceuticals: Radiochemistry and Applications.* Chichester, J. Wiley and Sons Ltd. 2003; 71–86.

11. Pike VW. PET radiotracers: crossing the blood–brain barrier and surviving metabolism. *Trends Pharmacol Sci.* 2009;**30**(8):431–40.

12. Nofzinger EA. Neuroimaging and sleep medicine. *Sleep Med Rev.* 2005;**9**(3):157–72.

13. Dang-Vu TT, Desseilles M, Petit D, *et al.* Neuroimaging in sleep medicine. *Sleep Med.* 2007;**8**(4):349–72.

14. Hamacher K, Coenen HH, Stöcklin G. Efficient stereospecific synthesis of no-carrier-added 2-[18F]-fluoro-2-deoxy-D-glucose using aminopolyether supported nucleophilic substitution. *J Nucl Med.* 1986;**27**(2):235–8.

15. Mock BH, Vavrek MT, Mulholland GK. Back-to-back "one-pot" [18F]FDG syntheses in a single Siemens-CTI chemistry process control unit. *Nucl Med Biol.* 1996;**23**(4):497–501.

16. Clark JC, Crouzel C, Meyer GJ, Strijckmans K. Current methodology for oxygen-15 production for clinical use. *Int J Rad Appl Instrum A.* 1987;**38**(8):597–600.

17. Clark JC, Aigbirhio FI. Chemistry of nitrogen-13 and oxygen-15. In Welch MJ, Redvanly CS, eds. *Handbook of Radiopharmaceuticals: Radiochemistry and Applications.* Chichester, J. Wiley and Sons Ltd. 2003;112–40.

18. Sajjad M, Liow JS, Moreno-Cantu J. A system for continuous production and infusion of [15O]H$_2$O for PET activation studies *Appl Radiat Isot.* 2000;**52**(2):205–10.

19. Wieland B, Schmidt DG, Bida G, *et al.* Efficient, economical production of oxygen-15 labeled tracers with low energy protons. *J Label Compd Radiopharm.* 1986;**23**:1214–16.

20. Powell J, O'Neil JP. Production of [15O] water at low-energy proton cyclotrons, *Appl Radiat Isot.* 2006;**64**(7):755–9.

21. Albin RL, Koeppe RA, Chervin RD, *et al.* Decreased striatal dopaminergic innervation in REM sleep behavior disorder. *Neurology.* 2000;**55**(9):1410–12.

22. Sudo Y, Suhara T, Honda Y, *et al.* Muscarinic cholinergic receptors in human narcolepsy. *A PET study. Neurology* 1998;**51**(5):1297–302.

23. Khan N, Antonini A, Parkes D, *et al.* Striatal dopamine D$_2$ receptors in patients with narcolepsy measured with PET and 11C-raclopride. *Neurology.* 1994;**44**(11):2102–4.

24. Humm JL, Rosenfeld A, Del Guerra A. From PET detectors to PET scanners. *Eur J Nucl Med Mol Imaging.* 2003;**30**(11):1574–97.

25. Hoffman EJ, Huang SC, Phelps ME, Kuhl DE. Quantitation in positron emission computed tomography: 4. Effect of accidental coincidences. *J Comput Assist Tomogr.* 1981;**5**(3):391–400.

26. Popescu LM, Lewitt RM, Matej S, Karp JS. PET energy-based scatter estimation and image reconstruction with energy-dependent corrections. *Phy Med Biol.* 2006;**51**(11):2919–37.

27. Casey ME, Nutt R. A multicrystal two dimensional BGO detector system for positron emission tomography. *IEEE Trans Nucl Sci.* 1986;**33**(1):460–3.

28. Brambilla M, Secco C, Dominietto M, *et al.* Performance characteristics obtained for a new 3-dimensional lutetium oxyorthosilicate-based whole-body PET/CT scanner with the National Electrical Manufacturers Association NU 2–2001 standard. *J Nucl Med.* 2005;**46**(12):2083–91.

29. Logan J. Graphical analysis of PET data applied to reversible and irreversible tracers. *Nucl Med Biol* 2000;**27**(7):661–70.

30. Shepp LA, Logan BF, Jr. Fourier reconstruction of a head section. *IEEE Trans Nucl Sci.* 1974;NS-**21**(3):21–43.

31. Hudson HM, Larkin RS. Accelerated image reconstruction using ordered subsets of projection data. *IEEE Trans Med Imaging.* 1994;**13**(4):601–9.

32. Qi J, Leahy RM. Iterative reconstruction techniques in emission computed tomography. *Phys Med Biol.* 2006;**51**(15):R541–78.

33. Zaidi H, Hasegawa B. Determination of the attenuation map in emission tomography. *J Nucl Med.* 2003;**44**(2):291–315.

34. Beyer T, Townsend DW, Brun T, *et al.* A combined PET/CT scanner for clinical oncology. *J Nucl Med.* 2000;**41**(8):1369–79.

35. Beyer T, Townsend DW. Putting 'clear' into nuclear medicine: a decade of PET/CT development. *Euro J Nucl Med Mol Imaging.* 2006;**33**(8):857–61.

36. Townsend DW. Dual-modality imaging: combining anatomy and function. *J Nucl Med.* 2008;**49**(6):938–55.

37. Brihaye C, Depresseux JC, Comar D. Radiation dosimetry for bolus administration of oxygen-15-water. *J Nucl Med.* 1995;**36**:651–6.

Fundamentals of single-photon emission computed tomography (SPECT) and SPECT/CT imaging

Mordechai Lorberboym

Introduction

Nuclear medicine imaging employs the administration of trace amounts of compounds labeled with radioactivity (radionuclides) that are used to provide diagnostic information in a wide range of disease states [1]. Special imaging instruments (e.g., gamma cameras, positron emission tomography (PET) scanners) detect the emitted photons from these nuclides following radioactive decay and provide non-invasive means to image physiological and pathological states within the body (Figure 6.1).

Detection of disease with anatomical imaging methods often requires gross structural changes to be apparent before the diagnosis is definitive. The reliance on anatomical information for diagnosis also makes it difficult to monitor the response of diseased and normal tissues in the critical post-therapy period. In comparison, radiotracer imaging methods such as single-photon emission computed tomography (SPECT) and PET are well suited to provide critical information about the functional, metabolic, and molecular status of tissues and organs.

SPECT is a technique widely used in nuclear medicine for the imaging of many organs including the skeleton, heart, lungs, kidneys, and brain, as well as for whole-body imaging [2, 3]. The study is obtained by moving a gamma camera on a gantry in a circular or elliptical orbit around the patient, obtaining information from different angles, which is then combined into a 3-dimensional (3D) volume. SPECT studies are normally viewed as a set of slices cut in the transaxial, sagittal, and coronal planes, with optional 3-dimensional interactive views. As opposed to 2-dimensional (2D) images, SPECT imaging provides higher contrast, depth information, and optional quantification.

Brain SPECT is used mainly for perfusion or receptor imaging of the brain. Frequently brain pathology will manifest itself as functional changes before anatomical changes have taken place. The use of tracers of cerebral perfusion and brain neurotransmitter systems has resulted in the development of a number of applications for brain SPECT in neurology and psychiatry [4–6]. Common indications include dementia, epilepsy, neurovascular disorders, parkinsonism, and following minor head trauma. It also has the potential to be a valuable research tool for the study of in vivo brain function.

Underlying principles

Instrumentation

SPECT technique is a non-invasive technique using a single gamma ray emission at particular energies, to provide 3D functional information with high sensitivity and specificity. Similar to all nuclear medicine imaging procedures, it is based on the injection of tracer amounts (nano- to picomoles) of a molecule labeled with a radioactive isotope [7]. Technetium-99m (^{99m}Tc) is the most commonly used radioactive tracer, because it emits readily detectable 140 keV gamma rays, and its half-life for gamma emission of 6 h is convenient for imaging.

Radioactive decay results in the emission of photons. The gamma camera converts the photons emitted by the patient into a light pulse and subsequently into a voltage signal. The signal is used to form an image of the distribution of the radionuclide. A collimator is inserted between the patient and the camera detectors to direct the stream of emitted photons into a beam such that each location on the detector is associated to a line in space along which the decay occurred – the line of response (LOR). In the clinical setting the most common is the parallel-hole collimator in which photons traveling perpendicular to the absorbing plate (and the detector) are able to pass through the apertures and are detected.

Low-energy high-resolution (LEHR) or low-energy ultrahigh-resolution (LEUHR) parallel-hole collimators are the most readily available collimator sets for brain imaging. Fan-beam collimators are generally preferred over parallel-hole collimators due to the advantageous trade-off between resolution and sensitivity.

The scintillation camera technology currently in use for clinical studies still relies on the technology invented by Hal Anger in 1957 [8, 9]. Newer materials used for the detection of photons in SPECT are cadmium zinc telluride (CZT) [10, 11] and silicon used for Compton collimation [12]. A SPECT camera using CZT provided 40% efficiency for stopping 140 keV ^{99m}Tc photons [10]. This system achieved a spatial resolution of 1.4 mm with a 0.5-mm-diameter pinhole collimator. The CZT technology is extremely compact and does not have the limitations of energy resolution and spatial resolution of conventional sodium iodide (NaI) technology. Four different innovations are practiced: solid-state detector technology with

Neuroimaging of Sleep and Sleep Disorders, ed. Eric Nofzinger, Pierre Maquet, and Michael J. Thorpy. Published by Cambridge University Press. © Cambridge University Press 2013.

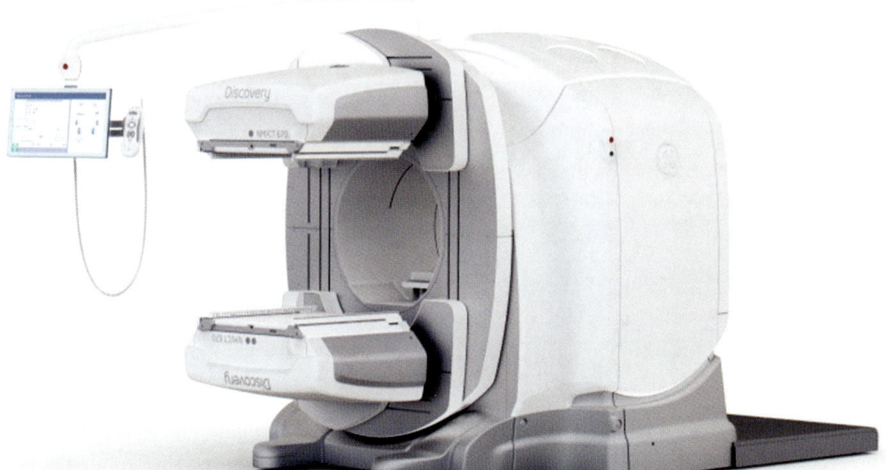

Figure 6.1 Current-generation SPECT/CT gamma camera.

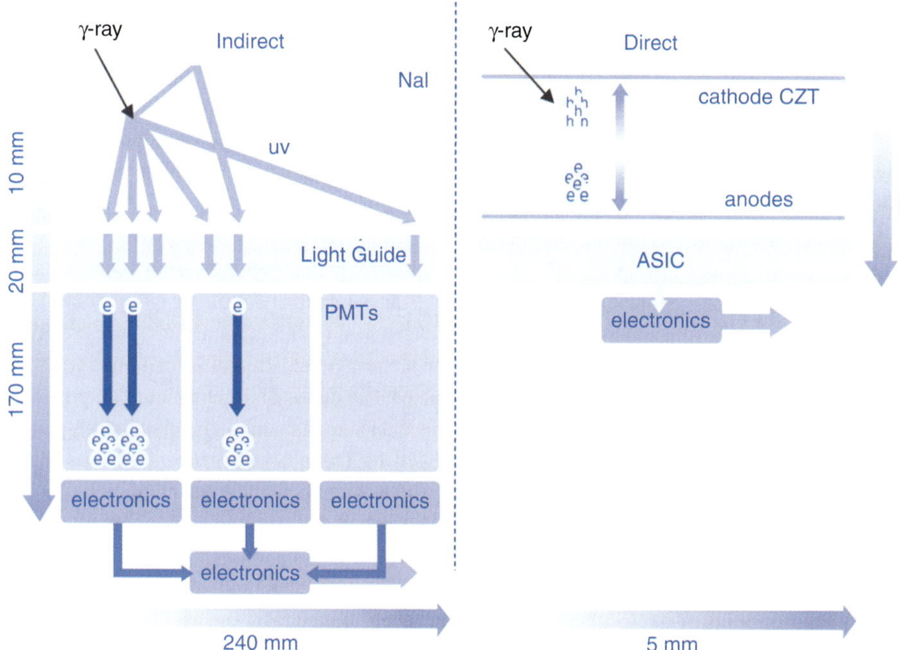

Figure 6.2 Indirect versus direct gamma ray conversion comparison. PMTs = photomultiplier tubes

its direct conversion of gamma rays into electronic signal (Figure 6.2) results in improved energy and spatial resolution. Stationary acquisition provides full volume scans with no moving parts. Focused collimation enables all views to focus on the area of interest resulting in high sensitivity capabilities, and tomographic reconstruction provides optimized image quality.

The improved technique provides clear images and reduces the probability of artifacts. Improved energy resolution can allow for simultaneous acquisitions of different isotopes, like ^{99m}Tc/^{201}Tl or ^{99m}Tc/^{123}I, resulting in fast, high-quality studies. At this early stage in their development, the use of solid-state and semiconductor detectors has focused on imaging of the heart [13, 14], breast [15], and other small organs [16]. Nevertheless, it is likely that as these newer detector technologies mature, they will become more robust in performance and

cost-effectiveness and therefore eventually replace the photomultiplier tube in radionuclide imaging detectors.

A silicon Compton camera is being investigated for non-collimated SPECT, to greatly increase the sensitivity of detecting photons from SPECT nuclides while attempting to maintain spatial resolution [17].

Radiopharmaceuticals

Brain perfusion imaging remains the most widely used and most important form of brain SPECT at present, particularly as a clinical tool. There are several physiological properties that radiopharmaceuticals must have to be useful for the measurement of brain perfusion by SPECT: they must cross the blood–brain barrier; they should have a high extraction fraction, and their initial distribution should be proportional to regional cerebral blood flow (rCBF). They should also be stable after preparation and they must be retained within the brain after initial distribution long enough for diagnostic tomographic images to be obtained [6, 18]. Ideally, tracer uptake should show no redistribution, so that the initial tracer uptake, reflecting rCBF at a fast time window after injection, remains almost unchanged for several hours.

Several radiopharmaceuticals are commercially available for brain perfusion SPECT. In Europe, the most widely used radiopharmaceuticals for rCBF SPECT are ^{99m}Tc-labeled compounds, ethyl cysteinate dimer (^{99m}Tc-ECD, Neurolite, DuPont) and hexamethylpropylene amine oxime (^{99m}Tc-HMPAO, Ceretec, GE Healthcare). Differences between the two commercially available radiopharmaceuticals, ^{99m}Tc-ECD and ^{99m}Tc-HMPAO, include in vitro stability, uptake mechanism, cerebral distribution [19], and dosimetry.

Mechanism of perfusion imaging

Brain perfusion imaging makes use of the tight autoregulation of brain perfusion. Areas of the brain undergoing increased neuronal activity consume increasing amounts of oxygen and metabolites. These areas therefore rapidly undergo a corresponding increase in perfusion. In turn areas of the brain that are less functionally active are perfused less. This close coupling of brain perfusion and metabolic function remains intact in the majority of physiological and pathological situations, with one or two notable exceptions [4, 20]. An image of cerebral perfusion thus indirectly reflects cerebral metabolism [3].

In normal brain tissue, the kinetic properties of the two common agents are very similar. They enter the brain cells due to their lipophilic nature and remain there due to conversion into hydrophilic compounds. After administration of the radiopharmaceutical intravenously, the highly lipophilic ^{99m}Tc-HMPAO rapidly and easily crosses the blood–brain (BBB) barrier in proportion to blood flow [21]. Once it has entered neuronal tissue, the radiopharmaceutical undergoes an interaction with the tripeptide glutathione, resulting in it undergoing a stereoisomeric change [22]. This new stereoisomer is hydrophilic and thus unable to wash back out of the neuronal tissue, and it is therefore trapped. For ^{99m}Tc-ECD retention, de-esterification is the crucial reaction leading to hydrophilic conversion. This entire process is complete after 1–2 min. The distribution of the radioactivity in the brain therefore provides a snapshot of brain perfusion during a brief period after the injection, despite the fact that the patient may undergo imaging hours later.

Differences in the retention mechanisms may account for some different behavior of the tracers in specific disorders such as subacute stroke, where ^{99m}Tc-ECD distribution seems to reflect metabolic activity more closely, whereas ^{99m}Tc-HMPAO is better correlated with cerebral perfusion [23].

Brain SPECT is not limited to the imaging of brain perfusion, but can also be used to image different known neurotransmitter systems involved in brain function. The most widely used radiopharmaceutical for clinical studies is ^{123}I-labeled

N-(3-fluoropropyl)-2-carbomethoxy-3-(4-iodophenyl) nortropane (^{123}I-FP-CIT) for differential diagnosis of Parkinson's disease. This ligand is a cocaine analog designed to bind to the dopaminergic presynaptic transporter. Uptake of this radiopharmaceutical therefore provides information about presynaptic function of the dopaminergic system, which is particularly useful for evaluating patients with parkinsonism. SPECT agents for serotonergic, noradrenergic, cholinergic, and gamma-aminobutyric acid (GABA)ergic receptor systems are in various stages of clinical trials.

Procedure

Brain SPECT is relatively simple to perform and is well tolerated by the majority of patients. Usually an intravenous access is established in advance so that no discomfort is felt at the time of radiopharmaceutical administration. The patient then lies comfortably in a quiet dimly lit room for approximately 30 min before receiving the radiopharmaceutical. Once the radiopharmaceutical has been administered, the patient continues to rest for a further 5–10 min, after which uptake in the brain should be complete. The usual range of administered activity in adults is 555–1110 MBq (typically 740 MBq) of either radiopharmaceutical.

Imaging is commenced at least 30 min after the radiopharmaceutical administration, to allow for further clearance of vascular background activity, further enhancing the image contrast. For best image quality a delay of 90 min is advocated although less practical in clinical settings [24]. The biodistribution of the radiopharmaceutical is unaffected by any cognitive, visual, or motor activity of the patient during this period as it is already trapped within the brain. Imaging should be completed within 4 h after injection. In the case of dopamine transporter imaging the procedure simply involves an intravenous injection of the radioligand followed by imaging at least 3 h later.

Depending on the imaging device, typical scan time for triple head cameras is around 20–25 min (e.g., 120 projections, 40 projections per head, 20–25 s/projection); for dual head cameras it is closer to 30 min (e.g., 120 projections, 60 projections per head, 30 s/projection). Imaging is performed with the patient lying supine on an imaging bed with the head normally resting in a specially designed head holder. The acquired information is then combined into a single 3D volume using one of a number of possible reconstruction algorithms. Corrections for attenuation of photons emitted from deeper brain structures, and for photon scatter may be employed. Finally image intensity is normalized and images may be viewed using a chosen color scale.

Reconstruction techniques

Until recently the conventional and the most extensively used reconstruction technique for SPECT imaging was filtered back-projection (FBP) [25–29]. Although FBP gained popularity as a very fast reconstruction technique there are limitations in the image quality produced. To a large extent this is due to the back-projection process and the necessary filtering, which accentuates noise and can result in streak artifacts. Iterative reconstruction has virtually replaced FBP reconstruction in routine clinical practice of SPECT imaging [30–36].

Iterative reconstruction

The most widely used reconstruction algorithm in emission tomography is the maximum likelihood expectation maximization algorithm (ML-EM) [37, 38] and its accelerated form based on ordered subsets (OS-EM) [39].

The ML-EM algorithm involves two steps repeated iteratively: (a) estimated projections are produced by forward-projection from the current object estimate for comparison with the measured projections; (b) the ratio of measured to estimated projections is then back-projected and used as a multiplicative correction of the current object estimate. This process is repeated until the estimated and measured projections are matched, resulting in a reconstruction of the activity distribution.

The major advantage of iterative reconstruction techniques is that they permit the emission and detection process to be accurately modeled. The final reconstructed noise tends to be much more acceptable than that present using FBP. More striking is the absence of streaking artifacts, which are common in noisy FBP studies, particularly when there is a focus of high activity. However, it must be noted that, as iteration number increases, noise increases. The main limitation in applying ML is the time required for processing, particularly when multiple iterations are computed. With improved speed of computers this is becoming less of a problem.

Iterative reconstruction methods such as ML-EM and OS-EM allow incorporation of mathematical models that may correct photon attenuation [40, 41], depth-dependent spatial resolution loss (also known as the "geometrical response") of the radionuclide collimator, and scatter. These compensation methods are becoming common for improving the spatial resolution, contrast, and signal-to-noise characteristics of SPECT imaging and quantitative brain SPECT imaging [42–44], including those obtained with SPECT/CT.

A new type of reconstruction algorithm, called median root prior (MRP), is designed especially for noise reduction. This method is not sensitive to the number of iterations [45] (Figure 6.3).

Image interpretation

Images are interpreted visually using all the data in the sets of slices and 3D rendering [5, 46]. Three-dimensional display of the data set may be helpful for more accurate topographic orientation in some clinical questions and to appreciate overall patterns of disease.

The normal adult brain shows bilaterally symmetric tracer distribution, with higher activity in temporal, parietal, and occipital (primary visual) cortices, basal ganglia, and thalami. Activity in the white matter and interhemispheric fissures is

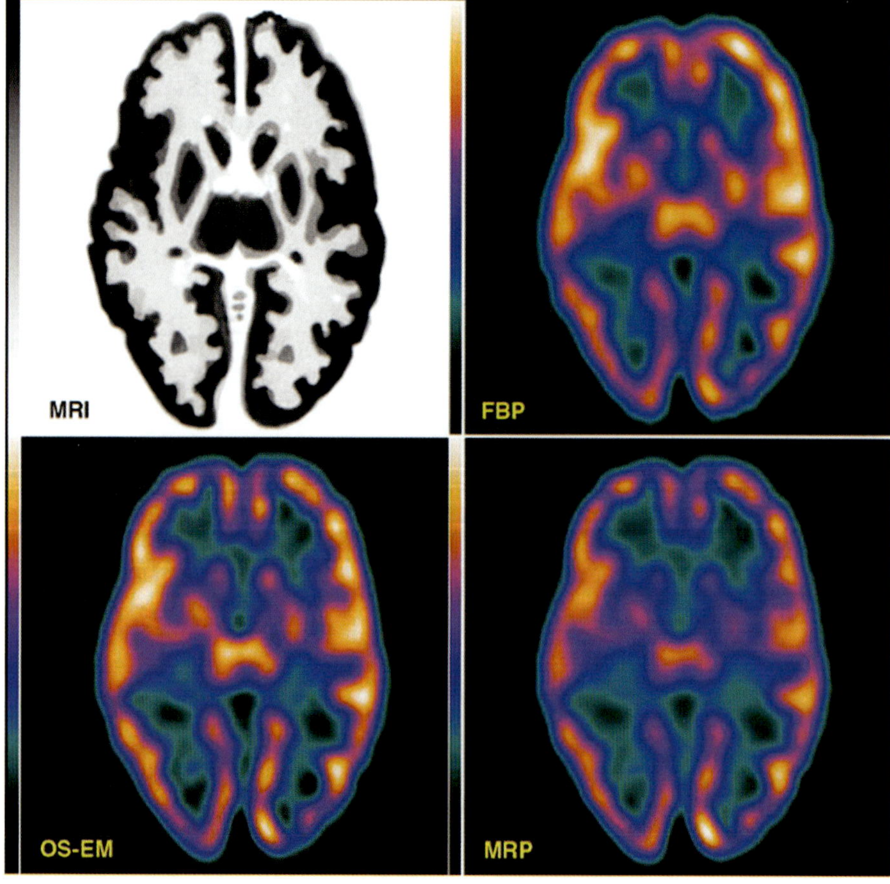

Figure 6.3 The middle slice of a brain phantom reconstructed by FBP, OS-EM, and MRP reconstruction methods. The MR image is taken from the same level as SPECT images. In the color images brighter colors (white, orange) represent higher perfusion, while the darker colors represent low perfusion (blue, green), or no perfusion (black). (Courtesy of Dr. Kauppinen [25].)

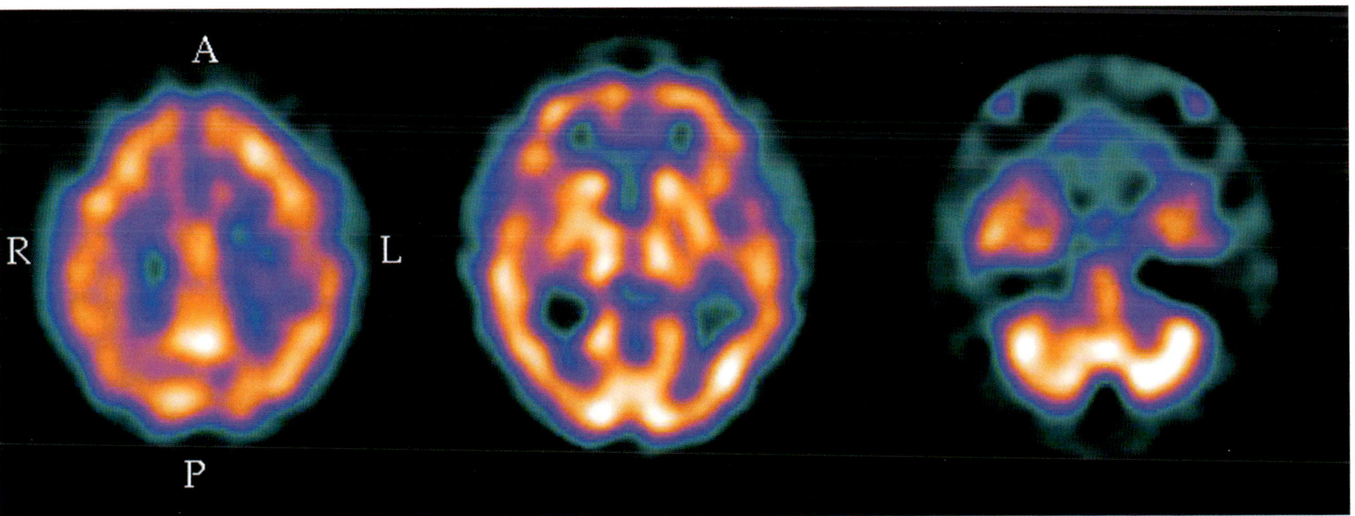

Figure 6.4 Representative transaxial slices from a normal perfusion brain SPECT using ^{99m}Tc-HMPAO showing higher activity in occipital (primary visual) cortices, basal ganglia, thalami, and cerebellum. Activity in the white matter and interhemispheric fissures is less, consistent with diminished cerebral perfusion in these regions.

less, consistent with diminished cerebral perfusion in these regions (Figure 6.4). Asymmetry in orthogonal slice representation may produce false abnormalities, which may be crucial in image interpretation, especially when looking for epileptic foci. Views other than standard reorientation may be helpful, e.g., sections parallel to the long axis of the temporal lobe in the evaluation of epilepsy and Alzheimer's disease.

Eyes open or closed may increase or decrease, respectively, the visual cortex activity by 30%. Motor and sensory stimuli have similar but asymmetric effects. Auditory stimuli effects are symmetric but less impressive. Abnormal findings include focal or regional areas of decreased or increased tracer uptake. Activation studies with brain SPECT have been performed and include visual stimulation, auditory stimulation, motor and sensory stimulation, memory tasks, pharmacological challenges and interventions, and investigation of complex cognitive tasks [47, 48].

Quantification

Quantification in terms of deviations of normal values or semiquantitatively assessing changes in follow-up studies is helpful in assisting visual interpretation [6]. Three general forms of image analysis are [23]:

Region-of-interest analysis: ROI techniques may be used to compare regional blood flow abnormalities with the rCBF of corresponding structures in the contralateral hemisphere or other reference regions (e.g., cerebellum, hemisphere, total brain).

Spatial normalization, comparison to normal databases, and voxel-based analysis: For assessment of normality, it is desirable to have a normal (age-matched) database available with the same radiopharmaceutical (^{99m}Tc-ECD or ^{99m}Tc-HMPAO), processed in the same way as patient studies (reconstruction, filtering, attenuation, and scatter correction), and preferably studied with the same type of

camera. Possible analysis methods include 3D surface projection algorithms, which are useful in cortical disease (several commercially available packages exist), or voxel-base statistical mapping such as SPM (statistical parametric mapping) [49, 50]. These methods allow an objective analysis of individual patient data compared to a normal database.

Subtraction analysis (after image count normalization to an appropriate reference region or the whole brain): This provides a tool for subtracting an activation study from a baseline study. SISCOM (subtraction ictal SPECT coregistered to MRI) is frequently used in ictal/interictal analysis of epilepsy patients [51, 52].

Applications of brain SPECT

Brain SPECT has a well-established role for a number of clinical indications (Table 6.1). Cerebral perfusion studies are mainly used in the evaluation of dementias, epilepsy, cerebrovascular disease, trauma, brain death, and to assist with neuropsychiatric evaluation.

Cerebrovascular disease

Perfusion SPECT provides valuable information in acute stroke with respect to complications, outcome, or choice of treatment strategy [53, 54]. The sensitivity and specificity of brain SPECT for stroke localization are 85.5% and 97.6%, respectively [55] (Figure 6.5). The sensitivity may decrease as the stroke evolves because of the luxury perfusion phenomenon, which starts between one and five days, leads to hyperemia (hyperperfusion) of the lesion, and may last as long as 20 days. Luxury perfusion may be easier to detect with ^{99m}Tc-HMPAO than with ^{99m}Tc-ECD [56]. False-negative brain SPECT findings in stroke are caused by lacunar or small cortical infarcts.

In chronic cerebrovascular disease rCBF SPECT with assessment of functional reserve capacity (using cerebrovascular dilator challenge) may guide decisions regarding vascular

Table 6.1. Common conditions investigated by SPECT imaging of the brain

Pathology	Mechanism	Tracer
Stroke	Perfusion	^{99m}Tc-HMPAO, ^{99m}Tc-ECD
	Blood–brain barrier	^{99m}Tc-DTPA
	Apoptosis	^{99m}Tc-HYNIC-annexin V
Dementia	Perfusion	^{99m}Tc-HMPAO, ^{99m}Tc-ECD
Epilepsy	Perfusion	^{99m}Tc-HMPAO, ^{99m}Tc-ECD
Trauma	Perfusion	^{99m}Tc-HMPAO, ^{99m}Tc-ECD
Parkinson's disease	Dopaminergic system	
	Presynaptic	
	dopamine transporter	^{123}I-FP-CIT, ^{123}I-β-CIT, ^{99m}Tc-TRODAT
	Postsynaptic	
	D_2 receptors	^{123}I-IBZM
	Perfusion	^{99m}Tc-HMPAO, ^{99m}Tc-ECD
Tumors	BBB	^{99m}Tc-Pertechnetate, ^{99m}Tc-DTPA
	Perfusion	^{99m}Tc-HMPAO, ^{99m}Tc-ECD
	Metabolism	201-Thallium, ^{99m}Tc-sestamibi
	Amino acid transport	^{123}I-IMT
Apoptosis		^{99m}Tc-HYNIC-annexin V
Psychiatric disorders	Perfusion	^{99m}Tc-HMPAO, ^{99m}Tc-ECD
Brain death	Flow and BBB	^{99m}Tc-DTPA
	Perfusion	^{99m}Tc-HMPAO, ^{99m}Tc-ECD
Neuroreceptors	GABAergic system	
	GABA$_A$/BZD receptor complex	^{123}I-iomazenil
	Serotonergic system	
	5-HT transporter (SERT)	^{123}I-ADAM

BZD = benzodiazepine.

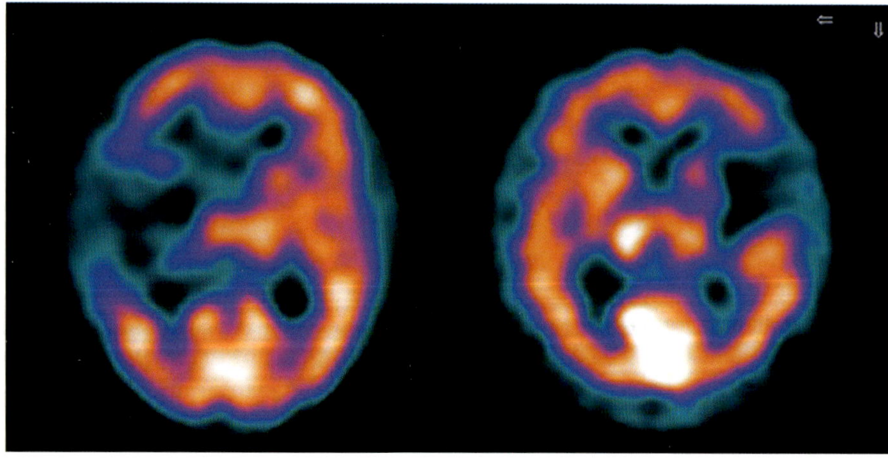

Figure 6.5 A 65-year-old male with a right middle cerebral artery (MCA) territory stroke (left) associated with severely diminished perfusion to the right basal ganglia and moderately diminished perfusion to the right thalamus. A 60-year-old female with a left MCA stroke (right).

surgery [55–57] and preoperative evaluation (e.g., during temporary balloon occlusion) for potential ischemia following carotid artery sacrifice [58, 59].

Focal or diffuse hypoperfusion or no perfusion is the most consistent finding in cerebrovascular disease, a direct consequence of local ischemia. Diaschisis, or decreased activity in a remote area, may be present, particularly in large strokes and usually as crossed cerebellar diaschisis. It is caused by disconnection of the cerebellar–corticopontine fibers as a consequence of ischemia or stroke. Hyperperfusion, or luxury perfusion, may be found in the evolution of strokes.

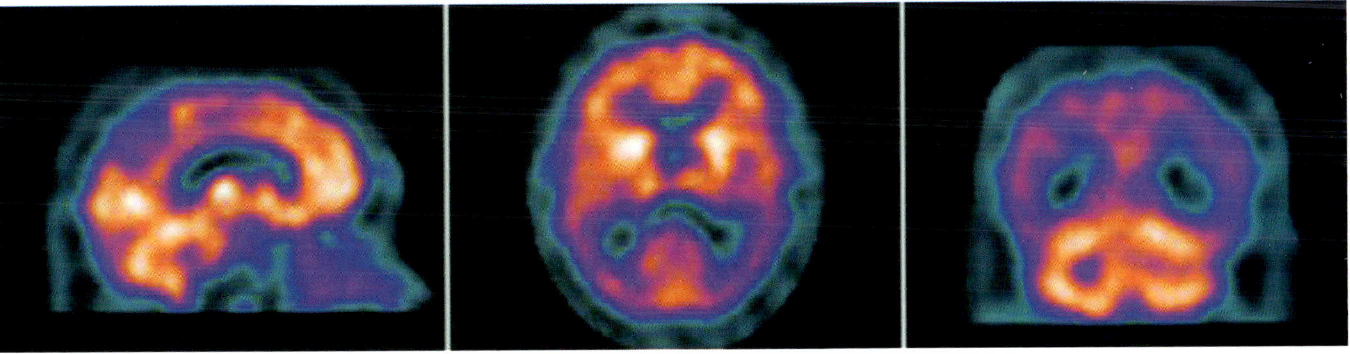

Figure 6.6 A 73-year-old male with Alzheimer's dementia. Perfusion SPECT using ^{99m}Tc-HMPAO shows markedly diminished perfusion in the posterior parietal cortex, temporal lobes, and precuneus.

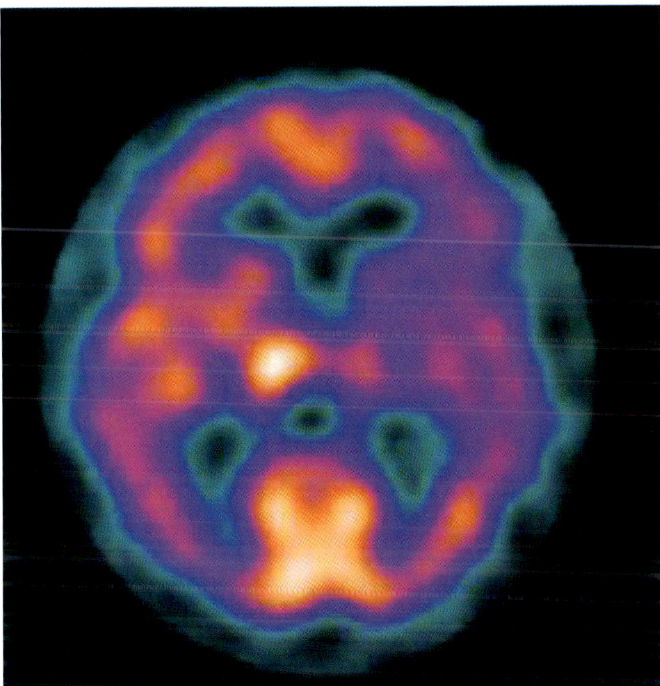

Figure 6.7 Multiple areas of diminished perfusion in cortical and subcortical regions associated with vascular dementia.

Dementias

Brain SPECT has been shown to demonstrate characteristic perfusion abnormalities with different types of dementia. Indications include the early detection and differential diagnosis of various forms of dementia [60], such as Alzheimer's disease [61], Lewy body dementia [62], Parkinson's disease with dementia [63], vascular dementia [64], and frontotemporal dementia [65]. In the pre-dementia phase of these diseases, known as mild cognitive impairment, SPECT can detect a functional deficit and thus guide prognosis [66].

Dementia of Alzheimer's type classically shows decreased perfusion in the temporoparietal regions bilaterally (Figure 6.6), although this may be unilateral, especially during the early stages of the disease [67]. As cases advance, the frontal cortex is also affected. Typically, primary sensorimotor cortex, visual cortex, subcortical structures such as basal ganglia and thalami, and the cerebellar lobes are spared.

Multiinfarct or vascular dementias (VDs) are the second cause of dementia in the elderly. In VD, impairment of intellectual function is caused by multiple infarcts that may occur unilaterally or bilaterally, are usually asymmetric, and may involve any part of the cerebral cortex. The history of one or more events can be disclosed, and the symptoms will have the characteristic temporal profile of such an event [4]. The cause of multiple small emboli is atherosclerotic disease, usually in the carotid artery or in the middle cerebral artery distribution. VD frequently coexists with Alzheimer's disease (AD).

Brain SPECT in these patients shows multiple focal areas of hypoperfusion that can affect cortical and subcortical structures (Figure 6.7) [68]. Motor and sensory cortices may also be involved. Underlying vascular abnormalities resulting in a decreased cerebrovascular reserve can be further elucidated by administering the cerebral vasodilator acetazolamide prior to the radiopharmaceutical.

Frontal lobe dementia (FD) is characterized by a special form of cerebral degeneration with atrophy circumscribed to frontal or temporal lobes involving both gray and white matter. Clinical diagnosis is difficult and structural and functional imaging play an important role in differential diagnosis. Symptoms usually include gradual onset of confusion with respect to place and time, anomia, slowness of comprehension, inability to cope with unusual problems, loss of tact, and changes in personality and behavior [69]. Brain SPECT usually shows symmetric hypoperfusion of the frontal and temporal lobes (Figure 6.8) [68] extending to the cingulate gyrus [70]. In the early phase of the disease, CT or MRI may show normal findings or only mild frontal cerebral atrophy, disproportionate to the degree of hypoperfusion.

AIDS dementia typically shows multifocal defects on brain SPECT [68]. This too can be useful for diagnosis and for the evaluation of therapy in this condition.

Epilepsy

A rapidly growing indication for brain SPECT is its use in refractory focal epilepsy for patients who are candidates for surgical resection of the epileptogenic focus [6, 71–75]. MRI imaging has led to a revolution in the management of these

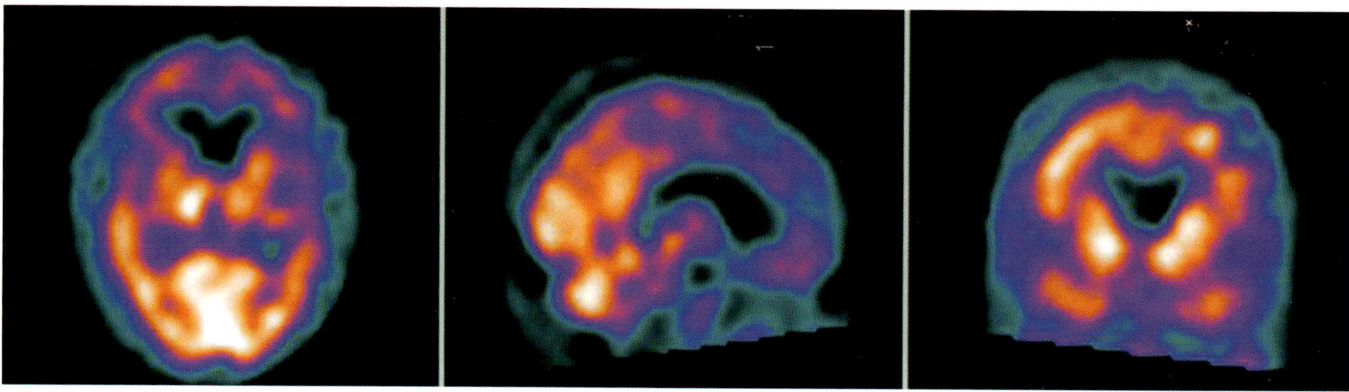

Figure 6.8 Symmetric hypoperfusion of the frontal and temporal lobes in frontotemporal dementia.

patients, but not all epileptogenic foci can be accurately localized with this modality. Similarly, not all anatomical foci are the cause of the patient's seizures [76]. The ability of perfusion brain SPECT to capture a snapshot representing a relatively short time window is particularly valuable with this technique and the use of ictal SPECT contributes greatly to the localization of the epileptogenic focus in these patients [77]. Injection of the radiopharmaceutical as soon as possible after the onset of the seizure demonstrates a focal area of increased uptake of activity at the site of the epileptogenic area. In contrast, a scan obtained between seizures shows no abnormality or even an area of decreased activity in this part of the brain. The detection of the epileptogenic focus can be further enhanced using Subtraction Ictal SPECT coregistered with MRI (SISCOM) [78]. This technique entails coregistering the two SPECT studies and subtracting the interictal image from the ictal image. The difference image can then be superimposed onto a coregistered anatomical MRI for accurate anatomical localization of the lesion. SISCOM is currently the most accurate imaging modality available for the detection and localization of these lesions.

Vasculitis

Another useful clinical application of perfusion brain SPECT is the diagnosis of cerebral vasculitis. This typically reveals a pattern of multifocal perfusion deficits, a common example being patients with systemic lupus erythematosus (SLE). Subtle clinical manifestations of neurolupus can make this a useful objective tool to assist the clinician in selected cases [79].

Head trauma

Brain SPECT is useful for the evaluation of patients with a history of previous head trauma in whom subtle neuropsychological deficits may be detected [80]. SPECT can show lesions in patients without anatomical abnormalities on CT or MRI [81–83]. Deficits may also be revealed sooner although the specificity of these lesions is low. Regardless of the type of injury (subdural hematoma, cerebral contusion, or subarachnoid hemorrhage), the images show focal, multifocal, or regional areas of hypoperfusion that correlate better with the clinical status of the patient than do structural images. The main value of this study is its high negative predicative value in those individuals who have normal studies [84].

Brain death

Scintigraphic assessment of the arrest of cerebral perfusion using a three-phase brain scan including a SPECT study with either ^{99m}Tc-HMPAO or ^{99m}Tc-ECD is an accurate technique to confirm brain death [85] (Figure 6.9). This technique is much more sensitive and specific compared to the previously used planar scans with non-diffusible agents.

Blood–brain barrier disruption

^{99m}Tc-diethylenetriamine penta-acetic acid (^{99m}Tc-DTPA) brain scintigraphy is using a non-diffusible tracer for evaluation of BBB permeability and it is the technique of choice for the assessment of BBB disruption. It has been used in the past to localize areas within the cranium which had been disrupted by infection, neoplasms, trauma, or stroke [86, 87]. ^{99m}Tc-DTPA SPECT imaging of the BBB combined with quantitative analysis in patients with acute stroke is significantly related to clinical outcome [88]. This technique may identify a subpopulation of patients at increased risk of neurological deterioration and it may assist in the follow-up and management of patients with acute stroke.

Brain tumors

Brain SPECT perfusion agents such as ^{123}I-iodoamphetamine (^{123}I-IMP), ^{99m}Tc-HMPAO, and ^{99m}Tc-ECD have not been useful for imaging primary brain tumors. Conflicting results have been obtained with perfusion tracers: in one study [89], 77% of patients with brain tumor showed an increased concentration of ^{99m}Tc-HMPAO and normal uptake of ^{99m}Tc-ECD. Metastatic lesions usually show decreased uptake of brain perfusion tracers. In contrast, brain SPECT with ^{201}Tl-thallous chloride and ^{99m}Tc-sestamibi have been useful in distinguishing radiation effects from residual or recurrent tumor, a distinction not possible with CT or MRI [90, 91].

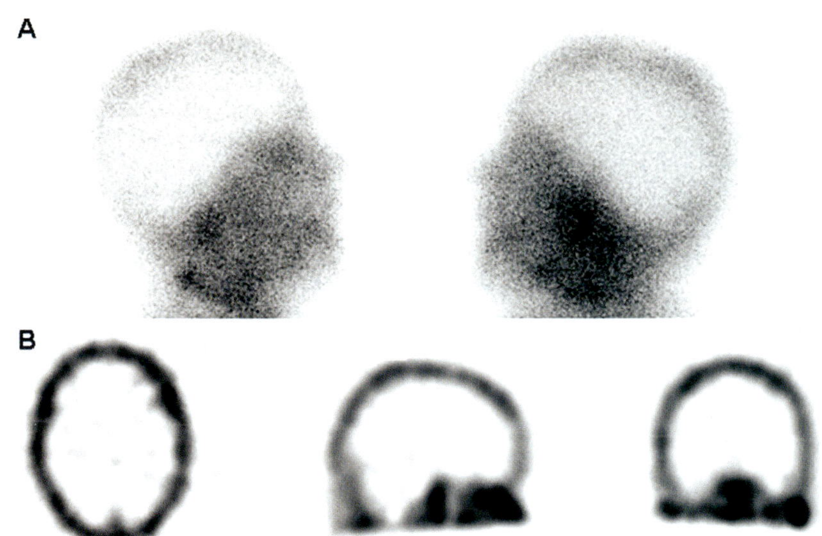

Figure 6.9 Lateral planar images (A) and representative SPECT images (B) of a 35-year-old female with brain death showing no brain activity in the cerebrum, cerebellum, and brainstem.

Apoptosis

Apoptosis is an essential component of normal human growth and development, frequently described as "programmed cell death" (PCD). Apoptosis causes susceptible cells to undergo a series of enzymatic and morphological changes encoded by the human genome. Apoptosis plays a significant role in the pathogenesis of many disorders, including malignancy, organ and bone marrow transplant rejection, and tumor response to chemotherapy and radiation [92].

Annexin V is an endogenous human protein which binds to membrane-bound phosphatidylserine (PS), a constitutive anionic membrane phospholipid [93]. PS is normally restricted to the inner leaflet of the plasma membrane lipid bilayer, but is exposed on the surfaces of cells as they undergo apoptosis.

SPECT studies show that it is possible to identify in-vivo regions of ischemic neuronal injury and neuronal stress using radiolabeled annexin V in patients suffering from an acute stroke [94]. Since apoptosis can be reversed in the early phases of the process, annexin imaging can play a major role in the selection of therapy in the initial period following stroke in adults (Figure 6.10).

Parkinsonism

Parkinson's disease is a degenerative condition characterized by tremor, hypokinesis, postural instability, and rigidity. Approximately 10% of Parkinson's disease patients develop dementia, with parietal, temporal, and occipital lobe hypoperfusion seen on brain SPECT studies. Demented Parkinson's disease patients and AD patients share a common pattern of marked posterior hypoperfusion, although the defects are more prominent and extensive in AD [95].

The clinical evaluation of patients with parkinsonism can be extremely challenging, even in expert hands [96]. The cocaine derivative ^{123}I-FP-CIT (DaTSCAN, GE Healthcare) is a sensitive marker of the degeneration of the dopaminergic nigrostriatal pathway. Studies have reported that SPECT imaging with ^{123}I-FP-CIT shows decreased uptake of dopamine transporter (DAT) ligands in patients with presynaptic parkinsonism [97, 98] (Figure 6.11).

DAT imaging enables the distinction of patients with Parkinson's disease, progressive supranuclear palsy (PSP), and multisystem atrophy (MSA) from those without dopaminergic deficits such as those with essential tremor [99].

Drug-induced parkinsonism (DIP) is clinically indistinguishable from Parkinson's disease and brain imaging with DAT can help the clinician to determine whether DIP is entirely drug-induced or an exacerbation of subclinical Parkinson's disease [100]. In addition functional imaging with ^{123}I-FP-CIT SPECT is highly recommended in patients with cerebrovascular disease who develop symptoms of vascular parkinsonism to confirm or exclude the existence of nigrostriatal dopaminergic degeneration [101]. Identifying a subset of patients with reduced ^{123}I-FP-CIT binding in the striatum is important for better treatment selection.

Although in general there is a good correlation between disease severity and striatal dopaminergic loss in Parkinson's disease [102, 103], there is a non-linear progression of Parkinson's disease, characterized by a more rapid decline in ligand uptake in the early stages of the disease, with subsequent slowing of the decline. Furthermore, in patients with advanced stages of the disease there are residual functional dopaminergic nerve terminals in the striatum, implying that even after very long disease course, the dopaminergic nigrostriatal projections are not totally lost [104].

Imaging of postsynaptic dopaminergic function using a radioligand such as ^{123}I-iodobenzamine (^{123}I-IBZM) can be useful to distinguish patients with Parkinson's disease in whom postsynaptic dopaminergic function is normal or even slightly increased, from patients with PSP and MSA in which it is abnormal [105].

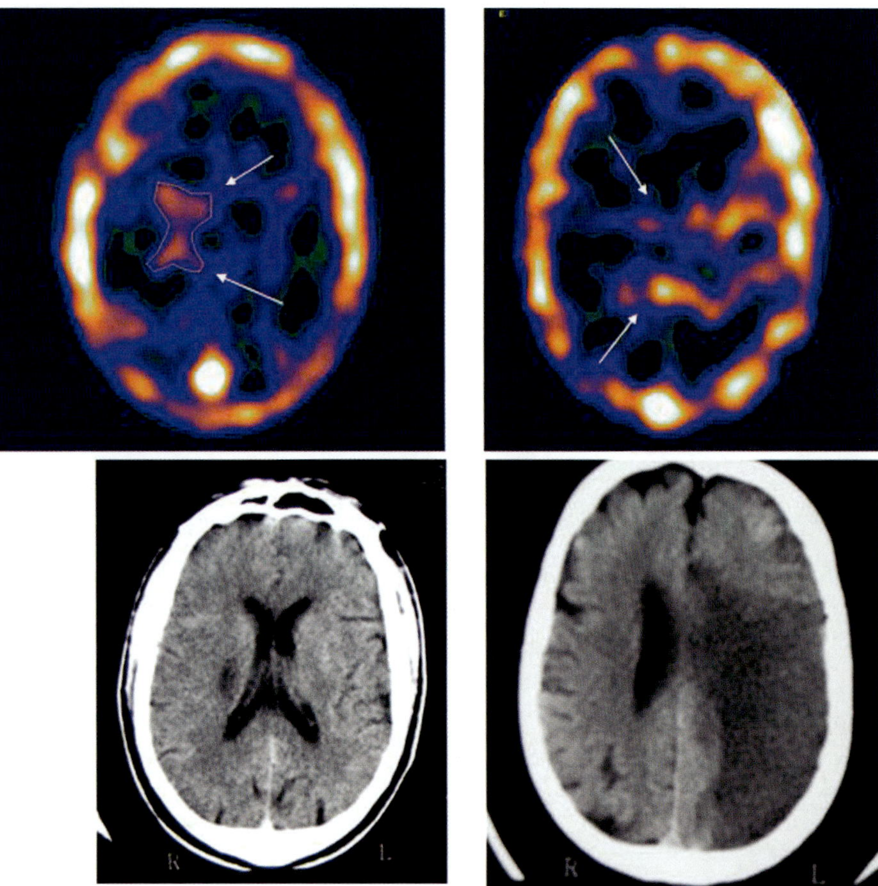

Figure 6.10 Annexin V brain SPECT in a patient with a right periventricular stroke (left), showing a wider distribution of annexin (top, arrows) compared to the CT findings (bottom). Another patient (right) with a cortical stroke localized to the left MCA region shows extensive stroke on CT (bottom) with selective uptake of annexin in the same region (top, arrows), crossing the midline.

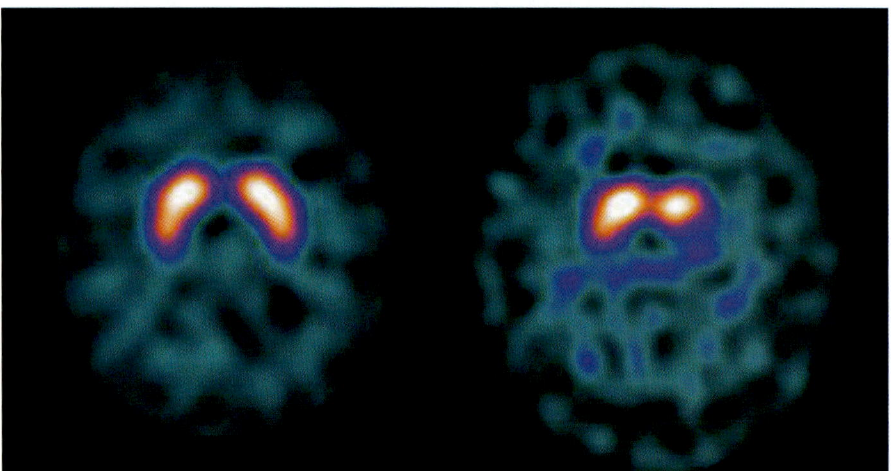

Figure 6.11 A dopamine transporter SPECT scan obtained after the administration of 185 MBq of ^{123}I-Ioflupane (DaTSCAN) showing normal striatal uptake in a patient with essential tremor (left) and markedly diminished uptake in the left putamen of a patient with an early stage Parkinson's disease (right). Brighter colors represent a higher ligand uptake.

Psychiatric disorders

Schizophrenia

Schizophrenia comprises a group of closely related disorders characterized by a particular type of disordered affect, behavior, and thinking [69]. Symptoms are usually categorized as positive or negative. Brain perfusion SPECT most frequently shows hypofrontality, especially during a specific task; perfusional changes in the basal ganglia, possibly related to the use of neuroleptic drugs; and temporal lobe hypoperfusion, usually on the left side and frequently associated with ipsilateral frontal lobe hypoperfusion [106]. Other disorders evaluated with a brain SPECT include unipolar depression, panic disorders, and substance abuse and dependence.

Sleep disorders

Brain imaging studies in patients with sleep disorders are still sparse [107]. In narcoleptic patients, structural and functional brain imaging studies have suggested the involvement of the hypothalamus in the pathophysiology of narcolepsy. Other neuroimaging studies have focused on the assessment of neurotransmission, especially acetylcholine (ACh), serotonin (5-HT), and dopamine (DA), and the effects of pharmacological treatment in narcoleptic patients. One SPECT study using ^{123}I-IBZM demonstrated an increase in postsynaptic D2-receptor binding in the striatum of seven drug-naïve narcoleptic patients (compared to seven controls) and a significant positive correlation of this binding with the incidence of sleep attacks and cataplexy [108]. By contrast, results from other ^{123}I-IBZM SPECT [109, 110], as well as from [^{11}C]raclopride [111, 112] and N-(3-[l8F] fluoropropyl)-spiperone (FPSP) [113] PET studies did not show such enhancement of D2 binding in the basal ganglia.

Results on striatal presynaptic DAT studies [114] do not consistently support a primary impairment of the DA system in narcolepsy.

Rapid eye movement (REM) sleep behavior disorder (RBD) occurs either as an idiopathic disease or in association with neurodegenerative diseases, particularly alpha-synucleinopathies [115]. Recent studies have demonstrated a reduction of striatal presynaptic DATs [116, 117] in idiopathic RBD (iRBD). Another study has also shown reduced cardiac ^{123}I-metaiodobenzylguanidine uptake in patients with iRBD, indicating the presence of sympathetic cardiac denervation [118]. An rCBF study using SPECT in patients with iRBD [119] found decreased rCBF in the parieto-occipital lobe (precuneus), limbic lobe, and cerebellar hemispheres in patients with iRBD, which is commonly seen in patients with Lewy body disease or MSA, suggesting that iRBD can be a presymptomatic stage of alpha-synucleinopathies.

Kleine–Levin syndrome (KLS) is characterized by recurrent periods of hypersomnia, compulsive hyperphagia, hypersexuality, and other behavioral/cognitive disturbances [120]. Reduced DAT availability in the asymptomatic phase of KLS as compared to controls was found [121]. A study using SPECT imaging with ^{99m}Tc-TRODAT-1 [122] found a greater reduction of DAT availability in the symptomatic than asymptomatic phase, implicating dopaminergic dysfunction in different phases of KLS.

Selective serotonin reuptake inhibitors have been associated with the risk of restless legs syndrome (RLS). A study that compared the availability of serotonin transporter (SERT) between 16 drug-naïve patients with RLS and 16 healthy controls using [123]I- FP-CIT SPECT [123] found that the availability of SERT was similar in the RLS group and the control group with regards to the pons and the medulla. However, the severity of RLS symptoms increased as the availability of SERT decreased.

Changes in rCBF in patients with obstructive sleep apnea-hypopnea syndrome (OSAHS) were investigated using ^{99m}Tc-ECD SPECT images of 27 patients with OSAHS and those of age- and sex-matched healthy volunteers [124]. SPM analysis showed that rCBF in patients with OSAHS was significantly reduced in bilateral parahippocampal gyri and in the right lingual gyrus, as compared with that of healthy volunteers.

SPECT as a research tool

Along with PET and functional magnetic resonance imaging (fMRI), brain SPECT is used extensively as a research tool. Brain function is evaluated at baseline, before and after pharmacotherapy or psychotherapy, and following a number of activation tasks to examine a large number of psychiatric conditions including depression, schizophrenia, anxiety disorders, and substance abuse. The use of powerful voxel-based tools such as SPM to analyze functional brain images in a standard stereotactic space has further enhanced the usefulness of these techniques [8].

SPECT CT

While radionuclide SPECT imaging is sensitive for disease detection, it also has limitations in spatial resolution and statistical quality [125–127]. Uptake of radiopharmaceuticals targeted at specific biochemical processes can occur in both diseased and normal sites and it is important to differentiate these sites to correctly evaluate the patient's status. The integration of SPECT and CT in a single imaging device facilitates anatomical localization of the radiopharmaceutical to differentiate physiological uptake from that associated with disease.

Dual-modality imaging occurs when the physician acquires functional (e.g., SPECT, PET) and anatomical (e.g., CT, MRI) images of a patient using separate systems. However, the process of acquiring and spatially correlating data from two or more imaging systems [128–132] is complicated and may be inaccurate. For these reason, dual-modality systems [133–137] are increasingly being used to acquire complementary image data with geometrical configurations that are as consistent to one another as possible. These systems can also facilitate attenuation correction of radionuclide data with patient-specific attenuation maps acquired from CT [138–141], and in correlating functional information from the radionuclide image with anatomical studies visualized with CT [135, 142]. The multi-modality image registration is also important in planning treatment options for radiation oncology and surgery [132, 142] and in quantitation of radiopharmaceutical uptake [143, 144] needed for radiation dosimetry [145].

For SPECT/CT and PET/CT, such imaging is performed with a system that acquires data from two image modalities supported on a single integrated gantry. The imaging study is performed with the patient remaining on the patient table and the data are translated from the CT scanner to the PET or SPECT system to acquire the correlated X-ray and radionuclide image data. The resulting dual-modality image data then can be transferred electronically to a common computer for data correction, reconstruction, display, integration, and analysis.

CT can be used to perform attenuation correction of radionuclide emission data since the CT image inherently represents an anatomical map of linear attenuation coefficients reconstructed at the effective energy of the X-ray beam [138, 139].

The improved signal-to-noise characteristics and multislice capability of the higher-power CT systems offer detailed anatomical information with improved spatial resolution, excellent soft-tissue contrast resolution, and sufficiently fast scan speed for applications with intravenous iodine contrast enhancement [146]. These characteristics are especially suitable for oncology [135, 147] where detailed anatomical localization is needed. Other investigators have reported using the higher-performance SPECT/CT systems for applications in orthopedics [148], infection and inflammation [149, 150], pulmonary function [151, 152], endocrinology [153], and the combining of myocardial perfusion imaging and coronary artery calcium scanning [154].

Concluding remarks

Although PET imaging is frequently considered the gold standard in functional brain imaging, SPECT is much more widely available, provides similar information (with different sensitivity and specificity), and may even have advantages over PET in localization of epileptogenic foci and in using multiple energy windows. Furthermore, the continual improvement and increasing availability of computer software enabling the accurate coregistration of structural and functional modalities (SPECT/CT) further benefits the clinician and researcher in extracting more information by synergistically combining imaging techniques.

SPECT and SPECT/CT is continuing to evolve with the introduction of new technologies that have the potential to improve performance beyond that possible with Anger's pioneering approach. Recent advances in detector technology that incorporate silicon photodiode or solid-state materials offer the potential for improved spatial resolution and energy resolution, with greater stability and more compact size, compared to conventional camera designs based on photomultiplier tube technology.

New cellular targets specific to a particular disease state are being identified. These targets are being used for diagnostic and therapeutic purposes and can be exploited further by designing biomarkers with the ability to evaluate the status of diseased tissue in vivo and avoiding invasive diagnostic procedures in humans.

References

1. Cherry SR, Sorenson JA, Phelps ME. *Physics in Nuclear Medicine*. 3rd edn. Philadelphia, Saunders, 2003.

2. Heneweer C, Grimm J. Clinical applications in molecular imaging. *Pediatr Radiol*. 2011;**41**:199–207.

3. Mariani G, Bruselli L, Kuwert T, *et al*. A review on the clinical uses of SPECT/CT. *Eur J Nucl Med Mol Imaging*. 2010;**37**:1959–85.

4. Warwick JM. Imaging of brain function using SPECT. *Metab Brain Dis*. 2004;**19**:113–23.

5. Camargo EE. Brain SPECT in neurology and psychiatry. *J Nucl Med*. 2001;**42**:611–23.

6. Kapucu OL, Nobili F, Varrone A, *et al*. EANM procedure guideline for brain perfusion SPECT using 99mTc-labelled radiopharmaceuticals, version 2. *Eur J Nucl Med Mol Imaging*. 2009;**36**:2093–102.

7. Accorsi R. Brain single-photon emission CT physics principles. *AJNR Am J Neuroradiol*. 2008;**29**:1247–56.

8. Seo Y, Mari C, Hasegawa BH. Technological development and advances in single-photon emission computed tomography/computed tomography. *Semin Nucl Med*. 2008;**38**:177–98.

9. Anger HO. Scintillation camera. *Rev Sci Instrum*. 1957;**29**:27–33.

10. Kim H, Furenlid LR, Crawford MJ, *et al*. SemiSPECT: a small-animal single-photon emission computed tomography (SPECT) imager based on eight cadmium zinc telluride (CZT) detector arrays. *Med Phys*. 2006;**33**:465–74.

11. Rowland DJ, Cherry SR. Small-animal preclinical nuclear medicine instrumentation and methodology. *Semin Nucl Med*. 2008;**38**:209–22.

12. Studen A, Burdette D, Chesi E, *et al*. First coincidences in pre-clinical Compton camera prototype for medical imaging. *Nucl Instrum Methods Phys Res Sect A*. 2004;**531**:258–264.

13. Kubo N, Mabuchi M, Katoh C, *et al*. Validation of left ventricular function from gated single photon computed emission tomography by using a scintillator-photodiode camera: a dynamic myocardial phantom study. *Nucl Med Commun*. 2002;**23**:639–43.

14. Kumita S, Tanaka K, Cho K. Assessment of left ventricular function using solid-state gamma camera equipped with a highly-sensitive collimator. *Ann Nucl Med*. 2003;**17**:517–20.

15. Hruska CB, O'Connor MK, Collins DA. Comparison of small field of view gamma camera systems for scintimammography. *Nucl Med Commun*. 2005;**26**:441–5.

16. Fukumitsu N, Tsuchida D, Ogi S, *et al*. Use of Digirad 2020tc Imager, a multi-crystal scintillation camera with solid-state detectors in one case for the imaging of autografts of parathyroid glands. *Ann Nucl Med*. 2001;**15**:533–6.

17. Seo H, Lee SH, Jeong JH, *et al*. Feasibility study on hybrid medical imaging device based on Compton imaging and magnetic resonance imaging. *Appl Radiat Isot*. 2009;**67**:1412–15.

18. Reba RC, Holman BL. Brain perfusion radiotracers. In: Diksic M, Reba RC, eds. *Radiopharmaceuticals and Brain Pathology Studied with PET and SPECT*. Boca Raton, CRC Press. 1991;35–9.

19. Inoue K, Nakagawa M, Goto R, *et al*. Regional differences between 99mTc-ECD and 99mTc-HMPAO SPECT in perfusion changes with age and gender in healthy adults. *Eur J Nucl Med Mol Imaging*. 2003;**30**:1489–97.

20. Lou H, Edvinsson L, Mackenzie ET. The concept of coupling blood flow to brain function: revision required? *Ann Neurol*. 1987;**22**:289–297.

21. Leonard JP, Nowotnik DP, Neirinckx RD. Technetium-99m-d,1-HM-PAO: a new radiopharmaceutical for imaging regional brain perfusion using SPECT-a comparison with iodine-123 HIPDM. *J Nucl Med*. 1986;**27**:1819–23.

22. Babich JW. Technetium-99m-HMPAO retention and the role of glutathione: the debate continues. *J Nucl Med*. 1991;**32**:1681–3.

23. Friedman NC, Burt RW. Cerebral perfusion imaging. In: Henkin RE, Bova D, Dillehay L, *et al*., eds. *Nuclear*

Medicine, 2nd edn. Philadelphia, Mosby-Elsevier. 2006;1255–81.

24. Thomsen G, de Nijs R, Hogh-Rasmussen E, *et al.* Required time delay from Tc-99m HMPAO injection to SPECT data acquisition: healthy subjects and patients with rCBF pattern. *Eur J Nucl Med Mol Imaging.* 2009;35:2212–19.

25. Kauppinen T, Koskinen MO, Alenius S, Vanninen E, Kuikka JT. Improvement of brain perfusion SPET using iterative reconstruction with scatter and non-uniform attenuation correction. *Eur J Nucl Med.* 2000;27:1380–6.

26. Brooks RA, Di Chiro G. Principles of computer assisted tomography (CAT) in radiographic and radioisotopic imaging. *Phys Med Biol.* 1976;21:689–732.

27. Larsson SA. Gamma camera emission tomography: development and properties of a multi-sectional emission computed tomography system. *Acta Radiol.* 1980;363:1–75.

28. Bracewell RN, Riddle AC. Inversion of fan-beam scans in radio astronomy. *Astrophys J.* 1967;150:427–34.

29. Ramachandran GN, Lakshminarayanan AV. Three-dimensional reconstruction from radiographs and electron micrographs: application of convolutions instead of Fourier transforms. *Proc Natl Acad Sci U S A.* 1971;68:2236–40.

30. Qi J, Leahy RM. Iterative reconstruction techniques in emission computed tomography. *Phys Med Biol.* 2006;51:R541–78.

31. Lewitt RM, Matej S. Overview of methods for image reconstruction from projections in emission computed tomography. *Proc IEEE.* 2003;91:1588–611.

32. Hutton BF, Nuyts J, Zaidi H. Iterative reconstruction methods. In: Zaidi H, ed. *Quantitative Analysis in Nuclear Medicine Imaging.* Singapore, Springer. 2006;107–40.

33. Defrise M, Kinchan PE, Michel CJ Image reconstruction algorithms in PET. In: Bailey DL, Townsend DW, Valk PE, Maisey MN, eds. *Positron Emission Tomography: Basic Sciences.* London, Springer-Verlag. 2005;63–91.

34. Lalush DS, Wernick MN. Iterative image reconstruction. In: Wernick M, Aarsvold J, eds. *Emission Tomography:*

The Fundamentals of PET and SPECT. San Diego, Academic Press. 2004;443–72.

35. Hutton BF. Recent advances in iterative reconstruction for clinical SPECT/PET and CT. *Acta Oncol.* 2011;50:851–8.

36. Natterer F. *The Mathematics of Computerized Tomography.* New York, Wiley, 1986.

37. Lange K, Carson RE. EM reconstruction algorithms for emission and transmission tomography. *J Comput Assist Tomogr.* 1984;8:306–16.

38. Shepp LA, Vardi Y. Maximum likelihood reconstruction for emission tomography. *IEEE Trans Med Imaging.* 1982;1:113–22.

39. Hudson HM, Larkin RS. Accelerated image reconstruction using ordered subsets of projection data. *IEEE Trans Med Imaging.* 1994;13:601–9.

40. Kalki K, Blankespoor SC, Brown JK, *et al.* Myocardial perfusion imaging with a combined x-ray CT and SPECT system. *J Nucl Med.* 1997;38:1535–40.

41. Gullberg GT, Huesman RH, Malko JA, Pelc NJ, Budinger TF. An attenuated projector-backprojector for iterative SPECT reconstruction. *Phys Med Biol.* 1985;30:799–816.

42. Almeida P, Ribeiro MJ, Bottlaender M, *et al.* Absolute quantitation of iodine-123 epidepride kinetics using single-photon emission tomography: comparison with carbon-11 epidepride and positron emission tomography. *Eur J Nucl Med.* 1999;26:1580–8.

43. Meikle SR, Hutton BF, Bailey DL. A transmission-dependent method for scatter correction in SPECT. *J Nucl Med.* 1994;35:360–7.

44. Axelsson B, Msaki P, Israelsson A Subtraction of Compton-scattered photons in single-photon emission tomography. *J Nucl Med.* 1984; 25:490–4.

45. Alenius S, Ruotsalainen U. Bayesian image reconstruction for emission tomography based on median root prior. *Eur J Nucl Med.* 1997;24:258–65.

46. *Procedure Guidelines Manual.* Reston, VA, *Society of Nuclear Medicine* 1999. 105–10.

47. Woods SW, Hegeman IM, Zubal G, *et al.* Visual stimulation increases technetium-99m-HMPAO distribution in human visual cortex. *J Nucl Med.* 1991;32:210–15.

48. Rivera-Luna H, Camargo EE, Sostre S, *et al.* 99m-Tc-HMPAO SPECT imaging identifies cerebral activation changes during the Stroop test [abstract]. *J Nucl Med.* 1991;32(Suppl):991.

49. Friston KJ. Introduction: experimental design and statistical parametric mapping. In: Frackowiak RSJ, Friston KJ, Frith C, eds. *Human Brain Function*, 2nd edn. New York: Academic Press; 2003: xii–xv.

50. McNally KA, Paige AL, Varghese G, *et al.* Localizing value of ictal-interictal SPECT analyzed by SPM (ISAS). *Epilepsia.* 2005;46:1450–64.

51. Kaiboriboon K, Lowe VJ, Chantarujikapong SI, Hogan RE. The usefulness of subtraction ictal SPECT coregistered to MRI in single- and dual-headed SPECT cameras in partial epilepsy. *Epilepsia.* 2002;43:408–14.

52. Dupont P, Van Paesschen W, Palmini A, *et al.* Ictal perfusion patterns associated with single MRI-visible focal dysplastic lesions: implications for the noninvasive delineation of the epileptogenic zone. *Epilepsia.* 2006;47:1550–7.

53. Masdeu JC, Irimia P, Asenbaum S, *et al.* EFNS guideline on neuroimaging in acute stroke. Report of an EFNS task force. *Eur J Neurol.* 2006;13:1271–83.

54. Mountz JM, Liu HG, Deutsch G. Neuroimaging in cerebrovascular disorders: measurement of cerebral physiology after stroke and assessment of stroke recovery. *Semin Nucl Med.* 2003;33:56–76.

55. Lee TH, Kim SJ, Kim IJ, *et al.* Statistical parametric mapping and statistical probabilistic anatomical mapping analyses of basal/acetazolamide Tc-99m ECD brain SPECT for efficacy assessment of endovascular stent placement for middle cerebral artery stenosis. *Neuroradiology.* 2007;49:289–98.

56. Lee HY, Paeng JC, Lee DS, *et al.* Efficacy assessment of cerebral arterial bypass surgery using statistical parametric mapping and probabilistic brain atlas on basal/acetazolamide brain perfusion SPECT. *J Nucl Med.* 2004;45:202–6.

57. Aso K, Ogasawara K, Sasaki M, *et al.* Preoperative cerebrovascular reactivity to acetazolamide measured by brain perfusion SPECT predicts development of cerebral ischemic lesions caused by microemboli during carotid

endarterectomy. *Eur J Nucl Med Mol Imaging*. 2009;**26**:294–301.

58. Lorberboym M, Pandit N, Machac J, *et al.* Brain perfusion imaging during preoperative temporary balloon occlusion of the internal carotid artery. *J Nucl Med*. 1996;**37**:415–19.

59. Sugawara Y, Kikuchi T, Ueda T, *et al.* Usefulness of brain SPECT to evaluate brain tolerance and hemodynamic changes during temporary balloon occlusion test and after permanent carotid occlusion. *J Nucl Med*. 2002;**43**:1616–23.

60. Devous MD, Sr. Functional brain imaging in the dementias: role in early detection, differential diagnosis, and longitudinal studies. *Eur J Nucl Med Mol Imaging*. 2002;**29**:1685–96.

61. Matsuda H. Role of neuroimaging in Alzheimer's disease, with emphasis on brain perfusion SPECT. *J Nucl Med*. 2007;**48**:1289–300.

62. Kemp PM, Holmes C. Imaging in dementia with Lewy bodies: a review. *Nucl Med Commun*. 2007;**28**:511–19.

63. Chang CC, Liu JS, Chang YY, *et al.* (99 m)Tc-ethyl cysteinate dimer brain SPECT findings in early stage of dementia with Lewy bodies and Parkinson's disease patients: a correlation with neuropsychological tests. *Eur J Neurol*. 2008;**15**:61–5.

64. Kato H, Yoshikawa T, Oku N, *et al.*, Statistical parametric analysis of cerebral blood flow in vascular dementia with small-vessel disease using ^{99m}Tc-HMPAO SPECT. *Cerebrovasc Dis*. 2008;**26**:556–62.

65. Le Ber I, Guedj E, Gabelle A, *et al.* Demographic, neurological and behavioural characteristics and brain perfusion SPECT in frontal variant of frontotemporal dementia. *Brain*. 2006;**129**:3051–65.

66. Johnson KA, Moran EK, Becker JA, *et al.* Single photon emission computed tomography perfusion differences in mild cognitive impairment. *J Neurol Neurosurg Psychiatry*. 2007;**78**:240–7.

67. Jobst KA, Barnetson LP, Shepstone BJ. Accurate prediction of histologically confirmed Altzheimer's disease and the differential diagnosis of dementia: the use of NINCDS-ADRDA and DSMIII-R criteria, SPECT, X-ray CT, and Apo E4 in medial temporal lobe dementias: Oxford project to investigate memory and ageing. *Int Psychogeriatr*. 1998;**10**:271–302.

68. Catafau AM. Brain SPECT in clinical practice. Part I: Perfusion. *J Nucl Med*. 2001;**42**:259–71.

69. Adams RD, Victor M, Ropper AH. *Principles of Neurology*, 6th edn. New York, NY, McGraw-Hill. 1997; 3–11, 94–113, 1046–1107, 1507–1529, 1544–1564.

70. Miller BL, Cummings JL, Villanueva-Meyer J, *et al.* Frontal lobe degeneration: clinical, neuropsychological, and SPECT characteristics. *Neurology*. 1991;**41**:1374–82.

71. Goffin K, Dedeurwaerdere S, Van Laere K, Van Paesschen W. Neuronuclear assessment of patients with epilepsy. *Semin Nucl Med*. 2008;**38**:227–39.

72. Van Paesschen W, Dupont P, Sunaert S, Goffin K, Van Laere K. The use of SPECT and PET in routine clinical practice in epilepsy. *Curr Opin Neurol*. 2007;**20**:194–202.

73. Van Paesschen W. Ictal SPECT. *Epilepsia*. 2004;**45**(Suppl 4):35–40.

74. Zaknun JJ, Bal C, Maes A, *et al.* Comparative analysis of MR imaging, ictal SPECT and EEG in temporal lobe epilepsy: a prospective IAEA multi-center study. *Eur J Nucl Med Mol Imaging*. 2008;**35**:107–15.

75. Patil S, Biassoni L, Borgwardt L. Nuclear medicine in pediatric neurology and neurosurgery: epilepsy and brain tumors. *Semin Nucl Med*. 2007;**37**:357–81.

76. Holmes MD, Dodrill CB, Ojemann LM, Ojemann GA. Five-year outcome after epilepsy surgery in nonmonitored and monitored surgical candidates. *Epilepsia*. 1996;**37**:748–52.

77. Spencer SS. The relative contribution of MRI, SPECT and PET imaging in epilepsy. *Epilepsia*. 1994;**35**(Suppl. 6): S72–89.

78. O'Brien TJ, So EL, Mullan BP, *et al.* Subtraction ictal SPECT coregistered to MRI improves clinical usefulness of SPECT in localizing the surgical seizure focus. *Neurology*. 1998;**50**:445–54.

79. Liu FY, Huang WS, Kao CH, *et al.* Usefulness of Tc-99m ECD brain SPECT to evaluate the effects of methylprednisolone pulse therapy in lupus erythematosis with brain involvement: a preliminary report. *Rheumatol Int*. 2003;**23**:182–5.

80. Abdel-Dayem HM, Abu-Judeh H, Kumar M, *et al.* SPECT brain perfusion abnormalities in mild or moderate traumatic brain injury. *Clin Nucl Med*. 1998;**23**:309–17.

81. Roper SN, Mena I, King WA, *et al.* An analysis of cerebral blood flow in acute closed-head injury using technetium-99m-HMPAO SPECT and computed tomography. *J Nucl Med*. 1991;**32**:1684–7.

82. Gray BG, Ichise M, Chung D-G, Kirsh JC, Franks W. Technetium-99m-HMPAO SPECT in the evaluation of patients with a remote history of traumatic brain injury: a comparison with x-ray computed tomography. *J Nucl Med*. 1992;**33**:52–8.

83. Lorberboym M, Lampl Y, Gerzon I, Sadeh M. Brain SPECT evaluation of amnestic ED patients after mild head trauma. *Am J Emerg Med*. 2002;**20**:310–13.

84. Ichise M, Chung DG, Wang P, *et al.* Technetium-99m-HMPAO SPECT, CT and MRI in the evaluation of patients with chronic traumatic brain injury: a correlation with neuropsychological performance. *J Nucl Med*. 1994;**35**:217–26.

85. Donohoe KJ, Frey KA, Gerbaudo VH, *et al.* Procedure guideline for brain death scintigraphy. *J Nucl Med*. 2003;**44**:846–51.

86. Barth A, Haldemann AR, Reubi JC, *et al.* Noninvasive differentiation of meningiomas from other brain tumours using combined 111 Indium-octreotide/99mtechnetium-DTPA brain scintigraphy. *Acta Neurochir Wien*. 1996;**138**:1179–85.

87. Inoue Y, Momose T, Machida K, *et al.* Delayed imaging of Tc-99m-DTPA-HSA SPECT in subacute cerebral infarction. *Radiat Med*. 1993;**11**:214–16.

88. Lorberboym M, Lampl Y, Sadeh M. Correlation of 99mTc-DTPA SPECT of the blood-brain barrier with neurologic outcome after acute stroke. *J Nucl Med*. 2003;**44**:1898–904.

89. Papazyan JP, Delavelle J, Burklard P, *et al.* Discrepancies between HMPAO and ECD SPECT imaging in brain tumors. *J Nucl Med*. 1997;**38**:592–6.

90. Lorberboym M, Estok L, Machac J, *et al.* Rapid differential diagnosis of cerebral toxoplasmosis and primary central nervous system lymphoma by

thallium-201 SPECT. *J Nucl Med.* 1996;**37**:1150–4.

91. Lorberboym M, Mandell LR, Mosesson RE, *et al.* The role of thallium-201 uptake and retention in intracranial tumors after radiotherapy. *J Nucl Med.* 1997;**38**:223–6.

92. Blankenberg FG, Katsikis PD, Tait JF, *et al.* In vivo detection and imaging of phosphatidylserine expression during programmed cell death. *Proc Natl Acad Sci U S A.* 1998;**95**:6349–54.

93. Zwaal RF, Schroit AJ. Pathophysiologic implications of membrane phospholipid asymmetry in blood cells. *Blood.* 1997;**89**:1121–32.

94. Lorberboym M, Blankenberg FG, Sadeh M, Lampl Y. In vivo imaging of apoptosis in patients with acute stroke: correlation with blood-brain barrier permeability. *Brain Res.* 2006;**1103**:13–19.

95. Spampinato U, Habert MO, Mas JL, *et al.* (99mTc)-HM-PAO SPECT and cognitive impairment in Parkinson's disease: a comparison with dementia of the Alzheimer type. *J Neurol Neurosurg Psychiatry.* 1991;**54**:787–92.

96. Hughes AJ, Daniel SE, Kilford L, and Lees AJ. Accuracy of clinical diagnosis of idiopathic Parkinson's disease: A clinicopathological study of 100 cases. *J Neurol Neurosurg Psychiatry.* 1992;**55**:181–4.

97. Tolosa E, Coelho M, Gallardo M. DAT imaging in drug-induced and psychogenic parkinsonism. *Mov Disord.* 2003;**18**(Suppl 7):S28–33.

98. Booij J, Speelman JD, Horstink MW, Wolters EC. The clinical benefit of imaging striatal dopamine transporters with [^{123}I]FP-CIT SPECT in differentiating patients with presynaptic parkinsonism from those with other forms of parkinsonism. *Eur J Nucl Med.* 2001;**28**:266–72.

99. Varrone A, Marek KL, Jennings D, Innis R-B, Seibyl JP. [(123)I]beta-CIT SPECT imaging demonstrates reduced density of striatal dopamine transporters in Parkinson's disease and multiple system atrophy. *Mov Disord.* 2001;**16**:23–32.

100. Lorberboym M, Treves TA, Melamed E, *et al.* [^{123}I]-FP/CIT SPECT imaging for distinguishing drug-induced parkinsonism from Parkinson's disease. *Mov Disord.* 2006;**21**:510–14.

101. Lorberboym M, Djaldetti R, Melamed E, Sadeh M, Lampl Y. ^{123}I-FP-CIT SPECT imaging of dopamine transporters in patients with cerebrovascular disease and clinical diagnosis of vascular parkinsonism. *J Nucl Med.* 2004;**45**:1688–93.

102. Seibyl JP, Marek K, Sheff K, *et al.* Iodine-123-beta-CIT and iodine-123-FPCIT SPECT measurement of dopamine transporters in healthy subjects and Parkinson's patients. *J Nucl Med.* 1998;**39**:1500–8.

103. Tissingh G, Bergmans P, Booij J, *et al.* Drug-naive patients with Parkinson's disease in Hoehn and Yahr stages I and II show a bilateral decrease in striatal dopamine transporters as revealed by [123I]beta-CIT SPECT. *J Neurol.* 1998;**245**:14–20.

104. Djaldetti R, Lorberboym M, Karmon Y, *et al.* Residual striatal dopaminergic nerve terminals in very long-standing Parkinson's disease: a single photon emission computed tomography imaging study. *Mov Disord.* 2011;**26**:327–30.

105. van Royen E, Verhoeff NF, Speelman JD, *et al* Multiple system atrophy and progressive supranuclear palsy. Diminished striatal D2 dopamine receptor activity demonstrated by ^{123}I-IBZM single photon emission computed tomography. *Arch Neurol.* 1993;**50**:513–16.

106. Woods SW. Regional cerebral blood flow imaging with SPECT in psychiatric disease: focus on schizophrenia, anxiety disorders and substance abuse. *J Clin Psychiatry.* 1992;**53**(Suppl):20–5.

107. Dang-Vu TT, Desseilles M, Schwartz S, Maquet P. Neuroimaging of narcolepsy. *CNS Neurol Disord Drug Targets.* 2009;**8**:254–263.

108. Eisensehr I, Linke R, Tatsch K, *et al.* Alteration of the striatal dopaminergic system in human narcolepsy. *Neurology.* 2003;**60**:1817–19.

109. Hublin C, Launes J, Nikkinen P, Partinen M. Dopamine D2-receptors in human narcolepsy: a SPECT study with ^{123}I-BZM. *Acta Neurol Scand.* 1994;**90**:186–9.

110. Staedt J, Stoppe G, Kogler A, *et al.* [123I] IBZM SPET analysis of dopamine D2 receptor occupancy in narcoleptic patients in the course of treatment. *Biol Psychiatry.* 1996;**39**:107–11.

111. Khan N, Antonini A, Parkes D, *et al.* Striatal dopamine D2 receptors in patients with narcolepsy measured with PET and 11C-raclopride. *Neurology.* 1994;**44**:2102–4.

112. Rinne JO, Hublin C, Partinen M, *et al.* Positron emission tomography study of human narcolepsy: no increase in striatal dopamine D2 receptors. *Neurology.* 1995;**45**:1735–8.

113. MacFarlane JG, List SJ, Moldofsky H, *et al.* Dopamine D2 receptors quantified in vivo in human narcolepsy. *Biol Psychiatry.* 1997;**41**:305–10.

114. Rinne JO, Hublin C, Nagren K, Helenius H, Partinen M. Unchanged striatal dopamine transporter availability in narcolepsy: a PET study with [11C]-CFT. *Acta Neurol Scand.* 2004;**109**:52–5.

115. Boeve BF, Silber MH, Saper CB, *et al.* Pathophysiology of REM sleep behaviour disorder and relevance to neurodegenerative disease. *Brain* 2007;**130**:2770–88.

116. Stiasny-Kolster K, Doerr Y, Moller JC, *et al.* Combination of idiopathic REM sleep behaviour disorder and olfactory dysfunction as possible indicator for alpha-synucleinopathy demonstrated by dopamine transporter FP-CIT-SPECT. *Brain* 2005;**128**:126–37.

117. Eisensehar I, Linke R, Noachtar S, *et al.* Reduced striatal dopamine transporters in idiopathic rapid eye movement sleep behaviour disorder. Comparison with Parkinson's disease and controls. *Brain* 2000;**123**:1155–60.

118. Miyamoto T, Miyamoto M, Inoue Y, *et al.* Reduced cardiac 123I-MIBG scintigraphy in idiopathic REM sleep behavior disorder. *Neurology* 2006;**67**:2236–8.

119. Hanyu H, Inoue Y, Sakurai H, *et al.* Regional cerebral blood flow changes in patients with idiopathic REM sleep behavior disorder. *Eur J Neurol.* 2011;**18**:784–8.

120. Arnulf I, Lin L, Gadoth N, *et al.* Kleine–Levin syndrome: a systematic study of 108 patients. *Ann Neurol.* 2008;**63**:482–93.

121. Hoexter MQ, Shih MC, Mendes DD, *et al.* Lower dopamine transporter density in an asymptomatic patient with Kleine–Levin syndrome. *Acta Neurol Scand.* 2008;**117**:370–3.

122. Huang YS, Lakkis C, Guilleminault C. Kleine-Levin syndrome: current status. *Med Clin North Am.* 2010;**94**:557–62.

123. Jhoo JH, Yoon IY, Kim YK, *et al.* Availability of brain serotonin

transporters in patients with restless legs syndrome. *Neurology*. 2010;**74**:513–18.

124. Joo EY, Tae WS, Han SJ, Cho JW, Hong SB. Reduced cerebral blood flow during wakefulness in obstructive sleep apnea-hypopnea syndrome. *Sleep*. 2007;**30**:1515–20.

125. Petersson J, Sánchez-Crespo A, Larsson SA, Mure M. Physiological imaging of the lung: single-photon-emission computed tomography (SPECT). *J Appl Physiol*. 2007;**102**:468–76.

126. Kessler RM. Imaging methods for evaluating brain function in man. *Neurobiol Aging*. 2003;**24**:S21–35; discussion S37–9.

127. Jaszczak RJ, Coleman RE, Lim CB. SPECT: single photon emission computed tomography. *IEEE Tran Nucl Sci*. 1980;NS-**27**:1137–53.

128. Loats H. CT and SPECT image registration and fusion for spatial localization of metastatic processes using radiolabeled monoclonals. *J Nucl Med*. 1993;**34**:562–6.

129. Maintz JB, Viergever MA. A survey of medical image registration. *Med Image Anal*. 1998;**2**:1–36.

130. Hill DL, Batchelor PG, Holden M, Hawkes DJ. Medical image registration. *Phys Med Biol*. 2001;**46**:R1–45.

131. Hutton BF, Braun M, Thurfjell L, Lau DYH. Image registration: an essential tool for Nuclear Medicine. *Eur J Nucl Med Mol Imaging*. 2002;**29**:559–77.

132. Kessler ML. Image registration and data fusion in radiation therapy. *Br J Radiol*. 2006;79 Spec No **1**:S99–108.

133. Hasegawa BH, Wong KH, Iwata K, *et al*. Dual-modality imaging of cancer with SPECT/CT. *Technol Cancer Res Treat*. 2002;**1**:449–58.

134. Townsend DW, Beyer T. A combined PET/CT scanner: the path to true image fusion. *Br J Radiol*. 2002;**75**:S24–30.

135. Keidar Z, Israel O, Krausz Y. SPECT/CT in tumor imaging: technical aspects and clinical applications. *Semin Nucl Med*. 2003;**33**:205–18.

136. Schillaci O, Simonetti G. Fusion imaging in Nuclear Medicine–applications of dual-modality systems in oncology. *Cancer Biother Radiopharm*. 2004;**19**:1–10.

137. Townsend DW, Yap JT, Carney JP, Hall NC. Developments in PET/CT: from concept to practice. *Med Phys*. 2004;**31**:1694(abst).

138. LaCroix KJ, Tsui BMW, Hasegawa BH, Brown JK, Investigation of the use of x-ray CT images for attenuation correction in SPECT. *IEEE Trans Nucl Sci*. 1994;**41**:2793–9.

139. Blankespoor SC, Wu X, Kalki K, *et al*. Attenuation correction of SPECT using x-ray CT on an emission-transmission CT system: myocardial perfusion assessment. *IEEE Trans Nucl Sci*. 1996;**43**:2263–74.

140. Kinahan PE, Townsend DW, Beyer T, Sashin D. Attenuation correction for a combined 3D PET/CT scanner. *Med Phys*. 1998;**25**:2046–53.

141. Kinahan PE, Hasegawa BH, Beyer T. X-ray-based attenuation correction for position tomography/computed tomography scanners. *Semin Nucl Med*. 2003;**33**:166–79.

142. Munley MT, Marks LB, Scarfone C, *et al*. Multi-modality nuclear medicine imaging in three-dimensional radiation treatment planning for lung cancer: challenges and prospects. *Lung Cancer*. 1999;**23**:105–14.

143. Liu A, Williams LE, Raubitschek AA. A CT assisted method for absolute quantitation of internal radioactivity. *Med Phys*. 1996;**23**:1919–28.

144. Da Silva AJ, Tang HR, Wong KH, *et al*. Absolute quantitation of regional myocardial uptake of ^{99m}Tc-sestamibi with SPECT: experimental validation in a porcine model. *J Nucl Med*. 2001;**42**:772–9.

145. Ellis RJ, Kaminsky DA. Fused radioimmunoscintigraphy for treatment planning 2006; Rev Urol. 8 Suppl 1:S11–19.

146. Boone JM, Multidetector CT: opportunities, challenges, and concerns associated with scanners with 64 or more detector rows. *Radiology*. 2006;**241**:334–7.

147. Krausz Y, Keidar Z, Kogan I, *et al*. SPECT/CT hybrid imaging with ^{111}In-pentetreotide in assessment of neuroendocrine tumours. *Clin Endocrinol (Oxf)*. 2003;**59**:565–73.

148. Horger M, Eschmann SM, Pfannenberg C, *et al*. The value of SPET/CT in chronic osteomyelitis. *Eur J Nucl Med Mol Imaging*. 2003;**30**:1665–73.

149. Bar-Shalom R, Yefremov N, Guralnik L, *et al*. SPECT/CT using ^{67}Ga and ^{111}In-labeled leukocyte scintigraphy for diagnosis of infection. *J Nucl Med*. 2006;**47**:587–94.

150. Filippi L, Schillaci O. SPECT/CT with a hybrid camera: a new imaging modality for the functional anatomical mapping of infections. *Expert Rev Med Devices*. 2006;**3**:699–703.

151. Suga K, Kawakami Y, Zaki M, *et al*. Clinical utility of co-registered respiratory-gated (^{99m})Tc-Technegas/MAA SPECT-CT images in the assessment of regional lung functional impairment in patients with lung cancer. *Eur J Nucl Med Mol Imaging*. 2004;**31**:1280–90.

152. Suga K, Kawakami Y, Iwanaga H, Tokuda O, Matsunaga N. Automated breath-hold perfusion SPECT/CT fusion images of the lungs. *AJR Am J Roentgenol*. 2007;**189**:455–63.

153. Tan KG, Bartholomeusz FD, Chatterton BE. Detection and follow up of biliary leak on Tc-99m DIDA SPECT-CT scans. *Clin Nucl Med*. 2004;**29**:642–3.

154. Rana JS, Rozanski A, Berman DS. Combination of myocardial perfusion imaging and coronary artery calcium scanning: potential synergies for improving risk assessment in subjects with suspected coronary artery disease. *Curr Atheroscler Rep*. 2011;**13**:381–9.

Fundamentals of transcranial B-mode sonography

Jana Godau and Daniela Berg

Introduction

Transcranial B-mode sonography (TCS), also named brain parenchyma sonography (BPS), is a relatively young method that has originally been applied in the diagnosis and intraoperative monitoring of solid brain tumors. More recently, it has been implemented in the diagnostic approach to Parkinson's disease (PD). Its relevance for evaluation of sleep disorders becomes especially evident at the overlap of movement disorders and sleep disorders, such as in restless legs syndrome (RLS) and rapid eye movement (REM) sleep behavior disorder (RBD).

Technical aspects

TCS requires application of a high-end ultrasound machine equipped with a 1.5–3.5 MHz ultrasound transducer the same as used for transcranial Doppler and duplex sonography (TCD). An overview of basic system settings is given in Table 7.1. TCS allows an axial spatial resolution of approximately 0.7 mm and a lateral resolution of approximately 1.05 mm, which is higher than in routine magnetic resonance imaging (MRI) [1].

Scanning procedure

For the standard examination, two different standardized planes are scanned through the posterior temporal bone window from both sides. The ultrasound probe is oriented parallel to the imagined orbitomeatal line (Figure 7.1).

First, the midbrain plane is visualized. It allows depiction of the butterfly-shaped mesencephalic brainstem which appears with low echogenicity surrounded by strongly echogenic basal cisterns. Within the midbrain three key structures can be differentiated which all appear moderately echogenic within the brainstem tissue. These structures include the substantia nigra (SN), brainstem raphe nuclei, and red nucleus (RN).

Table 7.1. Transcranial B-mode sonography (TCS) system settings

System	High-end
Ultrsound transducer	1.5–3.5 Mhz phased array
Penetration depth	14–16 cm
Dynamic range	45–60 dB
Contour amplification	Medium-high
Image persistence	High
Image rate	Low
Postprocessing parameters	Moderate suppression of low echo signals
Time gain compensation	Adjust as needed
Image brightness	Adjust as needed

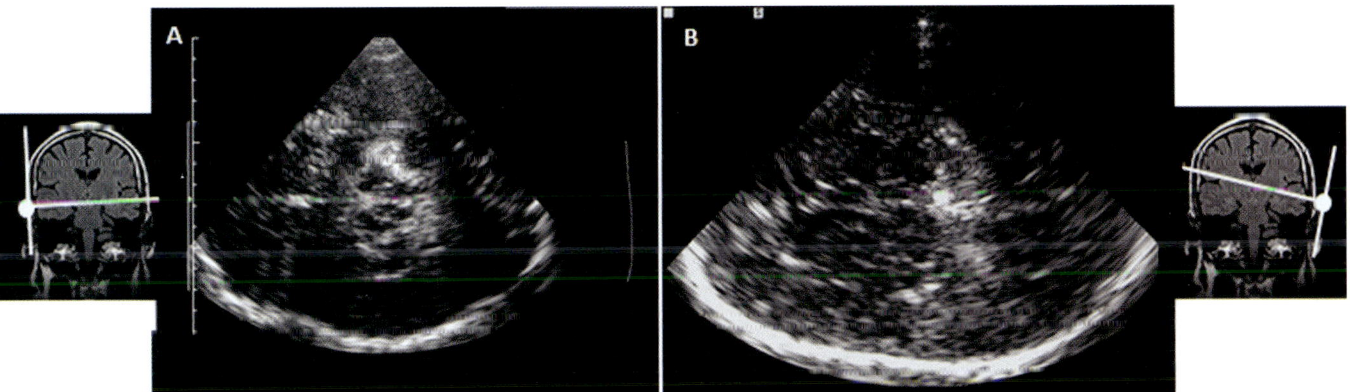

Figure 7.1 Scanning planes. (A) Mesencephalic plane comprising the hypoechogenic butterfly-shaped midbrain which is surrounded by strongly echogenic basal cisterns. (B) Plane of the third ventricle allowing assessment of the ventricular system (low echogenicity) and the basal ganglia which are isoechogenic to the surrounding tissue.

Neuroimaging of Sleep and Sleep Disorders, ed. Eric Nofzinger, Pierre Maquet, and Michael J. Thorpy. Published by Cambridge University Press. © Cambridge University Press 2013.

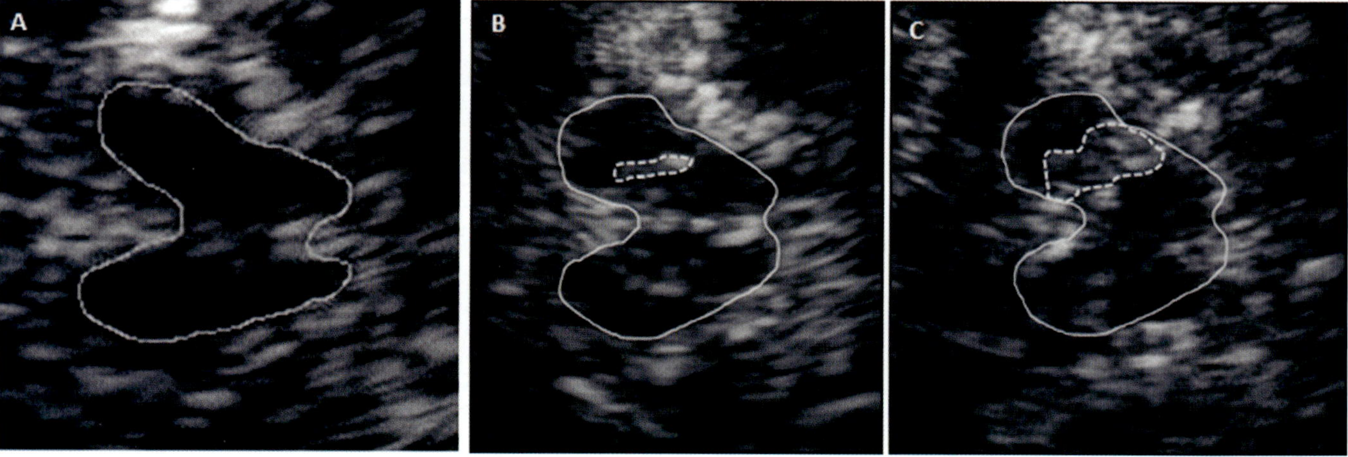

Figure 7.2 Substantia nigra (SN). (A) SN hypoechogenicity, the SN cannot be distinguished from the brainstem tissue. (B) Normal SN echogenicity, the SN appears mildly echogenic within the midbrain. (C) Marked SN hyperechogenicity, the echogenic area covers a large portion of the midbrain peduncles. The continuous line indicates the midbrain borders. The spaced line encircles the ipsilateral SN area of echogenicity.

The second scanning plane is the third ventricle plane, which can be reached by tilting the ultrasound probe slightly upwards (approximately 10–20°). In addition to the third ventricle, also the anterior horns of the lateral ventricles, and the basal ganglia including the caudate (CN) and the lentiform nucleus (LN) can be distinguished.

In addition to these two standard planes also the plane of the cella media of the lateral ventricles (tilting the probe approximately 30–40°) and the cerebellar plane (rotating the probe about 40°) can be reached from the midbrain plane. These allow assessment of a number of additional structures including cerebellar hemispheres and cerebellar nuclei, fourth ventricle, hippocampus, frontal and parietal lobes. These have, however, not yet been implemented in the standard assessments. A more detailed description of the scanning procedure can for example be found in publications by Walter and colleagues [2] and Skoloudik and Walter [3].

Evaluation of structures

By convention and due to the resolution of the ultrasound waves in proximity of the probe, structures that are close to the midline (i.e., brainstem structures) are assessed from the ipsilateral side whereas structures that are located distant to the midline (i.e., LN) are examined from the contralateral side [4].

Many structures are rated semiquantitatively according to their degree of echogenicity. These include the SN, RN, CN, and LN. The degree of echogenicity may vary between "iso-echogenic to the surrounding tissue," which means that the structure cannot be distinguished, and "mildly, moderately, or markedly hyperechogenic." CN and LN usually appear iso-echogenic to the surrounding tissue, hyperechogenicity indicates an abnormal finding. SN and RN usually appear mildly hyperechogenic; abnormalities of these structures may therefore include both increased and decreased degrees of echogenicity.

In addition to the semiquantitative rating, SN echogenicity can also be evaluated quantitatively by manually encircling the area of SN echogenicity at its largest expansion (Figure 7.2). SN areas which exceed the 90th percentile of the normal population on at least one side are referred to as increased SN echogenicity or "SN hyperechogenicity." The cutoff value normally ranges from 0.20 to 0.25 cm², depending on the applied ultrasound system [5]. SN areas which are below the 10th percentile of the normal population are referred to as decreased SN echogenicity or "SN hypoechogenicity." In order to accommodate for higher inaccuracy when measuring very small areas, the sum area of both sides has been taken for the assessment of cutoff values in the case of SN hypoechogenicity. Hence, the cutoff value for SN hypoechogenicity corresponds to a sum area of both sides of or below 0.20 cm² (approximately 0.10 cm² per side) [6].

The brainstem raphe normally appears as a continuous echogenic midline in the area of the lower mesencephalon. It is rated semiquantitatively as either "normal" or "reduced echogenicity." Reduced echogenicity is determined when the echogenic midline structure is either interrupted or absent (Figure 7.3). An interrupted or absent raphe structure is also referred to as "raphe hypoechogenicity" [7].

The width of the third ventricle is rated quantitatively. It is determined by the distance between its two strongly echogenic ependymal linings. The width of the third ventricle depends on age and correlates well with MRI and computed tomography (CT) measurements [8]. Third ventricle widths are considered to be abnormal when values > 6 mm (age < 65 years) or > 7.5 mm (age ≥ 65 years) are measured [5].

Application in sleep disorders

Most data on TCS in disorders associated with insomnia or parasomnias have been evaluated from the movement disorder perspective and did not address diagnosis or differential diagnosis of sleep disorders directly. Therefore, one needs to be careful with the interpretation of the data. However, some interesting findings indicate that TCS might be valuable for the evaluation of sleep disorder patients with suspected RLS, depressive disorder, or RBD.

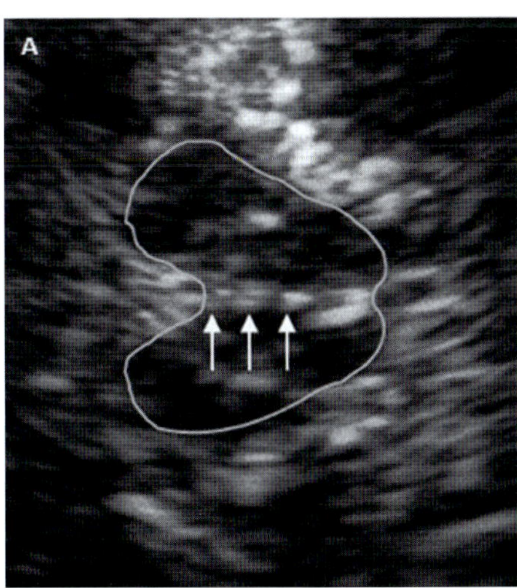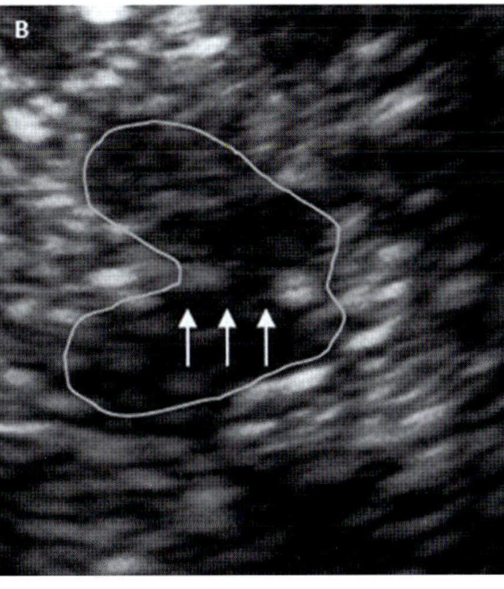

Figure 7.3 Brainstem raphe. (A) Normal raphe echogenicity (continuous midline, arrows). (B) Raphe hypoechogenicity with interrupted (or absent) midline structure. The continuous line indicates the midbrain borders.

Restless legs syndrome (RLS)

RLS can be described as a combined sensory, movement, and sleep disorder. It is characterized by an irresistible urge to move the legs and sometimes other body parts which occurs or worsens at rest and can be relieved by moving around. It is usually accompanied by sensory discomfort, and often nightly involuntary rhythmic periodic limb movements (PLM). RLS usually occurs or worsens at bedtime and is often associated with insomnia.

The typical ultrasound picture of RLS includes SN hypoechogenicity as the key feature, often associated with raphe hypoechogenicity and moderate to marked RN hyperechogenicity [9].

SN hypoechogenicity as a common feature among patients with idiopathic RLS was first described in 2005 [10]. It has been found to be a fairly sensitive (82–89%) and specific (83–86%) marker for idiopathic RLS with a positive predictive value of 94%, and was also found in about 60% of patients with symptomatic RLS [6, 9]. SN hypoechogenicity is associated with reduced brain iron content as measured by MRI (turbo spin-echo sequence), a causative relationship is likely, but could not be proven so far [11].

RN hyperechogenicity is present in about 60% of patients with idiopathic and symptomatic RLS. The pathophysiological relevance of this finding is yet unclear [9].

Raphe hypoechogenicity is a common feature in primary depressive disorders (see below). It can be found in approximately 73% of patients with RLS, both in idiopathic and symptomatic subtypes [9]. These numbers are higher than the percentage of RLS patients actually suffering from a concomitant depressive disorder (22.4–36.9%) [12, 13], which might indicate that raphe hypoechogenicity might also be directly related to RLS.

Regarding *differential diagnosis* of RLS and other disorders with predominant leg discomfort, the value of TCS seems to be rather low, as also about 60% of patients with neuropathic pain show the same sonographical picture as RLS patients [14]. Also patients with other neuropathic disorders such as Friedreich ataxia commonly exhibit SN hypoechogenicity, which is sometimes but not always associated with clinical RLS [15].

No data are currently available on the differential diagnostic capacity of TCS features for RLS versus other sources of insomnia. Still, in the assessment of a patient with disturbed sleep, TCS as an additional diagnostic instrument may help to support the clinical impression of an underlying RLS.

Depressive disorders

Raphe hypoechogenicity is a characteristic feature of primary depressive disorders, found in 50–60% of patients with depression [16, 17]. One study also suggested that raphe hypoechogenicity may also be an indicator for positive response to treatment with selective serotonin reuptake inhibitors (SSRIs), although these results lack a prospective design [16]. Regarding clinical associations, the data are not consistent, ranging from no correlation between raphe echogenicity and severity of depressive symptoms [18] to a clear association of more severe depressive symptoms with more pronounced raphe hypoechogenicity [19].

The predictive value of raphe hypoechogenicity for depression has not been evaluated so far. However, one might assume that the presence of raphe hypoechogenicity in a sleep disorder patient with suspected depression might support the diagnosis of an underlying primary depressive disorder.

REM sleep behavior disorder (RBD)

RBD is a parasomnia characterized by dream-enacting behavior often associated with violent dream contents and nightmares. The dream-enacting behavior is caused by a lack of muscular inactivation during the REM sleeping stage. RBD can occur symptomatically in the frame of other sleep disorders such as narcolepsy, but most cases are considered as idiopathic.

Interestingly, in the course of 5–12 years 16.4–52.4% of the patients with idiopathic RBD (iRBD) develop a neurodegenerative disorder including PD, atypical Parkinsonian syndromes

(APS), and most frequently dementia [20, 21]. TCS has proven to be a valuable tool for the diagnosis and differential diagnosis of PD, even in the very early and preclinical phase, when the diagnostic key symptoms are not yet present [22].

The typical feature of PD is *SN hyperechogenicity* with a cumulated sensitivity of 91% (82–98%) and a cumulated specificity of 92% (70–100%) in eight studies with 611 patients and 574 controls [23]. SN hyperechogenicity in a healthy person aged 50 years or older is associated with a 17.8-fold increased risk to develop PD within the next three years [24]. In a person already experiencing potential yet unspecific non-motor features of PD such as hyposmia the relative risk to develop PD may even be higher [25]. The presence of LN hyperechogenicity combined with signs of brain atrophy such as an enlarged third ventricle may be an indicator for an underlying APS [26]. An enlarged third ventricle may also be an early indicator for cognitive decline and dementia [27].

Thirty-seven percent of patients with iRBD exhibit SN hyperechogenicity [28], whereas patients with symptomatic RBD such as in narcolepsy do not exhibit this feature [29]. Data on other sonographical features of patients with iRBD have not been published so far. As prospective studies using TCS in RBD cohorts are lacking, it is also still unclear whether iRBD patients with SN hyperechogenicity will really develop PD more often than those with normal SN echogenicity.

Therefore, if supported by prospective data, it may well be that sonographic abnormalities in patients with iRBD may help to identify subjects who are at an increased risk to develop a neurodegenerative disorder. In the future, this may help to initiate an early neuroprotective treatment in these patients to potentially delay or prevent the onset of typical clinical features.

Summary

Transcranial B-mode sonography (TCS) is a widely available, non-invasive and cost-effective diagnostic instrument. A large amount of data indicates that it is especially valuable for the diagnosis and differential diagnosis of movement disorders. Only few data are available regarding application in sleep disorders; therefore its applicability is still limited. However, in a patient complaining about disturbed sleep a TCS demonstrating SN hypoechogenicity, raphe hypoechogenicity, and RN hyperechogenicity may help to support a suspected diagnosis of RLS. Raphe hypoechogenicity as a single feature may point towards an underlying primary depressive disorder. Finally, in patients with iRBD TCS might be a valuable tool to identify subjects at risk of eventually developing a neurodegenerative disorder. Here, SN hyperechogenicity as an early marker for PD seems to be most important.

References

1. Walter U, Kanowski M, Kaufmann J, *et al.* Contemporary ultrasound systems allow high-resolution transcranial imaging of small echogenic deep intracranial structures similarly as MRI: a phantom study. *Neuroimage.* 2008;**40**:551–8.

2. Walter U, Behnke S, Eyding J, *et al.* Transcranial brain parenchyma sonography in movement disorders: state of the art. *Ultrasound Med Biol.* 2007;**33**:15–25.

3. Skoloudik D, Walter U. Method and validity of transcranial sonography in movement disorders. *Int Rev Neurobiol.* 2010;**90**:7–34.

4. Berg D, Becker G. Perspectives of B-mode transcranial ultrasound. *Neuroimage.* 2002;**15**:463–73.

5. Berg D, Behnke S, Walter U. Application of transcranial sonography in extrapyramidal disorders: updated recommendations. *Ultraschall Med.* 2006;**27**:12–19.

6. Godau J, Schweitzer KJ, Liepelt I, *et al.* Substantia nigra hypoechogenicity: definition and findings in restless legs syndrome. *Mov Disord.* 2007;**22**:187–92.

7. Becker G, Struck M, Bogdahn U, *et al.* Echogenicity of the brainstem raphe in patients with major depression. *Psychiatry Res* 1994;**55**:75–84.

8. Kern R, Perren F, Kreisel S, *et al.* Multiplanar transcranial ultrasound imaging: standards, landmarks and correlation with magnetic resonance imaging. *Ultrasound Med Biol.* 2005;**31**:311–15.

9. Godau J, Wevers AK, Gaenslen A, *et al.* Sonographic abnormalities of brainstem structures in restless legs syndrome. *Sleep Med.* 2008;**9**:782–9.

10. Schmidauer C, Sojer M, Seppi K, *et al.* Transcranial ultrasound shows nigral hypoechogenicity in restless legs syndrome. *Ann Neurol.* 2005;**58**:630–4.

11. Godau J, Klose U, Di Santo A, *et al.* Multiregional brain iron deficiency in restless legs syndrome. *Mov Disord.* 2008;**23**:1184–7.

12. Banno K, Delaive K, Walld R, *et al.* Restless legs syndrome in 218 patients: associated disorders. *Sleep Med.* 2000;**1**:221–9.

13. Winkelmann J, Prager M, Lieb R, *et al.* "Anxietas tibiarum". Depression and anxiety disorders in patients with restless legs syndrome. *J Neurol.* 2005;**252**:67–71.

14. Godau J, Manz A, Wevers AK, *et al.* Sonographic substantia nigra hypoechogenicity in polyneuropathy and restless legs syndrome. *Mov Disord.* 2009;**24**:133–137.

15. Synofzik M, Godau J, Lindig T, *et al.* Transcranial sonography reveals cerebellar, nigral, and forebrain abnormalities in Friedreich's ataxia. *Neurodegener Dis.* 2011;**8**:470–5.

16. Walter U, Prudente-Morrissey L, Herpertz SC, *et al.* Relationship of brainstem raphe echogenicity and clinical findings in depressive states. *Psychiatry Res.* 2007;**155**:67–73.

17. Berg D, Supprian T, Hofmann E, *et al.* Depression in Parkinson's disease: brainstem midline alteration on transcranial sonography and magnetic resonance imaging. *J Neurol.* 1999;**246**:1186–93.

18. Becker G, Becker T, Struck M, *et al.* Reduced echogenicity of brainstem raphe specific to unipolar depression: a transcranial color-coded real-time sonography study. *Biol Psychiatry.* 1995;**38**:180–4.

19. Budisic M, Karlovic D, Trkanjec Z, *et al.* Brainstem raphe lesion in patients with major depressive disorder and in patients with suicidal ideation recorded on transcranial sonography. *Eur Arch Psychiatry Clin Neurosci.* 2010;**260**:203–8.

20. Postuma RB, Gagnon JF, Vendette M, *et al.* Quantifying the risk of neurodegenerative disease in idiopathic REM sleep behavior disorder. *Neurology.* 2009;**72**:1296–300.

21. Schenck CH, Bundlie SR, Mahowald MW. Delayed emergence of a parkinsonian disorder in 38% of 29 older men initially diagnosed with idiopathic rapid eye movement sleep behaviour disorder. *Neurology.* 1996;**46**:388–93.

22. Gaenslen A, Unmuth B, Godau J, *et al.* The specificity and sensitivity of transcranial ultrasound in the differential diagnosis of Parkinson's disease: a prospective blinded study. *Lancet Neurol.* 2008;**7**:417–24.

23. Godau J, Berg D. Role of transcranial ultrasound in the diagnosis of movement disorders. *Neuroimaging Clin N Am.* 2010;**20**:87–101.

24. Berg D, Seppi K, Behnke S, *et al.* Enlarged substantia nigra hyperechogenicity and risk for Parkinson disease: a 37-month 3-center study of 1847 older persons. *Arch Neurol.* 2011;**68**:932–7.

25. Liepelt I, Behnke S, Schweitzer K, *et al.* Pre-motor signs of PD are related to SN hyperechogenicity assessed by TCS in an elderly population. *Neurobiol Aging.* 2009;**32**:1599–606.

26. Behnke S, Berg D, Naumann M, *et al.* Differentiation of Parkinson's disease and atypical parkinsonian syndromes by transcranial ultrasound. *J Neurol Neurosurg Psychiatry.* 2005;**76**:423–5.

27. Wollenweber FA, Schomburg R, Probst M, *et al.* Width of the third ventricle assessed by transcranial sonography can monitor brain atrophy in a time- and cost-effective manner – results from a longitudinal study on 500 subjects. *Psychiatry Res.* 2011;**191**:212–16.

28. Stockner H, Iranzo A, Seppi K, *et al.* Midbrain hyperechogenicity in idiopathic REM sleep behavior disorder. *Mov Disord.* 2009,**24**.1906–09.

29. Unger MM, Moller JC, Ohletz T, *et al.* Transcranial midbrain sonography in narcoleptic subjects with and without concomitant REM sleep behaviour disorder. *J Neurol.* 2009;**256**:874–7.

Fundamentals of magnetoencephalography

Jeffrey David Lewine, Nitin Bangera, and Bruce J. Fisch

Introduction

Magnetoencephalography (MEG) is a non-invasive method for measuring the weak magnetic fields generated by the brain's electrical activity. In most situations, MEG results are integrated with spatially aligned magnetic resonance data to produce magnetic source localization images that provide a roadmap of structural–functional relationships with millimeter and millisecond precision. Of course, there is a wide range of methods now available for non-invasive evaluation of brain function, including positron emission tomography (PET), single-photon emission computed tomography (SPECT), functional magnetic resonance imaging (fMRI), and electroencephalogram (EEG), so it is important that clinicians and research scientists understand the advantages and limitations of MEG within the context of these other methods [1, 2].

MEG holds two distinct advantages over non-invasive functional imaging methods in neuroradiology. First, MEG provides a direct measure of brain electrophysiology that is not available through the other methods. In PET, SPECT, and fMRI, measurements are made of fluctuations in brain metabolism and hemodynamics. These changes are secondary and tertiary to electrophysiological activity, and as such, they provide only indirect insight into the neurophysiological changes of primary interest in most studies of brain function. The situation is especially complicated because the precise nature and dynamics of the coupling between brain electrophysiology, metabolism, and blood flow remains poorly understood. Caution is essential when drawing neuro-functional inferences from hemodynamic data, especially in clinical populations where disease processes and pharmacological agents may alter coupling mechanisms. For example, patients with long-standing diabetes often show reduced fMRI signals relative to control subjects, but this appears, at least in part, to be a reflection of altered glucose metabolism and decreased vascular compliance [3].

The second critical advantage of MEG relative to neuro-radiological tools is its exquisite temporal resolution. Information processing by the brain takes place on a time scale of milliseconds, and only electromagnetic methods can track this with adequate fidelity. The magnetic field pattern recorded over the head changes instantaneously with changes in the underlying pattern of the brain's neuroelectric activity. In contrast, the temporal resolution of PET, SPECT, and fMRI is severely limited – not so much by the speed at which *images* can be acquired (echo-planar MRI systems can acquire blood oxygen level-dependent (BOLD) fMRI images as fast as every 20–40 ms) – but rather, by the time-constants of the physiological processes being measured. Activity-dependent changes in brain hemodynamics are inherently sluggish and they take several seconds to develop. So, increasing the speed of hemodynamic imaging is unlikely to yield a significant increase in resolution of the true temporal sequence of brain activity supporting critical cognitive skills.

Only the method of EEG provides an alternative direct and temporally precise non-invasive measure of electrophysiological activity. In practice, and as elucidated below, MEG and EEG are differentially affected by the biophysical properties of the brain, skull, and scalp. As such, they offer potentially complimentary information on human brain function, and in most modern MEG studies, EEG is also recorded [4, 5].

MEG technology has both practical and theoretical limitations. On the practical side, MEG machines are few and far between, with fewer than 100 MEG units world-wide. Also, the machines are very expensive to purchase (~$2.5 million) and maintain (~$200K/year for liquid helium and service contract); and successful operation requires a diverse technical team with expertise in neuroscience, biophysics, and biomedical engineering. Fortunately, with adequate resources, these limitations can be overcome.

The theoretical limitations of MEG are thereby more problematic. These relate to (1) a lack of sensitivity to certain configurations of neuronal currents and (2) limitations for solving the "inverse problem" of identifying a unique profile of intracranial currents that generate an extracranially recorded magnetic field pattern. More details on these limitations are given in subsequent sections, along with a description of the real-world consequences (and lack thereof) of these limitations in different situations. Importantly, despite these limitations, MEG can, in appropriately identified clinical and research situations, provide unique and critically important information on brain function in both health and disease. Through the combined efforts of basic science researchers and clinicians, MEG has recently found its footing in the clinical arena, with Medicaid, Medicare, and most private insurance companies now providing reimbursement for MEG procedures related to presurgical localization of epileptic foci in patients with medically refractory seizures, and for presurgical functional mapping of eloquent cortical areas in patients with tumors, arteriovenous malformations, and epilepsy [5, 6]. There is also a rich body of literature focusing on the use of MEG to evaluate other clinical conditions (e.g., schizophrenia, autism, stroke, dementia), and for addressing key issues in basic neuroscience related to specification of neuronal networks supporting language, attention, memory, and other cognitive skills [7]. Several investigative teams are also using MEG to evaluate the underlying neurobiology of sleep. In this chapter, we will outline basic aspects of MEG technology, provide an example of how the method is used clinically, and finally describe how MEG is being used in sleep research.

Basic principles of MEG: Overview

As first described by Oersted in 1837, all time-varying electrical currents generate a surrounding magnetic field. Following the remarkable 1963 demonstration by Baule and McFee that a hand-wound, two million turn induction coil could be used to non-invasively record the magnetic signal generated by the aggregate electrical activity of heart cells, attention turned towards the possible measurement of the brain's neuromagnetic signature. Possibility became reality in 1968 when David Cohen at Massachusetts Institute of Technology used an induction coil and signal averaging techniques to measure the neuromagnetic correlate of the brain's alpha rhythm [8].

The single most critical event for MEG technology was the development of the point-contact SQUID by Zimmerman and colleagues [9]. A SQUID is a Superconducting Quantum Interference Device. SQUIDs are able to detect minute fluctuations in magnetic flux. Using this superconducting technology, magnetic counterparts of the brain's spontaneous awake and sleeping neuroelectric activities (e.g., alpha, beta, delta, theta, mu, and gamma rhythms, sleep spindles, and vertex waves) can now be readily identified without need for signal averaging. MEG can also be used to characterize abnormal brain signals such as those associated with epilepsy and other neurological disorders. Furthermore, through application of signal averaging procedures, one can isolate stimulus-evoked and event-related neuromagnetic signals generated by electrophysiological activity in primary, secondary, and association cortical regions.

The basic principles of MEG are outlined in many articles and books [2, 7, 10–12] and are summarized in Figure 8.1. Current flow, be it in wires, or neurons, generates a surrounding magnetic field that can be measured with SQUID-coupled induction coils. A key to MEG experiments is adequate sampling of the spatial pattern of the magnetic field at each instant in time. Present day whole-head biomagnetometer systems utilize 148–306 sensors arrayed about the head and contained within a cryogenically insulated dewar filled with liquid helium. The pattern of the magnetic field is a reflection of the intracranial currents that generate it. Using simplifying mathematical assumptions (e.g., a dipole-in-a-sphere model), inferences can be drawn as to the location of the relevant neuronal currents. MEG information can be then integrated with MRI data to provide magnetic source localization images that demarcate regions of active brain tissue.

In considering the application of MEG to research and clinical problems, a detailed understanding of the relevant neurophysiology and biophysics is important. Several physiological and biophysical factors influence the relative contributions of different cellular currents to extracranially recorded neuromagnetic signals. Relevant factors include the current configuration within individual cells, the extent to which synchronous activity in nearby cells allows for summation of magnetic fields, the distance of the active population relative to the sensors, the geometry and conductivity profile of cranial tissues (e.g., brain, skull, and scalp), and also the orientation of the relevant currents.

For example, currents associated with action potentials make a minimal contribution to the extracranial field because action currents are characterized by a leading edge of depolarization and a trailing tail of hyperpolarization. This configuration is that of a current quadrapole, and at a distance, the magnetic field generated by the lead edge is almost completely canceled by that associated with the tail. In contrast, dendritic currents initiated at distal spines potentially give rise to strong neuromagnetic fields, although the extracranial field generated by a single neuron is negligible and below the sensitivity level of currently available detectors. Summation of activity across many, many neurons is therefore needed to generate a detectable signal. Realistically, the signals that we are able to record reflect synchronous activity in >100 000 neurons occupying at least a few millimeters of tissue. In considering this situation, it is important to note that summation of magnetic fields is highly dependent on the relative orientation of the critical neuronal elements. Just as there are open- and closed-field configurations for EEG, so too are there open- and closed-field configurations for MEG. For example, the structure of the cortex is such that synchronous activity in the apical dendrites of a patch of commonly oriented pyramidal cells can give rise to a large neuromagnetic signal. In contrast, synchronous activity in stellate cells of the amygdala will give only a very weak signal outside of the head because of the distance to the detectors and the variable orientation of the magnetic fields generated by nearby dendritic elements which leads to cancellation of the signal [13, 14].

Whereas the scalp-recorded EEG is a reflection of current sources and sinks that neuronal currents generate within the extracellular medium, MEG signals are mostly a direct reflection of intracranial currents, with volume conducted extracellular currents making only a minor contribution that is dependent on skull geometry. Thus, the "lead-field" in MEG is more spatially restricted than that in EEG, a factor which provides MEG with somewhat better spatial resolution than EEG [14–16]. Both the EEG and MEG are influenced by the geometry and electrical properties of cranial tissues, but the affects are more prominent in EEG. Specifically, the low conductivity of the skull causes significant attenuation, spatial distortion, and spread of the electrical potential profile, and this can only be accounted for if one has detailed information on the relative geometry and conductivity of the various tissues of the

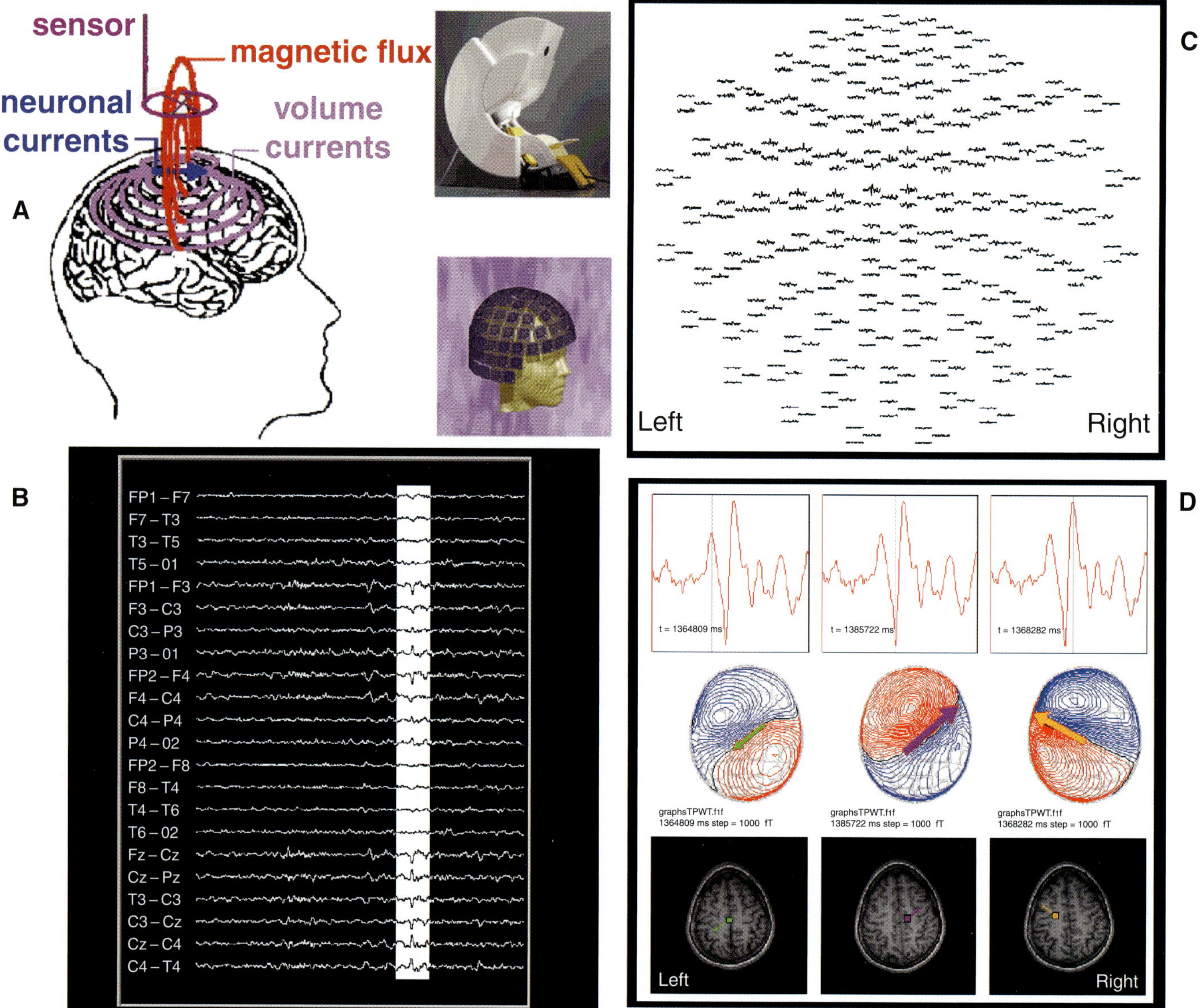

Figure 8.1 Basic Principles of MEG. (A) current flow within the apical dendrites of pyramidal neurons oriented parallel to the skull give rise to a magnetic field that can be detected using super-cooled sensors contained within a cryogenic dewar. (B) ten seconds of EEG recorded during sleep showing vertex waves. (C) MEG data corresponding to the vertex wave highlighted in the lower left panel. For the sensor layout, left channels are on the left. Frontal channels are at the top of the display, occipital channels are at the bottom, temporal lobe channels are lateral, and central/vertex channels are in the middle. The largest MEG deflection is seen in the left fronto-central channels. (D) during the 150 ms duration of the vertex wave, three distinct peaks are identified. Each is associated with a different dipolar pattern. For the iso field contour maps, red shows emerging flux and blue shows entering flux. Corresponding magnetic source localization images are shown. The activity begins in the left cingulate cortex, spreads to the right parasagittal cingulate region, and ends in the left supplementary motor area. Note that magnetic source localization images are presented as right-on-right to allow for easier comparison with the isofield contour maps.

cranium. In contrast, the magnetic signal passes through the skull and scalp with minimal attenuation and distortion. Indeed, to the extent that the skull is spherical, it has no influence on the extracranial magnetic signal, and even fairly significant distortions from sphericity have only minor affects.

A major advantage and disadvantage of MEG relates to orientation selectivity. In EEG, the scalp-recorded electrical potential pattern is a reflection of summated current sources and sinks associated with currents generated by pyramidal cells of radial, tangential, and oblique orientations relative to the skull. Radial currents make the greatest contribution, but EEG sees the entire cortical matrix. In contrast, to the extent that a dendritic current is completely radial to the skull, no recordable magnetic signal is generated outside of the head. In practice, less than 10% of the cortex shows a completely radial orientation, but the MEG is clearly heavily dominated by activity in pyramidal cells aligning sulci, with minimal contributions from gyral caps. In a sense, MEG is a spatially filtered version of EEG, in which some aspects of the core neurophysiological signal are emphasized (e.g., tangential current components) at the expense of others (e.g., radial current components). As a result, MEG can see certain things more simply and clearly, but at the expense of other aspects of the data. It is therefore highly recommended that EEG always be recorded in conjunction with MEG. MEG will provide a clear picture of the tangential component of activity of pyramidal cells, but EEG is needed to capture radial activity.

A final issue with MEG technology relates to the factors that influence the ability of the method to accurately localize the spatial position of those populations of brain cells that give rise to recorded signals. In MRI, PET, and SPECT, the techniques for relating the measured signals back to their spatial location of origin are relatively well established and straightforward. This is not quite true for MEG. For a given pattern of electrical currents flowing within the brain, the pattern of the magnetic field generated in the extracranial space is exactly defined by a set of "forward" calculations using Maxwell's equations and the Biot–Savart Law. In contrast, the "inverse problem" of specifying that set of intracranial currents which produces a particular set of extracranial magnetic field measurements is ill-posed.

To make the inverse problem mathematically tractable, the electrical conductivity profile of the head must be modeled and inverse solutions to the problem must be constrained with respect to the nature of allowable current configurations. For example, when considering the 20 ms component of the magnetic field pattern recorded from the brain after electrical stimulation of the median nerve, it is common to model the head as a homogeneous spherical volume conductor, and to presume that the recorded magnetic activity can be modeled as though it were generated by a relatively simple current configuration – an equivalent, point-source, current dipole. This simple biophysical model is often used for purposes of source localization, even though it is recognized that the field pattern actually reflects a very complex pattern of underlying neuronal currents. Once the "dipole-in-a-sphere" assumptions are made, mathematical algorithms can then be used to identify the location, orientation, and strength of that equivalent current dipole (^{99m}Tc-ECD) which best accounts (in a statistical sense) for the recorded field pattern. The location of this ^{99m}Tc-ECD is then taken as indicative of the location of the population of brain cells that actually generated the magnetic signals.

To the extent that the model assumptions are valid, MEG sources can be localized with excellent spatial precision. For the described case of median nerve stimulation, the modeled MEG source for the magnetic field pattern at 20 ms post-stimulus, consistently localizes to the primary somatosensory cortex (area 3b) of the postcentral gyrus. As validated by invasive electrophysiological studies, non-invasive MEG provides for excellent spatial localization (within a few millimetres) of that part of the cortex initially activated by median nerve stimulation [17, 18].

In more complex situations, such as those involving MEG signals associated with higher-order cognitive events, more complex models of the underlying current configurations must be used to provide an adequate account of brain electrophysiology. The challenge, of course, is that inappropriate modeling will lead to an incorrect interpretation of the data.

Fortunately, as outlined in subsequent sections, methods for assessing the general adequacy of a source model are available, and MEG can be applied with confidence to the spatiotemporal analysis of a wide range of normal and pathological patterns of brain activity.

EEG, like MEG, is plagued by an ill-posed inverse problem that compromises specification of the brain regions that generate particular EEG signals. The EEG problem is somewhat more difficult to manage than that for MEG. The brain, cerebrospinal fluid, skull, and scalp each demonstrate different electrical conductivities. For evaluation of MEG data, these differences can be mostly ignored, because of reasonable spherical symmetry for the cranium and the concentric nature of the different tissues. In EEG, each conductivity barrier distorts the flow of volume currents, so without detailed knowledge of the exact shape and electrical properties of the skull and scalp, it is difficult to manage the inverse problem and specify the locations of EEG sources with sub-centimeter precision.

Magnetic signals fall rapidly with distance from a source, so the magnetic signal recorded at each point over the head mostly reflects only nearby neuronal populations. In contrast, the EEG signal recorded at any given electrode can be significantly influenced by distant activity. As a consequence, it is rare that single dipole models are applicable to EEG data. For example, three dipole sources with overlapping time course are required to account for the neuroelectric potential pattern at 20 ms after stimulation of the median nerve [19]. The practical problem with this situation is that multiple dipole solutions are often unstable, with confidence in the spatial position of any particular source becoming less and less as the number of dipoles increases. In most cases, EEG source locations can be specified only to within 1–2 cm. The blindness of MEG to distant and radial sources is both its curse and blessing. Not everything is seen, but what is seen is seen clearly. MEG data are often easily interpretable and solutions are stable and statistically robust.

MEG clinical example

In the clinical arena, MEG is most commonly used for presurgical planning purposes with the goal of localizing epileptogenic regions in patients with medically refractory seizures. In many of these cases, MEG provides unique clinical information that alters clinical care in a positive manner [20, 21]. Epilepsy surgery patients also provide a unique opportunity for cross-validation of MEG source modeling strategies, because in many cases, structural lesions may be seen, and in some, direct intracranial recording data are available. Figure 8.2 shows a clinical epilepsy example. Data are from a 23 year-old female with a history of complex partial seizures since 8 years of age. Clinic events are characterized by head turning to the right, babbling speech, and postictal lethargy. Multiple MRI examinations including an evaluation using a 3 T machine were all read as within normal limits. Interictal EEG showed bifrontal/mesial spikes, right > left. Ictal EEG suggested mesial frontal seizure onset. Interictal SPECT showed left temporal hypoperfusion, while an ictal SPECT showed right anterior/inferior frontal hyperperfusion.

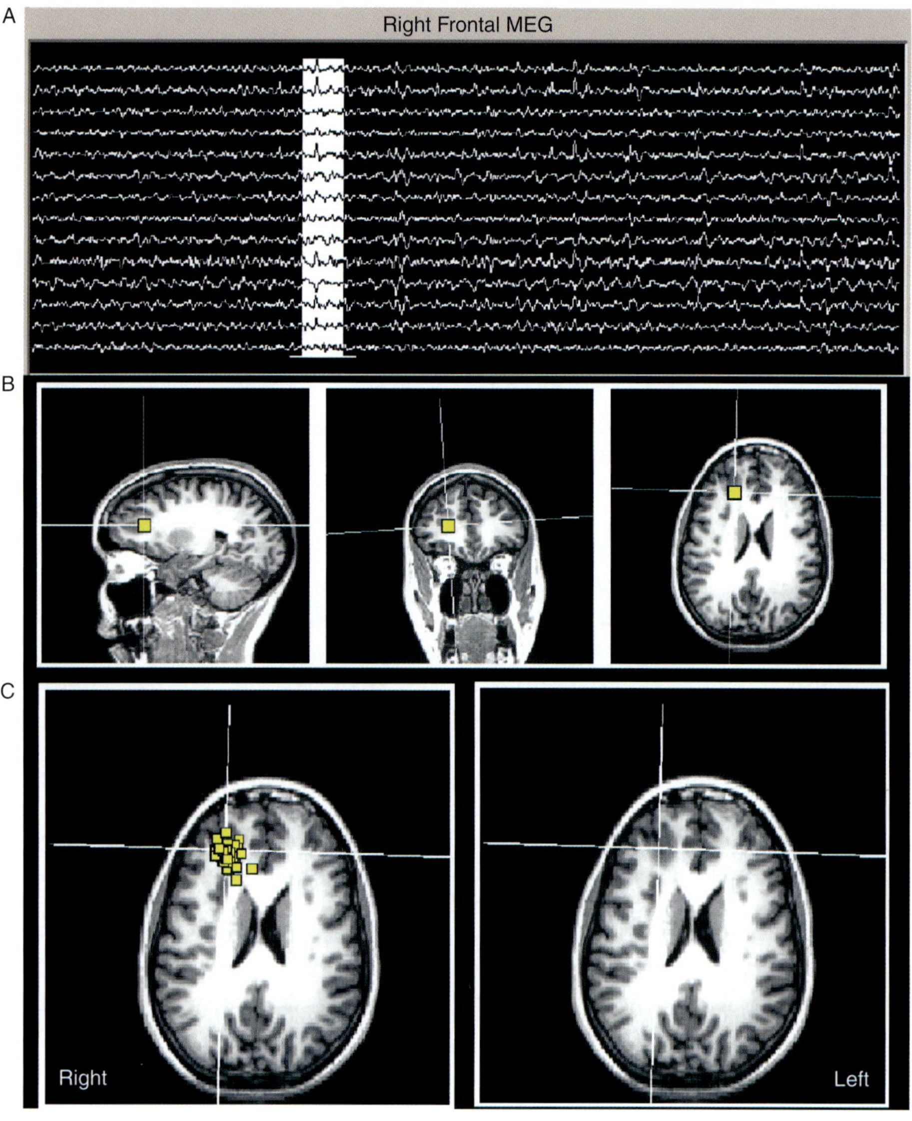

Figure 8.2 Clinical case example. (A) representative 10 seconds of right frontal MEG data from a 23-year-old female with a history of complex partial seizures since 8 years of age. MEG shows frequent right frontal spikes and sharp waves. (B) yellow box shows the location of the best-fitting dipole source for the epileptic spike highlighted in the upper panel. (C) yellow boxes show source locations for the multiple spikes recorded during a 20-min period. There is clear spatial clustering of source locations in the right prefrontal cortex. A review of the corresponding MRI reveals a coincident region of cortical dysplasia. Magnetic source localization images are presented in radiographic, left-on-right views. It is noteworthy that all prior MRI examinations, including the presented one, had been initially read by a neuroradiologist as within normal limits.

EEG recorded simultaneous with whole-head MEG showed medial frontal spikes. The MEG showed spikes that lead the EEG spikes by about 5 ms and which were clearly lateralized to the right frontal lobe. For each spike, a dipole-in-a-sphere model accounted for more than 80% of the variance in the recorded magnetic field pattern. The locations of the best-fitting equivalent current dipoles across spikes were very similar and indicative of a focal epileptogenic zone in the right frontal lobe. The MEG zone was concordant with the anterior/superior region of ictal SPECT activity. Review of the MRI data, within the context of the MEG data, led to discovery of a previously unidentified region of cortical thickening that was coincident with the MEG spike zone.

This patient subsequently underwent invasive phase II video monitoring with bifrontal cortical electrode grids and bi-temporal depth probes. The monitoring confirmed that the MEG identified interictal spike zone was in fact the interictally active and the seizure onset zone. Resective surgery was performed in the epileptogenic zone as originally identified by MEG and the patient has been seizure free for more than 2.5 years.

MEG in sleep research

Since the initial development of EEG technology in the 1930s, much has been learned about the general phenomenology of human sleep, but there remains a relative lack of specific information on the detailed intracranial events that give rise to surface-recorded EEG sleep signals, including vertex waves, sleep spindles, and slow waves. Invasive monitoring studies in animals (and occasionally in humans) show an important role for thalamocortical interactions in generating these events, but detailed characterization of cortical source configurations in man are mostly lacking.

The use of MEG in sleep research is still at an early stage, with fewer than 20 relevant publications, but even these initial studies are revealing novel information on the distribution and physiology of relevant cortical processes. As subjects transition into phase I sleep, MEG, like EEG, shows a loss of alpha activity and a general shift in the background towards slower signals. In stage II sleep, neuromagnetic correlates of vertex waves, K-complexes, and spindles can be seen. In the EEG, the topographic configuration of vertex waves is relatively stable for a given subject with a clear central (Cz) maximum. The situation in MEG is more complicated. In MEG, the activity profile is quite variable across even temporally nearby vertex wave events. Sometimes, vertex waves show a single stable generator, with a particular vertex wave showing origins in any one of a number of regions. On the other hand, there is sometimes evidence of local and sometimes transcallosal propagation of activity (as was illustrated in Figure 8.1), with the duration of the signal at each generative zone being shorter than that recorded in the EEG at Cz. That is to say, the neuroelectric signal seems to reflect the temporal and spatial envelop of a discrete sequential series of local events in the MEG. Brain regions implicated in the generation of vertex waves include parasagittal aspects of the pre- and postcentral gyri, midline and lateral supplementary motor areas, and the cingulate cortex. In some cases there may also be involvement in the dorsolateral prefrontal cortex and the inferior parietal lobule. Quite remarkably, 50% of EEG vertex waves show complex magnetic field patterns indicative of asynchronous activity of multiple bilateral and within hemisphere generators, as illustrated in Figure 8.3. It is noteworthy that the variable and complex field topography of the neuromagnetic correlates of vertex waves appears to be a cardinal characteristic. This is actually quite useful in studies of parietal and frontal lobe epilepsies, where spikes in the EEG may have a potential pattern very similar to that seen for vertex waves such that differentiation of spikes from normal sleep activity becomes problematic. Spatial clustering of the sources of sharp transients in the MEG provides a clue that the observed activity is a reflection of a consistent epileptogenic zone rather than the shifting and variable profile of vertex waves.

Sleep spindles are often considered to be a hallmark manifestation of thalamocortical synchronization processes. Occurring predominantly in stage II sleep, spindles typically occur as waxing-and-waning 10–16 Hz oscillations, typically lasting 0.5–3.0 s. The functional role of spindles remains somewhat underspecified, but they have been implicated in learning and memory consolidation [22], regulation of arousal [23], cortical development [24], and thalamic gating [25].

EEG-recorded spindles are generated at multiple cortical sites as a reflection of the intrinsic properties and interactions between inhibitory cells in the thalamic reticular nucleus and bursting thalamocortical relay neurons. Early EEG studies further suggest a high degree of synchrony across electrodes, with spindle synchronization thought to be controlled by neocortical feedback mechanisms [26]. However, whereas spindles were once thought to be a unitary, prototypical reflection of thalamocortical interactions, there is mounting evidence from MEG and other methods to indicate that they are actually a rather diverse phenomenon. For example, detailed EEG studies [22, 27, 28] demonstrate that at least two spindle generators may be active, as indicated by the presence of fast versus slow spindles with different topographies (i.e., fast: 13–15 Hz, mostly centro-parietal; slow: 11–13 Hz, mostly frontal). MEG studies support a dichotomy for fast and slow spindles and indicate additional levels of diversity. For example, studies using

simultaneous EEG and MEG have found that, while the majority of spindles are seen in both modalities, it is not uncommon to find spindles that appear only in MEG; or only in EEG. Furthermore, in most cases, source analysis of MEG spindles has found that asynchronous activity in multiple generative zones is necessary to account for the field pattern [29–31]. The exact number of generators remains somewhat unclear and varies from spindle to spindle, although there seem to be four primary sources, located bilaterally in fronto-central and deep parietal-central regions.

In situations where the number of generators is four or more, it may be useful to analyze MEG data using alternative distributed source models that allow for extended regions of activation throughout the brain. The most commonly used method is dynamic statistical parametric mapping (DSPM), which allows for MEG/EEG integrated source modeling and also comparative separate modeling (see Figure 8.4). As developed by Dale and colleagues, DSPM uses an inverse solution derived from a minimum-norm procedure [32]. In the minimum-norm solution, dipole elements are allowed at each of several thousand calculation vertices, and the sum-of-the-squares of the current values across all vertices is minimized. In DSPM, the source space is constrained to lie in the cortex [32]. The source strength estimate at each location is then normalized for noise-sensitivity, with statistical significance rather than dipole moment actually plotted. This normalization results in a relatively uniform point spread function between different dipole locations.

Using this method, it has now become clear that there may also be additional temporal lobe and occipital-temporal generators contributing to spindles. Most importantly, the data confirm the prior MEG suggestion of multiple discrete generation zones with temporal/phase offsets between regions, and perhaps a posterior-anterior gradient in spindle generation. In considering the MEG evidence of multiple asynchronous generators and the partly contrary scalp EEG data suggestive of a high level of synchrony, there are two possible explanations. First, it may be that the apparent synchrony in the EEG is an artifact of low density recordings, volume conduction, and/or the spatial smearing effects of the skull. Alternatively, it might be that there are additional synchronous generators that dominate the EEG signal but are minimally contributory to MEG because of their depth or radial orientation. Examination of simultaneous MEG and EEG data by Dehghani and colleagues mostly favors the later possibility because the amplitude of actually recorded spindles in the EEG is about 50× larger than would be expected based on the neuroelectric profile that would be produced by MEG identified sources alone [33–35]. Also, direct modeling of the EEG data suggests that the EEG has different generator locations than the MEG and that there is highly synchronous activity across the EEG generators (see Figure 8.4). The data thereby suggest that MEG and EEG reflect different spindle mechanisms, perhaps related to activities modulated by the thalamic core (MEG) versus the matrix (EEG).

To date, no studies have explicitly focused on MEG correlates of slow waves during stage III sleep, although some studies

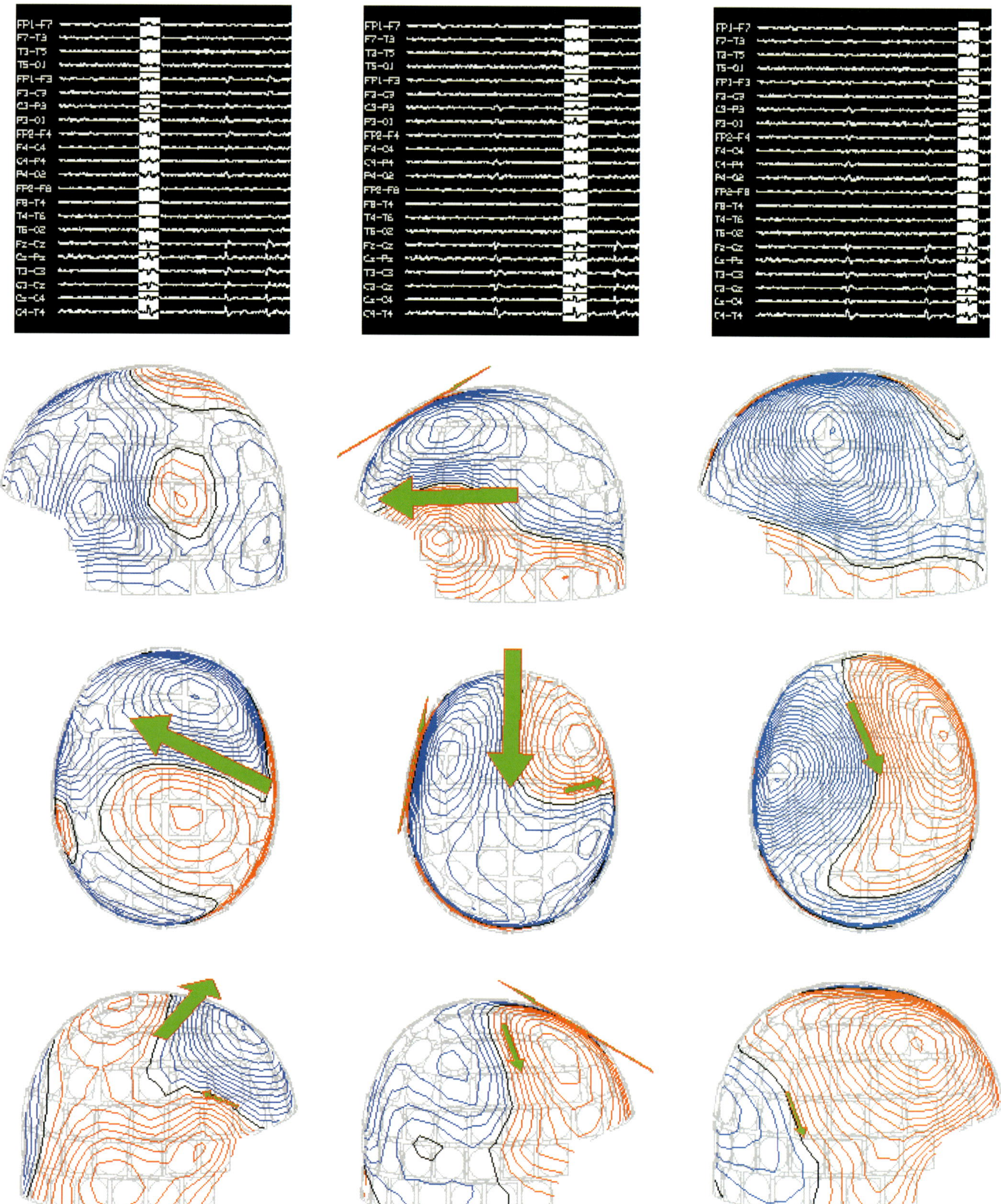

Figure 8.3 MEG correlates of vertex waves. The MEG correlates of EEG identified vertex waves often show diverse and complicated magnetic field patterns that are highly variable from event to event. More than 50% of vertex waves show evidence of contributions from multiple generative regions.

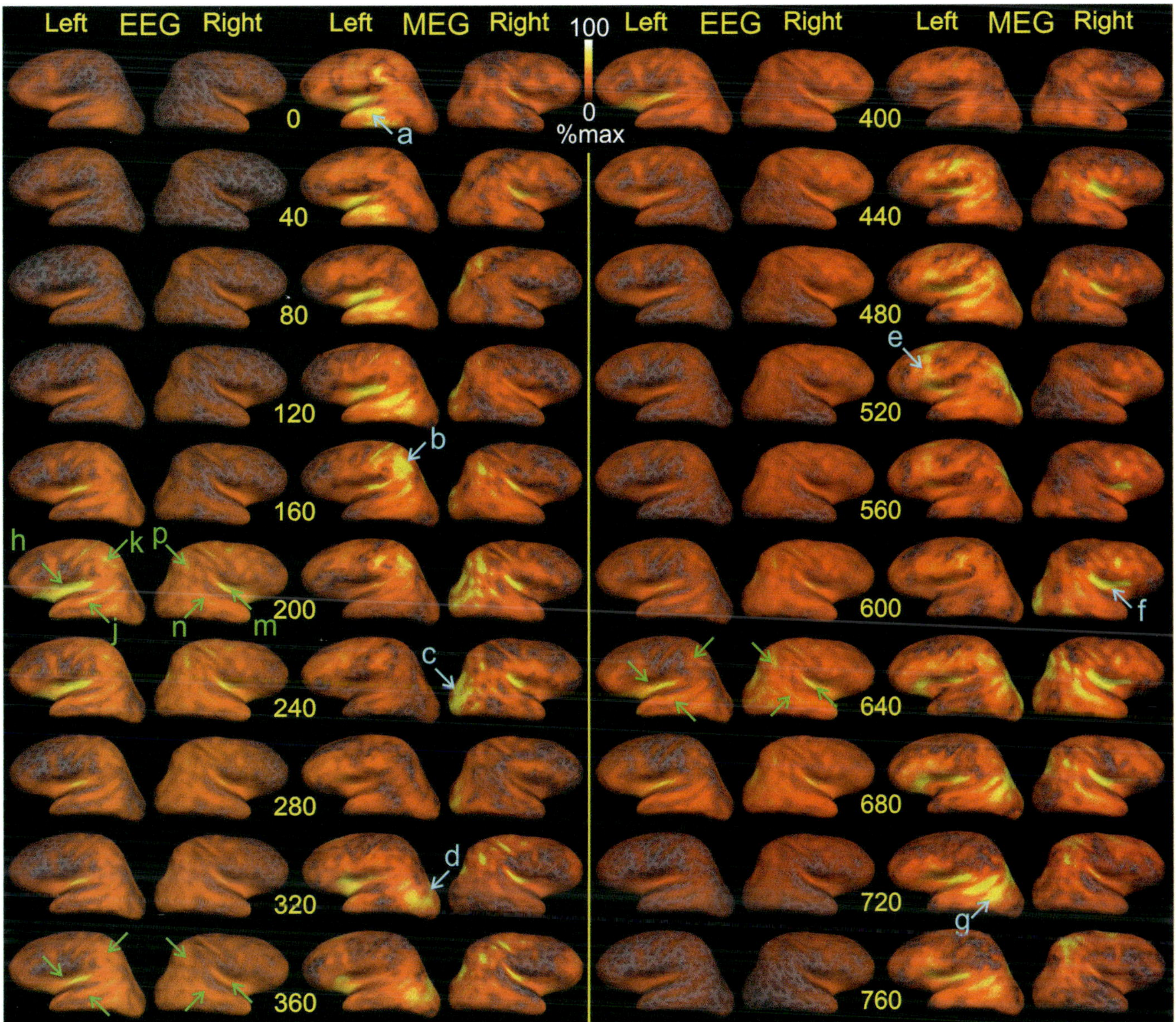

Figure 8.4 Dynamic spatiotemporal patterns of spindling: contrasting DSPM solutions from MEG and EEG to simultaneous data, as mapped on the cortical surface throughout the duration of a spindle. Time proceeds from top to bottom in each column, with successive snapshots separated by 40 ms. The left four columns show activity from 0 to 360 ms, and the right four columns from 400 to 760 ms, of the same spindle discharge. Note that activation peaks are not synchronous in MEG and EEG, nor are they in the same locations. MEG is highly variable across time, with successive peaks of activity (see blue arrows) in left temporal at 0 ms (**a**), left parietal at 160 (**b**), right occipital at 240 (**c**), left occipital at 320 (**d**), left frontal at 520 (**e**), right insula at 600 (**f**), and left occipitotemporal at 720 (**g**). In contrast, EEG-derived source localizations appear more bilaterally symmetrical and consistent over time. For example, at 200 ms, relatively high activation is estimated to the left and right insula (**h, m**), superior temporal sulcus (**j, n**), and parietal lobe (**k, p**). Very similar activation is seen at 360 and 640 ms (see green arrows). Estimated ^{99m}Tc-ECD strength is plotted on the subject's cortex after expansion to reveal sulcal (dark gray) as well as gyral (light gray) cortex.

make mention of MEG slow waves during sleep [36]. In general, the data indicate that MEG slow-wave signals during sleep are not amenable to simple source models (this is contrary to the situation for slow waves associated with pathophysiological activity associated with brain lesions, where simple dipole modeling can be viable). The data suggest that multiple brain regions are involved in the generation of sleep slow waves, with asynchronous, overlapping activity in the insula, cingulate cortex, frontal and parietal lobes, perhaps with an anterior-posterior propagation bias. In our experience, the source profile is highly variable from event to event, even in the same subject.

The final area of sleep research where MEG is starting to provide some new inputs relates to the neurobiological events that precede eye movements during rapid eye movement (REM) sleep. Using an iterative minimum norm method known as magnetic field tomography [37], Ioannides and colleagues [38] have found multiple circuits to be active prior to each REM saccade. Starting 400–600 milliseconds before a REM saccade, activity changes can be seen in the bilateral pontine nuclei and also in the frontal eye fields. Interestingly, a second circuit, not directly related to initiation of saccades is also seen to show altered activity in the last 100 ms leading to a REM saccade.

This circuit involved several brain regions including orbital frontal cortex, the amygdale and parahippocampal gyri, and the pontine nuclei. In a separate study focusing on the analysis of beta and gamma band activity during pre-REM sleep versus phasic-REM sleep versus tonic-REM sleep, Corsi-Cabrera and colleagues found evidence for broadly increased power in pre- and phasic-REM periods relative to tonic-REM [39]. During pre-REM and phasic-REM there is also evidence of decreased temporal coupling between left frontal executive areas and parietal sensory areas, and increased right-frontal to midline coupling, relative to tonic-REM periods. These data suggest that phasic activity during REM sleep is associated with complex modulation of multiple brain circuits.

In summary, MEG is starting to play an increased role in the understanding of how brain circuits are modulated during sleep, with the most significant insights coming in relationship to the origins of sleep spindles and the complex modulation of neural interactions during REM sleep.

References

1. Orrison WW, Lewine JD, Sanders JA, Hartshorne MF, eds. *Functional Brain Imaging*. St. Louis, Mosby Yearbook, 1995.

2. Toga A, Mazziotta JC. *Brain Mapping: The Methods*, 2nd edn. San Diego, Academic Press, 2002.

3. Wessels AM, Rombouts SA, Simsek S, *et al.* Microvascular disease in type 1 diabetes alters brain activation: a functional magnetic resonance imaging study. *Diabetes.* 2006;**55**:334–40.

4. Tanaka N, Hamalainen MS, Ahlfors SP, *et al.* Propagation of epileptic spikes reconstructed from spatiotemporal magnetoencephalographic and electroencephalographic source analysis. *Neuroimage.* 2010;**50**:217–22.

5. Bagic A, Knowlton RC, Rose DF, *et al.* American Clinical Magnetoencephalography Society clinical practice guideline 1: recording and analysis of spontaneous cerebral activity. *J Clin Neurophysiol.* 2011;**28**:348–54.

6. Burgess RC, Funke ME, Bowyer SM, *et al.* American Clinical Magnetoencephalography Society clinical practice guideline 2: presurgical functional brain mapping using magnetic evoked fields. *J Clin Neurophysiol.* 2011;**28**:355–61.

7. Hansen PC, Kringelbach ML, Salmelin R. *MEG: An Introduction to Methods*. Oxford, Oxford University Press, 2010.

8. Cohen D. Magnetoencephalography, Evidence of magnetic fields produced by alpha rhythm currents. *Science.* 1968;**161**:784–6.

9. Zimmerman JE, Thiene P, Harding JT. Design and operation of stable rf-biased super-conducting quantum interference devices and a note on the properties of perfectly clean metal contacts *J Appl Phys.* 1970; **41**:1572–80.

10. Hari R, Ilmoniemi RJ. Cerebral magnetic fields. *Crit Rev Biomed Eng.* 1986;**14**:93–126.

11. Lewine JD, Orrison WW. Magnetoencephalography and magnetic source imaging, In: Orrison WW, Lewine JD, Sanders JA, Hartshorne MF, eds. *Functional Brain Imaging*. St Louis, Mosby Yearbook. 1995;369–418.

12. Papanicolaou A, ed. *Clinical Magnetoencephalography and Magnetic Source Imaging*. Cambridge, Cambridge University Press, 2009.

13. Okada Y. Neurogenesis of evoked magnetic fields. In: Williamson SJ, Romani GL, Kaufman L, *et al.*, eds. *Biomagnetism, An Interdisciplinary Approach*. New York, Plenum Press. 1983;399–408.

14. Hamalainen M, Hari R, Ilmoniemi RJ, *et al.* Magnetoencephalography: theory, instrumentation, and applications to noninvasive studies of the working brain. *Rev Mod Phys.* 1993;**65**:413–98.

15. Cohen D, Cuffin N, Yunokuchi K, *et al.* MEG versus EEG localization test using implanted sources in the human brain. *Ann Neurol.* 1990;**28**:811–17.

16. Mosher JC, Spencer ME, Leahy RM, *et al.* Error bounds for EEG and MEG dipole source localization. *Electroencephalogr Clin Neurophysiol.* 1993;**86**:303–21.

17. Ganslandt O, Fahlbusch R, Nimsky C, *et al.* Functional neuronavigation with magnetoencephalography: outcome in 50 patients with lesions around the motor cortex. *J Neurosurg.* 1999;**91**:73–9.

18. Roberts TP, Ferrari P, Perry D, *et al.* Presurgical mapping with magnetic source imaging: comparisons with intraoperative findings. *Brain Tumor Pathol.* 2000;**17**:57–64.

19. Buchner H, Adams L, Knepper A, *et al.* Preoperative localization of the central sulcus by dipole source analysis of early somatosensory evoked potentials and three-dimensional magnetic resonance imaging. *J Neurosurg.* 1994;**80**:849–56.

20. Knowlton RC. The role of FDG-PET, ictal SPECT, and MEG in epilepsy surgery evaluation. *Epilepsy Behav.* 2006;**8**:91–101.

21. Sutherling WW, Mamelak AN, Thyerlei D, *et al.* Influence of magnetic source imaging for planning intracranial EEG in epilepsy. *Neurology.* 2008;**71**:990–6.

22. Schabus N, Gruber G, Parapatics S, *et al.* Sleep spindles and their significance for declarative memory consolidation. *Sleep* 2004;**27**:1478–85.

23. Destexhe A, Sejnowski TJ. Interactions between membrane conductances underlying thalamocortical slow-wave oscillations. *Physiol Rev.* 2003;**83**:1401–53.

24. Khazipov R, Sirota A, Leinekugel X, *et al.* Early motor activity drives spindle bursts in developing somatosensory cortex. *Nature.* 2004;**432**:758–61.

25. Steriade M. The corticothalamic system in sleep. *Front Biosci* 2003;**8**:878–99.

26. Contreras D, Destexhe A, Sejnowski, *et al.* Spatiotemporal patterns of spindle oscillations in cortex and thalamus. *J Neurosci.* 1997;**17**:1179–96.

27. De Gennaro L, Ferrara M. Sleep spindles: an overview. *Sleep Med Rev.* 2003;**7**:423–40.

28. Gibbs FA, Gibbs EL. *Atlas of Electroencephalography*. Cambridge, Addison Wesley Press, 1950.

29. Lu ST, Kajola M, Joutisniemi SL, *et al.* Generator sites of spontaneous MEG activity during sleep. *Electroencephalogr Clin Neurophysiol.* 1992;**82**:182–96.

30. Shih JJ, Weisend MP, Davis JT, *et al.* Magnetoencephalographic characterization of sleep spindles in humans. *J Clin Neurophysiol.* 2000;**17**:224–31.

31. Urakami Y. Relationships between sleep spindles and activities of cerebral cortex as determined by simultaneous EEG and MEG recording. *J Clin Neurophysiol.* 2008;**25**:13–24.

32. Dale AM, Liu AK, Fischl BR, *et al.* Dynamic statistical parametric mapping: combining fMRI and MEG for high-resolution imaging of cortical activity. *Neuron.* 2000;**26**:55–67.

33. Dehghani N, Cash SS, Rossetti AO, *et al.* Magnetoencephalography demonstrates multiple asynchronous generators during human sleep spindles. *J Neurophysiol.* 2010;**104**:179–88.

34. Dehghani N, Cash SS, Halgren E. Emergence of synchronous EEG spindles for asynchronous MEG spindles. *Hum Brain Mapp.* 2011;**32**:2217–27.

35. Dehghani N, Cash SS, Chen CC. *et al.* Divergent cortical generators of MEG and EEG during human sleep spindles suggested by distributed source modeling. *Plos One.* 2010;**5**(7):1–11.

36. Simon NR, Mandhanden I, Lopes da Silva FH. A MEG study of sleep. *Brain Res.* 2000;**860**:64–76.

37. Ionnides AA. Real-time human brain function: observations and inferences from single trial analysis of magnetoencephalographic signals. *Clin Electroencephalogr.* 2001;**32**:98–111.

38. Ionnides AA, Corsi-Cabrera M, Fenwick P, *et al.* MEG tomography of human cortex and brainstem activity in waking and REM sleep saccades. *Cereb Cortex.* 2004;**14**:56–72.

39. Corsi-Cabrera M, Guevara MA, Del Rio-Portilla Y. Brain activity and temporal coupling related to eye movements during REM sleep: EEG and MEG results. *Brain Res.* 2008;**1235**:82–91.

Fundamentals of low-resolution brain electromagnetic tomography

Peter Anderer and Bernd Saletu

Introduction

The electroencephalogram (EEG) is the core measurement in studying sleep. By means of the scalp-recorded EEG, brain activity can be monitored non-invasively throughout the night. As published by Rechtschaffen and Kales in 1968 [1], a central EEG channel (C3-A2 or C4-A1) is obligatory for sleep scoring in humans. Due to the high temporal resolution of the EEG, microstructures of sleep, such as slow waves, K-complexes, sleep spindles, vertex sharp waves, or sawtooth waves, can be identified and separated from alpha bursts, microarousals, or artifacts. To allow these discriminations, the sampling rate of the EEG recording has to be sufficiently high to enable the identification of waveform, amplitude, frequency, and duration of the events with adequate accuracy. A time resolution in the range of milliseconds, for instance, is necessary to discriminate a K-alpha complex (indicating an arousal) from a K-complex with a superimposed sleep spindle (indicating consolidated sleep).

While the value of the high temporal resolution of the EEG is unequivocally accepted, that of its spatial resolution is still underestimated. In 2007, the American Academy of Sleep Medicine (AASM) published the AASM manual for the scoring of sleep and associated events, recommending as a minimum requirement for sleep scoring two additional EEG channels, one frontal lead (F4-A1) and one occipital lead (O2-A1) [2]. According to the AASM rules, which are meant to replace the Rechtschaffen and Kales rules for scoring sleep stages, the occipital derivation should be used for identifying alpha activity and the frontal derivation for identifying K-complexes and slow-wave activity. In the process of adapting our automated sleep staging system Somnolyzer 24 × 7 – which in 2005 had been developed for scoring sleep according to Rechtschaffen and Kales [3] – to the new AASM rules, we performed a stage transition analysis to evaluate step by step the effects the change of the rules had on sleep staging [4]. On average, the inclusion of the occipital lead for detecting alpha activity affected only 2–3 epochs per recording. In these rare cases, epochs changed from stage S1 to stage W, since the occipital alpha activity was not detectable at central leads. In the vast majority of cases, however, alpha was detectable not only at occipital, but also at central leads and thus the inclusion of the occipital lead had only a minor effect on sleep stage scoring. More epochs were

affected by the addition of the frontal lead as epochs with slow waves (just) below 75 μV at central leads may change from S2 to N3 if their amplitudes are above 75 μV at frontal leads. As a consequence, an average of 19 epochs per recording changed from S2 to N3. The exact influence of the change in the scoring rules depends on individual EEG characteristics, such as the anterior-posterior gradient of slow-wave amplitudes or densities of sleep spindles and K-complexes on the one hand and arousal density and alpha topography on the other. In summary, standard sleep recordings with frontal, central, and occipital EEG leads exploit only small parts of the spatial information available in scalp-recorded EEG.

The addition of a parietal EEG electrode makes it possible to evaluate brain topography along the anterior-posterior axis by re-referencing the EEG leads to bipolar derivations (e.g., F3-C3, C3-P3, P3-O1). Such fronto-occipital EEG power gradients in the sleep of young healthy subjects demonstrated topographic power shifts at non-rapid eye movement (NREM)–REM sleep transitions as well as across and within NREM periods [5]. Since the regional EEG power spectra showed state-related and frequency-specific differences, the study highlighted the additional information that may be gained by a – thorough, rather limited – spatial analysis of sleep EEG data. As early as in 1993, a topographic study performed by our group with 18 EEG leads showed an increase in delta power (which was most pronounced frontally) and a decrease in alpha power (which was most pronounced parieto-occipitally) from sleep stage S1 to S4 [6]. A follow-up study demonstrated that not only slow waves, but also sleep spindles are not uniformly distributed across the scalp. We showed that slow sleep spindles were generally distributed over anterior and fast sleep spindles over parietal regions [7]. These early topographic studies indicated that the neuronal processes underlying the sleep EEG differ between brain regions, supporting the hypothesis of local aspects of sleep.

Consequently, a comprehensive sleep analysis should include spatial information. Today, a number of sleep recording systems allow the acquisition of data from multiple EEG channels and thus, limiting factors for increasing the number of electrodes are subjects' comfort, the time necessary for applying the electrodes, and the increasing time and effort required for artifact handling. In 2004, Huber *et al.* [8]

Neuroimaging of Sleep and Sleep Disorders, ed. Eric Nofzinger, Pierre Maquet, and Michael J. Thorpy. Published by Cambridge University Press. © Cambridge University Press 2013.

published a study using a 256-channel EEG recording system with an electrode cap for revealing local changes in slow-wave activity in a night after a learning task of rotation adaptation. The high-density EEG analysis revealed a remarkably stable slow-wave activity that was most pronounced over frontal regions, confirming our early topographic delta distribution obtained with 18 electrodes. However, Huber *et al.* described the recordings with high-density EEGs as quite uncomfortable for the subjects, and thus the cap was removed after 2 h in order to prevent disturbed sleep and the consequent influence on the learning task [8]. In a more recent study, a high-density 256-channel EEG was recorded successfully over the entire night in healthy subjects as well as in schizophrenia patients [9]. The reported measures of sleep maintenance (defined as the percentage of total sleep time related to time in bed after sleep onset) were 91% for both healthy subjects and schizophrenia patients, which indicates that it is possible to measure high-density EEG without significantly disturbing sleep. Thus, caps and electrodes with improved comfort and systems combining polysomnographic (PSG) and high-density EEG devices are now available and will hopefully stimulate new studies on the spatial analysis of sleep EEG.

Irrespective of the number of channels and the method used for analyzing sleep EEG data, the significance of the results critically depends on the treatment of artifacts. It is obvious that analysis of data contaminated by artifacts can lead to spurious results. In sleep EEG data, simple artifact elimination methods based on the definition of a threshold for maximal EEG amplitudes, as frequently used in evoked potential studies for instance, are certainly not appropriate. As part of the EU-funded project SIESTA, we reviewed in detail types and treatment of artifacts in the sleep EEG [10]. A reliable and valid artifact processing strategy should include: (1) high-quality recording techniques in order to minimize the occurrence of avoidable artifacts (e.g., technical artifacts); (2) artifact minimization procedures in order to minimize the loss of data by estimating the interference of different artifacts in the EEG recordings, thus allowing the calculation of the "corrected" EEG (e.g., ocular and electrocardiogram (ECG) artifacts); and finally (3) artifact identification procedures in order to define and eliminate epochs contaminated by remaining artifacts (e.g., movement and muscle artifacts).

Methodological aspects of low-resolution brain electromagnetic tomography

Scalp distributions of EEG amplitudes and power are ambiguous and thus cannot be interpreted directly in terms of brain electrical generators. Even for high-density EEG recordings, an infinite number of different generator distributions may explain the scalp-recorded data. Thus, the challenge for source localization methods is to provide a unique solution to this inverse problem (i.e., estimate the unknown current density distribution on the basis of the measured scalp potential distribution), yielding a physiologically meaningful generator distribution without prior knowledge of the number, location, or orientation of the sources.

In addition, scalp distributions of EEG amplitudes and power are reference-dependent. While the aforementioned anterior distribution of slow spindles and the posterior distribution of fast spindles was observed in referential recordings versus mastoid electrodes [7], bipolar recordings found fast spindles in anterior and slow in posterior derivations [5]. Thus, a source localization method has to consider this so-called "reference electrode problem" as well, which means that the inverse solution has to be independent of the arbitrary choice of the reference electrode.

Low-resolution brain electromagnetic tomography (LORETA) devised by Pascual-Marqui *et al.* in 1994 was one of the first attempts to solve both the inverse problem and the reference electrode problem [11]. The latter was addressed by re-referencing the EEG data to an average reference, which corresponds to explicitly modeling the reference electrode in the equation of the forward problem (i.e., determine the potential field at the scalp for a given cortical current source density distribution). For a mathematical proof that the use of the average reference solves the reference electrode problem, see [12]. The first attempt to overcome the inverse problem for EEG data was the minimum norm solution, as published in 1984 by Hämäläinen and Ilmoniemi [13]. This method uses the Tikhonov regularization for selecting the solution with minimum power and is denoted as unweighted or classical minimum norm estimate (MNE). This solution, however, is limited to problems where the sources are assumed to be restricted to superficial areas of the cortex, since the method significantly misplaces deep sources [14]. LORETA, however, is able to localize deep sources as well by minimizing the squared three-dimensional (3D) spatial Laplacian operator to determine the unique solution. This results in the solution with maximal smoothness [11]. In a review of methods for solving the EEG inverse problem, Pascual-Marqui showed with simulation data using 148 electrodes and 818 uniformly distributed voxels that LORETA achieved an average localization error of 1 grid unit uniformly at all depths [14]. The author showed further that smooth sources could be precisely estimated, while – due to the inherent characteristics of the LORETA method – point sources were estimated as blurred, but correctly localized images, and the deeper the actual source, the more blurred is the LORETA solution [14]. In the same paper, the author compared five inverse solutions (minimum norm, weighted minimum norm, Backhaus and Gilbert, weighted resolution optimization [WROP] and LORETA) by testing localization errors in the estimation of single and multiple sources and concluded that only LORETA was able to correctly localize the sources in 3D space [14].

The assumption of LORETA that the smoothest of all possible inverse solutions is most plausible is consistent with the notion that the major contribution to the scalp-recorded potential field is made by simultaneously and synchronously active neighboring neurons. Extracranial recordings of EEG and magnetoencephalography (MEG) are predominantly generated by cortical pyramidal neurons, which are oriented perpendicularly to the cortical surface and undergo postsynaptic potentials (PSPs). The magnitude of the recorded extracranial signal is a result of the spatial summation of the impressed current density induced by highly synchronized PSPs occurring in large clusters of neurons [15].

Meanwhile LORETA has received considerable validation from studies combining it with other more established localization methods, such as functional magnetic resonance imaging (fMRI) (e.g., [16]), structural MRI (e.g., [17]), and positron emission tomography (PET) (e.g., [18]). Further LORETA validation has been based on accepting as ground truth the localization findings obtained from implanted depth electrodes, with a number of studies in epilepsy (e.g., [19]) and cognitive event-related potentials (e.g., [20]). It is important to note that LORETA does not postulate one or a small number of point sources, but approximates the current density distribution throughout the full brain volume. Thus, LORETA is thought to dissociate an unknown number of multiple, distributed sources which may be simultaneously active.

Already the first implementation of LORETA using a 3-shell spherical head model with a regular 3D grid of 1153 voxels within the upper hemisphere revealed for the auditory N1 component – which topographically shows the maximal amplitude at the vertex – the expected activation of the right and left auditory cortex [21]. In the LORETA version presented in 1999 by Pascual-Marqui [14, 22], LORETA is based on realistic head geometry and solution space is restricted to cortical gray matter and the hippocampus, as determined in the digitized Probability Atlas (Brain Imaging Center, Montreal Neurological Institute), based on the Talairach human brain atlas [23]. A voxel is included in the solution space if its probability of being gray matter is higher than 33%, and higher than its probability of being either white matter or cerebrospinal fluid. LORETA images represent the power (i.e., squared magnitude of computed intracerebral current density) in 2394 voxels with a grid size of 7 mm. Using this implementation of LORETA we identified two symmetric local maxima of the N1 source distribution in the left and right primary auditory cortices at Talairach coordinate [−59,−32,8] in the left superior temporal lobe (Brodmann area BA 42) and [60,−32,15] in the right superior temporal lobe (BA 42), which is in accordance with intracranial studies on the auditory N1 sources [24].

In LORETA studies on the sources of the auditory odd-ball P300, we identified P300 generators in bilateral dorso- and ventrolateral prefrontal, bilateral middle/superior temporal, and bilateral posterior superior temporal/inferior parietal regions as well as in medial frontal regions, the posterior cingulate cortex, and the precuneus [20, 24]. With the exception of the medial temporal generators located in the hippocampal and perirhinal cortex, LORETA revealed similar P300 sources as described by Halgren et al. [25] based on 4000 intracranial recording sites. Indeed, the medial temporal depth P3b generators are unlikely to make a major contribution to the scalp-recorded P300. They are probably masked by volume conduction effects or other neocortical P300 generators, and/or behave like a closed dipole field so that the local synaptic currents cancel each other [26]. One has to be aware that only cortical activities that make major contributions to the scalp-recorded EEG can be estimated by source localization.

This has to be considered not only in the interpretation of electrophysiological neuroimaging results, but also in studies comparing the various neuroimaging methods as well as in multi-modal neuroimaging approaches. Not all active sources in the brain make a traceable contribution to the scalp-recorded potential distribution.

On the other hand, brain sources that do contribute to the scalp-recorded EEG may be detected non-invasively by means of electrophysiological neuroimaging methods. Based on these high time-resolution intracranial signal estimates, in a recent paper Pascual-Marqui et al. presented a method for assessing interactions in the brain [12]. Measures of linear dependence (coherence) and non-linear dependence (phase synchronization) between the current source density time series are determined and decomposed into instantaneous and lagged components to considerably reduce non-physiological contributions due to volume conduction and low spatial resolution in the connectivity measures. Since connectivity matrices estimating the "similarity" between the time-varying current source density estimates for all possible voxel-pairs lead to a hardly comprehensible dimension, the authors suggest applying graph-theoretical methods or independent components and singular value decomposition methods for summarizing and interpreting connectivity data [12]. Revealing interactions between the various brain regions will significantly help to understand the changes in the functional connectivity of the brain during sleep and consciousness.

While up to now LORETA, which minimizes the squared 3D spatial Laplacian operator, has been by far the most frequently applied method for source localization based on the scalp-recorded EEG, numerous other methods have been developed for solving the inverse problem, some of them attempting to reduce the blurring size to better identify focal sources, some of them trying to reduce the localization error to a minimum, some of them including temporal information to achieve stable estimates over time, and others combining different methods to exploit the respective advantages of the methods.

In 2002, Pascual-Marqui presented standardized low-resolution electromagnetic tomography (sLORETA) and showed that under ideal conditions (low measurement noise) this method has a localization error of zero [27]. Based on the classical minimum norm solution, which by itself has a large localization error for deeper sources, sLORETA computes standardized current density by dividing the current density in each voxel by the square root of its estimated variance. The variance is defined by using a functional analysis formulation based on the covariance matrix, which receives contributions from noise in the scalp measurements and from neuronal generator noise. This standardization results in unitless z-values for each voxel, instead of current density values in $\mu A/mm^2$. The performance of sLORETA in respect to localization error, spatial spread, and estimated activity values was compared with minimum norm and the Dale method [28]. While the Dale method standardizes the current source density estimates based only on measurement noise, sLORETA takes into account the actual source noise as well. In both noise-free and noisy simulations, sLORETA outperformed the two other methods [27]. Two independent groups replicated that sLORETA has no localization bias in the absence of measurement noise [29, 30]. In this sense, sLORETA is an improvement of the classical LORETA version and due to improved localization properties all validation results obtained with LORETA also serve as a validation for sLORETA. Furthermore, sLORETA has been validated in simultaneous EEG/fMRI studies (e.g., [31]) and in an EEG localization study of epilepsy [32].

A comprehensive review of methods for solving the inverse problem in EEG source analysis presents 16 methods, including MNE, weighted minimum norm estimates (WMNE), MNE with focal underdetermined system solution (FOCUSS), LORETA, LORETA with FOCUSS, sLORETA, variable resolution electrical tomography (VARETA), quadratic regularization and spatial regularization (S-MAP) using dipole intensity gradients, spatio-temporal regularization (ST-MAP), spatio-temporal modeling, the Backus–Gilbert method, WROP, the local autoregressive average (LAURA), as well as shrinking methods and multiresolution methods such as S-MAP with iterative focusing, shrinking LORETA-FOCUSS (SLF), standardized shrinking LORETA-FOCUSS (SSLOFO) and adaptive standardized LORETA/FOCUSS (ALF) [33]. The authors performed a Monte-Carlo analysis to compare 4 out of the 16 methods (WMNE, LORETA, sLORETA, and SLF) with different noise levels and different simulated source depths using 32 electrodes and 755 voxels. As compared to the other methods tested, the best solution in terms of both localization error and ghost sources was achieved by regularized sLORETA, the second best by regularized LORETA. A ghost source was defined as a local maximum in the current source density distribution which was not actually present in the simulated scenario. Regularization is a kind of extra smoothing of the source distribution and there are various methods to automatically determine the optimal regularization parameter (for a review see [33]). In the results presented above, Tikhonov regularization was used and the optimal value for the regularization parameter was found using the L-curve method [33]. In a paper evaluating eight different cortical source localization methods available in CURRY software, including moving dipoles, minimum norm, and LORETA, Yao and Dewald [34] used the realistic boundary element method (BEM) with 3306 triangles with a size of 7 mm for the brain compartment and 163 scalp electrodes. On the basis of simulated data they concluded that LORETA had the best source localization ability of all tested methods [34]. The same superiority of LORETA over moving dipoles and minimum norm was seen for somatosensory evoked-potentials as well as upper-limb motor related potentials, which resulted in physiologically meaningful source distributions, based on 163-channel EEG recordings coregistered with the subjects' MRI data after determining the position of each electrode by a 3D magnetic digitizer [34].

In a further development in 2007, Pascual-Marqui used an iterative approximation procedure to solve the inverse problem by estimating the coefficients of the weight matrix providing a solution which has zero localization errors when tested with point sources anywhere in the brain under no-noise conditions [35]. He denoted this discrete, 3D distributed, linear, weighted minimum norm inverse solution as exact low-resolution brain electromagnetic tomography (eLORETA). It should be emphasized that the localization properties of any linear 3D inverse solution (i.e., tomography) can always be determined by the localization errors to simulated point sources. If such a tomography has a localization error of zero to such point sources located anywhere in the brain, then, except for low spatial resolution, the tomography will correctly localize any arbitrary 3D distribution. This is due to the principles of linearity and superposition. The particular weights used in eLORETA endow the tomography with the property of exactly localizing test point sources, yielding images of current density with exact localization, albeit with low spatial resolution (i.e., neighboring neuronal sources will be highly correlated). It is also important to emphasize that eLORETA has no localization bias even in the presence of structured noise. In this sense, eLORETA is an improvement compared with the previously developed LORETA and sLORETA. Moreover, like LORETA, eLORETA provides source orientation estimates that were not available in sLORETA. Due to its improved localization properties, the validation data for LORETA and sLORETA serve also as validation for eLORETA. In the eLORETA implementation developed by Pascual-Marqui, computations are made in a realistic head model with the 3-dimensional solution space restricted to cortical gray matter, as determined by the probabilistic Talairach atlas [36]. The intracerebral volume is divided into 6239 voxels at 5 mm spatial resolution. Thus, eLORETA images represent the electric activity at each voxel in neuroanatomical Montreal Neurological Institute (MNI) space as the exact magnitude of the estimated current density in $\mu A/mm^2$. In a simulation study using a realistic head model with 71 electrodes and 7002 cortical voxels, Pascual-Marqui et al. [12] presented performance features of eLORETA as compared with two other regularized weighted minimum norm solutions under non-ideal (signal-to-noise ratio 10) and ideal (no noise) conditions. In all performance measures (e.g., average localization error to 7002 test point sources with random orientation, average percent of voxels with higher activation than the actually active voxel) eLORETA outperformed the classical minimum norm solution [13] as well as the depth-weighted minimum norm solution as described by Lin et al. [37]. In the same paper, the authors presented validation results where eLORETA was applied to EEG recordings under right visual field pattern-reversal checkerboard stimulation, central visual field stimulation with white words on a black screen, auditory stimulation with short tone bursts, and somatosensory stimulation of the right hand. The eLORETA results showed correct localization of the respective visual, auditory, and somatosensory cortices [12].

As described above, sophisticated methods have been developed to solve the inverse problem. Also concerning the forward models improvements have been made. The sphere head volume models have been replaced by realistic head models. If the exact 3D position of each electrode is measured, co-registration with the subject's individual MRI data is possible. Moreover, the boundary element method (BEM) or finite element method

(FEM) based on a subject's MRI data may be used to define the individualized volume conductor model [34].

Applying LORETA to sleep EEG data

In 2001, we published the first study that applied LORETA to sleep EEG data [38]. We selected artifact-free epochs with sleep spindles (Figure 9.1) and determined LORETA power in the frequency domain via the EEG cross-spectral matrix. For details concerning the computation of frequency-domain electric neuronal generators, see [39]. LORETA revealed cortical spindle sources predominantly medially in the frontal and parietal lobe. Weaker bilateral frontal and parietal sources showed a left-hemispheric predominance (Figure 9.2A). Interestingly, the prefrontal sources (Brodmann areas 9 and 10) oscillated with a frequency below 13 Hz, and the precuneus sources (Brodmann area 7), with a frequency above 13 Hz (Figure 9.2B). The finding that different brain regions were involved in the generation of slow and fast spindles was confirmed by means of a non-parametric single-threshold test on the basis of the theory for randomization and permutation test developed by Holmes *et al.* [40] for functional neuroimaging experiments. It should be noted that statistical methods developed for other functional neuroimaging data such as fMRI or PET are also well suited for LORETA data as they face similar challenges, i.e., multiple comparisons of strongly dependent

data, The above-described localized cortical brain regions for spindles are directly connected with adjacent parts of the dorsal thalamus where sleep spindles are generated. Our results of simultaneously active frontal and parietal sleep spindle sources oscillating at different frequencies were confirmed in further studies using multichannel matching pursuit [41] or independent component analysis [42] to reveal sleep spindle characteristics in a first step and perform LORETA on the obtained spindle components thereafter.

Interestingly, the cortical generators localized for delta waves in slow-wave sleep (SWS) (Figures 9.3 and 9.4) showed considerable overlap with the spindle generators [43]. Indeed, with increasing hyperpolarization of thalamocortical cells, spindles are gradually replaced by intrinsically generated delta rhythms [44]. The reported LORETA sources for delta waves in the medial prefrontal cortex spreading to the anterior cingulate and the orbitofrontal cortex and in the precuneus were perfectly in line with decreases in cortical regional cerebral blood flow during SWS revealed by PET [45]. Thus, the LORETA data further support the idea of local aspects of sleep, since both the prefrontal cortex and the precuneus are particularly active during wakefulness and thus might have a greater need for recuperation [45]. Indeed, the cortical areas involved in both SWS and spindle generation show considerable overlap with the brain's default mode network. This functional network was identified as a set of

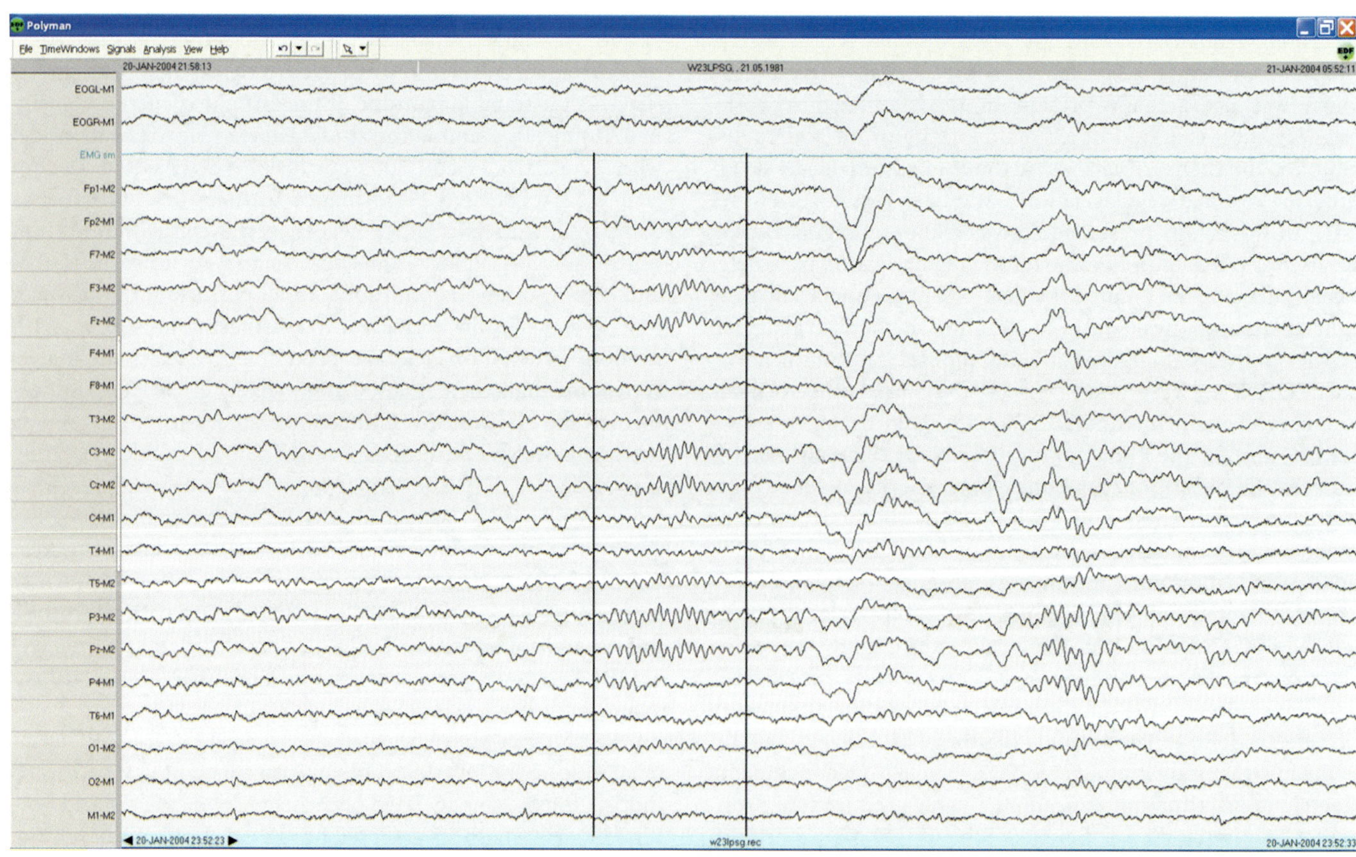

Figure 9.1 Example of a 10-s sleep EEG recorded in stage 2. The left and right electrooculogram (EOG) channels, the chin EMG channel, and 20 EEG channels are plotted with a scaling of ±50 µV. A 1.25-s artifact-free epoch with spindle activity is marked. Note that the EEG channels have to be re-referenced versus average reference prior to source analysis.

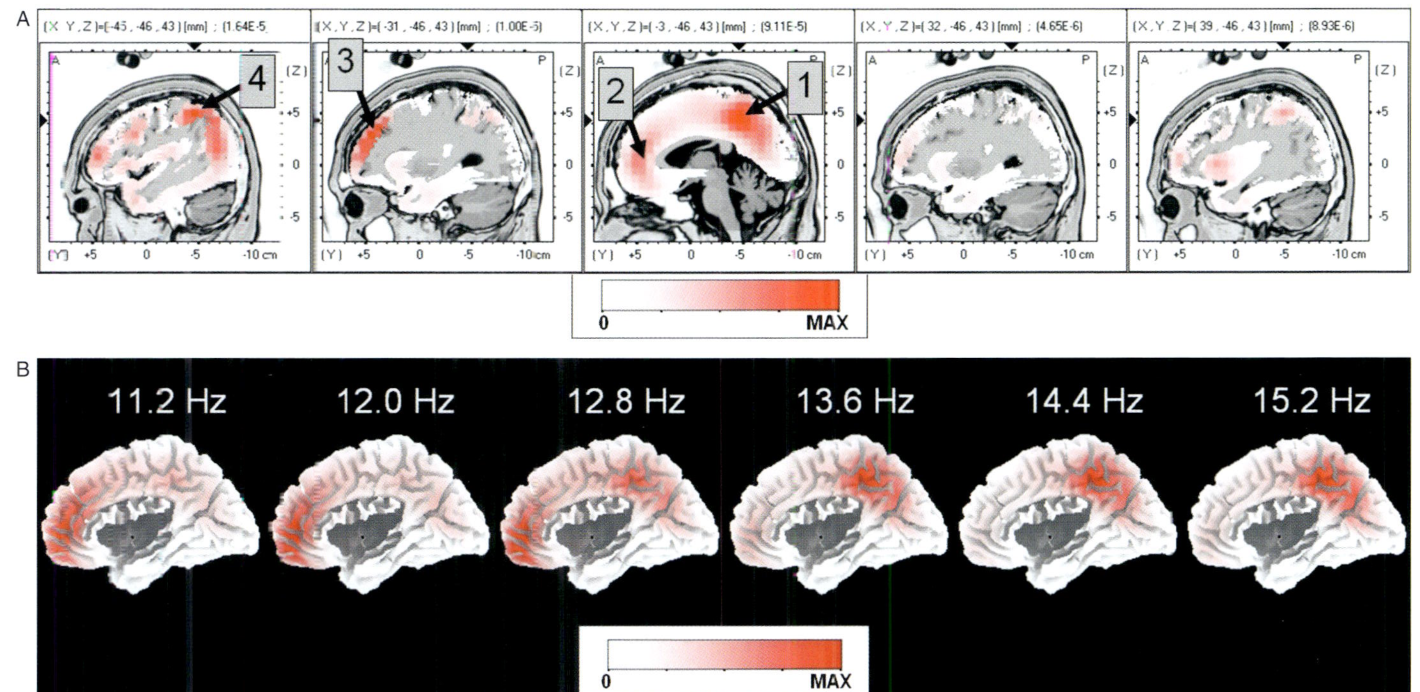

Figure 9.2 LORETA images of spindle power. The color scale depicts differences in LORETA power between spindle and control epochs (i.e., artifact-free 1.25-s epochs in stage 2 without spindles or K-complexes). One hundred and forty-four spindle epochs from 10 young healthy subjects (3 males, 7 females, aged 20–35 years) were included in the analysis. LORETA-KEY software (http://www.uzh.ch/keyinst/loreta.htm) was used for computation and display of LORETA power. For further details on the study, see [38]. (A) LORETA images of spindle power in the frequency band 11.2–15.2 Hz. Saggital slices in Talairach space are seen from left (A: anterior; P: posterior). The first two local maxima are seen medially at $X = -3$ mm (maximum$_1$: BA 7, precuneus; maximum$_2$: BA 9, 10, 32, 24, medial prefrontal, and anterior cingulate). Maximum$_3$ is located left dorsolaterally prefrontally at $X = -31$ mm (BA 9, 10, 46, 45) and maximum$_4$ left inferiorly parietally at $X = -45$ mm (BA 40). The corresponding maxima in the right hemisphere are significantly smaller. A local maximum is defined as a voxel with negative power gradients in all directions. The scaling factor for $X = -45$ mm and $X = 30$ mm is 2.3, for $X = -31$ mm and $X = 32$ mm is 2.9, and for $X = -3$ mm is 9.1 (in 10^{-5} μA^2/mm^4). (B) LORETA images of spindle power at discrete frequencies. The surface-rendered images of the right medial surface are seen from left. The images are scaled individually for each frequency bin in 10^{-5} μA^2/mm^4 (11.2 Hz: 2.6; 12.0 Hz: 4.7; 12.8 Hz: 10.1; 13.6 Hz: 26.7; 14.4 Hz: 14.1; 15.2 Hz: 2.0). Below 13 Hz, the frontal source is predominant, above 13 Hz the parietal.

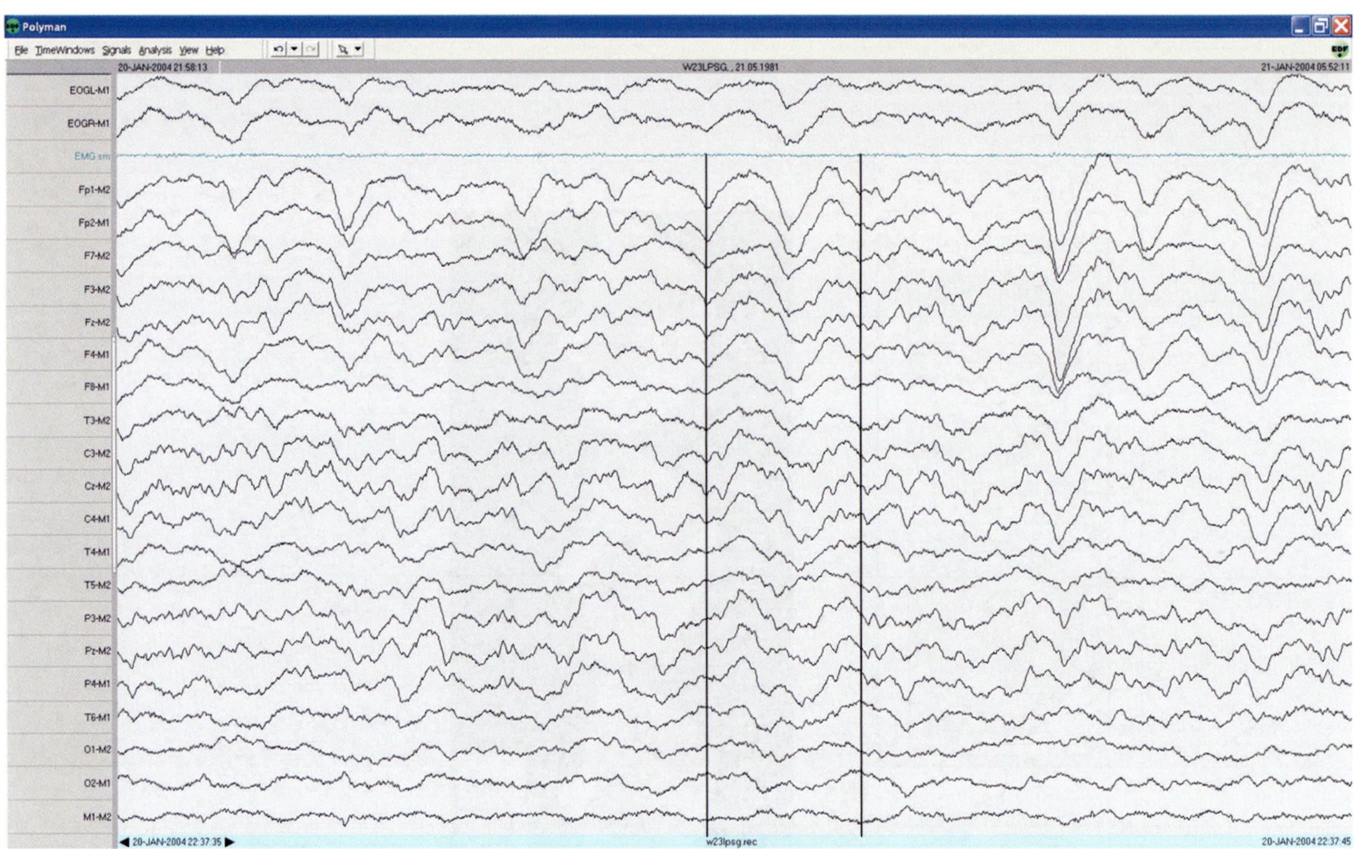

Figure 9.3 Example of a 10-s sleep EEG recorded in stage 4. The left and right EOG channels, the chin EMG channel, and 20 EEG channels are plotted with a scaling of ±50 μV. A 1.25-s artifact-free epoch with slow-wave activity is marked. Note that the EEG channels have to be re-referenced versus average reference prior to source analysis.

brain regions continuously active during resting states in wake for monitoring the external environment, social cognition, and memory, which undergo task-dependent deactivations as measured by fMRI and PET [46]. These findings are in line with the hypothesis that slow waves and spindles are involved in short-term plasticity, strengthening of synaptic contacts, and communication between different parts of the brain and thus in processes underlying consolidation of memory [44]. A recent study on the involvement of spindle sources in visuomotor learning by means of sLORETA further supports the hypothesis that the thalamocortical network underlying the generation of spindles may contribute to the synaptic plasticity that occurs during sleep [47]. sLORETA revealed significant increases in fast spindle activity in the left frontal and parietal areas in the night after learning as compared to a control night. Interestingly, these increases in the left hemisphere are consistent with our previously described left-hemispheric dominance of sleep spindles [38].

The medial frontal source of delta waves was also observed by Ferri *et al.* in the cyclic alternating pattern (CAP) subtype A1 characterized by slow-wave activities [48]. For CAP subtype A3, which is characterized by faster waves, including the alpha frequency band, LORETA revealed midline and hemispheric activations in the parietal and occipital areas. This is in line with the putative posterior distribution of the alpha generators in wakefulness.

Two recent studies applied sLORETA to EEG data obtained during REM sleep. In both, event-related potentials time-locked to the onset of rapid eye movements during REM sleep were investigated, with the first study focusing on sLORETA sources of a negativity preceding the eye movement [49], the second on sources of a positive component approximately 200 ms after the eye movement (P200r) [50]. The studies were intended to contribute to the understanding of the role of rapid eye movements during REM sleep. The current sources of the pre-REM negativity were observed in various brain regions including the medial prefrontal and anterior cingulate, parahippocampal cortex and right premotor cortex. The authors suggested that emotion-, memory-, and motor-related brain activity might occur before rapid eye movements in REM [49]. The sources of the P200r were located in brain regions known to be involved in visuomotor processing (left premotor area, left primary motor and sensory cortices, left inferior parietal lobule, and bilateral occipital areas). According to the authors the data provide evidence that rapid eye movements during REM sleep and saccades during wakefulness involve different neuronal networks [50].

In a study on source modeling of sleep slow waves by Murphy *et al.*, sLORETA was applied to a high-density 256-channel sleep-EEG recording and compared to LORETA, LAURA, and the Bayesian minimum norm [51]. In a pre-study, the authors validated different source localization methods by analyzing slow waves evoked by transcranial magnetic

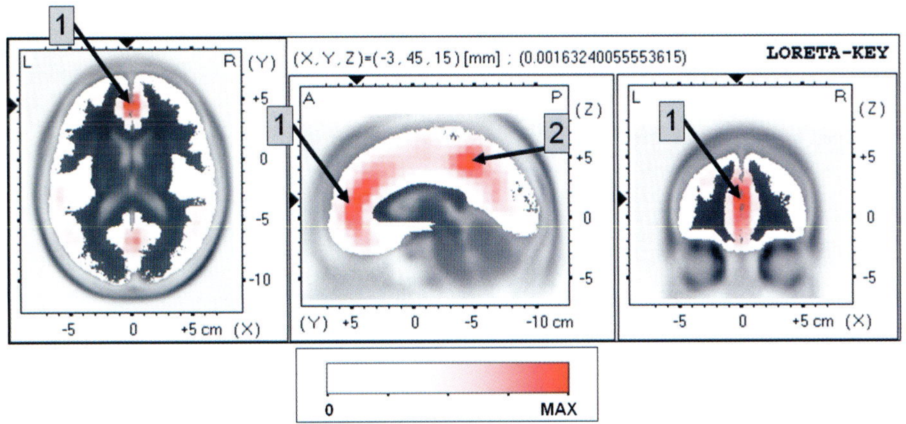

Figure 9.4 LORETA images of slow waves in the frequency band 0.8–4.0 Hz. The color scale depicts LORETA power and is scaled between 0 and 1.6×10^{-3} $\mu A^2/mm^4$. Two hundred and forty slow-wave epochs from 10 young healthy subjects (3 males, 7 females, aged 20–35 years) were included in the analysis. The axial slice left is seen from above, nose up; the sagittal slice in the middle is seen from left and the coronal slice right is seen from rear. X, Y, Z are Talairach coordinates: X from left (L) to right (R); Y from posterior (P) to anterior (A); Z from basal to dorsal. The frontal source (maximum$_1$) involves the medial prefrontal cortex (BA 9 and 10) and spreads into the anterior cingulate (BA 32 and 24) and orbitofrontal cortex (BA 11). The parietal source (maximum$_2$) is located in the precuneus (BA 7). For further details on the study, see [43].

stimulation (TMS) in NREM sleep stage 2. Irrespective of the source localization method used, TMS-triggered slow waves spread through source space in a stereotyped pattern – a pattern so robust that the source model of any individual TMS-triggered slow wave closely resembled the averaged source model. Next, they applied source modeling to individual slow waves during NREM stages 3 and 4 of the first sleep cycle and found that each slow wave showed a unique pattern of propagation across the cortex. Thus, the results clearly speak against a single subcortical substrate of slow waves. Even though every voxel was included in the generation of at least one slow wave, they identified two hot spots, one centered at the lateral sulcus and the other in the medial cingulate gyrus. Concerning the propagation of slow waves, source localization methods revealed that slow waves often travel along the anterior-posterior axis via the cingulate cortices. Interestingly, slow waves preferentially involve certain brain areas (inferior, medial, and middle frontal gyrus; insula, anterior, and posterior cingulate gyrus; and the precuneus), but avoid others (visual and sensory cortices and the fusiform gyrus). These findings are in accordance with our previously reported LORETA sources of slow waves (Figure 9.4). While in our data the maximal anterior LORETA source for slow waves was located in the medial prefrontal cortex, the activity spread considerably into neighboring parts of the frontal lobe and the anterior cingulate. Further statistics will be necessary to reveal the exact extent of this source. Most interesting from a methodological point of view is the finding that all four source localization methods used in the study by Murphy *et al.* (LAURA, LORETA,

sLORETA, and the Bayesian minimum norm) revealed similar results [51], which speaks for the robustness of the source localization methods.

Conclusions

Cortical source localization based on the scalp-recorded EEG is the only way to non-invasively investigate cortical activities during undisturbed sleep with high temporal and spatial resolution. Various methods have been developed and validated with simulated and real data to solve the ill-posed inverse problem. Further studies evaluating and comparing the localization properties of these inverse solutions dependent on spatial sampling (number and exact position of electrodes), head volume conductor models (e.g., based on averaged MRI or subjects' MRI), and the method for determining regularization parameters would be highly appreciated. However, the aforementioned similar findings for various inverse solutions and the physiologically meaningful results obtained not only for high-density but also for rather low-density EEG recordings strongly suggest the immediate utilization of these methods in functional neuroimaging of sleep and sleep disorders. LORETA was applied to reveal changes in brain activity due to chronic hypoxia in patients with obstructive sleep apnea syndrome (OSAS) [52, 53]. Examples for the application of LORETA to the EEG and cognitive event-related potentials of narcolepsy patients and its role in the assessment of therapeutic effects in these patients are summarized by Saletu and Saletu-Zyhlarz in Chapter 29 of this book.

References

1. Rechtschaffen A, Kales A. *A Manual of Standardized Terminology, Techniques and Scoring System for Sleep Stages of Human Subjects*. Public Health Service, U.S. Goverment Priting Office, 1968.

2. Iber C, Ancoli-Israel S, Chesson A, *et al.* for the American Academy of Sleep Medicine. *The AASM Manual for the Scoring of Sleep and Associated Events: Rules, Terminology and Technical Specifications*, 1st edn Westchester, Illinois, American Academy of Sleep Medicine, 2007.

3. Anderer P, Gruber G, Parapatics S, *et al.* An E-health solution for automatic sleep classification according to Rechtschaffen and Kales: validation study of the Somnolyzer 24x7 utilizing the Siesta database. *Neuropsychobiology*. 2005;51:115–33.

4. Anderer P, Moreau A, Woertz M, *et al.* Computer-assisted sleep classification according to the standard of the American Academy of Sleep Medicine: validation study of the AASM version of the Somnolyzer 24x7. *Neuropsychobiology*. 2010;62:250–64.

5. Werth E, Achermann P, Borbély AA. Fronto-occipital EEG power gradients in human sleep. *J Sleep Res.* 1997;**6**:102–12.

6. Zeitlhofer J, Anderer P, Obergottsberger S, *et al.* Topographic mapping of EEG during sleep. *Brain Topogr.* 1993;**6**:123–9.

7. Zeitlhofer J, Gruber G, Anderer P, *et al.* Topographic distribution of sleep spindles in young healthy subjects. *J Sleep Res.* 1997;**6**:149–55.

8. Huber R, Ghilardi MF, Massimini M, *et al.* Local sleep and learning. *Nature.* 2004;**430**:78–81.

9. Ferrarelli F, Peterson MJ, Sarasso S, *et al.* Thalamic dysfunction in schizophrenia suggested by whole-night deficits in slow and fast spindles. *Am J Psychiatry.* 2010;**167**:1339–48.

10. Anderer P, Roberts S, Schlögl A, *et al.* Artifact processing in computerized analysis of sleep EEG – a review. *Neuropsychobiology.* 1999;**40**:150–7.

11. Pascual-Marqui RD, Michel CM, Lehmann D. Low resolution electromagnetic tomography: a new method for localizing electrical activity in the brain. *Int J Psychophysiol.* 1994;**18**:49–65.

12. Pascual-Marqui RD, Lehmann D, Koukkou M, *et al.* Assessing interactions in the brain with exact low-resolution electromagnetic tomography. *Philos Transact A math Phys Eng Sci.* 2011;**369**:3768–84.

13. Hämäläinen MS, Ilmoniemi RJ. *Interpreting Measured Magnetic Fields of the Brain: Estimates of Current Distributions.* Technical Report TKK-F-A559, Helsinki University of Technology, 1984.

14. Pascual-Marqui RD. Review of methods for solving the EEG inverse problem. *Int J Bioelectromagn.* 1999;**1**:75–86.

15. Silva LR, Amitai Y, Connors BW. Intrinsic oscillations of neocortex generated by layer 5 pyramidal neurons. *Science.* 1991;**251**:432–5.

16. Vitacco D, Brandeis D, Pascual-Marqui R, *et al.* Correspondence of event-related potential tomography and functional magnetic resonance imaging during language processing. *Hum Brain Mapp.* 2002;**17**:4–12.

17. Worrell GA, Lagerlund TD, Sharbrough FW, *et al.* Localization of the epileptic focus by low-resolution electromagnetic tomography in patients with a lesion demonstrated by MRI. *Brain Topogr.* 2000;**12**:273–82.

18. Zumsteg D, Wennberg RA, Treyer V, *et al.* H2(15)O or 13NH3 PET and electromagnetic tomography (LORETA) during partial status epilepticus. *Neurology.* 2005;**65**:1657–60.

19. Zumsteg D, Friedman A, Wieser HG, *et al.* Propagation of interictal discharges in temporal lobe epilepsy: correlation of spatiotemporal mapping with intracranial foramen ovale electrode recordings. *Clin Neurophysiol.* 2006;**117**:2615–26.

20. Anderer P, Saletu B, Semlitsch HV, *et al.* Non-invasive localization of P300 sources in normal aging and age-associated memory impairment. *Neurobiol Aging.* 2003;**24**:463–79.

21. Anderer P, Pascual-Marqui RD, Semlitsch HV, *et al.* Differential effects of normal aging on sources of standard N1, target N1 and target P300 auditory event-related brain potentials revealed by low resolution electromagnetic tomography (LORETA). *Electroencephalogr Clin Neurophysiol.* 1998;**108**:160–74.

22. Pascual-Marqui RD, Lehmann D, Koenig T, *et al.* Low resolution brain electromagnetic tomography (LORETA) functional imaging in acute, neuroleptic-naïve, first-episode, productive schizophrenia. *Psychiatry Res.* 1999;**90**:169–79.

23. Talairach J, Tournoux P. *Co-Planar Stereotaxic Atlas of the Human Brain.* Stuttgart, Thieme, 1988.

24. Anderer P, Saletu B, Saletu-Zyhlarz G, *et al.* Brain regions activated during an auditory discrimination task in insomniac postmenopausal patients before and after hormone replacement therapy: low-resolution brain electromagnetic tomography applied to event-related potentials. *Neuropsychobiology.* 2004;**49**:134–53.

25. Halgren E, Matinkovic K, Chauvel P. Generators of the late cognitive potentials in auditory and visual oddball tasks. *Electroencephalogr Clin Neurophysiol.* 1998;**106**:156–64.

26. Smith ME, Halgren E, Sokolik M, *et al.* The intracranial topography of the P3 event-related potential elicited during auditory oddball. *Electroencephalogr Clin Neurophysiol.* 1990;**76**:235–48.

27. Pascual-Marqui RD. Standardized low-resolution brain electromagnetic tomography (sLORETA): technical details. *Methods Find Exp Clin Pharmacol.* 2002;**24**(Suppl C):5–12.

28. Dale AM, Liu AK, Fischl BR, *et al.* Dynamic statistical parametric mapping: combining fMRI and MEG for high-resolution imaging of cortical activity. *Neuron.* 2000;**26**:55–67.

29. Sekihara K, Sahani M, Nagarajan SS. Localization bias and spatial resolution of adaptive and non-adaptive spatial filters for MEG source reconstruction. *Neuroimage.* 2005;**25**:1056–67.

30. Greenblatt RE, Ossadtchi A, Pflieger ME. Local linear estimators for the bioelectromagnetic inverse problem. *IEEE Trans Signal Processing.* 2005;**53**:3403–12.

31. Olbrich S, Mulert C, Karch S, *et al.* EEG-vigilance and BOLD effect during simultaneous EEG/fMRI measurements. *Neuroimage.* 2009;**45**:319–32.

32. Rullmann M, Anwander A, Dannhauer M, *et al.* EEG source analysis of epileptiform activity using a 1 mm anisotropic hexahedra finite element head model. *Neuroimage.* 2009;**44**:399–410.

33. Grech R, Cassar T, Muscat J, *et al.* Review on solving the inverse problem in EEG source analysis. *J Neuroeng Rehab.* 2008;**5**:25.

34. Yao J, Dewald PA. Evaluation of different cortical source localization methods using simulated and experimental EEG data. *Neuroimage.* 2005;**25**:269–92.

35. Pascual-Marqui RD. Discrete, 3D distributed, linear imaging methods of electric neuronal activity. Part 1: exact, zero error localization. arXiv:0710.3341 [math-ph], 2007-October-17. http://arxiv.org/pdf/0710.3341. (Accessed August 22, 2012.)

36. Lancaster JL, Woldorff MG, Parsons LM, *et al.* Automated Talairach Atlas labels for functional brain mapping. *Hum Brain Mapp.* 2000;**10**:120–31.

37. Lin FH, Witzel T, Ahlfors SP, *et al.* Assessing and improving the spatial accuracy in MEG source localization by depth-weighted minimum-norm estimates. *Neuroimage.* 2006;**31**:160–71.

38. Anderer P, Klösch G, Gruber G, *et al.* Low-resolution brain electromagnetic tomography revealed simultaneously

active frontal and parietal sleep spindle sources in the human cortex. *Neuroscience.* 2001;**103**:581–92.

39. Frei E, Gamma A, Pascual-Marqui R, *et al.* Localization of MDMA-induced brain activity in healthy volunteers using low resolution brain electromagnetic tomography (LORETA). *Hum Brain Mapp.* 2001;**14**:152–65.

40. Holmes AP, Blair RC, Watson JDG, *et al.* Nonparametric analysis of statistical images from functional mapping experiments. *J Cereb Blood Flow Metab.* 1996;**16**:7–22.

41. Durka PJ, Matysiak A, Martinez Montes E, *et al.* Multichannel matching pursuit and EEG inverse solutions. *J Neurosci Methods.* 2005;**148**:49–59.

42. Ventouras EM, Ktonas PY, Tsekou H, *et al.* Independent component analysis for source localization of EEG sleep spindle components. *Comput Intell Neurosci.* 2010;**2010**: 329436.

43. Anderer P, Gruber G, Saletu B, *et al.* Non-invasive electrophysiological neuroimaging of sleep. In: Hirata K, ed. *Recent Advances in Human Brain Mapping.* Amsterdam, Elsevier. 2002; 795–800.

44. Steriade M, Amzica F. Slow sleep oscillation, rhythmic K-complexes, and their paroxysmal developments. *J Sleep Res.* 1998;7(Suppl 1):30–5.

45. Maquet P. Functional neuromapping of normal human sleep by positron emission tomography. *J Sleep Res.* 2000;**9**:207–31.

46. Raichle ME, Snyder AZ. A default mode of brain function: a brief history of an evolving idea. *Neuroimage.* 2007;**37**:1083–90.

47. Tamaki M, Matsouka Z, Nittino H, *et al.* Activation of fast sleep spindles at the premotor cortex and parietal areas contributes to motor learning: a study using sLORETA. *Clin Neurophysiol.* 2009;**120**:878–86.

48. Ferri R, Bruni O, Miano S, *et al.* Topographic mapping of the spectral components of the cyclic alternating patter (CAP). *Sleep Med.* 2005;**6**:29–36.

49. Abe T, Ogawa K, Nittono H, *et al.* Neural generators of brain potentials before rapid eye movements during human REM sleep: a study using sLORETA. *Clin Neurophysiol.* 2008;**119**:2044–53.

50. Ogawa K, Abe T, Nittono H, *et al.* Phasic brain activity related to the onset of rapid eye movements during rapid eye movement sleep: study of event-related potentials and standardized low-resolution brain electromagnetic tomography. *J Sleep Res.* 2010;**19**:407–14.

51. Murphy M, Riedner BA, Huber R, *et al.* Source modeling sleep slow waves. *Proc Natl Acad Sci U S A.* 2009;**106**:1608–13.

52. Lee HK, Park DH, Shin HS, *et al.* Comparison of low resolution electromagnetic tomography imaging between subjects with mild and severe obstructive sleep apnea syndrome: a preliminary study. *Psychiatry Investig.* 2008;**5**:45–51.

53. Toth M, Faludi B, Wackermann J, *et al.* Characteristics in brain electrical activity due to chronic hypoxia in patients with obstructive sleep apnea syndrome (OSAS): a combined EEG study using LORETA and omega complexity. *Brain Topography.* 2009;**22**:185–90.

Methodology of combined EEG and fMRI

Helmut Laufs and Karsten Krakow

Motivation for EEG-combined fMRI recordings during sleep

Simultaneous recording of electroencephalogram (EEG) and functional magnetic resonance imaging (fMRI) (EEG-fMRI) was developed motivated by the wish of epileptologists to localize with MRI paroxysmal interictal epileptiform discharges [1, 2]. In classical "cognitive" fMRI studies via a specifically designed paradigm, brain function is externally manipulated in order to test a hypothesis about the identification of task-related fMRI activation patterns. In contrast, EEG-fMRI studies allow the investigation of spontaneously occurring brain activity observable with EEG in combination with or in the absence of external stimulation [3]. This spontaneous activity extends from epileptic spikes to sleep paroxysms such as spindles, K-complexes, and vertex sharp waves but also to ongoing EEG oscillations characteristic for wakefulness and different sleep stages [4–12].

Hence, extending EEG-fMRI recordings to polysomnographic recordings during fMRI (Figure 10.1) especially in conditions with fluctuating vigilance (e.g., resting state or sleep studies) allows the exact assignment of epochs of fMRI to sleep stages [13], and the correlation of sleep paroxysmal events with fMRI. Based on this, two basic scenarios can be imagined: (1) sleep physiology per se is the subject of primary interest, i.e., blood oxygen level-dependent (BOLD) signal maps can be generated revealing the anatomical structures underlying sleep physiological (EEG) phenomena; (2) the EEG exclusively serves vigilance state classification, i.e., when neuronal processing as measured with fMRI is the subject of interest as function of vigilance state [14–17]. Similarly, changes in the functional architecture of the brain across sleep have been the objective of recent studies [18–24].

Most EEG-fMRI sleep studies so far have focused on sleep physiology serving as the basis for the understanding of the pathology of intrinsic sleep disorders such as idiopathic insomnia, narcolepsy, and obstructive sleep apnea. Extending previous neuroimaging work, due to its temporal sensitivity, EEG-fMRI will allow the study of brief or transient changes reflected in the polysomnographic measures, such as cataplectic attacks, sleep paralysis, individual respiratory events, sleep stage transitions, and potentially hypnagocic hallucinations [25, 26].

Of course, an important fundamental question is whether it is possible to sleep in an MRI bore during fMRI and if so, which sleep stage is reached and for what amount of time. We tried to derive an answer from our own collective of subjects who were scanned in the evening hours (between 8 and 10 pm) but were not sleep deprived (Figure 10.2). Data were lost because of excessive motion [27], subjects aborting the EEG-fMRI experiment, and technical or human error in approximately 10% of cases, each, leaving 70% of data sets for analysis. Of these, as can be expected in healthy subjects, nobody reached rapid eye movement (REM) sleep, but about a third of the subjects entered deep sleep (N3) for up to 30 min (of 50 min total recording time). This underlines the feasibility of recording sleep in the scanner without sleep deprivation. In summary, based on our cohort assuming a data loss of 30%, about a quarter of the scanned subjects can be expected to reach an average of 5 min of N3 sleep.

Methodological aspects

The following sections will cover practical aspects when planning and conducting a simultaneous EEG-fMRI experiment. First, the choice of hardware to provide patient safety and comfort, while delivering high quality EEG and fMRI data, is discussed. Second, we examine the choice of post-processing methods applied to the electrophysiological data for scanner- and subject-induced artifact reduction.

The signal transduction chain (Figure 10.3) of the electrophysiological signal of interest (e.g., EEG, electromyogram (EMG), skin impedance) starts at the subject's surface where electrodes make skin contact with the aid of a conductive gel or paste which should not dry during extended sleep recordings. The currents generated by synchronously active and parallel oriented pyramidal neurons will cause a potential between EEG electrodes which then generate current flow into the amplifier facilitating signal digitization followed by computerized recording and processing. The signal is relayed between the electrode and amplifier through wires. Either, these (metallic) wires reach from inside the scanner bore to the outside of the electromagnetically shielded scanner room, in which conventional EEG amplification and digitization hardware can be used as long as it provides sufficient amplitude range and sampling

Neuroimaging of Sleep and Sleep Disorders, ed. Eric Nofzinger, Pierre Maquet, and Michael J. Thorpy. Published by Cambridge University Press. © Cambridge University Press 2013.

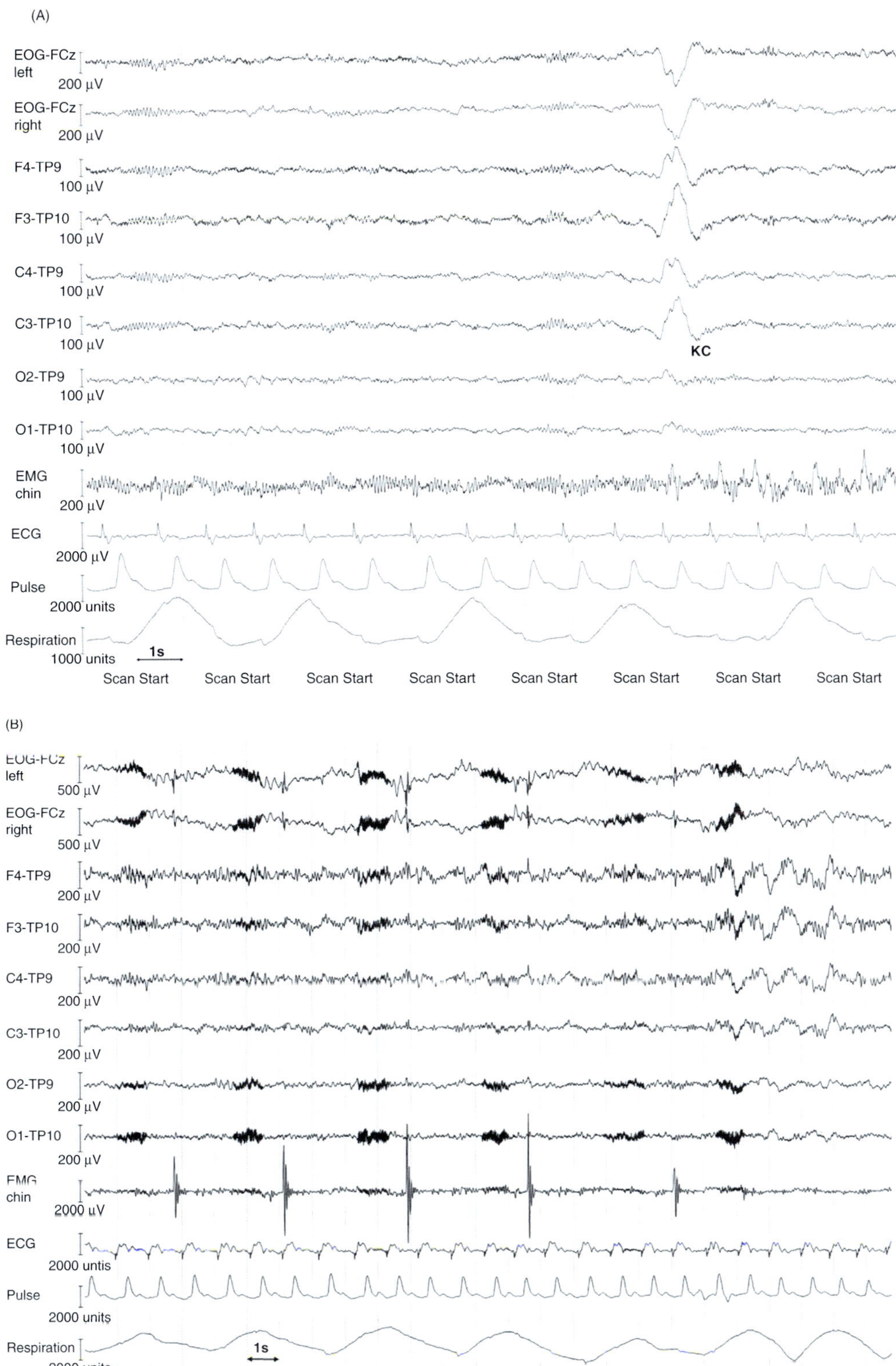

Figure 10.1 Example polysomnography recording. (A) Exemplary channels of the polysomnography data acquired during fMRI scanning show several sleep spindles before one K-complex (KC) during stage N2 sleep. Frontal, central, occipital EEG channels are referenced to mastoid-near temporal parietal (TP) channels, EOG to the frontal centro-central channel (following AASM criteria). Pulse and respiration channels have arbitrary units. Scan start markers indicate fMRI volume acquisitions (time of repetition is 2 s). EEG channels are filtered at 0.5 Hz (Butterworth 0 Phase, low cutoff). (B) Example of a subject at the end of a rapid eye movement sleep epoch with transition to N2 sleep showing low amplitude chin EMG activity with brief bursts of summed muscle action potentials in temporal correlation with snoring which causes the approximately 1-s epochs of high-frequency artifact on the EEG and EOG channels with every respiratory cycle. Settings and markers are the same as in panel A.

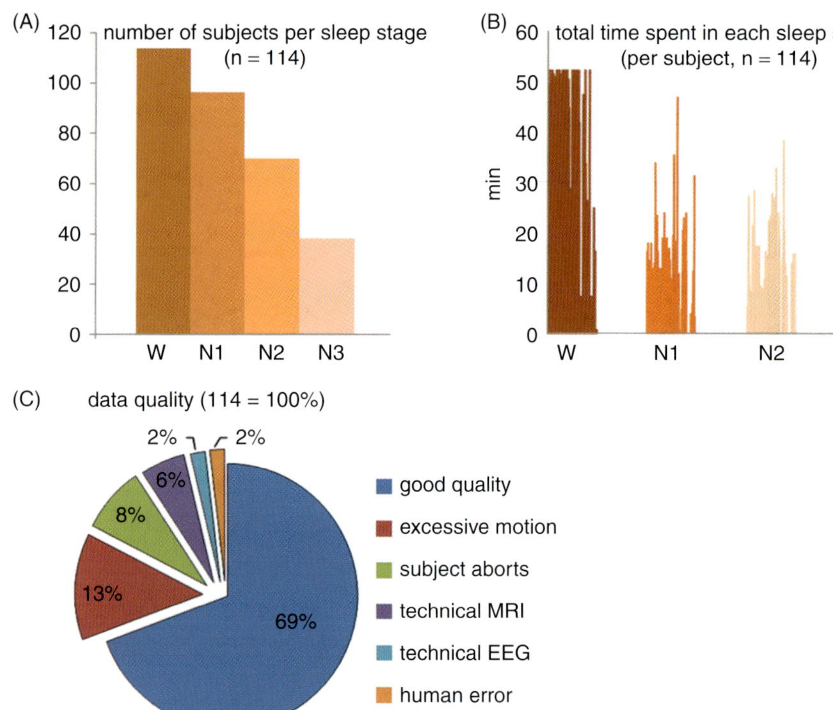

Figure 10.2 (A) Sleep depth. Number of subjects (n = 114) exhibiting at least one epoch (30 s) of the given sleep stages (W: 114; N1: 96; N2: 70; N3: 38). Subjects were not sleep deprived and were scanned in the early evening. (B) Time spent in each epoch. Each subject is represented by one vertical bar per sleep stage indicating the number of min spent in the respective sleep stage(s). Mean ± standard deviation [min]: W: 29 ± 17; N1: 10 ± 8; N2: 8 ± 9, N3: 5 ± 9. (C) Data quality. Of the 114 data sets (100%), 79 (69%) can be considered of high quality, while 15 (13%) were affected by motion events requiring special modeling strategies [27], 9 (8%) data sets were incomplete due to subjects aborting the scan, 7 (6%) and 2 (2%) data sets had to be discarded because of technical MRI and EEG problems, respectively. Two (2%) data sets were lost due to experimenter error.

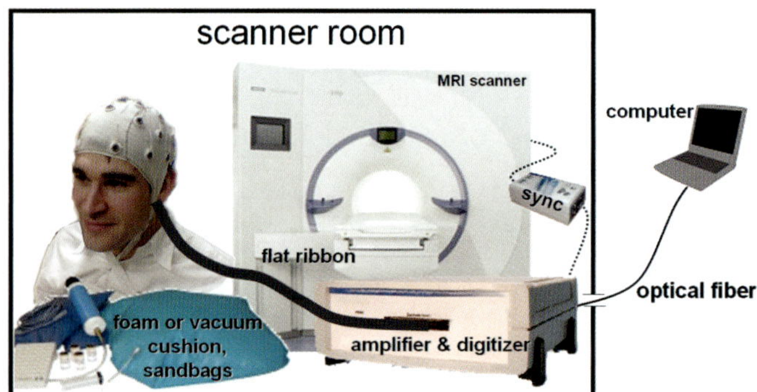

Figure 10.3 Schematic of an example EEG-fMRI experimental setup. EEG ring electrodes with current limiting safety resistors are woven into a cap. Their bundled wires converge into a flat ribbon cable which connects to the battery-driven amplifier and digitizer, which is usually positioned at the head end of the scanner bore; a second amplifier and digitizer, e.g., for EMG recordings, is positioned near the subject's lower extremities. The digitizer is connected to the MRI scanner clock via a synchronization device [41]. A fiber optical cable transmits the digitized electrophysiological signals through the wave guide to a recording computer outside the scanner room. A foam or vacuum cushion serves subject comfort and reduces head motion [40]. (Figure modified, with permission from Elsevier, from Laufs H, Daunizeau J, Carmichael DW, Kleinschmidt A, 2007. Recent advances in recording electrophysiological data simultaneously with magnetic resonance imaging. *Neuroimage.* **40**: 515–28.)

rate. Or, preferably, the signal is amplified and digitized within or near the scanner bore before leaving the scanner room through optical fibers [28]. This has the advantages of both increased signal fidelity and patient safety.

Materials should be non-ferrous (wires are mostly copper or carbon), and all equipment introduced into the shielded MRI room must not emit RF (radio frequency) in the scanner frequency band [29] such that scanner functionality, image quality, and subject safety are not compromised [30, 31]. Obviously, the electrophysiology recording equipment needs to remain operational within the MR scanner environment and during scanner operation [29]. Gold electrodes [32] or ring-mounted sintered Ag/AgCl ring electrodes including safety resistors are commonly used and have good artifact characteristics.

Artifacts are caused on the EEG due to induction of the MR scanners switching gradients. The artifact results from a complex combination of factors including the field strength (and so frequency), orientation, positioning of the recording equipment relative to the RF coil, and the geometric relationship between the magnetic field gradients relative to the electrophysiological equipment. When recording limb EMG during polysomnography, for example, increasing distance between the recording locations and the magnet isocenter does not necessarily translate into reduced artifact (despite decreasing field strength) because the field homogeneity decreases and hence motion will cause greater artifact than in the homogeneous field.

Sleep pathology-associated motion, artifact due to snoring, or apnea-induced changes to the neurovascular coupling [33] require special consideration, as do pharmacological manipulations [34].

EMG recordings during fMRI are particularly affected by artifact induced by motion in the static field because even during isometric contractions (i.e., muscle contraction without gross limb movement) some degree of electrode movement in the field is inevitable. True bipolar recordings are advantageous as artifact common to closely positioned electrodes is already reduced prior to correction [35, 36]. Other polygraphic measurements required for sleep recordings like respiration and pulse oximetry can be recorded via respective MR-compatible pneumatic and optic devices as provided by most scanner manufacturers [4].

Subject safety issues pertain to current flow and heating within the body, which is usually greatest close to the electrodes. The time-varying (switching) magnetic field gradients induce voltages in electrodes and leads. Current will flow within tissue potentially causing stimulation, electric shock, and tissue damage. Movement of an electric circuit (wire loop) in the static magnetic field will cause current flow and could cause injury via the same mechanisms [37]. Sleep studies naturally require prolonged scanning periods. Scanner heating over time needs to be avoided for both patient safety and data quality reasons. Consequently, appropriate coil and sequence selection are required [38]. To prevent data loss, it is worthwhile making sure that the accumulating large amount of data can be handled by the recording systems.

Directing special effort at subject comfort – especially during prolonged sleep experiments – is warranted for increasing the tolerance of the subject and thus also limiting head motion. Using a vacuum head cushion [39] has been found to minimize both motion-induced artifacts on the images as well as motion-induced currents contaminating the electrophysiological signal. Alternatively, foam cushions with some spatial inertia ("memory") provide high patient comfort and a good degree of head fixation.

Raw data quality remains essential despite sophisticated gradient and pulse artifact reduction algorithms. The generic setup outlined above should be adapted to and optimized for every scanner, electrophysiological recording equipment, and site.

All artifact reduction methods benefit from hardware synchronization of EEG sampling with the MR sequence [40].

Two important types of artifacts in electrophysiological recordings originate specifically from the MR scanner, manifesting as induced voltages that add linearly to the EEG signal and thus obscure the biological signal of interest (Figure 10.4). (1) MRI scanning ("imaging artifact"): this is usually the largest in amplitude (in the order of mV) but the most stable over time [28]. Its origin has already been discussed above: the time varying electromagnetic fields induce currents resulting in artificial voltages in the recorded electrophysiological data; (2) cardiac pulsation ("pulse artifact") [41]: This is understood to be due to heartbeat-related movements (systolic pulsation) of the head or of electrodes in the vicinity of blood vessels, or of the blood itself caused by

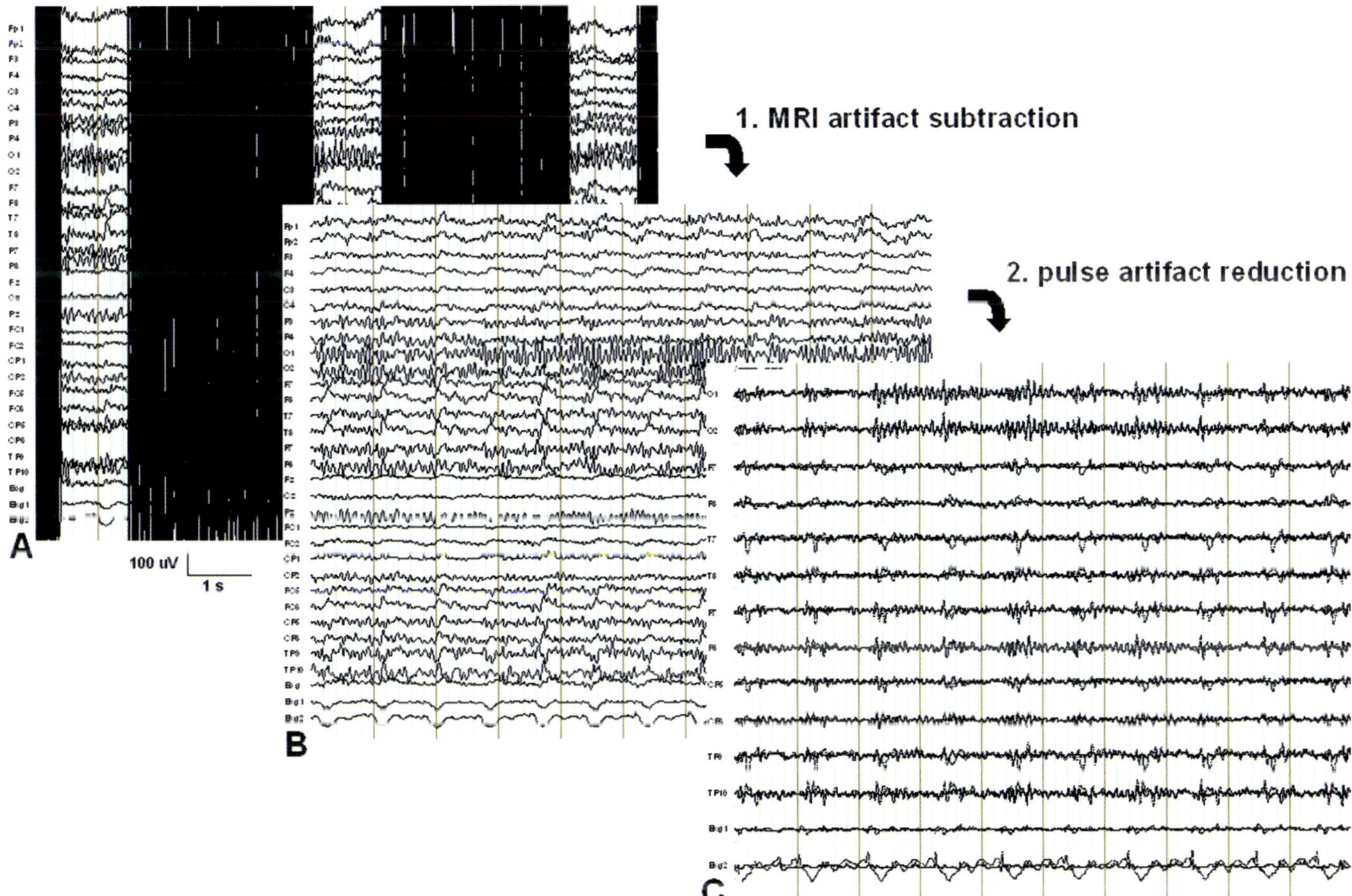

Figure 10.4 Schematic of preprocessing stages of MRI and pulse artifact affected EEG. (A) Segment (10 s) of a 32 channel electrophysiological recording during "interleaved" fMRI acquisition (for didactic purposes) with about 3 s of imaging per acquired volume followed by a gap in scanning of about 1 s duration; (B) the same segment after channel-wise subtraction of a template MRI artifact obtained by averaging [28]; (C) identical segment (dotted lines) after channel-wise pulse artifact reduction (solid line) via subtraction of an ECG-locked sliding average [42]. (With permission from Elsevier from Laufs H, Daunizeau J, Carmichael DW, Kleinschmidt A, 2007. Recent advances in recording electrophysiological data simultaneously with magnetic resonance imaging. Neuroimage. **40**: 515–28.)

systolic acceleration and abrupt diastolic directional change of blood flow in large body vessels and – arguably [42] – due to fluctuations of the Hall-voltage due to the pulsatile arterial blood flow [43].

The scanner-generated imaging artifact is theoretically the most straightforward one to remove owing to its periodicity. All currently available artifact subtraction methods exploit this regularity. However, since the regularity is not perfect, neither are the correction algorithms. Due to the scanner artifact's huge amplitude compared to the biological EEG signal (about a factor of 1000 for a standard set-up), even slight imperfections of the artifact correction leave the quality of the corrected EEG compromised. In the absence of the perfect algorithm, a suitable method needs to be identified for each specific application.

The principle of the first MRI scanner artifact reduction method was based on determining a template artifact waveform by time-locked averaging to the periodic MR acquisition [2]. This procedure is based on the rationale that those components of the recorded signal, which are not time-locked to image acquisition, should average to zero. Because of the additive property of the theoretically constant imaging artifact, averaging results in a template which can be subtracted from the data and thus recover the biological signal (and noise), artifact drifts can be partly addressed by sliding average formation and subsequent linear filtering and, theoretically, adaptive noise cancellation [28, 44].

Other approaches to imaging artifact correction have been suggested that also rely on the (*a-priori* knowledge of the) specific sequence-related artifact shape, its determination using principle component analysis and subsequent respective artifact fitting and filtering steps. Combining different methods can prove very efficient (for review see [45]). However, the correction of artifacts in EMG signals currently remains challenging [35, 46], and algorithms will have to be developed accounting for artifact as a function of both electromagnetic field changes and simultaneous relative subject (electrode) movement therein.

The pulse artifact often requires more attention than the imaging artifact due to its biological origin and variability [41] adding a spatio-temporally complex, non-stationary signal to the EEG [47].

Methods for pulse artifact subtraction resemble those discussed for the imaging artifact: due to its periodic nature, the average subtraction approach can be applied [42]. However, the periodicity of this biological artifact is subject to heart rate variability and drift artifacts, leading to greater instability of the pulse artifact compared to the imaging artifact. This is the reason why a sliding average approach with or without additional weighting [36, 41, 43, 48] or the use of several artifact templates per channel is beneficial [49]. In sleep studies, pulse artifact correction algorithms should also cope with systematic variability in heart rate, e.g., dependent on sleep stage [50, 51].

Other methods use channel-wise ECG-locked temporal principal component analysis (PCA) [49, 52], or PCA of representative epochs of data building a spatial filter to remove pulse artifact-related components [39]. The question

of the selection and refinement of the components to remove is a problem inherent to data driven approaches. Similarly for independent component analysis (ICA), which can be used to further process the averaged pulse-contributed signal [42] or to determine and remove related components [39, 42, 49, 53, 54]. Again, combining different approaches can be advantageous [55], but because of the non-stationary aspect of the signal, the use of statistical procedures such as ICA and PCA is limited [47].

Analysis strategies

Two empirical approaches have been mainly used to integrate fMRI and EEG data; first, using fMRI for the better determination of the source of the measured electrical EEG signal and second, trying to find the common neural "origin" of both the EEG and fMRI signals in a broader sense [3]. The first approach is usually based on averaged EEG event-related responses used with fMRI-derived activations to constrain EEG source localization [56]. The second relates more generally to the identification of a functional state of the brain associated with specific EEG

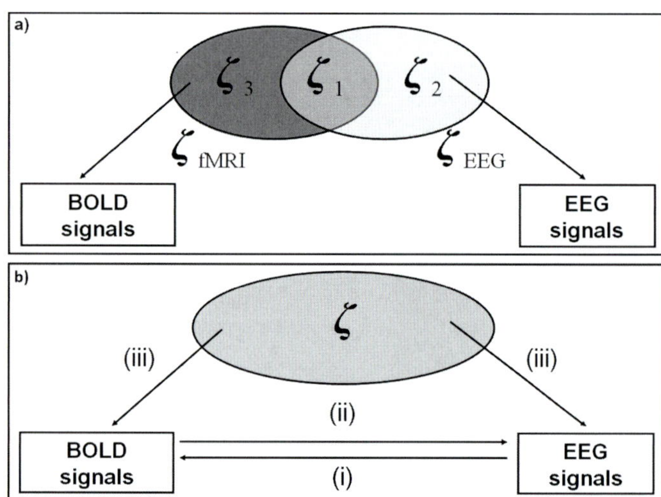

Figure 10.5 Computational neurophysiology. Formalization of theoretical EEG-fMRI coupling-uncoupling (a) and EEG-fMRI integration approaches (b) (adapted from [67]; with permission from Elsevier (a) Daunizeau J, Grova C, Marrelec G, Mattout J, Jbabdi S, Pelegrini-Issac M Lina JM, Benali H, 2007. Symmetrical event-related EEG/fMRI information fusion in a variational Bayesian framework. *Neuroimage*. **36**: 69–87 and (b) Kilner JM, Mattout J, Henson R, Friston KJ, 2005. Hemodynamic correlates of EEG: a heuristic. *Neuroimage*. **28**: 280–6). The "neurovascular brain activity" ζ can be understood as two non-orthogonal subspaces ζ_{EEG} and ζ_{fMRI} that correspond to the part of ζ that contributes to EEG and fMRI data sets, respectively [68]. The intersection ζ_1 of ζ_{EEG} and ζ_{fMRI} defines the "common substrate" of neuronal activity. Conversely, ζ_2 (ζ_3, respectively) denotes the subspace of neuronal activity detected by EEG (fMRI) that does not contribute to fMRI (EEG) measurements. Any multimodal information integration approach will be beneficial for inferring the common substrate ζ_1. This means that asymmetrical EEG-fMRI approaches systematically bias their estimate of ζ_1 by introducing information from ζ_{EEG} ((i): EEG to fMRI approaches, i.e., integration through prediction as in EEG-fMRI epilepsy studies) or ζ_{fMRI} ((ii): fMRI to EEG approaches, i.e., integration through constraints). In contradistinction, symmetrical EEG-fMRI fusion approaches rely on a joint EEG-fMRI generative model, which allows the estimation of ζ_1 to be derived from an optimal balance between EEG and fMRI-derived information (((iii): integration through forward models in which a joint parameter estimation is performed minimizing the difference between the measured and the modeled (predicted) EEG and fMRI signals).

features, e.g., sleep graphic elements [7–9, 57], that can be used to interrogate the simultaneously measured fMRI data, e.g., in the form of an EEG-based general linear model. Analysis of ongoing EEG-MRI activity during different sleep stages has revealed changes in relative BOLD signal amplitudes [58, 59], functional connectivity [21, 60–62] as well as changes due to different forms of stimulation [15, 16, 63, 64] and demonstrate that fMRI signal changes can indicate changes in brain function characterized by EEG reflecting different vigilance states [11, 12]. This is opposed to EEG-correlated fMRI activations representing the electrical sources of the measured EEG phenomena [3].

At the theoretical level, three perspectives on the combination of electrophysiology with fMRI have been discussed [65, 66]: integration through (1) prediction; (2) constraints; (3) fusion with forward models. These are explained in Figure 10.5.

Summary

EEG in combination with a fast whole-brain imaging method such as fMRI is an ideal tool to study sleep. The EEG can serve to classify the spontaneously occurring neuronal activity, e.g., into different sleep stages, and is sensitive to brief events (e.g., graphic elements). EEG-defined epochs can be characterized using different fMRI analysis strategies, e.g., functional connectivity analyses. Brief events leaving a trace in brain hemodynamics can be assigned topographical activity patterns by means of event-related analysis. The associated BOLD-topographical patterns, or "networks," can then be interpreted in the context of the vast (fMRI) literature on human brain function leading to a better understanding of sleep pathophysiology.

The main associated technical challenges have been successfully addressed both in terms of acquisition and post-processing of the inevitably artifact-laden data. EMG recordings are feasible but await further improved artifact reduction methods dealing with motion in the magnetic field.

Acknowledgements

This work was funded by the Bundesministerium für Bildung und Forschung (grant 01 EV 0703) and the Landes-Offensive zur Entwicklung Wissenschaftlich-ökonomischer Exzellenz (Neuronale Koordination Forschungsschwerpunkt Frankfurt). I thank Astrid Morzelewski for help with preparing the figures and everybody contributing to this work, especially Sergey Borisov, Kolja Jahnke, Frederic von Wegner. This chapter uses various, partly modified, excerpts and figures, with permission from Elsevier, from Laufs H, Daunizeau J, Carmichael DW, Kleinschmidt A, Recent advances in recording electrophysiological data simultaneously with magnetic resonance imaging. *Neuroimage* 2007;**40**:515–28.

References

1. Laufs H, Duncan JS. Electroencephalography/functional MRI in human epilepsy: what it currently can and cannot do. *Curr Opin Neurol.* 2007;**20**(4):417–23.

2. Laufs H. A personalized history of EEG-fMRI integration. *Neuroimage.* 2012;**62**(2):1056–67.

3. Laufs H. Endogenous brain oscillations and related networks detected by surface EEG-combined fMRI. *Hum Brain Mapp.* 2008;**29**(7):762–9.

4. Laufs H, Walker MC, Lund TE, 'Brain activation and hypothalamic functional connectivity during human non-rapid eye movement sleep: an EEG/fMRI study'–its limitations and an alternative approach. *Brain.* 2007;**130**(Pt 7):e75; author reply e6.

5. Mochring J, Coropceanu D, Galka A, et al. Improving sensitivity of EEG-fMRI studies in epilepsy: the role of sleep-specific activity. *Neurosci Lett.* 2011;**505**(2):211–15.

6. Tyvaert L, Levan P, Grova C, Dubeau F, Gotman J. Effects of fluctuating physiological rhythms during prolonged EEG-fMRI studies. *Clin Neurophysiol.* 2008;**119**(12):2762–74.

7. Jahnke K, von Wegner F, Morzelewski A, et al. To wake or not to wake? The two-sided nature of the human K-complex. *Neuroimage.* 2012;**59** (2):1631–8.

8. Schabus M, Dang-Vu TT, Albouy G, et al. Hemodynamic cerebral correlates of sleep spindles during human non-rapid eye movement sleep. *Proc Natl Acad Sci U S A.* 2007;**104**(32):13164–9.

9. Caporro M, Haneef Z, Yeh HJ, et al. Functional MRI of sleep spindles and K-complexes. *Clin Neurophysiol.* 2012;**123**(2):303–9.

10. Wehrle R, Czisch M, Kaufmann C, et al. Rapid eye movement-related brain activation in human sleep: a functional magnetic resonance imaging study. *Neuroreport.* 2005;**16**(8):853–7.

11. Laufs H, Holt JL, Elfont R, et al. Where the BOLD signal goes when alpha EEG leaves. *Neuroimage.* 2006;**31**(4):1408–18.

12. Olbrich S, Mulert C, Karch S, et al. EEG-vigilance and BOLD effect during simultaneous EEG/fMRI measurement. *Neuroimage.* 2009;**45**(2):319–32.

13. AASM. *The AASM Manual for the Scoring of Sleep and Associated Events: Rules, Terminology and Technical Specifications.* Chicago: American Academy of Sleep Medicine, 2007.

14. Czisch M, Wehrle R, Kaufmann C, et al. Functional MRI during sleep: BOLD signal decreases and their electrophysiological correlates. *Eur J Neurosci.* 2004;**20**(2):566–74.

15. Czisch M, Wetter TC, Kaufmann C, et al. Altered processing of acoustic stimuli during sleep: reduced auditory activation and visual deactivation detected by a combined fMRI/EEG study. *Neuroimage.* 2002;**16**(1):251–8.

16. Portas CM, Krakow K, Allen P, et al. Auditory processing across the sleep-wake cycle: simultaneous EEG and fMRI monitoring in humans. *Neuron.* 2000;**28** (3):991–9

17. Bergmann TO, Molle M, Diedrichs J, Born J, Siebner HR. Sleep spindle related reactivation of category-specific cortical regions after learning face-scene associations. *Neuroimage.* 2012;**59** (3):2733–42.

18. Larson-Prior LJ, Power JD, Vincent JL, et al. Modulation of the brain's functional network architecture in the

transition from wake to sleep. *Prog Brain Res.* 2011;**193**:277–94.

19. Larson-Prior LJ, Zempel JM, Nolan TS, *et al.* Cortical network functional connectivity in the descent to sleep. *Proc Natl Acad Sci U S A.* 2009;**106** (11):4489–94.

20. Sämann PG, Tully C, Spoormaker VI, *et al.* Increased sleep pressure reduces resting state functional connectivity. *MAGMA.* 2010;**23** (5–6):375–89.

21. Horovitz SG, Braun AR, Carr WS, *et al.* Decoupling of the brain's default mode network during deep sleep. *Proc Natl Acad Sci U S A.* 2009;**106** (27):11376–81.

22. Andrade KC, Spoormaker VI, Dresler M, *et al.* Sleep spindles and hippocampal functional connectivity in human NREM sleep. *Neuroscience.* 2011;**31**(28):10331–9.

23. Koike T, Kan S, Misaki M, Miyauchi S. Connectivity pattern changes in default-mode network with deep non-REM and REM sleep. *Neurosci Res.* 2011;**69** (4):322–30.

24. Sämann PG, Wehrle R, Hoehn D, *et al.* Development of the brain's default mode network from wakefulness to slow wave sleep. *Cereb Cortex.* 2011;**21** (9):2082–93.

25. Dang-Vu TT, Desseilles M, Schwartz S, Maquet P. Neuroimaging of narcolepsy. *CNS Neurol Disord Drug Targets.* 2009;**8** (4):254–6.

26. Desseilles M, Dang-Vu T, Schabus M, *et al.* Neuroimaging insights into the pathophysiology of sleep disorders. *Sleep.* 2008;**31**(6):777–94.

27. Lemieux L, Salek-Haddadi A, Lund TE, Laufs H, Carmichael D. Modelling large motion events in fMRI studies of patients with epilepsy. *Magn Reson Imaging.* 2007;**25**(6):894–901.

28. Allen PJ, Josephs O, Turner R. A method for removing imaging artifact from continuous EEG recorded during functional MRI. *Neuroimage.* 2000;**12** (2):230–9.

29. Ives JR, Warach S, Schmitt F, Edelman RR, Schomer DL. Monitoring the patient's EEG during echo planar MRI. *Electroencephalogr Clin Neurophysiol.* 1993;**87**(6):417–20.

30. Angelone LM, Potthast A, Segonne F, *et al.* Metallic electrodes and leads in simultaneous EEG-MRI: specific absorption rate (SAR) simulation studies. *Bioelectromagnetics.* 2004;**25** (4):285–95.

31. Angelone LM, Vasios CE, Wiggins G, Purdon PL, Bonmassar G. On the effect of resistive EEG electrodes and leads during 7 T MRI: simulation and temperature measurement studies. *Magn Reson Imaging.* 2006;**24** (6):801–12.

32. Krakow K, Allen PJ, Symms MR, *et al.* EEG recording during fMRI experiments: image quality. *Hum Brain Mapp.* 2000;**10**(1):10–15.

33. Wibral M, Muckli L, Melnikovic K, *et al.* Time-dependent effects of hyperoxia on the BOLD fMRI signal in primate visual cortex and LGN. *Neuroimage.* 2007;**35** (3):1044–63.

34. Iannetti GD, Wise RG. BOLD functional MRI in disease and pharmacological studies: room for improvement? *Magn Reson Imaging.* 2007;**25**(6):978–88.

35. Richardson MP, Grosse P, Allen PJ, Turner R, Brown P. BOLD correlates of EMG spectral density in cortical myoclonus: description of method and case report. *Neuroimage.* 2006;**32** (2):558–65.

36. Goldman RI, Stern JM, Engel J, Jr., Cohen MS. Acquiring simultaneous EEG and functional MRI. *Clin Neurophysiol.* 2000;**111**(11):1974–80.

37. Lemieux L, Allen PJ, Franconi F, Symms MR, Fish DR. Recording of EEG during fMRI experiments: patient safety. *Magn Reson Med.* 1997;**38**(6):943–52.

38. Nöth U, Laufs H, Stoermer R, Deichmann R. Simultaneous electroencephalography-functional MRI at 3 T: an analysis of safety risks imposed by performing anatomical reference scans with the EEG equipment in place. *J Magn Reson Imaging.* 2012;**35** (3):561–71.

39. Bénar C, Aghakhani Y, Wang Y, *et al.* Quality of EEG in simultaneous EEG-fMRI for epilepsy. *Clin Neurophysiol.* 2003;**114**(3):569–80.

40. Mandelkow H, Halder P, Boesiger P, Brandeis D. Synchronization facilitates removal of MRI artifacts from concurrent EEG recordings and increases usable bandwidth. *Neuroimage.* 2006;**32**(3):1120–6.

41. Allen PJ, Polizzi G, Krakow K, Fish DR, Lemieux L. Identification of EEG events in the MR scanner: the problem of pulse artifact and a method for its subtraction. *Neuroimage.* 1998;**8**(3):229–39.

42. Nakamura W, Anami K, Mori T, *et al.* Removal of ballistocardiogram artifacts from simultaneously recorded EEG and fMRI data using independent component analysis. *IEEE Trans Biomed Eng.* 2006;**53**(7):1294–308.

43. Ellingson ML, Liebenthal E, Spanaki MV, *et al.* Ballistocardiogram artifact reduction in the simultaneous acquisition of auditory ERPS and fMRI. *Neuroimage.* 2004;**22**(4):1534–42.

44. Wan X, Iwata K, Riera J, Kitamura M, Kawashima R. Artifact reduction for simultaneous EEG/fMRI recording: adaptive FIR reduction of imaging artifacts. *Clin Neurophysiol.* 2006;**117** (3):681–92.

45. Laufs H, Daunizeau J, Carmichael DW, Kleinschmidt A. Recent advances in recording electrophysiological data simultaneously with magnetic resonance imaging. *Neuroimage.* 2008;**40**(2):515–28.

46. van Duinen H, Zijdewind I, Hoogduin H, Maurits N. Surface EMG measurements during fMRI at 3T: accurate EMG recordings after artifact correction. *Neuroimage.* 2005;**27** (1):240–6.

47. Debener S, Mullinger KJ, Niazy RK, Bowtell RW. Properties of the ballistocardiogram artifact as revealed by EEG recordings at 1.5, 3 and 7 T static magnetic field strength. *Int J Psychophysiol.* 2008;**67**(3):189–99.

48. Sijbers J, Michiels I, Verhoye M, *et al.* Restoration of MR-induced artifacts in simultaneously recorded MR/EEG data. *Magn Reson Imaging.* 1999;**17** (9):1383–91.

49. Niazy RK, Beckmann CF, Iannetti GD, Brady JM, Smith SM. Removal of FMRI environment artifacts from EEG data using optimal basis sets. *Neuroimage.* 2005;**28**(3):720–37.

50. Leclercq Y, Schrouff J, Noirhomme Q, Maquet P, Phillips C. FMRI artefact rejection and sleep scoring toolbox. *Comput Intell Neurosci.* 2011;**2011**:598206.

51. Snisarenko AA. The cardiac rhythm during waking and the various periods of sleep. *Hum Physiol.* 1978;**4**(1):79–83.

52. Negishi M, Abildgaard M, Nixon T, Constable RT. Removal of time-varying gradient artifacts from EEG data

acquired during continuous fMRI. *Clin Neurophysiol.* 2004;**115**(9):2181–92.

53. Srivastava G, Crottaz-Herbette S, Lau KM, Glover GH, Menon V. ICA-based procedures for removing ballistocardiogram artifacts from EEG data acquired in the MRI scanner. *Neuroimage.* 2005;**24**(1):50–60.

54. Mantini D, Perrucci MG, Cugini S, *et al.* Complete artifact removal for EEG recorded during continuous fMRI using independent component analysis. *Neuroimage.* 2007;**34**(2):598–607.

55. Debener S, Strobel A, Sorger B, *et al.* Improved quality of auditory event-related potentials recorded simultaneously with 3-T fMRI: removal of the ballistocardiogram artifact. *Neuroimage.* 2007;**34**(2):587–97.

56. Daunizeau J, Grova C, Mattout J, *et al.* Assessing the relevance of fMRI-based prior in the EEG inverse problem: a Bayesian model comparison approach. *IEEE Trans Sign Proc.* 2005;**53**(9):3461–72.

57. Stern JM, Caporro M, Haneef Z, *et al.* Functional imaging of sleep vertex sharp transients. *Clin Neurophysiol.* 2011;**122**(7):1382–6.

58. Fukunaga M, Horovitz SG, van Gelderen P, *et al.* Large-amplitude, spatially correlated fluctuations in BOLD fMRI signals during extended rest and early sleep stages. *Magn Reson Imaging.* 2006;**24**(8):979–92.

59. Horovitz SG, Fukunaga M, de Zwart JA, *et al.* Low frequency BOLD fluctuations during resting wakefulness and light sleep: a simultaneous EEG-fMRI study. *Hum Brain Mapp.* 2008;**29**(6):671–82.

60. Spoormaker VI, Schroter MS, Gleiser PM, *et al.* Development of a large-scale functional brain network during human non-rapid eye movement sleep. *J Neurosci.* 2010;**30**(34):11379–87.

61. Kaufmann C, Wehrle R, Wetter TC, *et al.* Brain activation and hypothalamic functional connectivity during human non-rapid eye movement sleep: an EEG/fMRI study. *Brain.* 2006;**129**(Pt 3):655–67.

62. Dang Vu TT, Schabus M, Desseilles M, *et al.* Spontaneous neural activity during human slow wave sleep. *Proc Natl Acad Sci U S A.* 2008;**105**(39):15160–5.

63. Born AP, Law I, Lund TE, *et al.* Cortical deactivation induced by visual stimulation in human slow-wave sleep. *Neuroimage.* 2002;**17**(3):1325–35.

64. Christmann C, Koeppe C, Braus DF, Ruf M, Flor H. A simultaneous EEG-fMRI study of painful electric stimulation. *Neuroimage.* 2007;**34**(4):1428–37.

65. Kilner JM, Mattout J, Henson R, Friston KJ. Hemodynamic correlates of EEG: a heuristic. *Neuroimage.* 2005;**28**(1):280–6.

66. Horwitz B, Poeppel D. How can EEG/MEG and fMRI/PET data be combined? *Hum Brain Mapp.* 2002;**17**(1):1–3.

67. Rosa MJ, Daunizeau J, Friston KJ. EEG-fMRI integration: a critical review of biophysical modeling and data analysis approaches. *J Integr Neurosci.* 2010;**9**(4):453–76.

68. Pieger PJ, Greenblatt RE. Nonlinear analysis of multimodal dynamic brain imaging data. *Int J Bioelectromagn.* 2001;**3**(1)Available at http://ijbem.k.hosei.ac.jp/2006-/volume3/number1/greenblatt/index.htm.)

Chapter

Neuroimaging of wakefulness

1

Frederic von Wegner and Helmut Laufs

Overview

Wakefulness is defined as a set of brain states compatible with responsiveness, action planning and execution, the ability to (re-) direct attention, and the processing of information in higher-order cortices. This contrasts brain states characterized by natural (sleep), artificial (general anesthesia), or pathological (coma) reductions of vigilance. The physiological transitions between wake and sleep states are regulated by the central nervous system including the hypothalamic orexin system, the limbic system as well as systems controlling reward and metabolism [1]. Detailed accounts of sleep-specific changes in neural activity as seen by functional magnetic resonance imaging (fMRI) and combined electroencephalography (EEG)-fMRI can be found in recent review articles [2, 3] and the preceding chapters of this book. In the wakeful state, the brain generates a large number of neural processes that interact as a complex regulatory network and which can be grouped into functional modules characterized by anatomical connectivity and covarying levels of neural activity. The scope of the present article is to report results on spontaneous brain activity during wakeful rest, i.e., a task-free condition, rather than to present an exhaustive enumeration of the wealth of processes occurring during wakefulness, such as sensory processing, speech, and homeostatic regulation. Given that the experimental setting underlying the resting state actually represents a non-condition, i.e., is defined by the absence of a specific task, the resting state concept remains cloudy. Methodologically, the present article focuses on findings obtained with EEG and fMRI, either acquired separately or simultaneously. While the EEG signal reflects the electrical activity of cortical neuronal populations in the kHz range, the blood oxygen level-dependent (BOLD) fMRI signal reflects hemodynamic changes associated with neural activity covering the whole brain at a low temporal sampling rate (usually < 1 Hz).

EEG of wakefulness

The EEG hallmark of relaxed wakefulness is the alpha rhythm, an amplitude-modulated 8–12 Hz oscillation with the largest amplitudes during a relaxed eyes-closed condition and at occipital electrodes. This rhythm was already described in the publication of the first EEG recordings in 1929 [4]. The amplitude of the alpha rhythm diminishes drastically and almost immediately upon eye opening or with the onset of a cognitive task [4]. This reduction in amplitude is interpreted as a desynchronization of the oscillatory generators, in other words, the generators oscillate synchronously during rest and desynchronize with the onset of processing. The alpha rhythm was considered an "idling rhythm" [5], indicating a default pattern of cortical activity when the corresponding area is task-free, but ready to react. A contrasting interpretation states that the negative correlation of alpha band amplitude and task engagement reflects an active inhibitory process [6]. During wakefulness, the main oscillations besides the alpha rhythm are the beta and gamma rhythms, related to a spectral peak in the 13–30 Hz range (beta frequency band) and a broadband activity in the 30–80 Hz range (gamma frequency band) of resting state EEG spectra [7]. Beta–gamma band activity is generally associated with attention and active cortical processing [7]. In order to describe the brain state of wakefulness, it is necessary to characterize related states such as drowsiness and sleep. Similar to eye opening or cognitive processing, the EEG correlate of transitions to states of reduced vigilance is the desynchronization of the occipital alpha rhythm and, to a lesser extent, the appearance of slower oscillations [8, 9]. During this transition to sleep, the EEG shows low-amplitude activity without distinct peaks in the frequency distribution. Studying the EEG of drowsy subjects reporting their subjective vigilance state, short periods of alpha desynchronization could be related to a floating sensation [9]. The authors concluded that, in the context of clinical studies, states of drowsiness should be avoided as they resemble certain pathological patterns. The similarity of low alpha amplitude patterns associated with reduced vigilance and those observed regularly in certain neuropsychiatric disorders was also discussed by Roth [10]. He noted that vigilance fluctuations are common during EEG recordings of healthy subjects and that the EEG of wakefulness is markedly non-stationary. The preceding discussion shows that alpha band amplitude cannot be interpreted as a vigilance marker on its own, as drowsiness on the one side and engagement in a cognitive task or in sensory processing on the other are likewise reflected by a marked decrease in occipital alpha activity. These results were summarized and quantified as a bell-shaped relationship between the vigilance level and alpha band amplitude by Ota *et al.* [11]. The transition from drowsiness to deeper sleep stages is marked by increased theta and delta band activity and the occurrence of

Neuroimaging of Sleep and Sleep Disorders, ed. Eric Nofzinger, Pierre Maquet, and Michael J. Thorpy. Published by Cambridge University Press. © Cambridge University Press 2013.

synchronization phenomena such as vertex sharp waves, sleep spindles, and K-complexes. A widely used set of EEG-based criteria to distinguish wake and sleep episodes is the reference manual for evaluation of clinical polysomnograms published by the American Association of Sleep Medicine [12]. A further subclassification of the transition states between wakefulness and light sleep is achieved by taking into account the fronto-occipital gradient of alpha power and the contribution of alpha band power to the total EEG power. Based on these classification schemes, a given time interval can be translated into a sequence of separate brain states with a length of (multiples of) 30 s. It is important to note that these are operational definitions of wake and sleep states designed to work with EEG recordings: the wake/sleep transition in terms of the subjective conscious experience, however, is not completely represented by these measures. Last but not least, it must be noted that wake and sleep states interact. Thus, the spatial patterns of BOLD activity during wakefulness are influenced by sleep homeostasis and, vice versa, the experiences during a wake period influence the brain activity during the subsequent sleep episode [13].

fMRI of wakefulness

In order to study spontaneous brain activity during wakefulness, and at the same time to minimize systematic confounds arising from task-related activations, a task-free condition is employed. The ensuing brain state is termed the "resting state." Resting state-specific activation patterns can be analyzed in different ways: (a) statistically contrasting the between-task (resting state) condition against the task condition ("reverse subtraction") yields a set of regions termed task-specific deactivations [14], (b) using data driven methods, mainly independent component analysis (ICA) to identify coherent and mutually independent activity patterns [15], (c) using non-fMRI modalities such as EEG-derived measures [16], surface electromyogram (EMG) [17], or other physiological measurements [18] as regressors in a generalized linear model of the BOLD signal. In the early years of resting state research, the search for task-specific deactivations yielded a set of brain regions termed the default mode network (DMN) [19], including the medial prefrontal cortex, the posterior cingulate cortex, the precuneus, and parts of the parietal cortex. The set of regions has been accredited special importance as it appears to be independent of the task against which the resting state condition is contrasted [20]. Complementary to the DMN, another, regionally non-overlapping network positively correlated to tasks was found and termed the anti-correlated network [14, 21]. Functionally, activity in the DMN has been related to the processing of internal or self-related information while the anti-correlated network has been associated with attention and working memory [20]. Closer inspection of DMN dynamics showed that DMN activity is reorganized, rather than deactivated during task initiation and performance [22] and that brain activity during relaxed wakefulness spontaneously switches between modes that were interpreted as an introspective (default) mode and an alert mode with the readiness to process changes in the internal or external environment [23]. Because of its link to self-related information processing, the role of the DMN during

wakefulness was investigated in a number of studies. The results of these studies showed that DMN activity at least partially reflects intrinsic patterns of brain activity unrelated to consciousness, as shown by intact DMN activity in states of reduced or absent consciousness (sleep, coma, anesthesia) [24]. Likewise, the combination of fMRI and fiber tract visualization using diffusion tensor imaging showed that the DMN as well as other resting state networks are reflected in the intrinsic white matter connectivity of the brain, i.e., that functional networks are at least partially determined by anatomy [25]. In accordance with these findings, correlated activity in the default mode regions cannot only be found during wakefulness but also across sleep stages. Tracking DMN functional connectivity during the wake-sleep transition and across sleep stages, however, it has been observed that cortico-cortical functional connectivity of DMN components decreases with increasing sleep depth and it has been suggested that these changes are functionally related to the simultaneous decrease in consciousness and external and internal awareness [26]. Similarly, analysis of DMN functional connectivity in deep sleep stages has shown that frontal areas functionally segregate from the parietal DMN areas compared to the functional connectivity pattern during wakefulness [27]. Apart from these findings, network integrity seems to be surprisingly stable across sleep stages [28, 29]. Behaviorally, it was found that activity in the DMN correlated with the subjective experience of mind wandering [30]. The EEG signature of mind wandering on the other hand is very similar to early sleep stages, showing increased power in the theta and delta frequency bands and simultaneous decreases in alpha and beta band power [31]. Thus, the switch from predominant alpha and beta band activity to theta and delta frequencies in the EEG does not appear to be equivalent to sleep onset, implying a loss of conscious mentation. To summarize, the mere existence of coherent activity in DMN components may not be a good indicator of the state of vigilance, whereas, e.g., the connectivity within the network may enhance our knowledge of the current brain state.

When extracting resting state networks from fMRI time series using ICA, it is generally observed that different subsystems of the brain spontaneously activate and deactivate without apparent external stimuli conditioning these systems to engage or disengage [15]. The identified subsystems were found to match networks characteristically involved in task processing, among them visual cortices, the auditory and sensorimotor systems, and the executive control network [15]. Using voxel-wise functional connectivity analysis, the set of networks representing functional brain modules could be reproduced, and further networks of still unknown functional relevance were described [32]. Comparing ICA components across sleep stages and between subjects, it was found that the principal resting state networks were consistent across subjects and that virtually all brain regions participate in spontaneous activity during wake and sleep [33]. It is still unclear how the temporal sequence of resting state maps evolves, which mechanisms determine the switches between different networks, and how they interact. Addressing these questions will certainly be the subject of future research, which might reveal different answers for different vigilance states.

Simultaneous EEG-fMRI of wakefulness

In the preceding paragraphs, two approaches to analyze resting state activity with fMRI were discussed, namely reverse subtraction (activity correlated with task deactivation) and ICA-based region analysis. A third way to explore resting state BOLD activity is to add information obtained with independent recording modalities, in particular EEG. When EEG and fMRI are recorded simultaneously (EEG-fMRI), fMRI activity patterns associated with EEG-defined brain states can be analyzed.

Relaxed wakefulness in the EEG is characterized by alpha and beta band oscillations. Using the instantaneous amplitude of the band-limited signals (the envelope of the oscillations) as regressors in generalized linear models of the BOLD signal, the brain regions showing a significant positive or negative correlation with the EEG regressor can be identified. Correlations between the EEG and the BOLD signals can either arise directly, i.e., when the brain region emitting the BOLD signal is at the same time as the source of the electrical activity recorded by the EEG, or they arise indirectly, when mediated by other neuronal structures or in case of a common source. Using the instantaneous alpha band power as a regressor, negative correlations with BOLD fluctuations are much more prominent than positive correlations. Negative correlations are widespread, but mainly concentrated in occipital regions [34–36]. It is important to note that this pattern occurs in a strict eyes-closed condition and can therefore not be explained by a combination of EEG desynchronization and processing of external visual information by occipital cortices as this occurs upon eye opening. Studies (statistically) isolating the effects of eye opening showed that alpha power modulation due to the open–close condition yields different BOLD maps than spontaneous (unrelated to the open–close state) alpha band fluctuations [37]. Further analyses revealed the existence of at least two characteristic subpatterns. While some experiments gave a bilaterally extended occipital pattern of negative correlations, others gave a bilateral frontoparietal pattern [38]. Spectral analysis of the EEG recordings showed that the frontoparietal pattern was associated with high beta and low theta band power whereas the occipital pattern occurred when the EEG contained significant theta band contributions and low beta power. Functionally, the frontoparietal pattern was interpreted as an attentional pattern. These results suggest two different states, an attentive state indicated by elevated beta power and an unattentive, possibly drowsy state indicated by low alpha activity and increased theta power [38]. Also in other studies, single-subject analyses showed a high variability between and even within subjects, and this variability was also reflected in different EEG frequency distributions [39] and sleep-related effects were discussed. Positive correlations between alpha band power and the BOLD signal, when found, were located in the thalamus, the insula, and the anterior cingulate [34, 40, 41]. Positive correlations in the thalamus are in accordance with classical and current models of alpha rhythm generation in thalamocortical circuits [42, 43]. In agreement with the idea that the occipital pattern may be related to vigilance drops, an identical map was found to be correlated to states of reduced vigilance by using an EEG-based vigilance classifier [44]. Furthermore, these states were associated with increased BOLD activity in the anterior cingulate and extended frontoparietal cortices, as well as decreased activity in the thalamus and small frontal areas [44]. The similarity of the results shows the actual relevance of vigilance fluctuations on the expression of BOLD activity patterns. Vigilance, e.g., as measured by EEG, should therefore be included in models of resting state brain activity, a strategy as of yet uncommonly pursued. Alpha oscillations alone, however, are not sufficient to characterize functional brain states during rest. Judging from cortical deactivations correlated to alpha band power, alpha oscillations were interpreted as a marker of inattention whereas activity in the beta frequency band was related to cognitive processes such as sensory perception [45]. As both high and low alpha band power can be accompanied by either high or low beta and high or low theta activity, alpha power alone is an unspecific and incomplete marker of the brain's resting state. Therefore, multifrequency models including the power modulations of all the main EEG frequency bands have been employed [46]. Based on the full EEG spectral information, after the elimination of the relatively high correlation between frequency bands the differential effects of single frequency bands can be analyzed. Using a different approach, Mantini and colleagues first extracted resting state networks with ICA and then computed the corresponding EEG frequency distributions. They found different spectral signatures for five typical resting state networks [47]. Concerning negative correlations with alpha band power, their findings are consistent with EEG driven analyses showing an occipital pattern in the presence of relevant contributions from theta and delta frequency bands, and the frontoparietal pattern in the presence of beta band activity [45]. fMRI maps similar to the classical resting state networks could also be reproduced using regressors computed from the temporal sequence of prototypical EEG topographic maps, termed EEG microstates [48, 49], reinforcing the claim of a link between resting state dynamics as seen by surface EEG patterns and fMRI. Eventually, a thorough analysis of EEG and fMRI patterns during wakeful rest yields a complex relationship where certain EEG patterns can be associated with different BOLD maps and vice versa [16]. Thus, both modalities represent different, but partially overlapping aspects of the same phenomenon, as opposed to an exact one-to-one correspondence of EEG and fMRI patterns.

Conclusions

During relaxed wakefulness the human brain exhibits non-stationary spontaneous activity reflecting a variety of brain states. Functional MR imaging in particular could demonstrate that spontaneously occurring activity patterns represent functional modules as expressed during the processing and execution of tasks. Since the early days of EEG research, it has been recognized that subjects during relaxed wakefulness exhibit episodes of drowsiness. The detection and classification of these drowsy states, however, is not as standardized as that of deeper sleep stages characterized by distinct EEG phenomena such as vertex sharp waves, spindles, or K-complexes. Desynchronization of the occipital alpha rhythm is an important EEG feature of early drowsiness or light sleep but at the same time it is not an unambiguous marker of reduced vigilance. Scalp EEG only incompletely reflects the brain state. Especially during drowsiness, a single EEG pattern can be associated with different subjective experience (alert, drowsy, unconscious). However, fMRI experiments including rest conditions bear the risk of relevant vigilance fluctuations that remain undetected unless EEG is recorded simultaneously. Considering the complex reorganization of cortical and subcortical neuronal activity observed during the descent to sleep, such vigilance-associated changes in the brain functional architecture can easily cover or be mistaken as those considered to arise due to the experimental condition. This can potentially generate false-positive results. In our own collective of healthy subjects participating in a resting state EEG-fMRI study, we have observed that 50% of the subjects present sleep episodes within the first 5 min of the recording. It is hence important to distinguish BOLD signal changes acquired during drowsiness or light sleep from those recorded during wakefulness in order to reduce the heterogeneity and increase the specificity of the obtained results. Additionally, the cognitive performance during a neuroimaging experiment is influenced by the wake-sleep cycle and is partially determined by the physiology of circadian dynamics including genetic factors [50, 51]. In conclusion, wakefulness is characterized by a complex interaction of neural processes that partially can be captured and operationally defined as different brain states by neuroimaging techniques. Spontaneous vigilance fluctuations are frequent and relevant because of associated global changes in neural activity and should thus be controlled for in neuroimaging experiments. The simultaneous recording of EEG with fMRI currently represents the most accurate and reliable method to assess an individual's vigilance state.

Acknowledgements

This work was funded by Bundesministerium für Bildung und Forschung (grant 01 EV 0703) and the Landes-Offensive zur Entwicklung Wissenschaftlich-ökonomischer Exzellenz (Neuronale Koordination Forschungsschwerpunkt Frankfurt).

References

1. Sakurai T. The neural circuit of orexin (hypocretin): maintaining sleep and wakefulness. *Nat Rev Neurosci.* 2007; **8**(3):171–81.

2. Dang-Vu TT, Schabus M, Desseilles M, *et al.* Functional neuroimaging insights into the physiology of human sleep. *Sleep.* 2010;**33**(12):1589–603.

3. Spoormaker VI, Czisch M, Maquet P, Jäncke L. Large-scale functional brain networks in human non-rapid eye movement sleep: insights from combined electroencephalographic/ functional magnetic resonance imaging studies. *Philos Transact A Math Phys Eng Sci.* 2011;**369**(1952):3708–29.

4. Berger H. On the electroencephalogram of man. *Electroencephalogr Clin Neurophysiol.* 1969; **Suppl 28**:37+.

5. Pfurtscheller G, Stancák A, Neuper C. Event-related synchronization (ERS) in the alpha band–an electrophysiological correlate of cortical idling: a review. *Int J Psychophysiol.* 1996;**24**(1–2):39–46.

6. Jensen O, Mazaheri A. Shaping functional architecture by oscillatory alpha activity: gating by inhibition. *Front Hum Neurosci.* 2010;**4**:186.

7. Freeman WJ. Origin, structure, and role of background EEG activity. Part 1. Analytic amplitude. *Clin Neurophysiol.* 2004;**115**(9):2077–88.

8. Loomis AL, Harvey EN, Hobart G. Potential rhythms of the cerebral cortex during sleep. *Science.* 1935;**81**(2111):597–8.

9. Davis H, Davis PA, Loomis AL, Harvey EN, Hobart G. Changes in human brain potentials during the onset of sleep. *Science.* 1937;**86**(2237):448–50.

10. Roth B. The clinical and theoretical importance of EEG rhythms corresponding to states of lowered vigilance. *Electroencephalogr Clin Neurophysiol.* 1961;**13**:395–9.

11. Ota T, Toyoshima R, Yamauchi T. Measurements by biphasic changes of the alpha band amplitude as indicators of arousal level. *Int J Psychophysiol.* 1996;**24**(1–2):25–37.

12. AASM. *The AASM Manual for the Scoring of Sleep and Associated Events: Rules, Terminology and Technical Specifications.* Chicago, American Academy of Sleep Medicine, 2007.

13. Jedidi Z, Rikir E, Muto V, *et al.* Functional neuroimaging of the reciprocal influences between sleep and wakefulness. *Pflügers Arch.* 2011;**463**:103–9.

14. Raichle ME, Snyder AZ. A default mode of brain function: a brief history of an evolving idea. *Neuroimage.* 2007;**37**(4):1083–90; discussion 1097–9.

15. Beckmann CF, DeLuca M, Devlin JT, Smith SM. Investigations into resting-state connectivity using independent component analysis. *Philos Trans R Soc Lond B Biol Sci.* 2005;**360**:1001–13.

16. Laufs H. Endogenous brain oscillations and related networks detected by surface EEG-combined fMRI. *Hum Brain Mapp.* 2008;**29**(7):762–9.

17. van Rootselaar AF, Renken R, de Jong BM, *et al.* fMRI analysis for motor paradigms using EMG-based designs: a validation study. *Hum Brain Mapp.* 2007;**28**(11):1117–27.

18. de Munck JC, Goncalves SI, Faes TJC, *et al.* A study of the brain's resting state based on alpha band power, heart rate and fMRI. *Neuroimage.* 2008;**42**(1):112–21.

19. Raichle ME, MacLeod AM, Snyder AZ, *et al.* A default mode of brain function. *Proc Natl Acad Sci U S A.* 2001;**98**(2):676–82.

20. Buckner RL, Andrews-Hanna JR, Schacter DL. The brain's default network: anatomy, function, and relevance to disease. *Ann N Y Acad Sci.* 2008;**1124**:1–38.

21. Fox MD, Raichle ME. Spontaneous fluctuations in brain activity observed with functional magnetic resonance imaging. *Nat Rev Neurosci.* 2007;**8**(9):700–11.

22. Fransson P. How default is the default mode of brain function? Further evidence from intrinsic BOLD signal

fluctuations. *Neuropsychologia.* 2006;**44**(14):2836–45.

23. Fransson P. Spontaneous low-frequency BOLD signal fluctuations: an fMRI investigation of the resting-state default mode of brain function hypothesis. *Hum Brain Mapp.* 2005;**26**(1):15–29.

24. Boly M, Phillips C, Tshibanda L, *et al.* Intrinsic brain activity in altered states of consciousness: how conscious is the default mode of brain function? *Ann N Y Acad Sci.* 2008;**1129**:119–29.

25. van den Heuvel MP, Mandl RCW, Kahn RS, Hulshoff Pol HE. Functionally linked resting-state networks reflect the underlying structural connectivity architecture of the human brain. *Hum Brain Mapp.* 2009;**30**(10):3127–41.

26. Saemann PG, Wehrle R, Hoehn D, *et al.* Development of the brain's default mode network from wakefulness to slow wave sleep. *Cereb Cortex.* 2011;**21**(9):2082–93.

27. Horovitz SG, Braun AR, Carr WS, *et al.* Decoupling of the brain's default mode network during deep sleep. *Proc Natl Acad Sci U S A.* 2009;**106**(27):11376–81.

28. Horovitz SG, Fukunaga M, de Zwart JA, *et al.* Low frequency BOLD fluctuations during resting wakefulness and light sleep: a simultaneous EEG-fMRI study. *Hum Brain Mapp.* 2008;**29**(6):671–82.

29. Larson-Prior LJ, Zempel JM, Nolan TS, *et al.* Cortical network functional connectivity in the descent to sleep. *Proc Natl Acad Sci U S A.* 2009;**106**(11):4489–94.

30. Mason MF, Norton MI, Van Horn JD, *et al.* Wandering minds: the default network and stimulus-independent thought. *Science.* 2007;**315**(5810):393–5.

31. Braboszcz C, Delorme A. Lost in thoughts: neural markers of low alertness during mind wandering. *Neuroimage.* 2011;**54**(4):3040–47.

32. Power JD, Cohen AL, Nelson SM, *et al.* Functional network organization of the human brain. *Neuron.* 2011;**72**(4):665–678.

33. Duyn J. Spontaneous fMRI activity during resting wakefulness and sleep. *Prog Brain Res.* 2011;**193**:295–305.

34. Goldman RI, Stern JM, Engel J, Cohen MS. Simultaneous EEG and fMRI of the alpha rhythm. *Neuroreport.* 2002;**13**(18):2487–92.

35. Laufs H, Kleinschmidt A, Beyerle A, *et al.* EEG-correlated fMRI of human alpha activity. *Neuroimage.* 2003;**19**(4):1463–76.

36. Moosmann M, Ritter P, Krastel I, *et al.* Correlates of alpha rhythm in functional magnetic resonance imaging and near infrared spectroscopy. *Neuroimage.* 2003;**20**(1):145–58.

37. Ben-Simon E, Podlipsky I, Arieli A, Zhdanov A, Hendler T. Never resting brain: simultaneous representation of two alpha related processes in humans. *PLoS One.* 2008;**3**:e3984.

38. Laufs H, Holt JL, Elfont R, *et al.* Where the BOLD signal goes when alpha EEG leaves. *Neuroimage.* 2006;**31**(4):1408–18.

39. Goncalves SI, de Munck JC, Pouwels PJW, *et al.* Correlating the alpha rhythm to BOLD using simultaneous EEG/fMRI: inter-subject variability. *Neuroimage.* 2006;**30**(1):203–13.

40. Feige B, Scheffler K, Esposito F, *et al.* Cortical and subcortical correlates of electroencephalographic alpha rhythm modulation. *J Neurophysiol.* 2005;**93**(5):2864–72.

41. Difrancesco MW, Holland SK, Szaflarski JP. Simultaneous EEG/functional magnetic resonance imaging at 4 Tesla: correlates of brain activity to spontaneous alpha rhythm during relaxation. *J Clin Neurophysiol.* 2008;**25**(5):255–64.

42. Lopes da Silva FH, Hoeks A, Smits H, Zetterberg LH. Model of brain rhythmic activity. The alpha-rhythm of the thalamus. *Kybernetik.* 1974;**15**(1):27–37.

43. Valdes PA, Jimenez JC, Riera J, Biscay R, Ozaki T. Nonlinear EEG analysis based on a neural mass model. *Biol Cybern.* 1999;**81**(5–6):415–24.

44. Olbrich S, Mulert C, Karch S, *et al.* EEG-vigilance and BOLD effect during simultaneous EEG/fMRI measurement. *Neuroimage.* 2009;**45**(2):319–32.

45. Laufs H, Krakow K, Sterzer P, *et al.* Electroencephalographic signatures of attentional and cognitive default modes in spontaneous brain activity fluctuations at rest. *Proc Natl Acad Sci U S A.* 2003;**100**(19):11053–8.

46. de Munck JC, Goncalves SI, Mammoliti R, Heethaar RM, Lopes da Silva FH. Interactions between different EEG frequency bands and their effect on alpha-fMRI correlations. *Neuroimage.* 2009;**47**(1):69–76.

47. Mantini D, Perrucci MG, Del Gratta C, Romani GL, Corbetta M. Electrophysiological signatures of resting state networks in the human brain. *Proc Natl Acad Sci U S A.* 2007; Aug;**104**(32):13170–5.

48. Britz J, Van De Ville D, Michel CM. BOLD correlates of EEG topography reveal rapid resting-state network dynamics. *Neuroimage.* 2010;**52**(4):1162–70.

49. Musso F, Brinkmeyer J, Mobascher A, Warbrick T, Winterer G. Spontaneous brain activity and EEG microstates. A novel EEG/fMRI analysis approach to explore resting-state networks. *Neuroimage.* 2010;**52**(4):1149–61.

50. Schmidt C, Collette F, Leclercq Y, *et al.* Homeostatic sleep pressure and responses to sustained attention in the suprachiasmatic area. *Science.* 2009;**324**(5926):516–19.

51. Vandewalle G, Archer SN, Wuillaume C, *et al.* Functional magnetic resonance imaging-assessed brain responses during an executive task depend on interaction of sleep homeostasis, circadian phase, and PER3 genotype. *J Neurosci.* 2009;**29**(25):7948–56.

Neuroimaging of phasic and non-phasic NREM activities

Thien Thanh Dang-Vu

Introduction

The majority of functional neuroimaging studies of normal human sleep have compared brain activity patterns between stages of sleep and wakefulness [1, 2]. Most of these studies resorted to positron emission tomography (PET) to describe the differences in either regional brain glucose metabolism (CMRglu) – with ^{18}F-fluorodeoxyglucose (^{18}F-FDG) – or regional cerebral blood flow (rCBF) – with ^{15}O-water ($H_2^{15}O$) – across the sleep/wake cycle. Likewise some functional magnetic resonance imaging (fMRI) studies, using a block-design, compared blood oxygen level-dependent (BOLD) responses between sleep stages, in particular non-rapid eye movement (NREM) sleep, and wakefulness [3].

The superior temporal resolution of fMRI allows assessing activations directly related to neural events within sleep stages. Sleep microarchitecture is indeed constituted by spontaneous brain oscillations, i.e., spindles and slow waves during NREM sleep [4]. These oscillations not only organize phasic brain activity during sleep, but also potentially modulate important functional properties of sleep. Electrophysiological data for instance suggest that spindles [5, 6] and slow waves [7] affect the processing of external stimulation during sleep, while behavioral studies consistently show some evidence for a role of these rhythms in sleep-dependent memory consolidation [8, 9]. Investigation of phasic NREM activities is thus of prime importance for the understanding of sleep regulation and functions.

The aim of the present chapter is to review functional brain imaging studies – using PET and fMRI – that have examined neural activity patterns between NREM sleep and wakefulness, and within NREM sleep in association with phasic neuronal oscillations. Recent fMRI data investigating the relationship between these rhythms and the processing of external stimulation during sleep will also be detailed.

Neuroimaging of NREM sleep as compared to wakefulness

Global and regional brain activity patterns characteristic of NREM sleep – taken as a whole – were obtained with PET (using $H_2^{15}O$ or ^{18}F-FDG) [10–15] and fMRI [3, 16]. These studies compared NREM sleep to REM sleep and/or wakefulness and showed a decrease in brain activity during NREM

sleep both at a global [14] and regional [1, 10] level. They are reviewed and discussed in detail elsewhere [1, 2].

PET studies found a global decrease of brain glucose metabolism during NREM sleep when compared to wakefulness. Quantitatively, this decrease was estimated at around 40% during slow-wave sleep (SWS; stage N3 of NREM sleep) compared to wakefulness [14]. This drop is in agreement with the concept of a homeostatic need for brain energy recovery. Subsequent PET studies then showed that this reduction was not homogeneously distributed. Indeed, regional decreases of CBF or CMRglu were located in the brainstem, thalamus, basal forebrain, basal ganglia, and cerebellum, as well as in associative cortices (prefrontal, anterior cingulate, precuneus) [1, 10–13] (Figure 12.1). One PET study also showed a relative increase of CMRglu during NREM sleep in the hippocampus after controlling for declines in absolute metabolism for the whole brain [15].

Brain structures that decreased their activity during NREM sleep include neuronal populations involved in arousal and awakening, as well as areas which are among the most active during wakefulness [1]. Their deactivation during NREM sleep is therefore in line with a facilitation of sleep-promoting processes and a local homeostatic regulation. In addition, structures such as the brainstem and thalamus are involved in the generation of NREM sleep oscillations (see below). At the cortical level, deactivation patterns were circumscribed to associative cortices, particularly in the ventromedial prefrontal cortex, encompassing the orbitofrontal and anterior cingulate gyri. These cortical areas are involved in many complex cognitive processes during wakefulness, such as decision-making and action monitoring, and are thus amongst the most solicited brain areas at wake. They are also major sites for the regulation of NREM sleep rhythms, in particular for slow-wave initiation [17]. In contrast, primary cortices were the least deactivated cortical areas during NREM sleep. The relative preservation of activity in these areas might allow them to remain responsive to external stimulation during sleep (see below).

Neuroimaging of NREM phasic activities

Brain activity during NREM sleep is not uniformly organized, but rather constituted by spontaneous and coalescent brain oscillations, mainly consisting of spindles and slow waves [4]. In humans, spindles appear on scalp electroencephalographic

Neuroimaging of Sleep and Sleep Disorders, ed. Eric Nofzinger, Pierre Maquet, and Michael J. Thorpy. Published by Cambridge University Press. © Cambridge University Press 2013.

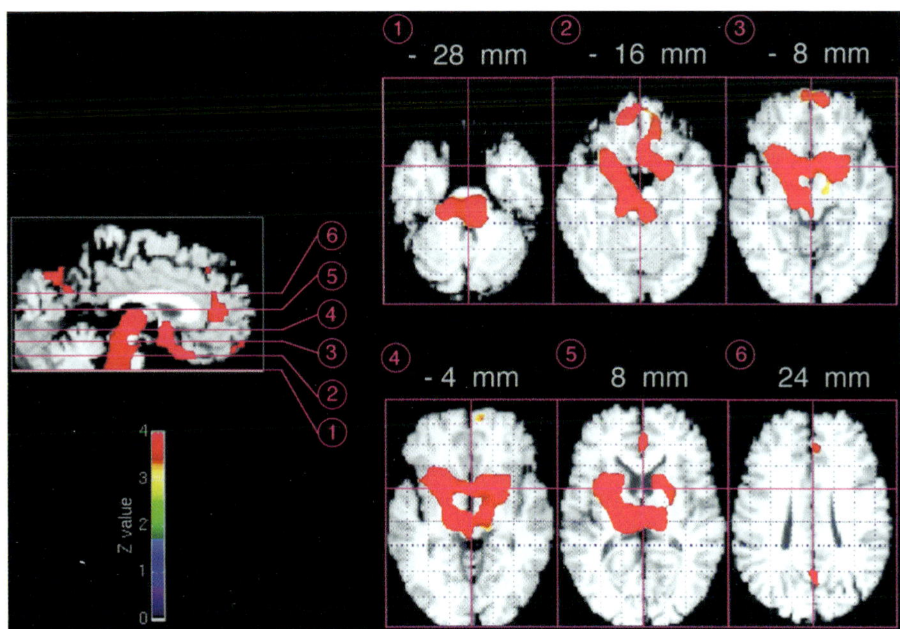

Figure 12.1 Neural correlates of NREM sleep. H$_2$^{15}O-PET study showing brain areas in which rCBF decreased during NREM sleep as compared to wakefulness and REM sleep. Image sections are displayed on different levels of the z-axis as indicated at the top of each picture. The color scale indicates the range of Z values for the activated voxels, superimposed on a canonical T1-weighted MRI image. Displayed voxels were significant at P < 0.05 after correction for multiple comparisons. (Adapted from Maquet P, Degueldre C, Delfiore G, Aerts J, Peters JM, Luxen A, Franck G. Functional neuroanatomy of human slow-wave sleep. *J Neurosci.* 1997;**17**(8):2807–12 with permission.)

(EEG) recordings as waxing-and-waning waves oscillating at a frequency of 11–15 Hz, and lasting more than 0.5 s [18]. Spindles are predominant during NREM sleep stage N2 but also persist in deeper stages of NREM sleep, during which they are progressively replaced by slow waves. The latter are defined as low frequency (0.5–4 Hz), high amplitude (peak-to-peak > 75 μV) waves prominent during SWS.

NREM sleep oscillations were initially described in electrophysiological studies in cats, as rhythms produced through the interplay of synaptic mechanisms and voltage-gated currents in thalamic and cortical structures [4]. Sleep spindle generation was shown to be tightly dependent on the thalamus [4]. In particular, a specific population of thalamic neurons located in the reticular nucleus were considered as "pacemakers" for spindle oscillations. Despite the observation that spindles can be generated within the thalamus in the absence of the cerebral cortex, it appears that the cortex is also critical for the initiation and termination of spindles [19]. The slow oscillation on the other hand was originally reported from intracellular recordings in anesthetized cats [20] and subsequently confirmed in naturally sleeping animals [21] and EEG recordings in humans [22]. Because it is absent in the thalamus of decorticated animals [23] but is still observed in the cerebral cortex after thalamectomy [24], the slow oscillation is considered as a cortically generated rhythm. The slow oscillation is composed of two phases: an "up" state characterized by neuronal depolarization and brisk firing, and a "down" state during which neurons are hyperpolarized and silent. The thalamus also plays an important and active role in shaping the slow oscillation [25]. This is the consequence of a synaptically induced effect of cortical discharges onto thalamic neurons during the neocortical slow oscillation [26, 27]. This synaptic reflection also facilitates the production of sleep spindles, resulting in the grouping of spindles by the slow oscillation up state [28].

In humans, NREM sleep rhythms were notably investigated by EEG topographical studies. Sleep spindles were shown to predominate on central and parietal leads with an average frequency of 14 Hz [29]. Less frequently, spindles can also be recorded on frontal derivations, at a slower mean frequency of 12 Hz. Slow waves can be recorded with EEG on almost any cortical area, and propagate in any direction, each wave following a unique pattern of propagation. However, they most often originate from frontal areas, reflecting current sources centered on the lateral sulci (e.g., insula), and propagate along the antero-posterior axis mediated by cingulate pathways [17, 30].

Altogether animal studies and human EEG recordings reported the cellular mechanisms and scalp topography of NREM sleep phasic activities, but they were not designed to highlight the neural networks consistently recruited by these oscillations at the whole-brain level. As detailed below, this topic was addressed by functional neuroimaging studies that allowed a non-invasive investigation of cortical and deep brain structures involved in the generation and modulation of spontaneous NREM sleep rhythms.

Neural correlates of sleep spindles

Functional neuroimaging studies of sleep spindles were conducted with PET and fMRI. Despite its limited temporal resolution, PET still allows correlation of rCBF values with EEG spectral power in the spindle frequency range as an indirect reflection of spindle waves. A negative correlation was thus found in six sleep deprived normal human volunteers between spindle EEG power and rCBF in the thalamus [31]. This result concurs with the central role of thalamic nuclei in the generation of spindles as demonstrated by animal studies. The negative direction of the correlation (i.e., the more spindle activity, the less perfusion in the thalamus) might be explained by the limited temporal resolution of PET: since spindles are coalesced with slow oscillation, the latter consisting of an alternation of neuronal hyperpolarization and depolarization, the negative pattern of correlation could be related to a more prominent metabolic impact of hyperpolarization phases over depolarization states when averaging rCBF across the entire scanning time. Another possibility is that the negative correlation would be directly related to electrophysiological mechanisms of spindle generation in the thalamus, e.g., the induction of inhibitory postsynaptic potentials in thalamocortical neurons. It should be noted that spindle EEG power might not be equated to spindles as discrete events: divergence between both measures were indeed observed [32].

Better temporal resolution of fMRI allows direct evaluation of brain activity patterns associated with the occurrence of spindle events. Fourteen healthy non-sleep-deprived volunteers were therefore scanned with simultaneous EEG and fMRI recordings during the first half of the night [33]. Spindles were detected offline on stages N2 and N3 EEG epochs after artifact correction, using an automatic detection algorithm: EEG signal was bandpass filtered in the 11–15 Hz range, and sleep spindles were detected on electrode Cz each time the root mean square (rms) of the filtered signal reached its 95th percentile [34]. The fMRI analysis then revealed the brain responses consistently associated with the occurrence of all detected spindles compared to the baseline activity of NREM

sleep stages N2–N3 on the selected epochs [33]. Significant brain responses time-locked to spindles were found in the thalamus (lateral and posterior parts), and in specific cortical areas including paralimbic (anterior cingulate cortex, insula) and neocortical (superior temporal gyrus) structures (Figure 12.2, central panels). Most importantly, all brain responses associated with spindles consisted of increases in BOLD signal compared to the baseline brain activity of sleep stages N2–N3. While PET data showed that NREM sleep – taken as a whole – is a state of brain deactivation compared to wakefulness, fMRI studies demonstrated that NREM sleep is also a state of transient and phasic increases of brain activity organized by sleep oscillations such as spindles. The activation of the thalamus is perfectly in line with the active role of this structure in spindle generation [4]. In addition a few cortical areas were identified as participating in the modulation of spindle sequences in humans. These cortical activations are well in agreement with computational data and intracellular recordings in animals showing the involvement of cortico-thalamic projections in the initiation and termination of spindles [19].

Since two spindle subtypes seem to emerge from topographical EEG studies – fast (centro-parietal) and slow (frontal)

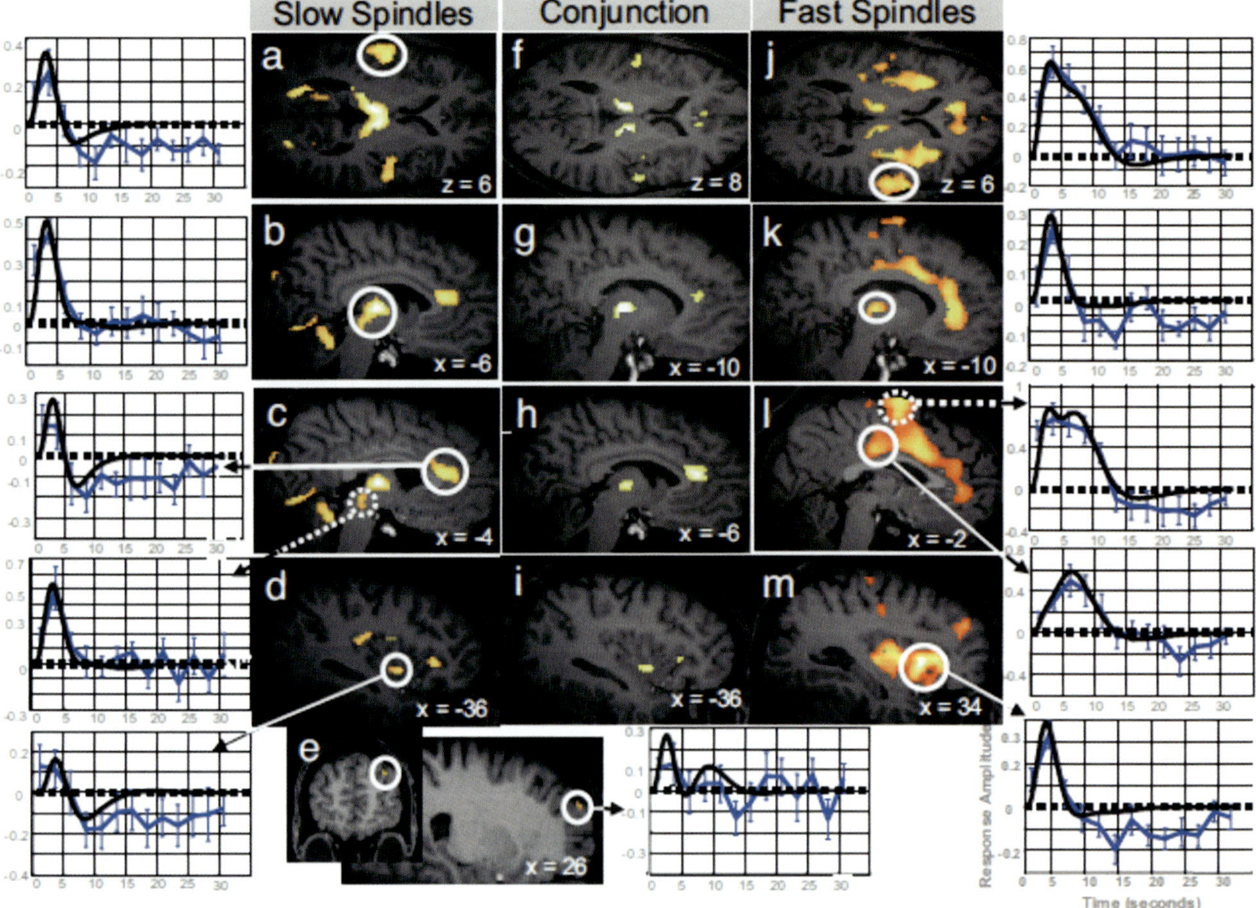

Figure 12.2 Neural correlates of spindles. This figure shows the fMRI responses associated with all sleep spindles (i.e., slow and fast; central panels, f–i), slow spindles (left panels, a–e), and fast spindles (right panels, j–m), as compared to the baseline brain activity of NREM sleep. Brain responses were significant at p <0.05, corrected for multiple comparisons on a volume of interest. The side panels show the time course (in seconds) of fitted response amplitudes (in arbitrary units) during spindles in the corresponding circled brain area. All responses consisted in regional increases of BOLD signal.(Adapted from [33]. Copyright (2007) National Academy of Sciences, U.S.A.)

spindles – fMRI studies also looked specifically at responses to these potential subtypes. Slow and fast spindles were thus detected using distinct bandpass filters on EEG channel Cz at 11–13 Hz and 13–15 Hz respectively [33]. Slow spindles displayed brain activations very close to the common spindle network (Figure 12.2, left panels). Fast spindles on the other hand showed a more diffuse cortical activation extending to somatosensory areas and mid-cingulate cortex (Figure 12.2, right panels) [33]. Contrasting brain responses elicited by the two subtypes of spindles revealed that fast spindles were associated with larger activation in precentral and postcentral gyri, medial prefrontal cortex and hippocampus. These results support the hypothesis of two spindle subtypes mediated by (partially) distinct neural networks. They also suggest specific roles for fast spindles: the activation of pre- and postcentral gyri potentially indicates a role in sensorimotor processing, and the activation of hippocampus and medial prefrontal cortex raises a possible contribution to sleep-related memory consolidation. Accordingly, another fMRI study demonstrated an increased functional connectivity between the hippocampal formation and neocortical areas during sleep stage N2, particularly in interaction with fast spindles [35]. In addition, brain regions activated during declarative learning were found reactivated during fast spindles of subsequent NREM sleep and in relation with spindle amplitude [36]. These data are in line with a possible transfer of information between hippocampus and neocortex during fast spindles.

Neural correlates of slow waves

The neural correlates of slow waves were also investigated using PET with correlations between rCBF and EEG spectral power in the delta frequency band (1.5–4 Hz) as a reflection of slow-wave activity [31]. Delta power was negatively correlated with rCBF in the thalamus, brainstem, cerebellum, anterior cingulate, and orbitofrontal cortex. Another $H_2^{15}O$-PET study, conducted on a larger sample and on non-sleep-deprived subjects, also found a negative correlation between rCBF and delta power in the ventromedial prefrontal cortex (including orbitofrontal and anterior cingulate gyrus) [37]. However, no correlation was found this time in the thalamus, brainstem, and cerebellum. Instead, other negative correlations were observed in the basal forebrain, putamen, insula, posterior cingulate gyrus, and precuneus. Although these results do not exclude a participation of the thalamus in the modulation of slow waves [25], they concur with the concept of slow wave as a cortically generated rhythm. These studies also confirm the prominent involvement of frontal and insular cortices in the initiation of slow-waves, as also shown by EEG data [17, 30]. As for the other brain areas, they belong to the set of neural structures found deactivated during NREM sleep compared to wakefulness [13], which suggests that the neural processes underlying slow-wave generation also shape the changes in brain perfusion across sleep stages. The negative pattern of the correlations might be due to a more pronounced influence of down states over up states when averaging the effects across scanning time.

In order to directly assess neural activations recruited by slow waves, 14 non-sleep-deprived volunteers were scanned with simultaneous EEG/fMRI following a procedure similar to the fMRI spindle study [33]. Slow waves were detected offline on the selected NREM sleep stage N3 epochs, using an automatic algorithm relying on amplitude (> 75 µV) and duration criteria applied on a bandpass-filtered (0.1–4 Hz) EEG signal [17, 18]. The analysis of fMRI data showed the brain responses consistently associated with the occurrence of all detected slow waves compared to the baseline activity of NREM sleep stage N3 on the selected epochs [38]. Significant brain responses were found in the frontal cortex (inferior and medial aspects), parahippocampal gyrus, precuneus, posterior cingulate cortex, brainstem, and cerebellum (Figure 12.3). All reported activations consisted in BOLD signal increases compared to the baseline brain activity of sleep stage N3, further confirming the persistence of phasic brain activity increases during the deepest stages of sleep. The frontal activation is in line with the frequent frontal site of initiation for slow waves from EEG studies [17]. The reported cortical activations are also corroborated by source modeling of high-density EEG data: large currents were indeed found in inferior and medial frontal areas, precuneus, and posterior cingulate cortex, in association with slow waves [30]. Brainstem activation, in the area of the pontomesencephalic tegmentum, appears more surprising given the well-known role of brainstem nuclei in arousal and awakening processes [4]. However, this area includes the locus coeruleus – a major noradrenergic nucleus – which was recently demonstrated to fire in phase with the cortical slow oscillation in naturally sleeping rats [39]. More precisely, locus coeruleus neurons preferentially fired during the transition from slow oscillation down to up state, thus potentially contributing to the cortical depolarization associated with slow waves.

The effect of wave amplitude was also evaluated by considering brain responses to medium- (75–140 µV) and high- (> 140 µV) amplitude slow waves respectively [38]. Medium-amplitude waves preferentially activated frontal areas, while high-amplitude waves were specifically associated with brainstem and parahippocampal activation. This suggests that a higher level of neuronal synchronization resulting in larger wave amplitude more consistently triggers the activation of mesio-temporal areas, which could potentially promote the offline consolidation of memories. Behavioral data indeed suggest a role for slow oscillations in declarative memory consolidation [8].

Interplay between NREM phasic activities and external stimulation processing during sleep

Among the major criteria that define sleep is the reversible lack of responsiveness to external stimulation. The brain is therefore commonly thought to be isolated from the environment in the descent to sleep, and particularly through the deepest stages of NREM sleep. In humans, a few functional neuroimaging studies investigated this topic by reporting the brain activations associated with acoustic stimulation during NREM sleep. An fMRI study found that sound-related activation in the thalamus

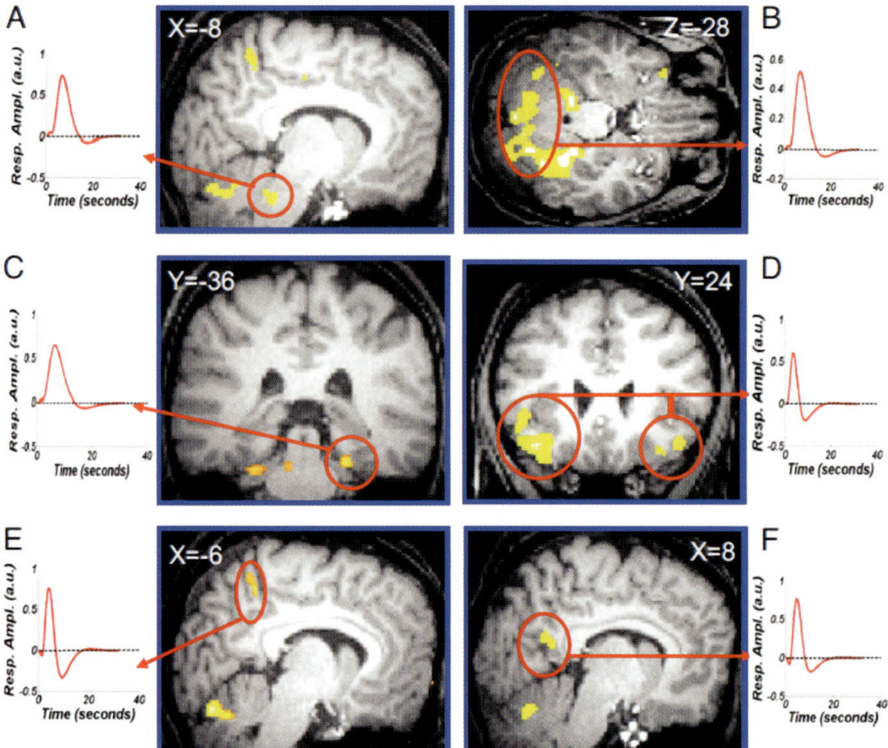

Figure 12.3 Neural correlates of slow waves. This figure shows the fMRI responses associated with slow waves, as compared to the baseline brain activity of NREM sleep. Brain responses were significant at p < 0.05, corrected for multiple comparisons on a volume of interest. Activations were located in the pons (A), cerebellum (B), parahippocampal gyrus (C), inferior frontal gyrus (D), precuneus (E), and posterior cingulate gyrus (F). The side panels show the time course (in seconds) of fitted response amplitudes (in arbitrary units) during slow waves in the corresponding circled brain area. All responses consisted in regional increases of BOLD signal. (Adapted from [40]. Copyright (2008) National Academy of Sciences, U.S.A.)

and auditory cortex persisted during NREM sleep [40]. In this study, two types of tones were presented: pure tones ("beep") and subject's own name. It was shown that the amygdala and prefontal cortex were more activated by the subject's own name than by pure tones, and more so during NREM sleep than during wakefulness. From this study, it appears that – in addition to being responsive to external stimulation – the sleeping brain might also be able to partially decode the content and emotional load of the stimulation. Results from a series of subsequent fMRI studies were, however, quite inconsistent with this finding: neural responses to acoustic stimulation were found decreased during NREM sleep as compared to wakefulness, in line with the concept of brain isolation from the environment during sleep [41, 42]. Moreover stimulus-related negative BOLD effects during NREM sleep were positively correlated with EEG power in the delta band, suggesting that "sleep-protective" deactivation is modulated by the level of neuronal synchronization [16]. In a study using visual stimulation during NREM sleep, brain activity decreases were also observed in the occipital cortex during stimulation [43].

Whether external stimulation during NREM sleep elicits a "sleep-protective" deactivation of primary sensory areas or on the contrary an activation of these areas reflecting a certain extent of cortical information processing thus remains controversial. However, none of these studies investigated the effects of ongoing neural activity – in particular NREM sleep oscillations – on the brain responses to environmental stimulation. Indeed it was shown in animals [44] and humans [45] that the processing of external sensory information is modulated by ongoing spontaneous brain activity. Representing the major spontaneous oscillations of NREM sleep, spindles and slow waves are

therefore in position to deeply modify the reactivity of large populations of neurons to external stimuli. This hypothesis is supported in humans by a few event-related potential (ERP) studies. When sounds were presented during spindles, the sleep-related increase of positive component P2 and decrease of negative component N1 were further enhanced [5, 6]. As for slow waves, it was shown that short and long latency components of somatosensory-evoked potentials were affected by the phase of the slow wave, increasing along the descending phase and decreasing along the positive slope [7]. ERP studies, however, did not unequivocally address the significance of these changes and were not designed to identify the neural structures involved in these processes.

In order to further explore this relationship between external stimulation and NREM sleep phasic activity, brain responses to pure tones delivered during NREM sleep were evaluated in a recent event-related fMRI study [46]. Pure tones ("beep," 400 Hz, 300 ms) were presented binaurally and randomly (70% probability of occurrence at each scan) during NREM sleep to 13 non-sleep-deprived young healthy volunteers, while simultaneous EEG/fMRI recording was acquired. Tones during NREM sleep (stages N2–N3) were classified offline according to their presentation outside (TN) or within detected spindles (TS) (Figure 12.4A). In agreement with Portas and colleagues [40], TN activated the primary auditory cortex and thalamus (Figure 12.4B, left panel), confirming that external stimulation is still processed in thalamocortical pathways during NREM sleep. Additional activations with TN were found in the brainstem (including areas compatible with the cochlear nuclear groups, the trapezoid bodies, and the superior olivary complex), cerebellum, middle frontal gyrus, precuneus,

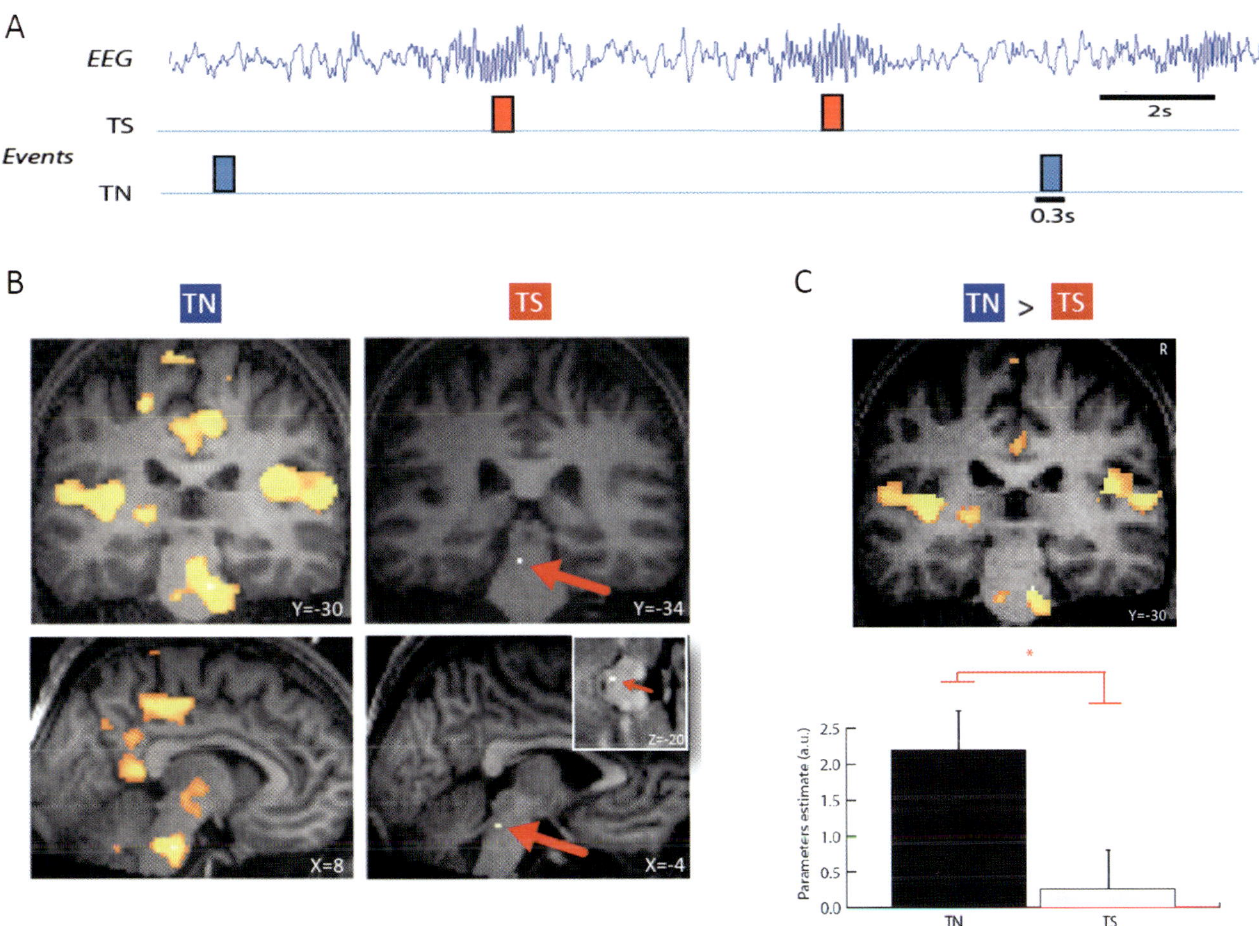

Figure 12.4 Spindles modulate the processing of auditory information during NREM sleep. (A) Tones were categorized according to their occurrence during NREM sleep stage N2–N3 within spindles (TS, red squares) or outside spindles (TN, blue squares). (B) The left panels show the fMRI responses associated with tones presented during NREM sleep in the absence of spindles (TN), including the primary auditory cortex, thalamus, brainstem, cerebellum, precuneus, and posterior cingulate gyrus. The right panels show the fMRI responses associated with tones presented within spindles (TS), confined to a small area of the brainstem (see arrow and inset). Brain responses were significant at $p < 0.05$, corrected for multiple comparisons on a volume of interest. (C) The top panel shows the fMRI responses significantly associated with TN, as compared to TS. The bottom panel shows the mean parameter estimates (arbitrary units ± SEM) for TN and TS in the primary auditory cortex (* $p \leq 0.05$). Larger responses were observed for TN as compared to TS in this area. (Adapted from [46]. Copyright (2011) National Academy of Sciences, U.S.A.)

and posterior cingulate gyrus. When brain responses associated with TS were examined, no significant activation was found, either in the primary auditory cortex or thalamus. Only a small area in the brainstem – encompassing the nuclei of the lateral lemniscus – was activated with TS (Figure 12.4B, right panel). The comparison between TN and TS showed that responses to TN were larger than those to TS in the primary auditory cortex (Figure 12.4C). These results therefore demonstrate that spindles affect the processing of external stimulation during sleep, reducing the consistency of transmission of sensory information to the cortex [46]. In other words, sleep spindles induce a distortion of sensory information, which results in isolating the cortex from the environment. This finding might contribute to explain the differences in sensitivity to noise during sleep across individuals. Another study accordingly showed that subjects with a higher density of spindles were more likely to preserve sleep stability when submitted to a variety of sounds during NREM sleep [47]. It is tempting to speculate which type of information is then processed during sleep spindles while the brain is

disconnected from the surrounding environment. Given the growing evidence that spindles are involved in sleep-dependent memory consolidation, it could be hypothesized that the brain functional isolation promoted by sleep spindles would facilitate the processing of endogenous information and thereby favor memory consolidation and brain plasticity.

In the same fMRI study, the relationship between auditory stimulation and slow waves was also explored [46]. It is well known that external stimulation during NREM sleep can trigger a slow wave on EEG recordings: such evoked slow waves, especially during stage N2, are also termed K-complexes. The functional significance of K-complexes remains debated; some authors suggesting that it reflects an arousal phenomenon, others a sleep-protective response, or finally a marker of sleep state (for review, see [48]). In order to address this question, tones delivered during NREM sleep (TN) were divided in two subcategories (TNK and TN0), according to whether or not TN was followed by an evoked K-complex [46]. Both TNK and TN0 were associated with the activation of the network recruited by

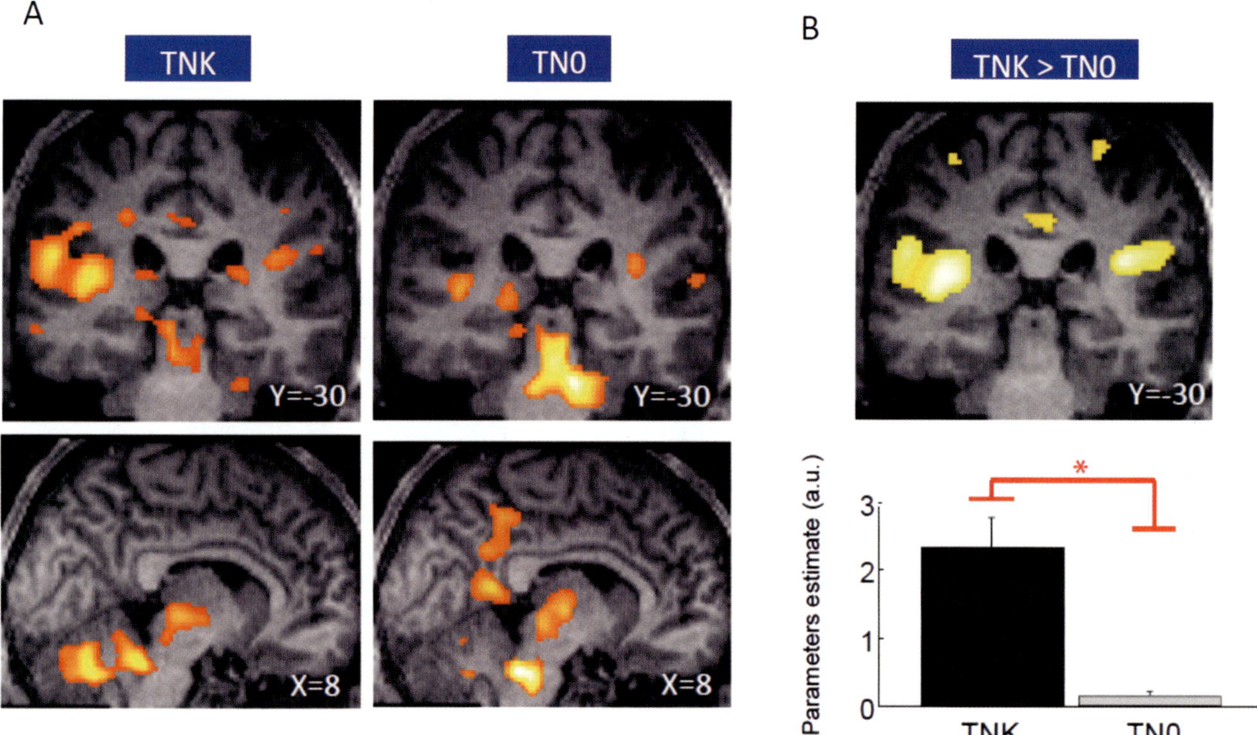

Figure 12.5 K-complexes and the processing of auditory information during NREM sleep. (A) Tones during NREM sleep stage N2–N3, outside spindles, were categorized according to the presence of a tone-induced K-complex (TNK) or not (TN0). The left panels show the fMRI responses associated with TNK, and the right panels those associated with TN0. For both TNK and TN0, those responses overlapped with areas recruited by TN (see Figure 12.4B). Brain responses were significant at p < 0.05, corrected for multiple comparisons on a volume of interest. (B) The top panel shows the fMRI responses significantly associated with TNK, as compared to TN0. The bottom panel shows the mean parameter estimates (arbitrary units ± SEM) for TNK and TN0 in the primary auditory cortex (* p ≤ 0.05). Larger responses were observed for TNK as compared to TN0 in this area. (Adapted from [46]. Copyright (2011) National Academy of Sciences, U.S.A.)

TN, i.e., primary auditory cortex, thalamus, brainstem, cerebellum, posterior cingulate gyrus, and precuneus (Figure 12.5A). The comparison between TNK and TN0, however, revealed larger responses in the primary auditory cortex with TNK (Figure 12.5B). Thus K-complex induced by sensory stimulation is associated with enhanced processing of the stimulus at the cortical level. These results are in agreement with those of a previous event-related fMRI study on 10 subjects using an acoustic oddball paradigm, which showed that rare tones followed by an evoked K-complex compared to those not followed by a K-complex were associated with the activation of various cortical areas including the auditory cortex [42]. Neuroimaging data therefore do not support the view of K-complex as an arousal phenomenon, but do not confirm either the concept of a sleep-protective inhibitory response to external stimulation. Instead these data demonstrate that stimulus-induced K-complex is in part reflected by a neural response specific to the sensory modality.

Conclusion

Functional neuroimaging data with combined EEG/fMRI have made possible the characterization of NREM sleep functional neuroanatomy beyond the conventionally defined sleep stages. From these studies, NREM sleep is not confined anymore to a mere state of brain rest and disconnection, but now appears as

an active state organized by phasic neural activities. These results, however, do not demonstrate that brain activity during NREM sleep overall reaches a level comparable to wakefulness. PET studies indeed consistently showed decreases in rCBF or CMRglu when comparing NREM sleep to wakefulness. Altogether PET and fMRI data rather suggest phasic increases of brain responses over a NREM sleep deactivated baseline activity.

Activations associated with sleep oscillations, as evidenced by functional neuroimaging, identify brain areas that are consistently recruited by these brain waves. They do not exclude the participation of other neural structures in the initiation or propagation of individual oscillations. High-density EEG studies for instance suggest that slow waves can originate from any cortical area, although preferential patterns of origin and propagation can be observed in agreement with brain imaging data [17, 30].

NREM sleep has classically been conceived as a state of brain isolation from the external world due to the blockade of incoming stimuli at the thalamic level. Recent functional neuroimaging results offer a contrasting view. On the one hand, they suggest that the sleeping brain is not disconnected from the environment but is still able to process sensory information at the thalamocortical level during NREM sleep. On the other hand, they demonstrate that spontaneous neural events in sleep, such as spindles, determine the fate of incoming external stimuli during sleep, and therefore might ultimately participate in the consolidation of previous experience. Beyond the impact of neuronal oscillations on the processing of sensory information, functional neuroimaging also shows that external stimulation during NREM sleep can in turn induce a stereotypical wave – the K-complex – that underlies larger stimulus-induced neural responses in primary sensory areas.

Acknowledgements

This research was supported by the Fonds National de la Recherche Scientifique (Belgium), the Fonds Léon Frédéricq (Belgium), the Belgian College of Neuropsychopharmacology and Biological Psychiatry, and the Canadian Institutes of Health Research.

References

1. Maquet P. Functional neuroimaging of normal human sleep by positron emission tomography. *J Sleep Res.* 2000;**9**(3):207–31.

2. Dang Vu TT, Desseilles M, Peigneux P, Laureys S, Maquet P. Sleep and sleep states: PET activation patterns. In: Squire LR, ed. *Encyclopedia of Neuroscience.* Oxford, Academic Press. 2009;955–61.

3. Kaufmann C, Wehrle R, Wetter TC, *et al.* Brain activation and hypothalamic functional connectivity during human non-rapid eye movement sleep: an EEG/fMRI study. *Brain.* 2006;**129** (Pt 3):655–67.

4. Steriade M, McCarley RW. *Brain Control of Wakefulness and Sleep.* New York, Springer, 2005.

5. Cote KA, Epps TM, Campbell KB. The role of the spindle in human information processing of high-intensity stimuli during sleep. *J Sleep Res.* 2000;**9**(1):19–26.

6. Elton M, Winter O, Heslenfeld D, *et.al.* Event-related potentials to tones in the absence and presence of sleep spindles. *J Sleep Res.* 1997;**6**(2):78–83.

7. Massimini M, Rosanova M, Mariotti M. EEG slow (approximately 1 Hz) waves are associated with nonstationarity of thalamo-cortical sensory processing in the sleeping human. *J Neurophysiol.* 2003;**89**(3):1205–13.

8. Marshall L, Helgadottir H, Molle M, Born J. Boosting slow oscillations during sleep potentiates memory. *Nature.* 2006;**444**(7119):610–13.

9. Schabus M, Gruber G, Parapatics S, *et al.* Sleep spindles and their significance for declarative memory consolidation. *Sleep.* 2004;**27**(8):1479–85.

10. Andersson JL, Onoe H, Hetta J, *et al.* Brain networks affected by synchronized sleep visualized by positron emission tomography. *J Cereb Blood Flow Metab.* 1998;**18**(7):701–15.

11. Braun AR, Balkin TJ, Wesenten NJ, *et al.* Regional cerebral blood flow throughout the sleep-wake cycle. An H2(15)O PET study. *Brain.* 1997;**120** (Pt 7):1173–97.

12. Kajimura N, Uchiyama M, Takayama Y, *et al.* Activity of midbrain reticular formation and neocortex during the progression of human non-rapid eye movement sleep. *J Neurosci.* 1999;**19** (22):10065–73.

13. Maquet P, Degueldre C, Delfiore G, *et al.* Functional neuroanatomy of human slow wave sleep. *J Neurosci.* 1997;**17**(8):2807–12.

14. Maquet P, Dive D, Salmon E, *et al.* Cerebral glucose utilization during sleep-wake cycle in man determined by positron emission tomography and [18]2-fluoro-2-deoxy-D-glucose method. *Brain Res.* 1990;**513**(1):136–43.

15. Nofzinger EA, Buysse DJ, Miewald JM, *et al.* Human regional cerebral glucose metabolism during non-rapid eye movement sleep in relation to waking. *Brain.* 2002;**125**(Pt 5):1105–15.

16. Czisch M, Wehrle R, Kaufmann C, *et al.* Functional MRI during sleep: BOLD signal decreases and their electrophysiological correlates. *Euro J Neurosci.* 2004;**20**(2):566–74.

17. Massimini M, Huber R, Ferrarelli F, Hill S, Tononi G. The sleep slow oscillation as a traveling wave. *J Neurosci.* 2004;**24** (31):6862–70.

18. Iber C, Ancoli-Israel S, Chesson AL, Quan SF. *The AASM Manual for the Scoring of Sleep and Associated Events.* Westchester, American Academy of Sleep Medicine, 2007.

19. Bonjean M, Baker T, Lemieux M, *et al.* Corticothalamic feedback controls sleep spindle duration in vivo. *J Neurosci.* 2011;**31**(25):9124–34.

20. Steriade M, Nunez A, Amzica F. A novel slow (< 1 Hz) oscillation of neocortical neurons in vivo: depolarizing and hyperpolarizing components. *J Neurosci.* 1993;**13**(8):3252–65.

21. Steriade M. Impact of network activities on neuronal properties in corticothalamic systems. *J Neurophysiol.* 2001;**86**(1):1–39.

22. Achermann P, Borbely AA. Low-frequency (< 1 Hz) oscillations in the human sleep electroencephalogram. *Neuroscience.* 1997;**81**(1):213–22.

23. Timofeev I, Steriade M. Low-frequency rhythms in the thalamus of intact-cortex and decorticated cats. *J Neurophysiol.* 1996;**76**(6):4152–68.

24. Steriade M, Nunez A, Amzica F. Intracellular analysis of relations between the slow (< 1 Hz) neocortical oscillation and other sleep rhythms of the electroencephalogram. *J Neurosci.* 1993;**13**(8):3266–83.

25. Blethyn KL, Hughes SW, Toth TI, Cope DW, Crunelli V. Neuronal basis of the slow (< 1 Hz) oscillation in neurons of the nucleus reticularis thalami in vitro. *J Neurosci.* 2006;**26** (9):2474–86.

26. Contreras D, Steriade M. Cellular basis of EEG slow rhythms: a study of dynamic corticothalamic relationships. *J Neurosci.* 1995;**15**(1 Pt 2):604–22.

27. Steriade M, Contreras D, Curro Dossi R, Nunez A. The slow (< 1 Hz) oscillation in reticular thalamic and thalamocortical neurons: scenario of sleep rhythm generation in interacting thalamic and neocortical networks. *J Neurosci.* 1993;**13** (8):3284–99.

28. Steriade M, Timofeev I. Neuronal plasticity in thalamocortical networks during sleep and waking oscillations. *Neuron.* 2003;**37**(4):563–76.

29. De Gennaro L, Ferrara M. Sleep spindles: an overview. *Sleep Med Rev.* 2003;**7**(5):423–40.

30. Murphy M, Riedner BA, Huber R, *et al.* Source modeling sleep slow waves. *Proc Natl Acad Sci U S A.* 2009;**106** (5):1608–13.

31. Hofle N, Paus T, Reutens D, *et al.* Regional cerebral blood flow changes as a function of delta and spindle activity

during slow wave sleep in humans. *J Neurosci.* 1997;**17**(12):4800–8.

32. Gais S, Molle M, Helms K, Born J. Learning-dependent increases in sleep spindle density. *J Neurosci.* 2002;**22**(15):6830–4.

33. Schabus M, Dang-Vu TT, Albouy G, *et al.* Hemodynamic cerebral correlates of sleep spindles during human non-rapid eye movement sleep. *Proc Natl Acad Sci U S A.* 2007;**104**(32):13164–9.

34. Molle M, Marshall L, Gais S, Born J. Grouping of spindle activity during slow oscillations in human non-rapid eye movement sleep. *J Neurosci.* 2002;**22**(24):10941–7.

35. Andrade KC, Spoormaker VI, Dresler M, *et al.* Sleep spindles and hippocampal functional connectivity in human NREM sleep. *J Neurosci.* 2011;**31**(28):10331–9.

36. Bergmann TO, Molle M, Diedrichs J, Born J, Siebner HR. Sleep spindle-related reactivation of category-specific cortical regions after learning face-scene associations. *Neuroimage.* 2012;**59**(3):2733–42.

37. Dang-Vu TT, Desseilles M, Laureys S, *et al.* Cerebral correlates of delta waves during non-REM sleep revisited. *Neuroimage.* 2005;**28**(1):14–21.

38. Dang-Vu TT, Schabus M, Desseilles M, *et al.* Spontaneous neural activity during human slow wave sleep. *Proc Natl Acad Sci U S A.* 2008;**105**(39):15160–5.

39. Eschenko O, Magri C, Panzeri S, Sara SJ. Noradrenergic neurons of the locus coeruleus are phase locked to cortical up-down states during sleep. *Cereb Cortex.* 2012;**22**(2):426–35.

40. Portas CM, Krakow K, Allen P, *et al.* Auditory processing across the sleep-wake cycle: simultaneous EEG and fMRI monitoring in humans. *Neuron.* 2000;**28**(3):991–9.

41. Czisch M, Wetter TC, Kaufmann C, *et al.* Altered processing of acoustic stimuli during sleep: reduced auditory activation and visual deactivation detected by a combined fMRI/EEG study. *Neuroimage.* 2002;**16**(1):251–8.

42. Czisch M, Wehrle R, Stiegler A, *et al.* Acoustic oddball during NREM sleep: a combined EEG/fMRI study. *PLoS One.* 2009;**4**(8):e6749.

43. Born AP, Law I, Lund TE, *et al.* Cortical deactivation induced by visual stimulation in human slow-wave sleep. *Neuroimage.* 2002;**17**(3):1325–35.

44. Arieli A, Sterkin A, Grinvald A, Aertsen A. Dynamics of ongoing activity: explanation of the large variability in evoked cortical responses. *Science.* 1996;**273**(5283):1868–71.

45. Boly M, Balteau E, Schnakers C, *et al.* Baseline brain activity fluctuations predict somatosensory perception in humans. *Proc Natl Acad Sci U S A.* 2007;**104**(29):12187–92.

46. Dang-Vu TT, Bonjean M, Schabus M, *et al.* Interplay between spontaneous and induced brain activity during human non-rapid eye movement sleep. *Proc Natl Acad Sci U S A.* 2011;**108**(37):15438–43.

47. Dang-Vu TT, McKinney SM, Buxton OM, Solet JM, Ellenbogen JM. Spontaneous brain rhythms predict sleep stability in the face of noise. *Curr Biol* 2010;**20**(15):R626–7.

48. Colrain IM. The K-complex: a 7-decade history. *Sleep.* 2005;**28**(2):255–73.

Functional connectivity in wakefulness and sleep

Victor I. Spoormaker and Michael Czisch

Functionally related networks of spontaneous fluctuations in the brain

In 1995, Biswal *et al.* [1] performed a functional magnetic resonance imaging (fMRI) study that was central to the development of fMRI functional connectivity analysis, with functional connectivity defined as the temporal coherence between neurophysiological signals measured in different brain regions [2]. Functional MRI activity analyses focus on the hemodynamic blood oxygen level-dependent (BOLD) signal response to an event or during a block of interest. Biswal *et al.* for instance performed a bilateral hand motor task and demonstrated activity in the left and right motor cortex, and in the supplementary motor area (SMA) [1]. However, they also noted the existence of spontaneous BOLD signal fluctuations during a run in which the subjects were instructed to simply rest and to refrain from any cognitive, language, or motor tasks as much as possible. When they correlated this spontaneous BOLD signal fluctuation during this resting state to all (measured) voxels in the brain, they observed a specific pattern of correlations in the ipsilateral and contralateral motor cortex, and the SMA [1]. This suggested that the spontaneous BOLD signal fluctuation has a neurophysiological origin.

Further research showed that these correlation maps of gray matter regions were confined to gray matter and did not occur in white matter or the cerebro spinal fluid, and that they were more specifically confined to gray matter regions sharing a similar behavioral function [3]. Motor cortex fluctuations correlated with ipsilateral, contralateral, and midline (pre-)motor areas, medial visual cortex fluctuations correlated with ipsi- and contralateral medial visual cortices, and the same applied to auditory cortices [4]. The application of independent component analysis (ICA) to fMRI data [5] further allowed model-free separation of multiple non-Gaussian sources and revealed the existence of multiple functionally related networks [6], which were through their acquisition in the resting-state referred to as resting state networks or simply resting networks. These resting networks were spatially consistent across subjects and importantly, across measurements in the resting state [7].

One intriguing feature of these slow fluctuations is their low frequency nature. Biswal *et al.* already reported a strong power in frequency bands lower than 0.1 Hz [1], with higher frequency

peaks representing heart rate or respiratory peaks. Here it is worth noting that the fMRI BOLD signal reflects a blurred and delayed hemodynamic response to neural events, which can cause higher frequency or broadband neural activity to become more pronounced in ultraslow frequencies (>0.1 Hz) in the BOLD signal akin to a low-pass filter [8]. However, such ultraslow fluctuations have also been detected by intracranial EEG and the correlation between fMRI BOLD signal fluctuations and physiological intracranial EEG fluctuations was moderate to high, indicating a potential electrophysiological source for these spontaneous BOLD signal fluctuations [9]. The coupling of intracranial EEG and spatial BOLD signal correlations was not only observed for intracranial EEG frequencies below 0.5 Hz, but also for delta (0.5–4.0 Hz) and gamma (>40 Hz) frequencies, although the latter coupling appeared vigilance-state dependent as it was observed in wakefulness and rapid eye movement (REM) sleep but not non-REM (NREM) sleep [9]. Such frequency coupling has recently been shown to occur throughout the human neocortex with the phase of lower frequency fluctuations affecting the amplitude of higher frequency bursts [10]. The fMRI signal may therefore well represent a slow cortical potential, as proposed by He and Raichle [11]; however, to date more research into the neurophysiological origins is required for such a conclusion.

Yet the consistency of fMRI signal correlations over subjects, time, and analysis methods strongly suggests a neurophysiological origin of the signal, and here it is important to realize that task-induced fMRI activity increases are typically a few percent points or less and that spontaneous fluctuations of similar strength may actually constitute the major part of the brain's energy consumption [3, 4]. Several resting networks have been described and can be divided into sensory/motor resting networks (e.g., sensorimotor, auditory, and visual networks) and into cognitive networks such as the dorsal and ventral attention networks, the frontoparietal networks and the "default mode network" (DMN) [6, 12]. The DMN, consisting of the medial prefrontal cortex, posterior cingulate, precuneus (and retrosplenial cortex and hippocampal complex), and the bilateral inferior parietal lobules, has received most attention because of its task-negative activity pattern and because of its proposed involvement in episodic memory retrieval [13], imagination of future outcomes [14], and internal versus external awareness [15], and its

---

Neuroimaging of Sleep and Sleep Disorders, ed. Eric Nofzinger, Pierre Maquet, and Michael J. Thorpy. Published by Cambridge University Press. © Cambridge University Press 2013.

possible role as a marker for psychiatric [16] and neurological disorders [17]. Moreover, an attention network is typically anti-correlated to the DMN: it shows the reverse time-course, which may represent a shift in cognition from internally oriented thoughts and mentations during rest to task-specific attention [4].

A relevant question is what happens to these resting networks in sleep, as their occurrence throughout sleep would indicate a disconnect of resting networks from cognition or even consciousness, and instead would suggest that if they have any function, this would be related to more general brain maintenance functions [3, 4]. Conversely, changes throughout sleep would suggest a vigilance-state dependency, and be indicative of a functional significance for cognition and consciousness. Here it is worth reiterating that specifically the DMN in relation to its anti-correlated attention network has been proposed critical to consciousness [15]. Interestingly, the DMN has been observed in anesthetized monkeys [18], which has often been used as an argument that the DMN is not relevant to consciousness. However, it is essential to note that this DMN presence in anesthetized monkeys considered posterior DMN nodes only, and that the typical human anterior–posterior midline coupling was not observed. In humans, as we will discuss later, anterior–posterior coupling is observed in wakefulness and light sleep but breaks down in deep sleep [19, 20]. Therefore, conclusions on the relationship between cognition and the DMN should not categorically look at whether it is "present" or "not present" but instead focus on spatial and temporal dynamics, and anti-correlations of the DMN.

Functionally related networks of spontaneous fluctuations in the brain in sleep

Previous EEG/fMRI studies have examined these resting networks also during sleep and reported that, in general, functional connectivity is maintained in light sleep. Horovitz *et al.* observed that DMN connectivity persisted in light sleep, and also found an increase in BOLD signal fluctuations in the visual and auditory cortices and the precuneus, among others [21]. An increase of activity in the left precuneus and bilateral inferior parietal lobules has been observed in early sleep stage 1 specifically [22]. Larson-Prior *et al.* reported no significant changes in functional connectivity in various sensory and cognitive resting networks from wakefulness to light sleep, while an increase in functional connectivity was observed in the dorsal attention network [12]. Sämann *et al.* [20] noted the continued presence of the DMN in light sleep (Figure 13.1), but with reduced contribution from the posterior cingulate, retrosplenial cortex, and parahippocampal gyri. These results are largely in line with EEG studies, which reported increased neocortical connectivity (EEG synchronization) in specific frequency bands during sleep [23–25]. At the same time, Sämann *et al.* observed a reduction in the anti-correlation between DMN and attention network regions already in light sleep [20], something that was corroborated by an analysis of Larson-Prior *et al.* [26].

A breakdown of intra-network connectivity was observed in slow-wave sleep, specifically in the correlation between the anterior and posterior nodes of the DMN [19, 20], with the posterior parietal areas maintaining or even strengthening their connectivity [19]. This long-distance breakdown of cortico-cortical connectivity in slow-wave sleep parallels a combined high-density EEG and transcranial magnetic stimulation (TMS) study during sleep [27], which reported that TMS-induced activation spread over the cortex during wakefulness but remained local in slow-wave sleep.

The breakdown in functional connectivity during slow-wave sleep is in accord with the fading of consciousness in NREM sleep [28], but the preservation or even increase in functional connectivity in light sleep stages appears more puzzling and counterintuitive. However, according to an information integration of consciousness, not the connectivity per se but the capacity of a network to integrate information is proposed critical for high complex cognitive functions such as consciousness [29]. This would mean that a possible increase in connectivity in light sleep could be compatible with fading consciousness if the network's capacity to integrate information would be reduced, which may occur due to exclusion of pivotal nodes (such as the thalamus) or increased randomness in the network. In order to examine such hypotheses, a focus on a large-scale functional brain network is required.

A large-scale functional brain network throughout sleep

Large-scale functional brain networks as derived from fMRI time-series can be examined by graph theoretical analysis; such analysis has revealed a small-world organization of human functional brain networks during wakefulness [30], with high local clustering and short path length [31] (see Table 13.1 for definitions). A small-world topology is a promising model for large-scale brain networks [32] as it supports both specialized processing in local clusters and integrated processing over the entire network [33]. Small-world properties of large-scale brain networks have helped in characterizing aging processes [34, 35], intelligence [36], psychiatric disorders like schizophrenia [37], and neurodegenerative disorders [38, 39].

In a recent study [40], we applied graph theoretical analysis on the correlations between extracted BOLD signal time-courses of atlas-defined cortical and subcortical regions [41] in wakefulness, light sleep stages 1 and 2 (S1, S2), and slow-wave sleep (SW), and we observed three patterns in the descent from wakefulness to SW. First, we found an increase in cortico-cortical connectivity in light sleep stages S1 and S2, but a strong reduction of cortico-cortical connectivity in SW. Second, thalamocortical correlation values sharply decreased in light sleep stage S1 and were partially restored in deeper sleep stages (Figure 13.2). Third, there was also a significant effect of sleep on small-world properties, in particular on local clustering values, which were highest in SW and lowest in S1 and S2 when compared to values of randomly rewired networks as a reference. Note that these differences all had a Bonferroni-corrected significance.

The decrease in thalamocortical correlation values was specific to light sleep stage 1. This stage has been proposed to signify a transition period rather than a sleep stage per se [42, 43];

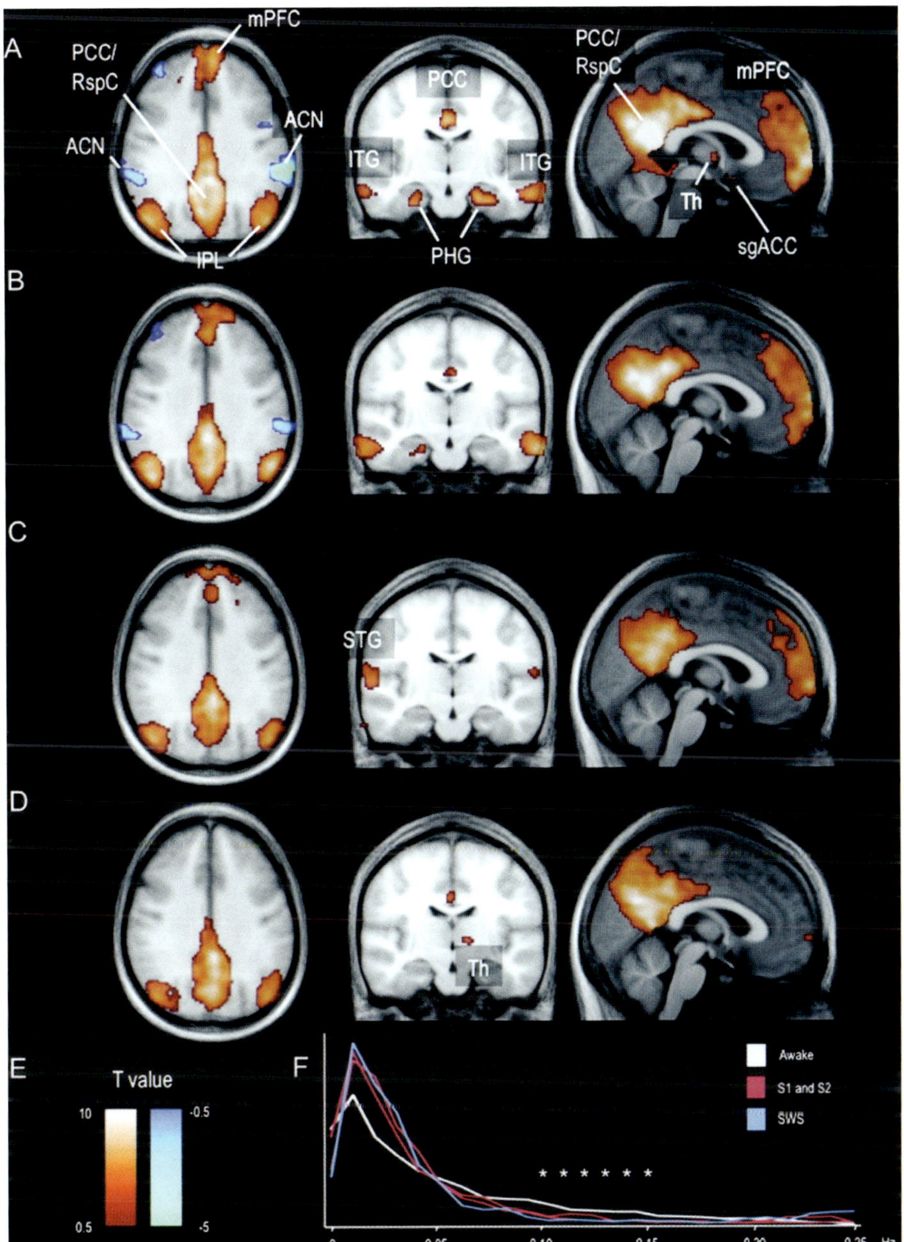

Figure 13.1 Default-mode network (DMN) connectivity (hot colors) with anti-correlated regions (cool colors) throughout wakefulness (A), light sleep stage 1 (B), light sleep stage 2 (C), and slow-wave sleep (D), with t-statistics (E), and temporal dynamics (F). Light sleep was characterized by a reduced contribution of the hippocampal complex to the DMN, reduced anti-correlations, and weakened although still detectable DMN connectivity. Slow-wave sleep was marked by a breakdown in correlations between anterior and posterior nodes of the DMN, and further tests revealed that these between-stage differences were significant at $p_{corr} < 0.05$. (Reproduced with kind permission from Oxford Journals, [20].) Pcc/RspC = posterior cingulate cortex/retrosptenial cortex; SgACC = subgenual anterior cingulate cortex; ACN = anti-correlated network; IPL = inferior parietal lobules; ITG = inferior temporal gyrus; PHG = parsahippocampal gyrus; TL = temporal lobe.

sleep stage 2 would reflect more consolidated sleep. Here the subclassification of stage 1 into early stage 1 sleep (stage 1a) and a deeper stage 1 sleep (stage 1b) may be informative, as auditory detection levels in stage 1a are comparable to waking levels whereas in stage 1b sleep they appear more reduced to levels typical for consolidated sleep [44]. An increase in thalamocortical correlation values in later sleep stages could be a consequence of sleep-specific phenomena either originating in the thalamus or mediated by the thalamus, such as sleep spindles [45, 46].

Moreover, the counterintuitive increase in cortico-cortical connectivity in light sleep is accompanied by a move towards randomness of the large-scale functional brain network. This is reflected in critical network properties such as the clustering coefficient that were closest to random network values in light sleep. The unspecific increase in functional connectivity in light sleep, paralleled with a more random network organization, limits its capacity to integrate information, in line with an information integration theory of consciousness [29]. In contrast, slow-wave sleep was characterized by a breakdown in cortico-cortical connectivity and by an increase in local clustering compared to random values. Although there were no significant differences for characteristic path length (topological distance between nodes), the correlation values of physical long-distance connections (> 75 mm) were sharply reduced in slow wave sleep. As a result, the large-scale functional brain network in slow-wave sleep demonstrated both high local clustering and fewer physical long-range connections, which reflects a move towards a regular network [47].

Hierarchy of the low-frequency network

We observed most pronounced changes in functional connectivity in higher-order association cortices [40], which is critical as these areas are typically involved in inter-modular whole-brain

Table 13.1. Definition of graph theoretical analysis

Term	Description	Graphical depiction
Degree	Number of connections (edges) per node in a graph/network	
Regular graph/ lattice	Graph in which each node has the same number of neighbors	
Random graph	Graph with randomly rewired edges	
Clustering coefficient	Extent to which a node's direct neighbors are connected with each other	
Path length	Shortest number of steps between two nodes in a network (1/efficiency)	
Small-world topology	Topology in which a network has an abundance of local connections and a few long-distance connections	
Modularity	Strength of partitioning of a network into different groups or communities	
Hierarchical clustering	Cluster analysis method that aims to generate a hierarchy of clusters typically displayed in a dendogram	
Hub	High-degree node	

integration rather than intra-modular processing. Interestingly, inter-modular hubs can show up as one separate cluster in a hierarchical cluster analysis [48]. Previous studies employing hierarchical clustering analysis on human functional brain networks have revealed a robust hierarchical organization in limbic, subcortical, and several neocortical clusters that have a functional and local proximity [49, 50], and we have observed a fair overlap between hierarchical clusters and reported resting-state networks in wakefulness [51]. There were 3 (out of 11) clusters indicative of such inter-modular integration in wakefulness, all consisting of long-range frontoparietal connectivity patterns. Because these frontoparietal regions are associated with some of the most

complex cognitive functions [52], we aimed to examine whether this inter-modular, frontoparietal connectivity would disintegrate in sleep [53].

A hierarchical cluster analysis indeed illustrated that frontoparietal clusters could be detected in wakefulness but not in deeper NREM sleep stages (Figure 13.3). This was quantitatively verified with a seed connectivity analysis in which we correlated the time-course of the left and right inferior parietal lobule to all voxels in the brain and observed reduced connectivity in all sleep stages compared to wakefulness in the medial superior frontal gyrus and dorsolateral prefrontal cortex. These frontoparietal clusters are the most likely candidates for inter-modular hubs

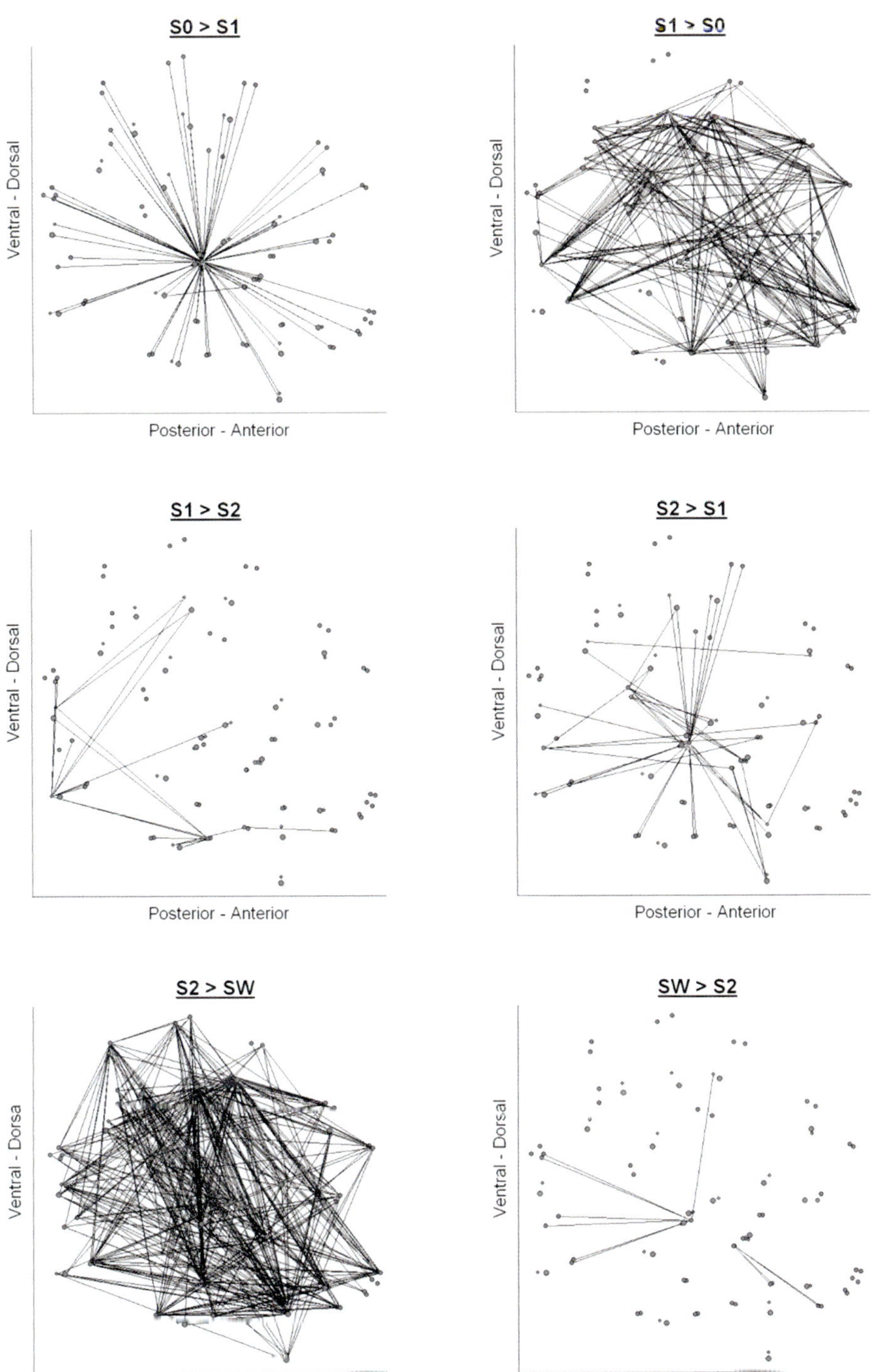

Figure 13.2 Differences in connections of 90 cortical and subcortical regions in the transition from wakefulness (S0) to light sleep stages 1 (S1) and 2 (S2) and slow-wave sleep (SW), with lines depicting a differential correlation value > |0.20| between two stages. Linear mixed models revealed that connectivity differences were robustly significant across sleep stages for neocortical regions but not for limbic/subcortical regions; the only subcortical region showing (Bonferroni corrected) significant differences across sleep stages was the thalamus. The reduction in thalamo-cortical correlation values in stage 1 sleep is illustrated in the upper left panel, and the lower left panel illustrates the reduction of neocortical connectivity in slow-wave sleep. There were no significant differences between stage 1 and 2 sleep. (Reproduced with kind permission from the Society for Neuroscience [60].)

[52], and their disintegration started already in sleep stage 1. This reduced connectivity is very dissimilar to the increase in func tional connectivity observed in light sleep stages [26, 40] and the increase in local connectivity in frontoparietal and visual networks, suggesting that a breakdown of long-distance frontoparietal connectivity may have functional significance. Whether reduced frontoparietal and thalamocortical connectivity are related remains an open question, but that may be likely due to the relay function of the thalamus in cortico-cortical connectivity [54]. We observed reduced connectivity of the inferior parietal lobule with other subcortical structures such as the caudate in sleep, which typically fluctuates with the thalamus in one subcortical network [6]. This appears in line with reduced frontoparietal–thalamus connectivity in propofol-induced anaesthesia [55]. In our data, we did observe reduced inferior parietal lobule–thalamus connectivity in sleep compared to wakefulness, but this did not survive whole-brain multiple test correction.

Slow-wave sleep showed a strong hierarchical clustering with a large number of local clusters, which was further supported by highest optimal modularity values in this sleep stage. Values were lowest for light sleep stages, with intermediate values for wakefulness, which is logical given the apparent randomization occurring

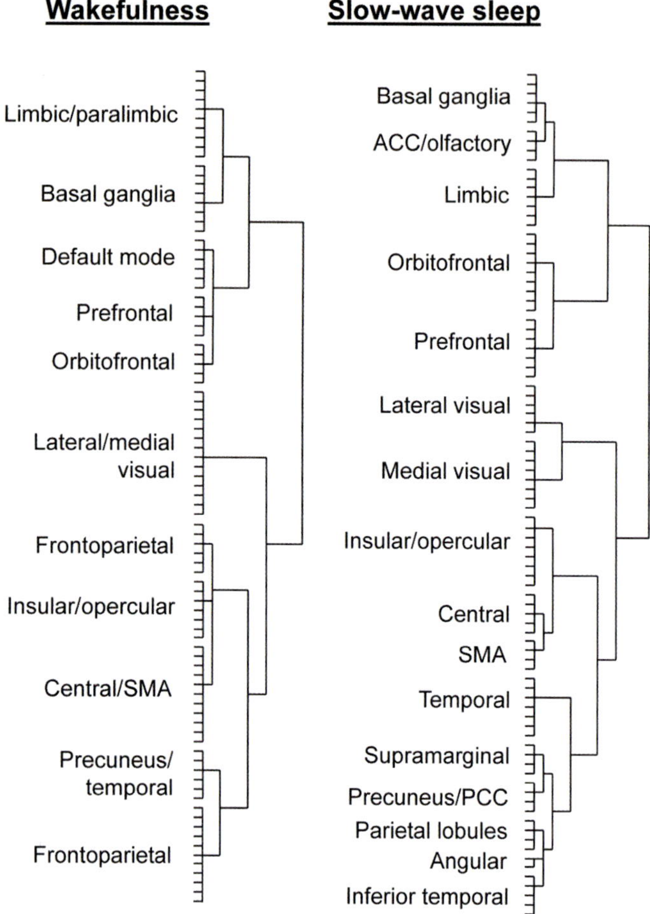

Figure 13.3 Hierarchy of a large-scale functional brain network in wakefulness and slow-wave sleep. Frontoparietal clusters were observed in wakefulness whereas slow-wave sleep was characterized by a high hierarchical clustering, resulting in multiple locally organized clusters. ACC = anterior cingulate cortex; PCC = posterior cingulate cortex; SMA = supplementary motor area.

in light sleep stages [40]. The increased community structure (and the more local hierarchical structure) in slow-wave sleep is indicative of a network optimal for processing information in segregated modules, and provides a context for previous reports on a reduction in anterior-posterior DMN coupling in slow-wave sleep [19, 20] together with a preserved or increased posterior node connectivity [19, 20, 56]. It is worth noting that between-stage differences in functional connectivity obtained through an anatomically based brain atlas [41] were corroborated by other brain atlases [53], including an atlas that used regions of interest with high functional connectivity in wakefulness [57].

Our findings show an increase in local community structure of a large-scale functional brain network with ongoing sleep that is accompanied by frontoparietal network disintegration. This resembles a move from sufficient global integration of separate clusters in wakefulness to poor global integration of separate clusters in slow-wave sleep. This dimensional transition from cluster synchrony to more global (but not full) synchrony has been modeled using the Kuramoto model of coupled oscillators applied to a structural brain connectivity matrix acquired with diffusion tensor imaging [58]. A particular subset of parameters was found to realistically simulate functional connectivity patterns according to the BOLD signal, for which subsets of nodes

synchronized (in local clusters) without global network synchronization [58]. It is possible that sleep reflects a move in parameter space resulting in less global synchrony in slow-wave sleep, with the sets of inter-modular frontoparietal hubs playing a critical role in this process.

Functional connectivity during phasic events in NREM sleep

The accurate detection of correlations requires a sufficient amount of time-points, which in combination with a typical repetition time of fMRI between 2 and 3 s means that several minutes of a particular vigilance state is needed for connectivity analyses. Given the typical fragmentation of sleep in the noisy and uncomfortable MR-scanner, finding a decent number of, e.g., 5-min long epochs in one sleep stage is a challenge in itself. Because of this, fMRI functional connectivity analyses have mostly focused on static sleep stages instead of phasic events during sleep, such as sleep spindles or slow waves.

However, if an event can be meaningfully modeled by the hemodynamic response function, as is the case for incidental spindles, one can analyze not only the activity associated with such phasic events but also the connectivity with other brain regions during such events. This can be done with a so-called psychophysiological interaction analysis, which in SPM software has been designed to evaluate how regions are differentially connected during a particular stimulus or task-block. Naturally one can replace the stimulus or task-block by a physiological event as detected in the EEG, as for instance a sleep spindle. It is important to realize that such interaction analyses are restricted to regions of interest, as it requires input from both stimulus (or physiological event) timing and from the spontaneous BOLD signal fluctuation in the region of interest. This spontaneous fluctuation can be assumed to be the hemodynamic response to neural events, and in a psycho- or physiophysiological interaction the BOLD signal is deconvolved in order to closer approximate the underlying neural activity in this region. This estimation of spontaneous neural activity is – together with the neurophysiological signal – used to generate a new variable, the psychophysiological interaction regressor. Depending on which contrast is entered during the construction, this regressor reflects increased connectivity during the neurophysiological event or during baseline.

In one recent study, we performed such an analysis with the spontaneous BOLD signal fluctuation in a hippocampal subregion, the subiculum, with fast sleep spindles as the physiological event of interest [59]. In line with previous studies focusing on regions showing increased activation in association with fast sleep spindles [45], there was increased activity in the anterior and posterior cingulate gyri and temporal cortices, but not in the hippocampus. This shows that the hippocampus itself does not show increased activity in response to fast spindles (Figure 13.4A). However, the hemodynamic response to the interaction regressor – i.e., the interaction between the subiculum time-course and sleep spindles – showed robust connectivity between the subiculum and widespread neocortical regions during spindles (Figure 13.4B). This analysis demonstrates a promising application of fMRI functional connectivity analyses;

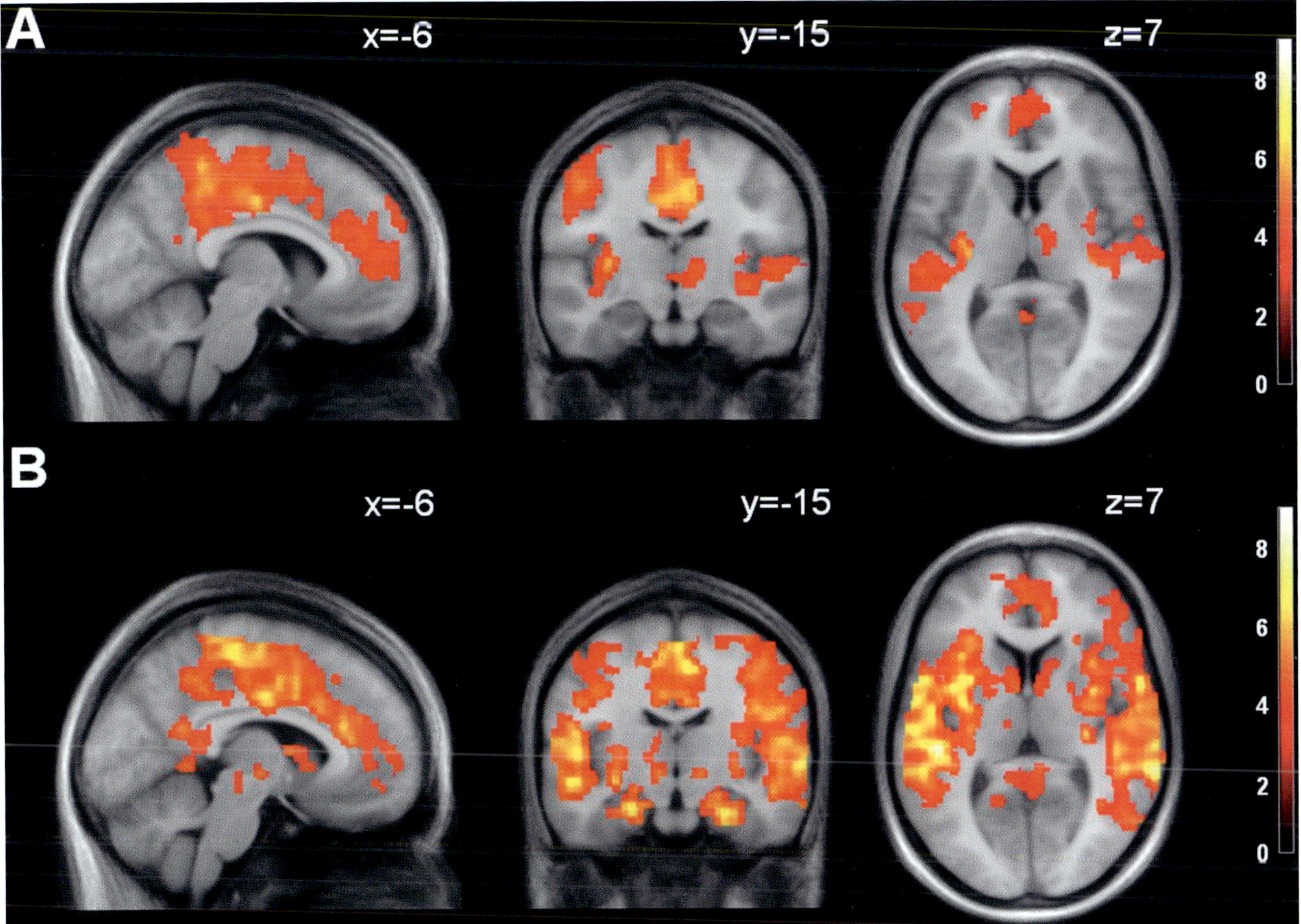

Figure 13.4 Regions with increased activity in association with individual sleep spindles (A) and regions with increased connectivity to the hippocampal subregion seed (subiculum) during sleep spindles (B), displaying a widespread connectivity pattern in neocortical regions. (Reproduced with kind permission from the Society for Neuroscience [57].)

regions may not show increased activation to a particular event even though they have increased connectivity patterns during the event, which may be relevant for hypotheses on hippocampal–neocortical transfer of information during sleep [60].

Note that in this study, there were no memory tasks performed before sleep, and therefore it is not possible to relate this increased connectivity with memory transfer; these results simply suggest an optimal state for hippocampal–neocortical connectivity (and possibly information transfer) during spindles. Another study focused on connectivity during sleep after face location association learning and observed increased functional connectivity in the fusiform gyrus during light sleep [61]. Moreover, connectivity between the fusiform gyrus and two clusters in the medial prefrontal cortex correlated with the pre- to post-sleep retention ratio of face-location associations. Such findings are promising and indicate an effect of learning on sleep, but caution in interpreting such results is warranted given the absence of a control group and the general increase in activity and connectivity of visual cortices in light sleep [19, 40, 62].

The connectivity results of the above studies have led some authors to suggest that connectivity analyses of sleep should be focused on phasic events rather than sleep stages; however, it is worth noting that phasic events cannot be studied from a whole-brain perspective. In our opinion, both analyses methods are needed in order to get a hypothesis-generating whole-brain overview, and then subsequentially to test specific hypotheses and regions in an approach focused on phasic events. Moreover, the former approach is more of interest for general information-theoretical models [28, 29] and the latter more for hypotheses on cognitive processes during sleep [60].

Overlap between functional connectivity and brain metabolism?

A final question to be addressed concerns the relationship between functional connectivity and brain metabolism [63] during sleep. There is considerable overlap between both measures, as is for instance illustrated by the overlap between fMRI activation patterns [64] and fMRI connectivity patterns in the transition from wakefulness to light sleep stage 1 [40]. Functional MRI activity analysis demonstrated deactivation of the bilateral thalamus during sleep stage 1 compared to wakefulness; the reverse contrast did not show any activation [64]. In our functional connectivity analysis [40], we could clearly see the reduction of thalamocortical connectivity that is presumably due to reduced thalamus activation (but not reduced correlations within the thalamus [26]). At the same time, we found increased cortical connectivity in sleep stage 1, in line with previous EEG and EEG/fMRI studies [12, 21, 23, 24]. This increased connectivity is not accompanied by increased activity; it simply reflects increased temporal synchrony between regions. In this manner, functional activity analysis revealed which region showed differential activity, and functional connectivity analysis showed what happened to the network when this critical node was removed. This demonstrates activity and connectivity are related but not the same, and that they describe two related but fundamentally different dimensions. However, to identify overlapping and differentiating information between functional connectivity and brain metabolism, more fine-grained analyses are needed preferably of multimodal neuroimaging data.

Conclusion

Although the neurophysiological origin of the fMRI BOLD signal is still poorly understood, spontaneous fMRI signal fluctuations show consistent spatial correlations in functionally related networks. The vigilance-state dependency of these functional connectivity patterns suggests a potential functional significance for cognition and cognitive processes. Functional connectivity of phasic events allows further spatial and temporal refinement of vigilance-state dependent connectivity patterns, and may be of special interest for phasic EEG events during sleep. Finally, although functional connectivity appears to overlap to a considerable extent with brain metabolism, these measures seem to represent correlated but different dimensions.

References

1. Biswal B, Yetkin FZ, Haughton VM, Hyde JS. Functional connectivity in the motor cortex of resting human brain using echo-planar MRI. *Magn Reson Med.* 1995;**34**:537–41.

2. Friston KJ, Frith CD, Liddle PF, Frackowiak RS. Functional connectivity: the principal-component analysis of large (PET) data sets. *J Cereb Blood Flow Metab.* 1993;**13**:5–14.

3. Fox MD, Raichle ME. Spontaneous fluctuations in brain activity observed with functional magnetic resonance imaging. *Nat Rev Neurosci.* 2007;**8**:700–11.

4. Fox MD, Snyder AZ, Vincent JL, *et al.* The human brain is intrinsically organized into dynamic, anticorrelated functional networks. *Proc Natl Acad Sci U S A.* 2005;**102**:9673–8.

5. Beckmann CF, DeLuca M, Devlin JT, Smith SM. Investigations into resting-state connectivity using independent component analysis. *Philos Trans R Soc Lond Biol Sci.* 2005;**360**:1001–13.

6. Damoiseaux JS, Rombouts SARB, Barkhof F, *et al.* Consistent resting-state networks across healthy subjects. *Proc Natl Acad Sci U S A.* 2006;**103**:13848–53.

7. Shehzad Z, Kelly AM, Reiss PT, *et al.* The resting brain: unconstrained yet reliable. *Cereb Cortex.* 2009;**19**:2209–29.

8. Niazy RK, Xie J, Miller K, *et al.* Spectral characteristics of resting state networks. *Prog Brain Res.* 2011;**193**:259–76.

9. He BJ, Snyder AZ, Zempel JM, *et al.* Electrophysiological correlates of the brain's intrinsic large-scale functional architecture. *Proc Natl Acad Sci U S A.* 2008;**105**:16039–44.

10. He BJ, Zempel JM, Snyder AZ, Raichle ME. The temporal structures and functional significance of scale-free brain activity. *Neuron.* 2010;**66**:353–69.

11. He BJ, Raichle ME. The fMRI signal, slow cortical potential and consciousness. *Trends Cogn Sci.* 2009;**13**:302–9.

12. Larson-Prior LJ, Zempel JM, Nolan TS, *et al.* Cortical network functional connectivity in the descent to sleep. *Proc Natl Acad Sci U S A.* 2009;**106**:4489–94.

13. Buckner RL, Andrews-Hanna JR, Schacter DL. The brain's default network: anatomy, function, and relevance to disease. *Ann N Y Acad Sci.* 2008;**1124**:1–38.

14. Andrews-Hanna JR, Reidler JS, Huang C, Buckner RL. Evidence for the default network's role in spontaneous cognition. *J Neurophysiol.* 2010;**104**:322–35.

15. Boly M, Phillips C, Tshibanda L, *et al.* Intrinsic brain activity in altered states of consciousness: how conscious is the default mode of brain function? *Ann N Y Acad Sci.* 2008;**1129**:119–29.

16. Greicius MD, Flores BH, Menon V, *et al.* Resting-state functional connectivity in major depression: abnormally increased contributions from subgenual cingulate cortex and thalamus. *Biol Psychiatry.* 2007;**62**:429–37

17. Greicius MD, Srivastava G, Reiss AL, Menon V. Default-mode network activity distinguishes Alzheimer's disease from healthy aging: evidence from functional MRI. *Proc Natl Acad Sci U S A.* 2004;**101**:4637–42

18. Vincent JL, Patel GH, Fox MD, *et al.* Intrinsic functional architecture in the anaesthetized monkey brain. *Nature.* 2007;**447**:83–6.

19. Horovitz SG, Braun AR, Carr WS, *et al.* Decoupling of the brain's default mode network during deep sleep. *Proc Natl Acad Sci U S A.* 2009;**106**:11376–81.

20. Sämann PG, Wehrle R, Hoehn D, *et al.* Development of the brain's default mode network from wakefulness to slow wave sleep. *Cereb Cortex.* 2011;**21**:2082–93.

21. Horovitz SG, Fukunaga M, de Zwart JA, *et al.* Low frequency BOLD fluctuations during resting wakefulness and light sleep: a simultaneous EEG-fMRI study. *Hum Brain Mapp.* 2008;**29**:671–82.

22. Picchioni D, Fukunaga M, Carr WS, *et al.* fMRI differences between early and late stage-1 sleep. *Neurosci Lett.* 2008;**441**:81–5.

23. Ferri R, Rundo F, Bruni O, *et al.* Small-world network organization of functional connectivity of EEG slow-wave activity during sleep. *Clin Neurophysiol.* 2007;**118**:449–56.

24. Ferri R, Rundo F, Bruni O, *et al.* The functional connectivity of different EEG bands moves towards small-world network organization during sleep. *Clin Neurophysiol.* 2008;**119**:2026–36.

25. Dimitriadis SI, Laskaris NA, Del Rio-Portilla Y, Koudounis G. Characterizing dynamic functional connectivity across sleep stages from EEG. *Brain Topogr* 2009;**22**:119–33.

26. Larson-Prior LJ, Power JD, Vincent JL, *et al.* Modulation of the brain's

functional network architecture in the transition from wake to sleep. *Prog Brain Res.* 2011;193:277–94.

27. Massimini M, Ferrarelli F, Huber R, *et al.* Breakdown of cortical effective connectivity during sleep. *Science.* 2005;309:2228–32.

28. Tononi G, Massimini M. Why does consciousness fade in early sleep? *Ann N Y Acad Sci.* 2008;1129:330–4.

29. Tononi G. An information integration theory of consciousness. *BMC Neurosci.* 2004;5:42.

30. Achard S, Salvador R, Whitcher B, *et al.* A resilient, low-frequency, small-world human brain functional network with highly connected association cortical hubs. *J Neurosci.* 2006;26:63–72.

31. Bullmore E, Sporns O. Complex brain networks: graph theoretical analysis of structural and functional systems. *Nat Rev Neurosci.* 2009;10:186–98.

32. Bassett DS, Bullmore E. Small-world brain networks. *Neuroscientist.* 2006;12:512–23.

33. Sporns O, Chialvo DR, Kaiser M, Hilgetag CC. Organization, development and function of complex brain networks. *Trends Cogn Sci.* 2004;8:418–25.

34. Meunier D, Achard S, Morcom A, Bullmore E. Age-related changes in modular organization of human brain functional networks. *Neuroimage.* 2009;44:715–23.

35. Supekar K, Musen M, Menon V. Development of large-scale functional brain networks in children. *PLoS Biol.* 2009;7:e1000157.

36. van den Heuvel MP, Stam CJ, Kahn RS, Hulshoff Pol HE. Efficiency of functional brain networks and intellectual performance. *J Neurosci.* 2009;29:7619–24.

37. Bassett DS, Bullmore E, Verchinski BA, *et al.* Hierarchical organization of human cortical networks in health and schizophrenia. *J Neurosci.* 2008;28:9239–48.

38. Stam CJ, de Haan W, Daffertshofer A, *et al.* Graph theoretical analysis of magnetoencephalographic functional connectivity in Alzheimer's disease. *Brain.* 2009;132:213–24.

39. Stam CJ. Use of magnetoencephalography (MEG) to study functional brain networks in neurodegenerative disorders. *J Neurol Sci.* 2010;289:128–34.

40. Spoormaker VI, Schröter MS, Gleiser PM, *et al.* Development of a large-scale functional brain network during human non-rapid eye movement sleep. *J Neurosci.* 2010;30:11379–87.

41. Tzourio-Mazoyer N, Landeau B, Papathanassiou D, *et al.* Automated anatomical labeling of activations in SPM using a macroscopic anatomical parcellation of the MNI MRI single-subject brain. *Neuroimage.* 2002;15:273–89

42. Johnson LC, Hanson K, Bickford RG. Effect of flurazepam on sleep spindles and K-complexes. *Electroencephalogr Clin Neurophysiol.* 1976;40:67–77.

43. Ogilvie RD, Simons IA, Kuderian RH, *et al.* Behavioral, event-related potential, and EEG/FFT changes at sleep onset. *Psychophysiology.* 1991;28:54–64.

44. Niiyama Y, Fujiwara R, Satoh N, Hishikawa Y. Endogenous components of event-related potential appearing during NREM stage 1 and REM sleep in man. *Int J Psychophysiol.* 1994;17:165–74.

45. Schabus M, Dang-Vu TT, Albouy G, *et al.* Hemodynamic cerebral correlates of sleep spindles during human non-rapid eye movement sleep. *Proc Natl Acad Sci U S A.* 2007;104:13164–9.

46. Steriade M, Contreras D, Amzica F. Synchronized sleep oscillations and their paroxysmal developments. *Trends Neurosci.* 1994;17:199–208.

47. Watts DJ, Strogatz SH. Collective dynamics of 'small-world' networks. *Nature.* 1998;393:440–2.

48. Pirgnano L, Diaz-Guitera A. Extracting topological Features from dynamical measures in netoworks of Kuranoto oscillators. *Phys Rev E.* 2012;85:036112

49. Ferrarini L, Veer IM, Baerends E, *et al.* Hierarchical functional modularity in the resting-state human brain. *Hum Brain Mapp.* 2009;30:2220–31.

50. Salvador R, Suckling J, Coleman MR, *et al.* Neurophysiological architecture of functional magnetic resonance images of human brain. *Cereb Cortex.* 2005;15:1332–42.

51. Gleiser PM, Spoormaker VI. Modelling hierarchical structure in functional brain networks. *Philos Transact A Math Phys Eng Sci.* 2010;368:5633–544.

52. Corbetta M, Shulman GL. Control of goal-directed and stimulus-driven attention in the brain. *Nat Rev Neurosci.* 2002;3:201 15.

53. Spoormaker VI, Gleiser PM, Czisch M. Frontoparietal connectivity and hierarchical structure of the brain's Functional network during sleep. *Front Neurol.* 2012;3:80.

54. Steriade M. Acetylcholine systems and rhythmic activities during the waking–sleep cycle. *Prog Brain Res.* 2004;145:179–96.

55. Boveroux P, Vanhaudenhuyse A, Bruno MA, *et al.* Breakdown of within- and between-network resting state functional magnetic resonance imaging connectivity during propofol-induced loss of consciousness. *Anesthesiology.* 2010;113:1038–53.

56. Koike T, Kan S, Misaki M, Miyauchi S. Connectivity pattern changes in default-mode network with deep non-REM and REM sleep. *Neurosci Res.* 2011;69:322–30.

57. Dosenbach NU, Nardos B, Cohen AL, *et al.* Prediction of individual brain maturity using fMRI. *Science.* 2010;329:1358–61.

58. Cabral J, Hugues E, Sporns O, Deco G. Role of local network oscillations in resting-state functional connectivity. *Neuroimage.* 2011;57:130–9.

59. Andrade KC, Spoormaker VI, Dresler M, *et al.* Sleep spindles and hippocampal functional connectivity in human NREM sleep. *J Neurosci.* 2011;31:10331–9.

60. Diekelmann S, Born J. The memory function of sleep. *Nat Rev Neurosci.* 2010;11:114–26.

61. van Dongen EV, Takashima A, Barth M, Fernández G. Functional connectivity during light sleep is correlated with memory performance for face-location associations. *Neuroimage.* 2011;57:262–70

62. Spoormaker VI, Czisch M, Maquet P, Jäncke L. Large-scale functional brain networks in human non-rapid eye movement sleep: insights from combined electroencephalographic/ functional magnetic resonance imaging studies. *Philos Transact A Math Phys Eng Sci.* 2011;369:3708–29.

63. Maquet P. Functional neuroimaging of normal human sleep by positron emission tomography. *J Sleep Res.* 2000;9:207–31.

64. Kaufmann C, Wehrle R, Wetter TC, *et al.* Brain activation and hypothalamic functional connectivity during human non-rapid eye movement sleep: an EEG/fMRI study. *Brain.* 2006;129:655–67.

Functional neuroimaging of human REM sleep

Christelle Meyer, Zayd Jedidi, Vincenzo Muto, Caroline Kussé, Mathieu Jaspar, Laura Mascetti, Ariane Foret, and Pierre Maquet

Introduction

The brain is able to generate three distinct functional modes: wakefulness, non-rapid eye movement (NREM) sleep, and rapid eye movement (REM) sleep. These modes alternate on a daily basis and differ in many aspects: the associated neural activity, neuromodulation, systemic physiology, behavioral and cognitive correlates. REM sleep probably remains the least understood of these three modes. It is defined by low-voltage, fast-frequency rhythms on electroencephalographic (EEG) recordings, rapid eye movements, and muscle atonia. In animals, it is further characterized by phasic potentials generated in the pons that propagate to a number of rostral areas, including the lateral geniculate nuclei and occipital cortex, referred to as pontine or ponto-geniculo-occipital waves. REM sleep is also clearly associated with reports of vivid dreams in humans.

Functional neuroimaging studies in animals and humans aimed at better understanding this peculiar cerebral mode are reviewed in this chapter. We start with evidence that brain activity during REM sleep is influenced by previous experience, suggesting the participation of REM sleep in memory consolidation. We conclude with comments on the difficulty in interpreting functional imaging of REM sleep in terms of neural correlates of dreaming.

Neuroimaging of sleep processes: functional neuroanatomy of REM sleep

Cerebral neurons typically adopt a tonic firing pattern during REM sleep which on average is as intense as during wakefulness [1]. Accordingly, cerebral energy metabolism [2] and blood flow [3] reach similar levels during REM sleep as during wakefulness. However, the distribution of regional brain activity differs considerably between REM sleep and wakefulness and, in humans, is characterized by three main features (Figure 14.1).

First, in agreement with neurophysiological studies in animals [4, 5], functional imaging studies in humans reported high activity in the brainstem and thalamic nuclei. In humans, the activation of the mesopontine tegmentum and thalamic nuclei has been systematically reported during REM sleep [6–8]. This pattern of activity is easily explained by the known neurophysiological mechanisms which generate REM sleep in animals [9]. Moreover, neuronal populations in the mesopontine tegmentum are the source of a major activating input to the thalamic nuclei during REM sleep [1, 10].

Second, high activity has been observed in limbic and paralimbic areas. This was suggested by earlier measurements of brain energy metabolism in animals [4, 5, 11]. In the forebrain, REM sleep is characterized by high activity levels in the amygdala, the hippocampal formation, and the anterior cingulate, orbitofrontal, and insular cortices [6–8]. In addition to these limbic and paralimbic areas, temporal and occipital cortices were also shown to be very active [8], although this result was less frequently reported [7]. Finally, the motor and premotor cortices were also very active during REM sleep [12].

Third, this limbic activation contrasts with a relative quiescence of the associative frontal and parietal cortices during REM sleep, relative to wakefulness [7, 8]. More precisely, the hypoactive areas were located bilaterally in the inferior and middle frontal gyrus as well as the posterior part of the inferior parietal lobule [13]. Interestingly, the superior frontal gyrus, the medial frontal areas, the intraparietal sulcus, and the superior parietal cortex were not less active in REM sleep than during wakefulness [13].

Not only the distribution of brain activity, but also its functional connectivity is modified during human REM sleep. The functional relationship between striate and extrastriate cortices, which is excitatory during wakefulness, was inverted during REM sleep [14]. Likewise, the functional relationship between the amygdala and the temporal and occipital cortices was different during REM sleep than during wakefulness or non-rapid eye movement (NREM) sleep [15].

The reasons that explain this unusual functional segregation and integration remain unclear. It is usually assumed that changes in neuromodulation might contribute to a modification of forebrain activity and responsiveness during REM sleep because REM sleep is characterized by a prominent cholinergic tone and a decrease in noradrenergic and serotonergic modulation [1]. However, objective evidence supporting this hypothesis is still lacking.

It was also assumed that the regional distribution during REM sleep is partly driven by phasic events concomitant to rapid eye movements, called pontine waves or ponto-geniculo-occipital waves. However, brain activity associated with bursts of saccades, supposed to be associated with pontine waves in

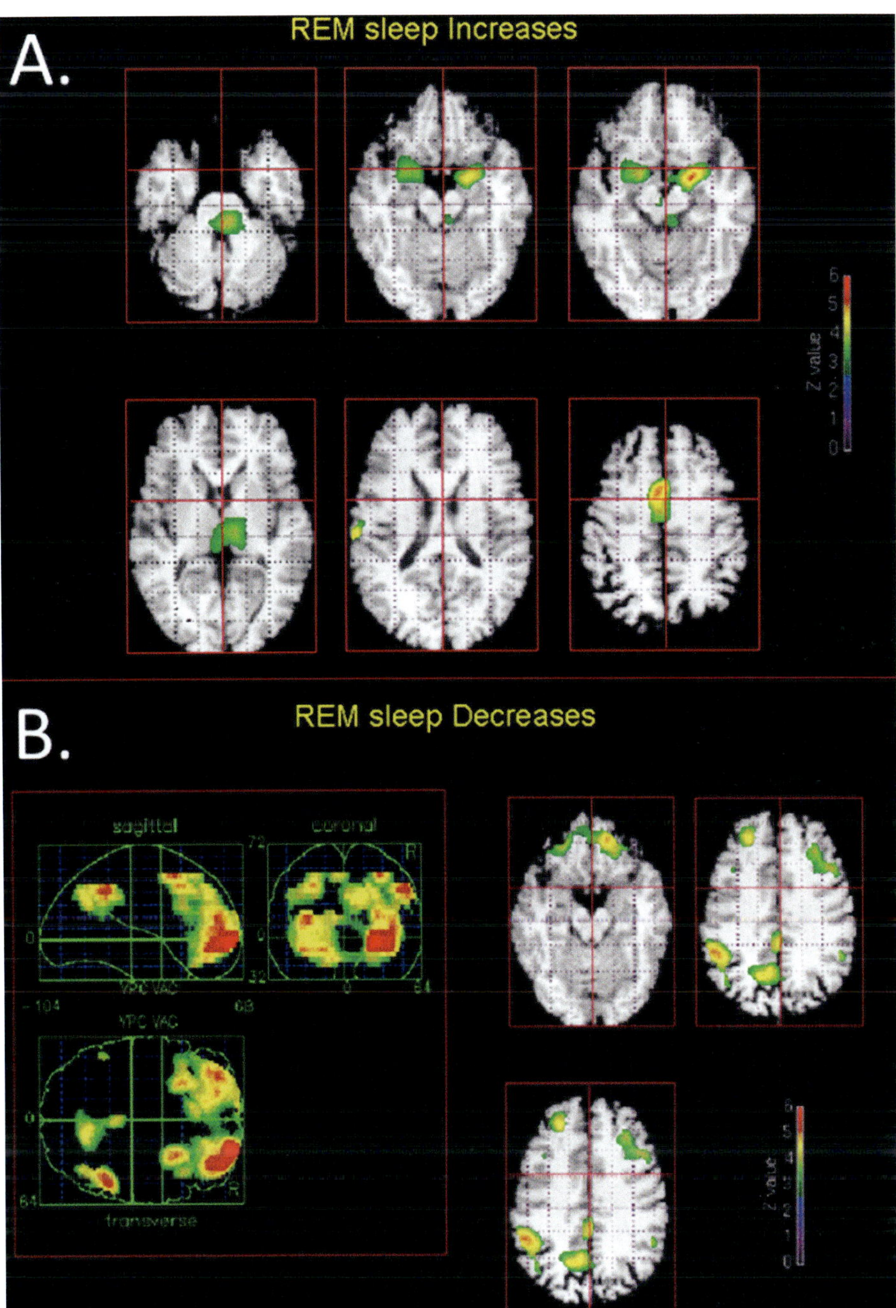

Figure 14.1 Functional neuroanatomy of human REM sleep, as assessed by H$_2$^{15}O-positron emission tomography [7]. (A) Increases in cerebral blood flow (CBF) during REM sleep, relative to wakefulness and slow-wave sleep. A significant increase in regional (CBF) (rCBF) is observed in the mesopontine tegmentum, the thalamic nuclei, both amygdalas, and the anterior cingulate cortex. (B) Decreases in CBF during REM sleep, relative to wakefulness and slow-wave sleep. A significant decrease is observed in the frontal and parietal associative cortices.

humans, showed a different distribution. Using positron emission tomography (PET) and cerebral blood flow (CBF) measurements, it was shown that the activity in the right geniculate body and the primary occipital cortex increased proportionally to the density of eye movements to a larger extent during REM sleep than during wakefulness [16]. Similar data were eventually reported with fMRI [17–19].

In consequence, the particular distribution of forebrain activity during REM sleep is not yet satisfactorily explained. It is reasonable to suggest that regulation centers in the hypothalamus, some of which have widespread projections on the forebrain [20], might be responsible for organizing forebrain activity during REM sleep.

Neuroimaging and dream correlates during REM sleep

To our knowledge, functional neuroimaging research specifically devoted to the characterization of dream correlates has been conducted only during REM sleep. Indeed, mentation during REM sleep is more abundant, vivid, and story-like and hence more detailed dream reports can be obtained from REM than from slow-wave sleep [21]. The particular pattern of cerebral activity observed during REM sleep (a high limbic contrasting with a low prefrontal and parietal activity) is usually assumed to correlate with, and possibly influence, the main characteristics of dreaming activity [7, 12, 21, 22].

Vision is the most prominent dreaming sensory modality, occurring almost in all dreams. This might be related to the activation of the occipital cortex. Indeed, PET studies revealed significant increases in regional CBF (rCBF) in extrastriate visual cortices, particularly within the ventral visual stream [8, 14]. The heterogeneous activation of ventral visual areas can be indicative of the bizarre properties of dreams [23]. In keeping with this hypothesis, visual imagery in dreams is absent in some patients with occipitotemporal lesions [24].

Motor behavior and movements probably activate motor-related brain areas during REM sleep. Indeed, rCBF measurements using PET have revealed a significant increase in activity of motor and supplementary motor areas during REM sleep (see control population in [12]).

On the other hand, affect and emotional intensification (anxiety, elation, anger) which are characteristically reported in dreams would be related to the significant activation of the limbic and paralimbic systems: amygdala, orbitofrontal cortex, and anterior cingulate cortex [7, 21, 22, 25]. Given the crucial role of the limbic system in the acquisition of emotional memories, the activation pattern in the amygdala and cortical areas provides a biological basis for the processing of some types of memory during REM sleep.

The activation of mesio-temporal areas would account for the memory content commonly found in dreams. However, this mesio-temporal activity occurs in the context of a relatively low activity of ventral prefrontal cortex, which is deemed participating in memory retrieval [26]. This pattern of regional brain activity would explain the peculiar aspects of episodic memory in dreams. Usually, "snips" of recent waking activity are frequently observed in dream reports. In contrast, although REM dreams can be very much story-like, complete waking life episodes, characterized by the association between specific locations, characters, objects, and actions, are seldom described as such in dream reports [27].

The relative quiescence of the anterior and ventral prefrontal areas might be related to other formal characteristics of dreams, such as temporal distortions, weakening of self-reflective control, and amnesia on awakening. The hypoactivation of the frontal lobe would explain that although the dreamer has access to "day residues," probably spontaneously generated by the coordinated activity of the mesio-temporal areas and the posterior cortices, the successful and comprehensive retrieval of a specific past episode is hindered. Low frontal activity would also account for the deficits in working memory, and executive functions that manifest themselves in dream reports from REM sleep awakenings [7, 21, 22, 25].

Brain plasticity during REM sleep

A growing body of data indicates that patterns of neural activity prevailing during sleep support offline processing of newly acquired information. In particular, one hypothesis assumes that the replay of learned neural activity patterns contributes to memory consolidation [28]. Recent research particularly emphasized the importance of NREM sleep oscillations, such as spindles or slow waves [29, 30], in the consolidation of recent memories. However, similar evidence exists during REM sleep [31], especially in humans [12].

The effect of motor sequence learning on subsequent REM sleep was evaluated using a probabilistic serial reaction time (SRT) task [32]. In this task, six permanent position markers are displayed on a computer screen above six spatially compatible response keys. On each trial, a black circle appears below one of the position markers, and the task consists of pressing as fast and as accurately as possible on the corresponding key. The next stimulus is displayed at another location after a 200 ms response–stimulus interval. Unknown to the subjects, the sequential structure of the material is manipulated by generating series of stimuli based on a probabilistic finite-state grammar that defines legal transitions between successive trials. To assess learning of the probabilistic rules of the grammar, there is a 15% chance, on each trial, that the stimulus generated based on the grammar (grammatical stimulus, G) is replaced by a non-grammatical (NG), random stimulus. Assuming that response preparation is facilitated by high predictability, predictable G stimuli should thus elicit faster responses than NG stimuli, but only if the context in which stimuli may occur has been encoded by participants. In this task, contextual sensitivity emerges through practice as a gradually increasing difference between the reaction times (RTs) elicited by G and NG stimuli occurring in specific contexts set by two to three previous trials at most [32].

A first group of subjects (group 1) were trained in the afternoon, then scanned during the post-training night, both during waking and in various sleep stages (i.e., stage 2, deep NREM sleep, and REM sleep), using ^{15}O-water ($H_2^{15}O$) PET [12]. A post-sleep training session verified that learning had occurred overnight. The analysis of PET data identified the brain areas more active in REM sleep than during resting wakefulness (Figure 14.2). To ensure that the post-training REM sleep rCBF distribution differed from the pattern of "typical" REM sleep, a second group of subjects (group 2), not trained to the task, were similarly scanned at night, both awake and during sleep. The analysis was aimed at detecting the brain areas that would be more active in trained than in non-trained subjects, during REM sleep as compared to resting wakefulness. And finally, to formally test that these brain regions, possibly reactivated during REM sleep, would be among the structures that had been engaged by executing and learning the task, a third group of subjects (group 3) were scanned during wakefulness both while they were performing the SRT task and at rest. The analysis identified the regions that would be *both* more active during REM sleep in the trained subjects (group 1) compared to the non-trained subjects (group 2) *and* activated during the execution of the task during waking (group 3), i.e., the regions reactivated in post-training REM sleep. The results showed that the bilateral cuneus and the adjacent striate cortex, the mesencephalon, and the left premotor cortex were both activated during the practice of the SRT task and during post-training REM sleep in subjects previously trained on the task, significantly more than in control subjects without prior training, suggesting a reactivation process which may have contributed to overnight performance improvement in the SRT task.

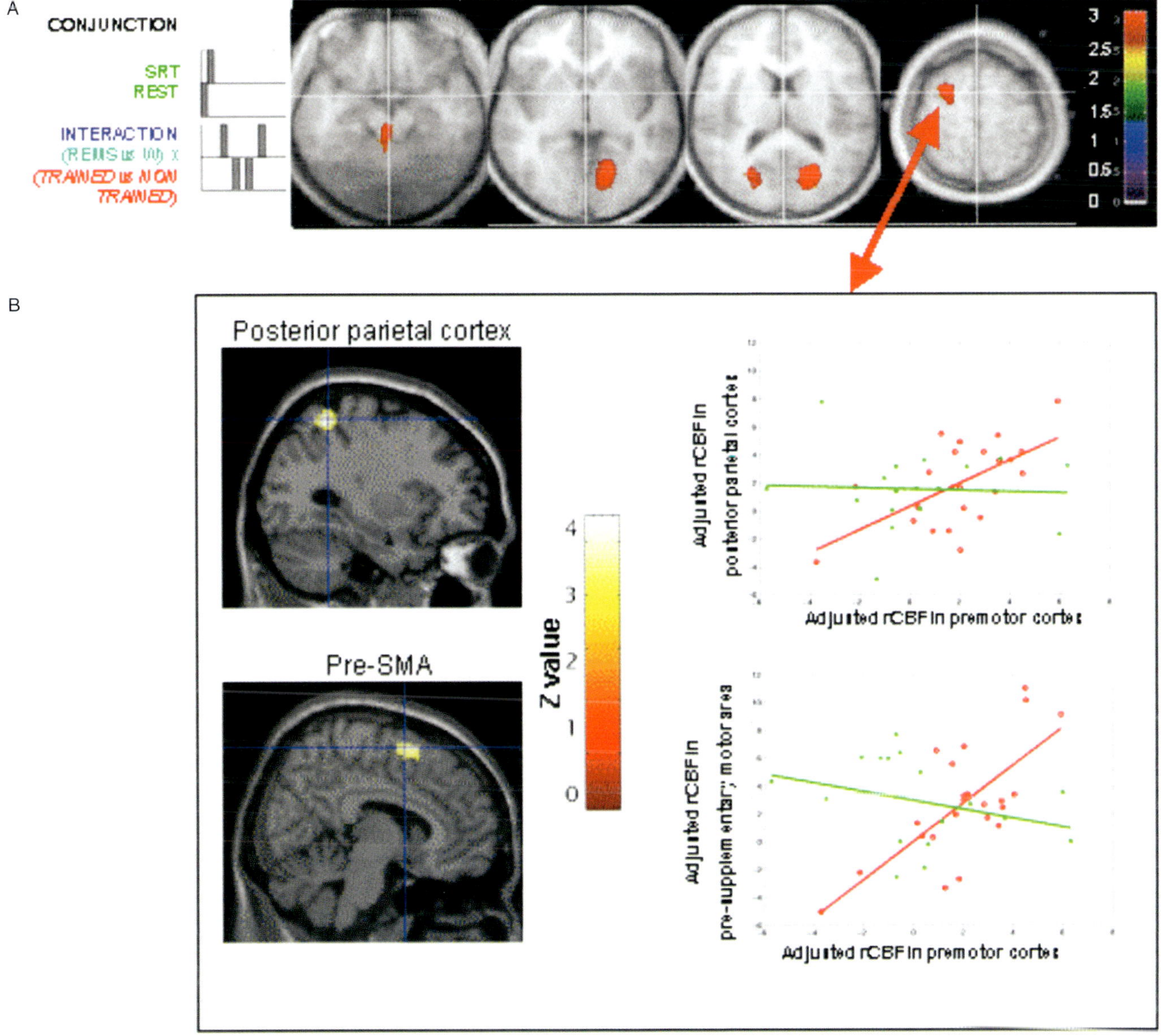

Figure 14.2 Experience-dependent changes in regional brain activity during REM sleep after motor sequence learning, as assessed by $H_2{}^{15}O$-positron emission tomography. (A) Brain areas that are more active during REM sleep after motor sequence learning [12]. (B) Increased functional connectivity of the premotor cortex with the parietal cortex and supplementary motor area during post-training REM sleep.

In addition, we reasoned that, if the reactivated regions participate in the processing of memory traces during REM sleep, they should establish or reinforce functional connections between parts of the network activated during the task. Consequently, such connections should be stronger, and the synaptic trafficking between network components more intense during post-training REM sleep than during REM sleep in non-trained subjects. Accordingly, we found that among the reactivated regions, the rCBF in the left premotor cortex was significantly more correlated with the activity of the pre-supplementary motor area (pre-SMA) and posterior parietal cortex during post-training REM sleep than during REM sleep in subjects without any prior experience with the task [33]. The demonstration of a differential functional connectivity during REM sleep between remote brain areas engaged in the practice of a previously experienced visuomotor task gave further support to the hypothesis that memory traces are replayed in the cortical network and contribute to the optimization of the performance.

It should be stressed that, in this first experiment, the conclusions were limited by the fact that it could not be specified whether the experience-dependent reactivation during REM sleep was related to the simple optimisation of a visuo-motor skill or to the high-order acquisition of the probabilistic structure of the learned material, or both. To test the hypothesis that the cerebral reactivation during post-training REM sleep reflects the reprocessing of high-order information about the sequential structure of the material to be learned, a new group of subjects (group 4) was scanned during sleep after practice on the same SRT task, but using a completely random sequence

[34]. The experimental protocol was identical in all respects to the trained group in our original study [12], except for the absence of sequential rules. Therefore, post-training rCBF differences during REM sleep between the subjects trained to the probabilistic SRT or to its random version should be related specifically to the reprocessing of the high-order sequential information. During post-training REM sleep, blood flow in left and right cunei increased more in subjects previously trained to a probabilistic sequence of stimuli than to a random one. Since both groups prior to sleep were exposed to identical SRT practice that differed only in the sequential structure of the stimuli, our result suggests that reactivation of neural activity in the cuneus during post-training REM sleep is not merely due to the acquisition of basic visuo-motor skills. Rather, it corresponds to the reprocessing of elaborated information about the sequential contingencies contained in the learned material.

If the material does not contain any structure, as is the case in the random SRT task, post-training REM sleep reactivation does not occur, or at least to a significantly lesser extent. These results are reminiscent of previous experiments. At the behavioral level, an increase in REM sleep duration was observed in rats following aversive conditioning in which a tone was paired with a footshock, but not after pseudo-conditioning in which the tone and the footshock were not paired [35]. Using a similar procedure at the systems level, tone-evoked responses were obtained in the medial geniculate nucleus [36] during REM sleep after a conditioning procedure initiated at wake, but not after pseudo-conditioning.

Moreover, during REM sleep, functional connections should be reinforced between the reactivated areas and cerebral structures specifically involved in sequence learning only after the practice of the probabilistic version of the task. Indeed, as compared to the practice of the random sequence, we observed that the cuneus establishes or reinforces functional connections with the caudate nucleus during REM sleep following probabilistic SRT practice. The cuneus, which participates in the processing of the probabilistic sequence both during SRT practice and post-training REM sleep, has been shown to be activated during sequential information processing in the waking state [37]. On the other hand, the striatum is known to play a main role in implicit sequence learning and specifically in the encoding of the temporal context set by the previous stimulus in the probabilistic SRT task [38]. The finding that the strength of the functional connections between cuneus and striatum is increased during post-training REM sleep suggests the involvement of the basal ganglia in the off-line reprocessing of implicitly acquired high-order sequential information.

Finally, a direct relationship between the pre-sleep learning performance and regional blood flow was found in the cuneus. In this region, the regional blood flow during post-training REM sleep is modulated by the level of high-order, but not low-order, learning attained prior to sleep. In other words, the neural activity recorded during REM sleep in brain areas already engaged in the learning process during wakefulness is related to the *amount of high-order learning* achieved prior to sleep. This latter result further supports the hypothesis that sleep is actively involved in the processing of recent memory traces.

Difficulty in the interpretation of imaging of REM sleep and dreams

Interpreting functional neuroimaging data in terms of dream activity is still at an embryonic stage. One must keep in mind that several basic assumptions have profound consequences on the interpretation of sleep neuroimaging studies, especially those that address the topic of the neural correlates of REM sleep and dreams.

During wakefulness, brain function is mainly driven by cognitive processes which can be readily elicited by experimental designs (perception, motor behavior, attention, memory, language, etc.). The interpretation of spontaneous waking activity is already more difficult because of the correlative nature of the relationships between ongoing mental representations and fluctuations of cerebral activity. For instance, it has been argued that the activity in the default mode network supports spontaneous inner thought processes, self-oriented representations, and expectations [39]. However, it is also known that activity fluctuations persist in this cerebral network under deep anesthesia in monkeys [40] and would primarily be explained by the structural backbone of brain connections [41]. Whether spontaneous fluctuations of activity in the default mode network is related to mental representations or basic brain physiology, or both in a given study cannot be certified without iteratively probing individual mental content [42, 43].

Similar hesitation prevails in the interpretation of sleep imaging, clearly a spontaneous state of brain activity. Whereas the understanding of evoked responses can be grounded on objective knowledge collected at the cellular level in animal studies [44], the interpretation of spontaneous ongoing brain activity is a blend of two possible explanations.

On the one hand, during sleep, regional brain function is primarily organized by specific sleep processes. For instance, during NREM sleep, a coalescence of oscillations organizes neural firing in specific temporal patterns (slow oscillation, delta rhythm, spindles). These oscillations are characterized by consistent regional brain responses [45, 46]. These processes are obviously different from those occurring during wakefulness in the same brain areas.

On the other hand, when sleep processes are associated with retrievable mental representations, e.g., dreams, one tends to argue that regional brain function is also organized by these mental processes (as reviewed above). In this context, it is assumed that information processing during sleep is regionally specific and respects the functional specialization known during wakefulness. In other words, it is assumed that dream content informs us on how regional brain function is organized during sleep [20]. This hypothesis is based on the reasonable postulate that brain specialization does not change between sleep and wakefulness and that structural brain connectivity, the main determinant of brain specialization, does not substantially change across vigilance states.

A more qualified assumption would be that brain activity associated with dreams results from genuine sleep processes taking place in a regionally specialized brain. As a consequence, describing the spatial distribution of brain activity during sleep provides only a partial view on the neural correlates of dreaming. For example: when lucid dreamers signal their dreams by sequences of saccades while being studied by functional neuroimaging, does it not seem trivial to observe a related increase in activity in the relevant motor areas [47]?

If brain specialization does not dramatically change between wakefulness and sleep, then what makes sleep and wakefulness so behaviorally different? It is clear that the main unknown resides in functional integration, namely how brain areas interact with each other during sleep. It is likely that interactions between functional brain units are profoundly modified by genuine sleep processes (slow oscillations, spindles, pontine waves, etc.), as suggested by transcranial magnetic stimulation during sleep [48]. Likewise, using functional magnetic resonance imaging in normal volunteers, a modification of the hierarchical organization of large-scale networks into smaller independent modules was observed during NREM sleep [49]. Such modifications in brain connectivity could hinder the brain's ability to integrate information and account for decreased consciousness during NREM sleep. Moreover, the dramatic change in neuromodulation that differentiates sleep states from wakefulness is another potential factor influencing functional brain integration [1].

Whereas some advances have been made in characterizing brain segregation during sleep, as reviewed above, yet very little is known about functional integration during sleep [50], especially REM sleep.

Conclusions

At present, although functional neuroimaging provides a general idea about the distribution of brain activity during NREM and REM sleep, it does not directly characterize the neural correlates of dreaming. This endeavor is difficult for various reasons: (1) reliable dream reports are not easy to obtain; (2) functional neuroimaging is still difficult to obtain during steady states of NREM or REM sleep; (3) the underlying mechanisms that activate the cortex during sleep are not comprehensively understood; and (4) the understanding of brain functional integration is still under development. Nevertheless, we are confident that, in the future, more progress will be made that will allow us to understand the neural mechanisms underlying dreaming even better.

Acknowledgements

Personal work cited in this review was supported by the Belgian Fonds National de la Recherche Scientifque (FNRS), the University of Liège and the Queen Elisabeth Medical Foundation (QEMF), and the Belgian Inter University Attraction Program (IUAP).

References

1. Steriade M, McCarley RW. *Brain Control of Wakefulness and Sleep*. New York, Kluwer Academic, 2005.

2. Maquet P, Dive D, Salmon E, *et al.* Cerebral glucose utilization during sleep-wake cycle in man determined by positron emission tomography and [18F] 2-fluoro-2-deoxy-D-glucose method. *Brain Res.* 1990;**513**(1):136–43.

3. Madsen PL, Holm S, Vorstrup S, *et al.* Human regional cerebral blood flow during rapid-eye-movement sleep. *J Cereb Blood Flow Metab.* 1991,**11**(3):502 7.

4. Ramm P, Frost BJ. Cerebral and local cerebral metabolism in the cat during slow wave and REM sleep. *Brain Res.* 1986;**365**(1):112–24.

5. Lydic R, Baghdoyan HA, Hibbard L, *et al.* Regional brain glucose metabolism is altered during rapid eye movement sleep in the cat: a preliminary study. *J Comp Neurol.* 1991;**304**(4):517–29.

6. Nofzinger EA, Mintun MA, Wiseman M, Kupfer DJ, Moore RY. Forebrain activation in REM sleep: an FDG PET study. *Brain Res.* 1997;**770** (1–2):192–201.

7. Maquet P, Peters J, Aerts J, *et al.* Functional neuroanatomy of human rapid-eye-movement sleep and dreaming. *Nature.* 1996;**383** (6596):163–6.

8. Braun AR, Balkin TJ, Wesenten NJ, *et al.* Regional cerebral blood flow throughout the sleep-wake cycle. An H2 (15)O PET study. *Brain.* 1997;**120**(Pt 7):1173–97.

9. Jones BE. Neurobiology of waking and sleeping. In: Montagna P, Chokroverty S, eds. *Sleep Disorders, Part I*, 3rd edn. Amsterdam, *Elsevier.* 2010; 131–49.

10. Steriade M, Datta S, Pare D, Oakson G, Curro Dossi RC. Neuronal activities in brain-stem cholinergic nuclei related to tonic activation processes in thalamocortical systems. *J Neurosci.* 1990;**10**(8):2541 59.

11. Ramm P, Frost BJ. Regional metabolic activity in the rat brain during sleep-wake activity. *Sleep.* 1983;**6**(3):196–216.

12. Maquet P, Laureys S, Peigneux P, *et al.* Experience-dependent changes in cerebral activation during human REM sleep. *Nat Neurosci.* 2000;**3**(8):831–6.

13. Maquet P, Ruby P, Maudoux A, *et al.* Human cognition during REM sleep and the activity profile within the frontal and parietal cortices: a reappraisal of functional neuroimaging data. In: Laureys S, ed. *Progess in Brain Research.* Amsterdam, *Elsevier.* 2005; 219–27.

14. Braun AR, Balkin TJ, Wesensten NJ, *et al.* Dissociated pattern of activity in visual cortices and their projections during human rapid eye movement sleep. *Science.* 1998;**279**(5347):91–5.

15. Maquet P, Phillips C. Functional brain imaging of human sleep. *J Sleep Res.* 1998;**7**(Suppl 1):42–7.

16. Peigneux P, Laureys S, Fuchs S, *et al.* Generation of rapid eye movements during paradoxical sleep in humans. *Neuroimage.* 2001;**14**(3):701–8

17. Wehrle R, Czisch M, Kaufmann *et al.* Rapid eye movement-related brain activation in human sleep: a Functional magnetic resonance imaging study. *Neuroreport.* 2005;**16**(8):853–7.

18. Hong CC, Marie JC, Pearlson GD, *et al.* FMRI evidence for multisensory recruitment associated with rapid eye movements during sleeps. *Hum Brain Mapp.* 2009;**30**(5): 1705–22.

19. Miyauchi S, Misaki M, Kan S, Fukunaga T, Koike T. Human brain activity time-locked to rapid eye movements during REM sleep. *Exp Brain Res.* 2009; **192**(4):657–67. Epub 2008 Oct 2.

20. Goutagny R, Verret L, Fort P, *et al.* Posterior hypothalamus and regulation of vigilance states. *Arch Ital Biol.* 2004;**142**(4):487–500.

21. Hobson JA, Pace-Schott EF, Stickgold R. Dreaming and the brain: toward a cognitive neuroscience of conscious states. *Behav Brain Sci.* 2000;**23** (6):793–842; discussion 904–1121.

22. Maquet P, Franck G. REM sleep and amygdala. *Mol Psychiatry.* 1997;**2** (3):195–6.

23. Schwartz S, Maquet P. Sleep imaging and the neuro-psychological assessment of dreams. *Trends Cogn Sci.* 2002;**6** (1):23–30.

24. Solms M. *The Neuropsychology of Dreams. A Clinico-Anatomical Study.* Mahwah, Lawrence Erlbaum Assocaites, 1997.

25. Maquet P. Functional neuroimaging of normal human sleep by positron emission tomography. *J Sleep Res.* 2000;**9**(3):207–31.

26. Rugg MD, Otten LJ, Henson RN. The neural basis of episodic memory: evidence from functional neuroimaging. *Philos Trans R Soc Lond B Biol Sci.* 2002;**357**(1424):1097–110.

27. Fosse MJ, Fosse R, Hobson JA, Stickgold RJ. Dreaming and episodic memory: a functional dissociation? *J Cogn Neurosci.* 2003;**15**(1):1–9.

28. Schwindel CD, McNaughton BL. Hippocampal-cortical interactions and the dynamics of memory trace reactivation. *Prog Brain Res.* 2011;193:163–77.

29. Diekelmann S, Born J. The memory function of sleep. *Nat Rev Neurosci.* 2010;**11**(2):114–26.

30. Huber R, Ghilardi MF, Massimini M, Tononi G. Local sleep and learning. *Nature.* 2004;**430**(6995):78–81.

31. Louie K, Wilson MA. Temporally structured replay of awake hippocampal ensemble activity during rapid eye movement sleep. *Neuron.* 2001;**29** (1):145–56.

32. Cleeremans A, McClelland JL. Learning the structure of event sequences. *J Exp Psychol Gen.* 1991;**120**(3):235–53.

33. Laureys S, Peigneux P, Phillips C, *et al.* Experience-dependent changes in cerebral functional connectivity during human rapid eye movement sleep. *Neuroscience.* 2001;**105**(3):521–5.

34. Peigneux P, Laureys S, Fuchs S, *et al.* Learned material content and acquisition level modulate cerebral reactivation during posttraining rapid-eye-movements sleep. *Neuroimage.* 2003;**20**(1):125–34.

35. Hennevin E, Leconte P. [The function of paradoxical sleep: facts and theories]. *Annee Psychol.* 1971;**71**(2):489–519.

36. Hennevin E, Maho C, Hars B, Dutrieux G. Learning-induced plasticity in the medial geniculate nucleus is expressed during paradoxical sleep. *Behav Neurosci.* 1993;**107**(6):1018–30.

37. Schubotz RI, von Cramon DY. Interval and ordinal properties of sequences are associated with distinct premotor areas. *Cereb Cortex.* 2001;**11**(3):210–22.

38. Peigneux P, Maquet P, Meulemans T, *et al.* Striatum forever, despite sequence learning variability: a random effect analysis of PET data. *Hum Brain Mapp.* 2000;**10**(4):179–94.

39. Raichle ME, Gusnard DA. Intrinsic brain activity sets the stage for expression of motivated behavior. *J Comp Neurol.* 2005;**493**(1):167–76.

40. Vincent JL, Patel GH, Fox MD, *et al.* Intrinsic functional architecture in the anaesthetized monkey brain. *Nature.* 2007;**447**(7140):83–6.

41. Honey CJ, Sporns O, Cammoun L, *et al.* Predicting human resting-state functional connectivity from structural connectivity. *Proc Natl Acad Sci U S A.* 2009;**106**(6):2035–40.

42. Christoff K, Gordon AM, Smallwood J, Smith R, Schooler JW. Experience sampling during fMRI reveals default network and executive system contributions to mind wandering. *Proc Natl Acad Sci U S A.* 2009;**106** (21):8719–24.

43. Stawarczyk D, Majerus S, Maquet P, D'Argembeau A. Neural correlates of ongoing conscious experience: both task-unrelatedness and stimulus-independence are related to default network activity. *PLoS One.* 2011;**6**(2): e16997.

44. Dang-Vu TT, Bonjean M, Schabus M, *et al.* Interplay between spontaneous and induced brain activity during human non-rapid eye movement sleep. *Proc Natl Acad Sci U S A.* 2011;**108** (37):15438–43.

45. Dang-Vu TT, Schabus M, Desseilles M, *et al.* Spontaneous neural activity during human slow wave sleep. *Proc Natl Acad Sci U S A.* 2008;**105**(39):15160–5.

46. Schabus M, Dang-Vu TT, Albouy G, *et al.* Hemodynamic cerebral correlates of sleep spindles during human non-rapid eye movement sleep. *Proc Natl Acad Sci U S A.* 2007;**104**(32):13164–9.

47. Dresler M, Koch SP, Wehrle R, *et al.* Dreamed movement elicits activation in the sensorimotor cortex. *Curr Biol.* 2011;**21**(21):1833–7.

48. Massimini M, Ferrarelli F, Huber R, *et al.* Breakdown of cortical effective connectivity during sleep. *Science.* 2005;**309**(5744):2228–32.

49. Boly M, Perlbarg V, Marrelec G, *et al.* Hierarchical clustering of brain activity during human non rapid eye movement sleep. *Proc Natl Acad Sci U S A.* 2012;**109** (15):5856–61.

50. Spoormaker VI, Czisch M, Maquet P, Jancke L. Large-scale functional brain networks in human non-rapid eye movement sleep: insights from combined electroencephalographic/functional magnetic resonance imaging studies. *Philos Transact A Math Phys Eng Sci.* 2011;**369**(1952):3708–29.

Complementarity of dream research and neuroimaging of sleep

Sophie Schwartz

Introduction

Sleep and dream research has recently been invigorated by the use of new methodologies, as well as by convergent data from complementary sources including neuroimaging studies of human sleep, clinical investigations of dreaming in brain-damaged patients, and the analysis of phenomenological characteristics of dream reports.

The aim of the present chapter is to show that dream reports contain valuable information about neural and cognitive processing during sleep. In particular, we propose that the characterization of sensory, cognitive, and emotional dream features, as well as the identification of typical bizarre elements in dreams may help specify how and what type of information is processed during sleep [1–3]. A systematic assessment of dream content can thus significantly contribute to the interpretation of functional imaging data recorded during sleep.

Below, we first consider the main difficulties that neuroscientists or clinicians may face when interpreting brain imaging data of human sleep. Next, we describe some reproducible cognitive and emotional features of dreams and show how they may orient the interpretation of patterns of brain activity recorded during sleep. Although dreaming may incorporate aspects of waking experiences, dreams are not replicas of real-life experiences. Instead, and as we then show, dreams contain many bizarre but typical features, which present similarities with specific neuropsychological deficits in neurological patients. Knowledge about brain damage underlying such deficits (during wakefulness) thus provides useful information about functional changes that may characterize normal human sleep, both at the brain and cognitive levels. Finally, we report some recent studies looking at the neural determinants of dream recall. In this chapter, we also suggest promising new ways of combining cognitive and neuroimaging experimental designs to better characterize cognitive or affective aspects of human sleep.

Interpreting neuroimaging data of human sleep: the problem

Non-invasive brain imaging methods have provided unprecedented insights into human brain functions. Likewise, descriptions of spontaneous brain activity across human sleep states have become increasingly complex and detailed. Yet, scientists may face several problems when attempting to interpret neuroimaging data of sleep, as illustrated by the following example. Let's imagine that we obtained a set of brain activity maps in people while they were sleeping in a scanner. We may want to compare the level of regional brain activity corresponding to different sleep/wake states, we could also identify changes in functional connectivity across distributed networks, we may also compare activity for different populations such as normal healthy controls and patients, etc. Any of these scenarios will result in statistics indicating differences for certain brain regions or networks, which will call for an interpretation. Several strategies can then be used to interpret such data.

A first approach is to link brain activation observed during human sleep to animal physiological and cellular data (Figure 15.1). For example, we may infer that increased activation of the amygdala during rapid eye movement (REM) sleep is a manifestation of the dense connections of the amygdala with typical sleep-regulating structures described in the animal literature, such as the pons and brainstem nuclei (see [4]; Figure 15.2A). Confirming (or disconfirming) that specific aspects of sleep at the cellular level in animals can translate into macroscopic neuroimaging data in humans is an important research objective. While this strategy has proven very successful as well as inspiring for neuroimaging studies, it could also be seen as having a confirmatory scope, with a relatively limited potential for discoveries. A second approach is to refer to what we know about the functions of different brain systems during wakefulness (Figure 15.1). In our example, we could relate the activation of the amygdala observed during REM sleep to the role of the amygdala in emotional processing and learning [5, 6]. Nevertheless, this interpretation remains speculative in the absence of a direct access to emotional responses during sleep (unlike neuroimaging studies of awake subjects). This is why additional physiological measures of emotional reactivity should be used, whenever available (e.g., skin conductance, heart rate variability, e.g., [7]). Yet, both these approaches appear particularly challenging for more subtle dimensions of emotional experience as well as for understanding higher-level cognitive functions in sleep. In this

Neuroimaging of Sleep and Sleep Disorders, ed. Eric Nofzinger, Pierre Maquet, and Michael J. Thorpy. Published by Cambridge University Press. © Cambridge University Press 2013.

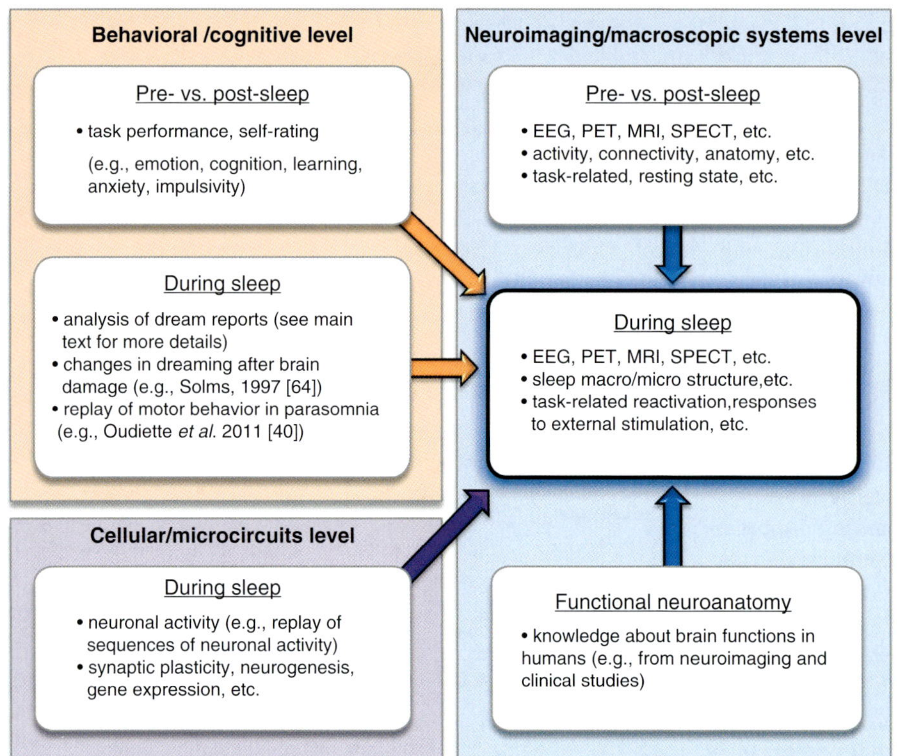

Figure 15.1 Examples of methods and data available in sleep research for interpreting brain imaging results from human sleep. Information about neural and cognitive processes during sleep may come from distinct sources and levels of description. Direct (during sleep) as well as indirect (e.g., pre- vs. post-sleep) measurements are represented. Arrows symbolize the contribution of various sources of information (e.g., dream data) to the interpretation of neuroimaging data collected during sleep.

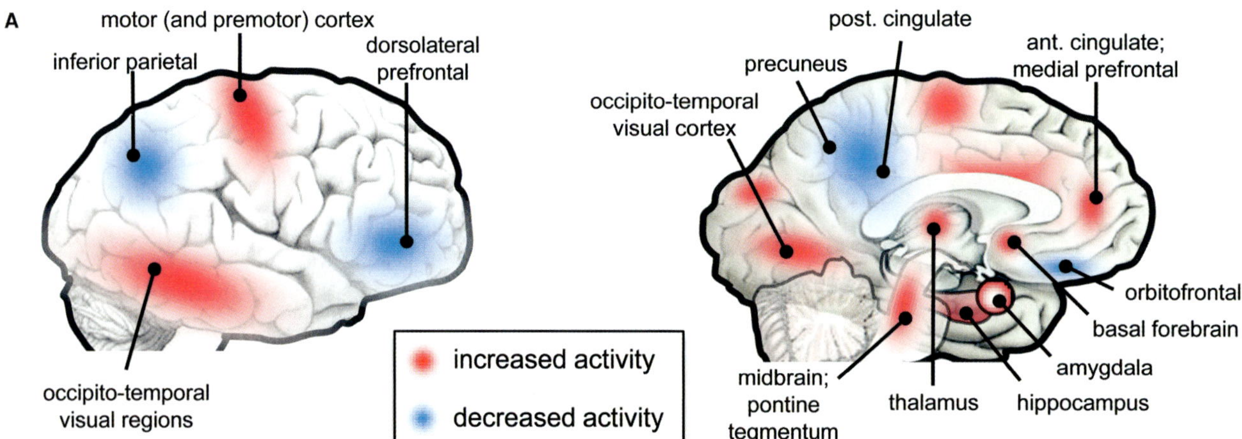

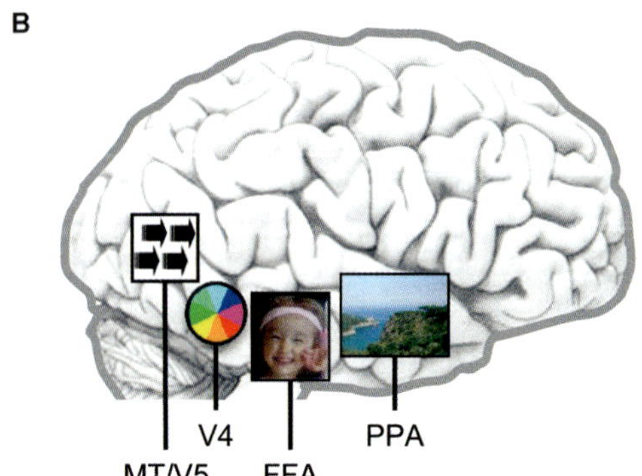

Figure 15.2 (A) Functional neuroanatomy of human REM sleep. Regions showing increased or decreased brain activity in the positron emission tomography (PET) studies reported in the main text. (Adapted with permission from Desseilles et al. [26] Conscious Cogn, 2011.) (B) Specialized brain regions for the processing of visual motion (MT/V5); colors (V4); layouts and landscapes (parahippocampal place area; PPA); face processing (fusiform face area; FFA). These regions are located within the occipital and temporal lobes.

context, dream reports represent an additional major source of information about cognitive and emotional processing during sleep (Figure 15.1). In our example, the interpretation of amygdala activation in terms of concomitant emotional processing during sleep would be supported by the high prevalence of intense negative emotions in dreams (see Distinct affective and cognitive dimensions in dream reports below), and by changes in dreamed emotions in conditions that modulate amygdala activity (e.g., pharmacological treatments, mood disorders, psychotherapy). Another attractive option is to use dedicated experimental protocols to indirectly probe cognition or emotion during sleep, for instance by using measures of waking performance in behavioral tasks (pre- and post-sleep behavioral measures; e.g., [8, 9]) or by presenting external stimuli during sleep (such as sounds, words, odors; e.g., [10–12]), with the assumption that observed changes in brain activity during sleep correspond to the active processing of information related to pre-sleep experience or external stimulation. A combination of such an experimental approach and the analysis of dream reports may be particularly promising for future studies [13].

We therefore propose that a thorough understanding of human sleep will require an interpretation of functional imaging data in terms of their concomitant cognitive processes, such as those revealed by the analysis of dream content.

Phenomenology of dreaming

In this section, we demonstrate that dream reports contain valuable information about the cognitive processes that contribute to their generation and that cognition during sleep can be inferred from common features found in dream reports from different individuals [1, 2, 14]. Here, we consider dream content as accurate descriptions of sensory, emotional, and cognitive experiences spontaneously generated during sleep. Accordingly, vivid visual imagery, emotional intensification, and illusion of reality would represent examples of the defining features of typical dream experiences. We suggest that frequent cognitive features of dreams inform about underlying brain functions, thus allowing the integration of dream data into a unified model of human sleep.

Methods to collect reliable dream data

Dreaming raises the following methodological problem, which is also shared by other manifestations of conscious processes: how can we study a phenomenon that is not directly and objectively observable, but only accessible through introspection? Introspection implies that we first look into our own mind and then report any thought, feeling, and sensation that we could discern. It is important to note that the difference between introspective data and objective data derived from overt behavioral responses is often overstated. Indeed, like introspective data, behavioral measurements in cognitive studies frequently rely on inspecting mental representations or sensations and making decisions about them [15, 16]. By the very fact that they constitute a form of memory recall, dream reports may also be influenced by several factors such as

forgetting, reconstruction mechanisms, verbal description difficulties, censorship, experimental demands, and lack of independent verification. The impact of each of these factors can be minimized by using appropriate strategies, in particular by a careful training of the participants at reporting their dreams (more information about these strategies in [2]). Different methods can be used to collect representative and reliable dream material such as home-based dream diaries, dream questionnaires measuring precise features of dream experience, and dreams collected after awakening from polysomnographically defined sleep stages. Finally, asking people to report their most recent dream, whether it was "last night, last week, or last month," can also provide valuable information about dream content, in particular to characterize dreams in specific populations ("most recent dream" method; [17]).

Statistical approach to dreaming

Humans have always been intrigued by the varieties of dream experiences. Indeed, the seemingly disorganized and bizarre aspects in dreams contrast with the consistency and reproducibility of certain dream features, including some of the most bizarre dreams. It is thus not surprising that scientific approaches to dreaming have been interested in measuring the frequency of specific dream contents. Here we suggest that frequent dream features must relate to recurrent patterns of brain activity during sleep.

In 1893, a first statistical investigation was conducted on 375 dream reports by Mary Calkins [18], who found a clear predominance of visual experiences in dreams (57%), followed by auditory experiences (37%), and then by gustatory and olfactory experiences (1%) (see [19] for similar results). By programming awakenings at different times in the night, she also observed that more dreams occurred during the late part of the night (between 4 and 8 am), and that these late dreams were more vivid (this observation was replicated in several recent studies; e.g., [20–22]). Much more recently, and almost at the same time as REM sleep was discovered, Hall and Van De Castle published an extensive manual for coding of the content of dream reports [23]. This classification system was initially designed to measure common features in a large sample of dream reports from healthy young students (e.g., people, objects, places, social interactions, activities, emotions, etc.) and provided normative values for different content categories, which have since then been used to study many different samples of dreams (e.g., [24]). Nowadays, scales and coding systems have become standard tools to quantify dream characteristics. This classification approach is very efficient for assessing specific content categories, such as different types of emotions or bizarre features in the dreams of healthy or patient populations, or when testing theoretically driven hypotheses (e.g., [25]). However, coding systems rely on the delimitation of a priori categories to be quantified and therefore purposefully dismiss a large portion of information in the data. They also require that dream reports are analyzed manually, which may become particularly time-consuming when processing large dream data sets. To overcome some of these limitations, we proposed to use lexical statistical methods on large samples of dreams [1, 2]. Such methods allowed us to identify recurrent patterns of dream content based on the distribution of words in the dream reports, without any a-priori coding of the dreams, as we describe in the next section.

Distinct affective and cognitive dimensions in dream reports

We applied multidimensional statistical methods to a large longitudinal dream diary containing 1770 dream reports as well as to the original dreams used by Hall and Van de Castle consisting in total of 1000 dreams from 50 male and 50 female students (data set available: www.dreambank.net; [23]). Our results revealed well-segregated and consistent cognitive dimensions in the dreams from different individuals (more details about these results can be found in [1, 26]).

For example, frightening experiences formed a highly consistent category of dream content, which was clearly separated from dream elements referring to affective and working concerns related to the sleeper's waking life because limbic circuits, in particular the amygdala, contribute to emotional and memory processing [5, 6, 27], amygdala activation during sleep [4, 28, 29] might provide a permissive condition for emotionally relevant elements of memory to be selectively reprocessed in sleep (Figure 15.2A) [30–33]. This is consistent with an overrepresentation of recent elements of real-life and social emotions in the dreams [34–36]. On the other hand, intense fear-related emotions in dreams associated with rather unfamiliar settings as compared to waking life suggest that enhanced activation of the amygdala could also contribute to the rehearsal of genetically programmed or "primitive" behavioral responses to threatening stimuli [25, 37, 38]. A careful analysis of dream data therefore suggests that amygdala activation during REM sleep may be interpreted as contributing to distinct memory functions. Because the replay of recent neuronal activity possibly predominates during slow-wave sleep [39, 40], the finding that current concerns are frequent in dreams would also motivate future studies looking at transient patterns of regional cerebral activity [41, 42] and at the specific distribution of affective contents in dreams across all sleep stages [22].

As another example, the same statistical analyses also revealed that different categories of dream reports are characterized by distinct types of visual processes, such as color vision versus motion perception, or landscapes and outdoor scenes versus familiar people (among other visual characteristics; Figure 15.2B). Dissociation between these different visual properties is consistent with well-known functional specializations in the human brain (e.g., color vision in V4; motion processing in MT/V5; layouts and landscapes in the parahippocampal place area [PPA]; face processing in the fusiform face area[FFA]). While activation of associative visual areas is common in REM sleep [29, 43, 44], the functional dissociations in dreamed visual content, as found here, suggest that activity within associative visual areas during sleep might be more heterogeneous than previously thought, while involving reproducible patterns of brain activity.

Importantly, consistent emotional and cognitive dissociations were found in independent sets of dream data. Thus, the categories of dream content reported here substantiate our initial hypothesis that typical or common features in dream reports provide new information about emotional and cognitive processes at play during sleep.

Neuropsychology of dream bizarreness

When compared to usual experiences of waking life, dreams present innumerable anomalies. In this section, we show that bizarre features in the dreams may reflect specific functional states of the sleeping brain. We propose that (a) some bizarre features reported in dreams present remarkable similarities with specific neuropsychological deficits observed in brain-damaged patients, and that (b) the lesional topography causing these deficits in patients provides useful information about brain regions activated or deactivated during normal sleep [2]. Below, we illustrate with a few examples how bizarre aspects of visual processing in dreams may resemble some neurological syndromes. Note that the existence of striking similarities between certain neuropsychological syndromes and typical dream productions suggests commonalities in their underlying brain organization, but this does not imply at all that sleep or dreaming is a pathological state.

Misidentification for faces

One common bizarre feature in dreams is the disruption in visual recognition, whereby a dreamed character or object is clearly recognized although its physical appearance is drastically modified in the dream [2, 45]. In dreams, such dissociations between appearance and meaning commonly occur for faces or characters. The following dream reported by a 25 year-old man after an experimental awakening from REM sleep illustrates a typical mismatch between the identity of a character and its appearance: "Ah yes, exactly, I had a talk with your colleague, but she looked differently, much younger, like someone I went to school with, perhaps a 13-year-old girl …" ([19], p. 71). Normal identification of faces relies on a specific network of specialized brain areas including the FFA (Figure 15.2B) for the visual extraction of facial traits, the amygdala for detection of emotional significance [46], and infero-temporal and prefrontal regions that provide semantic information about particular people. Delusional misidentification or hyperidentification for people corresponds to a well-known neurological condition (sometimes called the Frégoli syndrome), whereby an unknown person face's is erroneously recognized as a familiar person, despite the lack of any obvious physical resemblance [47–49]. Brain lesions in this disorder may encompass temporo-occipital regions and the prefrontal cortex [47, 50, 51]. As exemplified by the dream excerpt above, misidentification for faces is a common feature of dream experience [45], which might relate to an activation of the FFA and temporal areas in the absence of selective reciprocal constraints between these regions, and in the absence of monitoring from prefrontal areas (whose activity is reduced during human sleep; [4, 29, 52]). Moreover, activation of limbic circuits during REM sleep may promote an abnormal bias in attributing a personal meaning or relevance to unknown faces [4, 29].

Misidentification for places

Misidentifications for places are also extremely frequent in dream reports, in which one place can be recognized as familiar in the absence of any apparent similitude to the corresponding original place. Neuroimaging studies in awake subjects have identified a specific brain area that is specialized for the processing of places and layouts, i.e., the PPA (just anterior to the FFA; Figure 15.2B). Delusional misidentification syndromes or "reduplicative paramnesia" for places can occur after temporal and prefrontal lesions, with a right hemisphere predominance [53–55]. Like the misidentifications for faces, misidentifications for places in dreams likely result from a disconnection between the PPA (mediating perceptual features), temporal regions (semantic information), and frontal regions (monitoring).

Other visual distortions

A non-exhaustive list of other typical visual distortions in dreams includes the multiplication of a visual percept in time ("palinopsia") or in space ("polyopia"), which is observed in patients with lesions in visual associative areas [56, 57], and abnormal visual size perception with apparent reduction ("micropsia") or increase ("macropsia") of the size of objects, previously reported after right occipital damage [58]. A typical example of macropsia is offered in the following excerpt from a dream of a 23-year-old woman (laboratory recording, awakening from REM sleep): "I was together with two boys, about 17 years old. They were fixing an enormous steak, a T-bone steak. I noticed how they had prepared it. It was a gigantic piece, one might have thought from an elephant, incredibly huge." ([19], p. 147). These distortions are present in a significant fraction of dream reports, suggesting that selective visual areas are hypoactivated or disconnected from other higher-level areas during this type of dream experiences. The loss of color saturation in visual perception ("achromatopsia") found in patients with occipital lesions in lingual and fusiform gyri [59] is also frequently found in dream imagery [60] and suggests a hypoactivation of occipital color areas (Figure 15.2B) or a disconnection between color regions and other visual or parietal regions subtending multimodal integration.

Interestingly, recent combined electroencephalogram (EEG) and TMS (Transcranial magnetic stimulation) studies have shown that functional connectivity across cortical regions is reduced during non-rapid eye movement (NREM) sleep but possibly restored during REM sleep [61, 62]. Although the functional dialog across brain regions during some sleep stages may be quantitatively comparable to that observed during wakefulness, cognitive dissociations in dream reports suggest some alterations of the functional integration of neural activity across regions, which may be due to decreased perceptual and physiological constraints (e.g., reduced sensory inputs, limited monitoring mechanisms, variations in neurotransmitters balance) during sleep as compared to wakefulness. The analysis of specific bizarre features in dreams might thus offer specific and useful constraints to the interpretation of functional imaging data collected during sleep.

Neural determinants of dream recall

Several studies are directly aimed at revealing the neural correlates of dreaming. In particular, selective disorders of dreaming may result from regionally specific brain damages [63, 64], showing a high degree of overlap with regions found to be activated during REM sleep, thus confirming the hypothesis that activation during REM sleep may, at least in part, support dreaming [3]. Lately, some studies looked at the EEG power spectra during periods of sleep preceding awakenings with and without dream recall [65, 66]. Although not always consistent, the results showed that changes in cortical oscillatory activity may predict successful dream recall, with more frequent recall when frontal theta is high during REM sleep and when NREM sleep oscillations are attenuated (e.g., lower frontal delta and higher temporal alpha). A preliminary study also used transcranial direct current stimulation during stage 2 sleep to directly modulate brain activity and dreaming, and found increased frequency of dreams with visual imagery during stimulation of posterior regions (and deactivation of frontal regions) [67]. These studies confirm that dreaming is not confined to periods of REM sleep and that dreaming may occur on variable backgrounds of neural activity over a night of sleep. While these studies point to a distribution of neural activation that may optimize consciousness and memory for dream experiences, links with specific dream contents still need further research. Related to this issue, a recent study investigated whether anatomical measures of the amygdala and hippocampus correlated with quantitative and qualitative aspects of dream reports in healthy subjects, and showed that the volume and mean diffusivity of the amygdala correlated with emotional and bizarre features in the dreams [68]. These findings demonstrate that individual differences in dream experiences are underlined by differences in brain structure. An important extension of this work will be to test how individual difference in dream content (and brain anatomy) covary with behavioral and brain measures during wakefulness (i.e., emotional responses and amygdala activity). This non-exhaustive selection of studies indicates very clearly that brain imaging methods can be used to investigate mental processes during sleep and their underlying neural substrate. Conversely, future studies are expected to show that dream characteristics may represent biomarkers of important brain functions, such as emotional regulation processes [26]. Thus, future studies of sleep in health and disease would benefit from collecting dreams in a systematic manner.

Conclusions

In the present chapter, we showed that the study of dreams provides meaningful and valuable information about cognitive and affective processes occurring during sleep. We first demonstrated that typical features in large dream samples can be identified using statistical methods and that these features are in good correspondence with known patterns of brain activity during sleep, in particular REM sleep. These analyses are based on the frequency of occurrence and degree of uniformity of dream contents, irrespective of whether the dreams mimicked real-life experiences or were extremely bizarre. We then showed that bizarre but common aspects in dreams have much in common with known neuropsychological syndromes. This approach has taken into account the typical pattern of activation during REM sleep (high limbic and low prefrontal/parietal activity), but it further suggests that sensory areas are heterogeneously activated (i.e., in different dreams) and that the functional connectivity between brain regions, including associative regions beyond early sensory cortices, may be modulated as well. Future research should objectively characterize these region- and episode-specific patterns of activation across all

sleep stages and help specify the hypothesized mechanisms that might explain them, such as ponto-geniculo-occipital activity [69] or experience-dependent cortico-limbic interplay [39, 70]. Unlike early brain imaging studies (most of them using PET) that were restricted to reporting mean levels of regional cerebral activity during distinct sleep stages, a few recent neuroimaging studies, in particular functional MRI studies, showed that it is now possible to capture more transient, dynamic changes of brain activity with a high anatomical resolution [41, 42, 71]. Altogether, this new, integrated approach to sleep and dreaming will undoubtedly contribute to redefining the links between brain processes and the varieties of dream experiences, and lead to a more comprehensive model of human brain function during sleep.

References

1. Schwartz S. What dreaming can reveal about cognitive and brain functions during sleep? A lexico-statistical analysis of dream reports. *Psychol Belg.* 2004;**44**(1):5–42.

2. Schwartz S, Maquet P. Sleep imaging and the neuro-psychological assessment of dreams. *Trends Cogn Sci.* 2002;**6**(1):23–30.

3. Hobson JA, Stickgold R, Pace-Schott EF. The neuropsychology of REM sleep dreaming. *Neuroreport.* 1998;**9**(3): R1–14.

4. Maquet P, Peters J, Aerts J, *et al.* Functional neuroanatomy of human rapid-eye-movement sleep and dreaming. *Nature.* 1996;**383**(6596):163–6.

5. Phelps EA, LeDoux JE. Contributions of the amygdala to emotion processing: from animal models to human behavior. *Neuron.* 2005;**48**(2):175–87.

6. Phan KL, Wager T, Taylor SF, Liberzon I. Functional neuroanatomy of emotion: a meta-analysis of emotion activation studies in PET and fMRI. *Neuroimage.* 2002;**16**(2):331–48.

7. Desseilles M, Vu TD, Laureys S, *et al.* A prominent role for amygdaloid complexes in the Variability in Heart Rate (VHR) during Rapid Eye Movement (REM) sleep relative to wakefulness. *Neuroimage.* 2006;**32** (3):1008–15.

8. Maquet P, Laureys S, Peigneux P, *et al.* Experience-dependent changes in cerebral activation during human REM sleep. *Nat Neurosci.* 2000;**3**(8):831–6.

9. Peigneux P, Laureys S, Fuchs S, *et al.* Are spatial memories strengthened in the human hippocampus during slow wave sleep? *Neuron.* 2004;**44**(3):535–45.

10. Portas CM, Krakow K, Allen P, *et al.* Auditory processing across the sleep-wake cycle: simultaneous EEG and fMRI monitoring in humans. *Neuron.* 2000;**28**(3):991–9.

11. Rasch B, Buchel C, Gais S, Born J. Odor cues during slow-wave sleep prompt declarative memory consolidation. *Science.* 2007;**315**(5817):1426–9.

12. Czisch M, Wehrle R, Stiegler A, *et al.* Acoustic oddball during NREM sleep: a combined EEG/fMRI study. *PloS One.* 2009;**4**(8):e6749.

13. Wamsley EJ, Tucker M, Payne JD, Benavides JA, Stickgold R. Dreaming of a learning task is associated with enhanced sleep-dependent memory consolidation. *Curr Biol.* 2010;**20**(9):850–5.

14. Hobson JA, Pace-Schott EF, Stickgold R. Dreaming and the brain: toward a cognitive neuroscience of conscious states. *Behav Brain Sci.* 2000;**23**(6):793–842; discussion 904–1121.

15. Cohen G. *Memory in the Real World.* 2nd edn. Hove, East Sussex, UK, Psychology Press, 1996.

16. Ericsson KA, Simon HA. Verbal reports as data. *Psychol Rev.* 1980;**87**(3):215–51.

17. Domhoff GW. *Finding Meaning in Dreams: A Quantitative Approach.* New York, NY, Plenum Press, 1996.

18. Calkins MW. Statistics of dreams. *Am J Psychol.* 1893;**5**:311–43.

19. Strauch I, Meier B. *In Search of Dreams: Results of Experimental Dream Research.*

Albany, NY, State University of New York Press, 1996.

20. Fosse R, Stickgold R, Hobson JA. Thinking and hallucinating: reciprocal changes in sleep. *Psychophysiology.* 2004;**41**(2):298–305.

21. Fosse R, Stickgold R, Hobson JA. Brain-mind states: reciprocal variation in thoughts and hallucinations. *Psychol Sci.* 2001;**12**(1):30–6.

22. Wamsley EJ, Hirota Y, Tucker MA, Smith MR, Antrobus JS. Circadian and ultradian influences on dreaming: a dual rhythm model. *Brain Res Bull.* 2007;**71**(4):347–54.

23. Hall CS, Van de Castle RL. *The Content Analysis of Dreams.* New York, Appleton-Century-Crofts, 1966.

24. Domhoff GW, Schneider A. New rationales and methods for quantitative dream research outside the laboratory. *Sleep.* 1998;**21**(4):398–404.

25. Valli K, Revonsuo A. The threat simulation theory in light of recent empirical evidence: a review. *Am J Psychol.* 2009;**122**(1):17–38.

26. Desseilles M, Dang-Vu TT, Sterpenich V, Schwartz S. Cognitive and emotional processes during dreaming: a neuroimaging view. *Conscious Cogn.* 2011;**20**(4):998–1008.

27. Vuilleumier P. How brains beware: neural mechanisms of emotional attention. *Trends Cogn Sci.* 2005;**9**(12):585–94.

28. Nofzinger EA, Mintun MA, Wiseman M, Kupfer DJ, Moore RY. Forebrain activation in REM sleep: an FDG PET study. *Brain Res.* 1997;**770**(1–2):192–201.

29. Braun AR, Balkin TJ, Wesensten NJ, *et al.* Regional cerebral blood flow throughout the sleep-wake cycle: An H$_2^{15}$O PET study. *Brain.* 1997;**120**:1173–97.

30. Hennevin E, Maho C, Hars B. Neuronal plasticity induced by fear conditioning is expressed during paradoxical sleep: evidence from simultaneous recordings in the lateral amygdala and the medial geniculate in rats. *Behav Neurosci.* 1998;**112**(4):839–62.

31. Pare D, Collins DR, Pelletier JG. Amygdala oscillations and the consolidation of emotional memories. *Trends Cogn Sci.* 2002;**6**(7):306–14.

32. Popa D, Duvarci S, Popescu AT, Lena C, Pare D. Coherent amygdalocortical theta promotes fear memory consolidation during paradoxical sleep. *Proc Natl Acad Sci U S A.* 2010;**107**(14):6516–19.

33. Sterpenich V, Albouy G, Darsaud A, *et al.* Sleep promotes the neural reorganization of remote emotional memory. *J Neurosci.* 2009;**29**(16):5143–52.

34. Hobson JA, Pace-Schott EF. The cognitive neuroscience of sleep: neuronal systems, consciousness and learning. *Nat Rev Neurosci.* 2002;**3**(9):679–93.

35. Schwartz S. Are life episodes replayed during dreaming? *Trends Cogn Sci.* 2003;7(8):325–7.

36. Schredl M, Hofmann F. Continuity between waking activities and dream activities. *Conscious Cogn.* 2003;**12**(2):298–308.

37. Revonsuo A. The reinterpretation of dreams: an evolutionary hypothesis of the function of dreaming. *Behav Brain Sci.* 2000;**23**(6):877–901; discussion 904–1121.

38. Jouvet M. Paradoxical sleep as a programming system. *J Sleep Res.* 1998;7(Suppl):1–5.

39. Diekelmann S, Born J. The memory function of sleep. *Nat Rev Neurosci.* 2010;**11**(2):114–26.

40. Oudiette D, Constantinescu I, Leclair-Visonneau L, *et al.* Evidence for the re-enactment of a recently learned behavior during sleepwalking. *PloS One.* 2011;**6**(3):e18056.

41. Schabus M, Dang-Vu TT, Albouy G, *et al.* Hemodynamic cerebral correlates of sleep spindles during human non-rapid eye movement sleep. *Proc Natl Acad Sci U S A.* 2007;**104**(32):13164–9.

42. Dang-Vu TT, Schabus M, Desseilles M, *et al.* Spontaneous neural activity during human slow wave sleep. *Proc Natl Acad Sci U S A.* 2008;**105**(39):15160–5.

43. Braun AR, Balkin TJ, Wesensten NJ, *et al.* Dissociated pattern of activity in visual cortices and their projections during human rapid eye movement sleep. *Science.* 1998;**279**(5347):91–5.

44. Maquet P. Functional neuroimaging of normal human sleep by positron emission tomography. *J Sleep Res.* 2000;**9**(3):207–31.

45. Kahn D, Stickgold R, Pace-Schott EF, Hobson JA. Dreaming and waking consciousness: a character recognition study. *J Sleep Res.* 2000;**9**(4):317–25.

46. Vuilleumier P, Armony JL, Driver J, Dolan RJ. Effects of attention and emotion on face processing in the human brain: an event-related fMRI study. *Neuron.* 2001;**30**(3):829–41.

47. Vuilleumier P, Mohr C, Valenza N, Wetzel C, Landis T. Hyperfamiliarity for unknown faces after left lateral temporo-occipital venous infarction: a double dissociation with prosopagnosia. *Brain.* 2003;**126**(Pt 4):889–907.

48. Forstl H, Almeida OP, Owen AM, Burns A, Howard R. Psychiatric, neurological and medical aspects of misidentification syndromes: a review of 260 cases. *Psychol Med.* 1991;**21**(4):905–10.

49. Young AH, Ellis HD, Szulecka TK, de Pauw KW. Face processing impairments and delusional misidentification. *Behav Neurol.* 1990;**3**(3):153–68.

50. Rapcsak SZ, Reminger SL, Glisky EL, Kaszniak AW, Comer JF. Neuropsychological mechanisms of false facial recognition following frontal lobe damage. *Cogn Neuropsychol.* 1999;**16**(3–5):267–92.

51. Hudson AJ, Grace GM. Misidentification syndromes related to face specific area in the fusiform gyrus. *J Neurol Neurosurg Psychiatry.* 2000;**69**(5):645–8.

52. Muzur A, Pace-Schott EF, Hobson JA. The prefrontal cortex in sleep. *Trends Cogn Sci.* 2002;**6**(11):475–81.

53. Benson DF, Gardner H, Meadows JC. Reduplicative paramnesia. *Neurology.* 1976;**26**(2):147–51.

54. Kapur N, Turner A, King C. Reduplicative paramnesia: possible anatomical and neuropsychological mechanisms. *J Neurol Neurosurg Psychiatry.* 1988;**51**(4):579–81.

55. Hakim H, Verma NP, Greiffenstein MF. Pathogenesis of reduplicative paramnesia. *J Neurol Neurosurg Psychiatry.* 1988;**51**(6):839–41.

56. Michel EM, Troost BT. Palinopsia: cerebral localization with computed tomography. *Neurology.* 1980;**30**(8):887–9.

57. Bender MB, Feldman M, Sobin AJ. Palinopsia. *Brain.* 1968;**91**(2):321–38.

58. Ceriani F, Gentileschi V, Muggia S, Spinnler H. Seeing objects smaller than they are: micropsia following right temporo-parietal infarction. *Cortex.* 1998;**34**(1):131–8.

59. Paulson H, Galetta S, Grossman M, Alavi A. Hemiachromatopsia of unilateral occipitotemporal infarcts. *Am J Ophthalmol.* 1994;**118**(4):518–23.

60. Rechtschaffen A, Buchignani C. The visual appearance of dreams. In: Antrobus JS, Bertini M, eds. *The Neuropsychology of Sleep and Dreaming.* Hillsdale, NJ, Lawrence Erlbaum Associates. 1992; 143–55.

61. Massimini M, Ferrarelli F, Huber R, *et al.* Breakdown of cortical effective connectivity during sleep. *Science.* 2005;**309**(5744):2228–32.

62. Massimini M, Ferrarelli F, Murphy M, *et al.* Cortical reactivity and effective connectivity during REM sleep in humans. *Cogn Neurosci.* 2010;**1**(3):176–83.

63. Doricchi F, Violani C. Dream recall in brain-damaged patients: a contribution to the neuropsychology of dreaming through a review of the literature. In: John S, Antrobus MB, eds. *The Neuropsychology of Sleep and Dreaming.* Lawrence Erlbaum Associates, Inc, Hillsdale, NJ, US; 1992; 99–129.

64. Solms M. *The Neuropsychology of Dreams: A Clinico-Anatomical Study.* Mahwah, NJ, Lawrence Erlbaum Associates, 1997.

65. Chellappa SL, Frey S, Knoblauch V, Cajochen C. Cortical activation patterns herald successful dream recall after NREM and REM sleep. *Biol Psychol.* 2011;**87**(2):251–6.

66. Marzano C, Ferrara M, Mauro F, *et al.* Recalling and forgetting dreams: theta and alpha oscillations during sleep predict subsequent dream recall. *J Neurosci.* 2011;**31**(18):6674–83.

67. Jakobson AJ, Fitzgerald PB, Conduit R. Induction of visual dream reports after transcranial direct current stimulation (tDCs) during Stage 2 sleep. *J Sleep Res.* 2012;**21**(4):369–79.

68. De Gennaro L, Cipolli C, Cherubini A, *et al.* Amygdala and hippocampus volumetry and diffusivity in relation to dreaming. *Hum Brain Mapp.* 2011;**32**(9):1458–70.

69. Peigneux P, Laureys S, Fuchs S, *et al.* Generation of rapid eye movements during paradoxical sleep in humans. *Neuroimage.* 2001;**14**(3):701–8.

70. Perogamvros L, Schwartz S. The roles of the reward system in sleep and dreaming. *Neurosci Behav Rev.* 2012;**36**(8):1934–51.

71. Bergmann TO, Molle M, Diedrichs J, Born J, Siebner HR. Sleep spindle-related reactivation of category-specific cortical regions after learning face-scene associations. *Neuroimage.* 2012;**59**(3):2733–42.

Chapter

16

Functional neuroimaging of sleep deprivation

Michael W. L. Chee and Robert Joseph Thomas

Introduction

Functional magnetic resonance imaging (fMRI) is a non-invasive and highly versatile tool to study neurobehavioral alterations associated with sleep deprivation (SD) as well as their underlying mechanisms. Here, we briefly review the techniques currently applied to study brain function during SD – as opposed to the consequence of SD, described in previous chapters. We provide a bird's-eye view of functional imaging studies performed on healthy young adult volunteers to date and comment on how this research has evolved our conceptualization of how SD modulates behavior. Subsequent chapters will discuss in depth how fMRI has been used to study attention (Chapter 17), decision-making (Chapter 18), and inter-individual differences in response to SD (Chapter 19).

Task-related fMRI is the most widely used technique for examining neurobehavioral alterations *during* SD [1–40] (Table 16.1). It measures relative change in blood oxygen level-dependent (BOLD) signal in capillaries and venules adjacent to neuronal clusters whose firing rate and, consequently, synaptic potentials are modulated by task performance. An increase in MR signal occurs as a result of a relatively disproportionate elevation in blood flow relative to oxygen consumption in response to sensory stimulation and/or task performance. In addition to task-related activation, the evaluation of task-related deactivation where signal changes fall below baseline levels [41] can be evaluated [1, 18, 25, 30] (Figure 16.1).

Correlating state-related alteration in BOLD signal with corresponding behavioral change under different levels of task load/difficulty affords better isolation of the cognitive process(es) underlying cognitive decline in SD. Ideally, this would be achieved by having the individual perform several tasks in the same scanning session, so that either different facets of a particular cognitive domain (e.g., sustained vs. selective attention) or several different cognitive domains [42, 43] can be evaluated simultaneously. Perhaps as a result of cost or logistical considerations, such studies have yet to be conducted despite the impressive list of cognitive domains studied with fMRI to date.

Although BOLD imaging serves as a proxy for relative changes in blood flow, it does not ascertain absolute blood flow. Quantification of blood flow may occasionally be useful, for example, to study time-on-task effects [44], and other phenomena whose observation requires signal stability over several minutes as opposed to several seconds. Such measurements can be obtained using a variety of arterial spin labeling

Table 16.1. fMRI studies involving sleep deprivation

Cognitive domain	Reference
Working memory	Bell-McGinty *et al.* (2004) [22] Habeck *et al.* (2004) [59] Chee & Choo (2004) [1] Caldwell *et al.* (2005) [24] Choo *et al.* (2005) [2] Mu *et al.* (2005a) [26] Mu *et al.* (2005b) [27] Chee *et al.* (2006) [4] Thomas and Kwong (2006) [39] Lim *et al.* (2007) [6] Luber et al (2008) [28] Vandewalle (2009) [35]
Attention (sustained or divided)	Portas et al. (1998) [40] Thomas *et al.* (2000) [56] Drummond *et al.* (2001) [58] Drummond *et al.* (2005) [25] Chee *et al.* (2008) [8] Tucker et al (2011) [31]
Attention (selective)	Mander et al. (2008) [33] Tomasi et al. (2009) [37] Volkow et al. (2009) [38] Chee and Tan (2010) [11] Chee *et al.* (2010) [12] Lim *et al.* (2010) [48] Chee *et al.* (2011) [15] Kong *et al.* (2011) [16]
Visual short-term memory	Chee & Chuah (2007) [5] Chuah and Chee (2008) [9]
Logical reasoning Inhibition (Go/No-Go) Risky decision-making	Drummond *et al.* (2004) [23] Chuah *et al.* (2006) [3] Venkatraman *et al.* (2007) [7] Venkatraman *et al.* (2011) [17]
Emotional processing	Sterpernich et al. (2007) [63] Yoo *et al.* (2007a) [29] Gujar *et al.* (2011) [32]
Verbal learning/Verbal episodic memory	Drummond *et al.* (2000) [20] Yoo *et al.* [2007b] [34] Chuah et al. (2009) [10]
Default mode/Resting state	Gujar (2010) [30] De Havas (2012) [18]

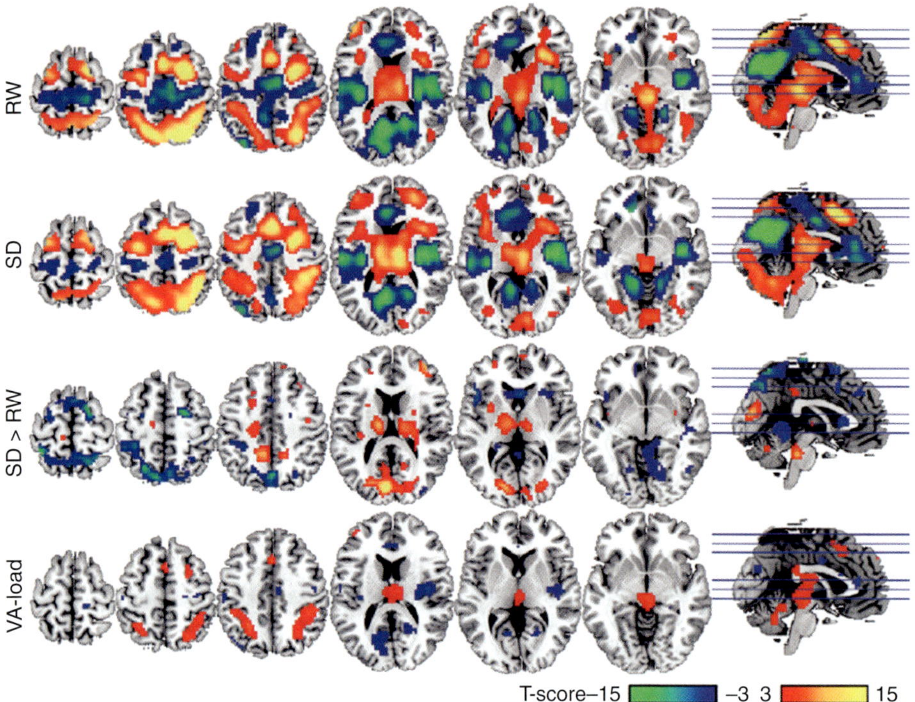

Figure 16.1 Task-related activation and deactivation, state and load contrasts in a visual tracking task. BOLD fMRI activation patterns for the main (rested wakefulness – RW, SD) and differential (SD > RW and visual attention – VA load) effects of visual attention using a ball-tracking task. In the first two rows, brain regions depicted in red-yellow show task-related activation (signal greater than during baseline) while those showing task-induced deactivation (signal less than during baseline) appear in blue-green. (Adapted from [37].)

(ASL) techniques that have different levels of precision [45, 46]. A general disadvantage of these methods limiting their wider use is inferior signal-to-noise ratio. Additionally, the requirement for block sampling also makes it impossible to perform event-related designs that are important in separating out trials where the subject may have been asleep [8].

The evaluation of functional connectivity, conducted by assessing signal covariation in pairs of regions, or by determining the extent to which signal in a "target" region interacts with that of a "seed" region according to state/task context, provides additional characterization of altered physiology. The latter method, known as psychophysiological interaction (PPI; [47]), has been applied in studies evaluating selective attention [12, 48], the processing of emotional pictures [29], as well as executive function/working memory [35].

In addition to fMRI studies designed to evaluate signal changes in response to task performance, it may be informative to evaluate "resting-state" activity [49, 50]. This refers to the identification of regions showing synchronous low frequency oscillations (0.1–0.01 Hz) in BOLD signal that are not time locked to task performance or sensory stimulation. Studies of this type in sleeping individuals have shown changes in connectivity within the default mode network (DMN) alluded to earlier [51, 52]. The first study evaluating resting state networks in the setting of SD found selective reductions in DMN functional connectivity and reduced anti-correlation with low frequency oscillations in the "task-positive" network [18], (Figure 16.2). Analyses of resting state data hold promise of being informative of alterations in brain function without requiring motivated performance on the part of a participant [53].

Related to functional connectivity, one can use MR to evaluate white matter connectivity but oddly, only one study to date has used diffusion tensor imaging to study sleep-deprived individuals [54].

Combining fMRI with other brain mapping tools requires instrumentation and technical sophistication available to relatively few teams. Combining electroencephalography (EEG) and fMRI in SD or sleep-related studies is primarily motivated by the need to monitor sleep stage [55] although the high temporal resolution of EEG is also well suited to study transient phenomena like lapsing. Functional MRI-guided repetitive transcranial magnetic stimulation (rTMS) has been used to evaluate the therapeutic potential of TMS in alleviating SD [28].

Evolution of studies: pioneering studies

The first functional imaging studies involving SD utilized positron emission tomography (PET) [40, 56]. One of these and the first fMRI studies were influenced by suggestions that the prefrontal cortex might be exquisitely sensitive to sleep loss [57]. As such, tasks like serial subtraction and verbal learning that were known to engage frontal lobe function were used [19, 20, 58]. Contrary to expectation, reduction in frontal lobe activation was observed only in the first of these fMRI studies [19]. Although performance generally declined, individuals with relatively preserved performance tended to have higher activation in the frontal and parietal regions following SD compared to the well-rested state in the verbal learning task [20] as well as in an experiment evaluating divided attention which incorporated verbal learning as one of the two tasks [58].

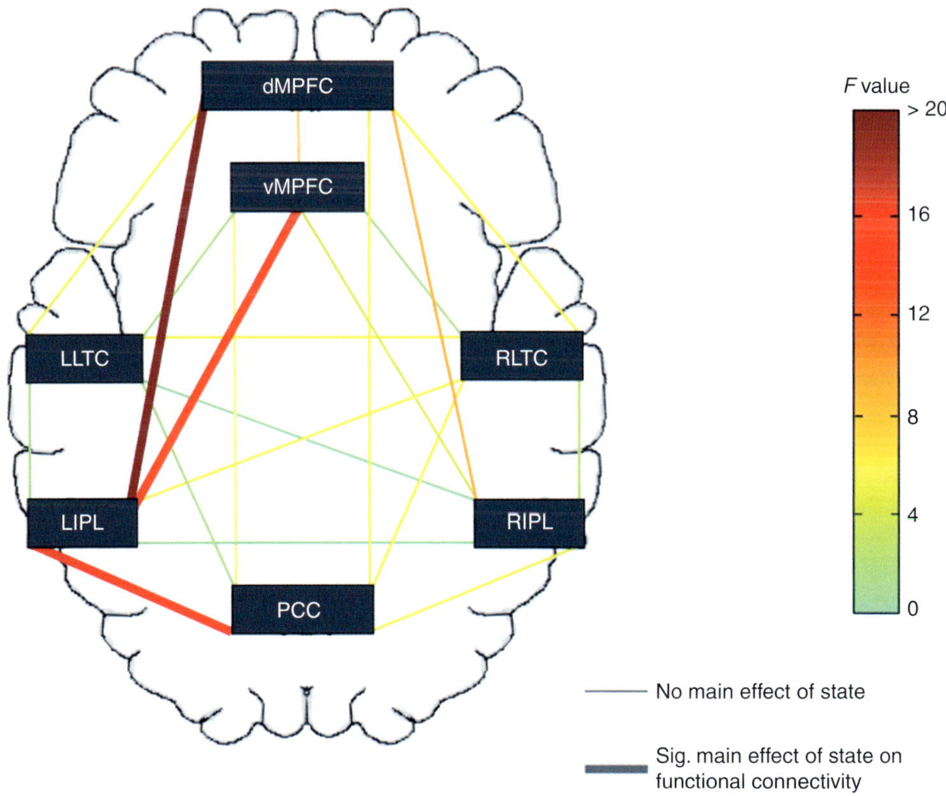

Figure 16.2 Main effect of state on default mode network functional connectivity. Schematic showing a significant main effect of state on DMN functional connectivity between three node pairs using a seed based analysis; left inferior parietal lobe (LIPL) and dorsal medial prefrontal cortex (dMPFC), LIPL and ventromedial prefrontal cortex (vMPFC), and LIPL and posterior cingulate cortex (PCC; Bonferroni corrected p < 0.05/21 = 0.002) (Used with permission from [18].)

Effects of task difficulty, cognitive domain tested, and inter-individual differences

Based on these initial findings, cognitive domain engaged and task difficulty were proposed as determinants of the neural response to SD [21]. This motivated subsequent studies probing working memory to examine the effect of manipulating task difficulty [1] or item load [2, 59]. While the specific areas most affected by SD differed somewhat across these studies, a common set of findings was a decrease in higher visual cortex and frontoparietal activation when performance declined during SD and contrastingly, relatively preserved activation when performance was maintained. The notion that increased task difficulty might elicit "compensatory" frontal activation was then independently demonstrated in a study evaluating logical reasoning [23].

As experience in fMRI cumulated with studies that recruited around 20 subjects each, it became evident that inter-individual differences in response to SD could be identified reliably. As discussed in Chapter 19, earlier studies suggested that a single imaging study conducted in the rested state might predict vulnerability to performance decline in the tested domain [4, 24, 26] whereas later studies were to discover that shifts in activation across state may be more reliable markers of inter-individual differences [9, 11].

A wealth of behavioral data collected on behavior in sleep-deprived persons suggests the loss of vigilance or sustained attention to be the most prominent deficit encountered in SD [14].

The failure of attention and the possible maladaptive consequences of endogenous efforts to sustain wakefulness in the face of mounting sleep pressure are elaborated in Chapters 17, 18, and 19. A cogent illustration of the vital role played by attention in supporting cognitive performance comes from an experiment originally designed to evaluate visual working memory capacity in SD [5]. The experiment is described in greater detail later, but its key finding was that during SD, even when memory capacity and perceptual load were not taxed, task-related activation in brain regions mediating top-down control of attention and visual perception in extrastriate visual cortex were significantly diminished. This indicated that a more global curtailment of processing resources rather than storage limitation was problematic. As both working memory and attention are intertwined processes [60] and engage similar cortical and subcortical areas [61], the parametric variation of visual memory and visual item load across multiple levels in two parallel sets of scans were instrumental in proving the point.

Additional studies probing the effects of SD on selective attention using visual tracking [37] or visual picture selection paradigms [48, 62] made convergent observations regarding the attenuation of top-down control of attention together with diminished engagement of the visual extrastriate cortex. In addition to such deficits in responding to stimuli, attenuated activation in the preparatory period prior to stimulus appearance has also been demonstrated [15].

While the effects of SD on cortical activation have been quite clearly delineated, its effects on subcortical activation are more complex. The thalamus, which plays an important role in mediating arousal and attention, shows decreased glucose metabolism across a block of time during SD [56]. However, in relation to individual events during SD, activation can be either higher or lower than during rested wakefulness depending on whether the volunteer is performing adequately or lapsing [8, 37].

Evaluating countermeasures

The majority of persons shows decline in cognitive performance even after 24 h of SD, and a natural extension of studies examining the neural correlates of such alterations in performance is to use imaging changes to track the efficacy of countermeasures. Functional MRI has been used to evaluate the effect of modafinil [39], a stimulant with multiple modes of action, and the cholinesterase inhibitor donepezil [9, 10], on healthy volunteers deprived of sleep for a single night. In both studies, the effect of drug in the well-rested state was negligible but was evident in the sleep-deprived state in some volunteers. In the donepezil trial, improvement was positively correlated with the magnitude of performance decline when undergoing SD on placebo in both short-term memory and episodic memory experiments in the same subjects. The smaller trial involving modafinil evidenced increases in both cortical and subcortical activation in volunteers sleep deprived on modafinil. Repetitive TMS was reported as improving verbal working memory in sleep-deprived volunteers when applied to the right "upper middle occipital" region [28] that was part of the network associated with SD induced performance impairment. Improvement correlated with the extent to which performance declined during SD in sham stimulations. Improvement during SD was not observed when the midline parietal region, also part of this network, and when the lower left middle occipital gyrus which was not part of the network were stimulated.

Affective aspects of behaviour: emotional processing and decision-making

Most of the tasks previously described engage an inter related frontoparietal network involved in the control of attention and the encoding of memories. These tasks do not evaluate affective changes that constitute an important aspect of behavioral alteration in SD. Brain structures involved in affective processes include the amygdala, striatum, ventromedial prefrontal cortex, and the insula. These structures can be expected to show alterations in activation during SD accompanying these behavioral shifts.

At the group level, SD enhanced responses to negative emotional pictures within the amygdala in one study [29]. In this study, individuals graded the emotionality of the faces. Reduced functional connectivity between the ventromedial prefrontal cortex and amygdala was observed (Figure 16.3A). In a second study [13], volunteers remembered neutral faces over a brief interval during which distractor pictures were presented. The distractors could be neutral, negative emotional, or noise patterns. Amygdala activation during the maintenance period was higher for emotional distractors than neutral distractors in both

states although maintenance activity was overall lower in the SD state for both conditions (Figure 16.3B). Face memoranda were less well maintained in working memory to the extent that SD reduced functional connectivity between ventromedial and dorsolateral frontal areas and the amygdala [13]. Responses to emotional stimuli during SD can thus be perturbed by disrupted transmission of control signals emanating from regions involved in valuation and/or cognitive control. Negative stimuli appear to be better recognized after SD than neutral or positive stimuli. The recollection of negative and positive stimuli evidenced greater functional connectivity between medial frontal regions and the hippocampus when subjects had a normal night of sleep compared to when they were sleep deprived [63]. Intriguingly, the recollection of negative stimuli was less affected than recollection of positive stimuli following SD, possibly as a consequence of greater amygdala activation during SD. This could represent the invoking of an alternative route for recollection that conserves the recollection of negative stimuli.

The bias towards processing emotional stimuli can sometimes extend to positive stimuli as well. SD caused volunteers to increase the number of neutral pictures that were rated positively [32]. This finding was related to enhanced hippocampal to medial frontal and hippocampal to orbitofrontal connectivity in the SD state providing yet another avenue of support for prior findings. It was postulated that changes in dopamine signaling in the SD state contributed to the change in functional connectivity, an idea reprised when discussing risky decision-making in SD in Chapter 18.

Suggestions for future functional imaging research in sleep deprived persons

A critical gap in our current knowledge of the mechanisms underpinning altered behavior in SD lies in the piecemeal use of functional imaging in this state whereby a single cognitive domain is tested in each subject. As elaborated in Chapters 18 and 19, behavioral studies show that SD may dissimilarly affect performance in different cognitive domains [42, 43]. It remains an open challenge to execute within-subject studies involving multiple, sensitive, short-duration tasks that probe dissociable cognitive domains even though viable protocols exist [64].

While total SD is convenient to study in a laboratory setting, most persons encounter the effects of sleep loss through chronic sleep restriction and sleep fragmentation [65]. Partial SD studies where sleep is restricted to between 3 and 6 hours of time in bed per night suggest that the relationship between hours of sleep and cognition is not linear [66, 67]. The rate of buildup of slow wave activity during sustained wakefulness and its dissipation following recovery sleep also does not correspond well with behavioral performance alteration, suggesting that different measures provide independent information regarding changes occurring in SD. It remains interesting to study how functional imaging changes evolve during partial SD [66] – such studies can provide new understanding of compensatory brain network dynamics during the process of chronic partial sleep restriction.

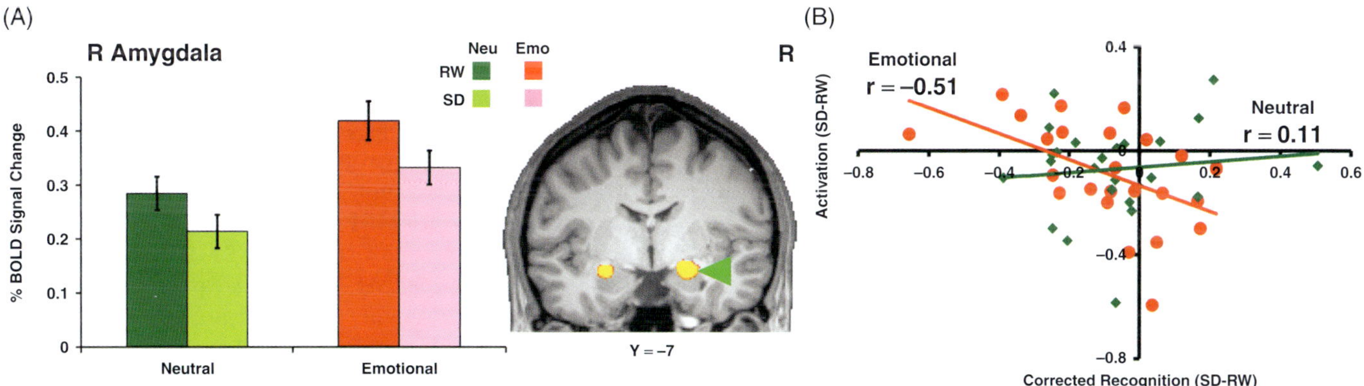

Figure 16.3 Functional imaging of responses to emotional pictures in sleep-deprived persons. (A) Functional connectivity between an amygdala seed (not shown) and ventromedial prefrontal cortex is decreased during SD compared to the well-rested /"sleep control" state (shown in yellow). (Adapted from [29]). (B) Right amygdala activity was elevated in response to emotional distracters relative to neutral distracters at rested wakefulness (RW). A state (rested wakefulness, sleep deprivation) by condition (neutral, emotional) repeated-measures ANOVA conducted on averaged activation within this region of interest indicated marginal decreases in amygdala activation following sleep deprivation. Critically, state-related change in amygdala activation correlated with the corresponding alteration of emotional distractibility while no parallel effect was present for neutral distracters. (Adapted from [13].)

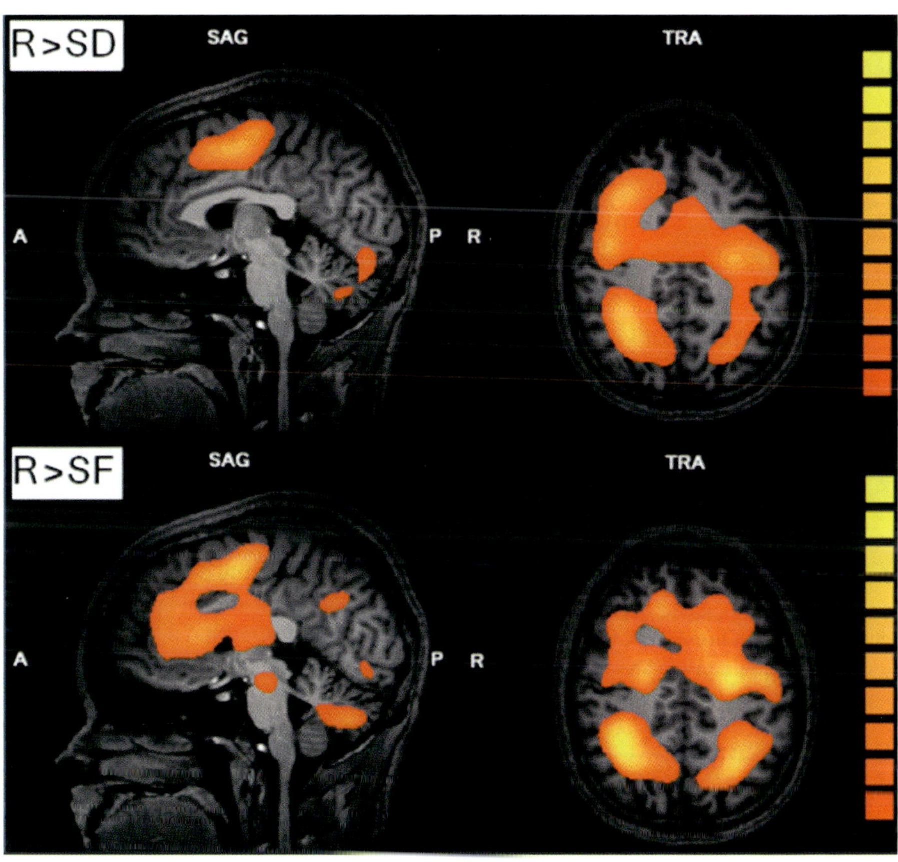

Figure 16.4 Effect of sleep deprivation and sleep fragmentation in healthy volunteers. Fixed effects subtraction images of 12 healthy subjects randomized to rested, sleep deprived (24 h) and sleep fragmented (single night auditory stimuli, 40–50 arousals/h of sleep) conditions, using a working memory 2-back block design task in a 3 tesla scanner. Note that while the patterns are similar, the sleep fragmentation contrast revealed a greater extent of activation difference. The performance decrement was also greater in the fragmented condition.

Preliminary data emerging from a laboratory-based study of a night of sleep fragmentation using auditory tones when healthy volunteers performed an n-back task suggest imaging alterations — reduced frontoparietal activation and increased thalamus activation, comparable to the effects of 28 h of total SD (Figure 16.4). Chronic sleep fragmentation experiments are extremely tedious to do, yet may provide new insights into the pathophysiology of conditions associated with interruptions of the ongoing continuity of sleep, such as pain, stress, and sleep apnea.

Imaging genomics seeks to identify genes that influence brain, cognition, and risk for disease (see Chapter 20). For example, the candidate gene approach was applied to study the effect of *Per 3^{5/5}* on n-back task performance in subjects undergoing total SD. Widespread relative reductions in task related activation were found in frontal, parietal, and occipital regions in this vulnerable group when they were sleep deprived [35]. The intriguing behavioral results were not replicated when a different set of sleep-restricted (not total SD) subjects were studied [68], leaving room for future studies to clarify.

SD provides a unique opportunity to perturb brain networks of healthy individuals in a manner that degrades performance in a reversible manner. Several similarities between the behavioral deficits in SD and cognitive aging have been highlighted [69, 70]. There are also functional imaging parallels that remain to be exploited in future studies [1, 71]. The attraction of this approach is that it may allow conspecific evaluation of cognitive enhancers in a relatively lower risk setting, keeping in mind that the target group of older adults may be less resilient to adverse effects should these occur.

The circadian system profoundly modulates brain function. During SD, cognitive performance during the biological night, as is a typical demand of shift-work, places both SD and circadian stress on neural function. The interaction of SD and circadian effects, including the effects of chronotype, could be a further target of functional neuroimaging studies, including the effect of countermeasures such as naps and stimulants.

Sleep inertia is the transient impairment of performance following an awakening from sleep. This phenomenon is particularly important during prolonged operational conditions, when napping may be a strategy used to counter sleep loss. The brain mechanisms of sleep inertia remain unknown, and offer an additional opportunity for functional neuroimaging.

Summary

Even a single night of SD can alter many aspects of behavior. Functional MRI has been used to evaluate the neural correlates of behavioral change in multiple cognitive domains. In addition to investigating alterations in task-related activation and deactivation, changes in functional connectivity can be probed. fMRI reliably detects and estimates the neural correlates of inter-individual differences in behavior following SD that can be incorporated into trials evaluating the efficacy of countermeasures. Among the many issues that require further exploration, it remains to study multiple tasks in the same subjects, to evaluate if partial SD and total SD evoke similar functional imaging changes.

Acknowledgements

This work was supported by grants awarded to MC from the Defence Science and Technology Agency Singapore (POD0713897) and the National Research Foundation Singapore (STaR Award) and USA National Heart Lung & Blood Institute grant K23HL004457 awarded to RJT.

References

1. Chee MW, Choo WC. Functional imaging of working memory after 24 hr of total sleep deprivation. *J Neurosci.* 2004;**24**(19):4560–7.

2. Choo WC, Lee WW, Venkatraman V, Sheu FS, Chee MW. Dissociation of cortical regions modulated by both working memory load and sleep deprivation and by sleep deprivation alone. *Neuroimage.* 2005;**25**(2):579–87.

3. Chuah YM, Venkatraman V, Dinges DF, Chee MW. The neural basis of interindividual variability in inhibitory efficiency after sleep deprivation. *J Neurosci.* 2006;**26**(27):7156–62.

4. Chee MW, Chuah YML, Venkatraman V, *et al.* Functional imaging of working memory following normal sleep and after 24 and 35 hours of sleep deprivation: correlations of fronto-parietal activation with performance. *Neuroimage.* 2006;**31**(1):419–28.

5. Chee MW, Chuah YM. Functional neuroimaging and behavioral correlates of capacity decline in visual short-term memory following sleep deprivation. *Proc Natl Acad Sci U S A.* 2007;**104**(22):9487–92.

6. Lim J, Choo WC, Chee MW. Reproducibility of changes in behaviour and fMRI activation associated with sleep deprivation in a working memory task. *Sleep.* 2007;**30**(1):61–70.

7. Venkatraman V, Chuah YM, Huettel SA, Chee MW. Sleep deprivation elevates expectation of gains and attenuates response to losses following risky decisions. *Sleep.* 2007;**30**(5):603–9.

8. Chee MW, Tan JC, Zheng H, *et al.* Lapsing during sleep deprivation is associated with distributed changes in brain activation. *J Neurosci.* 2008;**28**(21):5519–28.

9. Chuah LY, Chee MW. Cholinergic augmentation modulates visual task performance in sleep-deprived young adults. *J Neurosci.* 2008;**28**(44):11369–77.

10. Chuah LY, Chong DL, Chen AK, *et al.* Donepezil improves episodic memory in young individuals vulnerable to the effects of sleep deprivation. *Sleep.* 2009;**32**(8):999–1010.

11. Chee MW, Tan JC. Lapsing when sleep deprived: neural activation characteristics of resistant and vulnerable individuals. *Neuroimage.* 2010;**51**(2):835–43.

12. Chee MW, Tan JC, Parimal S, Zagorodnov V. Sleep deprivation and its effects on object-selective attention. *Neuroimage.* 2010;**49**(2):1903–10.

13. Chuah LY, Dolcos F, Chen AK, *et al.* Sleep deprivation and interference by emotional distracters. *Sleep.* 2010;**33**(10):1305–13.

14. Lim J, Dinges DF. A meta-analysis of the impact of short-term sleep deprivation on cognitive variables. *Psychol Bull.* 2010;**136**(3):375–89.

15. Chee MW, Goh CS, Namburi P, *et al.* Effects of sleep deprivation on cortical activation during directed attention in the absence and presence of visual stimuli. *Neuroimage.* 2011;**58**(2):595–604.

16. Kong D, Soon CS, Chee MW. Reduced visual processing capacity in sleep deprived persons. *Neuroimage.* 2011;**55**(2):629–34.

17. Venkatraman V, Huettel SA, Chuah LY, Payne JW, Chee MW. Sleep deprivation biases the neural mechanisms underlying economic preferences. *J Neurosci.* 2011;**31**(10):3712–18.

18. De Havas JA, Parimal S, Soon CS, Chee MW. Sleep deprivation reduces default mode network connectivity and anti-correlation during rest and task performance. *Neuroimage.* 2012;**59**(2):1745–51.

19. Drummond SP, Brown GG, Stricker JL, *et al.* Sleep deprivation-induced

reduction in cortical functional response to serial subtraction. *Neuroreport.* 1999;**10**(18):3745–8.

20. Drummond SP, Brown GG, Gillin JC, *et al.* Altered brain response to verbal learning following sleep deprivation. *Nature.* 2000;**403**(6770):655–7.

21. Drummond SP, Brown GG. The effects of total sleep deprivation on cerebral responses to cognitive performance. *Neuropsychopharmacology.* 2001;**25**(5 Suppl):S68–73.

22. Bell-McGinty S, Habeck C, Hilton HJ, *et al.* Identification and differential vulnerability of a neural network in sleep deprivation. *Cereb Cortex.* 2004;**14**(5):496–502.

23. Drummond SP, Brown GG, Salamat JS, Gillin JC. Increasing task difficulty facilitates the cerebral compensatory response to total sleep deprivation. *Sleep.* 2004;**27**(3):445–51.

24. Caldwell JA, Mu Q, Smith JK, *et al.* Are individual differences in fatigue vulnerability related to baseline differences in cortical activation? *Behav Neurosci.* 2005;**119**(3):694–707.

25. Drummond SP, Bischoff-Grethe A, Dinges DF, *et al.* The neural basis of the psychomotor vigilance task. *Sleep.* 2005;**28**(9):1059–68.

26. Mu Q, Mishory A, Johnson KA, *et al.* Decreased brain activation during a working memory task at rested baseline is associated with vulnerability to sleep deprivation. *Sleep.* 2005;**28**(4):433–46.

27. Mu Q, Nahas Z, Johnson KA, *et al.* Decreased cortical response to verbal working memory following sleep deprivation. *Sleep.* 2005;**28**(1):55–67.

28. Luber B, Stanford AD, Bulow P, *et al.* Remediation of sleep-deprivation-induced working memory impairment with fMRI-guided transcranial magnetic stimulation. *Cereb Cortex.* 2008;**18**(9):2077–85.

29. Yoo SS, Gujar N, Hu P, Jolesz FA, Walker MP. The human emotional brain without sleep–a prefrontal amygdala disconnect. *Curr Biol.* 2007;**17**(20):R877–8.

30. Gujar N, Yoo SS, Hu P, Walker MP. The unrested resting brain: sleep deprivation alters activity within the default-mode network. *J Cogn Neurosci.* 2010;**22**(8):1637–48.

31. Tucker AM, Rakitin BC, Basner RC, *et al.* fMRI activation during failures to respond key to understanding performance changes with sleep deprivation. *Behav Brain Res.* 2011;**218**(1):73–9.

32. Gujar N, Yoo SS, Hu P, Walker MP. Sleep deprivation amplifies reactivity of brain reward networks, biasing the appraisal of positive emotional experiences. *J Neurosci.* 2011;**31**(12):4466–74.

33. Mander BA, Santhanam S, Saletin JM, Walker MP. Wake deterioration and sleep restoration of human learning. *Curr Biol.* 2011;**21**(5):R183–4.

34. Yoo SS, Hu PT, Gujar N, Jolesz FA, Walker MP. A deficit in the ability to form new human memories without sleep. *Nat Neurosci.* 2007;**10**(3):385–92.

35. Vandewalle G, Archer SN, Wuilleume C, *et al.* Functional magnetic resonance imaging-assessed brain responses during an executive task depend on interaction of sleep homeostasis, circadian phase, and PER3 genotype. *J Neurosci.* 2009;**29**(25):7948–56.

36. Mander BA, Reid KJ, Davuluri VK, *et al.* Sleep deprivation alters functioning within the neural network underlying the covert orienting of attention. *Brain Res.* 2008;**1217**:148–56.

37. Tomasi D, Wang RL, Telang F, *et al.* Impairment of attentional networks after one night of sleep deprivation. *Cereb Cortex.* 2009;**19**(1):233–40.

38. Volkow ND, Tomasi D, Wang GJ, *et al.* Hyperstimulation of striatal D2 receptors with sleep deprivation: implications for cognitive impairment. *Neuroimage.* 2009;**45**(4):1232–40.

39. Thomas RJ, Kwong K. Modafinil activates cortical and subcortical sites in the sleep-deprived state. *Sleep.* 2006;**29**(11):1471–81.

40. Portas CM, Rees G, Howseman AM, *et al.* A specific role for the thalamus in mediating the interaction of attention and arousal in humans. *J Neurosci.* 1998;**18**(21):8979–89.

41. McKiernan KA, Kaufman JN, Kucera-Thompson J, Binder JR. A parametric manipulation of factors affecting task-induced deactivation in functional neuroimaging. *J Cogn Neurosci.* 2003;**15**(3):394–408.

42. Leproult R, Colecchia EF, Berardi AM, *et al.* Individual differences in subjective and objective alertness during sleep deprivation are stable and unrelated. *Am J Physiol Regul Integr Comp Physiol.* 2003;**284**(2):R280–90.

43. Van Dongen HP, Baynard MD, Maislin G, Dinges DF. Systematic interindividual differences in neurobehavioral impairment from sleep loss: evidence of trait-like differential vulnerability. *Sleep.* 2004;**27**(3):423–33.

44. Lim J, Wu WC, Wang J, *et al.* Imaging brain fatigue from sustained mental workload: an ASL perfusion study of the time-on-task effect. *Neuroimage.* 2010;**49**(4):3426–35.

45. Buxton RB. Quantifying CBF with arterial spin labeling. *J Magn Reson Imaging.* 2005;**22**(6):723–6.

46. Aguirre GK, Detre JA, Zarahn E, Alsop DC. Experimental design and the relative sensitivity of BOLD and perfusion fMRI. *Neuroimage.* 2002;**15**(3):488–500.

47. Friston KJ, Buechel C, Fink GR, *et al.* Psychophysiological and modulatory interactions in neuroimaging. *Neuroimage.* 1997;**6**(3):218–29.

48. Lim J, Tan JC, Parimal S, Dinges DF, Chee MW. Sleep deprivation impairs object-selective attention: a view from the ventral visual cortex. *PLoS One.* 2010;**5**(2):e9087.

49. Biswal B, Yetkin FZ, Haughton VM, Hyde JS. Functional connectivity in the motor cortex of resting human brain using echo-planar MRI. *Magn Reson Med.* 1995;**34**(4):537–41.

50. Beckmann CF, DeLuca M, Devlin JT, Smith SM. Investigations into resting-state connectivity using independent component analysis. *Philos Trans R Soc Lond B Biol Sci.* 2005;**360**(1457):1001–13.

51. Horovitz SG, Braun AR, Carr WS, *et al.* Decoupling of the brain's default mode network during deep sleep. *Proc Natl Acad Sci U S A.* 2009;**106**(27):11376–81.

52. Sämann PG, Tully C, Spoormaker VI, *et al.* Increased sleep pressure reduces resting state functional connectivity. *MAGMA.* 2010;**23**(5–6):375–89.

53. Cole DM, Smith SM, Beckmann CF. Advances and pitfalls in the analysis and interpretation of resting-state fMRI data. *Front Syst Neurosci.* 2010;**4**:8.

54. Rocklage M, Williams V, Pacheco J, Schnyer DM. White matter differences predict cognitive vulnerability to sleep deprivation. *Sleep.* 2009;**32**(8):1100–3.

55. Rasch B, Buchel C, Gais S, Born J. Odor cues during slow-wave sleep prompt declarative memory consolidation. *Science.* 2007;**315**(5817):1426–9.

56. Thomas M, Sing H, Belenky G, *et al.* Neural basis of alertness and cognitive performance impairments during sleepiness. I. Effects of 24 h of sleep deprivation on waking human regional brain activity. *J Sleep Res.* 2000;**9**(4):335–52.

57. Horne JA. Human sleep, sleep loss and behaviour. Implications for the prefrontal cortex and psychiatric disorder. *Br J Psychiatry.* 1993;**162**:413–19.

58. Drummond SP, Gillin JC, Brown GG. Increased cerebral response during a divided attention task following sleep deprivation. *J Sleep Res.* 2001;**10**(2):85–92.

59. Habeck C, Rakitin BC, Moeller J, *et al.* An event-related fMRI study of the neurobehavioral impact of sleep deprivation on performance of a delayed-match-to-sample task. *Brain Res Cogn Brain Res.* 2004;**18**(3):306–21.

60. Awh E, Vogel EK, Oh SH. Interactions between attention and working memory. *Neuroscience.* 2006;**139**(1):201–8.

61. Corbetta M, Shulman GL. Control of goal-directed and stimulus-driven attention in the brain. *Nat Rev Neurosci.* 2002;**3**(3):201–15.

62. Chee MWL, Tan JC, Parimal S, Zagorodnov V. Sleep deprivation and its effects on object-selective attention. *Neuroimage.* 2010;**49**(2):1903–10.

63. Sterpenich V, Albouy G, Boly M, *et al.* Sleep-related hippocampo-cortical interplay during emotional memory recollection. *PLoS Biol.* 2007;**5**(11):e282.

64. Drobyshevsky A, Baumann SB, Schneider W. A rapid fMRI task battery for mapping of visual, motor, cognitive, and emotional function. *Neuroimage.* 2006;**31**(2):732–44.

65. Goel N, Rao H, Durmer JS, Dinges DF. Neurocognitive consequences of sleep deprivation. *Semin Neurol.* 2009;**29**(4):320–39.

66. Van Dongen HP, Maislin G, Mullington JM, Dinges DF. The cumulative cost of additional wakefulness: dose-response effects on neurobehavioral functions and sleep physiology from chronic sleep restriction and total sleep deprivation. *Sleep.* 2003;**26**(2):117–26.

67. Belenky G, Wesensten NJ, Thorne DR, *et al.* Patterns of performance degradation and restoration during sleep restriction and subsequent recovery: a sleep dose-response study. *J Sleep Res.* 2003;**12**(1):1–12.

68. Goel N, Banks S, Mignot E, Dinges DF. PER3 polymorphism predicts cumulative sleep homeostatic but not neurobehavioral changes to chronic partial sleep deprivation. *PLoS One.* 2009;**4**(6):e5874.

69. Harrison Y, Horne JA, Rothwell A. Prefrontal neuropsychological effects of sleep deprivation in young adults – a model for healthy aging? *Sleep.* 2000;**23**(8):1067–73.

70. Tucker AM, Stern Y, Basner RC, Rakitin BC. The prefrontal model revisited: double dissociations between young sleep deprived and elderly subjects on cognitive components of performance. *Sleep.* 2011;**34**(8):1039–50.

71. Kong D, Soon CS, Chee MW. Functional imaging correlates of impaired distractor suppression following sleep deprivation. *Neuroimage.* 2012;**61**(1):50–5.

Neuroimaging of attention and alteration of processing capacity in sleep-deprived persons

Michael W. L. Chee and Christopher L. Asplund

Introduction

The human brain is an extremely sophisticated information processing system that allows us to perceive, learn, reflect, and respond flexibly in a myriad of situations. Despite this ability, at any given moment, even with something as seemingly mundane as crossing a busy street, we encounter more perceptual information than can be effectively processed. Competing with internal thoughts and the goals we set for ourselves are multiple bystander conversations, information from signs and billboards, as well as environmental sounds. Attention allows us to allocate our limited processing resources such that we can selectively perceive and respond to a subset of these stimuli in a timely fashion.

Attention itself has multiple components, reflecting the different environmental challenges we face. For example, when one deploys attention to search for targets in a given task, appropriate preparation for and anticipation of upcoming targets can improve response speed and accuracy. One may also need to suppress distractor items to optimally process these targets. Conversely, it can be advantageous to register unanticipated but possibly behaviorally relevant stimuli. Accomplishing such monitoring without compromising the primary task requires residual capacity to process peripheral information, capacity that may be unavailable if the primary task is difficult. Finally, to complete any real-life job, all of the processes above need to be repeated or maintained across time, requiring the effortful deployment of sustained attention over minutes or hours (vigilance).

Human factors research has deeply characterized how sleep deprivation (SD) affects sustained attention or vigilance but has shed little light on the neural mechanisms underlying these phenomena. In contrast, research on selective attention, including physiological and imaging studies, has scrutinized the neural mechanisms underlying the selection of what to process, where to direct focus, and when to deploy attention. For example, neurons in frontoparietal regions that mediate controlled processing fire faster, and elicit greater functional magnetic resonance imaging (fMRI) signal, when stimuli or locations are actively attended [1, 2]. These control regions provide top-down biases for sensory neurons, increasing firing rates in sensory neurons that detect task-relevant stimuli or features [3] while concurrently reducing the firing rates of neurons sensitive to currently irrelevant objects or features [4].

Although attention's effects and mechanisms are well studied in rested and alert individuals, only recently have experiments begun to reveal how attention varies across states, such as during SD. In this chapter, we review how different facets of attention and information processing are compromised in sleep-deprived persons. We illustrate both the link between behavioral alterations and concurrently observed shifts in task-related fMRI signal as well as how imaging can reveal alterations in processing not evident in overt behavior. We also examine how state-related shifts in task-related fMRI signal can be used to identify inter-individual differences in vulnerability to SD.

The majority of the SD studies summarized in this review used a similar general experimental procedure, logic, and analysis, so we relate key aspects here. Healthy college-aged adults were recruited after a briefing session and a qualifying week where sleep pattern and duration were verified. Each volunteer underwent two fMRI sessions separated by at least a week, one during rested wakefulness (RW) circa 8:30 am and another following 24 h of SD starting around 6:00 am. The term "sleep deprivation" is used here as shorthand for a combination of the effects of sustained wakefulness and of being tested shortly after the nadir of the circadian cycle, when psychomotor performance is poor [5, 6]. The specific test times were chosen because most young adults start their workday around 8:30 am and most accidents arising from vigilance failures occur around 6:00 am following a night of total SD [7].

Cognizance of inter-individual differences in responses to SD [8, 9] motivated the use of within-subject designs in our studies, as well as examination of the relationship between shifts in behavioral performance and corresponding shifts in functional imaging parameters. fMRI analysis was confined to correct responses, or in the case of block designs, blocks with >80% correct responses to exclude periods of sustained sleep.

Effects of sleep deprivation on selective attention

Selectively attending to a specific location [1, 10, 11], feature [12], or object [13] is a central aspect of many attention experiments. While these different types of selective attention can be behaviorally dissociated, the attentional control regions that support them overlap considerably [13, 14]. Across different paradigms,

Neuroimaging of Sleep and Sleep Disorders, ed. Eric Nofzinger, Pierre Maquet, and Michael J. Thorpy. Published by Cambridge University Press. © Cambridge University Press 2013.

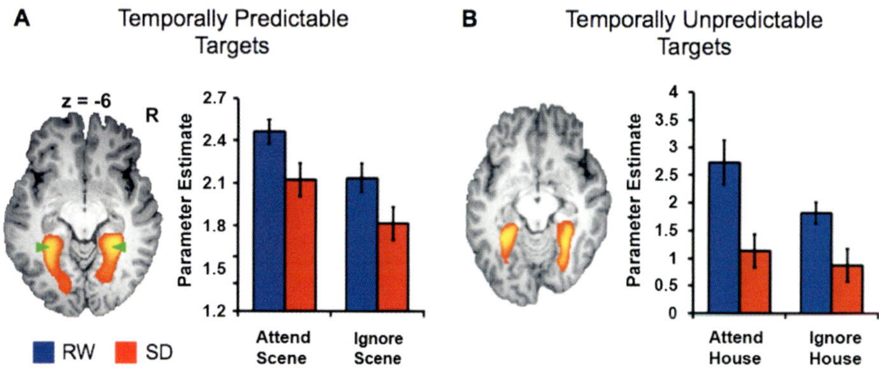

Figure 17.1 Effect of sleep deprivation on attentional selectivity may be modified by temporal predictability of targets. (A) When targets were temporally predictable, there was a main effect of attention and a main effect of state on parahippocampal place area activation. Selectivity of attention was preserved in both states. (B) When targets were temporally unpredictable, there was the expected interaction between state and attention on selectivity. (Adapted from Chee et al. [19]; Lim et al. [18].)

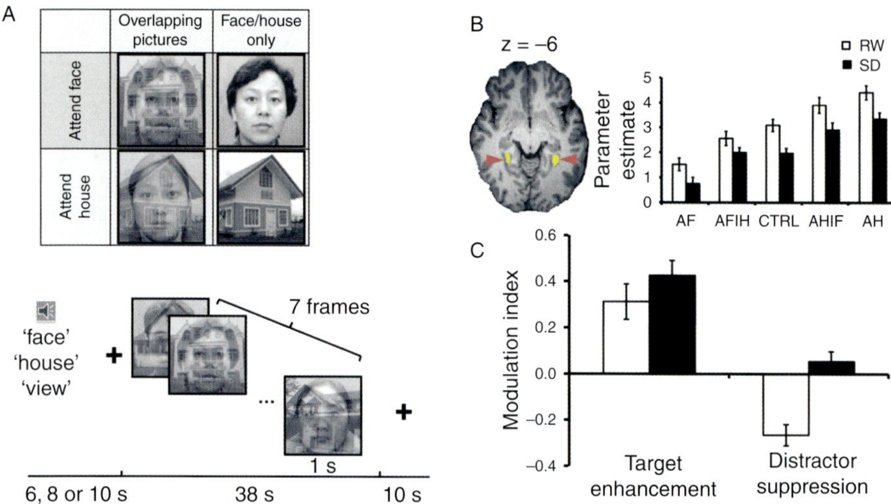

Figure 17.2 Sleep deprivation results in attenuated suppression of distractors. (A) Schematic of the experimental design showing examples of each of the four task conditions: attend face (AF), attend face ignore house (AFIH), attend house (AH), and attend house ignore face (AHIF). (B) State affected activation in parahippocampal place area in all conditions. Passive viewing served as the control condition (CTRL) . (C) Enhancement of attended houses was relatively preserved but suppression of distractor houses was impaired during sleep deprivation. (Adapted from Kong et al. [22].)

attended stimuli elicit greater dorsal fronto-parietal activation than do non-attended stimuli. The magnitude of this activation is generally reduced in sleep-deprived persons [15, 16], but this effect itself does not imply altered attentional selectivity.

The effects of state on attentional selectivity can be assessed, however, by examining category-specific activations in the ventral visual cortex. For well-rested subjects, trials in which scenes rather than faces are attended elicit higher activation [4] as well as more pronounced repetition suppression [17] in the parahippocampal place area (PPA). The size of the signal difference between attended and non-attended trials indicates selectivity (Figure 17.1). Selectivity was reduced in sleep-deprived persons, but only when the to-be-attended house stimuli were temporally unpredictable [18]. When face and house stimuli were alternated in a predictable manner, SD led to an overall reduction in activity but no change in selectivity [19]. The finding that SD's effects on selective attention may be more pronounced when stimuli are temporally unpredictable is consistent with similar effects found with vigilance in the well-rested state [20]. Regardless of this temporal predictability, SD decreased the functional connectivity between the intraparietal sulcus (IPS), an attentional control region, and the PPA [18, 19], confirming that dorsal frontoparietal activation was driving the attention effects in sensory cortex and suggesting that this might be the source of reduced selectivity.

Distractor suppression

Complimenting attention's enhancement effects is its ability to suppress irrelevant distractors. This ability is impaired by SD. For example, sleep-deprived persons showed more frequent lapses and head turns when performing the Psychomotor Vigilance Task (PVT) in the presence of a distracting movie [21]

There is also neural evidence of reduced distractor suppression. When subjects had to respond to a target house (or face) in a series of superimposed face/house images, not only did attention increase PPA activity when that target was a house, it suppressed activity in the same region when houses were distractors [22]. In sleep-deprived individuals, this suppression effect was weaker whereas the enhancement was relatively preserved (Figure 17.2). Attenuated distractor suppression has also been observed in studies involving healthy elderly persons [23, 24]. In some instances, these persons demonstrate relatively preserved enhancement of specific targets presented without distractors, just as Kong et al. observed in sleep-deprived individuals [22].

Peripheral perceptual processing capacity

In several imaging experiments assessing behavioral alterations in sleep-deprived persons, reduced task-related activation has been found to correlate with performance decline. Interestingly, attenuation of brain activation at different task loads [25] or levels of perceptual difficulty [26] has been observed even with correct trials, suggesting that a portion of the higher task-related activation observed after a normal night of sleep might correspond to "spare information processing capacity." This additional capacity might provide for redundancy in information processing or the encoding of environmental supports that could compensate for processing drop-outs arising from local sleep. Supporting this hypothesis, maintained or increased task-related activation during SD often corresponds with less compromised or maintained task performance [16, 26, 27].

The implied spare processing capacity associated with relatively higher task-related activation in the rested state could also have utility in processing stimuli presented outside the focus of attention. Here, the perceptual load theory of attention [28] provides a useful framework for evaluating SD-induced change in visual information processing. According to this model, focusing attention on a task-relevant stimulus inhibits the processing of task-irrelevant distractors to the extent that available perceptual processing capacity is engaged in processing the task-relevant stimulus. Conversely, if the task-relevant stimulus places low demands on the perceptual system, spare capacity becomes available to perceive the unattended distractors [29–31]. Notably, targets and distractors in these experiments do not spatially overlap, with a central target and peripheral distractors, allowing for serial processing of each. This situation is akin to keeping the traffic warden crossing the road in the center of our atttentional focus while still being able to detect a wayward child who strays onto the road after everyone else has crossed.

The degree of processing devoted to unattended distractors can be inferred from the magnitude of fMRI signal suppression related to distractor repetition, as this imaging measure scales with the extent to which these are perceived [32]. Critically, when faces are task-relevant and background scenes are distractors (Figure 17.3), the relative insensitivity of the PPA to faces permits activation associated with the distracting scenes to be evaluated without being significantly confounded by face stimulus-related signal. Examining how perceptual load interacts with state to influence repetition suppression can thus reveal how SD affects visual processing capacity.

To test the hypothesis that SD reduces visual processing capacity, participants were instructed to detect repeated faces in successive composite pictures comprising face photographs at the center of a larger background scene [32]. Perceptual load was manipulated by altering the clarity of the central faces. To assess repetition suppression, the accompanying background scenes were either novel or repeated and MR signal in the PPA was measured. One would expect to find preserved repetition suppression for distractor scenes irrespective of load during RW but reduced repetition suppression for the high perceptual load condition in SD.

Reduced visual perceptual processing capacity in sleep-deprived young adults was inferred from finding attenuated repetition suppression to place scenes when the perceptual load associated with central attended faces was high but not when the perceptual load was low [33]. This conclusion is founded on the premise that the magnitude of repetition suppression indexes functionally relevant information processing. Prior functional imaging studies have shown that higher repetition suppression to be related to memory strength [34], and superior navigational ability [35].

We also found significant associations between state-related decline in fusiform face area (FFA) activation, performance accuracy, and repetition suppression in the PPA. Such correlations have also been found in several studies, where SD-vulnerable individuals showed a greater decline in task-related activation when sleep deprived [25, 26, 36]. As only correct responses

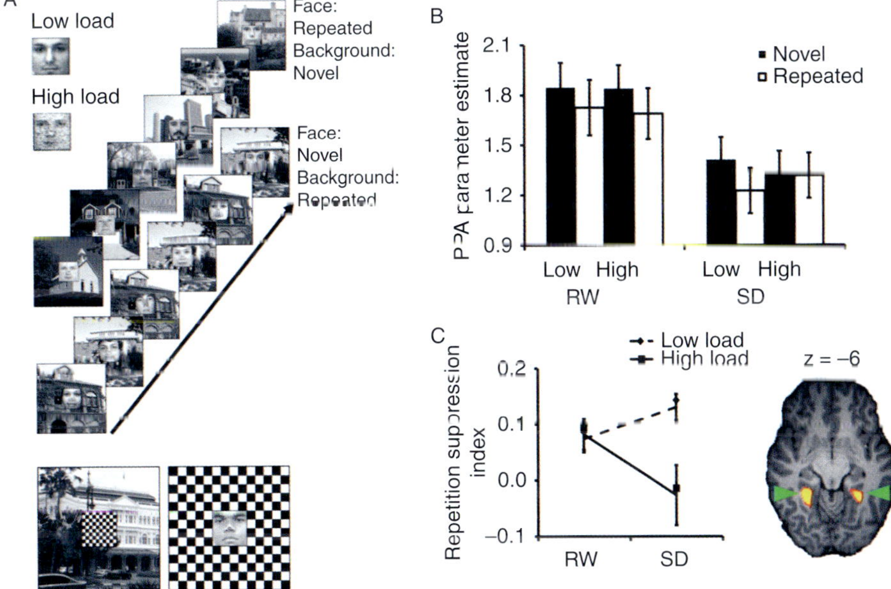

Figure 17.3 Evaluating perceptual processing capacity. (A) Each trial consisted of a series of six scene–face composite pictures, each shown for 500 ms, followed by a 500 ms checkerboard mask (not shown in figure). Faces were either undistorted (low-load condition) or degraded with salt and pepper noise (high-load condition). Surrounding each face were either alternately repeated (lower series) or completely non-repeated background scenes (upper series). After all frames had been presented, participants were given 3000 ms to indicate whether any face was repeated (upper series). A fixation cross was shown for 9000 ms before the next trial began. (B) Activation in the PPA corresponding to the different task conditions in each of the two states. (C) Repetition suppression index during SD was reduced in the high-load but not low-load condition showing a significant state-by-load interaction. (Adapted from Kong et al. [33].)

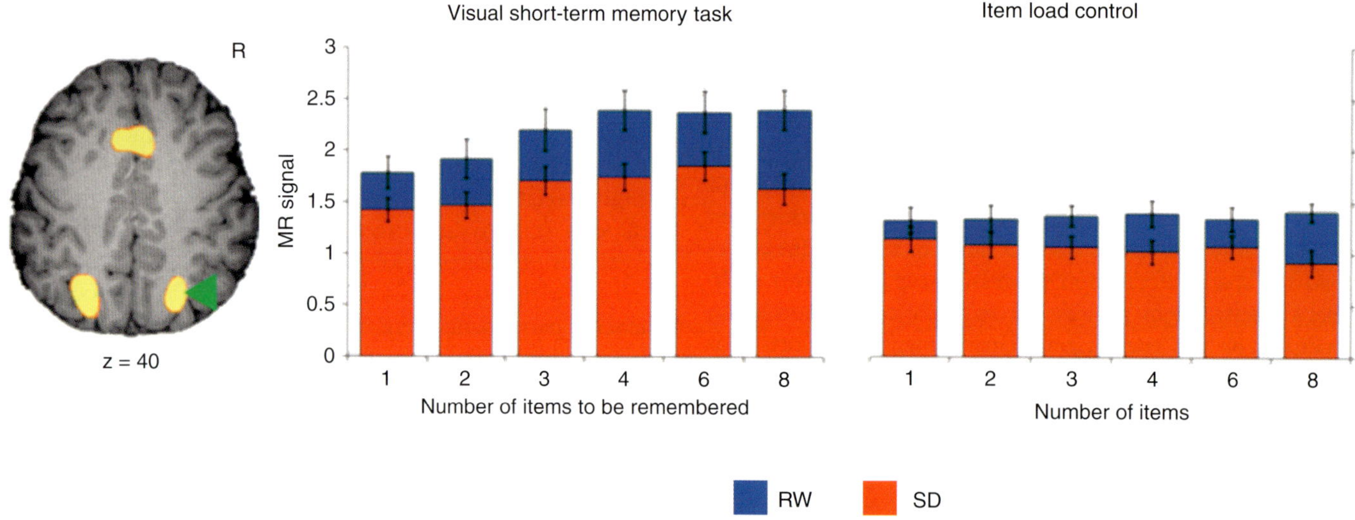

Figure 17.4 Deficits in attention underlie functional imaging changes when visual short-term memory is tested in the sleep-deprived state. Task-related activation of the intraparietal sulcus increases with memory load – but not visual item load when memory is not engaged – in both RW and SD. In the sleep-deprived state, even when visual short-term memory is not taxed (e.g., low test item load or no load on memory), decrements in activation are observed. This implicates a fundamental deficit in attention rather than one of storage capacity or memory. (Adapted from Chuah and Chee [25].)

were analyzed in these experiments, trials where reduced activation could be attributed to volunteers falling asleep were excluded. While mindful of the neural efficiency model, which suggests that efficient brains activate *less* to successfully accomplish a given task [37], we suggest instead that the relatively higher mean task-related activation during RW has functional value [38]. A crucial point in this argument is that the relevant comparison concerns activation elicited by the same person performing the identical task but under two different states.

These findings also provide a parsimonious reinterpretation of prior data that suggested persons with higher task-related activation during RW were more resistant to SD [39, 40]. Reexamination of these studies and others that have followed [19, 25, 26] indicate that it is not the higher level of activation in RW that is predictive of performance decline, but rather how much activation declines following SD.

Visual short-term memory

Maintaining a sensory representation for several seconds is crucial for enabling goal-directed behavior and is a core feature of attention [41]. This function is served by visual short-term memory (VSTM). VSTM, however, is severely capacity-limited, with individuals able to store about four visual items [42]. As test items only need to be stored for a few seconds and retrieved without internal manipulation, varying the size of the storage array allows one to identify and evaluate the neural substrate of storage capacity.

Such a paradigm was employed to evaluate the effect of SD on VSTM [15]. After a normal night of sleep, the superior parietal region showed an increase in activation with greater storage array size but relative indifference to a control in which the array size was altered without mnemonic demands. If SD were to affect storage alone, one would expect activation associated with short-term retention to be reduced with increasing memory set sizes. Instead, there were SD-induced reductions in

parietal activation at all set sizes. Both this region and visual extrastriate cortex, which was sensitive to set size even when recall was not required, showed attenuated activation even to singleton stimuli (Figure 17.4). These findings provided striking evidence that reduced top-down attention from the parietal lobe was responsible for activation and performance decline following SD.

This finding was replicated using an event-related version of the same task [25], a design that afforded restriction of analyses to correctly answered trials. Additionally, it was found that the cholinesterase inhibitor donepezil altered parietal and occipital activation in a manner that correlated with the extent to which state-related change in performance was modulated by the drug. Cholinergic augmentation can facilitate performance by exerting effects on memory and attention [43]. As parieto-occipital signal was modulated at all set sizes rather than selectively affecting larger set sizes, it would appear that donepezil improves SD performance *predominantly* by enhancing attention.

Lapses of attention resulting from loss of top-down control

Of the various cognitive domains studied in short-term total SD, "simple attention" – sustained attention or vigilance deployed to detect and respond to salient events – appears to be prominently affected. Failures of such attention are termed "lapses" and can be described operationally as slow responses, specifically those slower than twice the mean response time for the task.

By taking into account response time deviations from the mean in each state, the association of delayed responding and brain activation can be estimated [44]. In addition to the expected reduction in mean task-related signal in fronto-parietal cortex in SD, the signal associated with slow responses in SD was reduced relative to comparably slow responses following a normal night of sleep [45]. Conversely, slow responding in both states resulted in signal elevation in frontoparietal regions, consistent with inefficient task processing (simply conceptualized as having to work at the same task for longer and therefore expending more computing resources, albeit inefficiently). Thus, SD reduces activity overall despite the fact that it contained lapses that give rise to elevated frontoparietal activity.

No significant change in activity was associated with delayed responding after a normal night of sleep in the extrastriate visual cortex. However, there was significant reduction of extrastriate signal with lapses following SD. This signal attenuation in extrastriate cortex contrasted with the relative preservation of primary visual cortex activation in SD. As the extrastriate cortex in humans is more sensitive to the modulatory effect of attention [2], one explanation for these findings is that extrastriate activity is reduced upon losing support from top-down control of sensory processing during lapses in SD. Alternatively, the extrastriate cortex may be more sensitive to the effects of sustained wakefulness and might be manifesting some form of "local sleep," as observed from a prior invasive primate electrophysiological study [46].

A separate experiment in which the contrast of the visual stimuli was varied helped clarify the effects of SD on the visual cortex [26]. Responding to stimuli with reduced image contrast and size increases frontoparietal activation [47]. If the sensory system were deficient in SD, and there was no loss of top-down control, one would expect very low contrast (and thus the perceptually most difficult) items to elicit a precipitous decline in visual cortex activation without affecting activation of top-down frontoparietal circuits necessary to enhance sensory processing. Alternatively, if the loss of top-down control were at fault, one would expect reduction in frontoparietal activation regardless of image contrast. The latter scenario was observed in SD-vulnerable subjects (as ascertained by the greater performance decline across state) and, as might be expected, these subjects also showed lower extrastriate activation at all levels of stimulus contrast, consistent with reduction in top-down drive on sensory processing [26]. Conversely, non-vulnerable subjects maintained frontoparietal activation and appeared to activate as if they were not sleep deprived.

Although in much of the above, we focused on changes in top-down control of attention, other factors that contribute to performance maintenance remain to be studied. For example, in both experiments where lapses were evaluated, the thalamus showed higher activation at the average response time, even during SD. These results were also noted in experiments in which working memory [16], target number detection [48], and visual tracking [49] were assessed during SD, and suggest that the thalamus may contribute to maintaining arousal in sleep-deprived persons who strive to stay awake.

Preparatory attention

In addition to modulating stimulus-related activation, attention may bias sensory cortical activation in the period *preceding* the appearance of stimuli at a given location. Such biasing can include baseline shifts in neural activity, which have been demonstrated using single-cell recordings in monkey visual cortex [50], event-related potentials [51], and fMRI [52, 53] in humans. Preparatory period baseline shifts in neural activity in multiple brain areas including sensory, motor, and cognitive control areas have been shown to predict trial-by-trial fluctuations in performance [52, 54]. Indeed, response errors may be anticipated by signal changes *preceding* the stimulus by as much as 20 s [55].

To examine the effects of SD on preparatory attention, volunteers performed target detection under two conditions in each state. In one condition, subjects were cued to covertly direct attention to a peripheral location, in anticipation of targets that appeared after variable periods [11]. In another condition, targets were not preceded by a cue and were not attended. The effects of SD were apparent when contrasting the magnitude of baseline shift and attentional modulation of stimulus-related activity across task condition and state. These effects were examined in both frontoparietal regions mediating attentional control and retinotopically mapped visual cortex.

Baseline increases evoked in the preparatory period prior to stimulus appearance were attenuated within the right frontal eye field, the right intraparietal sulcus, and all retinotopically mapped visual areas in SD relative to the rested state [56]. Attenuation of visual cortex activation in SD occurred in early and higher visual cortices when a stimulus was anticipated but absent. In contrasting this attenuation of visual cortex activation was selective for extrastriate cortex in the presence of a stimulus, regardless of whether it was attended. As the former signal alterations occurred in the absence of visual stimulation, they provided unequivocal evidence that SD affects cortical regions mediating endogenous attention (Figure 17.5).

Reduced functional circuits: sleeping when awake in the sleep-deprived state

A parsimonious surmise from the studies described above is that there is a reduction in the number of functional neuronal circuits available to process visual information during SD. By "functional circuit," we mean an assembly of neurons that contribute to a given task. A given task will recruit many such circuits in a redundant manner. We hypothesize that during SD, the number of these circuits is reduced, perhaps falling below a critical number required to perform the task. This change would then lead to a reduction in neural signals as well as poorer behavioral performance.

This idea has neurophysiological support: a recent electrophysiological study showed that neurons can go into an "off" state in awake but sleep deprived animals that appear to continue to pursue goal-directed behavior [57]. This finding is also consonant with the notion that "local sleep" can occur following sustained wakefulness [58]. The propensity for neuronal columns entering this state is compounded by performing simple tasks that result in the same circuit being utilized repeatedly, enhancing "use-dependent" effects. (See Chapter 19 for further discussion of this idea.)

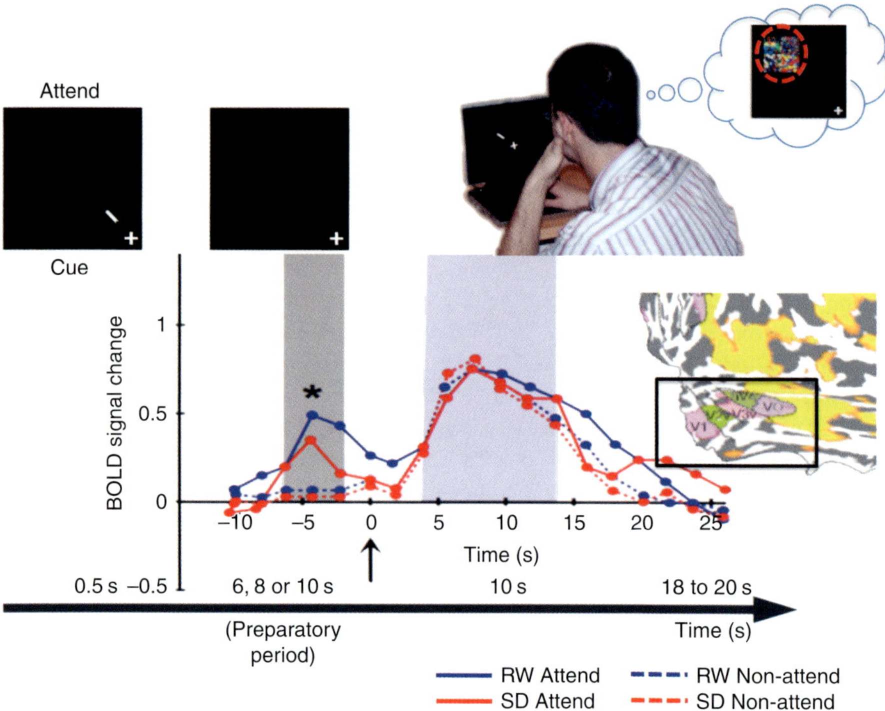

Figure 17.5 Examining preparatory attention and stimulus-driven effects on visual cortex activation (V1). In each state (RW and SD) volunteers performed under two different task conditions. In the attend condition, they prepared to respond to a difficult peripheral target that appeared in the upper left-hand quadrant of the visual field 6° peripheral to a central fixation cross. Targets appeared after a 6, 8, or 10 s preparatory period. During this period, exercise of top-down control of attention activates the visual cortex (inset) in a topographically specific manner. Within primary visual cortex (V1) preparatory activity is significantly reduced in the sleep-deprived state but stimulus-driven activity is not affected. (Adapted from Chee *et al.* [56].)

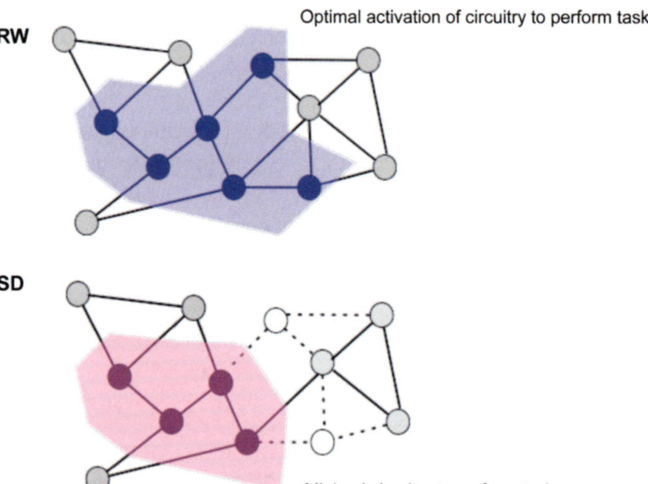

Figure 17.6 Schematic illustrating how "off" state neurons in awake but sleep-deprived individuals may affect performance. Each node represents a neuron and each line edge, a functional connection. During RW, "neurons" in the area shaded blue are activated. They represent the optimal level of activation of neural circuits recruited to perform the task. During SD, some "neurons" in this network (those represented by open circles) go into an "off" state, leaving only a critical minimal circuitry to execute the task (area shaded pink). This could lead to less efficient processing, or if more neurons enter the "off" state, a brief inability to respond. The gray "neurons" indicate how other neurons not immediately affected during task performance may be peripherally affected by the "off" neurons going offline. (Adapted from Chee *et al.* [56].)

Hence following SD, the minimum number of neural circuits needed to complete a given task successfully may not be reached, leading to a behavioral failure. Recall that SD caused attenuated parietal and extrastriate activation at all levels of VSTM or item load [15] even with correct responses, suggesting that redundant neural activation may occur when we respond to stimuli when *not* sleep deprived. Such additional activation may be important in ensuring optimal performance in well-rested persons, perhaps by coding peripheral information or ensuring sufficient redundancy so as to protect against random errors in information processing. Conversely, in the sleep-deprived state, during correct responses, a critical minimum activation may suffice in fulfilling immediate task goals but barely – leading to overall less accurate and slower performance (Figure 17.6).

Conclusion

Deficits in attention are a central mechanism through which performance in higher cognitive domains such as memory may be affected in SD. Reduced engagement of frontoparietal regions that mediate top-down control of attention has been demonstrated in experiments evaluating VSTM, preparatory attention, and selective attention. Either independently or consequentially to this, visual extrastriate cortex activation is markedly reduced, particularly during lapses of attention. Reductions in processing capacity are linked to diminished processing of peripheral visual stimuli on one hand and increased susceptibility to central distractors on the other. Future research into mechanisms of diminished processing capacity in SD should further consider the contributions of changes in intrinsic connectivity [59, 60] and alterations in default mode network behavior [15, 61, 62].

Acknowledgements

This work was supported by grants awarded to MC from the Defence Science and Technology Agency Singapore (POD0713897) and the National Research Foundation Singapore (STaR Award).

References

1. Corbetta M, Shulman GL. Control of goal-directed and stimulus-driven attention in the brain. *Nat Rev Neurosci*. 2002;**3**(3):201–15.

2. Kastner S, Ungerleider LG. Mechanisms of visual attention in the human cortex. *Annu Rev Neurosci*. 2000;**23**:315–41.

3. Desimone R, Duncan J. Neural mechanisms of selective visual attention. *Annu Rev Neurosci*. 1995;**18**:193–222.

4. Gazzaley A, Cooney JW, McEvoy K, Knight RT, D'Esposito M. Top-down enhancement and suppression of the magnitude and speed of neural activity. *J Cogn Neurosci*. 2005;**17**(3):507–17.

5. Doran SM, Van Dongen HP, Dinges DF. Sustained attention performance during sleep deprivation: evidence of state instability. *Arch Ital Biol*. 2001;**139**(3):253–67.

6. Graw P, Krauchi K, Knoblauch V, Wirz-Justice A, Cajochen C. Circadian and wake-dependent modulation of fastest and slowest reaction times during the psychomotor vigilance task. *Physiol Behav*. 2004;**80**(5):695–701.

7. Horne JA, Reyner LA. Sleep related vehicle accidents. *BMJ*. 1995;**310**(6979):565–7.

8. Leproult R, Colecchia EF, Berardi AM, *et al*. Individual differences in subjective and objective alertness during sleep deprivation are stable and unrelated. *Am J Physiol*. 2003;**284**(2):R280–90.

9. Van Dongen HP, Baynard MD, Maislin G, Dinges DF. Systematic interindividual differences in neurobehavioral impairment from sleep loss: evidence of trait-like differential vulnerability. *Sleep*. 2004;**27**(3):423–33.

10. Hopfinger JB, Buonocore MH, Mangun GR. The neural mechanisms of top-down attentional control. *Nat Neurosci*. 2000;**3**(3):284–91.

11. Kastner S, Pinsk MA, De Weerd P, Desimone R, Ungerleider LG. Increased activity in human visual cortex during directed attention in the absence of visual stimulation. *Neuron*. 1999;**22**(4):751–61.

12. Liu T, Slotnick SD, Serences JT, Yantis S. Cortical mechanisms of feature-based attentional control. *Cereb Cortex*. 2003;**13**(12):1334–43.

13. Serences JT, Schwarzbach J, Courtney SM, Golay X, Yantis S. Control of object-based attention in human cortex. *Cereb Cortex*. 2004;**14**(12):1346–57.

14. Wojciulik E, Kanwisher N. The generality of parietal involvement in visual attention. *Neuron*. 1999;**23**(4):747–64.

15. Chee MW, Chuah YM. Functional neuroimaging and behavioral correlates of capacity decline in visual short-term memory after sleep deprivation. *Proc Natl Acad Sci U S A*. 2007;**104**(22):9487–92.

16. Chee MWL, Choo WC. Functional imaging of working memory after 24 hr of total sleep deprivation. *J Neurosci*. 2004;**24**(19):4560–7

17. Yi D-J, Chun MM. Attentional modulation of learning-related repetition attenuation effects in human parahippocampal cortex. *J Neurosci*. 2005;**25**(14):3593–600.

18. Lim J, Tan JC, Parimal S, Dinges DF, Chee MW. Sleep deprivation impairs object-selective attention: a view from the ventral visual cortex. *PLoS One*. 2010;**5**(2):e9087.

19. Chee MWL, Tan JC, Parimal S, Zagorodnov V. Sleep deprivation and its effects on object-selective attention. *Neuroimage*. 2010;**49**(2):1903–10.

20. Langner R, Willmes K, Chatterjee A, Eickhoff SB, Sturm W. Energetic effects of stimulus intensity on prolonged simple reaction-time performance. *Psychol Res*. 2010;**74**(5):499–512.

21. Anderson C, Horne JA. Sleepiness enhances distraction during a monotonous task. *Sleep*. 2006;**29**(4):573–6.

22. Kong D, Soon CS, Chee MW. Functional imaging correlates of impaired distractor suppression following sleep deprivation. *Neuroimage*. 2012;**61**(1):50–5.

23. Gazzaley A, Cooney JW, Rissman J, D'Esposito M. Top down suppression deficit underlies working memory impairment in normal aging. *Nat Neurosci*. 2005;**8**(10):1298–300.

24. Darowski ES, Helder E, Zacks RT, Hasher L, Hambrick DZ. Age-related differences in cognition: the role of distraction control. *Neuropsychology*. 2008;**22**(5):638–44.

25. Chuah LY, Chee MW. Cholinergic augmentation modulates visual task performance in sleep-deprived young adults. *J Neurosci*. 2008;**28**(44):11369–77.

26. Chee MW, Tan JC. Lapsing when sleep deprived: neural activation characteristics of resistant and vulnerable individuals. *Neuroimage*. 2010;**51**(2):835–43.

27. Drummond SP, Meloy MJ, Yanagi MA, Orff HJ, Brown GG. Compensatory recruitment after sleep deprivation and the relationship with performance. *Psychiatry Res*. 2005;**140**(3):211–23.

28. Lavie N. Perceptual load as a necessary condition for selective attention. *J Exp Psychol Hum Percept Perform*. 1995;**21**(3):451–68.

29. Pessoa L, Padmala S, Morland T. Fate of unattended fearful faces in the amygdala is determined by both attentional resources and cognitive modulation. *Neuroimage*. 2005;**28**(1):249–55.

30. Forster S, Lavie N. High perceptual load makes everybody equal: eliminating individual differences in distractibility with load. *Psychol Sci*. 2007;**18**(5):377–81.

31. Rees G, Frith CD, Lavie N. Modulating irrelevant motion perception by varying attentional load in an unrelated task. *Science*. 1997;**278**(5343):1616–19.

32. Yi D-J, Woodman GF, Widders D, Marois R, Chun MM. Neural fate of ignored stimuli: dissociable effects of perceptual and working memory load. *Nat Neurosci*. 2004;**7**(9):992–6.

33. Kong D, Soon CS, Chee MW. Reduced visual processing capacity in sleep deprived persons. *Neuroimage*. 2011;**55**(2):629–34.

34. Turk-Browne NB, Yi DJ, Chun MM. Linking implicit and explicit memory: common encoding factors and shared representations. *Neuron*. 2006;**49**(6):917–27.

35. Epstein RA, Higgins JS, Thompson-Schill SL. Learning places from views: variation in scene processing as a function of experience and navigational ability. *J Cogn Neurosci*. 2005;**17**(1):73–83.

36. Lim J, Choo WC, Chee MW. Reproducibility of changes in behaviour and fMRI activation associated with sleep deprivation in a working memory task. *Sleep*. 2007;**30**(1):61–70.

37. Rypma B, Prabhakaran V. When less is more and when more is more: the

mediating roles of capacity and speed in brain-behavior efficiency. *Intelligence.* 2009;**37**(2):207–22.

38. Chuah LY, Chong DL, Chen AK, *et al.* Donepezil improves episodic memory in young individuals vulnerable to the effects of sleep deprivation. *Sleep.* 2009;**32**(8):999–1010.

39. Mu Q, Mishory A, Johnson KA, *et al.* Decreased brain activation during a working memory task at rested baseline is associated with vulnerability to sleep deprivation. *Sleep.* 2005;**28**(4):433–46.

40. Chee MWL, Chuah LYM, Venkatraman V, *et al.* Functional imaging of working memory following normal sleep and after 24 and 35 h of sleep deprivation: correlations of fronto-parietal activation with performance. *Neuroimage.* 2006;**31** (1):419–28.

41. Chun MM. Visual working memory as visual attention sustained internally over time. *Neuropsychologia.* 2011;**49** (6):1407–9.

42. Luck SJ, Vogel EK. The capacity of visual working memory for features and conjunctions. *Nature.* 1997;**390** (6657):279–81.

43. Everitt BJ, Robbins TW. Central cholinergic systems and cognition. *Annu Rev Psychol.* 1997;**48**:649–84.

44. Weissman DH, Roberts KC, Visscher KM, Woldorff MG. The neural bases of momentary lapses in attention. *Nat Neurosci.* 2006;**9**(7):971–8.

45. Chee MWL, Tan JC, Zheng H, *et al.* Lapsing during sleep deprivation is associated with distributed changes in brain activation. *J Neurosci.* 2008;**28** (21):5519–28.

46. Pigarev IN, Nothdurft HC, Kastner S. Evidence for asynchronous development of sleep in cortical areas. *Neuroreport.* 1997;**8**(11):2557–60.

47. Marois R, Chun MM, Gore JC. A common parieto-frontal network is recruited under both low visibility and high perceptual interference conditions. *J Neurophysiol.* 2004;**92**(5):2985–92.

48. Portas CM, Rees G, Howseman AM, *et al.* A specific role for the thalamus in mediating the interaction of attention and arousal in humans. *J Neurosci.* 1998;**18**(21):8979–89.

49. Tomasi D, Wang RL, Telang F, *et al.* Impairment of attentional networks after 1 night of sleep deprivation. *Cereb Cortex.* 2009;**19**(1):233–40.

50. Luck SJ, Chelazzi L, Hillyard SA, Desimone R. Neural mechanisms of spatial selective attention in areas V1, V2, and V4 of macaque visual cortex. *J Neurophysiol.* 1997;**77**(1):24–42.

51. Grent-'t-Jong T, Woldorff MG. Timing and sequence of brain activity in top-down control of visual-spatial attention. *PLoS Biol.* 2007;**5**(1):e12.

52. Sapir A, d'Avossa G, McAvoy M, Shulman GL, Corbetta M. Brain signals for spatial attention predict performance in a motion discrimination task. *Proc Natl Acad Sci U S A.* 2005;**102** (49):17810–15.

53. Stokes M, Thompson R, Nobre AC, Duncan J. Shape-specific preparatory activity mediates attention to targets in human visual cortex. *Proc Natl Acad Sci U S A.* 2009;**106**(46):19569–74.

54. Pessoa L, Kastner S, Ungerleider LG. Neuroimaging studies of attention: from modulation of sensory processing to top-down control. *J Neurosci.* 2003;**23** (10):3990–8.

55. Eichele T, Debener S, Calhoun VD, *et al.* Prediction of human errors by maladaptive changes in event-related brain networks. *Proc Natl Acad Sci U S A.* 2008;**105**(16):6173–8.

56. Chee MW, Goh CS, Namburi P, *et al.* Effects of sleep deprivation on cortical activation during directed attention in the absence and presence of visual stimuli. *Neuroimage.* 2011;**58** (2):595–604.

57. Vyazovskiy VV, Olcese U, Hanlon EC, *et al.* Local sleep in awake rats. *Nature.* 2011;**472**:443–7.

58. Krueger JM, Rector DM, Roy S, *et al.* Sleep as a fundamental property of neuronal assemblies. *Nat Rev Neurosci.* 2008;**9**(12):910–19.

59. De Havas JA, Parimal S, Soon CS, Chee MW. Sleep deprivation reduces default mode network connectivity and anti-correlation during rest and task performance. *Neuroimage.* 2012;**59** (2):1745–51.

60. Sämann PG, Tully C, Spoormaker VI, *et al.* Increased sleep pressure reduces resting state functional connectivity. *MAGMA.* 2010;**23**(5–6):375–89.

61. Gujar N, Yoo SS, Hu P, Walker MP. The unrested resting brain: sleep deprivation alters activity within the default-mode network. *J Cogn Neurosci.* 2010;**22** (8):1637–48.

62. Drummond SP, Bischoff-Grethe A, Dinges DF, *et al.* The neural basis of the psychomotor vigilance task. *Sleep.* 2005;**28**(9):1059–68.

Economic decision-making and the sleep-deprived brain

Vinod Venkatraman, Scott A. Huettel, Camilo Libedinsky, and Michael W. L. Chee

Introduction

As acceptable temporal boundaries of business and social activities gradually disappear with pervasive connectivity, an increasing number of persons will be called upon to make decisions at times that our predecessors reserved for sleep. In the last decade, there has been a surge in interest in the neural underpinnings of decision-making, particularly when individuals are faced with risk [1, 2]. Yet, despite the steady increase in numbers of persons who make decisions following chronic or acute sleep loss, there remains relatively little work about how sleep deprivation (SD) alters decision-making.

Risky decisions are those where the outcomes of one or more potential choices are probabilistic; that is, different outcomes might occur with known or estimated probabilities (e.g., gambling on roulette). The broad appeal, detailed characterization, ease of experimental design, and ready incentive compatibility have made risky decision-making a common target for research in decision neuroscience or "neuroeconomics" [1, 3, 4]. Moreover, risky decisions often must be made under conditions of reduced sleep (and/or other deleterious states), as in the cases of emergency personnel, physicians, financial markets, and even policy makers. For these reasons, an improved understanding of risky decision-making in sleep-deprived persons could have important real-world consequences.

Economic and neural models of decision-making under risk

Research into how risky choices are made has a rich history starting with the early insights of Pascal and Bernoulli [5], through axiomatic formalizations of von Neumann and Morgenstern [6] and Savage [7], to recent explorations of biases by Kahneman, Tversky, and many others [8–12].

Traditional expectation-based models assume that individuals integrate information across outcomes and probabilities. These models are often *compensatory*, which means that different outcome characteristics can compensate (i.e., trade off) for each other in decision-making. In a canonical example of compensatory decision-making, an individual must choose between one option that has a high probability of winning a small amount and a second option that has a low probability of winning a large amount. The most popular of compensatory risky choice models is the *expected utility* model where options are evaluated on their desirability or "utility." The utility of each outcome is multiplied by its probability of occurring, and the preferred option is the one for which this product is the highest [5, 6].

A deficiency of compensatory models is that they assume that individuals process and integrate all available information. In reality, we are constrained by processing capacity limitations (see Chapter 17), especially when under time pressure [13]. A viable alternative to compensatory models is the adaptive use of simplifying *heuristics*, defined as decision strategies that use only a subset of available information in making decisions. Heuristic strategies are fast, frugal, and non-compensatory [9, 12]. In an experiment we describe later, we illustrate that behavior observed following SD is better described by changes in the adaptive heuristic framework than by deficiencies in the computations of a compensatory strategy.

Neuroeconomic studies that seek to understand the neural mechanisms underlying economic decision-making often target a particular decision variable (e.g., loss aversion), incorporate that variable into a model function (e.g., prospect theory), manipulate the level of that variable across a range of stimuli (e.g., monetary gambles), and then identify aspects of brain function that track changes in that variable [1, 14]. Using this approach, researchers have identified potential neural underpinnings of nearly all of the core variables present in standard descriptive economic models, including value of monetary rewards, probability, risk, ambiguity, and probability weighting, among others [15–20]. Though early frameworks of risky choice lacked any consideration of emotion or affect, a growing body of evidence has demonstrated that affective content influences both the mechanism [21, 22] and the outcome of decisions [11, 23]. Across numerous recent studies, especially within neuroscience, there are striking examples of the interplay of cognition and emotion, typically with emotional content pushing individuals away from the normatively rational choice [22, 24–27]. But other recent research calls into question this simple dual-systems model of decision-making, suggesting instead that decision-making reflects the complex interplay between brain systems for setting up decision heuristics and those for processing decision variables [28, 29]. The complexity of current neural models of decision making suggests several routes through which SD may alter the choice process. In the following sections, we review

Neuroimaging of Sleep and Sleep Disorders, ed. Eric Nofzinger, Pierre Maquet, and Michael J. Thorpy. Published by Cambridge University Press. © Cambridge University Press 2013.

some of the behavioral evidence for altered choices following SD, and then consider the potential neural mechanisms.

Influence of behavioral studies on decision-making in sleep-deprived persons

Researchers with a background in human factors research conducted most of the early behavioral studies on decision-making in sleep-deprived persons. A number of these studies evaluated "naturalistic decision-making" in operational settings. For example, a key finding of the naturalistic decision-making framework is that sleep-deprived or fatigued decision-makers seize the first non-rejectable course of action instead of evaluating all available options [30]. While informative of operational behavior, such studies do not afford a more insightful analysis of the underpinnings of behavioral change – although they may serve as a launch pad for such inquiry. In neuroeconomic decision-making parlance, this behavior might correspond to a tendency to revert to adaptive use of heuristics in this state.

As SD can impair aspects of behavior mediated by the frontal lobes [31], such as flexible thinking, working memory, and executive function [31–34], early behavioral studies frequently attributed deficits in the overall quality of decision-making to frontal lobe dysfunction and in particular, the dorsolateral prefrontal cortex [35, 36]. Prominent among tasks that probe frontal lobe dysfunction is the Iowa Gambling Task (IGT), in which subjects choose between decks that vary in the frequency and magnitude of payoffs. In an early study, sleep-deprived participants persisted in choosing from the higher risk decks and exhibited a reduced concern for negative consequences [36], a behavior that had remarkable similarity to participants with orbitofrontal damage [37]. In a follow-up study using the IGT, Killgore and colleagues found similar effects but only after 49.5 h of SD [38]. The sleep-deprived participants in this study appeared to have difficulty weighting immediate short-term benefits against long-term consequences.

An alternative explanation for these findings relates to framing bias [39–41]. Participants in this task were asked to maximize winnings, which represents a positive frame of reference (i.e., a focus on positive outcomes). Low-risk decks provide greater certainty as their outcomes follow a more stable and predictable pattern, resulting in a greater number of positive outcomes. While normal adults demonstrate risk-aversion after being stung by losses, sleep-deprived participants were less sensitive to such framing biases. Importantly, while these findings are often interpreted as evidence for increased risk-seeking behavior following SD, they only provide an indirect assessment of risk, since outcome probabilities were not declared.

McKenna *et al.* sought to understand the effects of SD on risk and framing using a lottery choice task [42]. Participants made a series of choices between two gambles with equal expected payoffs but different risk levels. Following 23 h of total SD participants were more willing to take risks when considering a gain but not when considering a loss. Therefore, whether an individual was willing to take more risks following SD depended on whether the decision was framed as a gain or a loss [42]. Similar to the IGT, individuals were more risk seeking when decisions were framed as a gain, but not when they were framed as a loss. However, it remained unclear whether and how lack of adequate sleep shapes the very preferences that guide decision-making under risk, independently of its more general effects on cognition.

Sleep deprivation leads to increased expectation of gains and reduced concern for losses

In the first of two imaging studies on risky decision-making described here [43], volunteers came to the laboratory following either a night of SD or of normal sleep and made repeated choices between gambles that varied in magnitude and level of uncertainty (Figure 18.1). When persons were sleep deprived,

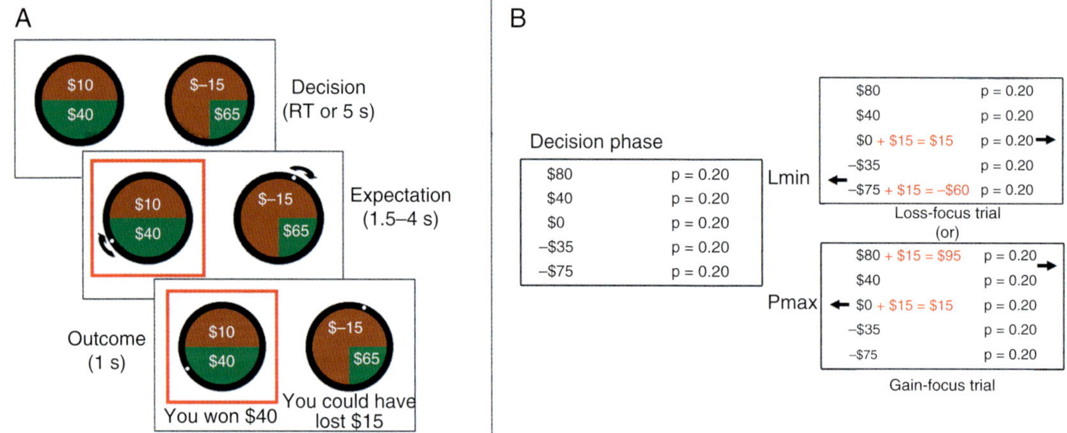

Figure 18.1 Schematic of risky choice tasks. (A) In the first study, participants were tested on a risky choice task involving three basic gamble types (certain [C], low-risk [LR] and high-risk [HR]) [43]. Certain gambles had only one fixed monetary reward, low-risk gambles consisted of two small, positive monetary rewards, and high-risk gambles had one large positive and one negative monetary reward. These gambles were combined as two pairs: C-LR and LR-HR, and subjects had to choose between the gambles with the objective of maximizing their winnings. The winnings from each gamble were revealed after a variable anticipation phase and subjects were paid a percentage of the amount they won on each trial. (B) In the second study, individuals were presented with a five-outcome complex mixed gamble in each trial that consisted of both gain and loss outcomes. They were then given an opportunity to improve each gamble by adding money to *one* of the outcomes in one of three ways: increasing the magnitude of the highest gain (Gmax), decreasing the magnitude of the worst loss (Lmin), or by improving the overall probability of winning (Pmax) by adding money to a central reference outcome. RT, reaction time. (Adapted from [43] and [56].)

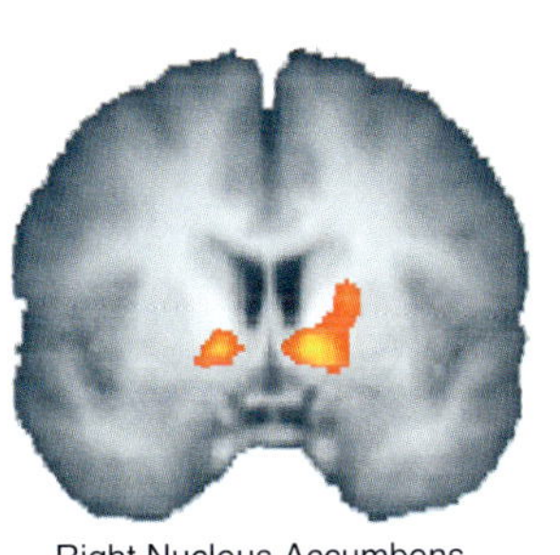

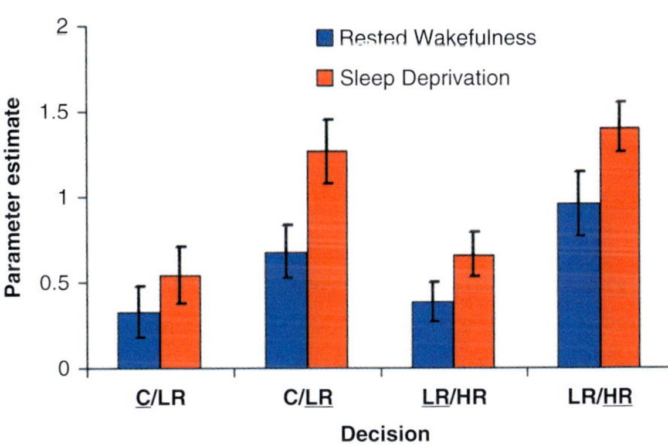

Figure 18.2 Activation in nucleus accumbens tracks enhanced optimism following SD. Choosing the riskier option was associated with increased activation in the nucleus accumbens during the decision phase in both states. There was a further significant increase in activation in this region following SD only for riskier choices, suggesting a greater expectation of being rewarded for these decisions when sleep deprived. (Adapted from [43].) SD = sleep deprivation.

decisions were made more slowly but risk preferences were unchanged from the rested wakeful state. However, there were significant effects of SD on the underlying brain activation. Trials where the riskier option was chosen were associated with greater nucleus accumbens activation when subjects were sleep deprived (Figure 18.2) compared to when they were well rested. Activation of the nucleus accumbens, a component of the ventral striatum, is modulated by the anticipation of reward outcomes and reward prediction errors [44–46]. SD also led to increased activation in the dorsal anterior cingulate, which has typically been associated with the control and monitoring of decision outcomes to guide future behavior [47–49]. As such, greater activation in this region might reflect the greater effort required to resolve conflict between maximization of expected value and minimization of regret.

Since each gamble was resolved to a gain or loss at the end of each trial, the effect of SD on emotional responses to decision outcome was evaluated by comparing activation associated with responses to loss and gain outcomes. A significant state-by-outcome interaction was present in the left anterior insula and left orbitofrontal cortex. Importantly, these regions showed reduced activation following SD only for losses. The insular cortex through its afferent and efferent connections to the medial and orbital prefrontal cortices, anterior cingulate, and amygdala is thought to evaluate the emotional significance of a stimulus and generate an appropriate affective response [25, 50]. The dorsal insula in particular has been associated with responding to punishment [51] while activity in the lateral orbitofrontal cortex appears to be sensitive to the magnitude of punishment [52].

The converse of the emotional high of being rewarded for a bet is being able to learn from negative outcomes. Reduced orbitofrontal activation to losses following SD could therefore indicate a state-dependent impairment of the learning of negative reward associations. Damage to the orbitofrontal cortex is thought to impair learning and the ability to reverse reward associations [53] by disrupting the ability to use emotional markers to guide decisions. Regret for poor decisions is one such emotional marker. In healthy adults, regret activates the lateral orbitofrontal cortex or ventromedial prefrontal cortex (vmPFC), reflecting learning to avoid subsequent bad decisions [21]. Therefore, one possibility is that SD leads to *reduced regret for losses* arising from risky decisions and hence an inability to effectively integrate feedback arising from negative consequences.

SD thus poses a dual threat to competent decision-making, by changing both the tendency toward risky decisions and the ability to learn from undesirable outcomes.

The primary limitation of this study was absence of a shift in decisions towards riskier choices even though the brain signals indicated that this might be imminent. One intriguing possibility is that imaging might be more sensitive than simple behavioral studies in detecting a cognitive phenomenon of interest serving as a leading indicator of shifts in preferences. Alternatively, SD-related alteration of risk preferences could have been masked by the tendency to maximize the overall probability of winning since this study only contrasted gambles with positive outcomes to mixed gambles involving both positive and negative outcomes [28, 54]. Further, separating decision and outcome phases in the imaging analysis could also be important as SD might interact with task context and feedback to influence neural responses and behavior. For example, as discussed earlier, the propensity to take higher risks in a gambling task can be modulated by decision frames [42]. Task differences may also reduce [55] or increase [38, 56] the likelihood of making a risky choice.

A second study [56] addressed some of these limitations using an incentive compatible risky choice task with complex multi-outcome mixed gambles [28]. Participants chose between different ways of improving a five-outcome mixed gamble across two states (Figure 18.1B). Across trials, the expected value relationship between the various options was varied. Different choices in this task reflected different strategic approaches to decision-making. For instance, choosing to improve the loss-minimizing (Lmin) option would be a risk averse strategy where individuals seek to diminish the effect of the worst loss should it occur. Conversely, improving the largest potential reward would be indicative of a gain-maximizing strategy (Gmax). The probability maximizing strategy (Pmax) focuses on maximizing the overall probability of winning while disregarding magnitude information about each individual outcome. Taken together, the richness of potential choices in this task allowed separating strategy-related and preference-related effects of SD. Decision and outcome phases were dissociated to decouple the effects of learning and feedback from decision valuation and preferences. In the decision phase, participants indicated their preferences without receiving feedback. In the outcome phase, a subset of gambles was resolved to gains and losses while subjects passively viewed these outcomes.

The proportions of Gmax or Lmin decisions, relative to Pmax decisions, were computed for the gain-focus and loss-focus trials respectively. Although there was no main effect of state (rested wakefulness [RW], SD) or choice (Gmax, Lmin), there was a significant state-by-choice interaction. Sleep-deprived participants exhibited an increased preference for Gmax choices in gain-focus trials, but a decreased preference for Lmin choices in loss-focus trials. Importantly, participants remained sensitive to the expected-value relationship between the two alternatives in both states, indicating that SD led to a change in preferences, not a simple increase in decision variability [56]. Hence, in contrast to the earlier study, there was evidence for a behavioral shift in preferences following SD whereby the same individual moved from defending against losses to chasing large gains in the absence of explicit post-trial feedback.

In the well-rested state, vmPFC activation correlated with the proportion of Gmax choices in gain-focus trials, while right anterior insula activation correlated with the proportion of Lmin choices in loss-focus trials. These findings concur with the previous studies associating insula activation with loss-averse behavior [22, 28, 57] and vmPFC activation with gain-seeking behavior [28, 58, 59]. SD led to increased activation in the vmPFC (Figure 18.3A), consistent with a shift towards gain-maximizing choices following SD. SD also resulted in reduced activation in the right anterior insula and dorsomedial prefrontal cortex during loss-focus trials (Figure 18.3B). Notably, these SD-induced changes in activation correlated with SD-induced changes in behavior. A reduced propensity to make Lmin choices

when sleep deprived correlated with reduced right anterior insula activation during these trials. Strikingly, SD did not affect dorsolateral prefrontal cortex activation in contrast to prior expectations emerging from behavioral studies [31, 38]. However, we did find SD-related decrease in anterior insula activation associated with loss-focus trials to correlate with SD-related increases in vmPFC activation during gain-focus trials.

Considering the results of the two risky choice studies together, SD appears to create an optimism bias whereby participants behaved as if positive consequences were more likely (or more valuable) and negative consequences less likely (or less harmful). As activation in the vmPFC and anterior insula is typically associated with salience of negative and positive outcomes respectively [22, 28, 60], one interpretation of the findings is that SD biases valuation by bringing about an increased attentional bias towards higher-ranked positive outcomes while concurrently reducing concern for losses.

During the outcome phase, where participants passively viewed gambles being resolved to an actual monetary gain or loss, there was increased activity in the ventral striatum and vmPFC for gains relative to losses following SD (Figure 18.4B). Consistent with the first study, SD was associated with marked attenuation of loss-related activation within the left anterior insula (Figure 18.4A). Finally, the decrease in activation of the left anterior insula for losses correlated with the increase in activation in the ventral striatum for gains. These findings are consistent with the hypothesis that lack of adequate sleep leads to increased sensitivity to positive reward outcomes with a corresponding diminished response to losses and negative consequences.

Relative shift in monetary and social valuation following sleep deprivation

Although the above studies indicate that SD affects economic preferences, little is known about the influence of social context on these mechanisms. Anderson and Dickinson used three different games involving bargaining and trust in the same individual to elucidate the effects of social context on preferences following RW and SD [61]. In each of these games, participants made simple monetary decisions on splitting a common pool of money with another anonymous partner, with real monetary consequences. In the bargaining games, sleep-deprived participants were willing to sacrifice monetary gains in order to reject unfair offers. Interestingly, these participants were also less likely to trust their anonymous partners in the trust game. How do these differences in social valuation translate into changes in economic preferences? How does the brain evaluate the relative value of different goods?

Recent studies suggest that decision preferences involving different types of goods reflect the subjective valuation of these different goods that have been converted into a standard signal, or "common neural currency" [62–66]. This common neural currency enables individuals to make decisions about nominally incommensurable rewards, as when exchanging money to obtain a desirable social interaction [63, 67]. Such common valuation signals have been demonstrated in vmPFC using fMRI and single-unit recording studies [63, 65, 68, 69].

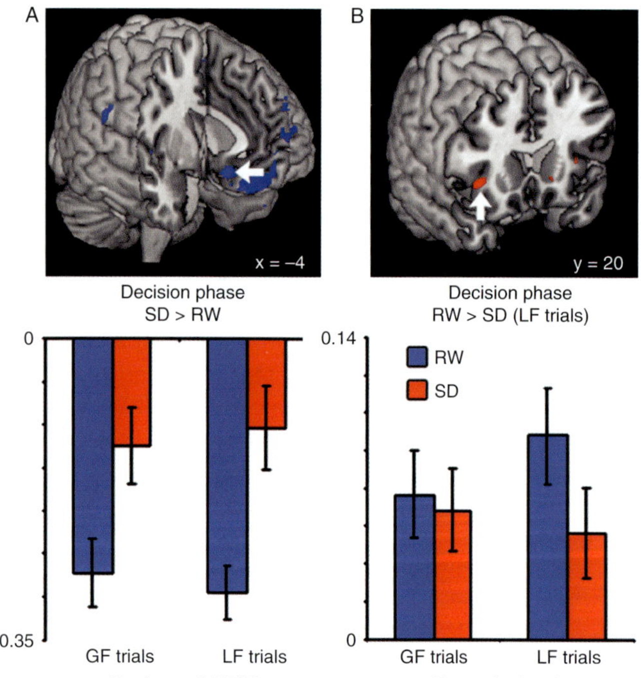

Figure 18.3 SD biases neural mechanisms underlying economic preferences. (A) SD resulted in increased activation (in this case, reduced deactivation) in the ventromedial prefrontal cortex for both gain- and loss-focus trials. (B) SD was also associated with reduced activation in the right anterior insula only for the loss-focus trials. (Adapted from [56].) RW = rested wakefulness; SD = sleep deprivation.

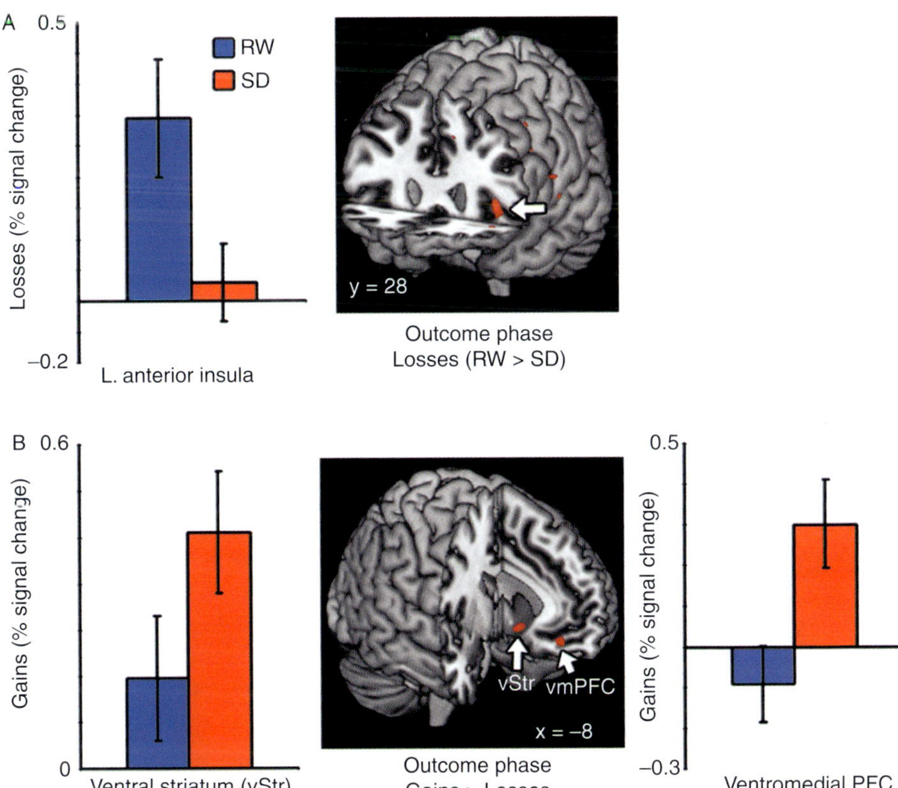

Figure 18.4 SD modulates neural sensitivity to reward outcomes. (A) Across both experiments, SD led to decreased activation in the left anterior insula for loss outcomes, compared to RW. (B) Additionally, in the second experiment, there was increased activation in the vmPFC and ventral striatum for gain outcomes following SD. (Adapted from [56].) RW = rested wakefulness; SD = sleep deprivation.

Interestingly, subjective valuation signals in the brain are generated even in the absence of overt decision-making [63, 70, 71]. Valuation can thus be appraised by incentive-compatible tasks that objectively reveal preferences without decisions. For example, in a monetary incentive delay (MID) task [44], volunteers are shown a monetary reward and informed that if they respond quickly enough to the upcoming target, they might receive that reward. Compared to a lesser-ranked reward, a higher-ranked one results in faster responses and greater activation of the ventral striatum. This task has been shown to work similarly with social and monetary rewards [72]. To determine if relative valuation for money and social rewards is altered by SD, male heterosexual volunteers performed both an MID and a social incentive delay task while undergoing fMRI [73]. These generated valuation signals following SD that could be compared and correlated with behavior.

Out of scanner, the same subjects performed an exchange task where they indicated how much they were willing to pay from an endowment to view an attractive female face in each state (RW and SD). Previous research had shown that male heterosexuals are consistent in their ratings for attractive female faces, enabling us to use this as a proxy for social reward [63]. Contrary to initial expectation, on aggregate, there was no significant shift in valuation in favor of either social or monetary rewards. However, reflecting individual differences, some volunteers became more willing to exchange money to view faces when sleep deprived while others shifted in the opposite direction.

Critically, vmPFC signal tracked these state-related individual differences (Figure 18.5). Across participants, the change in

an individual's relative activation to monetary and to social rewards in the vmPFC between SD and RW correlated with the change in that individual's exchange behavior in the two states [73]. This added support for the vmPFC being a region that indexes subjective valuation regardless of context – it generates a valuation signal that tracks different values of a single good, differences in goods, and now also different values of different goods across state.

Brain regions involved in social reward valuation, such as the amygdala, altered their responses to social rewards during SD in a manner that also correlated with the shift in vmPFC decision value signals. The latter finding suggests that the changes in vmPFC activation could be a result of state-related alteration of inputs from the amygdala and other regions mediating affective processes.

Shifts in risky decision-making and vigilance are uncorrelated

Strikingly, the shifts in economic preferences in the multiple-outcome gambling experiment as well as relative valuation for social and monetary stimuli were independent of the effects of SD on psychomotor vigilance, consistent with the suggestion that effects of SD vary according to cognitive domain [74]. This point is relevant for the increasing number of persons seeking to maintain performance when sleep deprived by taking stimulants. Stimulants may improve vigilance but may have minimal influence (or even negative effects) on other aspects of cognition, such as decision-making [55, 75–77]. Our findings that SD shapes

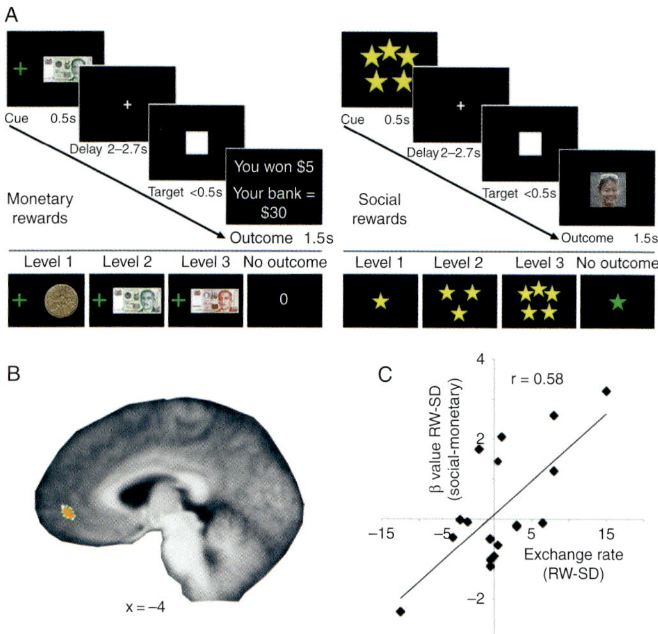

Figure 18.5 Regions carrying decision value signals in both RW and SD. (A) Trial structure of the incentive delay task. Male, heterosexual young adults viewed a cue (0.5 s) predictive of reward type and magnitude. Monetary rewards (left panel) ranged from $1 to $10. A monetary reward control predicted $0. Social rewards (right panel) ranged from 1-star (unattractive) to 5-stars (very attractive), based on ratings from an independent group of participants. A social reward control condition predicted the picture of a scrambled face. After a variable delay (2–2.7 s) a visual target (white square) appeared (< 0.5 s). Participants were instructed to respond as quickly as possible to the visual target. After the response, an outcome screen (1.5 s) revealed their reward: money or picture of a face if the response was fast enough, or no money or the picture of a scrambled face if the response was too slow. Reaction time thresholds were defined for each subject and each cue independently in a practice run that preceded the task, such that on average participants succeeded in 60% of the trials. (B) A region in the vmPFC showed a significant correlation between exchange rate and difference between activation in response to social and monetary rewards in both RW and SD. (C) Change in decision value signals across states (RW–SD, *y* axis) correlated significantly with change in exchange rate (RW–SD, *x* axis). (Adapted from [73].) RW = rested wakefulness; SD = sleep deprivation.

similar behavioral performances of these two groups in the IGT introduced earlier. An alternative view suggests that lack of adequate sleep influences valuation of inputs. Since the vmPFC plays an important role in the computation of a decision value, effects of SD on this region may lead to biases in the underlying computation value and hence poor decisions, both in a social and economic context.

We conjectured that changes in dopamine neurotransmission following SD might affect decision-making in that state. Positron emission tomography imaging with [^{11}C]raclopride suggests that sleep-deprived persons show elevated dopamine transmission in the striatum and thalamus. This change in dopamine transmission is thought to contribute to maintaining wakefulness, albeit somewhat unsuccessfully given the concurrent decline in visual attention as volunteers engaged in task performance [78, 79]. As levodopa administered to healthy young adults can transiently elevate subjective ratings of pleasantness [80], as well as increased impulsivity [81], we speculate that the optimism bias observed in SD could be a by-product of attempts to sustain wakefulness by elevating dopamine levels. The varying extent to which this is successful in a given individual might then account for the dissociation between vigilance and shift in risk preference.

This conjecture relating to "optimism bias" is supported by an experiment where healthy subjects were shown neutral or positive emotional pictures [82]. Sleep-deprived persons assigned more positive ratings to the same set of mixed neutral and positive pictures than non-sleep-deprived persons. This was associated with selectively elevated neural signals to positive pictures in the amydala, insula, and fusiform gyri. Altered connectivity between the ventrotegmental area and amydala as well as insula were also observed.

Summary

SD may affect the way we make risky decisions by altering preferences, specifically shifting our bias towards selecting higher-gain outcomes. Neuroimaging has shed light on the neural mechanisms underlying these changes in risk preference: increased gain chasing was associated with higher activation in the vmPFC, and decreased loss aversion was mirrored by lower activation in the anterior insula. This optimism bias may require specific task contexts to uncover as it is not seen in all experiments involving SD. At the present time, it does not appear that SD affects relative value signals associated with monetary and a form of social reward. A compelling conjecture is that alterations in risky decision-making may reflect alterations in dopamine signaling that may help maintain wakefulness but have maladaptive effects in the form of altered preferences.

decision preferences independent of its effects on vigilance cautions that the traditional countermeasures may be ineffective in ameliorating the decision biases engendered by limited sleep.

A region of particular interest across all studies presented here has been the vmPFC. The vmPFC has been shown to be instrumental in computing value as well as in supporting processes related to learning from reward and punishment [2, 53, 58]. One explanation for the effects of SD on vmPFC activation, as observed in a more lateral region in our first risky choice study, is that SD could hamper the integration of feedback when making decisions, consistent with the role of this region in learning. Under this view, the effects of SD are often compared to patients with lesions in the vmPFC, particularly based on

References

1. Platt ML, Huettel SA. Risky business: the neuroeconomics of decision making under uncertainty. *Nat Neurosci.* 2008;**11**(4):398–403.

2. Rangel A, Camerer C, Montague PR. A framework for studying the neurobiology of value-based decision making. *Nat Rev Neurosci.* 2008;**9**(7):545–56.

3. Glimcher PW, Rustichini A. Neuroeconomics: the consilience of brain and decision. *Science.* 2004;**306** (5695):447–52.

4. Sanfey AG, Loewenstein G, McClure SM, Cohen JD. Neuroeconomics: cross-currents in research on decision-making. *Trends Cogn Sci.* 2006;**10**(3):108–16.

5. Bernoulli D. Specimen theoriae novae de mensura sortis. *Commentarii Academiae Scientarum Imperialis Petropolitanae.* 1738;**5**:175–92.

6. von Neumann J, Morgenstern O. *Theory of Games and Economic Behavior.* Princeton, NJ, Princeton University Press, 1944.

7. Savage LJ. *Foundations of Statistics.* New York, Wiley, 1954.

8. Slovic P, Lichtenstein S. The relative importance of probabilities and payoffs in risk-taking. *J Exp Psychol Monograph Suppl.* 1968;**72**:1–18.

9. Tversky A, Kahneman D. Judgment under uncertainty: heuristics and biases. *Science.* 1974;**185**:1124–31.

10. Kahneman D, Tversky A. Prospect theory: an analysis of decision under risk. *Econometrica.* 1979;**47**(2):263–91.

11. Loewenstein GF, Weber EU, Hsee CK, Welch N. Risk as feelings. *Psychol Bull.* 2001,**127**(2):267–86.

12. Gigerenzer G, Goldstein DG. Reasoning the fast and frugal way: models of bounded rationality. *Psychol Rev.* 1996;**103**(4):650–69.

13. Simon HA. A Behavioral model of rational choice. *Quart J Econ.* 1955;**69**:99–118.

14. Tom SM, Fox CR, Trepel C, Poldrack RA. The neural basis of loss aversion in decision-making under risk. *Science.* 2007;**315**(5811):515–18.

15. Knutson B, Fong GW, Bennett SM, Adams CM, Hommer D. A region of mesial prefrontal cortex tracks monetarily rewarding outcomes: characterization with rapid event-related fMRI. *Neuroimage.* 2003;**18**(2):263–72.

16. Yacubian J, Glascher J, Schroeder K, et al. Dissociable systems for gain- and loss-related value predictions and errors of prediction in the human brain. *J Neurosci.* 2006;**26**(37):9530–7.

17. Huettel SA, Stowe CJ, Gordon EM, Warner BT, Platt ML. Neural signatures of economic preferences for risk and ambiguity. *Neuron.* 2006;**49**(5):765–75.

18. Hsu M, Bhatt M, Adolphs R, Tranel D, Camerer CF. Neural systems responding to degrees of uncertainty in human decision-making. *Science.* 2005;**310**(5754):1680–3.

19. Hsu M, Krajbich I, Zhao C, Camerer CF. Neural response to reward anticipation under risk is nonlinear in probabilities. *J Neurosci.* 2009;**29**(7):2231–7.

20. Berns GS, Capra CM, Chappelow J, Moore S, Noussair C. Nonlinear neurobiological probability weighting functions for aversive outcomes. *Neuroimage.* 2008;**39**(4):2047–57.

21. Coricelli G, Critchley HD, Joffily M, et al. Regret and its avoidance: a neuroimaging study of choice behavior. *Nat Neurosci.* 2005;**8**(9):1255–62.

22. Kuhnen CM, Knutson B. The neural basis of financial risk taking. *Neuron.* 2005;**47**(5):763–70.

23. Lerner JS, Small DA, Loewenstein G. Heart strings and purse strings: carryover effects of emotions on economic decisions. *Psychol Sci.* 2004;**15**(5):337–41.

24. Damasio AR. The somatic marker hypothesis and the possible functions of the prefrontal cortex. *Philos Trans R Soc Lond Biol Sci.* 1996;**351**(1346):1413–20.

25. Sanfey AG, Rilling JK, Aronson JA, Nystrom LE, Cohen JD. The neural basis of economic decision-making in the Ultimatum Game. *Science.* 2003;**300**(5626):1755–8.

26. Shiv B, Loewenstein G, Bechara A. The dark side of emotion in decision-making: when individuals with decreased emotional reactions make more advantageous decisions. *Brain Res Cogn Brain Res.* 2005;**23**(1):85–92.

27. De Martino B, Kumaran D, Seymour B, Dolan RJ. Frames, biases, and rational decision-making in the human brain. *Science.* 2006;**313**(5787):684–7.

28. Venkatraman V, Payne JW, Bettman JR, Luce MF, Huettel SA. Separate neural mechanisms underlie choices and strategic preferences in risky decision making. *Neuron.* 2009;**62**(4):593–602.

29. Venkatraman V, Payne JW, Huettel SA. Neuroeconomics of risky decisions: from variables to strategies. In: Delgado MR, Phelps EA, Robbins TW, eds. *Decision Making, Affect and Learning.* Oxford, Oxford University Press. 2011;153–72.

30. Kaempf GL, Klein G, Thordsen ML, Wolf S. Decision making in complex naval command and control environments. *Hum Factors.* 1996;**38**:220–31.

31. Harrison Y, Horne JA. The impact of sleep deprivation on decision making: a review. *J Exp Psychol Appl.* 2000;**6**(3):236–49.

32. Pilcher JJ, Huffcutt AI. Effects of sleep deprivation on performance: a meta-analysis. *Sleep.* 1996;**19**(4):318–26.

33. Durmer JS, Dinges DF. Neurocognitive consequences of sleep deprivation. *Semin Neurol.* 2005;**25**(1):117–29.

34. Roehrs T, Greenwald M, Roth T. Risk-taking behavior: effects of ethanol, caffeine, and basal sleepiness. *Sleep.* 2004;**27**(5):887–93.

35. Linde L, Edland A, Bergstrom M. Auditory attention and multiattribute decision-making during a 33 h sleep-deprivation period: mean performance and between-subject dispersions. *Ergonomics.* 1999;**33**(5):696–713.

36. Harrison Y, Horne JA. One night of sleep loss impairs innovative thinking and flexible decision making. *Organ Behav Hum Decis Process.* 1999,**78**(2):128–45.

37. Bechara A, Tranel D, Damasio H. Characterization of the decision-making deficit of patients with ventromedial prefrontal cortex lesions. *Brain.* 2000;**123**(Pt 11):2189–202.

38. Killgore WD, Balkin TJ, Wesensten NJ. Impaired decision-making following 49 h of sleep deprivation. *J Sleep Res.* 2006;**15**(1):7–13.

39. Kahneman D, Frederick S. Frames and brains: elicitation and control of response tendencies. *Trends Cogn Sci.* 2007;**11**(2):45–6.

40. Tversky A, Kahneman D. The framing of decisions and the psychology of choice. *Science.* 1981;**211**(4481):453–8.

41. Tversky A, Kahneman D. Rational choice and the framing of decisions. *J Bus.* 1986;**59**(4):S251–78.

42. McKenna BS, Dickinson DL, Orff HJ, Drummond SP. The effects of one night of sleep deprivation on known-risk and ambiguous-risk decisions. *J Sleep Res.* 2007;**16**(3):245–52.

43. Venkatraman V, Chuah YM, Huettel SA, Chee MW. Sleep deprivation elevates expectation of gains and

attenuates response to losses following risky decisions. *Sleep*. 2007;**30**(5):603–9.

44. Knutson B, Adams CM, Fong GW, Hommer D. Anticipation of increasing monetary reward selectively recruits nucleus accumbens. *J Neurosci*. 2001;**21**(RC159):1–5.

45. Knutson B, Cooper JC. Functional magnetic resonance imaging of reward prediction. *Curr Opin Neurol*. 2005;**18**(4):411–17.

46. Knutson B, Fong GW, Adams CM, Varner JL, Hommer D. Dissociation of reward anticipation and outcome with event-related fMRI. *Neuroreport*. 2001;**12**(17):3683–7.

47. Rushworth MFS, Walton ME, Kennerley SW, Bannerman DM. Action sets and decisions in the medial frontal cortex. *Trends Cogn Sci*. 2004;**8**(9):410–17.

48. Botvinick MM. Conflict monitoring and decision-making: reconciling two perspectives on anterior cinfulate function. *Cogn Affect Behav Neurosci*. 2007;**7**:365–6.

49. Botvinick MM, Rosen ZB. Anticipation of cognitive demand during decision-making. *Psychol Res*. 2009;**73**(6):835–42.

50. Ernst M, Nelson EE, Jazbec S, *et al*. Amygdala and nucleus accumbens in responses to receipt and omission of gains in adults and adolescents. *Neuroimage*. 2005;**25**(4):1279–91.

51. Paulus MP, Rogalsky C, Simmons A, Feinstein JS, Stein MB. Increased activation in the right insula during risk-taking decision making is related to harm avoidance and neuroticism. *Neuroimage*. 2003;**19**(4):1439–48.

52. O'Doherty JP, Critchley H, Deichmann R, Dolan RJ. Dissociating valence of outcome from behavioral control in human orbital and ventral prefrontal cortices. *J Neurosci*. 2003;**23**(21):7931–9.

53. Rolls ET, Hornak J, Wade D, McGrath J. Emotion-related learning in patients with social and emotional changes associated with frontal lobe damage. *J Neurol Neurosurg Psychiatry*. 1994;**57**(12):1518–24.

54. Payne JW. It is whether you win or lose: the importance of the overall probabilities of winning or losing in risky choice. *J Risk Uncertainty*. 2005;**30**(1):5–19.

55. Killgore WD, Grugle NL, Killgore DB, *et al*. Restoration of risk-propensity during sleep deprivation: caffeine, dextroamphetamine, and modafinil. *Aviat Space Environ Med*. 2008;**79**(9):867–74.

56. Venkatraman V, Huettel SA, Chuah LY, Payne JW, Chee MW. Sleep deprivation biases the neural mechanisms underlying economic preferences. *J Neurosci*. 2011;**31**(10):3712–18.

57. Paulus MP, Frank LR. Ventromedial prefrontal cortex activation is critical for preference judgments. *Neuroreport*. 2003;**14**(10):1311–15.

58. Bechara A, Damasio H, Damasio AR. Emotion, decision making and the orbitofrontal cortex. *Cereb Cortex*. 2000;**10**(3):295–307.

59. Tobler PN, O'Doherty JP, Dolan RJ, Schultz W. Reward value coding distinct from risk attitude-related uncertainty coding in human reward systems. *J Neurophysiol*. 2007;**97**(2):1621–32.

60. Preuschoff K, Quartz SR, Bossaerts P. Human insula activation reflects risk prediction errors as well as risk. *J Neurosci*. 2008;**28**(11):2745–52.

61. Anderson C, Dickinson DL. Bargaining and trust: the effects of 36-h total sleep deprivation on socially interactive decisions. *J Sleep Res*. 2010;**19**(1 Pt 1):54–63.

62. Montague PR, Berns GS. Neural economics and the biological substrates of valuation. *Neuron*. 2002;**36**(2):265–84.

63. Smith DV, Hayden BY, Truong TK, *et al*. Distinct value signals in anterior and posterior ventromedial prefrontal cortex. *J Neurosci*. 2010;**30**(7):2490–5.

64. Izuma K, Saito DN, Sadato N. Processing of social and monetary rewards in the human striatum. *Neuron*. 2008;**58**(2):284–94.

65. Kim H, Shimojo S, O'Doherty JP. Overlapping responses for the expectation of juice and money rewards in human ventromedial prefrontal cortex. *Cereb Cortex*. 2011;**21**(4):769–76.

66. Rademacher L, Krach S, Kohls G, *et al*. Dissociation of neural networks for anticipation and consumption of monetary and social rewards. *Neuroimage*. 2010;**49**(4):3276–85.

67. Lin A, Adolphs R, Rangel A. Social and monetary reward learning engage overlapping neural substrates. *Soc Cogn Affect Neurosci*. 2012;**7**(3):274–81.

68. Padoa-Schioppa C, Assad JA. Neurons in the orbitofrontal cortex encode economic value. *Nature*. 2006;**441**(7090):223–6.

69. Chib VS, Rangel A, Shimojo S, O'Doherty JP. Evidence for a common representation of decision values for dissimilar goods in human ventromedial prefrontal cortex. *J Neurosci*. 2009;**29**(39):12315–20.

70. Lebreton M, Jorge S, Michel V, Thirion B, Pessiglione M. An automatic valuation system in the human brain: evidence from functional neuroimaging. *Neuron*. 2009;**64**(3):431–9.

71. Tusche A, Bode S, Haynes JD. Neural responses to unattended products predict later consumer choices. *J Neurosci*. 2010;**30**(23):8024–31.

72. Carter RM, Macinnes JJ, Huettel SA, Adcock RA. Activation in the VTA and nucleus accumbens increases in anticipation of both gains and losses. *Front Behav Neurosci*. 2009;**3**:21.

73. Libedinsky C, Smith DV, Teng CS, *et al*. Sleep deprivation alters valuation signals in the ventromedial prefrontal cortex. *Front Behav Neurosci*. 2011;**5**:70.

74. Van Dongen HP, Baynard MD, Maislin G, Dinges DF. Systematic interindividual differences in neurobehavioral impairment from sleep loss: evidence of trait-like differential vulnerability. *Sleep*. 2004;**27**(3):423–33.

75. Gottselig JM, Adam M, Retey JV, *et al*. Random number generation during sleep deprivation: effects of caffeine on response maintenance and stereotypy. *J Sleep Res*. 2006;**15**(1):31–40.

76. Killgore WD, Lipizzi EL, Kamimori GH, Balkin TJ. Caffeine effects on risky decision making after 75 hours of sleep deprivation. *Aviat Space Environ Med*. 2007;**78**(10):957–62.

77. Huck NO, McBride SA, Kendall AP, Grugle NL, Killgore WD. The effects of modafinil, caffeine, and dextroamphetamine on judgments of simple versus complex emotional expressions following sleep deprivation. *Int J Neurosci*. 2008;**118**(4):487–502.

78. Volkow ND, Wang GJ, Telang F, *et al*. Sleep deprivation decreases binding of [11C]raclopride to dopamine D2/D3 receptors in the human brain. *J Neurosci*. 2008;**28**(34):8454–61.

79. Volkow ND, Tomasi D, Wang G-J, *et al*. Hyperstimulation of striatal D2

receptors with sleep deprivation: implications for cognitive impairment. *Neuroimage.* 2009;**45**(4):1232–40.

80. Sharot T, Shiner T, Brown AC, Fan J, Dolan RJ. Dopamine enhances expectation of pleasure in humans. *Curr Biol.* 2009;**19**(24):2077–80.

81. Pine A, Shiner T, Seymour B, Dolan RJ. Dopamine, time, and impulsivity in humans. *J Neurosci.* 2010;**30**(26):8888–96.

82. Gujar N, Yoo SS, Hu P, Walker MP. Sleep deprivation amplifies reactivity of brain reward networks, biasing the appraisal of positive emotional experiences. *J Neurosci.* 2011;**31**(12):4466–74.

Functional imaging of inter-individual differences in response to sleep deprivation

Michael W. L. Chee and Hans P. A. Van Dongen

Introduction

An important long-term goal of studying inter-individual differences in responses to sleep deprivation (SD) is to elucidate phenotypes that predict how an individual will perform in an operational setting after being sleep deprived. SD results in response slowing, reduced accuracy, and increased performance variability and response lapses [1]. Major factors modulating these phenomena include: cumulative duration of sustained wakefulness [2], time of day [3, 4], time on task [1, 5], stimulant use [6], and the type of cognitive/behavioral test [7–9]. Other factors to consider include posture [10], physical activity [11], light exposure [12], and chronotype [13, 14].

Even after controlling for these major factors, substantial inter-individual differences in behavioral performance after SD have been observed. Such variation in performance is magnified with the accumulation of SD, as evidenced by increased gaps in performance between the most and least affected persons [9, 15]. These inter-individual differences appear stable across different testing episodes [7–9] but different cognitive domains are not similarly affected [8, 9, 16]. Individuals most severely affected on one cognitive test may not be the same ones most severely affected on another test [7]. Although studies have found that affected behavioral measures clustered along at least three dimensions [9, 16], tentatively classified as subjective measures, objective measures of sustained attention, and objective measures of cognitive processing ability, it remains unclear how to best group cognitive tests in order to optimally predict real-world declines in operational performance.

Some guidance regarding test grouping comes from a recent meta-analysis of studies evaluating behavior in sleep-deprived persons, which found that "simple attention" was the most severely affected domain, followed by working memory and speed of processing [17]. This result may be skewed by limitations in the scope of prior research on neurobehavioral performance in sleep-deprived persons. Indeed, contemporary notions of how cognition is affected by SD are largely driven by experiments examining vigilant attention or human factors experiments evaluating "real-world tasks." The latter generally do not readily decompose into neuropsychological constructs that enable systematic and principled elucidation of the mechanisms underlying altered behavior [18].

With this caveat in place, the high weight placed on tests of sustained attention and vigilance, particularly when speeded responses are required, is likely well justified. The impact of SD on vigilant attention has been robustly demonstrated in multiple studies [1]. Attention may be broadly defined as the set of capacities that enables us to select a particular target task or stimulus and stick to it, even in the face of distraction. As such, many "higher cognitive functions" are likely to be dependent on adequate attention. Encoding of memories, even short-term memories, will be hindered if a person is insufficiently attentive. Executive functions engaged when "thinking flexibly" and acting contrary to habitual, pre-potent responses require us to be attentive. As such, some researchers consider deficits in attention as the central mechanism underlying failures in other cognitive domains [17].

At the present time it remains that the relative importance of different mechanisms enabling sustained attention is somewhat unclear. Deficits could arise from faulty arousal that is driven by subcortical structures like the brainstem and thalamus [19, 20]. Alternatively, loss of selective focus could result from loss of "top-down control" mediated by frontoparietal control systems [21–24]. Most recently it was proposed that sustained attention may fail in a "bottom-up" fashion as neuronal groups intensively engaged in task performance exhibit local sleep-like states that temporarily render them unresponsive [5, 25]. Finally, deficient attention could arise from a combination of mechanisms – for example, sensory systems that are "shut-down" as a result of insufficient "arousal" might fail to provide bottom-up signals to capture top-down control of attention [26]. There is evidence that fluctuation in vigilant attention over a timescale of tens of seconds may reflect oscillations in the brain's responsiveness to external stimuli [27, 28].

Findings from the cognitive aging literature might be informative regarding the gaps in the spectrum of neurobehavioral tests used in sleep-deprived persons [29]. In general it appears that tests where performance is facilitated by use of prior knowledge or experience, tests which do not involve time pressure, or those which do not require flexible thinking are those less affected by age [30]. Although the analogy between deficits related to aging and those related to SD has

Neuroimaging of Sleep and Sleep Disorders, ed. Eric Nofzinger, Pierre Maquet, and Michael J. Thorpy. Published by Cambridge University Press. © Cambridge University Press 2013.

caveats [31], there appear to be parallels between behavior in aging and behavior in sleep-deprived persons that remain to be exploited.

Using functional imaging to investigate inter-individual differences in response to sleep deprivation

As outlined in Chapters 16 and 17, functional imaging – being a physiological measure – evaluates changes not evident from observing behavior alone. For example, when selectively attending to a target colocated with distractors, evaluating higher visual cortex activation can inform how well the brain is achieving the behavioral goals of target enhancement and distractor suppression [32]. As illustrated later shifts in brain activation between well-rested and sleep-deprived states often correlate with behavioral alterations. These shifts can be used to assess the effects of countermeasures against SD. In select instances, imaging changes may be leading indicators in that changes in brain activation precede behavioral alterations [33]. Some studies, reviewed below, suggest that activation levels recorded after normal sleep may predict how a person would respond to future episodes of SD [34–36], although the direction of what is beneficial may vary with the task [37].

Prior to reviewing functional imaging assessments of inter-individual differences, we should first consider their reproducibility across test sessions. Early reproducibility experiments using functional magnetic resonance imaging (fMRI) typically invoked simple sensori motor paradigms [38–40] or examined the extent of hemispheric lateralization of specialized functions such as language [41]. Later experiments tested reproducibility in higher-level cognitive functions, for example an evaluation of the long-term reliability of fMRI over a year using a classification-learning paradigm [42]. This study showed task-related activation in midbrain and fronto-striatal regions to exhibit intra-class correlation coefficients (ICCs) ranging from 0.76 to 0.99, indicating high to excellent reproducibility.

In another investigation, more specific to the current context, 19 young adults were studied four times using a working memory task, twice following rested wakefulness after a normal night of sleep and twice after 24 h of SD [43]. Bilateral parietal, left prefrontal, and anterior cingulate activations in paired well-rested and sleep-deprived sessions were significantly correlated (correlations ranged from 0.6 to 0.8; Figure 19.1) and were similar in magnitude for both states. Critically, the shift in activation across states was also significantly correlated across test sessions but only for the left parietal region. ICCs were computed to demonstrate that the between-subject variances in activation across sessions were greater than the within-subject variances. ICC values for single-session, region-based analyses ranged from 0.58 to 0.69 in the bilateral parietal, left prefrontal, and anterior cingulate regions. The ICCs for state-related shifts in activation within the left and right parietal regions of interest (ROIs) were 0.49 and 0.46, respectively. These findings provide assurance that repeated fMRI evaluations across states can elicit reproducible imaging responses that can be used to evaluate inter-individual differences.

The search for an imaging predictor of performance when sleep deprived

Ideally, a probe that could uncover one's susceptibility to performance decline with SD without the individual having to be sleep deprived is needed. In a seminal study of this topic [36, 44], 33 subjects were evaluated after a normal night of sleep and again after 30 h of SD using a Sternberg-type working memory task. Frontoparietal regions were recruited to perform the task in the well-rested state. However, contrary to an influential hypothesis that the frontal lobes should be more affected by SD [45], bilateral posterior parietal areas were found to show greater decline in activation after SD in all subjects. To examine whether brain activation patterns were different in persons who showed a greater decline in performance accuracy and those who did not, the imaging findings of the ten best and ten worst performers were compared. Activation in the well-rested state and after SD, as well as the change across states were analyzed. The key finding was that individuals who evidenced greater "global activation" in the well-rested scan were more resistant to performance degradation.

This point was reiterated in a "real-world" comparison involving eight fighter pilots whereby those with greater "global" activation performed better in the flight simulator after SD [34]. It should be pointed out, however, that "global" activation was derived from the aggregation of activation primarily arising from frontoparietal areas. Critically, in the parent study, the largest state-related shifts in activation were observed in the posterior parietal cortex, and overall, vulnerable persons showed greater *shifts* in activation across states in the left frontal region.

In another study, using a different working memory task, a group of 28 volunteers underwent three fMRI scan sessions – after normal sleep and following about 24 h as well as 35 h of SD [35]. Persons with higher frontoparietal activation in the well-rested state were more resistant to performance decline after SD. This held up in a correlational approach as well as in a tertile split of volunteers where the top and bottom performing thirds were compared. Slightly at variance with earlier findings, parietal activation was more robustly correlated with behavior than frontal activation.

These findings have been interpreted in the context of cognitive reserve theory, which originated from healthy cognitive aging studies. The theory attributes better cognitive resilience to having more cognitive resources to begin with or having the capacity to engage alternative neural resources as needs arise [46]. Prior functional imaging studies found that individuals with higher working memory spans [47], fluid intelligence [48], or better working memory accuracy [49] engage the prefrontal and parietal regions to a greater extent than poorer performers. These studies attributed their findings to greater recruitment of attentional resources in better performers [48, 49]. Adapting the cognitive reserve theory to working memory experiments in sleep-deprived young adults,

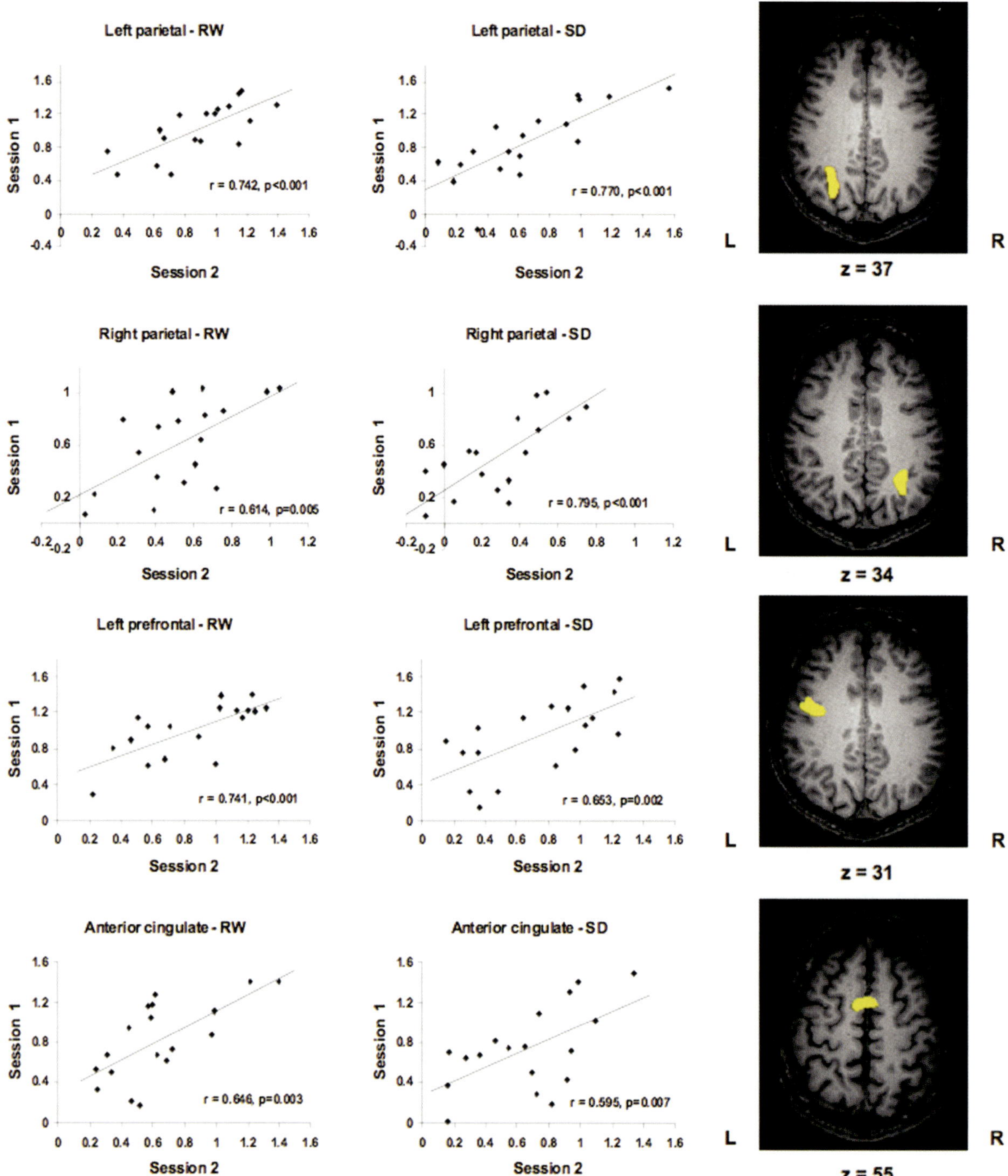

Figure 19.1 Correlations of parameter estimates of activation in task-related regions of interest for session 1 and session 2 in a working memory experiment during rested wakefulness (RW) and following sleep deprivation (SD). (Reproduced from [43].)

it has been postulated that persons resilient to SD have greater reserve in the form of higher task-related activation of fronto-parietal areas prior to SD.

Against the simple surmise that more activation in the rested state is better, studies that did not involve SD found lower prefrontal activation to be associated with better performance [50]. Reports linking lesser activation to better performance attribute their findings to "greater efficiency" of task performance, evidenced by faster, and sometimes also more accurate, responses in association with lower cortical activation. This line of reasoning finds support in studies involving healthy elderly individuals [51] and patients with schizophrenia [52, 53].

To illustrate the difficulty in predicting vulnerability to SD with a single fMRI measurement, when executive function was tested using the Go/No-Go task individuals with relatively *less* right ventrolateral prefrontal and insula activation in the rested state showed greater activation of these areas when sleep deprived [37]. These persons showed *less reduction in inhibitory efficiency when sleep deprived*, consistent with them being more efficient in the rested state. This could have left them with executive processing resources to compensate for the reduced tonic activation of ventrolateral prefrontal and anterior insula areas during SD. The anterior insula/ventrolateral prefrontal cortex contributes to pre-potent response inhibition in well-rested persons. Such an explanation is also consistent with the notion of "cognitive reserve" except that in this illustration, less rather than greater activation in the baseline state signals greater reserve.

Shifts in activation across states as a marker of inter-individual variability

The seemingly contradictory findings regarding the benefit of greater activation in areas of the brain led us to examine whether evaluating shifts in activation across states would prove a more reliable marker of inter-individual variability in behavior. The utility of this approach was first broached indirectly in a study evaluating verbal working memory using letters. The regional covariance approach used found that a larger decline in activation across several regions – "pattern expression" – correlated with lower performance accuracy following SD [54]. The reduction in pattern expression with SD for each subject was related to the magnitude of the change in performance on the memory task. Decreases in "pattern expression" within brain areas involved in spatial attention and visual processing correlated with reduced recognition accuracy, increased intra-individual variability in reaction time, and increased lapsing. The same researchers performed another experiment using non-verbalizable figures, and similarly found reduced pattern expression to relate to performance decrements [55].

In a selective attention task involving Navon figures [21, 22] we assessed response lapsing in sleep-deprived subjects. Faster correct responses were associated with *lower* frontoparietal activation than slower correct responses, independent of state. SD was associated with a mean level of activation that was lower than that following normal sleep. This was explained by suggesting that on average, fewer circuits may be available for task processing in the SD state (See Chapter 17 for an elaboration of this idea). Critically, when *less vulnerable* individuals underwent SD, they showed either comparable or greater activation of frontoparietal areas compared with the rested state *when they showed response lapses* [21].

The utility of assessing *shifts in activation* across well-rested and sleep-deprived conditions to predict inter-individual differences in response to SD was further corroborated in a pair of experiments evaluating the cholinesterase inhibitor donepezil as a countermeasure against SD. With both the visual short-term memory [23] and episodic memory [24] tasks, a larger drop in intraparietal sulcus activation across states predicted a larger performance decline during SD. Improvement of performance in the SD condition with donepezil as compared to placebo correlated with greater state-related shifts in activation while on the drug (Figure 19.2). In keeping with the notion that

optimal levels of neurotransmitter activation correspond to an inverted U-shaped function, persons who showed greater decline in performance on placebo when sleep-deprived tended to be those who benefited from donepezil, whereas for those relatively unaffected by SD, there was a trend towards deterioration with donepezil [23, 24].

Collectively, this group of studies indicates that better preserved recruitment of cortical areas involved in the control of attention or executive processes during SD differentiates more or less vulnerable persons – supporting the focus placed on studying attention in previous behavioral studies. Additionally, they illustrate that measuring activation changes across state in two sessions may provide a more reliable marker of individual vulnerability to SD than making inferences based on a single baseline scan.

Roles of subcortical areas and the default mode network in influencing sleep-deprived performance

The thalamus plays an important part in mediating both arousal and attention, which in turn have substantial effects on behavioral performance. Relay and reticular neurons in the thalamus exhibit marked changes in firing during the transition from wakefulness to sleep [56]. The pulvinar and medio-dorsal thalamic nuclei are the targets of top-down influences of attention [57]. At the group level, many studies (19–22, 54) have shown that, counterintuitively, the thalamus is more strongly activated after a normal night of sleep than following SD (Figure 19.3). However, while showing a trend, inter-individual differences in thalamic activation do not appear to predict performance decline. Thalamic activation is less reliably reproducible across scan sessions than fronto-parietal activation [43]. These findings may relate to the more complex dynamics of trial-to-trial modulation of thalamic activation in sleep deprived persons, whereby normal performance during SD is associated with activation higher than observed following normal sleep whereas response lapses during SD result in a precipitous fall in thalamic activation [21].

Rather than task-related activation [58], some parts of the brain consistently show task-related deactivation (i.e., falling below baseline). Signal alterations of this sort typically occur in the brain's "default mode network" – brain regions active in the absence of overt task performance and whose activity is diminished by engagement of attention and/or controlled processing [59]. Decreases in task-related deactivation (Figure 19.4) have been reported in several studies [60–63]. However, this effect is not as robust as what has been observed regarding shifts in the frontoparietal attention network (unpublished data relating to [35, 64]). Reduced intrinsic connectivity between the precuneus, a major node of the default mode network, and other nodes in this network has been observed following SD, but thus far, there has been no correlation with shifts in behavior [65]. There is ample potential for more studies in this area.

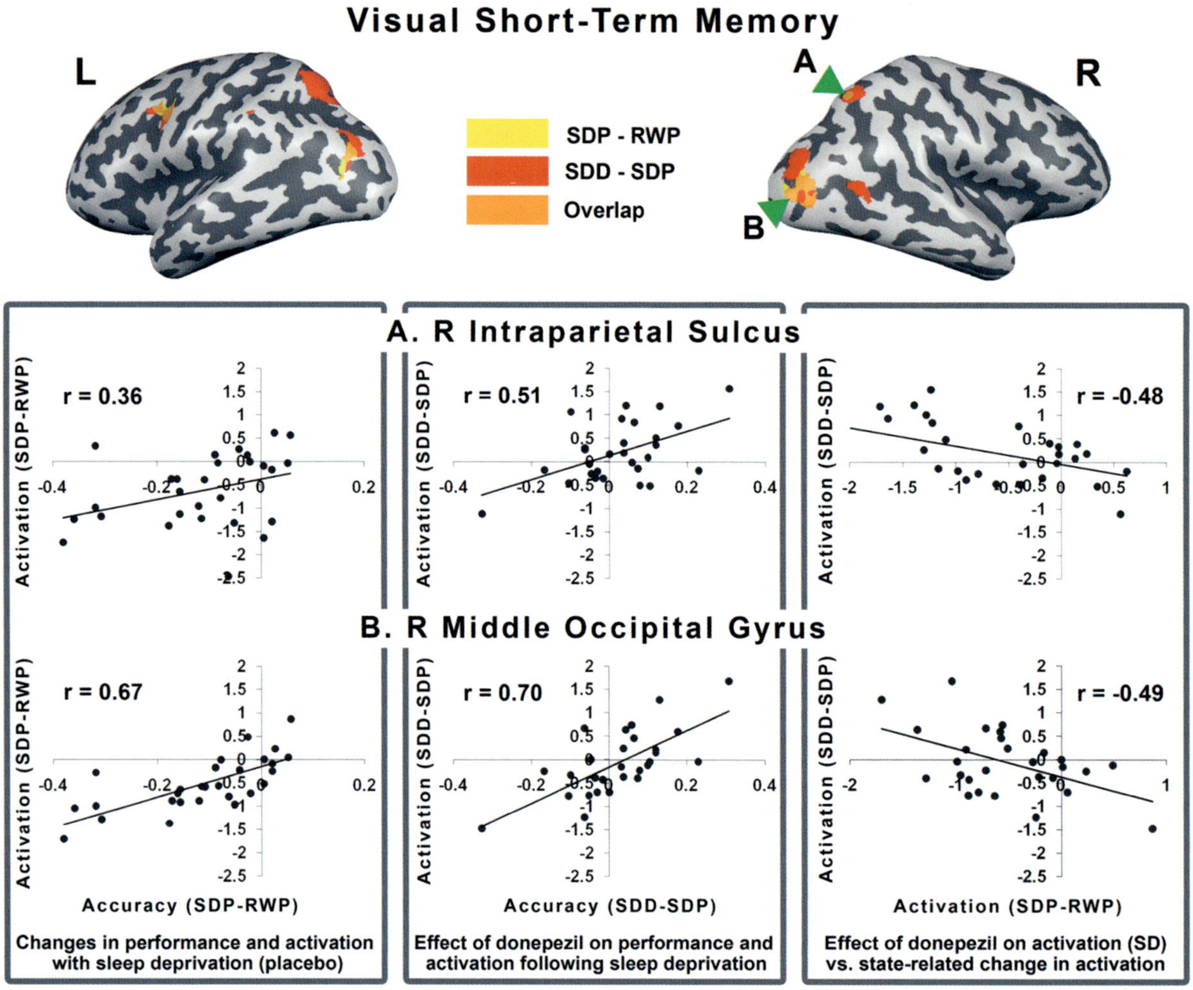

Visual Short-Term Memory

Figure 19.2 Upper panel: the inflated brains show regions where activation tracked behavior decline following sleep deprivation (SD) in the placebo condition (yellow). Regions where activation tracked the effect of donepezil in the setting of SD are shown in red. The overlap of these regions appears in orange and data for the correlation plots that ensue were obtained from these regions. Lower panel: The left-most graphs show the correlation between behavioral change elicited by SD in the placebo condition and the corresponding change in activation. The middle graphs show the correlation between how donepezil modulated performance and activation in the context of SD. The right-most graphs show the negative correlation between donepezil-induced changes in activation in the context of SD with SD-induced changes in activation when subjects were on placebo. All correlations were significant at p < 0.05. (Reproduced from [23].)

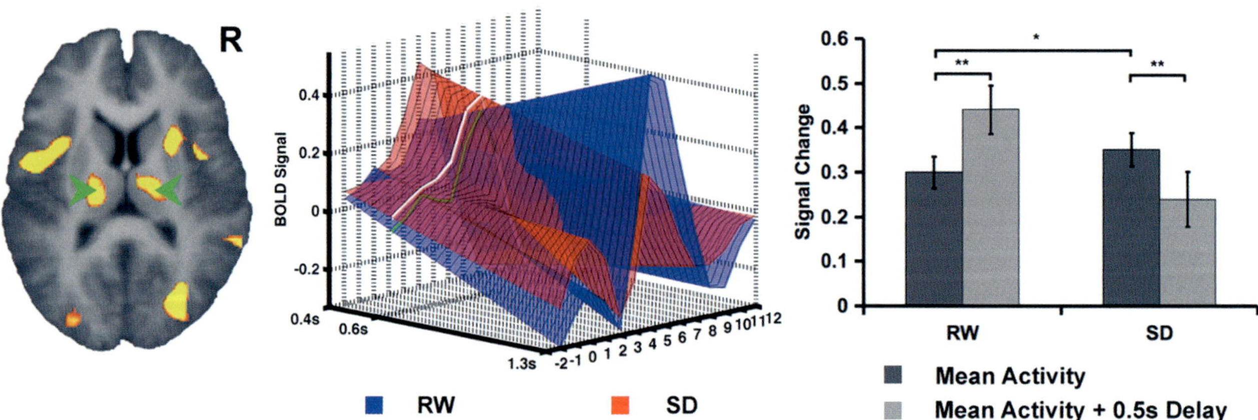

Figure 19.3 Three-dimensioned-plot showing the results of trial-by-trial modeling of fMRI signal in the thalamus. fMRI signal evolution for retention times (RTs) ranging from 0.2 s faster than mean RT for a given individual to 0.7 s slower than mean RT are displayed. The signal time course at the mean RT is marked in green. Responding at the average response time during SD elicited a higher signal than in RW but lapses (defined as mean RT + 0.5 s for that state) in SD significantly attenuated task-related thalamic activation. This contrasted with RW where lapses were associated with significantly greater peak fMRI signal. Error bars represent standard error of the mean. * p < 0.01, ** p < 0.001. (Reproduced from [22].)

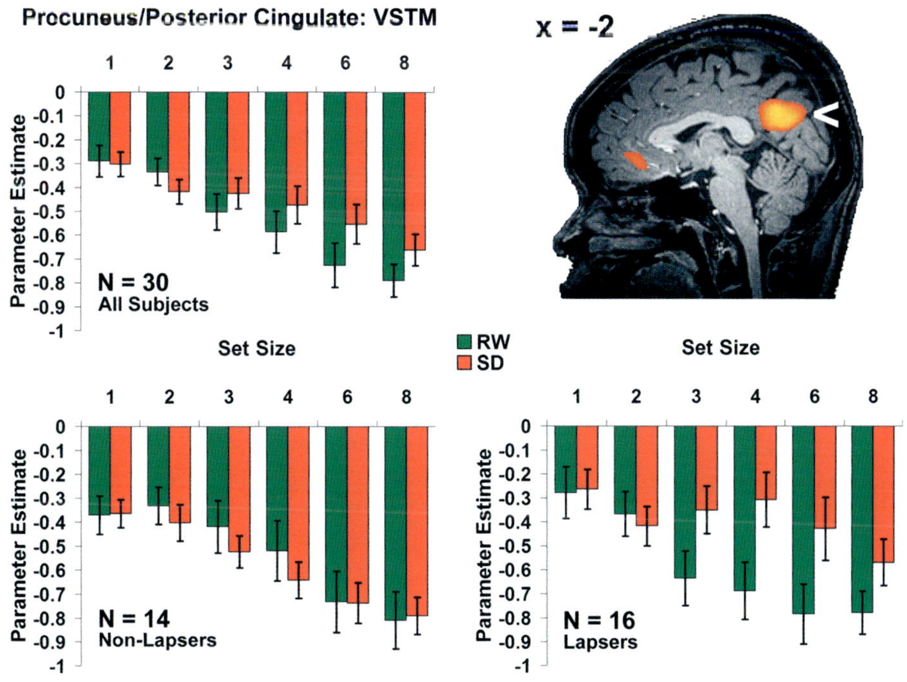

Figure 19.4. Activation in the precuneus/posterior cingulate cortex (PC/PCC) for the visual short-term memory task as a function of set size and state for 30 participants. There was a strong deactivation effect of set size. The effect of state was not significant when all participants were analyzed as a group. However, when a comparison was made between participants who responded to at least 95% of the trials on the visual short-term and visual array control tasks following sleep deprivation (non-lapsers; N = 14) with lapsers (N = 16), there was a significant interaction of state, set size, and group. This interaction reflects the finding that there was less deactivation following SD for those who lapsed more when sleep deprived, and that this effect was present mainly at higher visual loads. (Reproduced from [62].)

Differentiation of the effects of sleep deprivation across different behavioral measures

As important as the maintenance of vigilance/sustained attention is, in a recent study the number of lapses in a psychomotor vigilance test (PVT) was nonetheless uncorrelated with shifts in risky decision-making [33, 66] or in preferences between monetary and social rewards [67]. These observations are consistent with earlier findings that SD does not affect behavior uniformly across tasks [7–9] and suggests that future imaging work studying inter-individual differences should incorporate several behavioral assays that test dissociable cognitive domains.

We speculate that the heterogeneity of performance differences following SD in different tasks relates to the extent that a task repetitively engages particular neural circuits resulting in use-dependent effects [5, 68]. Tasks that tax sustained attention are typically stereotypical, require speeded responses, and do not allow much latitude in terms of strategy. In short they can be thought of re-engaging the sensory as well as frontoparietal circuits mediating top-down control of attention in a limited but repetitive manner. According to use dependent models of sleep homeostasis, this will increase the likelihood of local sleep occurring in these circuits [69]. In vivo recordings of "local sleep" in behaving animals have shown this phenomenon in both visual [70] and frontoparietal regions that can mediate top-down control of attention [71]. Hence, both sensory encoding and cognitive control regions may contribute to performance degradation for simple, repetitive tasks [72, 73], although most functional imaging evidence tends to support the latter as the dominant mechanism [26].

In contrast, more complex decision making tasks, where different strategies (see Chapter 18) may be engaged, allow some latitude regarding which neural circuits are engaged and, as such, are potentially less at risk of use-dependent effects. This may explain the mixed findings on the effects of SD in these domains.

Conclusion

Functional MRI provides a reproducible, non-invasive, and flexible means to study inter-individual variation in performance impairment in the setting of SD. Task-related fMRI has found that shifts in frontoparietal and sensory cortex activation across states are reliable correlates of behavioral change. Indeed, the observation of reduced activation of brain regions mediating attention underscores why attention has been so frequently studied in prior behavioral studies. Such alterations in task-related activation may relate to use-dependent local sleep induced by recurrent activation of particular neural circuits. However, why alterations of thalamic and default mode area activity are more variable in SD and how this relates to individual differences remains to be further investigated. Similarly, whether intrinsic connectivity might prove useful in differentiating more and less SD vulnerable persons remains an exciting realm to explore.

Acknowledgements

This work was supported by grants awarded to MC from the Defence Science and Technology Agency Singapore (POD0713897) and the National Research Foundation Singapore (STaR Award), and in part by a contract awarded to HVD from the US Office of Naval Research (N00014–11-C-0592) through Pulsar Informatics Inc.

References

1. Doran SM, Van Dongen HPA, Dinges DF. Sustained attention performance during sleep deprivation: evidence of state instability. *Arch Ital Biol.* 2001;**139**(3):253–67.

2. Van Dongen HPA, Maislin G, Mullington JM, Dinges DF. The cumulative cost of additional wakefulness: dose-response effects on neurobehavioral functions and sleep physiology from chronic sleep restriction and total sleep deprivation. *Sleep.* 2003;**26**(2):117–26.

3. Graw P, Kräuchi K, Knoblauch V, Wirz-Justice A, Cajochen C. Circadian and wake-dependent modulation of fastest and slowest reaction times during the psychomotor vigilance task. *Physiol Behav.* 2004;**80**(5):695–701.

4. Dijk DJ, Duffy JF, Czeisler CA. Circadian and sleep/wake dependent aspects of subjective alertness and cognitive performance. *J Sleep Res.* 1992;**1**(2):112–17.

5. Van Dongen HPA, Belenky G, Krueger JM. Investigating the temporal dynamics and underlying mechanisms of cognitive fatigue. In: Ackerman PL, ed. *Cognitive Fatigue: Multidisciplinary Perspectives on Current Research and Future Applications.* Washington, DC, American Psychological Association. 2011; 127–47.

6. Wesensten NJ, Killgore WD, Balkin TJ. Performance and alertness effects of caffeine, dextroamphetamine, and modafinil during sleep deprivation. *J Sleep Res.* 2005;**14**(3):255–66.

7. Frey DJ, Badia P, Wright KP, Jr. Inter- and intra-individual variability in performance near the circadian nadir during sleep deprivation. *J Sleep Res.* 2004;**13**(4):305–15.

8. Leproult R, Colecchia EF, Berardi AM, *et al.* Individual differences in subjective and objective alertness during sleep deprivation are stable and unrelated. *Am J Physiol.* 2003;**284**(2):R280–90.

9. Van Dongen HPA, Baynard MD, Maislin G, Dinges DF. Systematic interindividual differences in neurobehavioral impairment from sleep loss: evidence of trait-like differential vulnerability. *Sleep.* 2004;**27**(3):423–33.

10. Caldwell JA, Prazinko B, Caldwell JL. Body posture affects electroencephalographic activity and psychomotor vigilance task performance in sleep-deprived subjects. *Clin Neurophysiol.* 2003;**114**(1):23–31.

11. Lubin A, Hord DJ, Tracy ML, Johnson LC. Effects of exercise, bedrest and napping on performance decrement during 40 hours. *Psychophysiology.* 1976;**13**(4):334–9.

12. Vandewalle G, Maquet P, Dijk DJ. Light as a modulator of cognitive brain function. *Trends Cogn Sci.* 2009;**13**(10):429–38.

13. Schmidt C, Collette F, Leclercq Y, *et al.* Homeostatic sleep pressure and responses to sustained attention in the suprachiasmatic area. *Science.* 2009;**324**(5926):516–19.

14. Kerkhof GA, Van Dongen HPA. Morning-type and evening-type individuals differ in the phase position of their endogenous circadian oscillator. *Neurosci Lett.* 1996;**218**(3):153–6.

15. Van Dongen HPA, Dinges DF. Sleep, circadian rhythms, and psychomotor vigilance. *Clin Sports Med.* 2005;**24**(2):237–49.

16. Van Dongen HPA, Caldwell JA, Jr., Caldwell JL. Individual differences in cognitive vulnerability to fatigue in the laboratory and in the workplace. *Prog Brain Res.* 2011;**190**:145–53.

17. Lim J, Dinges DF. A meta-analysis of the impact of short-term sleep deprivation on cognitive variables. *Psychol Bull.* 2010;**136**(3):375–89.

18. Whitney P, Hinson JM. Measurement of cognition in studies of sleep deprivation. *Prog Brain Res.* 2010;**185**:37–48.

19. Portas CM, Rees G, Howseman AM, *et al.* A specific role for the thalamus in mediating the interaction of attention and arousal in humans. *J Neurosci.* 1998;**18**(21):8979–89.

20. Tomasi D, Wang RL, Telang F, *et al.* Impairment of attentional networks after 1 night of sleep deprivation. *Cereb Cortex.* 2009;**19**(1):233–40.

21. Chee MWL, Tan JC. Lapsing when sleep deprived: neural activation characteristics of resistant and vulnerable individuals. *Neuroimage.* 2010;**51**(2):835–43.

22. Chee MWL, Tan JC, Zheng H, *et al.* Lapsing during sleep deprivation is associated with distributed changes in brain activation. *J Neurosci.* 2008;**28**(21):5519–28.

23. Chuah LY, Chee MWL. Cholinergic augmentation modulates visual task performance in sleep-deprived young adults. *J Neurosci.* 2008;**28**(44):11369–77.

24. Chuah LY, Chong DL, Chen AK, *et al.* Donepezil improves episodic memory in young individuals vulnerable to the effects of sleep deprivation. *Sleep.* 2009;**32**(8):999–1010.

25. Van Dongen HPA, Belenky G, Krueger JM. A local, bottom-up perspective on sleep deprivation and neurobehavioral performance. *Curr Top Med Chem.* 2011;**11**(19):2414–22.

26. Chee MWL, Goh CS, Namburi P, *et al.* Effects of sleep deprivation on cortical activation during directed attention in the absence and presence of visual stimuli. *Neuroimage.* 2011;**58**(2):595–604.

27. Makeig S, Jung TP. Tonic, phasic, and transient EEG correlates of auditory awareness in drowsiness. *Brain Res.* 1996;**4**(1):15–25.

28. Makeig S, Jung TP, Sejnowski TJ. Awareness during drowsiness: dynamics and electrophysiological correlates. *Can J Exp Psychol.* 2000;**54**(4):266–73.

29. Harrison Y, Horne JA, Rothwell A. Prefrontal neuropsychological effects of sleep deprivation in young adults–a model for healthy aging? *Sleep.* 2000;**23**(8):1067–73.

30. Park DC, Polk TA, Mikels JA, Taylor SF, Marshuetz C. Cerebral aging: integration of brain and behavioral models of cognitive function. *Dialogues Clin Neurosci.* 2001;**3**(3):151–65.

31. Tucker AM, Stern Y, Basner RC, Rakitin BC. The prefrontal model revisited: double dissociations between young sleep deprived and elderly subjects on cognitive components of performance. *Sleep.* 2011;**34**(8):1039–50.

32. Kong D, Soon CS, Chee MWL. Functional imaging correlates of impaired distractor suppression following sleep deprivation. *Neuroimage.* 2012;**61**(1):50–5.

33. Venkatraman V, Chuah YM, Huettel SA, Chee MWL. Sleep deprivation elevates expectation of gains and

attenuates response to losses following risky decisions. *Sleep.* 2007;**30**(5):603–9.

34. Caldwell JA, Mu Q, Smith JK, *et al.* Are individual differences in fatigue vulnerability related to baseline differences in cortical activation? *Behav Neurosci.* 2005;**119**(3):694–707.

35. Chee MWL, Chuah YML, Venkatraman V, *et al.* Functional imaging of working memory following normal sleep and after 24 and 35 hours of sleep deprivation: correlations of fronto-parietal activation with performance. *Neuroimage.* 2006;**31**(1):419–28.

36. Mu Q, Mishory A, Johnson KA, *et al.* Decreased brain activation during a working memory task at rested baseline is associated with vulnerability to sleep deprivation. *Sleep.* 2005;**28**(4):433–46.

37. Chuah YM, Venkatraman V, Dinges DF, Chee MWL. The neural basis of interindividual variability in inhibitory efficiency after sleep deprivation. *J Neurosci.* 2006;**26**(27):7156–62.

38. Cohen MS, DuBois RM. Stability, repeatability, and the expression of signal magnitude in functional magnetic resonance imaging. *J Magn Reson Imaging.* 1999;**10**(1):33–40.

39. McGonigle DJ, Howseman AM, Athwal BS, *et al.* Variability in fMRI: an examination of intersession differences. *Neuroimage.* 2000;**11**(6 Pt 1):708–34.

40. Yetkin FZ, McAuliffe TL, Cox R, Haughton VM. Test-retest precision of functional MR in sensory and motor task activation. *AJNR Am J Neuroradiol.* 1996;**17**(1):95–8.

41. Rutten GJ, Ramsey NF, van Rijen PC, van Veelen CW. Reproducibility of fMRI-determined language lateralization in individual subjects. *Brain Lang.* 2002;**80**(3):421–37.

42. Aron AR, Gluck MA, Poldrack RA. Long-term test-retest reliability of functional MRI in a classification learning task. *Neuroimage.* 2006;**29**(3):1000–6.

43. Lim J, Choo W-C, Chee MWL. Reproducibility of changes in behaviour and fMRI activation associated with sleep deprivation in a working memory task. *Sleep.* 2007;**30**(1):61–70.

44. Mu Q, Nahas Z, Johnson KA, *et al.* Decreased cortical response to verbal working memory following sleep deprivation. *Sleep.* 2005;**28**(1):55–67.

45. Harrison Y, Horne JA. The impact of sleep deprivation on decision making: a review. *J Exp Psychol Appl.* 2000;**6**(3):236–49.

46. Stern Y. What is cognitive reserve? Theory and research application of the reserve concept. *J Int Neuropsychol Soc.* 2002;**8**(3):448–60.

47. Osaka N, Osaka M, Kondo H, *et al.* The neural basis of executive function in working memory: an fMRI study based on individual differences. *Neuroimage.* 2004;**21**(2):623–31.

48. Gray JR, Chabris CF, Braver TS. Neural mechanisms of general fluid intelligence. *Nat Neurosci.* 2003;**6**(3):316–22.

49. Pessoa L, Gutierrez E, Bandettini P, Ungerleider L. Neural correlates of visual working memory: fMRI amplitude predicts task performance. *Neuron.* 2002;**35**(5):975–87.

50. Smith EE, Geva A, Jonides J, *et al.* The neural basis of task-switching in working memory: effects of performance and aging. *Proc Natl Acad Sci U S A.* 2001;**98**(4):2095–100.

51. Cabeza R, Anderson ND, Locantore JK, McIntosh AR. Aging gracefully: compensatory brain activity in high-performing older adults. *Neuroimage.* 2002;**17**(3):1394–402.

52. Callicott JH, Mattay VS, Verchinski BA, *et al.* Complexity of prefrontal cortical dysfunction in schizophrenia: more than up or down. *Am J Psychiatry.* 2003;**160**(12):2209–15.

53. Egan MF, Goldberg TE, Kolachana BS, *et al.* Effect of COMT Val108/158 Met genotype on frontal lobe function and risk for schizophrenia. *Proc Natl Acad Sci U S A.* 2001;**98**(12):6917–22.

54. Habeck C, Rakitin BC, Moeller J, *et al.* An event-related fMRI study of the neurobehavioral impact of sleep deprivation on performance of a delayed-match-to-sample task. *Brain Res.* 2004;**18**(3):306–21.

55. Bell-McGinty S, Habeck C, Hilton HJ, *et al.* Identification and differential vulnerability of a neural network in sleep deprivation. *Cereb Cortex.* 2004;**14**(5):496–502.

56. Steriade M, McCarley RW. Changing concepts of mechanisms of waking and sleep states. In: *Brain Control of Wakefulness and Sleep.* New York, Kluwer Academic. 2005; 1–33.

57. LaBerge D. *Attentional Processing: The Brain's Art of Mindfulness.* Cambridge, MA, Harvard University Press, 1995.

58. McKiernan KA, Kaufman JN, Kucera-Thompson J, Binder JR. A parametric manipulation of factors affecting task-induced deactivation in functional neuroimaging. *J Cogn Neurosci.* 2003;**15**(3):394–408.

59. Raichle ME, MacLeod AM, Snyder AZ, *et al.* A default mode of brain function. *Proc Natl Acad Sci U S A.* 2001;**98**(2):676–82.

60. Chee MWL, Choo WC. Functional imaging of working memory after 24 hr of total sleep deprivation. *J Neurosci.* 2004;**24**(19):4560–7.

61. Gujar N, Yoo SS, Hu P, Walker MP. The unrested resting brain: sleep deprivation alters activity within the default-mode network. *J Cogn Neurosci.* 2010;**22**(8):1637–48.

62. Chee MWL, Chuah YM. Functional neuroimaging and behavioral correlates of capacity decline in visual short-term memory following sleep deprivation. *Proc Natl Acad Sci U S A.* 2007;**104**(22):9487–892.

63. Drummond SPA, Bischoff-Grethe A, Dinges DF, *et al.* The neural basis of the psychomotor vigilance task. *Sleep.* 2005;**28**(9):1059–68.

64. Chee MWL, Tan JC, Zheng H, *et al.* Lapsing during sleep deprivation is associated with distributed changes in brain activation. *J Neurosci.* 2008;**28**(21):5519–28.

65. De Havas JA, Parimal S, Soon CS, Chee MWL. Sleep deprivation reduces default mode network connectivity and anti-correlation during rest and task performance. *Neuroimage.* 2012;**59**(2):1745–51.

66. Venkatraman V, Huettel SA, Chuah LY, Payne JW, Chee MWL. Sleep deprivation biases the neural mechanisms underlying economic preferences. *J Neurosci.* 2011;**31**(10):3712–18.

67. Libedinsky C, Smith DV, Teng CS, *et al.* Sleep deprivation alters valuation signals in the ventromedial prefrontal cortex. *Front Behav Neurosci.* 2011;**5**:70.

68. Krueger JM, Tononi G. Local use-dependent sleep; synthesis of the new paradigm. *Curr Top Med Chem.* 2011;**11**(19):2490–2.

69. Rector DM, Topchiy IA, Carter KM, Rojas MJ. Local functional state differences between rat cortical columns. *Brain Res.* 2005;**1047**(1):45–55.

70. Pigarev IN, Nothdurft HC, Kastner S. Evidence for asynchronous development of sleep in cortical areas. *Neuroreport.* 1997;**8**(11):2557–60.

71. Vyazovskiy VV, Olcese U, Hanlon EC, et al. Local sleep in awake rats. *Nature.* 2011;**472**:443–7.

72. Rakitin BC, Tucker AM, Basner RC, Stern Y. The effects of stimulus degradation after 48 hours of total sleep deprivation. *Sleep.* 2012;**35**(1):113–21.

73. Ratcliff R, Van Dongen HPA. Diffusion model for one-choice reaction-time tasks and the cognitive effects of sleep deprivation. *Proc Natl Acad Sci U S A.* 2011;**108**(27):11285–90.

Neuroimaging the interaction between circadian and homeostatic processes

Gilles Vandewalle and Christina Schmidt

Introduction

In human beings, wakefulness and its associated cognitive processes are typically maintained for 16 continuous hours before sleep is initiated for about 8 hours. The fine tuning and timing of this sleep/wake cycle and the maintenance of cognitive abilities for such prolonged periods are achieved through interactions between circadian and homeostatic processes [1]. Sleep homeostasis is characterized by an increase or dissipation of sleep pressure as wakefulness extends or sleep progresses, respectively. The mechanisms involved in this hourglass-like process are still debated but animal research suggests that it arises from use-dependent sleep-promoting substances (adenosine [2] and cytokine [3]) during wakefulness and their dissipation during sleep. Accordingly, sleep homeostasis has been related to experience-dependent increases of brain synaptic strength [4]. Encephalographic (EEG) spectral power in the sleep slow wave activity range (SWA; 0.5–4 Hz) and in the waking theta band (4–8 Hz) have been shown to depend predominantly on prior history of sleep and wakefulness and are classically used as markers for sleep homeostasis [1]. Importantly, sleep-homeostatic-related changes at the physiological level are accompanied with prominent modulations in cognitive functions, such that cognitive performance deteriorates with increasing sleep pressure [5].

Combined evidence indicates, however, that, over a 24-h period, cognitive performance does not linearly decrease with increasing amounts of time spent awake, as would be expected by a pure influence of sleep homeostasic processes. Neurobehavioral performance is also regulated by a second, circadian, process, generating an endogenous nearly 24 h sleep/wake oscillation [1]. The circadian process originates in the suprachiasmatic nuclei (SCN) of the anterior hypothalamus, which is considered as the circadian master clock in most living organisms.

The time window of maximal circadian wake promotion has been defined as the *wake maintenance zone* [6], occurring just before the evening rise of endogenous melatonin secretion (typically around 2100 h in a standard 2300 h–0700 h sleep schedule) [7]. While the endogenous scheduling of the wake maintenance zone to the end of the habitual waking day seems paradoxical at first glance, it makes sense when considering it in combination with the temporal evolution of the homeostatic process throughout the habitual 24-h sleep/wake cycle. For instance, it is the very high circadian-based propensity for wakefulness that prevents us falling asleep early in the evening hours when homeostatic sleep pressure is high and strongly encourages sleep. Likewise, the circadian clock also promotes sleep (i.e., circadian increase in sleep tendency) as the biological night progresses, thus counteracting the decrease in sleep propensity associated with accumulated sleep and allowing the maintenance of a consolidated 8-h sleep episode. Although still putative, a sense of this circadian sleep-promoting signal can be found in the circadian regulation of rapid eye movement (REM) sleep and sleep spindles, which are most prominent at the end of the night [7].

Ultimately, when applied to cognitive functions, performance deteriorations associated with increasing sleep pressure are countered by the circadian wake-promoting signal during a normal waking day, allowing the achievement of appropriate cognitive control. However, if wakefulness is extended into the biological night, the circadian signal promotes sleep and thus no longer opposes increasing homeostatic sleep pressure, such that under conditions of extended wakefulness, cognitive performance is jeopardized, most strongly at the end of the night [1].

Although it is becoming evident that the interaction between the circadian signal and sleep homeostasis governs our ability to maintain efficient cognitive functions [1], the brain mechanisms involved remain poorly understood. First evidence comes from a positron emission tomography (PET) study, investigating changes in brain glucose metabolism between morning and evening acquisitions [8]. Compared to the morning, evening quiet wakefulness was associated with increased metabolism in hypothalamic and brainstem structures, putatively encompassing several sleep/wake or arousal-promoting nuclei. Decreased metabolism was also found at the cortical level in the temporal and occipital lobes. While these results clearly suggest that brain state changes during a normal day to maintain wakefulness, the study design did not allow disentangling what changes were associated with circadian and sleep homeostatic processes or their interaction. In addition, time resolution of PET acquisitions considerably limited the cognitive interpretation of such findings.

In this chapter, we will focus on two recent studies capitalizing on inter-individual differences in response to increased sleep homeostasis and misalignment between the circadian signal and sleep to better characterize the brain mechanisms involved in the maintenance of wakefulness and associated cognitive processes. Indeed, even though the interplay between circadian and homeostatic sleep/wake regulatory processes aspires to stability within a given state throughout the 24-h cycle, there exist fine grained fluctuations over the waking state which may be exaggerated by inter-individual differences in the orchestration of the underlying processes [9].

Time-of-day-dependent modulations in cognitive brain responses of extreme chronotypes

Extreme chronotypes are characterized by marked differences in their preferred timing for sleep and wakefulness, as well as optimal times of day to perform cognitively demanding tasks. This is confirmed by objective measures of performance, which undergo a relative decline in morning types and a relative increase in evening types throughout a normal waking day [10]. Morning and evening types differ in circadian phase and, for some of them, by a difference in the phase angle between the circadian signal and the sleep episode (e.g., wake time is closer to the maximal circadian sleep promotion in evening types) [11]. Importantly, chronotypes can also differ with respect to sleep homeostasis. Compared to evening types, morning types present higher power in the SWA range of the sleep EEG during the first non-rapid eye movement (NREM) sleep cycle, even if studied according to their preferred sleep-wake schedule of each subject. Throughout the night, both types then return to similar SWA levels [12, 13]. This indicates a faster build up of sleep need during a normal waking day in extreme morning types with a steeper decline during the night.

Taking advantage of these characteristic differences, a first study explored cerebral responses in prospectively recruited extreme morning and evening chronotypes at different time points within the day, while performing a psychomotor vigilance task (PVT) in a functional magnetic resonance imaging (fMRI) environment. The PVT has been repeatedly used to delineate circadian and homeostatic influences on cognitive performance [14]. It probes the ability to sustain attention over prolonged periods of time [15], a fundamental form of attention onto which many other cognitive processes build [16]. Neural correlates of two behavioral variables were considered: global alertness, as measured by average reaction times to the task (higher than the 10th percentile and lower than the 90th percentile, i.e., without bias from abnormally fast or slow reaction times and lapses), and optimal alertness, which can be phasically recruited above the normal level and is measured by comparing overall fastest reaction times to the task (lower than the 10th percentile) to average reaction times [17]. Brain responses were acquired 1.5 h and 10.5 h after wake-up time, i.e., in the subjective morning and early evening.

Only small differences between chronotypes were observed in the morning session, when homeostatic sleep pressure is low.

Conversely, during the evening hours, when the circadian system promotes wakefulness in order to counteract increasing homeostatic sleep pressure, global alertness was associated with increased thalamic responses in morning as compared to evening types. The observed response was located in a dorsal-median part compatible with the anterior part of the pulvinar, the activation of which has been shown to be increased following total sleep deprivation [18], as well as by using light exposure as an external activating factor [19]. In this perspective, pulvinar responses have been suggested to mediate the impact of arousal change on cognition (see also Chapter 21, p. 175). These results indicate that morning types maintain brain function and compensate for higher sleep pressure conditions through thalamic recruitment, while evening types do not need such compensating mechanisms at that time of day.

When looking at optimal alertness, extreme evening types were characterized by higher task-related responses in an anterior region of the hypothalamus encompassing notably the SCN, and in a posterior part of the brainstem confirmed to be compatible with the locus coeruleus by a follow-up investigation within an independent group using high-resolution T1-turbo spin echo images (T1-TSE) sensitive to neuromelanin-related contrasts [20] (Figure 20.1). The locus coeruleus constitutes the major source of norepinephrine of the brain and has widespread thalamic and cortical connections so that it can potentially modulate higher-order cognitive functions. The SCN and locus coeruleus are functionally connected and have been proposed as main actors for the generation of circadian wake promotion [21]. Thus, the known improved cognitive ability of evening chronotypes towards the end of a normal waking day may result from their capacity to recruit these interacting subcortical structures above normal levels.

Globally, the results suggest that evening types, which present less amounts of accumulated homeostatic sleep pressure at the end of a normal waking day, are more able to recruit arousal-promoting brain structures to maintain optimal alertness even with increasing homeostatic sleep pressure. A feedback mechanism of sleep homeostasis onto hypothalamic structures such as the SCN has been formerly proposed in rodents [22]. Reminiscent to this finding, evening optimal alertness-related activity in the anterior hypothalamus was higher for lower amounts of slow wave activity during the first NREM sleep cycle of the preceding night (significant inverse correlation). In that perspective, it may be assumed that performance of morning types would deteriorate in the evening through a negative impact of sleep pressure on the master circadian clock that is not compensated by the increase in average-alertness-related thalamic activation. Conversely, it may be through a decreased ability of anterior hypothalamic activity to counteract sleep pressure that morning types undergo greater performance decrement.

The next question which arises is to know whether those sleep/wake regulatory processes similarly or differentially account for differences in more demanding cognitive processing and their neuronal correlates. In this perspective, cognitive interference is crucial for maintaining a coherent stream of thought and thus represents a cognitive aspect required for

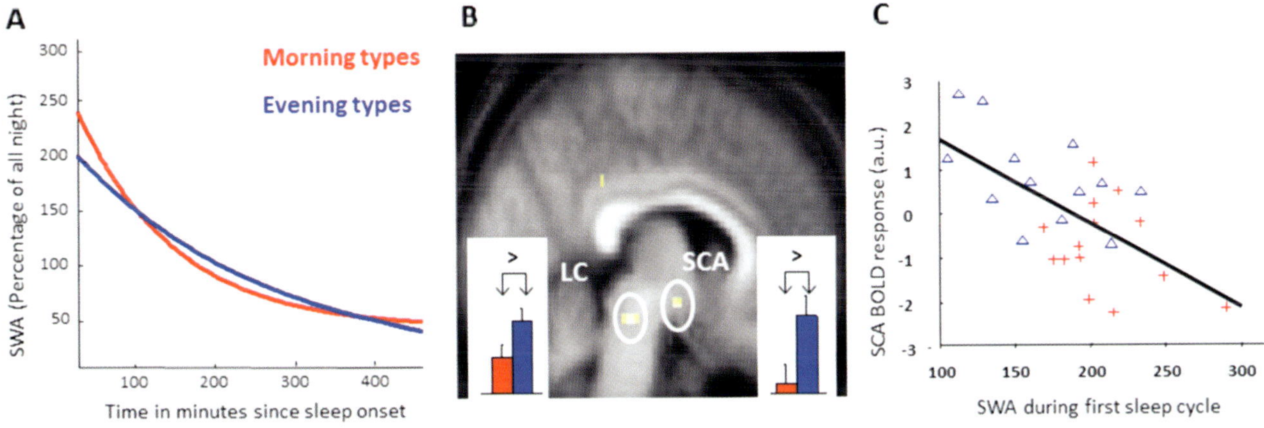

Figure 20.1 Morning and evening chronotypes differ in their brain responses to an attentional task and SWA. (A) Exponential decay function ($SWAt = SWA\infty + SWA0 \cdot e^{-rt}$) adjusted on relative SWA in sleep cycles (NREM sleep) measured from the central frontal derivation for all-night EEG of the night preceding the evening scan acquisition. (B) Increased task-related response in the dorsal pontine tegmentum and the anterior hypothalamus, compatible with the locus coeruleus (LC) and suprachiasmatic area (SCA) respectively, in evening as compared to morning chronotypes during the subjective evening for optimal sustained attention during the performance of a Psychomotor Vigilance Task. Corresponding activity estimates (arbitrary units) are displayed for event indicators of fast (< Percentile 10) reaction times. (C) Regression analysis of the relation between estimated blood oxygen level-dependent (BOLD) responses during optimal task performance in the SCA region and the amount of SWA during the first sleep cycle in the preceding night (r = 0.54, p < 0.05, n = 27). Red crosses: morning types, blue triangles: evening types. (Copied with permission from [9] and [13].)

behaving suitably in many daily life functions [23, 24]. In the context of the same study design, the neural bases of performance maintenance in chronotypes was also assessed with the Stroop paradigm [25], which challenges continuous control over conflicting information. Within this framework, we observed that chronotypes differ in daily fluctuations of interference-related cortical responses [26]. More precisely, results showed that interference-related hemodynamic responses are maintained or even increased in evening types from the subjective morning to the subjective evening in a set of brain areas playing a pivotal role in successful cognitive inhibition, whereas they decreased in morning types under the same conditions.

Importantly, during the evening hours again, activity in a posterior hypothalamic region, putatively involved in sleep wake regulation, correlated in a chronotype-specific manner with SWA at the beginning of the night, speaking again in favor of a differential expression of subcortical-driven wake-promoting signals throughout a normal waking day. Note that the cluster of activation was located more posterior than the anterior hypothalamic area detected in our previous report based on optimal performance measure on PVT [13]. Interestingly, the present area was close to the region reported to show a decrease in gray matter concentration in narcoleptic patients, relative to controls, and identified by the authors of this study as the posterior-lateral hypothalamus [27].

Time-of-day and sleep loss-associated changes in cognitive brain responses in two *PERIOD3* genotypes

The second study detailed in this chapter used a genetic trait as a means to characterize the regulation of cognitive performance throughout a normal waking day and following total sleep deprivation [28]. A variable-number-of-tandem-repeat (VNTR)

polymorphism in the coding region of the clock gene *PERIOD3* (*PER3*) was reported to present a weak association with chronotype [29]. Individuals homozygous for the long version of the gene, $PER3^{5/5}$, were more likely to be morning types, while $PER3^{4/4}$ individuals were more likely to be evening types, suggestive of an involvement of the gene in circadian and/or sleep homeostasis regulation. In fact this polymorphism has now been shown to predict homeostatic sleep regulation and individual vulnerability to sleep loss [1]. $PER3^{5/5}$ individuals present a higher level of theta power activity as early as after 8 h of wakefulness and throughout the remaining of a 40 h constant routine sleep deprivation protocol, and present higher delta power activity during the first NREM cycle of both baseline normal and recovery sleep [30–32].

With respect to cognitive performance, $PER3^{5/5}$ individuals undergo greater difficulties when confronted with extended neuropsychological testing throughout prolonged wakefulness, with very limited changes in the evening, after a normal waking day, but dramatic deteriorations in the morning during sleep loss [30]. This appears to be particularly the case for tasks involving executive functions [33]. In fact, a recent model suggests that differences between cognitive performance profiles of $PER3^{4/4}$ and $PER3^{5/5}$ (and by extension possibly between extreme evening and morning chronotypes) can be explained by a non-linear interaction between circadian and homeostatic signals [1] (Figure 20.2). In the evening, this results in only slight performance decrement, but the non-linearity of this interaction can be particularly sensed in the morning hours, when the circadian sleep-promoting signal amplifies the difference in homeostatic sleep pressure such that performance deteriorates disproportionally in $PER3^{5/5}$ individuals.

To characterize the cerebral correlates underlying these circadian and homeostatic interaction patterns in cognitive performance, $PER3^{4/4}$ and $PER3^{5/5}$ individuals were prospectively recruited to participate in four fMRI recordings separated

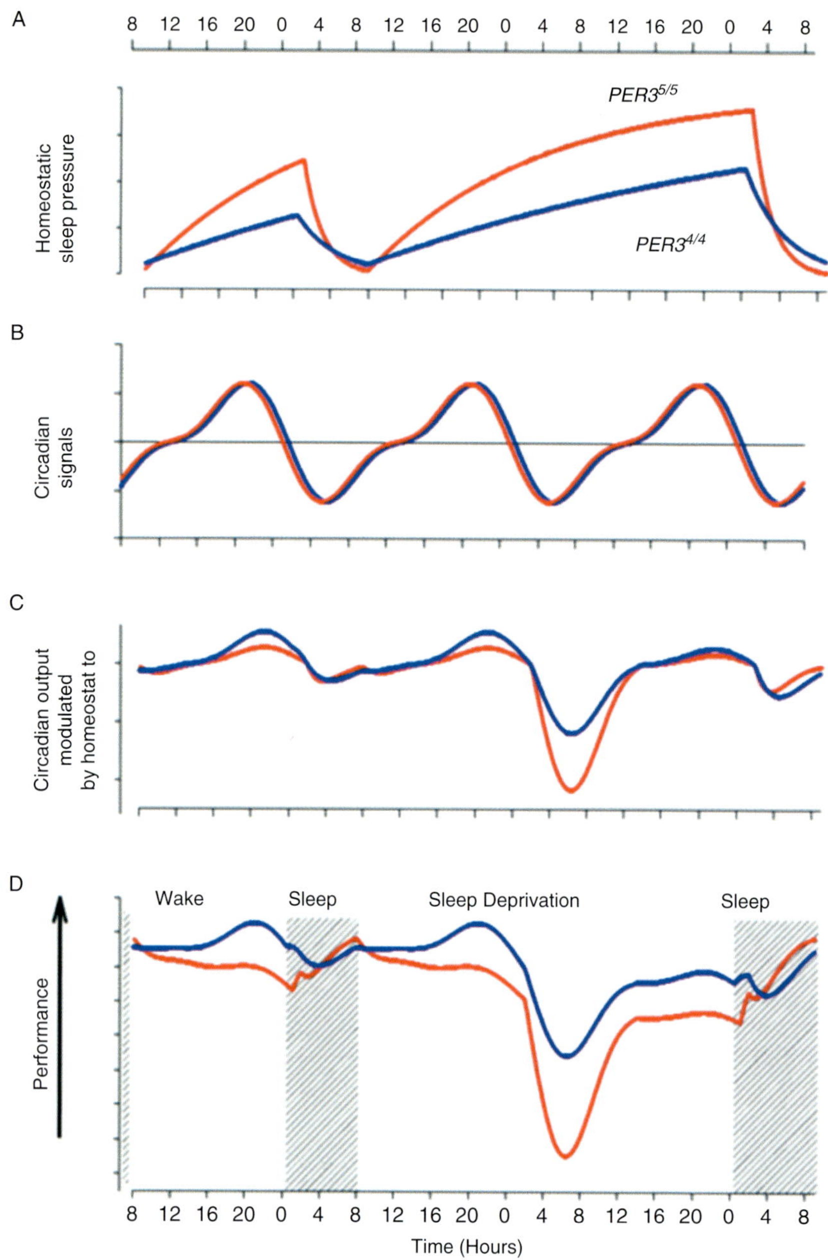

Figure 20.2 Impact of the interaction between circadian and homeostatic sleep regulations on performance in populations homozygous for one of the two forms of the *PERIOD3* VNTR polymorphism. (A) As compared with *PER3*[4/4] (blue), *PER3*[5/5] (red) individuals present a faster build up and a quicker dissipation of homeostatic sleep pressure during wakefulness and sleep, respectively, as indicated by slow wave activity measure (based on data from [30] and reproduced from [32]). (B) *PER3*[4/4] and *PER3*[5/5] do not appear to differ in term of circadian phase as indicated by melatonin, cortisol, and *PER3* mRNA measures (based on data from [30] and reproduced from [28]). Note that the circadian signal increasingly promotes wakefulness during the day (positive values, above horizontal line) and increasingly promotes sleep during the night (negative value, bellow horizontal line). (C) Theoretical modulation of the circadian signal by homeostatic sleep pressure in both *PER3* genotypes. The difference in sleep homeostatic sleep pressure results in a limited difference in the output of this interaction during a normal waking day. The output of the interaction affects much more negatively wakefulness of *PER3*[5/5] in the absence of overnight sleep, particularly in the early morning hours when the circadian system maximally promotes sleep. (D) Composite measures of performance in both *PER3* genotypes, based on extended neuropsychological test batteries [30]. Performance profile closely follow theoretical interaction between circadian and sleep homeostasis processes depicted in C. This model could speculatively be applied to extremes morning and evening chronotypes, which also differ in term of homeostatic sleep pressure built up [12] (but also they sometimes differ in term of circadian phase angle with sleep [11]). (Copied with permission from [1].)

in two experimental segments, which were identical except for the presence or absence of sleep during the night separating fMRI recordings. Brain responses to an auditory 3-back task were recorded in darkness (for data acquired with light administration see Chapter 21). This cognitive task probes executive functioning and requires continuous information updating and comparing in working memory in addition to basic attentional processes [24]. Recordings were carried out in the morning, shortly after the maximum of the circadian sleep-promoting signal, and in the evening, 2 h before sleep time, within the "wake-maintenance zone." Task duration was kept short so that brain activity could be recorded before the emergence of significant behavioral differences that would have biased fMRI results. Similarly to the chronotypes study, the focus of the study was brain function, not behavior.

Results show that from the morning to the evening of a normal waking day, *PER3*[4/4] individuals did not show any significant changes in brain responses to the task, while *PER3*[5/5] individuals presented a decreased activation in an area of the posterior dorsolateral prefrontal cortex (DLPFC). The limited performance change previously reported over the course of a normal waking day in both genotypes [30] thus seems to be mirrored by a small variation in the brain capacity to recruit brain regions for ongoing cognitive processes.

When then comparing both morning sessions, acquired at the same circadian phase, but after 1.5 h or 25 h of wakefulness, *PER3*[5/5] subjects presented widespread and numerous decreased activations during sleep loss in several areas of the temporal, occipital, and parietal cortices as well as bilaterally within the

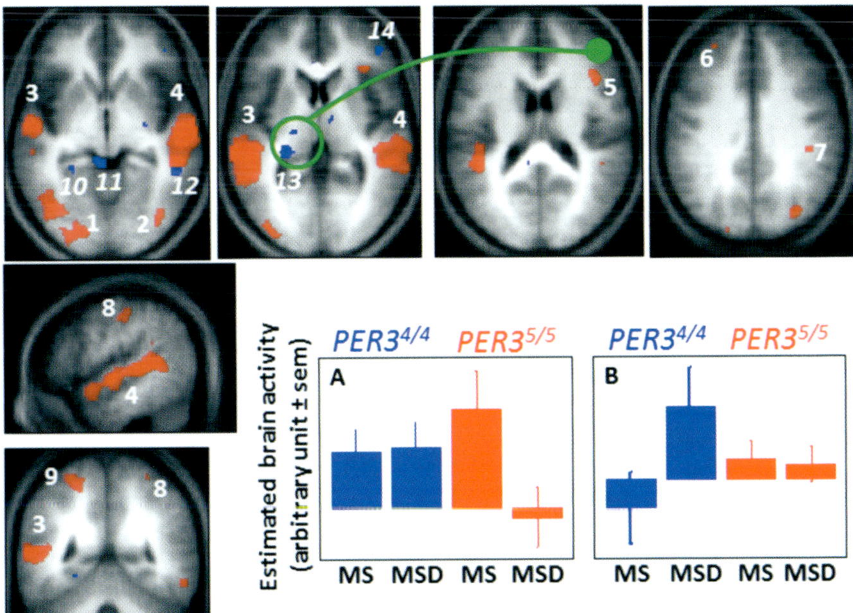

Figure 20.3 Difference between $PER3^{4/4}$ and $PER3^{5/5}$ individuals in the sleep loss-induced changed in brain responses to a working memory task. When comparing brain responses to an auditory 3-back task in the morning after a night of sleep (MS; 1.5 h of wakefulness) and in the morning after a night of sleep deprivation (MSD; 25h of wakefulness), $PER3^{5/5}$ individuals undergo marked decreases in activation in several brain areas of the occipital (1, 2) and temporal (3, 4) cortices, and of the dorsolateral prefrontal (5, 6) and parietal cortex (7–9), while $PER3^{4/4}$ individuals maintain brain responses in these areas (and do no present significant decreased activations in any brain regions). A representative profile of this brain activity change is displayed in panel A (similar profiles were observed for red areas 1–9). In contrast, when comparing the same sessions, $PER3^{4/4}$ individuals present increased activations (blue) in the parahippocampus (10), superior colliculus (11), temporal cortex (12), pulvinar (13), and ventrolateral prefrontal cortex (14), while no increased activation is observed in these regions in $PER3^{5/5}$ (and in any other brain regions). A representative profile of this brain activity change is displayed in panel B (similar profiles were observed for blue areas 10–14). A significant psychophysiologic interaction (PPI), indicative of modification in functional connectivity, was observed between the pulvinar and dorso-ventrolateral cortex (green) in the morning during sleep loss in $PER3^{4/4}$ but not in $PER3^{5/5}$ individuals (significant difference between genotypes; unpublished result). This suggests it is through tightened interaction between both brain areas that $PER3^{4/4}$ individuals are able to maintain better cognitive performance following sleep loss. A significant negative association was found between overnight change in brain response in the pulvinar (green circle) and self-reported daytime propensity to fall asleep in everyday life across all the subjects of the study (irrespective of genotype), further suggesting a central role for the pulvinar in wakefulness regulation. (Adapted with permission from [28].)

DLPFC, including the same DLPFC area deactivated during a normal waking day (Figure 20.3). In contrast, $PER3^{4/4}$ still did not present any decreased brain responses to the task, but rather recruited supplemental brain areas in the temporal cortex, superior colliculus, and, importantly, in the anterior ventro-lateral prefrontal cortex (VLPFC), and in the dorso-posterior thalamus in an area compatible with the pulvinar. In sharp contrast again, $PER3^{5/5}$ did not significantly recruit any additional brain areas to perform the task.

The observed task-related temporal and parietal activity decreases in the $PER3^{5/5}$ participants during the morning session after sleep loss is congruent with previously elaborated hypotheses of a reduction in attention and sensory processing following sleep deprivation [34]. Likewise, occipital activation reductions in the absence of visual inputs support a reduction of top-down parietal and prefrontal regulation on this sensory cortex. Finally, the supplemental areas recruited to perform the task in $PER3^{4/4}$ participants following sleep deprivation are probably part of a "compensatory" mechanism already evoked in some sleep deprivation studies of non-genotyped samples [35, 36]. These results strongly suggest that it is the ability or inability to trigger compensations and maintain brain responses under adverse circadian and sleep homeostasis circumstances that underlies vulnerability of cognitive brain functions to sleep loss.

In a next step, brain responses to the task in the morning following sleep deprivation were compared to the responses recorded the preceding evening, after 14 h of wakefulness. Under these conditions, differences in sleep pressure are intermediate but the change in the circadian signal is almost maximal. Analyses revealed increased compensatory activations in $PER3^{4/4}$ and decreased activations in $PER3^{5/5}$ in the same cortical and subcortical regions than those observed when comparing the two morning sessions. Importantly, these activation profiles were even more widespread, especially the decreased activation for the $PER3^{5/5}$ individuals. If sleep homeostasis was primarily responsible for differences observed between morning sessions acquired after sleep and sleep deprivation, differences should be reduced when comparing the morning session after sleep deprivation to the evening session after a normal waking day. This is not what the results showed, with little change over the course of a normal waking day and dramatic differences overnight. Likewise, if the circadian signal was solely responsible for changes in cognitive brain responses, then a difference should only be present when comparing morning to evening sessions, which was obviously not the case.

A putative scenario of the brain mechanisms regulating wakefulness in response to changes in the interaction between circadian and sleep homeostasis processes

According to a recent model of cognition the VLPFC plays a key role in higher cognitive control and is involved in complex neurobehavioral processes [37]. The recruitment of the VLPFC in $PER3^{4/4}$ participants may therefore reflect a switch to a more appropriate cognitive strategy to achieve the task under sleep loss conditions. In contrast, because of their higher vulnerability to increasing sleep pressure, $PER3^{5/5}$ individuals are not able to recruit this brain area after sleep deprivation and seem, moreover, unable to maintain activation in the DLPFC area also pivotal for successful cognitive control [37]. This suggests that the ability to recruit the LPFC represents a key factor for determining inter-individual differences in the neurobehavioral vulnerability to sleep loss.

But how is this prefrontal recruitment achieved? Simple psychophysiological interactions revealed that the functional connectivity between the pulvinar and the VLPFC was significantly enhanced following sleep deprivation in $PER3^{4/4}$ but not in $PER3^{5/5}$ individuals, indicating that information flow between these two areas was tightened when compensating for adverse circadian and sleep homeostasis conditions (green line, Figure 20.3; Vandewalle, Archer, Wuillaume, et al., unpublished result, 2009). In this perspective, the thalamus may constitute a subcortical site through which circadian and sleep homeostasis interaction affects cognition and alertness [21]. This assumption is strengthened by supplemental analysis indicating a significant negative association between overnight change in task-related pulvinar brain responses and daytime propensity to fall asleep in everyday life across all the subjects of the study (i.e., irrespective of genotype). Upstream effects within the brainstem (e.g., locus coeruleus) or hypothalamus could participate in this thalamic activity profile [13].

In addition, although not formally demonstrated, the investigation using the VNTR $PER3$ polymorphism could indicate that the magnitude of the changes in brain response to the task over a normal waking day is larger in $PER3^{5/5}$, particularly in higher associative prefrontal and parietal areas, important for the ongoing cognitive process (Figure 20.4). This suggests that $PER3^{5/5}$ may have greater circadian amplitude in brain activity (but a similar circadian phase).

Overall an "inverted U" shape profile which would differ between individuals more or less vulnerable to sleep loss could explain the results summarized in this chapter. In all individuals, accumulation of sleep pressure would initially be associated with activation of arousal-related thalamic regions, and higher-order prefrontal areas when higher cognitive processes are involved, followed by decreased activation in these regions once circadian and sleep homeostasis conditions become too adverse. $PER3^{5/5}$, and morning chronotypes, putatively characterized by greater circadian amplitude, would be fitter to perform during the day, particularly in the morning, but would "pay" this morning-oriented performance through a faster

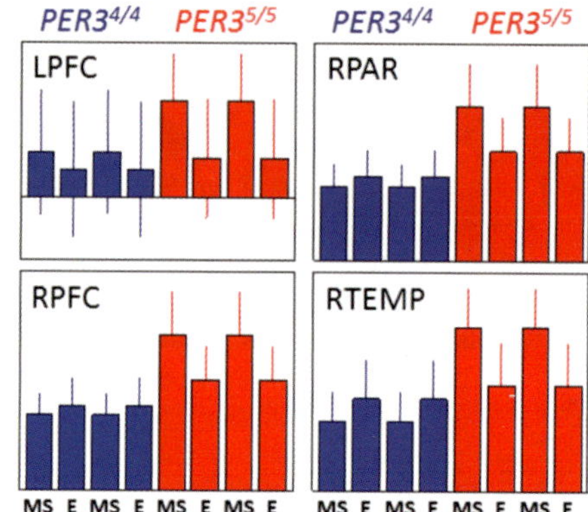

Figure 20.4 $PER3^{5/5}$ individuals may have greater circadian amplitude in their brain responses than $PER3^{4/4}$ individuals. Double plots of the brain responses to an auditory working 3-back task from a morning session after sleep (MS; 1.5 h of wakefulness) to an evening session after a normal waking day (E; 14 h of wakefulness). The data suggest that the amplitude in brain responses change could be greater in $PER3^{5/5}$ than in $PER3^{4/4}$ individuals notably in the left (LPFC) and right (RPFC) prefrontal cortex, and in the right parietal (RPAR) and temporal (RTEMP) cortices. The difference between morning and evening session is, however, only significant for LPFC in $PER3^{5/5}$ (significant difference between genotypes). (Based on data from [28].)

homeostatic sleep pressure buildup such that their cognitive resources would undergo faster decrement. To maintain wakefulness during normal waking, they would then recruit compensatory areas such as the pulvinar earlier than $PER3^{4/4}$ or extreme evening chronotypes. In the morning following a night without sleep, $PER3^{4/4}$, and putatively evening chronotypes, would still have available resources to recruit the pulvinar and LPFC and reduce performance deterioration in these adverse conditions. In contrast, $PER3^{5/5}$, and morning chronotypes, would be overridden by the adverse interaction output between high homeostatic sleep pressure and circadian sleep promotion.

Conclusions and perspectives

The scenario proposed in the preceding section remains speculative and should now be investigated in more detail to track homeostatic and circadian influences on cognitive brain functions. Constant routine and forced desynchrony protocols would allow a continuous investigation of their interaction at different times over the 24-h cycle [7, 38]. With this approach, one could specifically investigate the contributions made by the two processes during both the so-called sleep- and wake-maintenance zones. Thus, it would be important to study the interaction of these processes at multiple time points, implying different *states* in populations presenting homogeneous or heterogeneous *traits*. Sleep pressure could be directly manipulated through sleep deprivation, sleep restriction, or sleep satiation protocols. Alternatively, the administration of different compounds, such as caffeine or light exposure, impinging on circadian and homeostatic sleep/wake regulation, could have the potential to further elucidate cognition-related cerebral correlates underlying circadian and sleep homeostatic interaction patterns. Other genetic polymorphisms that have been reported to impact on sleep homeostasis (global modification in the amount of slow-wave sleep), including genes for adenosine deaminase [39] and DQB1*0602 [40], should be investigated in the same perspective. In addition, because the brain regions affected by changes along the sleep-homeostasis-and-circadian axis are most certainly task-specific, a wider spectrum of cognitive domains should be explored.

To sum up, the neuroanatomical basis and functional domains of circadian rhythmicity and sleep homeostasis are thought to be different. However, as mentioned above, both processes participate in the regulation of sleep and waking performance and should therefore interact at some levels in the central nervous system [41]. In fact, a molecular basis for the interaction of circadian and homeostatic processes in sleep-wake regulation has been proposed recently [42]. The two fMRI studies detailed here first bring evidence that this interaction also influences higher-order cognition-related cortical and subcortical brain functions. They further identified chronotypes and the *PER3* VNTR polymorphism as potential phenotypic and genetic markers of inter-individual differences in the vulnerability to adverse homeostatic sleep pressure and circadian misalignment [13, 28]. These markers are likely to be responsible for part of the variability previously observed in studies where the emphasis was on inter-individual differences in brain responses to sleep loss (see Chapter 19).

References

1. Dijk DJ, Archer SN. PERIOD3, circadian phenotypes, and sleep homeostasis. *Sleep Med Rev*. 2010;**14**:151–60.

2. Basheer R, Strecker RE, Thakkar MM, Mc Carley RW. Adenosine and sleep-wake regulation. *Prog Neurobiol*. 2004;**73**:379–96.

3. Krueger JM. The role of cytokines in sleep regulation. *Curr Pharm Des*. 2008;**14**:3408–16.

4. Tononi G, Cirelli C. Sleep function and synaptic homeostasis. *Sleep Med Rev*. 2006;**10**:49–62.

5. Banks S, Dinges DF. Behavioral and physiological consequences of sleep restriction. *J Clin Sleep Med*. 2007;**3**:519–28.

6. Strogatz SH, Kronauer RE, Czeisler CA. Circadian pacemaker interferes with sleep onset at specific times each day: role in insomnia. *Am J Physiol*. 1987;**253**:R172–8.

7. Dijk DJ, Czeisler CA, Contribution of the circadian pacemaker and the sleep homeostat to sleep propensity, sleep structure, electroencephalographic slow waves, and sleep spindle activity in humans. *J Neurosci*. 1995;**15**:3526–38.

8. Buysse DJ, Nofzinger EA, Germain A, *et al*. Regional brain glucose metabolism during morning and evening wakefulness in humans: preliminary findings. *Sleep*. 2004;**27**:1245–54.

9. Cajochen C, Chellappa S, Schmidt C. What keeps us awake? The role of clocks and hourglasses, light, and melatonin. *Int Rev Neurobiol*. 2010;**93**:57–90.

10. Schmidt C, Collette F, Cajochen C, Peignlux P. A time to think: circadian rhythms in human cognition. *Cogn Neuropsychol*. 2007;**24**:755–89.

11. Mongrain V, Cariner J, Dumont M. Circadian and homeostatic sleep regulation in morningness-eveningness. *J Sleep Res*. 2006;**15**:162–6.

12. Mongrain V, Dumont M. Increased homeostatic response to behavioral sleep fragmentation in morning types compared to evening types. *Sleep*. 2007;**30**:773–80.

13. Schmidt C, Collette F, Leclerq Y, *et al*. Homeostatic sleep pressure and responses to sustained attention in the suprachiasmatic area. *Science*. 2009;**324**:516–19.

14. Dorrian J, Rogers NL, Dinger DF. Psychomotor vigilance performance: A neurocognitive assay sensitive to sleep loss. In Kushida C, ed. *Sleep Deprivation: Clinical Issues, Pharmacology, and Sleep Loss Effects*. New York, Marcel Dekker. 2005;39–70.

15. Dinges DF, Powell JW. Microcomputer analyses of performance on a portable, simple visual RT task during sustained operations. *Behav Res Methods Instrum Comp*.1985;**17**:625–55.

16. Raz A, Buhle J. Typologies of attentional networks. *Nat Rev Neurosci*. 2006;**7**:367–79

17. Graw P, Kräuchi K, Knoblauch V, Wirz-Justice A, Cajochen C. Circadian and wake-dependent modulation of fastest and slowest reaction times during the psychomotor vigilance task. *Physiol Behav*. 2004;**80**:695–701

18. Portas CM, Rees G, Howseman AM, *et al*. A specific role for the thalamus in mediating the interaction of attention and arousal in humans. *J Neurosci*. 1998;**18**:8979–89.

19. Vandewalle G, Balteau E, Phillips C, *et al*. Daytime light exposure dynamically enhances brain responses. *Curr Biol*. 2006;**16**:1616–21.

20. Schmidt C, Peigneux P, Maquet P, Phillips C. Response to comment on "Homeostatic sleep pressure and responses to sustained attention in the suprachiasmatic area". *Science*. 2010;**328**:309.

21. Aston-Jones G, Cohen JD, An integrative theory of locus coeruleus-norepinephrine function: adaptive gain and optimal performance. *Annu Rev Neurosci*. 2005;**28**:403–50.

22. Deboer T, Détári L, Major JH. Long term effects of sleep deprivation on the mammalian circadian pacemaker. *Sleep*. 2007;**30**:257–62.

23. Collette F, Van der Linden M, Laureys S, *et al*. Exploring the unity and diversity of the neural substrates of executive functioning. *Hum Brain Mapp*. 2005;**25**:409–23.

24. Collette F, Hogge M, Salmon E, Van der Linden M. Exploration of the neural substrates of executive functioning by functional neuroimaging. *Neuroscience*. 2006;**139**:209–21.

25. Stroop JR. Studies of interference in serial verbal reactions. *J Exp Psychol*. 1935;**18**:643–62.

26. Schmidt C, Peigneux P, Leclerq Y, *et al*. Circadian preference modulates the neural substrate of conflict processing across the day. *PLoS One*. 2012;**7**:e29658.

27. Draganski B, Geisler P, Hajak G, *et al*. Hypothalamic gray matter changes in narcoleptic patients. *Nat Med*. 2002;**8**:1186–8.

28. Vandewalle G, Archer SN, Wuillaume C, *et al*. Functional magnetic resonance

imaging-assessed brain responses during an executive task depend on interaction of sleep homeostasis, circadian phase, and *PER3* genotype. *J Neurosci*. 2009;**29**:7948–56.

29. Archer SN, Robilliand Dc, Skene DJ, *et al*. A length polymorphism in the circadian clock gene Per3 is linked to delayed sleep phase syndrome and extreme diurnal preference. *Sleep*. 2003;**26**:413–15.

30. Viola AU, Archer SN, James LM, *et al*. *PER3* polymorphism predicts sleep structure and waking performance. *Curr Biol*. 2007;**17**:613–18.

31. Goel N, Banks S, Mignot E, Dinges DF *PER3* polymorphism predicts cumulative sleep homeostatic but not neurobehavioral changes to chronic partial sleep deprivation. *PLoS One*. 2009;**4**:e5874.

32. Vandewalle G, Archer SN, Wuillaume C, *et al*. Effects of light on cognitive brain responses depend on circadian phase and sleep homeostasis. *J Biol Rhythms*. 2011;**26**:249–59.

33. Groeger JA, Viola AM, Lo JC, *et al*. Early morning executive functioning during sleep deprivation is compromised by a PERIOD3 polymorphism. *Sleep*. 2008; **31**:1159–67.

34. Chee MW, Chuah LY. Functional neuroimaging insights into how sleep and sleep deprivation affect memory and cognition. *Curr Opin Neurol*. 2008;**21**:417–23.

35. Drummond SP, Brown GG, Salamat JS, Gillin JC. Increasing task difficulty facilitates the cerebral compensatory response to total sleep deprivation. *Sleep*. 2004;**27**:445–51.

36. Chee MW, Choo WC. Functional imaging of working memory after 24 hr of total sleep deprivation. *J Neurosci*. 2004; **24**:4560–7.

37. Koechlin E, Hyafil A. Anterior prefrontal function and the limits of human decision-making. *Science*. 2007;**318**:594–8.

38. Duffy JF, Dijk DJ. Getting through to circadian oscillators: why use constant routines? *J Biol Rhythms*. 2002;**17**:4–13.

39. Retey JV, Adam M, Honeggar E, *et al*. A functional genetic variation of adenosine deaminase affects the duration and intensity of deep sleep in humans. *Proc Natl Acad Sci U S A*. 2005;**102**:15676–81.

40. Goel N, Banks S, MIgnot E, Dinger DF. DQB1*0602 predicts interindividual differences in physiologic sleep, sleepiness, and fatigue. *Neurology*. 2010;**75**:1509–19.

41. Dijk DJ, Franker P. Interaction of sleep homeostasis and circadian rhythmicity: dependent or independent systems? In: Kryger MH, Dement W, Roth T, eds. *Principles and Practice of Sleep Medicine*. St. Louis, Elsevier, Saunders. 2005;418–35.

42. Franken P, Dijk DJ. Circadian clock genes and sleep homeostasis. *Eur J Neurosci*. 2009;**29**:1820–29.

Neuroimaging the effects of light on non-visual brain functions

Gilles Vandewalle and Derk-Jan Dijk

Light exposure is the major environmental factor regulating sleep and wakefulness

Light is necessary for image formation by the visual system, but is also essential for the regulation of numerous non-image-forming functions [1, 2]. Light is responsible for the synchronization of circadian rhythms to the external world and is able to alter the timing of these rhythms. Circadian rhythmicity is present in many processes, most notably in thermoregulation, endocrine and cardiovascular functions, sleep, alertness, and cognitive abilities. Light indirectly affects all these aspects in the long term, through its impact on circadian rhythms. Lack of light has also a negative impact on mood and repeated daily exposure to light is recommended as a therapy in seasonal affective disorders. These effects on mood, are possibly mediated through an impact on circadian rhythmicity [3]. In addition to these long-term effects, light also evokes strong and acute alterations in alertness, sleep propensity, attention, cognitive performance, cognitive brain function, body temperature, heart rate, melatonin and cortisol secretion, gene expression, and pupil constriction [1, 2, 4, 5]. Since most of the long-term and acute non-image-forming impacts of light either directly or indirectly affect the quality of sleep and wakefulness, light exposure emerges as a powerful environmental factor regulating our 24-h lives (Figure 21.1).

Analyses of the effects of light on cognition showed that the effects on performance are acute and encompass executive processes, such as inhibition, shifting and updating, memory processes, including working memory and long-term memory, and attention. Thus light has a broad impact on major aspects of cognition associated with wakefulness [1, 5–9] Light exposure during wakefulness has also been reported to acutely reduce electroencephalogram (EEG) delta, theta, and alpha activity as well as slow eye movements, which are all correlates of sleepiness and attention deficits [5, 9, 10]. This provides a first indication of the mechanisms involved in the effects of light on non-image-forming brain functions.

In this chapter, we will describe the physiological bases of the impact of light on non-image-forming functions before summarizing recent neuroimaging investigations that substantially increased our understanding of the brain mechanisms involved. The data show that light has a widespread impact on many brain functions and that this effect depends on the brain region and the ongoing process considered as well as on the duration and intensity of the light exposure, and time of day. The effects of light are also modulated by the health status and genotype of the participants.

The non-image-forming functions of light are mediated by a photoreception system sensitive to blue light

It has been shown in several species, including rodents, macaques, and humans, that light affects non-image-forming functions even in the absence of rods and cones, the classical visual photoreceptors [4]. This implies that another photoreceptor is involved. In addition, the ability of light to suppress melatonin secretion and subjective sleepiness, to increase body temperature, heart rate, and objective measures of alertness, and to shift circadian phase has been reported to be greatest with exposure to shorter wavelength light (at around 460–480 nm; blue light), which is at odds with the maximal sensitivity of the classical cone-driven photopic (~550 nm – green) and rod-driven scotopic (~505 nm – blue-green) photoreception systems [1, 2, 4, 5].

Intrinsically photosensitive retinal ganglion cells (ipRGC) expressing the photopigment melanopsin constitute a novel class of photoreceptors only marginally involved in vision, but deeply implicated in the non-image-forming functions of light [4]. Melanopsin is necessary for the intrinsic light response with a maximal sensitivity to wavelengths around 480 nm (blue light). Melanopsin-expressing ipRGCs constitute the only channel through which light affects non-image-forming functions but they receive inputs from rods and cones which modulate their overall response to light. Light responses depend therefore on the state of each class of photoreceptors so that the strength and wavelength sensitivity of the impact of light on non-image-forming functions vary with irradiance level and duration of light exposure and prior light history [4].

Melanopsin-expressing ipRGCs project to the lateral geniculate nucleus and the superior colliculus, and these projections are likely to contribute to vision, but also possibly to non-image-forming functions of light [4]. IpRGCs also project to the hypothalamus, particularly the suprachiasmatic nucleus (SCN), site of the master circadian clock, and the dorsomedial

Neuroimaging of Sleep and Sleep Disorders, ed. Eric Nofzinger, Pierre Maquet, and Michael J. Thorpy. Published by Cambridge University Press. © Cambridge University Press 2013.

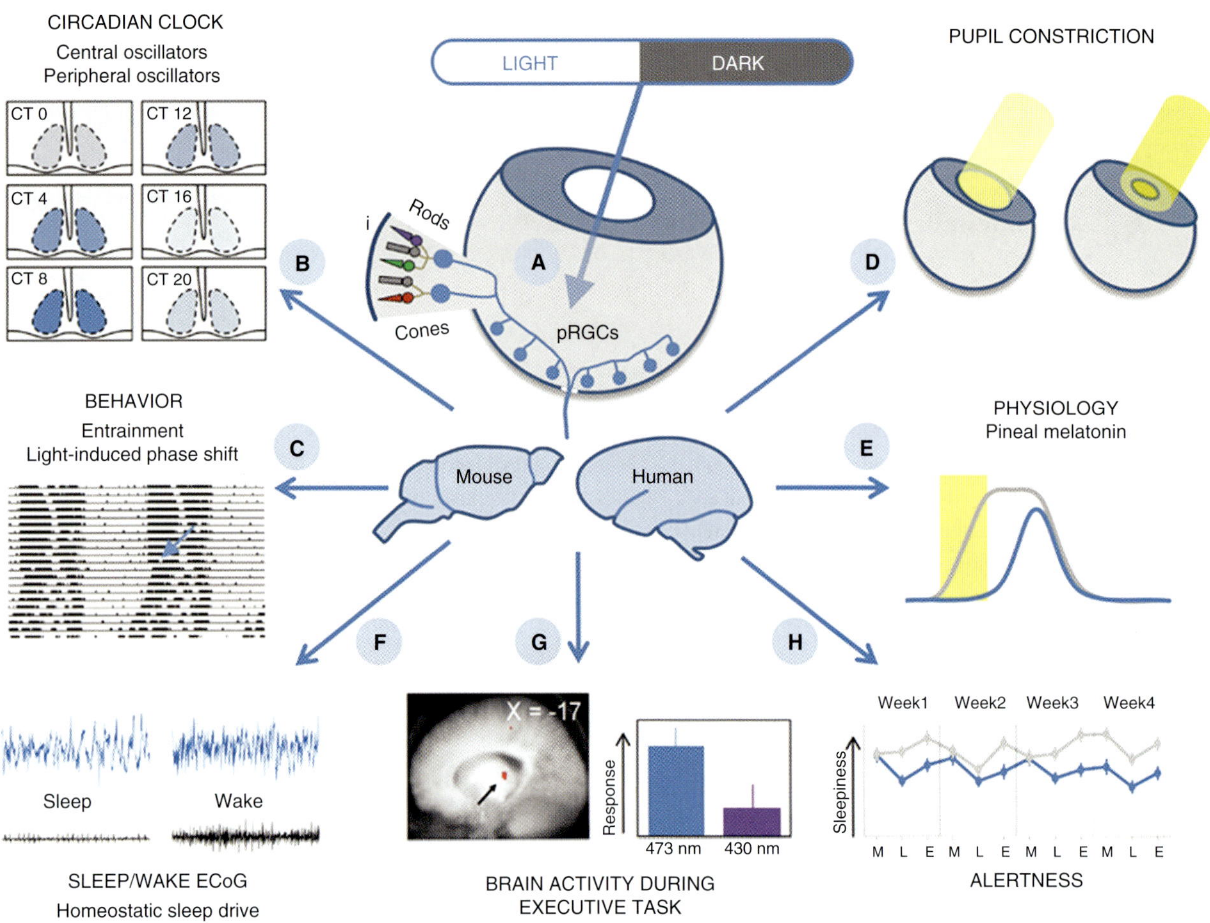

Figure 21.1 The broad non-image-forming functions of light. A diffuse network of melanopsin-expressing intrinsically photosensitive retinal ganglion cells (ipRGCs) are maximally sensitive to blue light (~480 nm) and receive input from rods and cones (A). These cells have direct projections to the SCN, site of the circadian master clock, and regulate circadian entrainment notably through influence on gene expression (B). Light also regulates locomotor activity and can shift circadian phase (C). IpRGC connections to the pretectum mediate pupil constriction (D), and indirect input via the SCN regulates the light-induced suppression of melatonin production in the pineal (E). ipRGCs also have direct projections to sleep regulatory structures such as the VLPO and thereby modulate sleep (F). Blue light can modify cognitive brain responses (G) and can improve alertness (H) during the morning, lunch time, and early evening. IpRGCs are also involved in rudimentary visual functions in rodents. (Figure copied from [2].) SCN = suprachiasmatic nucleus; VLPO = ventrolateral preoptic area; ECoG = electrocorticography.

hypothalamus (DMH), involved notably in feeding behavior and relay between the SCN and the brainstem locus coeruleus (LC) [4, 11]. A direct projection of ipRGCs to the ventrolateral preoptic area (VLPO), and the lateral hypothalamus (LH), containing orexin neurons may mediate effects on sleep regulation [4]. Projections of ipRGCs also include the pretectum within the posterior pretectal nucleus and olivary pretectal nucleus (OPN), mediating pupillary constriction, and the lateral habenula, implicated in reward processing [4]. Finally, sparse projections to the medial amygdala, involved in emotion regulation, have been reported [12]. These widespread and numerous projections are an essential component of the brain mechanisms through which light can exert a potent and diverse impact on non-image-forming functions.

Widespread impact of light on brain functions

A recent series of neuroimaging studies in young and healthy participants investigated the impact of light on cognition, initially using positron emission tomography (PET) [13], and functional magnetic resonance imaging (fMRI) in five subsequent experiments [14–18]. The experiments were designed so that the non-image-forming role of light could be examined with as little contamination as possible from its role in image formation. All studies administered light while subjects were performing tasks in the auditory modality. In other words, care was taken not to use tasks that directly depended on the visual system. The light was administered using large uniform diffusive surfaces, thereby minimizing activation of image-forming processes. Light stimuli were long (40 s to 20 min) and the effects of these stimuli were assessed during and after exposure. Comparisons were made between light of different wavelength, i.e., blue (473 nm and 480 nm), green (527 nm and 550 nm), or violet (430 nm), but equal photon density. This type of light exposure and assessments of its effects is very different from classical visual research in which the emphasis is on transient visual responses to small brief and contrasted stimuli.

Results demonstrated that light had a strong influence on the brain responses to an oddball paradigm task [13, 14], which mainly recruits attention, and to an n-back task [15–17], which involves continuous updating and comparing of information in working memory in addition to attention. More recently, brain responses to an emotional task, which requires the processing of negative and neutral prosody, were also reported to be affected by light exposure [18]. This latter observation extends the known acute non-image-forming role of light to the emotional domain and opens new perspectives as to how light affects mood and emotions in the long term.

These studies showed that light affected subcortical areas involved in alertness regulation. These areas included the hypothalamus, in an area encompassing the SCN and VLPO, while subjects were engaged in an oddball task [13]. Another area of the hypothalamus compatible with the DMH and paraventricular nucleus of the hypothalamus (PVNH), both involved in emotional responses, was affected by exposure to light specifically during the processing of negative auditory emotional stimulations (not for neutral stimuli) [18]. The dorsoposterior thalamus, in an area compatible with the pulvinar, was repeatedly shown to be affected by light exposure while performing an oddball and n-back tasks. Furthermore, an area of the brainstem compatible with the LC was affected during an n-back task [14–18]. Light also influenced responses of the hippocampus and amygdala, which are involved in long-term memory and emotion regulation.

At the cortical level, light affected areas involved in attention regulation during the exposure but also for several minutes during the darkness period immediately following light exposure [19]. Light-induced increases in activation were also observed in the occipital and temporal sensory cortices, likely through an increase of the top-down influence from parietal and frontal areas. Areas involved in updating and comparing of information in working memory were also affected [20]. These areas include the insula, the intraparietal sulcus (IPS) and supramarginal gyrus in the parietal cortex, and the dorso- (DLPFC) and ventrolateral prefrontal (VLPFC) cortex and frontopolar cortex (FPC) in the prefrontal cortex. According to a recent model of cognition [21], FPC and VLPFC are at the apex of the hierarchy of executive control and are involved in the more complex processes. Light appears therefore able to affect the frontoparietal repetition loop involved in working memory including those prefrontal areas at the top of executive control. Finally, the voice area of the temporal cortex was acutely affected by light exposure specifically for the processing of negative prosody stimulations [18].

The data show that light is able to trigger widespread modulations of brain activity in subcortical and cortical areas involved in the ongoing cognitive process. The distribution of affected areas is task-dependent and can include areas at the top of executive control, or crucial for attention, but also structures at the core of emotional responses, or essential for alertness regulation.

Wavelength-dependent modulation of brain responses

Behavioral studies have shown that, similarly to other non-image-forming functions, blue or blue-enriched light have a superior impact on cognitive performance, as compared to green light or standard white light [1, 5–9]. In accordance with these behavioral studies, brain responses to auditory n-back or emotional tasks were shown to be stronger with blue light exposure (473 nm or 480 nm, to which melanopsin ipRGCs and the non-image-forming system is maximally sensitive) compared to green light (527 nm, to which M-cones are maximally sensitive, and 550 nm to which the photopic visual system is maximally sensitive) and violet light (430 nm, to which S-cones are maximally sensitive) [15–18]. These wavelength-dependent effects were detected in subcortical areas including the hypothalamus (DMH- or PVNH-compatible area), in the brainstem (LC-compatible area), and pulvinar, but also in the IPS, DLPFC, VLPFC, FPC, as well as within the amygdala, hippocampus, insula, and temporal cortex voice-sensitive area. The superiority of blue light was observed during exposures lasting as little as 40–60 s and exposures lasting up to 18 min. In the amygdala and hippocampus the superiority of blue light compared to green light (527 nm) can already be observed at light onset, which is an event independent of cognition [16].

These results show that the impact of light on non-image-forming function is wavelength-dependent. The superiority of blue light suggests that the classical photopic visual system is not primarily responsible for the modulation of non-image-forming brain responses and is compatible with a major contribution from melanopsin-expressing ipRGCs [4, 22]. These observations do not exclude contributions from cones, while a contribution from rods remains to be investigated. Rods have been shown to contribute to the non-image-forming function of light at a higher irradiance level than their upper functional limit for vision [4, 22].

Duration-, intensity-, and task difficulty-dependent impact of light

Although no dose–response studies have been carried out, greater doses of light appear to induce stronger modulations. Twenty min of bright white light triggered significant effects on brain responses, which could be detected for up to 10 min after light off [13, 14], while significant differential effects of blue and green could only be detected during an 18-min exposure, which contained at least 100 times fewer photons, and not during the darkness period following light exposures [15]. Moreover when reducing light duration to less than a minute, brain responses to a 2-back task were mainly detected in subcortical areas including the pulvinar and a brainstem (LC-compatible) area, with little significant impact on the cortex [16]. This indicates that light-induced modulation of brain activity can be detected in subcortical areas when light is not yet significantly affecting the cortex.

In a subsequent investigation, impacts on the cortex were more numerous and widespread when using a much more difficult 3-back task (in which the current item has to be compared to the item presented three items earlier, instead of two) [17], suggesting that the effects of light were not only dependent on light intensity and duration, in addition to its wavelength, but also on the difficulty of the ongoing process, with more significant cortical modulation for more demanding tasks.

Significant behavioral impacts were only found with a higher amount of light (16 to 20 min of bright white light) [13, 14]. This supports the assumption that significant changes in brain responses precede significant behavioral changes and that it is only when the impact on brain function is strong enough that it is translated into behavioral changes. This assumption is supported by behavioral studies, which used similar wavelength and irradiance levels but for much longer durations, and found significant performance increase on task recruiting attention and executive functions [1, 5–9].

The interaction between circadian and sleep homeostasis signals modulates the impact of light

The first PET investigation of the impact of light on non-image-forming cognitive brain functions was conducted at night [13], while the subsequent fMRI studies were conducted during the daytime [14–18]. An impact of light on brain function was detected both at night and during the day. However, differences between PET and fMRI and between protocols limit the information that can be obtained from comparisons between these night and day experiments. Recent data show that time of day (morning vs. evening) and the associated changes in the interaction between circadian phase and homeostatic sleep pressure modulates the impact of light on cognitive brain function [17].

As already mentioned, the impact of light appears to be particularly pronounced under challenging conditions, which can be encountered while performing a difficult task, but also when the interaction between circadian and sleep homeostasis signals jeopardizes brain function. When comparing two fMRI sessions acquired in the morning at the same circadian phase, after a night of sleep and a night of sleep deprivation, respectively, it is in the latter condition that more widespread and more numerous light-induced modulations were observed [17]. Compared with green light (527 nm), 1 min of blue light (473 nm) could significantly increase brain responses to a 3-back task in the FPC, DLPFC, premotor cortex, and IPS, in the morning after a night of sleep or after a night of sleep deprivation. However, following sleep loss, effects were more numerous and widespread, so that they became significant bilaterally in prefrontal and parietal cortex and also included the insula (bilaterally) and the pulvinar.

Surprisingly, no differential impact of blue and green light on brain responses could be detected with a 1-min exposure in the evening, in the so-called wake-maintenance zone (i.e., when the circadian signal maximally promotes wakefulness [23] – see Chapter 20), following a normal waking day [17]. This implies that when the endogenous drive for wakefulness is high, there is a relative decrease in the capacity of light to modulate brain activations. It appears that the interaction between circadian and sleep homeostasis, which governs our ability to maintain proper waking brain function ([23] – see Chapter 20), also has a

dramatic influence on the ability of light to affect brain responses. Indeed, if homeostatic sleep pressure alone was influencing light impact, intermediate effects should be detected in the evening, as compared with effects in morning sessions after sleep and after sleep loss. In other words, light is not as stimulating in the evening, when brain responses are already maximally stimulated endogenously by the circadian system, and more light would be required to induce significant effects at this circadian phase. This assumption is supported by data showing significant impact of light on performance in the evening wake-maintenance zone using a similar irradiance level and wavelength of blue light but much longer exposures [8].

The impact of light depends on genotype

A variable number of tandem repeat (VNTR) polymorphism in the coding region of the gene *PERIOD3* (*PER3*) predicts a difference in the buildup of homeostatic sleep pressure and individual vulnerability to the impact of sleep loss on cognitive performance [23]. One genotype ($PER3^{5/5}$) has a faster increase of sleep pressure and is more vulnerable to sleep loss, as compared to the other ($PER3^{4/4}$) (see Chapter 20). While the impact of light in the evening wake maintenance zone did not differ between the genotypes, blue light significantly increased brain responses in the morning following sleep loss only in $PER3^{5/5}$ individuals, and in the morning following a night of sleep only in $PER3^{4/4}$ individuals [17]. This constitutes the first identification, both in human and animal research, of a genetic marker of individual differences in the impact of light on non-image-forming functions.

The difference between *PER3* genotypes with respect to their response to light may be related to differences in the endogenous drive for wakefulness. Because the buildup of homeostatic sleep pressure is slower in $PER3^{4/4}$ individuals they are less affected by the combination of sleep loss and an adverse circadian phase, i.e., the morning hours. $PER3^{4/4}$ individuals are therefore able to trigger endogenous compensatory brain mechanisms that maintain brain responses and recruit supplemental areas to perform a 3-back task even in the absence of light [24] (see Chapter 20). In contrast, the combination of sleep loss and an adverse circadian phase induces major reductions of activations across all parts of the cortex in $PER3^{5/5}$ individuals. Light appears therefore less able to stimulate brain responses in individuals already under great endogenous stimulation. It will provide more benefits to the genotype which is not able to maintain brain responses endogenously and is most challenged by the circadian and sleep homeostasis conditions. In addition, $PER3^{5/5}$ individuals are more likely to be morning chronotypes and to prefer performing in the morning hours [23]. The circadian amplitude in brain responses may be larger in morning types (see Chapter 20) so that in the morning following sleep they would be in optimal endogenous conditions to perform and could not benefit as much from an external light stimulation. $PER3^{4/4}$ individuals, which represent 45–50% of the general population and are more likely to be evening chronotypes, would benefit more from light in the morning after a night of sleep and significant effects could be detected. This hypothesis is in agreement with the previous studies, which were carried out in the morning shortly after sleep and found significant impact of light on brain responses in non-genotyped samples [14–16].

Light modifies the functional organization of the brain

Simple psychophysiological interaction analyses provided further insight on how light is able to modulate ongoing brain activity. While performing a 3-back task recruiting attention, working memory, and executive function, blue light increases the functional connectivity between the pulvinar and DLPFC, premotor cortex, and IPS, as well between the DLPFC and IPS (unpublished analyses of [17]). During an emotional auditory task using voice stimulation, the light-activated network is different and comprises the hypothalamus (DMH- or PVNH-compatible location), amygdala, and the voice-sensitive area of the temporal cortex [18]. The latter result was specific for the processing of emotional stimuli and was not observed for neutral stimuli. These data show that (blue) light modifies information flow between areas essential for a given ongoing task and suggest that the interactions between brain areas are optimized.

Summary and scenario of the brain mechanisms

In accordance with animal research, the neuroimaging results presented here are compatible with a scenario in which light would first influence subcortical structures involved in arousal regulation before significantly affecting the cortical areas involved in the ongoing non-image-forming process (Figure 21.2). These subcortical structures include the hypothalamus, within the SCN, but also possibly the VLPO, DMH, and PVNH. The SCN and DMH could in turn transfer light information to numerous brain sites through their numerous projections, which include the brainstem LC, to which they are functionally connected [11]. The LC constitutes the major source of norepinephrine of the organism and has a broad impact on alertness and cognition through its numerous projections to the thalamus and most of the cortex. However, other (aminergic) nuclei of the ascending arousal system could possibly be recruited as well. A pulvinar-compatible area of the thalamus appears also to be recruited at light onset but also throughout the 60 s to 20 min of exposure. The pulvinar, which has been suggested to mediate the impact of alertness on cognition ([24, 25] – see Chapter 20), is a major relay between cortical areas and an impact of light in that area could facilitate information flow within the cortex, as suggested by functional connectivity changes identified for a task involving attention, working memory, and executive functions. If sufficient, this subcortical impact would then significantly affect the cortical area recruited for the ongoing task, which could in turn affect behavior. Behavioral measures would only be significantly affected after prolonged light exposure either because the cortical impact requires time for the effect to be transferred to behavior or because behavioral measures are less sensitive than neuroimaging techniques, or probably both.

Several factors modulate the effects described in this scenario including light intensity, duration, and wavelength, and possibly task difficulty. The interaction between circadian and

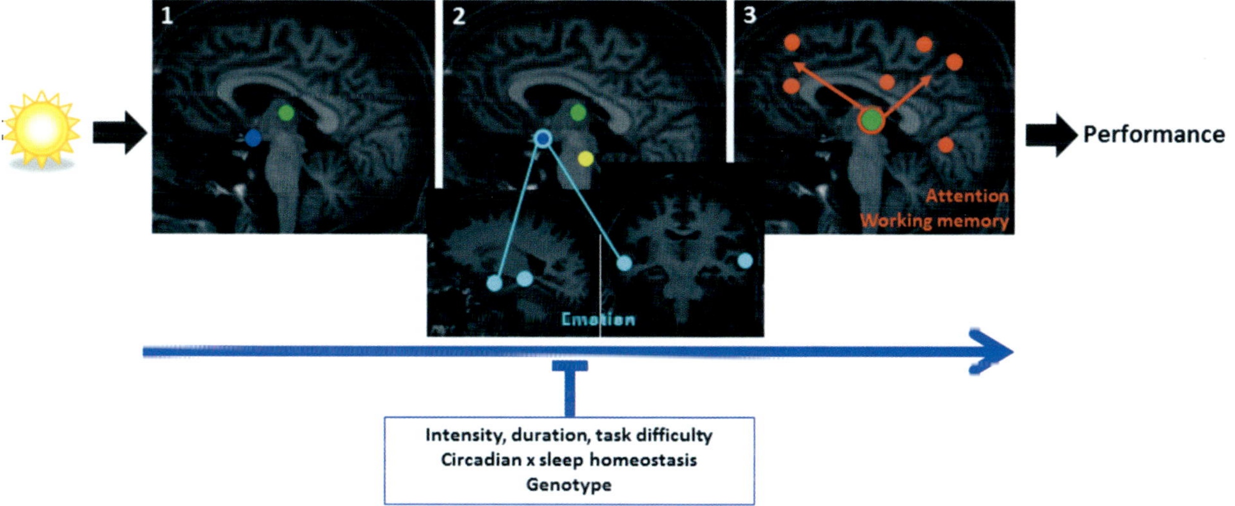

Figure 21.2 Schematic representation of the brain mechanisms involved in the non-image-forming impact of light on cognitive brain responses. (1) Responses at light onset are found within the hypothalamus (blue) and pulvinar (green) (and amygdala and hippocampus, not shown); (2) within the first seconds of the exposure, responses are found mainly in subcortical and cortical structures involved in alertness regulation (hypothalamus, brainstem (yellow), pulvinar); (3) late responses are detected at the cortical level in areas involved in the ongoing cognitive process and can subsequently affect performance. For attention/working memory/executive tasks (red) a network of areas around the pulvinar and including prefrontal and parietal areas appear to mediate the impact of light on alertness and cognition. For emotional responses to vocal stimuli (light blue), the network involves the hypothalamus, amygdala, and voice-sensitive area of the temporal cortex. Light seems to have a swifter impact on emotional cortical responses than attentional/working memory/executive responses. The impact of light is stronger with higher intensity, longer duration, and shorter wavelength (blue) light exposures, and seems also more pronounced when the participant performs a more difficult cognitive task. Time of day and the associated changes in the interaction between circadian and sleep homeostasis signals and *PERIOD3* genotype modulate the impact of light. (Adapted with permission from [5].)

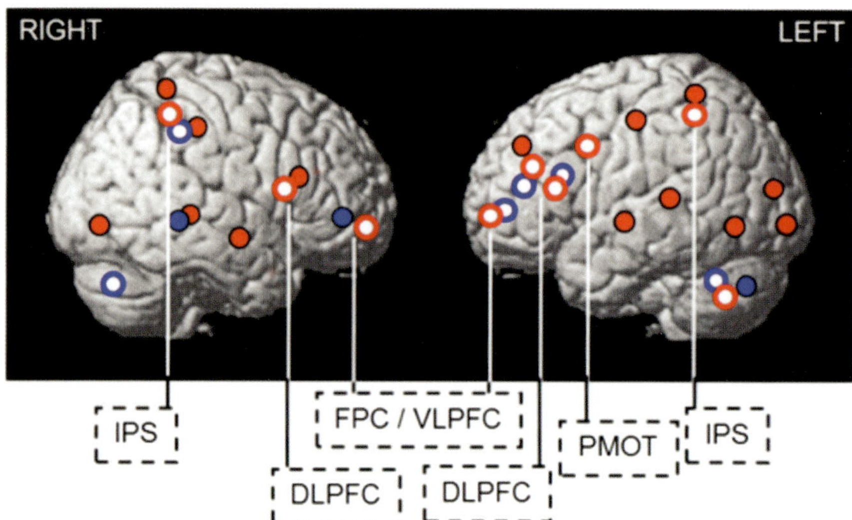

Figure 21.3 Blue light increases cognitive brain responses in locations showing in darkness decreased activation in $PER3^{5/5}$ or compensatory recruitment in $PER3^{4/4}$ following sleep loss. Compensatory increase in activation in the morning hours after 25 hours of wakefulness in $PER3^{4/4}$ (blue solid), found notably in the ventrolateral prefrontal cortex, temporal cortex, cerebellum, and thalamus (thalamus not shown). Decreases in activation in the morning hours after 25 hours of wakefulness in $PER3^{5/5}$ (red solid), observed notably in the occipital, temporal, parietal, and lateral prefrontal cortices. Blue light-induced increase in activations after 25 hours of wakefulness in $PER3^{5/5}$ (red open) (thalamus not shown). Blue light-induced increase in activity after 1.5 hours of wakefulness in $PER3^{4/4}$ (blue open). DLPFC = ventrolateral/dorsolateral prefrontal cortex; FPC/VLPFC = frontopolar/ventrolateral prefrontal cortex; IPS = intraparietal sulcus; PMOT = premotor cortex. (Copied with permission from [17].)

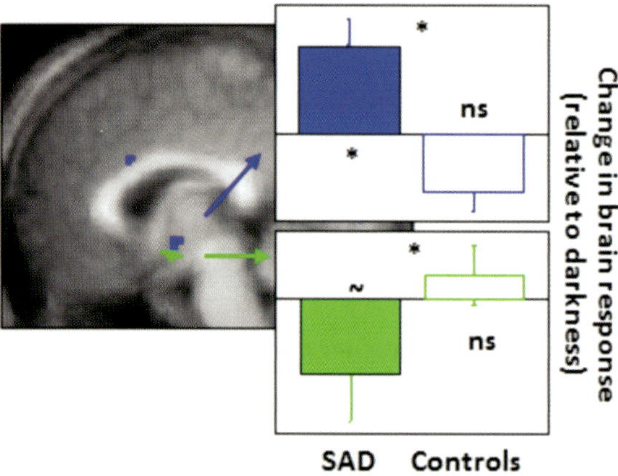

Figure 21.4 Hypothalamic responses to light as a neurobiological substrate of SAD. The impact of blue and green light exposure on the brain responses to auditory emotional stimuli is significantly different in the hypothalamus (LH- or PVNH-compatible area) of patients with SAD compared with healthy controls. Graphs: change in brain response under blue (480 nm) and green (550 nm) light exposures. (Modified with permission from [26].) *p < 0.05 after correction for multiple comparisons within a group or between group; ~p = 0.07 after correction for multiple comparisons; ns = not significant.

Importantly, the impact of light appears to be related to the activation pattern in the absence of light. For an auditory 3-back task, an impact of light is found in areas that undergo decreased activations or compensatory recruitment during sleep loss in darkness, particularly higher associative areas (Figure 21.3) [17, 24]. It seems therefore that there is an overlap between the endogenous brain mechanisms regulating wakefulness during a normal waking day and following sleep loss, and the mechanisms triggered by an external activating agent such as exposure to light.

Hypothalamic response to light as a neurobiological marker of psychiatric status

Seasonal affective disorder (SAD) is a major depressive disorder with a recurrent seasonal occurrence and most probably related to the lack of light exposure in fall/winter [3]. It has been suggested that the ability of light therapy to improve mood in SAD relates to abnormal circadian regulation or abnormal retinal physiology in patients [3]. The therapeutic effects of light may also be mediated through its acute ability to recruit a specific network of brain areas involved in emotional responses. This could in turn result in a better emotional regulation and improved mood.

Data acquired in patients suffering from SAD show that a posterior area of the hypothalamus, presumably including the LH containing orexin neurons, or the PVNH, present increased activations to emotional vocal stimulation under blue light (480 nm) illumination, but decreased activation under exposure to green light (550 nm) (Figure 21.4) [26]. These effects were not observed in healthy controls (significant difference between patients and controls). Since the hypothalamus, and particularly the LH, contributes to emotion, sleep/wake, and metabolism regulation, which are all disrupted to some extent in SAD, these light-induced activations may be of some interest. However, further research is required to elucidate whether this abnormal hypothalamic response to light constitutes a neurobiological indicator of how lack of light triggers SAD or

sleep homeostasis signals and *PER3* genotype can amplify or diminish the non-image-forming impact of light on cognitive brain function. The impact of light is also task specific and is primarily detected in areas involved in the ongoing process. The type of cognitive function is also a crucial determinant of the effect of light. For attention, working memory, and executive functions light effects appear to be mediated through a network in which the pulvinar plays a central role but which also includes prefrontal and parietal higher associative areas. For tasks triggering emotional responses, effects within cortical areas specially devoted to decoding the emotional content of a particular type of stimulus (e.g., the voice-sensitive area of the temporal cortex for voice stimulation) appear to be quick and mediated through a network based on hypothalamus and amygdala interactions.

how light therapy leads to remission, or if it is a secondary marker of a more central phenomenon.

Conclusions and perspectives

The data reviewed here indicate that exposure to light has a powerful impact on brain activity recruited by diverse aspects of cognition, so that the quality of brain functions associated with wakefulness are modulated. Several lines of evidence now suggest that exposure to light also affects subsequent sleep such that increased blue light exposure during the day can improve nocturnal sleep quality [27] and too much light in the evening disrupts sleep [28]. These effects are likely to be mediated by melanopsin, and sleep and the circadian system are so sensitive to light that ordinary room light exposure in the evening will impact circadian physiology and subsequent sleep [6, 27, 29]. This appears particularly relevant since melanopsin ipRGCs have been shown not only to acutely affect sleep and wakefulness, but also to have an impact on sleep homeostasis: melanopsin depletion in rodents reduced slow wave sleep rebound after sleep deprivation [30].

Understanding how light can be used to improve wakefulness and be modified to positively affect sleep could be of great interest for several segments of the general population: shift workers and jet-lagged people, sleeping and waking at the wrong circadian time; older and middle-aged people, with earlier wake times, decreased sleep quality [31], and

less able to shift their circadian phase in response to light [32]; Alzheimer patients, who benefit from light and melatonin administration [33]; or psychiatric patients for whom light therapy ameliorates symptoms, as demonstrated for an increasing number of disorders [3, 34]. Currently, requirements for indoor lighting are primarily focused on visual acuity but should also consider the non-image-forming functions of light so that we are not "blue-light deprived," particularly in winter, when our exposure to blue light decreases [35].

Acknowledgements

We thank the members of the Cyclotron Research Centre of the University of Liège and of the Functional Neuroimaging Unit and Center for Advanced Research in Sleep Medicine of the University of Montreal for their help in realizing the studies reviewed here. These studies were supported by the Belgian Fonds National de la Recherche Scientifique (FNRS), Fondation Médicale Reine Elisabeth (FMRE), University of Liège, Interuniversity Attraction Pole (PAI/IAP) P6/29, by the Wellcome Trust-GR069714MA, and Canadian Institute for Health Research. GV is supported by the FNRS. DJD has received research support from Philips Lighting (the Netherlands) but this research is distinct from the neuroimaging data reviewed in this chapter. The authors declare no other competing conflicts of interest.

References

1. Chellappa SL, Gordijn MC, Cajochen C. Can light make us bright? Effects of light on cognition and sleep. *Prog Brain Res.* 2011;**190**:119–33.

2. Dijk DJ, Archer SN. Light, sleep, and circadian rhythms: together again. *PLoS Biol.* 2009;**7**:e1000145.

3. Westrin A, Lam RW. Seasonal affective disorder: a clinical update. *Ann Clin Psychiatry.* 2007;**19**:239–46.

4. Schmidt TM, Chen SK, Hattar S. Intrinsically photosensitive retinal ganglion cells: many subtypes, diverse functions. *Trends Neurosci.* 2011;**34**:572–80.

5. Vandewalle G, Maquet P, Dijk DJ. Light as a modulator of cognitive brain function. *Trends Cogn Sci.* 2009;**13**:429–38.

6. Cajochen C, Frey S, Anders D, *et al.* Evening exposure to a light-emitting diodes (LED)-backlit computer screen affects circadian physiology and cognitive performance. *J Appl Physiol.* 2011;**110**:1432–8.

7. Chellappa SL, Steiner R, Blattner P, *et al.* Non-visual effects of light on melatonin, alertness and cognitive performance: can blue-enriched light keep us alert? *PLoS One.* 2011;**6**:e16429.

8. Cajochen C, Munch M, Kobialka S, *et al.* High sensitivity of human melatonin, alertness, thermoregulation, and heart rate to short wavelength light. *J Clin Endocrinol Metab.* 2005;**90**:1311–16.

9. Lockley SW, Evans EE, Scheer FAJL, *et al.* Short-wavelength sensitivity for the direct effects of light on alertness, vigilance, and the waking electroencephalogram in humans. *Sleep.* 2006;**29**:161–8.

10. Cajochen C, Zeitzer JM, Czeisler CA, *et al.* Dose-response relationship for light intensity and ocular and electroencephalographic correlates of human alertness. *Behav Brain Res.* 2000;**115**:75–83.

11. Aston-Jones G, Cohen JD. An integrative theory of locus coeruleus-norepinephrine function: adaptive gain and optimal performance. *Annu Rev Neurosci.* 2005;**28**:403–50.

12. Hattar S, Kumar M, Park A, *et al.* Central projections of melanopsin-expressing retinal ganglion cells in the mouse. *J Comp Neurol.* 2006;**497**:326–49.

13. Perrin F, Peigneux P, Fuchs S, *et al.* Nonvisual responses to light exposure in the human brain during the circadian night. *Curr Biol.* 2004;**14**:1842–6.

14. Vandewalle G, Balteau E, Phillips C, *et al.* Daytime light exposure dynamically enhances brain responses. *Curr Biol.* 2006;**16**:1616–21.

15. Vandewalle G, Gais S, Schabus M, *et al.* Wavelength-dependent modulation of brain responses to a working memory task by daytime lightexposure. *Cereb Cortex.* 2007;**17**:2788–95.

16. Vandewalle G, Schmidt C, Albouy G, *et al.* Brain responses to violet, blue, and green monochromatic light exposures in humans: prominent role of blue light and the brainstem. *PLoS One.* 2007;**2**:e1247.

17. Vandewalle G, Archer SN, Wuillaume C, *et al.* Effects of light on cognitive brain responses depend on circadian phase and sleep homeostasis. *J Biol Rhythms.* 2011;**26**:249–59.

18. Vandewalle G, Schwartz S, Grandjean D, *et al.* Spectral quality of light modulates emotional brain responses in humans. *Proc Natl Acad Sci U S A.* 2010;**107**:19549–54.

19. Corbetta M, Shulman GL. Control of goal-directed and stimulus-driven attention in the brain. *Nat. Rev. Neurosci..* 2002;**3**:201–15.

20. Collette F, Hogge M, Salmon E, *et al.* Exploration of the neural substrates of executive functioning by functional neuroimaging. *Neuroscience.* 2006;**139**:209–21.

21. Koechlin E, Hyafil A. Anterior prefrontal function and the limits of human decision-making. *Science.* 2007;**318**:594–8.

22. Lall GS, Revell VL, Momiji H, *et al.* Distinct contributions of rod, cone, and melanopsin photoreceptors to encoding irradiance. *Neuron.* 2010;**66**:417–28.

23. Dijk DJ, Archer SN. PERIOD3, circadian phenotypes, and sleep homeostasis. *Sleep Med Rev.* 2010;**14**:151–60.

24. Vandewalle G, Archer SN, Wuillaume C, *et al.* Functional magnetic resonance imaging-assessed brain responses during an executive task depend on interaction of sleep homeostasis, circadian phase, and PER3 genotype. *J Neurosci.* 2009;**29**:7948–56.

25. Portas CM, Rees G, Howseman AM, *et al.* A specific role for the thalamus in mediating the interaction of attention and arousal in humans. *J Neurosci.* 1998;**18**:8979–89.

26. Vandewalle G, Hebert M, Beaulieu C, *et al.* Abnormal hypothalamic response to light in seasonal affective disorder. *Biol Psychiatry.* 2011;**70**:954–61.

27. Viola AU, James LM, Schlangen LJ, *et al.* Blue-enriched white light in the workplace improves self-reported alertness, performance and sleep quality. *Scand J Work Environ Health.* 2008;**34**:297–306.

28. Santhi N, Thorne HC, van der Veen DR, *et al.* The spectral composition of evening light and individual differences in the suppression of melatonin and delay of sleep in humans. *J Pineal Res.* 2011;**53**:47–59.doi: 10.1111/j.1600–079X.2011.00970.x.

29. Gooley JJ, Chamberlain K, Smith KA, *et al.* Exposure to room light before bedtime suppresses melatonin onset and shortens melatonin duration in humans. *J Clin Endocrinol Metab.* 2011;**96**:E463–72.

30. Tsai JW, Hannibal J, Hagiwara G, *et al.* Melanopsin as a sleep modulator: circadian gating of the direct effects of light on sleep and altered sleep homeostasis in Opn4(-/-) mice. *PLoS Biol.* 2009;**7**:e1000125.

31. Gaudreau H, Morettini J, Lavoie HB, *et al.* Effects of a 25-h sleep deprivation on daytime sleep in the middle-aged. *Neurobiol Aging.* 2001;**22**:461–8.

32. Duffy JF, Zeitzer JM, Czeisler CA. Decreased sensitivity to phase-delaying effects of moderate intensity light in older subjects. *Neurobiol Aging.* 2007;**28**:799–807.

33. Riemersma-van der Lek RF, Swaab DF, Twisk J, *et al.* Effect of bright light and melatonin on cognitive and noncognitive function in elderly residents of group care facilities: a randomized controlled trial. *JAMA.* 2008;**299**:2642–55.

34. Terman M, Terman JS. Light therapy for seasonal and nonseasonal depression: efficacy, protocol, safety, and side effects. *CNS Spectr.* 2005;**10**:647–63.

35. Thorne HC, Jones KH, Peters SP, *et al.* Daily and seasonal variation in the spectral composition of light exposure in humans. *Chronobiol Int.* 2009;**26**:854–66.

Memory systems, sleep, and neuroimaging

Steffen Gais and Monika Schönauer

Introduction

An increasing number of studies have investigated the relation between sleep and memory in the last decade. Although there has been a long controversy, most current publications agree that sleep enhances consolidation in both the declarative and the procedural domain of memory [1, 2]. Declarative memory, which is the memory for facts and events, was the main focus of memory research for a long time, and an abundance of studies on sleep and declarative memory exist [3]. Only much later, nearly 80 years after the first report of a link between sleep and memory, a groundbreaking study by Avi Karni and colleagues showed in humans that post-training sleep also had an effect on consolidation of perceptual skill memory [4]. Since then, a great number of studies have shown robust effects of sleep on non-declarative memory consolidation [5].

Although the relation between sleep and memory is already an old topic that has been investigated by several generations of scientists [6–9], there are still many fundamental questions, which are left unanswered, e.g.:

- Which types of memory are affected by sleep, and do these effects occur only under specific conditions?
- Are all types of memory modified by sleep in the same way or are there multiple mechanisms by which sleep can affect memory?
- How do memory-related traces in the brain change across sleep? Are such changes of a qualitative or of a quantitative nature?

Whereas the first question can largely be answered by behavioral experiments, especially the second and the third question have been investigated by use of brain imaging. Given that it is no longer the issue of whether sleep affects memory, the subject of foremost relevance has become which mechanisms underlie the observed effects on memory consolidation. While there are already a number of studies providing ideas about what sleep does to a previously learned memory, we are still a long way from definitively answering these questions. In this chapter, we will look at how different memory systems are influenced by sleep. We will see that functional imaging can tell us much about covert processes which are sometimes hard to detect when looking at behavioral measures alone. In some cases,

functional imaging can even provide clues about underlying memory processes in the absence of behavioral effects, and thus point us to an amazing ability of the brain to compensate deficits in one memory system with increased activity in other systems. Considering the question of brain mechanisms of memory allows us to answer remaining questions relevant to our conceptualization of memory systems.

Over a long time, our understanding of how sleep affects memory has evolved [10]. Because most animal studies relate to hippocampus-dependent memories, most comprehensive models also pertain to these forms of memory. In the following, we will therefore mainly describe the currently most-widely accepted model of consolidation of hippocampus-dependent memory. The central notion of this model is the idea of two complementary learning systems. Basically, it is assumed that new memories are quickly encoded by a fast-learning hippocampal memory system. Then, over time, the to-be-remembered information is reinstated repeatedly, e.g., by reminiscence, and introduced into slower-learning neocortical structures [11]. Such a two-stage memory has several advantages. On the one hand, because old, consolidated knowledge is not stored in the same circuits as new information, it is relatively robust against interference, which otherwise could potentially disturb or overwrite similar or contradicting facts. Nonetheless, this system is able to acquire such information quickly during a single presentation, without the need for repeated rehearsal. On the other hand, a two-step process allows the extraction of importance and structure from the underlying experiences. Because of the need for repetition and integration into existing memory networks, only that information which is used and assimilable will enter long-term memory storage. The process of transferring new information between and integrating it into different memory systems has been called systems memory consolidation. Systems consolidation, as opposed to synaptic consolidation, does not simply involve strengthening connections in those parts of the brain which participated in learning, but by its nature requires a change in the representation of the memory itself. Because information storage in neural networks is intimately linked to the structure and function of the storing network, a neocortical trace must be different from a hippocampal one. Systems consolidation will therefore not only strengthen, but also change memory.

Neuroimaging of Sleep and Sleep Disorders, ed. Eric Nofzinger, Pierre Maquet, and Michael J. Thorpy. Published by Cambridge University Press. © Cambridge University Press 2013.

Sleep, in this framework of dual declarative memory storage systems, provides an offline condition during which systems consolidation can occur free of external interference [10]. Several models exist regarding what happens to a memory trace in the course of consolidation. Mainly, it is assumed that three processes occur during this period: reactivation, reorganization, and reprocessing. First, the recently learned memory must become activated again. This can happen in the form of active remembering during wakefulness, but in that case it is accompanied by a conscious experience. Sleep, on the other hand, can provide additional rehearsal to a new memory without the need for conscious experience. In this state, memories can be repeatedly replayed, maybe even in a more efficient, time-compressed form, thus providing additional rehearsal and strengthening of its trace [12]. Additionally, reactivation is thought to lead not only to a reinforcement of those synapses already strongly involved in the memory representation, but also to integration of new networks into existing neuronal representations. This process can be seen as a kind of transfer or reorganization of the memory trace, because new (mainly neocortical) areas of the brain are included in the memory network while others (mainly hippocampal) lose their importance for this specific memory. Such a transfer of information will probably usually not result in an identical copy of the memory, but lead to changes in the memory itself. Integration into new circuits will change the importance of specific aspects of what is remembered. More general aspects with more links to existing knowledge might become accentuated whereas other aspects might be abandoned. It is even possible that new connections are formed, thus reprocessing and changing the memory, leading to a new, perhaps more useful representation. Individual aspects of this model have been supported experimentally in animal and human studies. Below, we will take a look at human functional magnetic resonance imaging (fMRI) studies which provide evidence that, in fact, memories are reactivated, reorganized, and reprocessed during sleep.

Reactivation

Reactivation in sleep was first shown in hippocampal cells of rats [13]. During sleep, hippocampal place cells show firing patterns that are similar to those seen during preceding learning episodes. Because neuronal activity in sleep depends on previous experience during wakefulness, it has been supposed that this might represent processing of newly learned information during sleep. The first study that demonstrated reactivation to exist in the human neocortex examined visuomotor skill learning with positron emission tomography (PET) imaging [14]. After practicing a probabilistic serial reaction time task, during 4 h, regional cerebral blood flow was measured during different stages of sleep and wakefulness. It was found, that the cuneus and the premotor cortex were more active during rapid eye movement (REM) sleep after task practice than during REM sleep in control subjects without practice. As both areas were also activated by training, these data confirm the findings in animals that the same networks involved in learning are later reactivated during offline consolidation periods. In a follow-up study using the same task, the authors also showed that the reactivation is related to the

underlying structure of the sequence and does not occur simply after practicing tapping random sequences [15]. Additionally, the level of initial acquisition of the skill was directly related to the increase in regional cerebral blood flow in the cuneus during subsequent REM sleep, thus suggesting a direct link between behavioral performance and cerebral reactivation. These results therefore support the idea that REM sleep reactivation is involved in the consolidation of the high-order information contained in the learned material, rather than being use-dependent processes related to fatigue.

It is also possible to investigate changes brought about by memory consolidation by a more indirect approach. Instead of directly measuring brain activity during the consolidation interval, changes in recall activity from pre- to post-sleep testing can be evaluated. Whereas the former is more easily implemented in PET studies, the latter is more suited to fMRI methods. One of the first fMRI studies revealing an impact of sleep on how procedural memory is stored was published by Maquet *et al.* [16]. In that study, subjects learned a visuomotor tracing skill. Performance on the task after three days was better when subjects slept during the first night after learning, than when they were sleep deprived during that one night. When looking at brain activity differences between sleeping and sleep-deprived subjects, only one region became apparent: the superior temporal sulcus, an area which is often seen related to movement perception. Because brain activity was measured after two recovery nights, this result cannot be due to acute fatigue, but must result from changes brought about by the consolidation process. Another study investigated a purely visual skill [17], a visual discrimination task, which is the only task shown to require sleep for post-training improvement (and not only benefits compared to periods of wakefulness) [18]. That study compared a consolidated versus a new skill condition. Here, the only difference between the two was found in the early processing areas of the visual cortex, specifically at the location activated by simple checkerboard stimulation of the corresponding area of the visual field. In the consolidated condition, subjects showed stronger activity in this particular area. Thus, both studies show increases of activity in task-related sensory areas. This is an indication that sleep-related improvement in these two tasks is locally restricted to areas directly related to stimulus processing. Another study using the same visual discrimination task found additional activity in parietal and temporal regions [19]. However, that study trained the subjects shortly before scanning, which can lead to fatigue-related deterioration in performance across both trained and untrained eyes [20]. These effects of fatigue are supposed to occur at a higher level of neuronal processing and might have resulted in the increased activity in these additional regions. Several other studies explored motor skill learning. The task most widely used to investigate sleep effects in this regard is the so-called "finger-tapping task." For this task, subjects learn to press a short 5-item sequence of keys with the fingers of their non-dominant hand. This task shows very robust sleep-related effects [21]. Several regions have consistently been found in relation to sleep: the primary motor cortex, the medial prefrontal lobe, the cerebellum, the ventral striatum, and, astonishingly, the

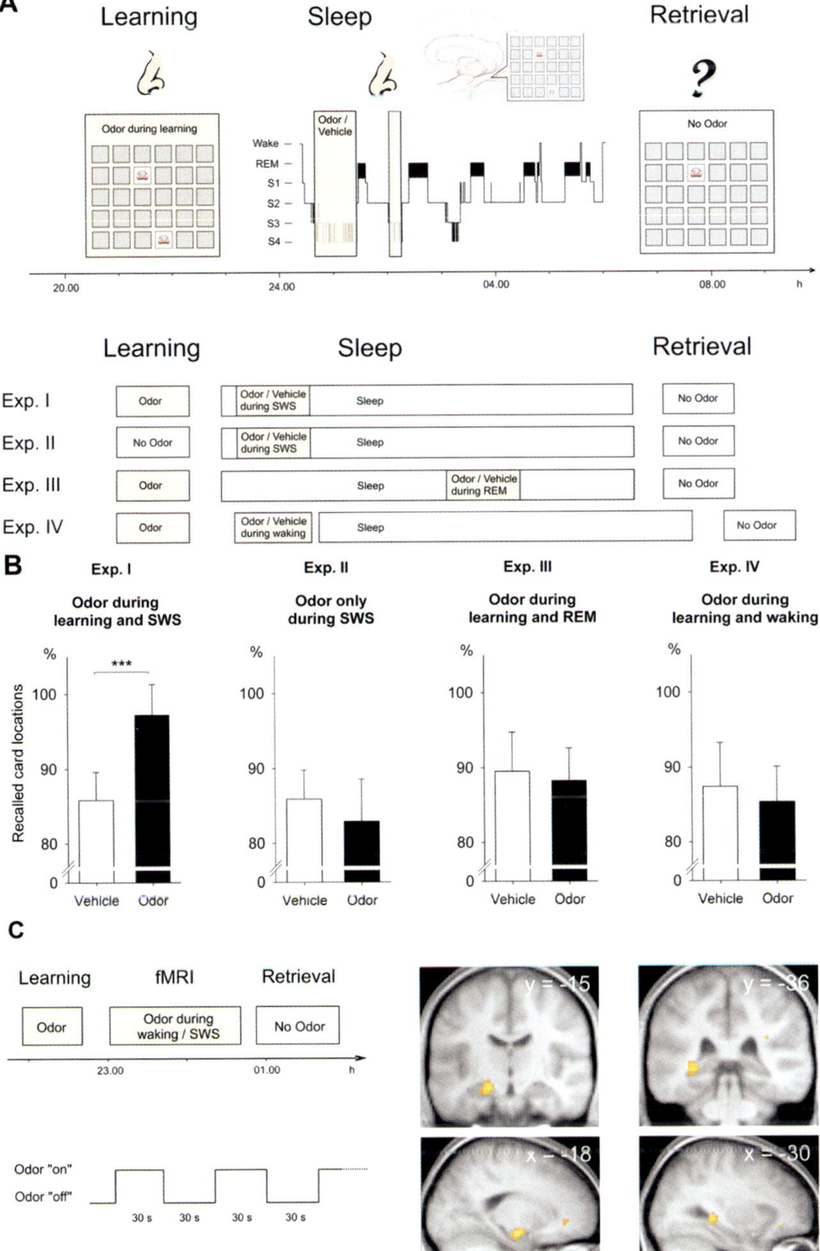

Figure 22.1 (A) Experimental design for examining reactivation of the declarative memory system during sleep. Subjects learned a spatial paired-association task in the presence of a context odor. The same odor was later also presented during slow-wave sleep (SWS) to reinforce memory reactivation. During later recall, the second card of each pair had to be located. In control conditions vehicle (odorless air) was presented during learning or reactivation, or the odor was not present during slow-wave sleep but was during wakefulness or REM sleep. (B) Behavioral results. Only when the odor was used as a context during learning and present during reactivation, an increase in behavioral performance was found. (C) fMRI experiment. The hippocampus was activated significantly by odor presentation in slow-wave sleep, indicating that the odor was indeed able to reactivate the declarative memory system during sleep. (Adapted with permission from [23].)

hippocampus [22]. Thus, with the exception of the hippocampus, these areas are motor-related and can support faster motor output and more precise mapping of movements. The hippocampus might underlie consolidation of the explicit order of the sequence. Again, this suggests that the effects of sleep on consolidation are mainly restricted to task-related brain areas, at least with respect to procedural memory systems.

For declarative memory, Rasch *et al.* [23] showed that reactivation exists in humans and has a functional relevance for memory. Subjects performed a spatial object location task before sleep in which they had to learn the positions of 15 pairs of cards presented as a rectangular field. Later, during recall, they were shown one of the cards and were asked to name the position of the corresponding other one. Throughout the whole learning session, a specific odor was presented as a context to the situation.

Then, the same odor was again present during sleep, in order to reinstate the specific context. In control experiments, the odor was presented during a period of wakefulness instead of sleep, or no odor was present during learning or during sleep. It could thus be tested whether the effect of the odor was due to it being a context of the learning session or whether it was due to its mere presence during sleep. It was also possible to test whether the effects of the odor were specific to its presentation in slow-wave sleep (see Figure 22.1 for a summary of methods and results). Odors do not have to pass the sensory gates of the thalamus and can therefore reach the cortical processing areas during sleep without waking the subject. Moreover, olfactory pathways have direct connections to the limbic system including the hippocampus; thus odors may activate memories more directly than other sensory modalities. Therefore, the reinstatement of the context odor during sleep was hypothesized to facilitate reactivation of the associated memories and lead to improved memory consolidation. The results of this study clearly showed that the odor in fact only improved memory consolidation when it was presented as a context during learning and when it was subsequently present again during sleep. These behavioral results already strongly support the idea that memory consolidation is based on reactivation of recent experiences during sleep. In an fMRI experiment, it was additionally shown that the odor presented during sleep after learning specifically activated the hippocampus. Context odor presentation thus led to reactivation of the hippocampus during sleep and, concurrently, to enhanced consolidation of a hippocampus-dependent memory task. The authors conclude that reactivation of memory-related brain areas during sleep can support memory consolidation.

Another way to demonstrate functional effects of reactivation was taken by Peigneux *et al.* [24]. They used a correlational approach o show that the amount of reactivation in the hippocampus during sleep is directly related to performance during memory retrieval the next day. They trained subjects on a virtual maze navigation task for four hours before sleep. Then, during following sleep, brain activity was measured using PET. In all subjects, hippocampal activity was higher than during wakefulness, relative to average brain activity. When directly comparing the training group to a control group without extensive task training, the hippocampus and parahippocampus were significantly more active after spatial learning. Moreover, when comparing the training group to a control group trained on a procedural memory task, hippocampal activity during slow-wave sleep was again higher after spatial learning. Finally, there was a strong positive correlation between hippocampal activity during sleep and performance increase during spatial memory recall the next morning. Together, the hippocampus seems to be more active than the rest of the brain during sleep, and it is more so after intense periods of spatial learning. The stronger this learning-related activity increase is during sleep, the better recall performance is on the next day, indicating that hippocampal reactivation during sleep directly relates to declarative memory consolidation.

Another recent study by Bergmann *et al.* looked particularly at the temporal aspects of reactivation during sleep using combined electroencephalography (EEG) and fMRI [25]. In particular, they explored the relationship between sleep spindles and memory reactivation. They used an image association task in which pairs of pictures of faces and scenes had to be remembered. This task activates a specific pattern of well-known brain areas including the fusiform face area, the occipital face area, the parahippocampal place area, and the hippocampus. It was therefore predicted that reactivation will occur in these areas during subsequent sleep. Specifically, reactivation was expected to occur during sleep spindles, because sleep spindles are thought to be related to memory processing [26]. They occur in temporal correlation with hippocampal sharp-wave ripple activity, which in turn has been shown to be related to memory processing [27, 28]. Measuring EEG and fMRI at the same time permitted the authors to focus on brain activity during the occurrence of sleep spindles. They found a number of cortical and subcortical regions in which activity correlated directly with sleep spindle amplitude, most prominently the hippocampus. Furthermore, they found that in task-specific areas (fusiform face area, the occipital face area, parahippocampal place area, and hippocampus) the correlation between fMRI activity and sleep spindle activity was learning specific and stronger than in a visuomotor control condition. Finally, hippocampal reactivation was correlated with task performance during learning. Thus, results showed that reactivation is restricted temporally to the occurrence of sleep spindles and regionally to areas active during learning.

Together, it seems that mainly those areas which are especially active during wakefulness before sleep are also reactivated during sleep. These can be sensory or motor areas, higher-level processing areas such as the fusiform face area or the parahippocampal place area, and memory-related areas such as the striatum, or the hippocampus. Reactivation can occur with declarative memory tasks as well as with procedural memory tasks. Most studies find stronger reactivation during slow-wave sleep, but some also see reactivation in REM sleep. To sum up, reactivation occurs during post-learning sleep, and it seems to be an important component of memory consolidation. In general, it has been found that it occurs in those brain regions most strongly related to the specific learning task.

Reorganization

As shown above, reactivation occurs during sleep in those brain areas directly participating in task performance. This is compatible with a view that synapses strengthened during previous learning subsequently have a higher statistical probability of firing than other synapses. This increased firing could then in turn further strengthen the synapse and later lead to improved memory recall. Reactivation could therefore support synaptic consolidation of memory traces. However, recent studies also provide more and more evidence for systems memory consolidation. This process requires the inclusion of new networks into existing memory representations or the loss of relevance of previously essential parts of the memory trace; thus, a shift in the brain representation of a memory. Studies investigating systems memory consolidation therefore look for changes in the pattern of brain activity over consolidation intervals. For declarative memory, the hippocampus is the focus of attention. According to the standard model of memory, the hippocampus is required for the initial storage of all kinds of declarative memory. After an extended period of consolidation, however, the memory becomes integrated into wider neocortical circuits and the hippocampus loses its role as the central memory store.

One of the first studies to show that the cortical representations of memories change with sleep over a consolidation period was done by Takashima and colleagues [29]. They used a picture recognition task to show changes of memory-related brain activity over a period of 90 days. Subjects studied one set of pictures on the first day of the experiment. After a 3-h rest period during which subjects were allowed to sleep, a new set of pictures was learned. Then, in an MR scanner, pictures from the first set, the second set, and new pictures were presented, and subjects had to do a recognition task. Brain activity for recent and remote pictures was compared. In addition to the 3-h condition, subjects performed the same procedure (learning new images followed by a recognition test including remote, recent, and new images in the MR scanner) after a 1-day, a 30-day, and a 90-day interval. The amount of slow-wave sleep during the rest period was correlated directly with recognition performance until day 30. In addition, slow-wave sleep correlated negatively with activity in the anterior hippocampus on day 1. Over the whole 90-day period, activity of remote versus recent images decreased in that area of the hippocampus while it increased in the medial prefrontal cortex. Findings thus indicate that, during the 90 days following learning, the hippocampus loses importance for picture recognition whereas the medial prefrontal cortex concurrently gains importance. This pattern of results is clearly compatible with a systems consolidation point of view. Particularly the medial prefrontal area has been proposed to take over the function of the hippocampus in consolidated memories [30]. There is also the reverse finding of stronger hippocampal activation with longer consolidation periods [31]. However, that study restricted analysis to a subgroup of better performing subjects, which might have led to a bias towards subjects who tried harder to remember and therefore also showed stronger brain activity.

A reduction of hippocampal activity over extended time periods has also been reported by Gais *et al.* [32], here as a function of sleep (S), compared to sleep deprivation (SD) (see Figure 22.2 for a summary of methods and results). In this study, subjects learned a paired-associate word list task and were then either sleep deprived for 24 h or allowed to sleep normally. Recall was tested two days later and six months later. Recall-related brain activity for words from the S and SD conditions were compared. Whereas after the short delay the hippocampus was significantly more active in the S than in the SD condition, after the six-month interval it was the medial prefrontal cortex that marked the difference between words from the S and SD conditions. Again, results are compatible with the view that over time, the hippocampus loses its function in favor of the medial prefrontal cortex. This conclusion is strengthened by the observation that the hippocampus is functionally connected to the medial prefrontal cortex at the two-day interval, i.e., both areas showed correlated activity in response to presentation of a recall stimulus. It is therefore well conceivable that, at first, the hippocampus, by reactivation, transmits information to the medial prefrontal cortex, which integrates this information slowly and, at a later time point, becomes sufficient for memory recall.

Similarly, Takashima and colleagues showed that by 24 h after learning a face-location association task a shift from a hippocampal to a neocortical representation occurs in the cortical memory trace, accompanied by an increase in cortico-cortical functional connectivity and a decrease in hippocampal involvement in the retrieval network [33]. Using the same face-location association task, van Dongen *et al.* [34] went one step further and investigated functional connectivity not only during retrieval, but also during sleep. They found that an increased functional connectivity between the fusiform gyrus and the medial prefrontal cortex during light sleep stages 1 and 2 could predict retention after the sleep interval. Thus, the common activity of these two areas could be a sign of a transfer of information between

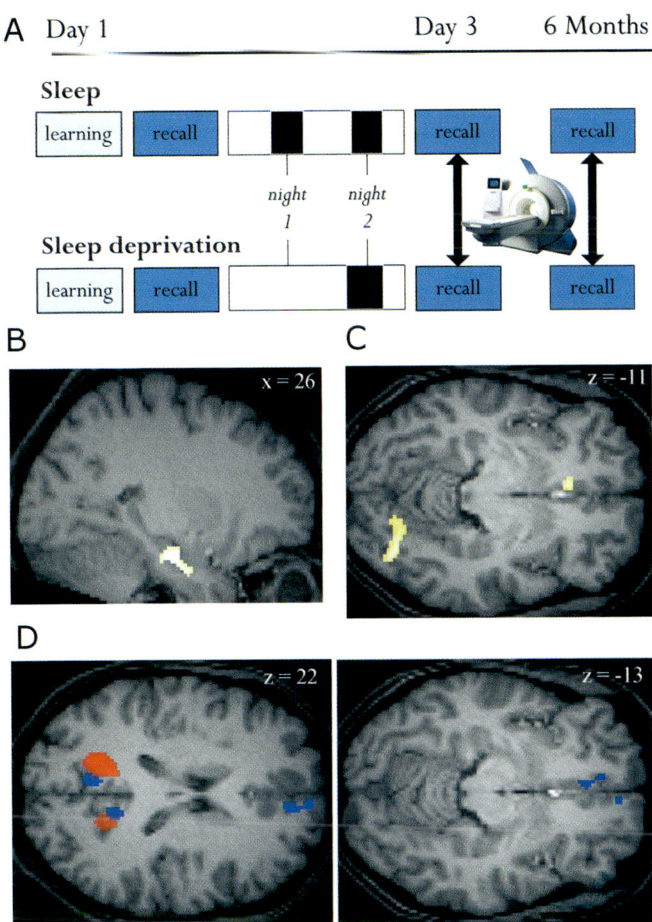

Figure 22.2 (A) Experimental design for examining hippocampal activity over extended time periods. Subjects learned a paired-associate word list task before sleeping (S) or staying awake for one night. During the second night subjects slept in both conditions in order to get rid of fatigue from the sleep deprivation (SD) night. On day 3 and after six months, subjects performed a cued recall of the word lists in the scanner. (B) Brain activity on day 3. Differences between S and SD conditions in brain activity related to correct word recall were found only in the anterior hippocampus. (C) Brain activity after six months. Differences between S and SD conditions in brain activity related to correct word recall were found only in the medial prefrontal cortex. (D) Functional connectivity on day 3. During pair recall on day 3, the precuneus showed correlated activity with the hippocampus in both S and SD conditions. The medial prefrontal cortex, however, showed a correlation with the hippocampus in the S condition. This region, which was functionally connected to the hippocampus during recall on day 3, was more active at the six-month interval for word pairs from the S than from the SD condition. (Adapted with permission from [32].)

them, leading to a stabilization of the memory and better recall performance after sleep. In line with this finding, functional connectivity increases between the hippocampal formation and neocortical regions during sleep, mainly in sleep stage 2, and specifically related to sleep spindles, suggesting an increased capacity for information transfer [35].

Not all types of declarative memory, however, are identical. Depending on the type of memory task, the changes in memory representation do not always occur in the same cortical areas. Orban *et al.* found that brain activity related to navigation in a virtual environment changes depending on sleep [36]. After a delay of three days, hippocampal activity was reduced during a place finding task compared to immediate performance, whereas activity in the caudate nucleus increased in the same contrast. Especially the activity in the caudate proved to be dependent on sleep. Subjects who slept during the first night after learning the navigation task showed significantly higher activity in the caudate nucleus three days later than subjects who stayed awake. Together, this study showed that not only hippocampal-neocortical, but also hippocampal-striatal reorganization can occur over sleep periods. Similar results, separating sleep-related changes in spatial and contextual memory have also been reported in another study using a similar navigation task [37]. Notably, both studies found differences in brain activity without differences in behavioral performance.

Emotional memory also shows specific changes in retrieval-related brain areas over sleep. In two studies Sterpenich and colleagues investigated neutral and emotional picture stimuli in a remember/know paradigm. They showed that three days after learning, the cortical response to recollection of emotionally negative items was larger in the hippocampus and several cortical areas, including the medial prefrontal cortex, in the sleep group than in the sleep-deprived group [38]. However, six months after learning, the hippocampus is no longer significantly activated in memory recollection, but the ventral medial prefrontal cortex and the precuneus are instead. In addition, functional connectivity also increased depending on sleep during the first night after learning [39]. Another study using emotional stimuli was done by Payne *et al.* [40]. These authors investigated memory for scenes with either emotional or neutral objects. Subjects had to perform a recognition task including old and new, emotionally negative and neutral stimuli during fMRI scanning 12 h after learning the stimuli. Whereas after daytime wakefulness negative stimuli activated a diffuse network of cortical regions, only a smaller set of mainly limbic regions was active after nighttime sleep. In particular, after a wake period lateral parietal and temporal areas of neocortex were more active, whereas after sleep the amygdala, medial prefrontal cortex, striatum, and thalamus showed higher activity. Regarding functional connectivity, a path analysis revealed a stronger effective connectivity within a network comprised of the amygdala, the hippocampus, fusiform gyrus, and ventromedial prefrontal cortex during retrieval after sleep than after wakefulness.

All these studies show that in addition to reactivation of memory-related brain areas, sleep also promotes reorganization of memory networks. In particular, many studies point to a reduction of hippocampal contribution to memory over time intervals in the range of days to months and a concurrent increase in recruitment of other memory-related areas, e.g., the medial prefrontal cortex and the striatum. This finding is consistent with the model of systems memory consolidation, which assumes that memory (either the information itself or some function required for retrieval) after initial acquisition is moved from a fast-learning hippocampal memory system to other slower-changing systems. It is assumed that this process happens during sleep or is at least enhanced by sleep. It is sometimes discussed whether the information itself or a kind of "index" or "pointer" to the information is stored, but effectively this does not change the concept of information transfer per se, because the pointer itself can be viewed as a kind of information (about which cortical nodes are involved in a specific memory). However, there is also another possible explanation for these findings. Instead of a transfer of information (or function) between brain areas, it is also possible that already to begin with multiple memory systems store traces of the information. Some of these traces decay with time or become stronger, e.g., by reactivation during sleep. This results in a shift in the brain regions participating in memory recall at different times after encoding, which can have the appearance of a transfer, without involving an actual relocation of information.

Reprocessing

Up to this point, we have mainly focused on memory as duplication of factual knowledge and previous events. There is, however, also another aspect of memory storage. Although we often believe that our memories reflect a true image of original events, this is generally not the case. Actually, memory is highly selective in what is retained and what is forgotten. Additionally, many memories are distorted or altered versions of the real events [41]. Thus, on the one hand, the brain has somehow to weigh the importance of memories in order to select which memories are retained and which ones are forgotten. On the other hand, memories have to be condensed, integrated with other memories, and reevaluated, and gaps in memory have to be filled in a meaningful way. There is evidence that at least some of these processes can be performed during sleep.

First, sleep can selectively strengthen some memories over others. Using a "directed forgetting" paradigm, Saletin *et al.* [42] showed that recall of items that were cued to be remembered were enhanced by sleep whereas items that were cued to be forgotten were not. In an fMRI study using the same paradigm, Rauchs *et al.* [43] also found that relevant items were remembered better after sleep than irrelevant items. fMRI showed that recall of remembered items compared to forgotten ones elicited stronger activity after sleep than after sleep deprivation. In addition, sleep engendered a common pattern of activity for relevant and irrelevant remembered items, something which did not happen when subjects stayed awake after learning. These studies provide evidence that the intention to remember items somehow changes the path consolidation takes during subsequent sleep, leading to different neuronal representations between sleep and sleep deprivation.

Apart from weighing the relevance of information, sleep can also process other aspects of our memories. There are many accounts of people who reportedly solved difficult problems during sleep, the most well known of which are those of Mendeleyev's invention of the periodic table of elements and Kekulé's discovery of the ring structure of benzene. In one of the first experimental studies investigating information processing during sleep, Wagner *et al.* [44] used a task that required subjects to form sequences of numbers according to a specific rule. This task could be solved in two ways. There was a standard solution, which took longer, but there existed also a shortcut solution, which allowed subjects to finish the task in a fraction of the time. Subjects were instructed to solve the task as quickly as possible. Most subjects were unable to find the shortcut within the few trials they had before a night time sleep or sleep-deprivation period. In the next morning, however, those subjects that were allowed to sleep during the night were much more likely to find the solution during another exposure to the task than sleep-deprived subjects. However, there was no difference between a sleep and a sleep-deprivation group who did not practice the task before sleep. Thus, the difference between groups was not due to acute effects of sleep deprivation on the task, but must be related to the previous engagement with the task. The authors suggest that the representation of the task is being transformed during sleep in a way that a solution can later be found more readily. In an imaging study, Darsaud *et al.* [45] investigated brain activity differences between subjects who solved this task and those who did not solve it. Already at training, future solvers and non-solvers differed in their cerebral responses. In future solvers, responses were observed in frontal and parietal cortical areas and in the insula. In contrast, non-solvers showed responses in the hippocampus. Moreover, the hippocampus was functionally connected with the basal ganglia in non-solvers and with the superior frontal sulcus in solvers, thus potentially biasing the participants' strategy towards implicit or controlled encoding processes, respectively. Most importantly, in solvers but not in non-solvers, response patterns were transformed overnight, enhancing responses in the ventral medial prefrontal cortex, an area also implicated in the consolidation of declarative memory. Together, these changes in brain activity suggest that hippocampal-prefrontal interaction can lead to improved explicit solutions in this task whereas hippocampal-basal ganglia interaction leads to implicit improvement, i.e., improved response times without explicit solutions to the task.

Obviously, looking for signs of reprocessing during sleep is the most difficult to do, because based on imaging data alone it is hard to distinguish from reorganization, and there are only few behavioral tasks that are designed to examine such changes. Still, it is important to remember that memory is not a one-to-one copy of reality, and that memory consolidation always involves reprocessing of the memory content. However, especially this area seems to require more in-depth studies.

Conclusion

It is long known that the brain representation of a memory changes over time. The functional imaging studies presented in this chapter indicate, that, at least in part, these changes relate to sleep. Different brain regions are active during memory recall depending on whether a subject slept or stayed awake after learning. Some of these differences can be found after a few hours, some develop over longer periods of up to several months. Functional connectivity also changes over time, depending on

sleep, perhaps designating very early which path a memory will take and which brain systems will be involved in its long-term storage. These changes over sleep periods are possibly the result of reactivation processes. Reactivation of task-related areas occurs during sleep, is not only fatigue-related but specific to the learning material, and correlates with later performance. Finally, there are some indications that sleep does not only strengthen existing memories, but also reprocesses and changes content and structure of the memories, making them more useful. It should, however, not be omitted that reactivation has also been found during periods of wakefulness in animals and in humans [46, 47]. It occurs for both declarative (hippocampus) and procedural (caudate) memories and can be seen during quiet wakefulness as well as during active wakefulness timed to an unrelated cognitive task. Whether reactivation has different purposes during sleep and wakefulness is currently unknown.

All things considered, present experiments allow us to conclude that sleep alters memory consolidation, and that the influence of sleep on later brain activity differs from that of comparable periods of wakefulness. However, when reconsidering some of the main questions asked at the beginning of the chapter, some of them do not have a definite answer, yet. All types of memory, declarative and procedural, spatial and contextual, neutral and emotional, have been found to depend on sleep; however, sometimes changes can only be found in brain activity, but not in behavioral performance. Activity in areas related to initial stimulus processing and learning seem to be activated rather at earlier points in time whereas later testing rather finds activity in previously uninvolved brain regions, speaking for both reactivation and reorganization of the memory representations, respectively. Thus, there seem to be different processes at work during sleep, perhaps interdependently. Yet, no specific brain area is related to consolidation during sleep. All areas related to stimulus processing and memory have been found at some stages of memory consolidation. Generally, it appears, however, that the hippocampus is rather involved soon after learning whereas other areas (striatum, medial prefrontal cortex) are involved in later stages. The changing activity pattern supports the notion that the memory trace is not only (quantitatively) strengthened, but also (qualitatively) changed during consolidation. Taken together, functional imaging studies on memory confirm that brain systems involved in memory storage reorganize during consolidation and that this transformation depends on sleep. The nature of these changes is not clear in detail, yet, and future studies will have to look in more detail into the different brain systems involved in memory storages.

References

1. Diekelmann S, Born J. The memory function of sleep. *Nat Rev Neurosci.* 2010;**11**:114–26.

2. Walker MP. A refined model of sleep and the time course of memory formation. *Behav Brain Sci.* 2005;**28**:51–64.

3. Rotenberg VS. Sleep and memory. II: Investigations on humans. *Neurosci Biobehav Rev.* 1992;**16**:503–5.

4. Karni A, Tanne D, Rubenstein BS, *et al.* Dependence on REM sleep of overnight improvement of a perceptual skill. *Science.* 1994;**265**:679–82.

5. Walker MP, Stickgold R. Sleep, memory, and plasticity. *Annu Rev Psychol.* 2006;**57**:139–66.

6. Heine R. Über wiedererkennen und rückwirkende hemmung. *Z Psychol.* 1914;**68**:161–236.

7. Van Ormer EB. Retention after intervals of sleep and waking. *Arch Psychol.* 1932; **21**:1–49.

8. Ekstrand BR, Barrett TR, West JN, *et al.* The effect of sleep on human long-term memory. In: Drucker-Colin RR, McGaugh JL, eds. *Neurobiology of Sleep and Memory.* New York, Academic Press. 1977;419–38.

9. Maquet P. The role of sleep in learning and memory. *Science.* 2001;**294**:1048–52.

10. Buzsáki G. Two-stage model of memory trace formation: a role for "noisy" brain states. *Neuroscience.* 1989;**31**:551–70.

11. McClelland JL, McNaughton BL, O'Reilly RC. Why there are complementary learning systems in the hippocampus and neocortex: insights from the successes and failures of connectionist models of learning and memory. *Psychol Rev.* 1995;**102**:419–57.

12. Euston DR, Tatsuno M, McNaughton BL. Fast-forward playback of recent memory sequences in prefrontal cortex during sleep. *Science.* 2007;**318**:1147–50.

13. Pavlides C, Winson J. Influences of hippocampal place cell firing in the awake state on the activity of these cells during subsequent sleep episodes. *J Neurosci.* 1989;**9**:2907–18.

14. Maquet P, Laureys S, Peigneux P, *et al.* Experience-dependent changes in cerebral activation during human REM sleep. *Nat Neurosci.* 2000;**3**:831–6.

15. Peigneux P, Laureys S, Fuchs S, *et al.* Learned material content and acquisition level modulate cerebral reactivation during posttraining rapid-eye-movements sleep. *Neuroimage.* 2003;**20**:125–34.

16. Maquet P, Schwartz S, Passingham R, *et al.* Sleep-related consolidation of a visuomotor skill: brain mechanisms as assessed by functional magnetic resonance imaging. *J Neurosci.* 2003;**23**:1432–40.

17. Schwartz S, Maquet P, Frith C. Neural correlates of perceptual learning: a functional MRI study of visual texture discrimination. *Proc Natl Acad Sci U S A.* 2002;**99**:17137–42.

18. Stickgold R, James L, Hobson JA. Visual discrimination learning requires sleep after training. *Nat Neurosci.* 2000;**3**:1237–8.

19. Walker MP, Stickgold R, Jolesz FA, *et al.* The functional anatomy of sleep-dependent visual skill learning. *Cereb Cortex.* 2005;**15**:1666–75.

20. Mednick SC, Arman AC, Boynton GM. The time course and specificity of perceptual deterioration. *Proc Natl Acad Sci U S A.* 2005;**102**:3881–5.

21. Walker MP, Brakefield T, Morgan A, *et al.* Practice with sleep makes perfect: sleep-dependent motor skill learning. *Neuron.* 2002;**35**:205–11.

22. Walker MP, Stickgold R, Alsop D, *et al.* Sleep-dependent motor memory plasticity in the human brain. *Neuroscience.* 2005;**133**:911–17.

23. Rasch B, Büchel C, Gais S, *et al.* Odor cues during slow-wave sleep prompt declarative memory consolidation. *Science.* 2007;**315**:1426–9.

24. Peigneux P, Laureys S, Fuchs S, *et al.* Are spatial memories strengthened in the human hippocampus during slow wave sleep? *Neuron.* 2004;**44**:535–45.

25. Bergmann TO, Molle M, Diedrichs J, *et al.* Sleep spindle-related reactivation of category-specific cortical regions after learning face-scene associations. *Neuroimage.* 2012;**59**:2733–42.

26. Gais S, Mölle M, Helms K, *et al.* Learning-dependent increases in sleep spindle density. *J Neurosci.* 2002;**22**:6830–4.

27. Clemens Z, Molle M, Eross L, *et al.* Fine-tuned coupling between human parahippocampal ripples and sleep spindles. *Eur J Neurosci.* 2011;**33**:511–20.

28. Girardeau G, Zugaro M. Hippocampal ripples and memory consolidation. *Curr Opin Neurobiol.* 2011;**21**:452–9.

29. Takashima A, Petersson KM, Rutters F, *et al.* Declarative memory consolidation in humans: a prospective functional magnetic resonance imaging study. *Proc Natl Acad Sci U S A.* 2006;**103**:756–61.

30. Frankland PW, Bontempi B. The organization of recent and remote memories. *Nat Rev Neurosci.* 2005;**6**:119–30.

31. Bosshardt S, Degonda N, Schmidt CF, *et al.* One month of human memory consolidation enhances retrieval-related hippocampal activity. *Hippocampus.* 2005;**15**:1026–40.

32. Gais S, Albouy G, Boly M, *et al.* Sleep transforms the cerebral trace of declarative memories. *Proc Natl Acad Sci U S A.* 2007;**104**:18778–83.

33. Takashima A, Nieuwenhuis IL, Jensen O, *et al.* Shift from hippocampal to neocortical centered retrieval network with consolidation. *J Neurosci.* 2009;**29**:10087–93.

34. van Dongen EV, Takashima A, Barth M, *et al.* Functional connectivity during light sleep is correlated with memory performance for face-location associations. *Neuroimage.* 2011;**57**:262–70.

35. Andrade KC, Spoormaker VI, Dresler M, *et al.* Sleep spindles and hippocampal functional connectivity in human NREM sleep. *J Neurosci.* 2011;**31**:10331–9.

36. Orban P, Rauchs G, Balteau E, *et al.* Sleep after spatial learning promotes covert reorganization of brain activity. *Proc Natl Acad Sci U S A.* 2006;**103**:7124–9.

37. Rauchs G, Orban P, Schmidt C, *et al.* Sleep modulates the neural substrates of both spatial and contextual memory consolidation. *PLoS One.* 2008;**3**:e2949.

38. Sterpenich V, Albouy G, Boly M, *et al.* Sleep-related hippocampo-cortical interplay during emotional memory recollection. *PLoS Biol.* 2007;**5**:e282.

39. Sterpenich V, Albouy G, Darsaud A, *et al.* Sleep promotes the neural reorganization of remote emotional memory. *J Neurosci.* 2009;**29**:5143–52.

40. Payne JD, Kensinger EA. Sleep leads to changes in the emotional memory trace: evidence from FMRI. *J Cogn Neurosci.* 2011;**23**:1285–97.

41. Loftus E. Our changeable memories: legal and practical implications. *Nat Rev Neurosci.* 2003;**4**:231–4.

42. Saletin JM, Goldstein AN, Walker MP. The role of sleep in directed forgetting and remembering of human memories. *Cereb Cortex.* 2011;**21**:2534–41.

43. Rauchs G, Feyers D, Landeau B, *et al.* Sleep contributes to the strengthening of some memories over others, depending on hippocampal activity at learning. *J Neurosci.* 2011;**31**:2563–8.

44. Wagner U, Gais S, Haider H, *et al.* Sleep inspires insight. *Nature.* 2004;**427**:352–5.

45. Darsaud A, Wagner U, Balteau E, *et al.* Neural precursors of delayed insight. *J Cogn Neurosci.* 2011;**23**:1900–10.

46. Carr MF, Jadhav SP, Frank LM. Hippocampal replay in the awake state: a potential substrate for memory consolidation and retrieval. *Nat Neurosci.* 2011;**14**:147–53.

47. Peigneux P, Orban P, Balteau E, *et al.* Offline persistence of memory-related cerebral activity during active wakefulness. *PLoS Biol.* 2006;**4**:e100.

Chapter

23

Imaging causes and consequences of insomnia and sleep complaints

Eus J. W. Van Someren, Ellemarije Altena, Jennifer R. Ramautar, Diederick Stoffers, Jeroen S. Benjamins, Sarah Moens, Eun Yeon Joo, Seung Bong Hong, and Ysbrand D. Van Der Werf

Introduction

The contents of the present volume, on *Neuroimaging of Sleep and Sleep Disorders,* leave no doubt on the relevance of a good night's sleep to support optimal brain function. For about one out of ten people, a good night's sleep is not easily accomplished. They complain of a prolonged latency to fall asleep, problems in maintaining sleep, early morning awakening, or non-restorative sleep. They moreover report significant daytime cognitive, emotional, social, or professional impairments as a consequence of their troubled sleep. If this situation occurs at least three times a week and for at least three months, they are likely to have the diagnosis of insomnia. In most sufferers, insomnia is a chronic condition. Half of the people experiencing insomnia today will still suffer from it next year. Insomnia can occur in isolation, but is also a very common comorbidity with other disorders. With a prevalence of 6–11% in the general population, insomnia is the most frequent complaint in general practice, psychological practice, and the sleep clinic alike. Insomnia is an all but trivial complaint, and its impact on society cannot be overemphasized; not only with respect to the number of people suffering, but also with respect to its consequences. While its prevalence increases up to ~40% with aging, it is becoming evident that insomnia significantly increases the risk of developing the most common mental and physical health problems of our aging society, including depression, cardiovascular disease, obesity, and the metabolic syndrome (reviewed in [1, 2]).

Despite the evident need to unravel its underlying brain mechanisms in order to treat insomnia effectively, studies investigating this are highly underrepresented. In particular, compared to the much less frequently occurring other sleep and psychiatric disorders, amazingly few studies have applied neuroimaging tools to better understand insomnia. The present review summarizes the few neuroimaging studies that have reported on insomnia. It includes some observations on neuroimaging correlates of poor sleep in elderly people and common sleep disturbances of old age. The scarcity of studies to summarize leaves room for the present review to suggest a number of avenues to explore using neuroimaging tools. These include both new views on possible brain mechanisms involved as well as suggestions to optimize the methodology of the direly needed future studies.

A first major question for imaging studies to address refers to the brain mechanisms involved in insomnia. What *causes* insomnia? What puts someone *at risk* of developing insomnia? What are the *neural correlates* of the experience of lying awake all night and suffering from that during daytime? A logical starting point to tackle these questions may be to investigate whether deviations exist in the neuronal networks and mechanisms involved in normal sleep regulation. The regulation of sleep and wakefulness is usually modeled with two underlying processes: a circadian "clock" process C and a homeostatic "hourglass" process S [3–5].

The central *clock* of our brain is located in the hypothalamic suprachiasmatic nucleus (SCN). It promotes sleep during one part of the 24-h day–night cycle and wakefulness during the other part [6]. The SCN affects sleep-regulatory systems of the brain indirectly, mostly via projections to the ventral subparaventricular zone (vSPZ) and from there to the dorsomedial hypothalamus (DMH), where clock signals are integrated with other inputs, including those associated with cognition from the prefrontal cortex and with emotion from the limbic system [7]. There is some support for involvement of deviant 24-h rhythm regulation in association with difficulties initiating or maintaining sleep in insomnia (reviewed in [8]). There is more conclusive support for a role of clock malfunction in the fragmented sleep that characterizes very old age and neurodegenerative diseases, notably Alzheimer's disease (e.g., [9–12]). Given the small size of the SCN, it is a difficult area to evaluate using brain imaging. Still, two recent functional magnetic resonance imaging (fMRI) studies showed a blood oxygen level-dependent (BOLD) signal increase in an area compatible with the SCN; one study in response to environmental light, known to be a stimulus of primary importance to the SCN [13], and the other study in association with sustained attention [14].

As compared to the identification of the SCN as the clock of the brain, the neuroanatomical contours of the *homeostatic component* are less well defined. The homeostatic component refers to an hourglass-like process. Sleep pressure increases homeostatically with the duration of wakefulness. While we sleep, this pressure dissipates [15–17]. With respect to the underlying mechanisms of the homeostatic buildup, important roles have been assigned to an increase in synaptic density

Neuroimaging of Sleep and Sleep Disorders, ed. Eric Nofzinger, Pierre Maquet, and Michael J. Thorpy. Published by Cambridge University Press. © Cambridge University Press 2013.

during wakefulness [18], to cytokines [19], and especially to adenosine [20]. Although possible deviations in these mechanisms have not been investigated in insomnia, genetic variance in adenosine deaminase is associated with sleep depth [21]. We are unaware of neuroimaging studies that have identified areas that activate or deactivate in congruence with the presumed underlying changes in "process S." However, one fMRI study showed an interaction effect between homeostatic sleep pressure, task-induced activation, and chronotype. BOLD activity in an SCN-compatible region increased during maintenance of attention in the evening, and more pronounced so in "evening types" than in "morning types" [14].

The model with the two components C and S, and their interactions, has been invaluable for our progress to understand how sleep is regulated. There is no doubt that these two components are necessary to understand the maintenance and transitions of sleep and wakefulness. This does not mean, however, that investigating only C- and S-related processes will be sufficient in order to uncover possible deviations that could underlie insomnia. Several *sleep-permissive and wake-promoting conditions* are monitored by the brain, and moderate the efficacy by which the clock and homeostat succeed to initiate and maintain sleep [22]. These include posture, thermal comfort, danger, nutritional status, pain, and stress. The brain needs to monitor whether these conditions are optimal prior to giving in to shutting off conscious perception of the environment, which would not be safe otherwise. These conditions are fully met in virtually all laboratory and clinical studies on insomnia. It has seldom been studied whether insomniacs might differ from good sleepers in their response to changes in these conditions, while there are indications this is where things may go wrong.

The most consistent observation on what may be wrong in insomniacs is their, so-called, state of "hyperarousal." Whether in the cognitive domain, the emotional domain, central nervous system activity, or autonomic nervous system activity, insomniacs seem to be in a state of increased arousal day and night (reviewed in [1]). Whereas a highly aroused state is profitable for an organism's survival in the case of thermal discomfort, danger, famine, pain, and stress, it is not conductive to falling asleep. Hyperarousal may thus become problematic if it fails to discontinue after the condition that elicited it has resolved. From this perspective, hyperarousal may be proposed as a common final path of maladaptation in the systems that evaluate sleep-permissive and wake-promoting factors.

In the review on neuroimaging studies on insomnia that will follow, the possible causal implications of the findings will be addressed in light of the three mechanisms discussed: mechanisms related to the clock, to the homeostat, and to the evaluation and processing of sleep-permissive and wake-promoting conditions.

A second major question for imaging studies to address refers to the *consequences* of insomnia for brain structure and function. How do chronic complaints of insomnia affect the brain and cognitive functioning? Because relatively few studies have addressed this question, we include some observations on the consequences of other sleep disorders and of experimental sleep disruption. A critical question to evaluate is whether

experimental sleep disruption is a valid model for insomnia. Also, it should be stated up front that it will require many more imaging studies to be more confident on whether observed abnormalities reflect either cause or consequence.

The remainder of this review discusses imaging studies in insomnia and in association with insomnia complaints in people not diagnosed with insomnia. This review includes studies applying structural and functional MRI, magnetic resonance spectroscopy (MRS), high-density electroencephalography, and transcranial magnetic stimulation (TMS). Studies that applied single-photon emission computed tomography (SPECT) and positron emission tomography (PET) in insomnia are discussed in great detail in Chapter 24. The studies here reviewed have reported almost exclusively on regions of the temporal lobe, frontal lobe, and parietal lobe. These cortical regions are of interest because of their key involvement in the cognitive domains that are most affected in insomnia and after sleep deprivation. Episodic memory and the executive functions of working memory and creative problem solving belong to the most reliably affected cognitive domains not only in insomnia [23] but also after sleep deprivation, which moreover most strongly affects sustained attention [24, 25]. The medial temporal lobe, including the hippocampus, and its interaction with the medial prefrontal cortex are key to episodic memory [26, 27]; the prefrontal cortex is essential to executive functioning; and the frontoparietal network supports sustained attention (reviewed in [28]). For each of these three cortical regions, and insofar as data are available and relevant, the subsequent sections review correlational data in primary insomnia, correlational data in other disorders and healthy controls, and sleep manipulation data. Because of a lack of data relating their function or structure to insomnia, the occipital lobe and subcortical regions are not discussed in separate paragraphs (but see Chapter 24 for PET and SPECT findings in these areas). For each lobe, the review systematically addresses differences between insomniacs and controls and correlations of insomnia symptom severity with brain changes in both insomniacs and people not diagnosed with insomnia. Subsequently, the findings are summarized and interpreted with respect to functional relevance, pitfalls, and conclusions on cause, risk factor, or consequence.

Temporal lobe

The temporal lobe can be divided into a superior, middle, and inferior temporal gyrus on the lateral surface; the ventral temporal cortex; the temporal pole; and the medial temporal gyrus, which is limbic cortex. By far, most studies that used structural MRI to evaluate regional differences in brain volume or gray matter density between insomnia and controls have reported on the medial temporal lobe. This part consists of anatomically related structures that are essential for the conscious memory of facts and events (declarative memory), including the hippocampus surrounded by the perirhinal, entorhinal, and parahippocampal cortices, as well as the more rostrally and dorsally located amygdala, which is central to emotional processing.

Group differences

Group differences between insomnia patients and controls without sleep problems have been evaluated in a number of studies on temporal lobe volume and gray matter density. Riemann *et al.* reported eight insomniacs to have a lower hippocampal volume than eight controls without sleep complaints [29]. Patients with a psychiatric disorder were carefully excluded from this study, which is important given the meta-analytic confirmation that insomnia frequently co-occurs with psychiatric disorders that themselves are associated with lower hippocampal volume [30–33]. Winkelman and colleagues could not confirm a reduced hippocampal volume in a group of 20 slightly younger insomnia patients, as compared to 15 controls [34]; neither did a manually delineated hippocampal volumetric study by Noh *et al.* [35] on 20 insomniacs and 20 matched controls. Using whole-brain voxel-based morphometry (VBM), the group of Seung Bong Hong found a reduction in superior temporal gyrus gray matter density in 27 insomniacs compared with 27 matched controls (data presented at the Worldsleep 2011 meeting [36]). Altena *et al.* also applied whole-brain VBM but did not find any medial temporal lobe gray matter density differences between 24 carefully selected insomniacs and 13 matched controls [37].

At present, we are aware of only one published report on the application of resting state MRI to study functional connectivity of medial temporal lobe structures in insomnia and controls. Focusing on the amygdala, Huang *et al.* found functional connectivity of the amygdala with the insula, striatum, and thalamus to be decreased and with the premotor and sensorimotor cortices to be increased [38].

A number of studies investigated the *correlation of complaints* with regional brain volume *within a group of insomniacs*. Winkelman *et al.* reported that poor sleep efficiency and increased wake after sleep onset were moderately associated with lower hippocampal volume in 20 insomniacs [34]. Within a group of 20 insomniacs Noh *et al.* found a strong negative correlation of hippocampal volume with the duration of insomnia, as well as a moderate correlation with the polysomnographically determined number of arousals from sleep [35]. A negative correlation of gray matter density in the inferior temporal gyrus with sleep onset latency was reported, with the most severe sleep onset problems experienced by those with the least inferior temporal gyrus gray matter [36].

In the resting state MRI study of Huang *et al.* the increased functional connectivity of the amygdala with the premotor cortex was most pronounced in those insomnia patients that showed the most severe complaints [38].

Correlations of sleep parameters with regional volumes of the temporal lobe have also been investigated in studies targeting *people without the diagnosis of insomnia*, either healthy or suffering from a different disorder. Neylan *et al.* investigated patients suffering from post-traumatic stress disorder and reported a negative correlation of the severity of insomnia complaints with hippocampal volume in the CA3/dentate gyrus subfield [39]. Two studies that have not yet appeared as full papers suggest an association of hippocampal volume with sleep parameters in people older than the age of 50, not selected on insomnia complaints. In older women, Hall *et al.* demonstrated a positive relation of hippocampus gray matter volume with reported sleep duration [40]. In unpublished data from our own group on 138 home-dwelling elderly people around the age of 70 years, medial temporal lobe atrophy showed a moderate correlation with fragmentation of sleep and wakefulness in the actigraphically determined activity rhythm [41].

Summary, interpretation, and functional relevance

Concertedly, the findings suggest that there may be an association of insomnia with hippocampal volume loss, be it either a weak one, or an inconsistent one that is present in some subtypes of insomnia only. The association may moreover be present in some sleep parameters only: findings are suggestive of compromised hippocampal volume in association with short and/or fragmented sleep. As will be discussed below, experimental sleep deprivation and fragmentation indeed both affect neuronal activity in the hippocampus. The volume reduction might be involved in the reported negative association of disturbed sleep with performance on memory tasks [42–44], confirmed in a meta-analysis [23].

Pitfalls

There are several pitfalls that need to be discussed in relation to hippocampal volume studies in insomnia. First, meta-analyses indicate hippocampal volume loss in depression [30], post-traumatic stress disorder [31], and schizophrenia [32]. Comorbid insomnia is highly prevalent in these disorders [33]. Most studies on hippocampal volume in insomnia thus rightfully excluded people diagnosed with a psychiatric syndrome. However, true matching of insomniacs and controls on relevant subclinical psychiatric *symptom scores* has seldom been accomplished, with the notable exception of the study by Altena *et al.* [37]. It may be valuable for future studies to investigate insomniacs with and without elevated scores on a psychiatric symptom scale such as depression, with each group matched by good sleeping controls likewise selected on the presence or absence of elevated scores. These types of studies may help elucidate whether hippocampal volume loss in insomnia is secondary to subclinical psychiatric symptoms. Interestingly, the association may be the other way around as well [37], i.e., that some volumetric changes in psychiatric disorders are secondary to the sleep problems that the patients usually suffer from.

Risk factor, cause?

There is little reason to propose that medial temporal lobe volume loss may predispose someone to develop insomnia. Although the expression of sleep is regulated by an extensive neuronal network comprising several nuclei and cortical areas, structures in the medial temporal lobe have never been proposed to be key to sleep regulation. Theoretically, input from the limbic system, to which the amygdala in the medial temporal lobe belongs, could modulate clock input at the level of the

DMH, where both these inputs are integrated with several others [7]. However, structural studies on insomnia never reported on amygdala volume, only on hippocampal volume. If the hippocampus is essentially involved in sleep regulation and insomnia complaints, disturbed sleep would be a commonly reported phenomenon in patients where part of the hippocampus was resected to alleviate epilepsy. As far as we have been able to track, not even case studies reporting such a consequence have appeared.

Consequence?

On the other hand, quite a number of observations suggest that disrupted sleep may be causally involved in the observed changes in hippocampal volume. In a 20-year longitudinal study of 48 postmenopausal women, the degree of gray matter loss in the right hippocampus was predicted by higher perceived stress at baseline [45]. Experimental sleep manipulation studies in healthy controls do support hippocampal sensitivity to disrupted sleep. Using fMRI, Yoo *et al.* demonstrated that one night of sleep deprivation leads to a suboptimal BOLD activation of the hippocampus during episodic memory encoding, and subsequently worse retention [46]. Van der Werf *et al.* showed that similar hippocampal and memory deficiencies already occur with a much milder sleep disruption that consisted of acoustic interruptions from slow-wave sleep [47]. Hippocampal sensitivity to sleep deprivation is confirmed by animal studies investigating hippocampal neurogenesis and cell proliferation [48, 49] and electrophysiological characteristics of neurons (reviewed in [50]).

Frontal lobe

The frontal cortex is the largest of the cortical lobes and is the cortical area lying anteriorly to the central sulcus; its general function is geared towards production of behavior rather than perception, which is related to the cortical regions lying posteriorly. Of the frontal cortex, the primary motor, premotor, and supplementary motor areas are involved in motor execution and do not belong to association cortex. The main connections are with the striatum and within and between the different parts of the motor cortical system. The remainder of the frontal cortex is called the prefrontal cortex, which covers part of the lateral convexity of the frontal lobe, the orbital surface, and medial cortex until its boundary with the limbic lobe. The superior and inferior prefrontal sulcus divide up the lateral prefrontal cortex into a superior, middle, and inferior prefrontal gyrus that are involved in various aspects of working memory, planning and programming of behavior, or complex problem solving; often these processes are collectively called executive or prefrontal functions. The main connections of these regions are with the other associational cortices, i.e., the parieto-occipitotemporal neocortex and the temporal pole. The ventral and medial prefrontal cortices appear to be more involved in emotional processing, reflected in relatively stronger connections with limbic structures such as the amygdala. Functional imaging studies have shown that especially the prefrontal areas decrease their activity during sleep, implying a possible functional interaction.

Group differences

Group differences between insomnia patients and controls without sleep problems have been evaluated in a number of studies on prefrontal volume, gray matter density, and functional activation (fMRI) as well as on the insomnia response to TMS. In the only published study to date using a whole-brain VBM analysis in clinically diagnosed insomniacs and matched controls, Altena *et al.* found insomnia patients to have a lower gray matter density in the orbitofrontal cortex (OFC) [37], as illustrated in Figure 23.1. This study not only excluded patients with a psychiatric disorder but went one step further to also exclude insomniacs with elevated, yet subclinical, depression

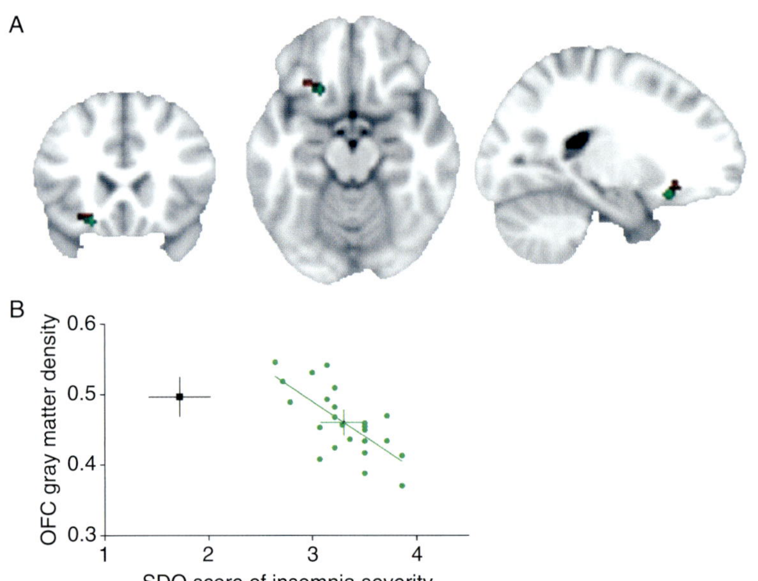

Figure 23.1 (A) Insomnia patients have a lower gray matter density in the left orbitofrontal cortex than controls, indicated by the red cluster. Regression analysis within the group of insomnia patients shows a strong negative relation between gray matter volume in the OFC and severity of insomnia measured by the SDQ-insomnia subscale. Green voxels indicate the OFC area, partly overlapping with the group difference cluster, where gray matter volume correlated significantly with severity of insomnia, with the strongest regression coefficient of b = −0.71 at voxel x = −20, y = 22, z = −14. Slices shown at these coordinates. OFC = orbitofrontal cortex. (B) Scatter plot with the SDQ insomnia subscale rating on the abscissa and the average value for gray matter density within the cluster, after controlling for age and total gray matter (GM) volume, on the ordinate. Individual insomnia patients are shown as green dots. The average of the controls is indicated by the black square. Error bars indicate the group 95% confidence intervals. (Adapted from Altena *et al.* [37].)

and anxiety ratings. A VBM study by the group of Seung Bong Hong, presented at the Worldsleep 2011 meeting, confirmed a reduction in orbitofrontal gray matter density in insomnia [36]. In this study, a reduction in frontal gray matter density was also found in the inferior and middle frontal gyri and the precentral gyrus. Riemann *et al.* on the other hand, found no volume differences in either orbitofrontal or dorsolateral selected regions of interest, which were manually delineated, in middle-aged insomnia patients [29].

Proton MRS (^{1}H-MRS) can be used to determine non-invasively gamma-aminobutynic acid (GABA) levels in the brain. Winkelman *et al.* estimated GABA in a central region of the brain of insomniacs that included not only parts of the frontal, temporal, parietal, and occipital cortex and white matter, but also the basal ganglia and thalamus [51]. Average brain GABA levels were a third lower in insomnia patients.

To date, only one published study used fMRI to investigate task-elicited activation in insomnia. Altena *et al.* report deviant prefrontal activation in insomnia patients performing fluency tasks [52]. They show less activation in task-related prefrontal regions (inferior frontal gyrus, medial prefrontal cortex) compared with controls without sleep complaints, as illustrated in Figure 23.2. Sleep therapy led to partial recovery. Remarkably, in spite of the hypoactivation, insomnia patients generated more words on both letter and category fluency tasks than matched controls without sleep complaints, suggestive of highly efficient compensatory mechanisms. Although compensatory activation in specific regions could not be detected [52], it may be that different subjects activate different brain regions, precluding the detection of a group effect. Further subtyping of insomnia, as well as larger samples, would seem necessary to map possibly different compensatory brain processes. The superior word fluency performance in insomnia deserves further attention. It might result from the hyperaroused state, or perfectionism, that characterizes many insomniacs [53–56]. It might also be involved in the tendency to ruminate, one of the most characteristic complaints of insomniacs (cf. [57]).

The use of high-density electroencephalography (EEG) allows for the mapping of scalp electrical activity to underlying sources in the brain. Szelenberger and Niencewiez measured high-density EEG during the Continuous Attention Test, a visual recognition task, and estimated source activation using low-resolution brain electromagnetic tomography (LORETA) [58]. Compared with controls, insomnia patients showed less event-related current density in the orbitofrontal, medial prefrontal, anterior cingulate, and premotor corties, as well as increased activation in the left dorsolateral prefrontal cortex (DLPFC). Notably, in agreement with the fMRI study of Altena *et al.* [52] mentioned above, differences in brain activation occurred in the absence of compromised performance.

The use of TMS allows for the non-invasive study of cortical excitability, interconnections, and balance between excitatory and inhibitory neurons [59, 60]. Motor cortical dysfunction is not a hallmark of poor sleep; yet, the motor cortex can be used as a model system for testing basic processes of cortical processing such as inhibition and facilitation. Using TMS, a painless and safe technique to deliver short-lived and focal stimulations to cortical regions of choice, it is possible to elicit visible responses from body parts when applying stimulation over the motor representation of the corresponding body part in the precentral gyrus [60]. When pulses are given in a paired fashion, also known as double-pulse stimulation, the first pulse acts to modulate the response to the second pulse. Depending on the duration of the interval between the pre-pulse and the test pulse, the modulation changes from inhibition (short inter-pulse intervals, i.e., < ~7 ms) to facilitation (longer inter-pulse intervals, i.e., ~7–15 ms). This allows the testing subjects with disorders of the nervous system or in specific conditions with respect to inhibitory and facilitatory interactions that reflect intracortical processes likely mediated by local pools of interneurons [61]. Van der Werf *et al.* have shown, using the double-pulse method over the primary motor cortex of the precentral gyrus, that patients with primary insomnia show a distinct difference compared with controls in their intracortical inhibition and facilitation [62], as illustrated in Figure 23.3.

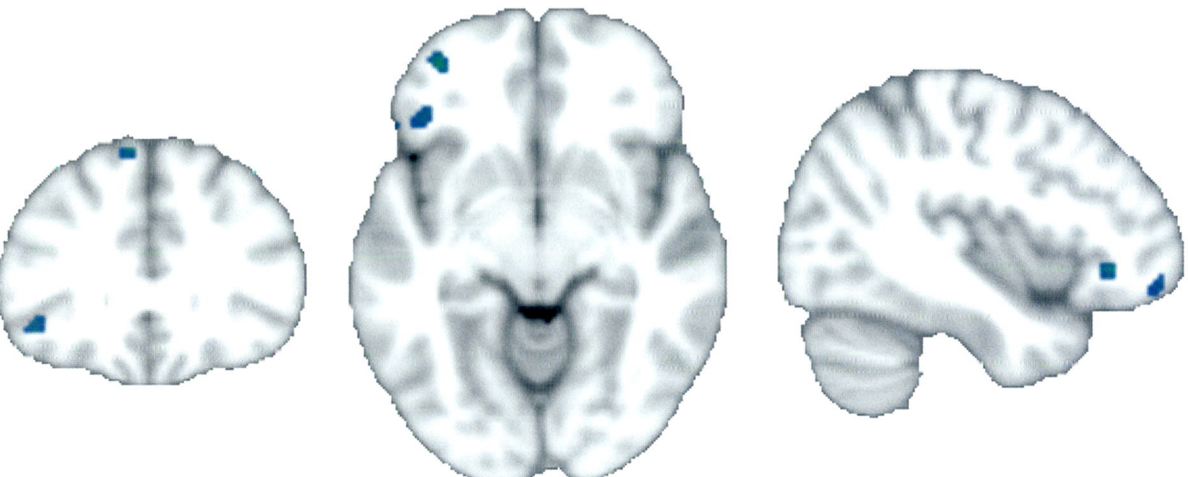

Figure 23.2 Lower activation in the left inferior frontal gyrus and medial prefrontal cortex (BA 44–45, BA 9) during word fluency in insomnia as compared to controls. Slices shown at x = −40, y = 30, z = −8. (Adapted from Altena *et al.* [52].)

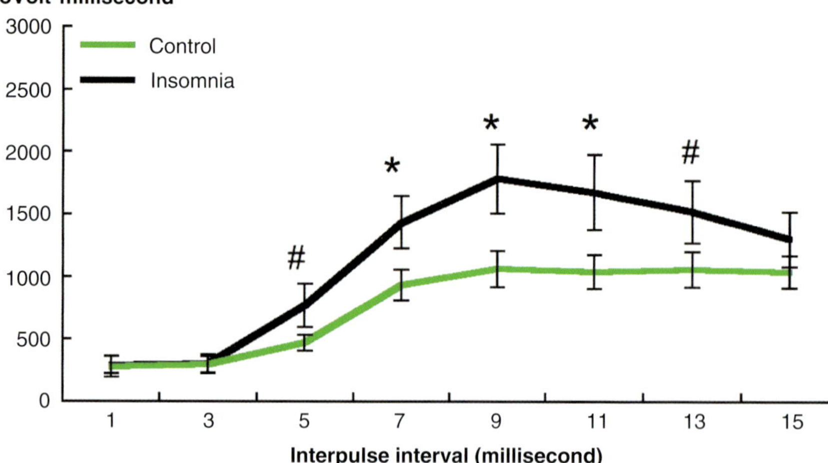

Figure 23.3 Insomnia patients show an increased response to double-pulse transcranial magnetic stimulation. The graph shows the area under the curve of the average motor-evoked potentials in response to double pulses with varying interpulse intervals. Notice the higher responses of insomnia patients across the different double-pulse types, yet the relative lessening of this exaggerated response at the higher inter pulse intervals, as described in Van der Werf *et al.* [62]. * Significant difference at $p \leq 0.05$; trend at $P = 0.10$.

Specifically, the patients showed exaggerated responses to the test pulses, but failed to show the relative facilitation with the longer inter-pulse intervals. Such exaggerated responses possibly reflect strong input–output relations in response to cortically applied stimuli, in accord with the idea of hyperarousal. They also suggest a cortical imbalance between excitatory glutamatergic and inhibitory GABA ergic neurotransmission.

Two studies investigated the *correlation of complaints* with frontal lobe gray matter density *within a group of insomniacs*. Interestingly, the orbitofrontal gray matter density reduction reported by Altena *et al.* showed a strong negative relation with insomnia severity; the most severe insomnia was experienced by those with the least orbitofrontal gray matter [37]. Winkelman *et al.* showed that average brain GABA levels were lower in insomnia patients with more severely disturbed sleep as indicated by their wake after sleep onset [51].

Only one study investigated the *correlation of insomnia complaints* with frontal lobe damage in *people without the diagnosis of insomnia*. In a group of 199 veterans who suffered brain damage from penetrating head injuries in the Vietnam war, computed tomography (CT) scans indicated that lesions in the 27 subjects with a score of 2 or greater on the Hamilton Anxiety Rating Scale (HAM-A) insomnia item were significantly more likely to include the left dorsomedial prefrontal cortex, located just superior and medial to the left insula [63]. Also worth mentioning is a stroke lesion study which showed that stroke patients with insula lesions more frequently suffer from typical insomnia complaints of anergia and tiredness than the control group of patients with stroke that did not affect the insula [64].

Summary, interpretation, and functional relevance

In summary, brain structural findings suggest that there may be an association of insomnia with a relatively low gray matter density, or damage, in prefrontal regions including the OFC, the inferior and middle frontal gyri, the dorsomedial prefrontal cortex, the insula, and the precentral gyrus. One ^{1}H-MRS study found less GABA in a central region of the brain of insomniacs that included not only parts of the frontal, temporal, parietal and occipital cortices, and white matter but also the basal ganglia and thalamus [51]. A functional study using fMRI reported hypoactivation of the inferior frontal gyrus and medial prefrontal cortex. A functional study using high-density EEG source mapping found hypoactivation of the orbitofrontal, medial prefrontal, anterior cingulate, and premotor cortices. This study was also the only one reporting enhanced activation in insomnia, which was limited to the left DLPFC. A functional study using TMS reported hyperexcitability of the precentral gyrus. As is the case for the medial temporal lobe deviations in insomnia, the associations are either weak ones, or inconsistent ones that are present in some subtypes of insomnia only. The reported changes in prefrontal structure and function might be involved in the reported negative association of disturbed sleep with executive functioning, notably working memory and creative problem solving in both insomnia [23] and sleep-deprived normal sleepers [24, 25].

Pitfalls

Pitfalls that need to be discussed in relation to insomnia studies on frontal structure and function are, as for the hippocampal volume studies, that frontal lobe deviations have frequently been reported in association with psychiatric disorders. It is thus of the utmost importance to verify whether reported associations with insomnia are not secondary to elevated scores on psychiatric symptom scales. Both the study of Koenigs *et al.* [63] and the study of Altena *et al.* [37] elegantly accounted for this potential pitfall.

Risk factor, cause?

The orbitofrontal cortical area where a lower gray matter density was reported in insomniacs is of key importance in the neuronal coding of the subjective experience of pleasure and comfort [65, 66], including thermal comfort judgments [67, 68]. Interestingly, the judgment of thermal comfort is compromised in insomniacs [69]. In line with the notion of sleep-permissive and wake-promoting conditions mentioned in the introduction, it is tempting to suggest that this structural and functional deficiency may leave sleep regulating structures void of a "green light for sleep" signal; from an evolutionary perspective it is not wise to lose consciousness if the environment is not comfortable. From this perspective, and supported by a lack of correlation with the duration of insomnia that would be expected if the OFC gray matter loss was a consequence of insomnia, it seems plausible to suggest that people at the lower end of the normal distribution of OFC gray matter density may have an increased risk of developing insomnia.

Dysfunction of the lateral orbital frontal circuit has also been associated with rumination, based on findings in obsessive–compulsive disorder (cf. [70]). Another area that is critically involved in rumination and "self-talk" is the left inferior frontal gyrus [71, 72]. Because rumination belongs to the most characteristic aspects of insomnia, further research into the involvement of the orbitofrontal [36, 37] and left inferior frontal gyrus [36, 37] abnormalities in insomnia are warranted. Moreover, the hyperactivation of the DLPFC in insomniacs shown by Szelenberger *et al.* [58] has also been seen during rumination in depressed patients [73].

Interestingly, the same sleep therapy that normalized prefrontal activation during word fluency [52] did not normalize the deviant cortical excitability shown using TMS [62]. This indicates that the abnormalities in cortical excitability are either more persistent and take longer to resolve, or alternatively could be another trait or endophenotype putting someone at risk of developing insomnia.

Consequence?

In a 20-year longitudinal study of 48 postmenopausal women, the degree of gray matter loss in the right OFC was predicted by higher perceived stress at baseline [45]. On the one hand, this may be interpreted as support for the possibility that structural changes in the OFC are not so much associated to sleep problems per se, but rather to an underlying sensitivity to stress, which then puts one at risk of developing insomnia. Several studies indeed indicate that the perception of stress, even more than the actual exposure to stress, is a trait-like risk factor for the development of insomnia [74–76]. On the other hand, the way by which stress sensitivity would induce structural brain changes is unresolved. Given the numerous studies that indicate derailment of neuronal function after sleep disruption, disturbed sleep could conceptually mediate at least part of the effect. Some animal work supports the possibility of functional consequences of sleep deprivation for prefrontal functioning, for example by interfering with the sleep-dependent gene expression that follows long-term potentiation [77].

Parietal lobe

The parietal cortex lies posterior to the central sulcus. Immediately postcentrally, the primary, secondary, and tertiary somatosensory cortices are found. Posterior to these, the deep horizontal intraparietal sulcus separates the superior and inferior parietal cortices. Together with the cortical fields lying inside the intraparietal sulcus these are areas that are globally involved in spatial processing and in converting visual information into constraints for movements, such as in tool use, but also in calculation and direction of (spatial) attention. The borders between the parietal cortex and the occipital and temporal cortices do not have clear landmarks; the region occupying the territory between the parietal, occipital, and temporal lobes is considered a transitional area between the three; it is neocortex and multimodal in nature, meaning it does not belong to any of the senses in particular. This is the parieto-occipitotemporal associational cortex of the brain that, together with the prefrontal cortex and the temporal pole, mediates higher-order cognitive processes.

Group differences

Group differences between insomnia patients and controls without sleep problems have been reported in two whole-brain VBM studies in clinically diagnosed insomniacs and matched controls. Altena *et al.* found insomnia patients to have a lower gray matter density in the anterior precuneus (BA 7) of the parietal cortex, extending to the transition area between the precuneus and primary somatosensory cortex in the postcentral gyrus [37]. An ongoing VBM study by the group of Seung Bong Hong, presented at the Worldsleep 2011 meeting, also found a reduction in gray matter density in the postcentral gyrus [36].

Summary, interpretation, and functional relevance

It would be of interest to evaluate the relevance of the reported low gray matter density in the precuneus [37] for activity in the default mode network (DMN), of which the precuneus is a key part. This brain network is active in the absence of task demands during restful waking as well as during sleep [78]. It is conceivable that a reduced gray matter density in an essential part of the DMN could result in a reduced capacity to disengage from external information processing, as has been reported in insomnia [79], and enter the resting state. Studies into resting state networks in insomnia are warranted.

The postcentral gyrus is the location of the primary somatosensory cortex, the main receptive area for input from the skin of the body signaling the senses of touch and temperature. Given the importance of skin temperature for sleep and alertness [80–83], as well as the deficiency in thermal comfort sensing in insomnia [84], further research into both primary (involving the postcentral gyrus) and higher-order (involving the OFC) temperature and thermal comfort sensing in insomnia is warranted. Too few data on the parietal lobe are available to justify a discussion on causes and consequences.

General conclusion

It is clear that neuroimaging has only just begun to investigate the brain of insomniacs. Very few of the abnormalities found can be related to the classical view of sleep regulation by a *clock* and a *homeostat*. Some of the findings are more compatible with abnormalities in the *monitoring of sleep-permissive and wake-promoting conditions*. Although interesting leads have been revealed, some inconsistency in the findings should be noted. We suggest these to be due to different phenotypes of insomnia. With a prevalence of about 10%, it is unlikely that a single diagnostic category suits the entire heterogeneous group of people wrestling with poor sleep. The situation may be compared to the diagnosis of dementia many years ago; by now we know that it is essential to differentiate between Alzheimer's, vascular, frontotemporal dementia, etc. Finding homogeneous subgroups of insomnia phenotypes may be essential [85] and now seems possible. Widespread Internet access allows for large-scale international studies applying questionnaires and computerized tasks to obtain a multivariate psychometric characterization of insomnia subtypes. Our group has developed a freely available tool for web-based assessment to facilitate introduction of this innovative research approach in worldwide cohort studies on insomnia. Subsequent application of neuroimaging tools to selected homogeneous subgroups rather than representative heterogeneous samples will strongly increase the likelihood of finding robust abnormalities. Areas and networks of major interest include especially those that are relevant to hyperarousal, to hedonic and emotional processing, to rumination, and to consciousness and making memories versus unawareness and forgetting of nocturnal awakenings. As will become even more clear in Chapter 24; on PET and SPECT studies in insomnia, neuroimaging has a high promise to reveal insights into the causes and consequences of insomnia, the first necessary steps towards a better treatment of a disorder that has such an enormous impact on so many people.

References

1. Riemann D, Spiegelhalder K, Espie C, *et al.* Chronic insomnia: clinical and research challenges–an agenda. *Pharmacopsychiatry.* 2011;**44**:1–14.

2. Baglioni C, Battagliese G, Feige B, *et al.* Insomnia as a predictor of depression: A meta-analytic evaluation of longitudinal epidemiological studies. *J Affect Disord.* 2011;**135**:10–19.

3. Borbély AA. A two process model of sleep regulation. *Hum Neurobiol.* 1982;**1**:195–204.

4. Daan S, Beersma DG, Borbely AA. Timing of human sleep: recovery process gated by a circadian pacemaker. *Am J Physiol.* 1984;**246**:R161–83.

5. Dijk DJ, Czeisler CA. Contribution of the circadian pacemaker and the sleep homeostat to sleep propensity, sleep structure, electroencephalographic slow waves, and sleep spindle activity in humans. *J Neurosci.* 1995;**15**:3526–38.

6. Mistlberger RE. Circadian regulation of sleep in mammals: role of the suprachiasmatic nucleus. *Brain Res Rev.* 2005;**49**:429–54.

7. Saper CB, Scammell TE, Lu J. Hypothalamic regulation of sleep and circadian rhythms. *Nature.* 2005;**437**:1257–63.

8. Lack LC, Gradisar M, Van Someren EJW, Wright HR, Lushington K. The relationship between insomnia and body temperatures. *Sleep Med Rev.* 2008;**12**:307–17.

9. Swaab DF, Fliers E, Partiman TS. The suprachiasmatic nucleus of the human brain in relation to sex, age and senile dementia. *Brain Res.* 1985;**342**:37–44.

10. Van Someren EJW, Riemersma-Van Der Lek RF. Live to the rhythm, slave to the rhythm. *Sleep Med Rev.* 2007;**11**:465–84.

11. Harper DG, Stopa EG, Kuo-Leblanc V, *et al.* Dorsomedial scn neuronal subpopulations subserve different functions in human dementia. *Brain.* 2008;**131**:1609–17.

12. Hu K, Van Someren EJW, Shea SA, Scheer FA. Reduction of scale invariance of activity fluctuations with aging and Alzheimer's disease: involvement of the circadian pacemaker. *Proc Natl Acad Sci U S A.* 2009;**106**:2490–4.

13. Vimal RL, Pandey-Vimal MU, Vimal LS, *et al.* Activation of suprachiasmatic nuclei and primary visual cortex depends upon time of day. *Eur J Neurosci.* 2009;**29**:399–410.

14. Schmidt C, Collette F, Leclercq Y, *et al.* Homeostatic sleep pressure and responses to sustained attention in the suprachiasmatic area. *Science.* 2009;**324**:516–19.

15. Achermann P, Dijk DJ, Brunner DP, Borbely AA. A model of human sleep homeostasis based on eeg slow-wave activity: quantitative comparison of data and simulations. *Brain Res Bull.* 1993;**31**:97–113.

16. Leemburg S, Vyazovskiy VV, Olcese U, *et al.* Sleep homeostasis in the rat is preserved during chronic sleep restriction. *Proc Natl Acad Sci U S A.* 2010;**107**:15939–44.

17. Van Someren EJW. Doing with less sleep remains a dream. *Proc Natl Acad Sci U S A.* 2010;**107**:16003–4.

18. Tononi G, Cirelli C. Sleep function and synaptic homeostasis. *Sleep Med Rev.* 2006;**10**:49–62.

19. Krueger JM, Clinton JM, Winters BD, *et al.* Involvement of cytokines in slow wave sleep. *Prog Brain Res.* 2011;**193**:39–47.

20. Porkka-Heiskanen T, Strecker RE, Thakkar M, *et al.* Adenosine: a mediator of the sleep-inducing effects of prolonged wakefulness. *Science.* 1997;**276**:1265–8.

21. Retey JV, Adam M, Honegger E, *et al.* A functional genetic variation of adenosine deaminase affects the duration and intensity of deep sleep in humans. *Proc Natl Acad Sci U S A.* 2005;**102**:15676–81.

22. Romeijn N, Raymann RJEM, Møst E, *et al.* Sleep, vigilance and thermosensitivity. *Pflügers Arch.* 2012;**463**:169–76.

23. Fortier-Brochu E, Beaulieu-Bonneau S, Ivers H, Morin CM. Insomnia and daytime cognitive performance: a meta-analysis. *Sleep Med Rev.* 2011;**16**:83–94.

24. Horne JA. Sleep loss and "divergent" thinking ability. *Sleep.* 1988;**11**:528–36.

25. Lim J, Dinges DF. A meta-analysis of the impact of short-term sleep deprivation on cognitive variables. *Psychol Bull.* 2010;**136**:375–89.

26. Frankland PW, Bontempi B. Fast track to the medial prefrontal cortex. *Proc Natl Acad Sci U S A.* 2006;**103**:509–10.

27. Takashima A, Petersson KM, Rutters F, *et al.* Declarative memory consolidation in humans: a prospective functional magnetic resonance imaging study. *Proc Natl Acad Sci U S A.* 2006;**103**:756–61.

28. Astill RG, van der Heijden KB, van Ijzendoorn MH, Van Someren EJW. Sleep, cognition and behavioral problems in school-aged children: a century of research meta-analyzed. *Psychol bull.* 2012; (in press).

29. Riemann D, Voderholzer U, Spiegelhalder K, *et al.* Chronic insomnia and MRI-measured hippocampal volumes: a pilot study. *Sleep.* 2007;**30**:955–8.

30. Videbech P, Ravnkilde B. Hippocampal volume and depression: a meta-analysis of MRI studies. *Am J Psychiatry.* 2004;**161**:1957–66.

31. Smith ME. Bilateral hippocampal volume reduction in adults with post-traumatic stress disorder: a meta-analysis of structural MRI studies. *Hippocampus.* 2005;**15**:798–807.

32. Nelson MD, Saykin AJ, Flashman LA, Riordan HJ. Hippocampal volume reduction in schizophrenia as assessed by magnetic resonance imaging: a meta-analytic study. *Arch Gen Psychiatry.* 1998;**55**:433–40.

33. Benca RM, Obermeyer WH, Thisted RA, Gillin JC. Sleep and psychiatric disorders. A meta-analysis. *Arch Gen Psychiatry.* 1992;**49**:651–68; discussion 669–70.

34. Winkelman JW, Benson KL, Buxton OM, *et al.* Lack of hippocampal volume differences in primary insomnia and good sleeper controls: an MRI volumetric study at 3 Tesla. *Sleep Med.* 2010;**11**:576–82.

35. Noh HJ, Joo EY, Kim ST, *et al.* The relationship between hippocampal volume and cognition in patients with chronic primary insomnia. *J Clin Neurol.* 2012;**8**:130–8.

36. Joo E, Hong SB. Gray matter changes in brains of primary insomnia. *Sleep Biol Rhythms.* 2011;**9**:253.

37. Altena E, Vrenken H, Van Der Werf YD, Van Den Heuvel OAV, Van Someren EJW. Reduced orbitofrontal and parietal gray matter in chronic insomnia: a voxel-based morphometric study. *Biol Psychiatry.* 2010;**67**:182–5.

38. Huang Z, Liang P, Jia X, *et al.* Abnormal amygdala connectivity in patients with primary insomnia: evidence from resting state fMRI. *Eur J Radiol.* 2012;**81**(6):1288–95.

39. Neylan TC, Mueller SG, Wang Z, *et al.* Insomnia severity is associated with a decreased volume of the ca3/dentate gyrus hippocampal subfield. *Biol Psychiatry.* 2010;**68**:494–6.

40. Hall MH, Soreca I, Matthews KA, Kuller LH, Gianaros PJ. Reported sleep duration and hippocampal gray matter volume in healthy women. *Sleep.* 2009;**32**:A3.

41. Van Someren EJW, Oosterman J, van Harten B, *et al.* Sleep-wake rhythm fragmentation predicts age-related medial temporal lobe atrophy. *J Sleep Res.* 2008;**17**:S71.

42. Backhaus J, Junghanns K, Born J, *et al.* Impaired declarative memory consolidation during sleep in patients with primary insomnia: influence of sleep architecture and nocturnal cortisol release. *Biol Psychiatry.* 2006;**60**:1324–30.

43. Oosterman J, Van Someren EJW, Vogels R, *et al.* Fragmentation of the rest-activity rhythm predicts age-related cognitive deficits. *J Sleep Res.* 2009;**18**:129–35.

44. Szelenberger W, Niemcewicz S. Severity of insomnia correlates with cognitive impairment. *Acta Neurobiol Exp (Warsz).* 2000;**60**:373.

45. Gianaros PJ, Jennings JR, Sheu LK, *et al.* Prospective reports of chronic life stress predict decreased gray matter volume in the hippocampus. *Neuroimage.* 2007;**35**:795–803.

46. Yoo SS, Hu PT, Gujar N, Jolesz FA, Walker MP. A deficit in the ability to form new human memories without sleep. *Nat Neurosci.* 2007;**10**:385–92.

47. Van Der Werf YD, Altena E, Schoonheim MM, *et al.* Sleep benefits subsequent hippocampal functioning. *Nat Neurosci.* 2009;**12**:122–3.

48. Guzman-Marin R, Suntsova N, Stewart DR, *et al.* Sleep deprivation reduces proliferation of cells in the dentate gyrus of the hippocampus in rats. *J Physiol.* 2003;**549**:563–71.

49. Tung A, Takase L, Fornal C, Jacobs B. Effects of sleep deprivation and recovery sleep upon cell proliferation in adult rat dentate gyrus. *Neurosci.* 2005;**134**:721–3.

50. Poe GR, Walsh CM, Bjorness TE. Cognitive neuroscience of sleep. *Prog Brain Res.* 2010;**185**:1–19.

51. Winkelman JW, Buxton OM, Jensen JE, *et al.* Reduced brain GABA in primary insomnia: preliminary data from 4T proton magnetic resonance spectroscopy (1H-MRS). *Sleep.* 2008;**31**:1499–506.

52. Altena E, Van Der Werf YD, Sanz-Arigita EJ, *et al.* Prefrontal hypoactivation and recovery in insomnia. *Sleep.* 2008;**31**:1271–6.

53. Bonnet MH, Arand DL. Hyperarousal and insomnia. *Sleep Med Rev.* 1997;**1**:97–108.

54. Vincent NK, Walker JR. Perfectionism and chronic insomnia. *J Psychosom Res.* 2000;**49**:349–54.

55. Pavlova M, Berg O, Gleason R, *et al.* Self-reported hyperarousal traits among insomnia patients. *J Psychosom Res.* 2001;**51**:435–41.

56. Lundh L-G, Broman J-E, Hetta J, Sanoonchi F. Perfectionism and insomnia. *Scand J Behav Ther.* 1994;**23**:3–18.

57. Jansson M, Linton SJ. The development of insomnia within the first year: a focus on worry. *Br J Health Psychol.* 2006;**11**:501–11.

58. Szelenberger W, Niemcewicz S. Event-related current density in primary insomnia. *Acta Neurobiol Exp (Warsz).* 2001;**61**:299–308.

59. Chen R. Studies of human motor physiology with transcranial magnetic stimulation. *Muscle Nerve suppl.* 2000;**9**:S26–32.

60. Kobayashi M, Pascual-Leone A. Transcranial magnetic stimulation in neurology. *Lancet Neurol.* 2003;**2**:145–56.

61. Kujirai T, Caramia MD, Rothwell JC, *et al.* Corticocortical inhibition in human motor cortex. *J Physiol.* 1993;**471**:501–19.

62. Van Der Werf YD, Altena E, Van Dijk KD, *et al.* Is disturbed intracortical excitability a stable trait of chronic insomnia? A study using transcranial magnetic stimulation before and after multimodal sleep therapy. *Biol Psychiatry.* 2010;**68**:950–5.

63. Koenigs M, Holliday J, Solomon J, Grafman J. Left dorsomedial frontal brain damage is associated with insomnia. *J Neurosci.* 2010;**30**:16041–3.

64. Manes F, Paradiso S, Robinson RG. Neuropsychiatric effects of insular stroke. *J Nerv Mental Dis.* 1999;**187**:707–12.

65. Kringelbach ML. The human orbitofrontal cortex: linking reward to

hedonic experience. *Nat Rev Neurosci.* 2005;**6**:691–702.

66. Kringelbach ML, Berridge KC. Towards a functional neuroanatomy of pleasure and happiness. *Trends Cogn Sci.* 2009;**13**:479–87.

67. Dunn BJ, Conover K, Plourde G, *et al.* Hedonic valuation during thermal alliesthesia. *Proceedings of the 16th Annual Meeting of the Organization for Human Brain Mapping, Barcelona, Spain,*2010.

68. Rolls ET, Grabenhorst F, Parris BA. Warm pleasant feelings in the brain. *Neuroimage.* 2008;**41**:1504–13.

69. Raymann RJ, Van Someren EJ. Diminished capability to recognize the optimal temperature for sleep initiation may contribute to poor sleep in elderly people. *Sleep.* 2008;**31**:1301–9.

70. Smith MT, Perlis ML, Chengazi VU, *et al.* Neuroimaging of NREM sleep in primary insomnia: a Tc-99-HMPAO single photon emission computed tomography study. *Sleep.* 2002;**25**:325–35.

71. Johnson DL, Wiebe JS, Gold SM, *et al.* Cerebral blood flow and personality: a positron emission tomography study. *Am J Psychiatry.* 1999;**156**:252–7.

72. Ray RD, Ochsner KN, Cooper JC, *et al.* Individual differences in trait rumination and the neural systems supporting cognitive reappraisal. *Cogn Affect Behav Neurosci.* 2005;**5**:156–68.

73. Cooney RE, Joormann J, Eugene F, Dennis EL, Gotlib IH. Neural correlates of rumination in depression. *Cogn Affect Behav Neurosci.* 2010;**10**:470–8.

74. Morin CM, Rodrigue S, Ivers H. Role of stress, arousal, and coping skills in primary insomnia. *Psychosom Med.* 2003;**65**:259–67.

75. Drake CL, Friedman NP, Wright KP, Jr., Roth T. Sleep reactivity and insomnia: genetic and environmental influences. *Sleep.* 2011;**34**:1179–88.

76. Basishvili T, Eliozishvili M, Maisuradze L, *et al.* Insomnia in a displaced population is related to war-associated remembered stress. *Stress Health.* 2012;**28**:186–92.DOI: 10.1002/smi.1421.

77. Romcy-Pereira RN, Erraji-Benchekroun L, Smyrniotopoulos P, *et al.* Sleep-dependent gene expression in the hippocampus and prefrontal cortex following long-term potentiation. *Physiol Behav.* 2009;**98**:44–52.

78. Fukunaga M, Horovitz SG, van Gelderen P, *et al.* Large-amplitude, spatially correlated fluctuations in bold fMRI signals during extended rest and early sleep stages. *Magn Reson Imaging.* 2006;**24**:979–92.

79. Bastien CH, Fortier-Brochu E, Rioux I, *et al.* Cognitive performance and sleep quality in the elderly suffering from chronic insomnia. Relationship between objective and subjective measures. *J Psychosom Res.* 2003;**54**:39–49.

80. Van Someren EJW. Sleep propensity is modulated by circadian and behavior-induced changes in cutaneous temperature. *J Therm Biol.* 2004;**29**:437–44.

81. Van Someren EJW. Mechanisms and functions of coupling between sleep and temperature rhythms. *Prog Brain Res.* 2006;**153**:309–24.

82. Raymann RJEM, Van Someren EJW. Time-on-task impairment of psychomotor vigilance is affected by mild skin warming and changes with aging and insomnia. *Sleep.* 2007;**30**:96–103.

83. Raymann RJEM, Swaab DF, Van Someren EJW. Skin deep: cutaneous temperature determines sleep depth. *Brain.* 2008;**131**:500–13.

84. Raymann RJEM, Van Someren EJW. Diminished capability to recognize the optimal temperature for sleep initiation may contribute to poor sleep in elderly people. *Sleep.* 2008;**31**:1301–9.

85. Van Someren EJW, Pollmächer T, Leger D, *et al.* The European insomnia network. *Front Neurosci.* 2009;**3**:436.

Functional neuroimaging of primary insomnia

Eric Nofzinger

Introduction

Insomnia is defined as the inability to fall asleep easily, to stay asleep, or to have quality sleep in an individual with adequate sleep opportunity [1–3]. In the USA, population-based estimates of either chronic or transient insomnia range from 10% to 40% of the population, or 30 to 120 million adults [4, 5]. Similar prevalence estimates have been reported in Europe and Asia [6]. Across studies, there are two age peaks: 45–64 years of age and 85 years and older. Women are 1.3 to 2 times more likely to report trouble sleeping than men, as are those who are divorced or widowed, and have less education. In the USA, the economic burden of insomnia approaches $100 billion, in direct healthcare costs, functional impairment, increased risk of mental health problems, lost productivity, worker absenteeism, and excess healthcare utilization [7–11]. It is recognized as a public health problem, contributing to more than twice the number of medical errors attributed to healthcare workers without insomnia episodes.

Clinically, insomnia patients describe overactive minds that don't turn off at night to allow them to sleep. This chapter will review brain imaging studies that comment on whether or not there is abnormal brain function in insomnia patients that may in some way relate to their difficulty sleeping. Interpretations will be aided by review of relevant preclinical studies of the neurobiology of sleep and recent neuroimaging studies in healthy humans across the sleep/wake cycle. The organization of this chapter will follow a systems neuroscience view of a hierarchical arousal network in the central nervous system (Figure 24.1). Abnormalities in any component of this interactive system may produce insomnia complaints. Finally, evidence will be presented as to the location where interventions may impact on regional brain function in insomnia patients.

Brainstem, hypothalamus, and basal forebrain

Preclinical research has identified the basic, or most primitive, circuits in the brain that are responsible for promoting arousal [12, 13]. A major component of this network is the brainstem reticular core, a diffuse network of predominantly glutamatergic long-projecting neurons and a smaller collection of presumed local circuit gamma-aminobutyic acid (GABA) neurons.

Additional components include a collection of nuclei in the brainstem tegmentum dorsal to the reticular formation that include cholinergic and monoaminergic (serotonergic, noradrenergic, and dopaminergic) neurons. These nuclei send rostral projections that parallel and are interconnected with those of the brainstem reticular core. Cholinergic nuclei are also clustered rostrally in the basal forebrain, including septal nuclei and the diagonal band of Broca. Recent attention has focused on the hypothalamus playing a significant role in arousal and in homeostasis. Specifically, the tuberomamillary histaminergic neurons and the perifornical hypocretin neurons in the posterior hypothalamus have extensive interconnections and interactions with the basic arousal systems.

Human sleep neuroimaging studies in healthy subjects support the involvement of these basic arousal networks in non-rapid eye movement (NREM) sleep. Blood flow has been shown to correlate negatively with the presence of NREM sleep in the pontine reticular formation [14–16], and in the basal forebrain/hypothalamus [14–16]. Reduction of activity in this network from waking to sleep is consistent with their role in promoting arousal and potentially in initiating sleep.

Human sleep neuroimaging studies in insomnia subjects support the involvement of these basic arousal networks in disturbances in NREM sleep. Nofzinger *et al.* [17] investigated the neurobiological basis of poor sleep in insomnia. Insomnia patients and healthy subjects completed regional cerebral glucose metabolic assessments during both waking and NREM sleep using ^{18}F-fluoro deoxy glucose positron emission tomography (^{18}F-FDG-PET). Healthy subjects reported better sleep quality than did insomnia subjects. The two groups did not differ on any measure of visually scored or automated measure of sleep. A group × state interaction analysis confirmed that insomnia subjects showed a smaller decrease than did healthy subjects in relative metabolism from waking to NREM sleep in the brainstem reticular core and hypothalamus (Figure 24.2) This study supports the concept that persistent activity in this basic arousal network may be responsible for the impaired objective and subjective sleep in insomnia patients.

In terms of interventions, the mechanism of action of sedative hypnotics may be primarily on these basic arousal systems. For example, Kajimura *et al.* [18] assessed regional cerebral blood flow during NREM sleep in response to triazolam, a

---

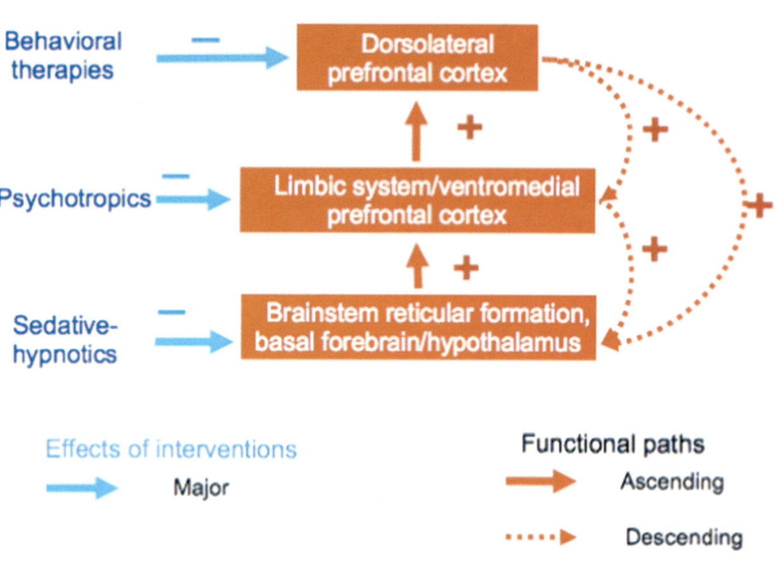

Figure 24.1 Hierarchical arousal networks in insomnia including impact of insomnia interventions.

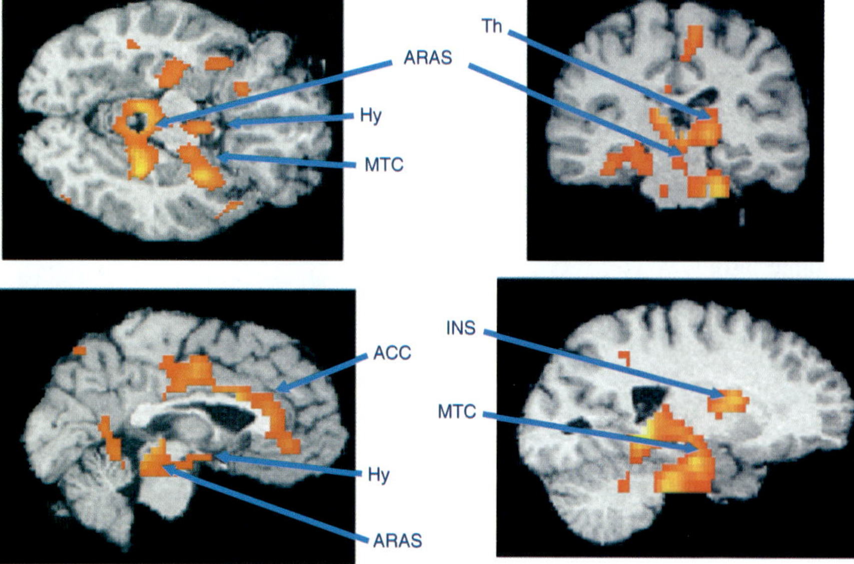

Figure 24.2 Brain regions where metabolic activity persists from waking to NREM sleep in insomnia patients relative to healthy controls. Th = thalamus; ARAS = asceding reticular activating system; Hy = hypothalamus; MTC = mesial temporal cortex; INS = insula; ACC = anterior cungulate cortex.

short-acting benzodiazepine sedative-hypnotic. They found that blood flow in the basal forebrain was lower during NREM sleep following triazolam administration than following placebo.

A recent study aimed to determine if eszopiclone, a non-benzodiazepine cyclopyrrolone, reversed the pattern of brain-stem, hypothalamus, and basal forebrain abnormalities found in insomnia patients [19]. In this study, 106 subjects were screened, 23 received in person assessments, and 12 met DSM-IV criteria for primary insomnia. Of these, 8 subjects (4 women/4 men, mean age + s.d. = 35 + 13 years) completed 2 weeks eszopiclone 3 mg qhs open label treatment. Pre- and post-treatment assessments included sleep diary, three nights of polysomnography, and waking and NREM sleep ^{18}F-FDG PET scans. Paired t-tests were performed on subjective and EEG sleep data. Voxel-based repeated measures ANCOVA (group = pre- vs. post, repeated measure = regional cerebral metabolism in waking and sleep, covarying for global metabolism) were performed on cerebral metabolic data. From pre- to post-treatment, insomnia patients showed improvements in all subjective measures of sleep, sleep quality, mood, and next morning alertness (e.g., Pittsburgh Sleep Quality Index Total = 11.9 + 2.5 pre- vs. 7.5 + 2.3 post-treatment, paired t(7) = 3.86, p = 0.006). Patients showed increases in stage 2 sleep and REM latency and decreases in stage delta sleep from pre- to post-treatment. Brain imaging analyses showed that the reduction in relative metabolism in an arousal network from waking to NREM sleep was greater following eszopiclone treatment than before. Specific regions included the pontine reticular formation and ascended into the midbrain, subthalamic nucleus, culmen of the cerebellum, and thalamus. Related neocortical areas showing this interaction included the orbitofrontal cortex, superior temporal lobe, right paracentral lobule of the posterior medial frontal lobe, right precuneus, dorsal cingulate gyrus, and portions of the frontal lobe (Figure 24.3). Comparisons involving only sleep, but not wake, revealed similar regions of post-treatment reductions in relative metabolism. These results demonstrate that eszopiclone reverses a pattern of central

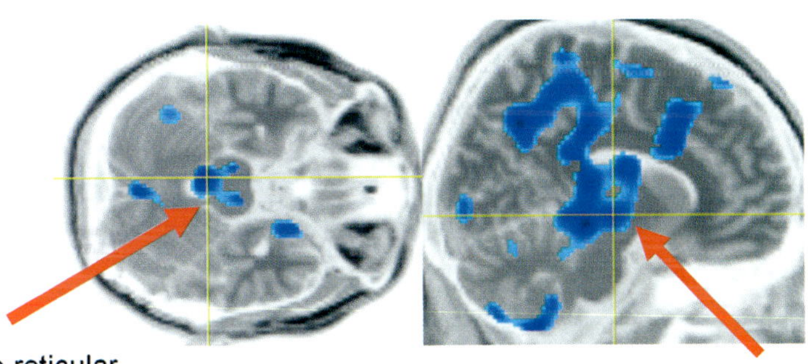

Figure 24.3 Regions where the decline in metabolism from waking to sleep is greater after two weeks, medication management with eszopiclone.

nervous system (CNS) hyperarousal in insomnia patients. This effect is most pronounced during NREM sleep, at a time when the concentration of eszopiclone in the brain, when given prior to sleep, should be highest. The inhibitory actions of eszopiclone, and likely similar non-benzodiazepine sedative-hypnotics and potentially the benzodiazepine sedative hypnotics, then, are likely responsible for the sedating properties that appear to be largely on a CNS arousal neural network within sleep that includes the pontine and midbrain reticular activating system.

Limbic and paralimbic system

Behaviorally, maintaining an alert brain serves broader functions than a simple homeostatic one related to sleep at night. It allows an individual to adapt in an efficient manner to a variety of salient events in real time while awake. Importantly, the basic biology of arousal can be modified by neural systems that regulate emotional and goal-directed behavior. These systems may play an important role in modulating or perpetuating the increased arousal of insomnia patients. This is especially true given the significant epidemiologic and neurobiological overlaps between insomnia and mental disorders.

The results of preclinical, healthy human and depressed human neuroimaging studies support the importance of two neural systems in emotional behavior [20]. A more ventrally located system, with important contributions from the amygdala, has been shown to be fundamental to the initial experience of emotions and to the automatic generation of emotional responses. The function of this system is a reactive one in response to emotional stimuli. Other structures related to this system include the anterior insula, ventral striatum, and ventral regions of the anterior cingulate cortex and ventral prefrontal cortex. A more dorsally located system, with important contributions from the dorsolateral prefrontal cortex (DLPFC), has been shown to be fundamental to the conscious, planned regulation of emotional behavior in light of future behavior. The function of this system is one of planning behavior in response to emotional stimuli. Other structures related to this system include the hippocampus, and dorsal regions of the anterior cingulate cortex. A primary structure in the ventral system is the amygdala. It has been shown to participate in the sensory component of emotional behavior and in the initial organization

of a reactive emotional response. In humans, the amygdala shows increased activation in response to a variety of emotional stimuli including fearful [21] and sad [22] faces, threatening words [23], and fearful vocalizations [24]. A reactive "motor" role for the amygdala includes the recruitment and coordinating of cortical arousal and vigilant attention for optimizing sensory and perceptual processing of stimuli associated with underdetermined contingencies [25].

Recent work shows that the amygdala is anatomically connected with and functionally modulates effects on the brainstem centers involved in arousal and sleep regulation [26, 27]. Similarly, other components of the ventral emotional system such as the ventral striatum, the subgenual anterior cingulate cortex and the ventromedial prefrontal cortex, are known to have both anatomical and functional relationships with brainstem centers thought to play a role in behavioral state regulation in addition to the primary roles they each play in cortical arousal [28, 29].

Human sleep neuroimaging studies support a role for the ventral emotional system in sleep processes. Blood flow has been shown to negatively correlate with the presence of NREM sleep in the anterior cingulated [14–16], the amygdala [16], and in the orbitofrontal cortex [14–16]. These changes suggest that components of the ventral emotion system play a role in modulating sleep or in the manifestation of sleep. Declining function in the amygdala raises the possibility that this structure modulates activity in core structures involved in regulating arousal.

Human sleep neuroimaging studies support the role for components of the ventral emotion system in pathological sleep associated with both depression and insomnia. Nofzinger et al. [30] used ^{18}F-FDG PET to define regional cerebral correlates of arousal in NREM sleep in 9 healthy and 12 depressed patients. They assessed electroencephalographic (EEG) power in the beta high frequency spectrum as a measure of cortical arousal. They then correlated beta power with metabolism in NREM sleep. They found that beta power negatively correlated with sleep quality. Further, beta power positively correlated with ventromedial prefrontal cortex metabolism in both a group of depressed and healthy subjects. They concluded that elevated function in the ventromedial prefrontal cortex, an area associated with obsessive behavior and anatomically linked with brainstem and hypothalamic arousal centers, may contribute to dysfunctional arousal. Nofzinger *et al.* [17] investigated the neurobiological basis of poor sleep in insomnia (referenced above, see Figure 24.2). Insomnia patients and healthy subjects completed regional cerebral glucose metabolic assessments during both waking and NREM sleep using ^{18}F-FDG PET. Healthy subjects reported better sleep quality than did insomnia subjects. A group × state interaction analysis confirmed that insomnia subjects showed a smaller decrease than did healthy subjects in relative metabolism from waking to NREM sleep in the insular cortex, amygdala, hippocampus, and anterior cingulate and medial prefrontal cortices. This study supports the notion that persistent overactivity in a limbic/paralimbic level of the arousal system contributes to the non-restorative sleep in insomnia patients.

Pharmacotherapy for insomnia may have some of its mechanism of action on these limbic and paralimbic structures, especially the antidepressant medications. When Kajimura *et al.* [18] assessed regional cerebral blood flow during NREM sleep in response to triazolam, they also found that blood flow in the amygaloid complexes, in addition to basal forebrain, was lower than following placebo. While not always consistent, several neuroimaging studies show that serotonergic antidepressants tend to lower, or inhibit, brain function (blood flow or metabolism) in the ventral limbic and paralimbic cortices including the amygdala [31, 32], perhaps via actions on 5-HT$_{1A}$ postsynaptic receptors, given their high density in these areas [33]. Inhibiting hyperarousal in this limbic/paralimbic emotional neural network could benefit insomnia patients.

Recent studies have focused on the role of sleep in memory consolidation, utilizing both cognitive neuroscience and brain imaging of the hippocampus. Nissen *et al.* [34] compared sleep-related consolidation of procedural memory in seven patients with primary insomnia and seven healthy controls. Performance on a mirror tracing task was measured before and after sleep. Performance in the mirror tracing task before sleep did not differ between the groups. Both groups performed significantly better in the recall condition after sleep. Healthy controls showed an improvement of 42.8% ± 5.8% in the mirror tracing draw time, whereas patients with insomnia showed an improvement of 20.4% ± 14.8% (multivariate analyses of variance test session × group interaction: F3,10 = 10.9, p = 0.002). These preliminary findings support the view that sleep-associated consolidation of procedural memories may be impaired in patients with primary insomnia.

Another study focused on morphology of the hippocampus in insomnia patients [35]. Morphometric analysis of magnetic resonance imaging (MRI) brain scans was used to investigate possible neuroanatomical differences between patients with primary insomnia and good sleepers. MRI images (1.5 tesla) of the brain were obtained from insomnia patients and good sleepers. MRI scans were analyzed bilaterally by manual morphometry for different brain areas including the hippocampus, amygdala, anterior cingulate, orbitofrontal, and dorsolateral prefrontal corties. Patients with primary insomnia demonstrated significantly reduced hippocampal volumes bilaterally compared with the good sleepers. None of the other regions of interest analyzed revealed differences between the two groups. While replication of

the findings in larger samples is needed to confirm the validity of the data, these pilot data raise the possibility that chronic insomnia is associated with alterations in brain structure. The integration of structural, neuropsychological, neuroendocrine, and polysomnographic studies is necessary to further assess the relationships between insomnia and brain function and structure.

One study suggested a role for the basal ganglia in the neurobiology of insomnia [36]. Patients with insomnia and good sleeper controls were studied polysomnographically for three nights with a whole-brain SPECT scan of NREM sleep on night 3. Tomographs of regional cerebral blood flow during the first NREM sleep cycle were successfully obtained. Contrary to expectations, patients with insomnia showed a consistent pattern of hypoperfusion across all eight preselected regions of interest, with particular deactivation in the basal ganglia (p = 0.006). The frontal medial, occipital, and parietal cortices also showed significant decreases in blood flow compared with good sleepers (p < 0.05). Subjects with insomnia had decreased activity in the basal ganglia relative to the frontal lateral cortex, frontal medial cortex, thalamus, and occipital and parietal cortices (p < 0.05). These preliminary results suggest that primary insomnia may be associated with abnormal CNS activity during NREM sleep that is particularly linked to basal ganglia dysfunction.

Thalamus and neocortex

In many respects, maintaining efficient thalamocortical activity during waking could be conceptualized as a primary function of sleep. The best way for the neocortex to maintain adequate daytime function is for an individual to sleep well at night. At the macroscopic level, sleep has been shown to discharge a wake-dependent sleep drive as measured by EEG spectral power in the delta frequency band. At the molecular and neuronal levels, hypothetical functions of sleep include the restoration of brain energy metabolism through the replenishment of brain glycogen stores that are depleted during wakefulness [37] and the downscaling of synapses that have been potentiated during waking brain function [38]. These restorative components of sleep are recognized to have regional selectivity. Slow-wave sleep rhythms have both thalamic and cortical components [39]. Decreases in brain activity from waking to NREM sleep are most pronounced in the frontoparietal cortex. An anterior dominance of EEG spectral power in the delta EEG spectral power range has also been reported [40]. A frontal predominance for the increase in delta power following sleep loss has also been reported [41]. This region of cortex plays a prominent role in waking executive functions which are preferentially impaired following sleep deprivation [42]. These sleep deprivation-induced cognitive impairments have been related to declines in frontal metabolism after sleep loss [43]. Further, recent topographic EEG studies during NREM sleep before and after training on a task revealed slow-wave activity increases in regions of cortex known to involve the task [44]. Evidence such as this, suggests that NREM sleep is important for prefrontal cortex function. As such, the alterations in NREM sleep in insomnia patients may relate to alterations in prefrontal cortex function.

Prefrontal cortex function may play a role in insomnia in several respects. As noted above, there are significant epidemiologic links between insomnia and disorders of emotion. The DLPFC is a primary structure in the dorsal emotional neural system. This structure has been shown to play an important role in executive function, including selective attention, planning, and effortful regulation of affective states [20]. The DLPFC maintains the representation of goals and the means to achieve them. It sends bias signals to other areas of the brain to facilitate the expression of task-appropriate responses in the face of competition with other responses [45]. Davidson *et al.* has emphasized the importance of left-lateralized prefrontal cortex regions in approach-related appetitive goals, and the right in behavioral inhibition and vigilant attention [25]. The DLPFC is not only responsible for recruiting or inhibiting limbic regions as appropriate for performing tasks (e.g., Davidson *et al.* [46]) but appears to be modulated by early limbic processing [47]. A related component of the dorsal emotional system is the dorsal anterior cingulate cortex [20]. This region has been associated with conflict-monitoring (e.g., it is particularly active during conditions when one must arbitrate quickly between two likely responses) [43]. Given its role in the executive aspects of emotional behavior, an abnormal increase in vigilant functions of the prefrontal cortex function could lead to insomnia, whereas deficient executive behavior could be a consequence of inadequate sleep resulting from insomnia.

Functional neuroimaging studies have revealed reliable global decreases in cerebral metabolism or blood flow from waking to NREM sleep (e.g., Nofzinger *et al.* [48]). Regionally, studies across several laboratories and using various imaging methods have demonstrated that between waking and NREM sleep there are relative reductions in activity in heteromodal association cortex in the frontal, parietal, and temporal lobes as well as in the thalamus. Sleep deprivation [43] is associated with global declines in absolute cerebral metabolism. Regionally, these declines are most notable in frontoparietal cortex and in the thalamus. Alertness and cognitive performance on a sleep deprivation-sensitive serial addition/subtraction test declined in association with the sleep deprivation-associated regional deactivations. These studies demonstrate that reductions in global brain function and especially in prefrontal cortex function are important for the restorative function of sleep. Inadequate sleep in insomniacs may lead to a deficit in prefrontal cortex function.

Nofzinger *et al.* [19] investigated regional cerebral glucose metabolism in insomnia patients and healthy subjects during both waking and NREM sleep using 18 F-FDG PET (referenced above). Insomnia subjects scored worse on measures of daytime concentration and fatigue consistent with prefrontal cortex impairment. Insomnia patients showed increased global cerebral glucose metabolism during sleep and wakefulness, suggesting an increased vigilant or attentive function of the neocortex consistent with hyperarousal. A group × state interaction analysis confirmed that insomnia subjects showed a smaller decrease than did healthy subjects in relative metabolism from waking to NREM sleep in the thalamus, and the anterior cingulate and medial prefrontal cortices, suggesting a persistence of

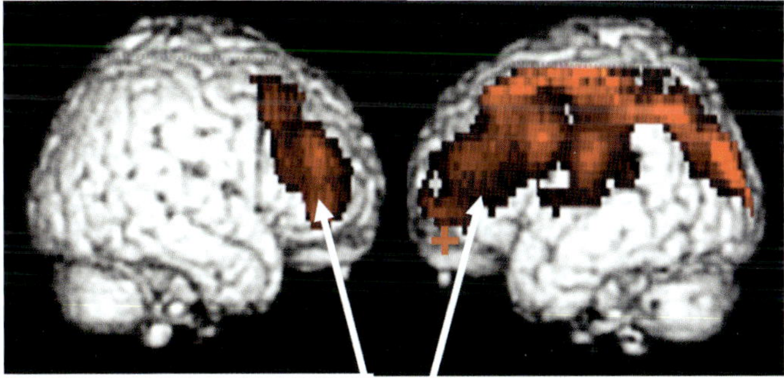

Prefrontal cortex

Figure 24.4 Regions of cortex demonstrating reduced metabolism in waking in insomnia patients relative to healthy subjects.

thalamocortical arousal even within sleep in insomnia patients (see Figure 24.2). While awake, in relation to healthy subjects, insomnia subjects showed relative hypometabolism in a broad region of the frontal cortex bilaterally; left hemispheric superior temporal, parietal, and occipital cortices; and the thalamus (see Figure 24.4]. Their daytime fatigue may reflect decreased activity in the prefrontal cortex that results from inefficient sleep.

A separate study showed that insomnia patients with high levels of arousal during sleep also had high levels of metabolic activity in the cortex [49]. Fifteen patients who met DSM-IV criteria for primary insomnia completed 1-week sleep diary (subjective) and polysomnographic (objective) assessments of wake after sleep onset (WASO) and regional cerebral glucose metabolic assessments during NREM sleep using ^{18}F-FDG PET. Whole-brain voxel-by-voxel correlations, as well as region-of-interest analyses, were performed between subjective and objective WASO and relative regional cerebral metabolism using the statistical software SPM2. Subjective WASO was significantly greater than objective WASO, but the two measures were positively correlated. Objective WASO correlated positively with the percentage of stage 2 sleep and negatively with the percentage of stages 3 and 4 sleep. Both subjective and objective WASO positively correlated with NREM sleep-related cerebral glucose metabolism in the pontine tegmentum and in thalamocortical networks in a frontal, anterior temporal, and anterior cingulate distribution. Increased relative metabolism in these brain regions during NREM sleep in patients with insomnia is associated with increased WASO measured either subjectively or objectively (Figure 24.5). These effects are related to the lighter sleep stages of patients with more WASO and may result from increased activity in arousal systems during sleep and/or to activity in higher-order cognitive processes related to goal-directed behavior, conflict monitoring, emotional awareness, anxiety, and fear. Such changes may decrease arousal thresholds and/or increase perceptions of wakefulness in insomnia.

Several interventions may alter activity in the prefrontal cortex in a beneficial manner for insomnia patients. For example, Lou *et al.* [50] assessed regional brain function associated with Yoga Nidra, a meditative state in which there is a loss of conscious control and an increased awareness of sensory experience. In their study, they found reduced blood flow during meditation in an attentional network that included the DLPFC

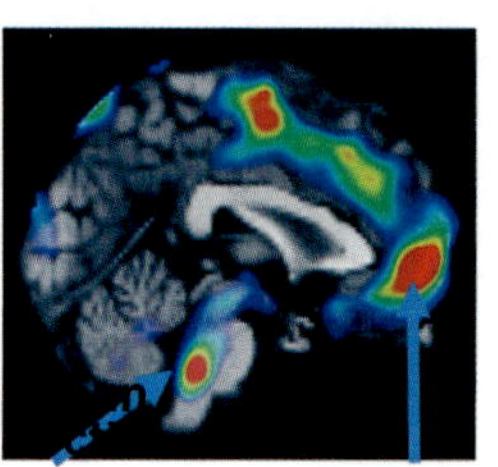
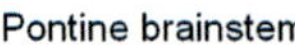
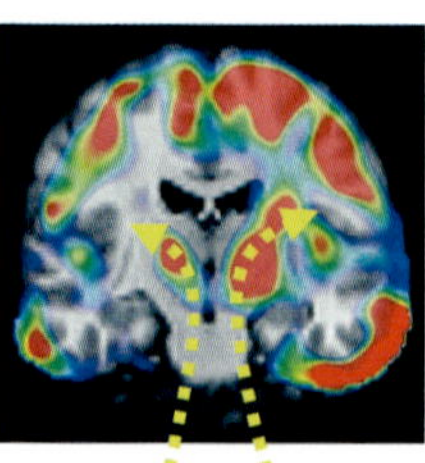

Figure 24.5 Brain regions where metabolic activity in sleep correlates with wakefulness after sleep onset in insomnia patients. ACC = anterior cingulate cortex.

and anterior cingulate cortex, as well as increased blood flow in posterior sensory and associative cortices associated with visual imagery. Cognitive approaches to the treatment of insomnia may have similar mechanisms of action in prefrontal areas. Serotonergically active antidepressants also increase brain function (blood flow or metabolism) in the dorsal paralimbic and dorsolateral prefrontal cortices [17, 37]. Increasing activity in the prefrontal cortex may reverse prefrontal deficits in insomnia patients, leading to improved daytime cognitive function. Alternatively, further increasing an already metabolically overactive prefrontal cortex may increase attentive and vigilant functions, thereby producing further insomnia, a not uncommon side effect of selective serotonium reuptake inhibitor (SSRI) therapy in either depressed or insomnia patients.

One study [51] documented prefrontal hypoactivation in insomnia as predicted from the background review above. Although subjective complaints about daytime cognitive functioning are an essential symptom of chronic insomnia, abnormalities in functional brain activation have not previously been investigated. This study investigated functional brain activation differences as a possible result of chronic insomnia, and the reversibility of these differences after non-medicated sleep therapy. Twenty-one insomniacs and 12 carefully matched controls underwent functional MRI (fMRI) scanning during the performance of a category and a letter fluency task. Insomniacs were randomly assigned to either a six-week period of non-pharmacological sleep therapy or a wait list period, after which fMRI scanning was repeated using parallel tasks. Task-related brain activation and number of generated words were considered as outcome measures. Compared to controls, insomnia patients showed hypoactivation of the medial and inferior prefrontal cortical areas (Brodmann Area 9, 44–45), which recovered after sleep therapy but not after a wait list period. These studies support the hypothesis that insomnia interferes in a reversible fashion with activation of the prefrontal cortical system during daytime task performance.

Another study assessed effects on frontal cortex function before and after treatment with cognitive behavior therapy for insomnia (CBTI) [52]. This preliminary study used ^{18}F-FDG PET to explore the effects of an eight-week course of CBTI on relative regional cerebral metabolic rate of glucose (rCMRglu) during morning wakefulness and NREM in five adults with primary insomnia. Post-treatment reductions in rCMRglu during wakefulness and NREM ($p < 0.05$) were observed in bilateral regions of dorsal frontoparietal and temporal cortices, thalami, basal ganglia, and limbic and paralimbic structures. These results suggest that CBTI is associated with reductions in relative rCMRglu during wakefulness and NREM in a limbic/paralimbic and neocortical distributed network involved in cognitive control of sleep/wake function.

Another study attempted to explore frontal cortex function in subsets of insomnia patients subtyped as either morning or evening chronotypes [53]. While insomnia is a well-established risk factor for the initial onset, recurrence, or relapse of affective disorders, the specific characteristics of insomnia that connote risk remain unclear. Insomnia patients with an evening chronotype may be one particularly high-risk group, perhaps due to alterations in positive affect and its related affective circuitry. This study explored this possibility by comparing diurnal patterns of positive affect and the activity of positive affect-related brain regions in morning and evening types with insomnia. They assessed diurnal variation in brain activity via the rCMRglu uptake by using ^{18}F-FDG PET during morning and evening wakefulness. The authors focused on regions in the medial prefrontal cortex and striatum, which have been consistently linked with positive affect and reward processing. As predicted, chronotypes differed in their daily patterns in both self-reported positive affect and associated brain regions. Evening types displayed diurnal patterns of positive affect characterized by phase delay and smaller amplitude compared to those of morning types with insomnia. In parallel, evening types showed a reduced degree of diurnal variation in the metabolism of both the medial prefrontal cortex and the striatum, as well as lower overall metabolism in these regions across both morning and evening wakefulness. Taken together, these preliminary findings suggest that alterations in the diurnal activity of positive affect-related neural structures may underlie differences in the phase and amplitude of self-reported positive affect between morning and evening chronotypes, and may constitute one mechanism for increased risk of mood disorders among evening-type insomniacs.

Frontal cerebral hypothermia as a treatment for insomnia

As noted above, recent advances have been made in the neurobiology of sleep and in the neurobiology of insomnia based on brain imaging studies of insomnia that can inform innovative non-pharmaceutical treatments for insomnia. While pharmaceutical interventions for insomnia have focused on hyperarousal in brainstem and hypothalamic arousal systems, it remains unknown as to whether an intervention designed to intervene at frontal hyperarousal may be beneficial in the treatment of insomnia. Considerable evidence suggests that sleep may serve a restorative function [54–57], especially involving the brain. An EEG marker of sleep homeostasis is EEG spectral power in the delta frequency range (1–4 Hz) [56, 58]. The homeostatic sleep drive may involve the restoration of brain energy metabolism through the replenishment of brain glycogen stores that are depleted during wakefulness [37, 59]. This function may have some regional specificity. A prefrontal dominance of EEG spectral power in the delta EEG spectral power range has been reported [40, 60, 61]. A prefrontal dominance for the increase in delta power following sleep loss has also been reported [41, 61–66). This region of cortex plays a prominent role in waking executive functions which are preferentially impaired following sleep deprivation [42, 43, 67–69].

As noted above, brain imaging studies also point to the prefrontal cortex as playing a role in the restorative aspects of sleep. In an ^{18}F-FDG PET) study, whole brain glucose metabolism declined significantly from waking to NREM sleep [48]. Relative decreases in regional metabolism from waking to NREM sleep were found in heteromodal frontal, parietal, and temporal cortices, and in the dorsomedial and anterior thalamus. These findings are consistent with a restorative role for NREM sleep largely in cortex that subserves essential functions in waking conscious behavior. In another study [70], changes in regional cerebral metabolism were identified that occur between usual NREM sleep and recovery NREM sleep following a night of sleep deprivation. In relation to baseline NREM sleep, subjects' recovery NREM sleep was associated with (1) increased slow wave activity (an electrophysiological marker of sleep drive); (2) global reductions in whole-brain metabolism; and (3) relative reductions in glucose metabolism in broad regions of the frontal cortex. Both these studies suggest that the restorative nature of sleep is subserved by reductions in brain metabolism and regionally with reductions in metabolism in the frontal regions. A medical device that alters metabolism in a pattern similar to that seen in healthy sleep or recovery sleep following sleep deprivation, therefore, may benefit insomnia patients.

As noted above "hyperarousal," involving various aspects of physiology, is one pathophysiological model of insomnia with considerable experimental support. Insomnia patients have been shown to have increased whole-brain metabolism across waking and sleep in relation to healthy subjects [17]; resting metabolic rate [71, 72], heart rate and sympathovagal tone in heart rate variability (HRV) [73, 74], cortisol secretion in the evening and early sleep hours [75,76], beta EEG activity during NREM sleep [77–81], increased levels of cortical glucose metabolism, especially in the prefrontal cortex, associated with higher levels of wakefulness after sleep onset [49]; impairments in the normal drop in core body temperature around the sleep onset period [82–85]; and cognitive hyperarousal resting on the presleep thoughts of insomnia patients [86–88], often described as "racing," unstoppable, and sleep-focused. Recent evidence also suggests that insomnia sufferers demonstrate selective attention directed toward sleep and bed-related stimuli [89, 90], which may lead to a self-reinforcing feedback loop of conditioned arousal, poor sleep, and impaired waking function [91, 92].

As noted above, brain imaging studies also lend support to the notion that the "brains" of insomnia patients, either primary insomnia, or secondary to other disorders, do not show the normal declines in metabolism in the frontal cortex from waking to sleep. An early ^{18}F-FDG PET study [17] showed that insomnia patients had increased whole-brain metabolism across waking and sleep and a persistence of metabolic activity from waking to sleep in a brainstem and hypothalamic arousal neural network. A recent analysis in a group of 18 primary insomnia patients and 18-age and gender-matched healthy good sleepers, replicated the increased whole brain metabolism in insomnia patients and further demonstrated that insomnia patients do not show the normal reductions in metabolic activity in frontoparietal cortex as do healthy good sleepers [93]. This general pattern has also been reported in secondary insomnias related to depression and to aging. Insomnia patients have demonstrated increases in beta EEG spectral power, a measure of cognitive arousal, that correlate with increased metabolism in the ventromedial prefrontal cortex during NREM sleep [30]. Severity of insomnia, as measured by either WASO or subjectively by the Pittsburgh Sleep Quality Index (PSQI), correlates positively with metabolism in the frontal cortex during sleep [49]. Evidence for improvements in sleep in insomnia patients has been associated with improvements in prefrontal cortex function as measured by functional neuroimaging [51]. These studies suggest that insomnia patients have brain hyperarousal that is preferential to the frontal cortex and consistent with their reports that they have trouble turning their minds off at night in order to get a good night's sleep. A decline in metabolism in the prefrontal cortex, therefore, appears to be important for the normal function of sleep and hypermetabolism in this region may interfere with this normal function of sleep in insomnia patients. These data suggest that interventions designed to reduce elevated metabolism in the prefrontal cortex may improve sleep in insomnia patients.

Reduction in brain metabolism by means of hypothermia is an established method in other medical disciplines, such as neurosurgery, emergency medicine, and anesthesiology, where this technique is used for its neuroprotective effects. Studies have shown that the application of a cooling stimulus to the scalp decreases brain temperature in the underlying cortex in both animals and humans. In a study in pigs, even a mild surface cooling of 15 °C was associated with cooling of the scalp and superficial brain to 35 °C [94]. In this study, there was a notable differential effect of surface cooling on superficial versus deep brain tissue, with superficial brain tissue cooled to a greater degree than deep brain tissue. In a human study [95], Wang *et al.*, were able to decrease surface brain temperatures by an average of 1.84 °C within 1 h of subjects wearing a whole head cooling helmet. Biomedical engineering models [96, 97] demonstrate that cooling of the brain gray matter can be achieved by selective head cooling on the surface. These lines of evidence support the concept that application of a cooling stimulus at the scalp will be associated with reductions in metabolism in the underlying cortex.

Cerebral hypothermia is an intervention that has previously been used to treat other medical disorders due to its neuroprotective effects [98–103]. Therapeutic hypothermia after global and focal ischemic and other neurotoxic events such as head trauma, stroke, and neuronal insult during cardiopulmonary surgery has shown beneficial results in controlled animal and human studies. Preclinical studies have shown many neuroprotective effects of brain cooling. These include: metabolism, pH, neurotransmitter levels, free fatty acids, blood–brain barrier, edema, glucose metabolism, cerebral blood flow, free radical activation, lipid peroxidation, calcium accumulation, protein synthesis, protein kinase-C activity, leukocyte accumulation, platelet function, *N-methyl-D-aspartate* (NMDA) neurotoxicity, growth factors, cytoskeletal proteins, calcium-dependent protein phosphorylation, heat shock protein, immediate early genes, nitric oxide synthase NOS activity, and matrix metalloproteinase MMP expression. It is conceivable that the neuroprotective benefits of cerebral hypothermia may aid patients with sleep disorders, including insomnia. Pathophysiologic models of the adverse events associated with sleep disorders are beginning to focus on the potential neuronal toxicity of having a sleep disorder [104, 105]. That this may occur in insomnia is suggested by findings of hypercortisolemia in insomnia patients in the evening and early hours of sleep [75, 76] and known adverse effects of hypercortisolemia on neuronal function [106]. One preliminary study has demonstrated reduced volumes of the hippocampus in insomnia patients [81]. This may be the result of neurotoxic factors.

Reducing hypermetabolism in the prefrontal cortex of insomnia patients during both the pre-sleep period and sleep may also reduce cognitive hyperarousal reported by insomnia patients [86–92]. Cerebral localization of this is hypothesized to occur in the prefrontal cortex given its role in executive function and ruminative cognitions. Application of a cooling stimulus to the frontal scalp area may also facilitate the normative changes in thermoregulation associated with sleep onset. Heat loss, via selective vasodilatation of distal skin regions as measured by the distal minus proximal skin temperature gradient (DPG), seems to be a crucial process for the circadian regulation of core body temperature CBT and sleepiness [107–109]. Increased DPG before lights off has been noted to promote a rapid onset of sleep, suggesting a link between thermoregulatory and arousal (sleepiness) systems [109, 110]. As noted above, impairments in the normal drop in core body temperature around the sleep onset period has been demonstrated in insomnia patients [82–85]. A device that produces heat loss, or a shifting of the balance of heat from the core to the periphery, therefore, may improve sleep in insomnia patients.

Two studies have utilized frontal cerebral hypothermia during sleep as a potential intervention in the treatment of insomnia. The first study aimed to determine if frontal cerebral hypothermia reduced frontal cerebral metabolism and core body temperature in insomnia patients [111]. Out of 148 subjects screened, 12 met DSM-IV criteria for primary insomnia, and 8 completed the study. Subjects wore a medical device on the scalp overlying the frontal cortex. The device delivered either a neutral temperature control or a mild hypothermic stimulus for 60 min before bedtime and during the first NREM cycle of sleep. Presentation of conditions was randomized and separated by a night of sleep. NREM sleep ^{18}F-FDG PET scans and core body temperature were assessed. Statistics included paired t-tests and ANCOVA.

Relative to control, the frontal hypothermic condition was associated with a relative reduction in metabolism in the underlying frontal and cingulate corties (t = 8.2; corrected p < 0.005; 3802 voxels). Five of eight insomnia patients showed reductions in whole-brain metabolism in the frontal hypothermic condition in relation to the control. In relation to the control, the frontal hypothermic condition was associated with an accelerated drop in core body temperature around the sleep onset period (group F = 3.68, one-tailed p = 0.03, time F = 53.6, p < 0.0001; group × time F = 1.7, one-tailed p = 0.10). Seventy-five percent of subjects subjectively reported benefits of the device, such as decreased distracting thoughts, facilitation of sleep maintenance, and/or refreshing sleep. Frontal cerebral hypothermia reduced brain metabolism during sleep especially in the frontal cortex in insomnia patients. Frontal cerebral hypothermia also facilitated the reduction in core body temperature at sleep onset in insomnia patients. These findings suggested that clinical trials were warranted to determine the efficacy of this intervention for chronic insomnia.

A second study aimed to determine whether all-night frontal cerebral thermal transfer (FCTT) in insomnia patients had a dose-dependent effect on improving sleep onset and sleep efficiency [112]. In this crossover study, order randomized between patients, subjects received all-night FCTT via a soft plastic cap fitted on the scalp and filled with circulating water. Conditions varied in the temperature of the circulating water, and, therefore, in thermal transfer intensities, and included: no device, and device with either neutral, moderate, or maximal cooling thermal transfer intensity. Out of 110 subjects screened, 12 met criteria for primary insomnia (9 women, mean age + sd = 44.6 + 12.5 years) and completed the study. Healthy age- and gender-matched subjects (n = 12) served as a reference. A repeated measures ANOVA revealed linear effects of thermal transfer intensities (2-night means) on sleep latency (p = 0.02; effect size = 0.45) and sleep efficiency (p = 0.05; effect size = 0.36). Sleep latency and sleep efficiency in insomnia patients in the maximum thermal transfer condition (13 + 7 min and 89 + 5%, respectively) did not differ from those of healthy age- and gender-matched sleepers (16 + 16 min and 89 + 7%, respectively). FCTT improved sleep latency and sleep efficiency in insomnia patients in a dose-dependent manner. In the maximum condition, sleep values in insomnia patients did not differ from healthy controls. These positive preliminary results of the effects of FCTT on EEG sleep latency and sleep efficiency in insomnia patients suggest the need for a large-scale clinical trial to determine if FCTT should be considered as a primary treatment for insomnia.

Summary

Cerebral metabolic studies, in light of preclinical work, suggest that there are hierarchical levels of arousal that may be disturbed in insomnia. Further, interventions may have their effects at different levels of a hierarchical arousal neural network. Traditional sedative-hypnotic approaches appear to target brainstem and hypothalamic arousal networks in insomnia patients while behavioral treatments and frontal cerebral hypothermia appear to target frontal hyperarousal in insomnia patients. Additional work is needed to clarify the degree to which alterations in these levels of arousal distinguish insomnia patients from those with other sleep disorders, or the degree to which distinct levels may be disturbed in individual patients. Additional work is also needed to match interventions for the treatment of insomnia with the levels of arousal that are unique to the individual patient. Importantly, brain imaging studies have helped to significantly advance our understanding of the neurobiology of hierarchical brain systems of arousal in insomnia and to advance more targeted treatment interventions directed to one or more levels of this hierarchical arousal network in insomnia patients.

References

1. Edinger JD, Bonnet MH, Bootzin RR, *et al.* Derivation of research diagnostic criteria for insomnia: report of an American Academy of Sleep Medicine Work Group. *Sleep.* 2004; **27**(8):1567–96.

2. American Academy of Sleep Medicine. *The International Classification of Sleep Disorders, Second Edition (ICSD-2): Diagnostic and Coding Manual.* Westcher, IL, American Academy of sleep Medicine, 2005.

3. American Psychiatric Association. *Diagnostic and Statistical Manual of Mental Disorders, Fourth Edition, Text Revision (DSM-IV-TR).* Washington, DC, American Psychiatric Association, 2000.

4. Ohayon MM. Epidemiology of insomnia: what we know and what we still need to learn. *Sleep Med Rev.* 2002;**6**(2):97–111.

5. Roth T, Roehrs T. Insomnia: epidemiology, characteristics, and consequences. *Clin Cornerstone.* 2003;**5**(3):5–15.

6. Soldatos CR, Allaert FA, Ohta T, Dikeos DG. How do individuals sleep around the world? Results from a single-day survey in ten countries. *Sleep Med.* 2005;**6**(1):5–13.

7. Schwartz S, McDowell Anderson W, Cole SR, Cornoni-Huntley J, Hays JC, Blazer D. Insomnia and heart disease: a review of epidemiologic studies. *J Psychosom Res.* 1999;**47**(4):313–33.

8. Riemann D, Voderholzer U. Primary insomnia: a risk factor to develop depression? *J Affect Disord.* 2003;**76**(1–3):255–9.

9. Breslau N, Roth T, Rosenthal L, Andreski P. Sleep disturbance and psychiatric disorders: a longitudinal epidemiological study of young adults. *Biol Psychiatry.* 1996;**39**(6):411–18.

10. Dryman A, Eaton WW. Affective symptoms associated with the onset of major depression in the community: findings from the US National Institute of Mental Health Epidemiologic Catchment Area Program. *Acta Psychiatr Scand.* 1991;**84**(1):1–5.

11. Weissman MM, Greenwald S, Nino-Murcia G, Dement WC. The morbidity of insomnia uncomplicated by psychiatric disorders. *Gen Hosp Psychiatry.* 1997;**19**(4):245–50.

12. Jones B. Anatomy and neurophysiology. In: Opp M, ed. *SRS Basics of Sleep Guide.* Westchester, IL, Sleep Research Society. 2005;57–64.

13. Henriksen S. Stimulants. In: Opp M, ed. *SRS Basics of Sleep Guide.* Westchester, IL, Sleep Research Society, 2005.

14. Braun AR, Balkin TJ, Wesenten NJ, *et al.* Regional cerebral blood flow throughout the sleep-wake cycle. An H2(15)O PET study. *Brain.* 1997;**120**:1173–97.

15. Hofle N, Paus T, Reutens D, *et al.* Regional cerebral blood flow changes as a function of delta and spindle activity during slow wave sleep in humans. *J Neurosci.* 1997;**17**(12):4800–8.

16. Maquet P, Degueldre C, Delfiore G, *et al.* Functional neuroanatomy of human slow wave sleep. *J Neurosci.* 1997;**17**(8):2807–12.

17. Nofzinger EA, Buysse DJ, Germain A, *et al.* Functional neuroimaging evidence for hyperarousal in insomnia. *Am J Psychiatry.* 2004;**161**(11):2126–8.

18. Kajimura N, Nishikawa M, Uchiyama M, *et al.* Deactivation by benzodiazepine of the basal forebrain and amygdala in normal humans during sleep: a placebo-controlled [15O]H2O PET study. *Am J Psychiatry.* 2004;**161**(4):748–51.

19. Nofzinger EA, Buysse D, Moul D, *et al.* Eszopiclone reverses brain hyperarousal in insomnia: evidence from [18]-FDG PET. *Sleep.* 2008;**31**:A232.

20. Phillips ML, Drevets WC, Rauch SL, Lane R. Neurobiology of emotion perception I: The neural basis of normal emotion perception. *Biol Psychiatry.* 2003;**54**(5):504–14.

21. Wright CI, Fischer H, Whalen PJ, *et al.* Differential prefrontal cortex and amygdala habituation to repeatedly presented emotional stimuli. *Neuroreport.* 2001;**12**(2):379–83.

22. Blair RJ, Morris JS, Frith CD, Perrett DI, Dolan RJ. Dissociable neural responses to facial expressions of sadness and anger. *Brain.* 1999;**122**:883–93.

23. Isenberg N, Silbersweig D, Engelien A, *et al.* Linguistic threat activates the human amygdala. *Proc Natl Acad Sci U S A.* 1999;**96**(18):10456–9.

24. Phillips ML, Young AW, Scott SK, *et al.* Neural responses to facial and vocal expressions of fear and disgust. *Proc Biol Sci.* 1998;**265**(1408):1809–17.

25. Davidson RJ, Kabat-Zinn J, Schumacher J, *et al.* Alterations in brain and immune function produced by mindfulness meditation. *Psychosom Med.* 2003;**65**(4):564–70.

26. Morrison AR, Sanford LD, Ross RJ. Initiation of rapid eye movement sleep: beyond the brainstem. In: Mallick BN, Inoue S, eds. *Rapid Eye Movement Sleep.* New York, Marcel Dekker. 1999;51–68.

27. Sanford LD, Ross RJ, Morrison AR. Serotonergic mechanisms in the amygdala terminate REM sleep. *Sleep Res.* 1995;**24**:54.

28. Semba K. The mesopontine cholinergic system: a dual role in REM sleep and wakefulness. In: Lydic R, Baghdoyan HA, eds. *Handbook of Behavioral State Control: Cellular and Molecular Mechanisms.* Boca Raton, CRC Press. 1999;161–80.

29. Sherin JE, Elmquist JK, Torrealba F, Saper CB. Innervation of histaminergic tuberomammillary neurons by GABAergic and galaninergic neurons in the ventrolateral preoptic nucleus of the rat. *J Neurosci.* 1998;**18**(12):4705–21.

30. Nofzinger EA, Price JC, Meltzer CC, *et al.* Towards a neurobiology of dysfunctional arousal in depression: the relationship between beta EEG power and regional cerebral glucose metabolism during NREM sleep. *Psychiatry Res.* 2000;**98**(2):71–91.

31. Mayberg HS, Brannan SK, Tekell JL, *et al*. Regional metabolic effects of fluoxetine in major depression: serial changes and relationship to clinical response. *Biol Psychiatry*. 2000;**48**(8):830–43.

32. Buchsbaum MS, Wu J, Siegel BV, *et al*. Effect of sertraline on regional metabolic rate in patients with affective disorder. *Biol Psychiatry*. 1997;**41**(1):15–22.

33. Tsukada H, Kakiuchi T, Nishiyama S, Ohba H, Harada N. Effects of aging on 5-HT(1A) receptors and their functional response to 5-HT(1a) agonist in the living brain: PET study with [carbonyl-(11)C]WAY-100635 in conscious monkeys. *Synapse*. 2001;**42**(4):242–51.

34. Nissen C, Kloepfer C, Nofzinger EA, *et al*. Impaired sleep-related memory consolidation in primary insomnia–a pilot study. *Sleep*. 2006;**29**(8):1068–73.

35. Riemann D, Voderholzer U, Spiegelhalder K, *et al*. Chronic insomnia and MRI-measured hippocampal volumes: a pilot study. *Sleep*. 2007;**30**(8):955–8.

36. Smith MT, Perlis ML, Chengazi VU, *et al*. Neuroimaging of NREM sleep in primary insomnia: a Tc-99-HMPAO single photon emission computed tomography study. *Sleep*. 2002;**25**(3):325–35.

37. Benington JH, Heller HC. Restoration of brain energy metabolism as the function of sleep. *Prog Neurobiol*. 1995;**45**(4):347–60.

38. Tononi G, Cirelli C. Sleep and synaptic homeostasis: a hypothesis. *Brain Res Bull*. 2003;**62**(2):143–50.

39. Steriade M, Amzica F. Coalescence of sleep rhythms and their chronology in corticothalamic networks. *Sleep Res Online*. 1998;**1**(1):1–10.

40. Werth E, Achermann P, Borbely AA. Brain topography of the human sleep EEG: antero-posterior shifts of spectral power. *Neuroreport*. 1996;**8**(1):123–7.

41. Cajochen C, Foy R, Dijk DJ. Frontal predominance of a relative increase in sleep delta and theta EEG activity after sleep loss in humans. *Sleep Res Online*. 1999;**2**(3):65–9.

42. Harrison Y, Horne JA. The impact of sleep deprivation on decision making: a review. *J Exp Psychol. Appl*. 2000;**6**(3):236–49.

43. Thomas M, Sing H, Belenky G, *et al*. Neural asis of alertness and cognitive performance impairments during sleepiness. I. Effects of 24 h of sleep deprivation on waking human regional brain activity. *J Sleep Res*. 2000;**9**(4):335–52.

44. Huber R, Ghilardi MF, Massimini M, Tononi G. Local sleep and learning. *Nature*. 2004;**430**(6995):78–81.

45. Miller EK, Cohen JD. An integrative theory of prefrontal cortex function. *Annu Rev Neurosci*. 2001;**24**:167–202.

46. Davidson RJ, Jackson DC, Kalin NH. Emotion, plasticity, context, and regulation: perspectives from affective neuroscience. *Psychol Bull*. 2000;**126**(6):890–909.

47. Perez-Jaranay JM, Vives F. Electrophysiological study of the response of medial prefrontal cortex neurons to stimulation of the basolateral nucleus of the amygdala in the rat. *Brain Res*. 1991;**564**(1):97–101.

48. Nofzinger EA, Buysse DJ, Miewald JM, *et al*. Human regional cerebral glucose metabolism during non-rapid eye movement sleep in relation to waking. *Brain*. 2002;**125**(Pt 5):1105–15.

49. Nofzinger EA, Nissen C, Germain A, *et al*. Regional cerebral metabolic correlates of WASO during NREM sleep in insomnia. *J Clin Sleep Med*. 2006;**2**(3):316–22.

50. Lou HC, Kjaer TW, Friberg L, *et al*. A 15O-H$_2$O PET study of meditation and the resting state of normal consciousness. *Hum Brain Mapp*. 1999;**7**(2):98–105.

51. Altena E, Van Der Werf YD, Strijers RL, Van Someren EJ. Sleep loss affects vigilance: effects of chronic insomnia and sleep therapy. *J Sleep Res*. 2008;**17**(3):335–43.

52. Milgrom O, Buysse D, Hall M, Nofzinger E, Germain A. Effect of CBTI on regional cerebral glucose metabolism during wakefulness and NREM sleep in adults with primary insomnia: a pilot study. (under review)

53. Hasler BP, Germain A, Nofzinger EA, *et al*. Chronotype and diurnal patterns of positive affect and affective neural circuitry in primary insomnia. *J Sleep Res*. 2012;**21**(5):515–26.

54. Feinberg I. Changes in sleep cycle patterns with age. *J Psychiatr Res*. 1974;**10**(3–4):283–306.

55. Borbely AA, Baumann F, Brandeis D, Strauch I, Lehmann D. Sleep deprivation: effect on sleep stages and EEG power density in man. *Electroencephalogr Clin Neurophysiol*. 1981;**51**(5):483–95.

56. Borbely AA. A two process model of sleep regulation. *Hum Neurobiol*. 1982;**1**(3):195–204.

57. Tobler II, Franken P, Trachsel L, Borbely AA. Models of sleep regulation in mammals. *J Sleep Res*. 1992;**1**(2):125–7.

58. Dijk DJ, Beersma DG, Daan S. EEG power density during nap sleep: reflection of an hourglass measuring the duration of prior wakefulness. *J Biol Rhythms*. 1987;**2**(3):207–19.

59. Petit JM, Tobler I, Allaman I, Borbely AA, Magistretti PJ. Sleep deprivation modulates brain mRNAs encoding genes of glycogen metabolism. *Eur J Neurosci*. 2002;**16**(6):1163–7.

60. De Gennaro L, Ferrara M, Curcio G, Cristiani R. Antero-posterior EEG changes during the wakefulness-sleep transition. *Clin Neurophysiol*. 2001;**112**(10):1901–11.

61. Finelli LA, Achermann P, Borbely AA. Individual 'fingerprints' in human sleep EEG topography. *Neuropsychopharmacology*. 2001;**25** (5 Suppl):S57–62.

62. Finelli LA, Baumann H, Borbely AA, Achermann P. Dual electroencephalogram markers of human sleep homeostasis: correlation between theta activity in waking and slow-wave activity in sleep. *Neuroscience*. 2000;**101**(3):523–9.

63. Cajochen C, Khalsa SB, Wyatt JK, Czeisler CA, Dijk DJ. EEG and ocular correlates of circadian melatonin phase and human performance decrements during sleep loss. *Am J Physiol*. 1999;**277**(3 Pt 2):R640–9.

64. Cajochen C, Knoblauch V, Krauchi K, Renz C, Wirz-Justice A. Dynamics of frontal EEG activity, sleepiness and body temperature under high and low sleep pressure. *Neuroreport*. 2001;**12**(10):2277–81.

65. Kingshott RN, Cosway RJ, Deary IJ, Douglas NJ. The effect of sleep fragmentation on cognitive processing using computerized topographic brain mapping. *J Sleep Res*. 2000;**9**(4):353–7.

66. Borbely AA. From slow waves to sleep homeostasis: new perspectives. *Arch Ital Biol*. 2001;**139**(1–2):53–61.

67. Horne JA. Human sleep, sleep loss and behaviour. Implications for the prefrontal cortex and psychiatric disorder. *Psychiatry*. 1993;**162**:413–19.

68. Horne J. Neuroscience. Images of lost sleep. *Nature*. 2000;**403**(6770):605–6.

69. Harrison Y, Horne JA, Rothwell A. Prefrontal neuropsychological effects of sleep deprivation in young adults–a model for healthy aging? *Sleep*. 2000;**23**(8):1067–73.

70. Johnson JJ, Nissen C, Germain A, Miewald JM, Nofzinger EA. Modulation of sleep homeostasis via sleep deprivation leads to reductions in glucose metabolism in the cerebral cortex during recovery sleep in humans: a repeated measures PET FDG study. *Sleep*. 2006;**29**:(Abstract).

71. Bonnet MH, Arand DL. 24-Hour metabolic rate in insomniacs and matched normal sleepers. *Sleep*. 1995;**18**(7):581–8.

72. Bonnet MH, Arand DL. Physiological activation in patients with Sleep State Misperception. *Psychosom Med*. 1997;**59**(5):533–40.

73. Bonnet MH, Arand DL. Heart rate variability in insomniacs and matched normal sleepers. *Psychosom Med*. 1998;**60**(5):610–15.

74. Hall M, Thayer JF, Germain A, *et al*. Psychological stress is associated with heightened physiological arousal during NREM sleep in primary insomnia. *Behav Sleep Med*. 2007;**5**(3):178–93.

75. Vgontzas AN, Bixler EO, Lin HM, Prolo P, Mastorakos G, Vela-Bueno A, *et al*. Chronic insomnia is associated with nyctohemeral activation of the hypothalamic-pituitary-adrenal axis: clinical implications. *J Clin Endocrinol Metab*. 2001;**86**(8):3787–94.

76. Rodenbeck A, Hajak G. Neuroendocrine dysregulation in primary insomnia. *Rev Neurol (Paris)*. 2001;**157**(11 Pt 2):S57–61.

77. Freedman RR. EEG power spectra in sleep-onset insomnia. *Electroencephalogr Clin Neurophysiol*. 1986;**63**(5).408–13.

78. Merica H, Blois R, Gaillard JM. Spectral characteristics of sleep EEG in chronic insomnia. *Eur J Neurosci*. 1998;**10**(5):1826–34.

79. Perlis ML, Smith MT, Andrews PJ, Orff H, Giles DE. Beta/Gamma EEG activity in patients with primary and secondary insomnia and good sleeper controls. *Sleep*. 2001;**24**(1):110–7.

80. Perlis ML, Merica H, Smith MT, Giles DE. Beta EEG activity and insomnia. *Sleep Med Rev*. 2001;**5**(5):363–74.

81. Krystal AD, Edinger JD, Wohlgemuth WK, Marsh GR. NREM sleep EEG frequency spectral correlates of sleep complaints in primary insomnia subtypes. *Sleep*. 2002;**25**(6):630–40.

82. Sewitch DE. Slow wave sleep deficiency insomnia: a problem in thermo-downregulation at sleep onset. *Psychophysiology*. 1987;**24**(2):200–15.

83. Morris M, Lack L, Dawson D. Sleep-onset insomniacs have delayed temperature rhythms. *Sleep*. 1990;**13**(1):1–14.

84. Gradisar M, Lack L, Wright H, Harris J, Brooks A. Do chronic primary insomniacs have impaired heat loss when attempting sleep? *Am J Physiol*. 2006;**290**(4):R1115–21.

85. van den Heuvel C, Ferguson S, Dawson D. Attenuated thermoregulatory response to mild thermal challenge in subjects with sleep-onset insomnia. *Sleep*. 2006;**29**(9):1174–80.

86. Harvey AG. Pre-sleep cognitive activity: a comparison of sleep-onset insomniacs and good sleepers. *The British Journal of Clinical Psychology*. 2000;**39** (Pt 3):275–86.

87. Nelson J, Harvey AG. An exploration of pre-sleep cognitive activity in insomnia: imagery and verbal thought. *J Clin Psychol*. 2003;**42**(Pt 3):271–88.

88. Wicklow A, Espie CA. Intrusive thoughts and their relationship to actigraphic measurement of sleep: towards a cognitive model of insomnia. *Behav Res Ther*. 2000;**38**(7):679–93.

89. Semler CN, Harvey AG. An investigation of monitoring for sleep-related threat in primary insomnia. *Behav Res Ther*. 2004;**42**(12):1403–20.

90. Semler CN, Harvey AG. Monitoring for sleep-related threat: a pilot study of the Sleep Associated Monitoring Index (SAMI). *Psychosom Med*. 2004;**66**(2):242–50.

91. Harvey AG. A cognitive model of insomnia. *Behav Res Ther*. 2002;**40**(8):869–93.

92. Perlis ML, Giles DE, Mendelson WB, Bootzin RR, Wyatt JK. Psychophysiological insomnia: the behavioural model and a neurocognitive perspective. *J Sleep Res*. 1997;**6**(3):179–88.

93. Buysse DJ. New adventures in sleep quality. Plenary presentation. *Sleep*. 2010.

94. Iwata O, Iwata S, Tamura M, *et al*. Early head cooling in newborn piglets is neuroprotective even in the absence of profound systemic hypothermia. *Pediatr Int*. 2003;**45**(5):522–9.

95. Wang H, Olivero W, Lanzino G, *et al*. Rapid and selective cerebral hypothermia achieved using a cooling helmet. *J Neurosurg*. 2004;**100**(2):272–7.

96. Diao C, Zhu L, Wang H. Cooling and rewarming for brain ischemia or injury: theoretical analysis. *Ann Biomed Eng*. 2003;**31**(3):346–53.

97. Zhu L, Diao C. Theoretical simulation of temperature distribution in the brain during mild hypothermia treatment for brain injury. *Med Biol Eng Comput*. 2001;**39**(6):681–7.

98. Sahuquillo J, Vilalta A. Cooling the injured brain: how does moderate hypothermia influence the pathophysiology of traumatic brain injury. *Curr Pharm Des*. 2007;**13**(22):2310–22.

99. McIlvoy LH. The effect of hypothermia and hyperthermia on acute brain injury. *AACN Clin Issues*. 2005;**16**(4):488–500.

100. Dietrich WD, Bramlett HM. Hyperthermia and central nervous system injury. *Prog Brain Res*. 2007;**162**:201–17.

101. Dietrich WD. The importance of brain temperature in cerebral injury. *J Neurotrauma*. 1992;**9** (Suppl 2):S475–85.

102. Iwata O, Thornton JS, Sellwood MW, *et al*. Depth of delayed cooling alters neuroprotection pattern after hypoxia-ischemia. *Ann Neurol*. 2005;**58**(1):75–87.

103. Qiu WS, Liu WG, Shen H, *et al*. Therapeutic effect of mild hypothermia on severe traumatic head injury. *Chin J Traumatol*. 2005;**8**(1):27–32.

104. Chiang AA. Obstructive sleep apnea and chronic intermittent hypoxia: a review. *Chin J Physiol*. 2006;**49**(5):234–43.

105. Gozal D. Obstructive sleep apnea in children: implications for the developing central nervous system. *Semin Pediatr Neurol*. 2008;**15**(2):100–6.

106. McEwen BS. Protective and damaging effects of stress mediators: central role of the brain. *J Neurosurg*. 2004;**100**:272–7.

107. Aschoff J. Internal-peripheral reciprocal action in thermoregulation. *Arch Phys Ther (Leipz)*. 1956;**8**:113–33.

108. Krauchi K, Wirz-Justice A. Circadian rhythm of heat production, heart rate, and skin and core temperature under unmasking conditions in men. *Am J Physiol*. 1994;**267**(3 Pt 2): R819–29.

109. Krauchi K, Cajochen C, Werth E, Wirz-Justice A. Functional link between distal vasodilation and sleep-onset latency? *Am J Physiol*. 2000;**278**(3): R741–8.

110. Krauchi K, Cajochen C, Werth E, Wirz-Justice A. Warm feet promote the rapid onset of sleep. *Nature*. 1999;**401**(6748):36–7.

111. Nofzinger EA, Miewald JM, Price J, Buysse DJ. Frontal cerebral hypothermia: a new approach to the treatment of insomnia. *Sleep*. 2009;**32**:A287.

112. Nofzinger EA, Buysse DJ. Frontal cerebral thermal transfer as a treatment for insomnia: a dose-ranging study. *Sleep*. 2011;**34**:A183.

Sleep neuroimaging in depression and schizophrenia

Eric Nofzinger

Background

Major depression is the leading cause of disability in the United States and worldwide, according to a study by the World Health Organization, the World Bank, and Harvard University [1]. Given its detrimental impact on behavior that leads to personal and societal productivity, it is imperative that the pathophysiology of the disorder is understood, with the ultimate goal being a translation of this information into effective new treatment strategies. Historical research, as well as emerging new data, suggests that the study of sleep neuroscience in depression will yield important insights into the pathophysiology of the disorder.

Effects of depression on EEG sleep

Extensive electroencephalographic (EEG) sleep studies have demonstrated increases in rapid eye movement (REM) sleep and changes in non-rapid eye movement (NREM) sleep in depression. In brief, depressed patients have difficulties falling asleep and staying asleep, and early morning awakenings [2–6]. In terms of REM sleep, depressed patients have a reduction in the latency to REM sleep, and increases in frequency of eye movements within a REM sleep period, or REM density [3, 5, 7, 8]. A genetic or familial basis for the REM sleep alterations in depression has received some support [9]. In terms of NREM sleep, depressed patients have reductions in stages 3 and 4, or delta, NREM sleep [3, 5, 7, 8], reductions in the amplitude or a reduction in the number of low frequency (0–4 Hz) delta waves during sleep [7, 10–16], and increased alpha [10] and beta [7, 17] high-frequency EEG spectral power. EEG sleep alterations predict poor response to psychotherapy but not medication therapy [18, 19]. Other studies have indicated that reduced REM latency and decreased delta EEG activity are associated with increased likelihood of, or decreased time until, recurrence of depression in patients treated with medications or psychotherapy [20]. Reduced REM latency is associated with increased response rates to pharmacotherapy [21], but not to psychotherapy [22, 23]. These early studies suggest neurobiological alterations in depressed patients, yet EEG sleep studies do not provide information on the neural networks that may be altered.

Neural systems related to REM and NREM sleep: preclinical studies

Extensive knowledge of the neural mechanisms of sleep/wake regulation is available from preclinical studies. Preclinical evidence shows that REM sleep is generated in the brainstem. The laterodorsal and pedunculopontine tegmental cholinergic nuclei (LDT and PPT) in the pontine reticular formation generate the phasic and tonic components of REM sleep [24–28]. A reciprocal interaction hypothesis proposes that these cholinergic nuclei are tonically inhibited by noradrenergic and serotonergic nuclei [29–37]. While early theories about the REM sleep disturbances in depression were brainstem based, relying heavily on these preclinical studies, they provided little information regarding the relationship of REM sleep to human behavior or why this relationship might be abnormal in depressed patients.

Preclinical studies show that NREM sleep is characterized by slower frequency, higher amplitude thalamocortical electrical oscillations [38]. These occur when there is a reduction in function in brain structures that control cortical arousal (see [39], for review). These include the ascending reticular activating system (ARAS) [40, 41], the pontine cholinergic nuclei, the midbrain raphe nuclei, the locus coeruleus, the midline and medial thalamus, the amygdala, the hypothalamus [41–51], and the basal forebrain-ventral striatum system [51–55]. The posterior hypothalamus includes hypocretin producing neurons that promote arousal via projections over the entire isocortex as well as to all other arousal systems noted above (see [56], for review). The anterior hypothalamus, including the ventrolateral preoptic area (VLPO), contains gamma-aminobutyric acid (GABA)ergic and galaninergic neurons that are active during sleep and are necessary for normal sleep. This region receives inputs from multiple brain systems that regulate arousal, autonomic, limbic, and circadian functions [57] and it sends inhibitory projections to arousal systems in the posterior hypothalamus and brainstem. As such, the VLPO may represent a "sleep switch" [58]. While these preclinical studies provide important information on the brain centers that are responsible for the generation of NREM sleep, they provide less information on the relationship of NREM sleep to emotional behavior or why this relationship might be abnormal in depressed patients.

Neuroimaging of Sleep and Sleep Disorders, ed. Eric Nofzinger, Pierre Maquet, and Michael J. Thorpy. Published by Cambridge University Press. © Cambridge University Press 2013.

NREM sleep and restoration of function in the prefrontal cortex

Considerable evidence suggests that NREM sleep may serve a restorative function [59–62]. An EEG marker of sleep homeostasis is EEG spectral power in the delta frequency range (1–4 Hz) [60, 63]. The homeostatic sleep drive may involve the restoration of brain energy metabolism through the replenishment of brain glycogen stores that are depleted during wakefulness [64, 65]. This function may have some regional specificity. A prefrontal dominance of EEG spectral power in the delta EEG spectral power range has been reported [66–68]. A prefrontal predominance for the increase in delta power following sleep loss has also been reported [67, 69–74]. This region of cortex plays a prominent role in waking executive functions which are preferentially impaired following sleep deprivation [75–79]. Evidence such as this suggests that NREM sleep is essential for optimal executive behavior and that the mechanism involves the prefrontal cortex. As such, the alterations in NREM sleep in depressed patients may lead to impaired restoration of prefrontal cortex function during NREM sleep.

Neural systems related to REM and NREM sleep: functional neuroimaging studies

Functional neuroimaging studies of sleep extend our preclinical understanding of the mechanisms of sleep/wake regulation by providing potential links between neural systems involved in emotional behavior and those involved in sleep. REM sleep has been shown to be an active brain state, in terms of blood flow and metabolism, that has been reliably associated with the selective activation of anterior limbic and paralimbic structures [5, 80–92].

Functional neuroimaging studies also showed that between waking and NREM sleep there is a global reduction in brain activity, including blood flow and metabolism [80, 81, 84, 93, 94], with relatively greater reductions in the heteromodal association cortex (frontal, parietal, and temporal regions) and in the thalamus [84, 93, 95–97] as well as in structures associated with cortical arousal such as the anterior cingulate, the pontine reticular formation, the basal forebrain/hypothalamus, the amygdala, and the orbitofrontal cortex. These observations suggest that NREM sleep is essential for the normal restoration of prefrontal cortex function and that the lighter NREM sleep of depressed patients may prevent this restoration in the prefrontal cortex. This may lead to waking hypofrontality and the associated deficits in cognitive function subserved by the prefrontal cortex.

The results of preclinical, healthy human and depressed human studies support the importance of two neural systems in emotional behavior [98, 99]. The roles of various structures and their pattern of abnormalities in depression are consistent with their involvement in broader neural systems. A more ventrally located system, with important contributions from the amygdala, has been shown to be fundamental to the initial experience of emotions and to the automatic generation of emotional responses. The function of this system is a reactive one in response to emotional stimuli. Other structures related to this system include the anterior insula, ventral striatum ventral regions of the anterior cingulate cortex, and the ventral prefrontal cortex. In general, these structures have increased activity in depressed patients in relation to healthy controls. A more dorsally located system, with important contributions from the dorsolateral prefrontal cortex (DLPFC), has been shown to be fundamental to the conscious, planned regulation of emotional behavior in light of future behavior. The function of this system is one of planning behavior in response to emotional stimuli. Other structures related to this system include the hippocampus and dorsal regions of the anterior cingulate cortex. In general, these structures have decreased activity in depressed patients in relation to healthy controls.

REM sleep imaging studies in depression

REM sleep is generated by brainstem mechanisms [30]. Functional neuroimaging studies demonstrate that REM sleep preferentially activates anterior limbic and paralimbic structures such as the amygdala and the anterior cingulated cortex in the absence of prefrontal activation [5, 83–86]. "Activation" of the limbic and paralimbic cortices in these studies refers to a relatively greater level of blood flow or metabolism during REM sleep in relation to a waking baseline condition. Given the lower functional activity of these structures in the preceding NREM period [84, 93, 95], one could conceptualize this as a "reactivation" of limbic and paralimbic cortex within REM sleep. The persistence of this waking vs. REM sleep pattern across blood flow and metabolic functional neuroimaging studies led to the notion that a waking vs. REM sleep functional neuroimaging paradigm may serve as a naturalistic probe of limbic and paralimbic function in patients with depression [5, 100]. Given the involvement of these structures in emotional regulation and motivated behavior, the alterations in REM sleep in depressed patients may reflect a functional alteration in these structures that may be central to the neurobiology of depression. Since depressed patients have increased REM sleep in relation to healthy subjects, depressed patients may exhibit a greater activation of the limbic and paralimbic cortices from waking to REM sleep relative to healthy subjects.

Three reports to date have addressed this question. A preliminary analysis of ^{18}F-fluorodeoxyglucose positron emission tomography (^{18}F-FDG PET) studies in six depressed patients [100] showed that depressed subjects showed greater increases from waking to REM sleep in relative metabolism in the tectal area and a series of left hemispheric areas including the sensorimotor cortex, inferior temporal cortex, uncal gyrus-amygdala, and subicular complex. Many of these structures are primary brainstem and limbic regions that are important in modulating emotional arousal. This pattern of wake-REM increases suggested that the increases in REM sleep in depressed patients may signal an increase in affective responsivity in depressed patients. In this preliminary report, in contrast to hypotheses, depressed patients did not show increases in relative metabolism in anterior paralimbic structures during REM sleep compared to waking. Subsequent analyses [101], however, suggested that the lack of increase from waking to in relative metabolism REM sleep in depressed patients may have been related to a ceiling effect, i.e., hypermetabolism in these structures during waking that could not be further increased in REM sleep.

Nofzinger *et al.* [102] completed a larger confirmatory analysis that included 24 depressed patients and 14 healthy subjects who underwent EEG sleep studies and regional cerebral glucose metabolism (rCMRglu) assessments during both waking and REM sleep using ^{18}F-FDG. Depressed patients showed greater REM sleep percent. Consistent with the hypothesis that depressed patients would show increased activation in limbic and anterior limbic structures from waking to REM, depressed patients showed greater increases in relative metabolism from waking to REM sleep than healthy subjects in the midbrain reticular formation including the pretectal area and in a larger region of anterior paralimbic cortex (see Figure 25.1). Additionally, depressed patients showed greater increases in relative metabolism from waking to REM sleep than healthy subjects in a broadly distributed region of predominantly left hemispheric dorsolateral prefrontal, parietal, and temporal cortices. This area included the frontal and parietal eye fields (FEF, PEF).

The first primary finding in this study was the increased activation of the brainstem reticular formation from waking to REM sleep in depressed patients. This is consistent with the model of an altered balance in brainstem monoaminergic (norepinephrine and serotonin) systems and brainstem acetylcholine neuronal systems in depressed patients as proposed by McCarley [103]. A second primary finding in this study was the increased activation of limbic and anterior paralimbic (hippocampus, basal forebrain/ventral pallidum, anterior cingulated, and medial prefrontal) cortices from waking to REM sleep in the depressed patients. The highest density of cholinergic axons is in core limbic structures such as the hippocampus and amygdala. Limbic and anterior paralimbic cortices also have high densities of inhibitory 5-HT$_{1A}$ postsynaptic receptors in relation to other areas of cortex. Behaviorly, increased activation of limbic and paralimbic cortices in depressed patients may reflect a susceptibility of depressed patients to experience stimuli in a more affectively intense, negative context, given the increased activation of these structures in response to negatively valenced stimuli or increased affective states. A third primary finding in this study was the relatively greater activation of executive cortex from waking to REM sleep in depressed patients. This may reflect a change in modulation of cortical function from monoaminergic during waking to cholinergic in REM sleep, coupled with a monoaminergic/cholinergic imbalance in depressed patients. Behaviorally, this may also reflect a greater involvement of executive function during REM sleep in depressed patients, perhaps in response to the increased affective state produced by the abnormal reactivation of limbic and paralimbic cortices during REM sleep in depressed patients.

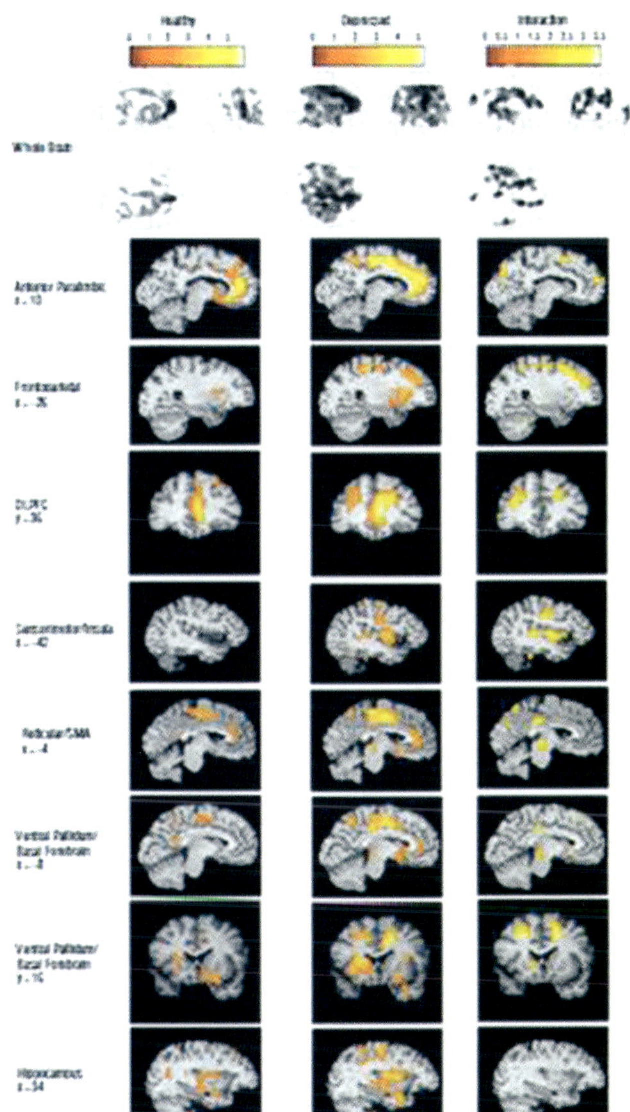

Figure 25.1 Waking to REM sleep activations in healthy subjects (column 1), depressed subjects (column 2), and interactions showing regions where the depressed subjects' wake to REM activations are greater than healthy subjects (column 3).

NREM sleep imaging studies in depression

Several reports to date have assessed regional brain function during NREM sleep in depressed patients to further clarify the neurobiology of these changes in NREM sleep. Ho *et al.* [104] assessed cerebral metabolism using the ^{18}F-FDG PET method in depressed and healthy men during the first NREM period and found increased whole-brain metabolism during NREM sleep in the depressed subjects. Regionally, these increases were most noticeable in the posterior cingulate, the amygdala, hippocampus, the occipital and temporal cortices, and the pons. Relative hypofrontality was noted in the patients, as well as reduced relative metabolism in the anterior cingulate, caudate, and medial thalamus in relation to the controls. On the basis of the increased overall brain metabolism, they interpreted these findings to suggest that depressed patients have "hyperarousal" during NREM sleep.

As noted above, several lines of evidence suggest that the homeostatic, or restorative, aspects of sleep are related to slow-wave NREM sleep and that this restorative aspect of sleep has some regional preference for more frontal regions of cortex. NREM sleep is associated with decreases in frontal, parietal, and temporal cortex metabolic activity compared to wakefulness. Depressed patients demonstrate "lighter" NREM sleep and waking hypofrontality. Therefore, Germain *et al.* [105] tested the hypothesis that depressed patients would show less of a decrease in frontal metabolism between waking and NREM sleep. They assessed 12 medication-free depressed patients and 13 healthy subjects using ^{18}F-FDG PET scans during pre-sleep wakefulness and during NREM sleep. Compared with healthy subjects, depressed patients showed less of a decrease in relative metabolism from pre-sleep wakefulness to NREM bilaterally in the laterodorsal frontal gyri, right medial prefrontal cortex, right superior and middle temporal gyri, and insula,

as well as right posterior cingulate cortex, lingual gyrus, striate cortex, cerebellar vermis, and left thalamus. These findings suggest that abnormal thalamocortical network function may underlie non-restorative sleep in depressed patients. Nofzinger *et al.* [106] hypothesized that depressed patients would show less of a decrease in frontal metabolism between waking and NREM sleep and that during NREM sleep, depressed patients would have increased activity in structures that promote arousal. They assessed EEG sleep and regional cerebral glucose metabolism (rCMRglu) assessments during both waking and NREM sleep using ^{18}F-FDG PET in depressed and healthy subjects. Depressed patients showed smaller decreases in relative metabolism in broad regions of the frontal, parietal, and temporal cortices from waking to NREM sleep (see Figure 25.2). Depressed patients showed larger decreases in relative metabolism in the left amygdala, anterior cingulate cortex, cerebellum, parahippocampal cortex, fusiform gyrus,

Healthy wake > NREM   Depressed wake > NREM

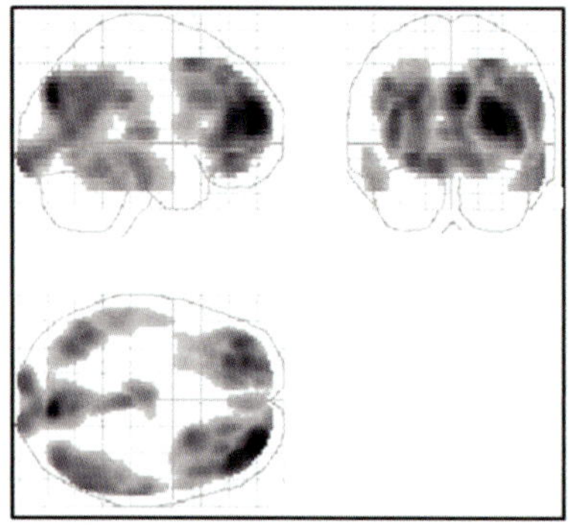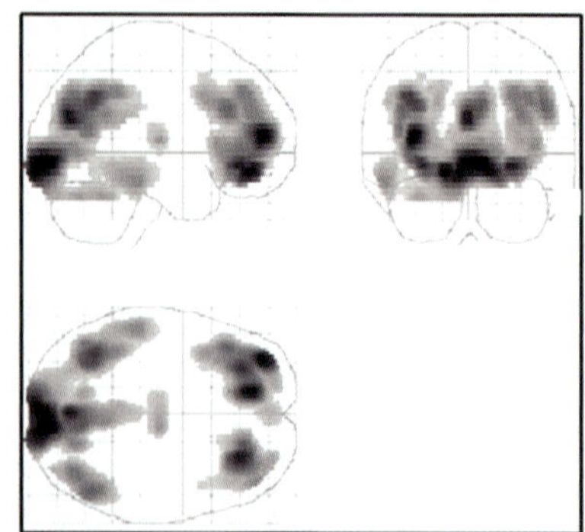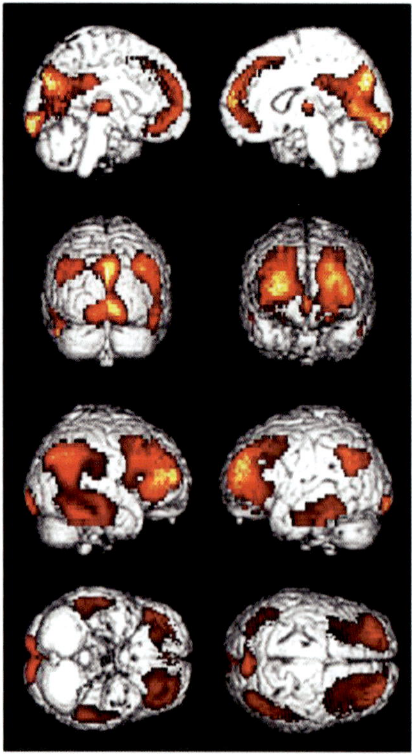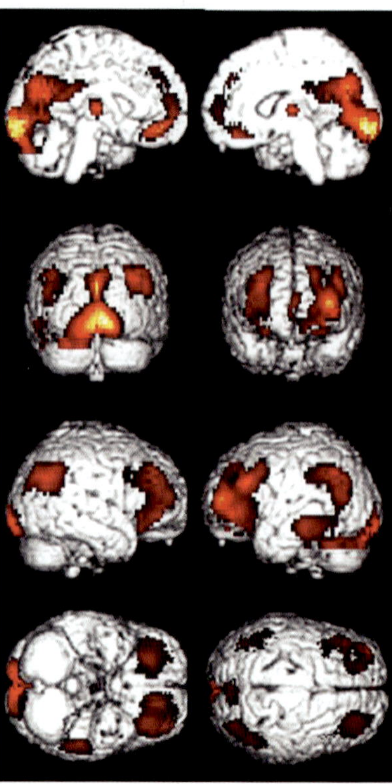

Figure 25.2 Column 1. Glass brain and 3D brain rendering images showing regions with significant declines in relative metabolism from waking to NREM sleep in healthy subjects. Regions include prefrontal cortex (28/54/20, tmax = 7.32, 5771 voxels); cuneus, precuneus, and left temporoparietal cortex (6/-78/32, tmax = 6.70, 3396 voxels); right temporoparietal cortex (56/-54/20, tmax = 4.78, 2305 voxels). Column 2. Glassbrain and 3D brain rendering images showing regions with significant declines in relative metabolism from waking to NREM sleep in depressed subjects, including cuneus, precuneus, and temporoparietal cortex (8/-90/-8, tmax = 7.60, 5303 voxels); left prefrontal cortex (-34/52/12, tmax = 6.95, 2500 voxels); right prefrontal cortex (26/36/-8, tmax = 6.08, 1325 voxels). (Note: all clusters reported are significant at p < 0.05, corrected; coordinates refer to local cluster maxima in Talairach x/y/z sections and tmax to the corresponding t-value).

and occipital cortex. However, in post-hoc analyses, depressed patients showed hypermetabolism in these areas during both waking and NREM sleep. They concluded that the smaller decrease in frontal metabolism from waking to NREM sleep is further evidence for a dynamic sleep/wake alteration in prefrontal cortex function in depression. Hypermetabolism in a ventral emotional neural system during waking in depressed patients persists into NREM sleep and may interfere with the normal production and function of sleep.

Sleep deprivation in depression

The notion of hyperarousal in paralimbic structures in depressed patients has received further support from an extensive literature describing the functional neuroanatomical correlates of the antidepressant response to sleep deprivation in depressed patients. These studies identify the anterior cingulate cortex as playing an important role in the response to sleep deprivation. Across studies, there is a general tendency for patients who have elevated baseline metabolism in the anterior cingulate cortex to have more favorable responses to sleep deprivation, and normalization of this increased function following sleep deprivation [107–113].

Relationship of sleep states to neural systems involved in emotional behavior

What is the relationship, then, between the effects of depression on sleep and the effects of depression on behavior in relation to the ventral and dorsal emotional neural systems? The patterns of neural activity found in REM and NREM sleep suggest that they are differentially related to the two neural systems involved in emotional behavior and that they may be abnormal in depressed patients. The activation of the amygdala and paralimbic cortex in REM sleep suggests that this state is related to the ventral neural system involved in emotional reactivity and

in the generation of automatic affective responses to emotionally salient material. The deactivation of the DLPFC in NREM sleep suggests that this state is related to the dorsal neural system. While the exact role for NREM sleep in the functioning of this system is not entirely known, impairments in both prefrontal cortex metabolism and in executive behavior following sleep deprivation suggest that NREM sleep is performing a restorative function for this dorsal neural system that is necessary for efficient waking executive function. Studies show that depressed patients do not deactivate the DLPFC as much as healthy subjects from waking to NREM sleep. Depressed patients, therefore, may not be restoring the DLPFC during NREM sleep. This may lead to both waking hypofrontality and impaired dorsal neural system function during waking.

Schizophrenia

Patients with schizophrenia are known to have severely disturbed subjective sleep. EEG sleep studies have largely supported alterations in NREM slow-wave sleep in schizophrenic patients. Slow-wave sleep is of particular interest to schizophrenia because of the implication of the prefrontal cortex in this disorder [114] and in the generation of slow-wave sleep [115]. Only one functional neuroimaging study has explored the relationship between some aspect of sleep and the pathophysiology of schizophrenia. Weiler et al. [116] compared cerebral metabolism between 49 awake schizophrenic patients, 30 awake controls, and 12 controls in REM sleep. The aim of the study was to determine if regional metabolism while awake in a psychotic disorder resembled healthy REM sleep, given some phenomenological similarities between the cognitions reported in dreaming and those in psychosis. No similarities were observed discounting the notion that schizophrenia represents an intrusion of REM sleep cognition into wakefulness. Additional functional neuroimaging studies of sleep in schizophrenia are needed.

References

1. Murray CJL, Lopez AD, Harvard School of Public Health, World Health Organization, World Bank. *The Global Burden of Disease: A Comprehensive Assessment of Mortality and Disability from Diseases, Injuries, and Risk Factors in 1990 and Projected to 2020.* Cambridge, MA, Published by the Harvard School of Public Health on behalf of the World Health Organization and the World Bank; Distributed by Harvard University Press, 1996

2. Buysse DJ, Reynolds CF, III, Monk TH, Berman SR, Kupfer DJ. The Pittsburgh Sleep Quality Index: a new instrument for psychiatric practice and research. *Psychiatry Res.* 1989;**28**(2):193–213.

3. Benca RM, Obermeyer WH, Thisted RA, Gillin JC. Sleep and psychiatric disorders: a meta-analysis. *Arch Gen Psychiatry.* 1992;**49**(8):651–68; discussion 669–70.

4. Nofzinger EA, Buysse DJ, Reynolds CF, 3rd, Kupfer DJ. Sleep disorders related to another mental disorder (nonsubstance/primary): a DSM-IV literature review. *J Clin Psychiatry* 1993;**54**(7):244–55; discussion 256–9.

5. Nofzinger EA, Mintun MA, Wiseman M, Kupfer DJ, Moore RY. Forebrain activation in REM sleep: an FDG PET study. *Brain Res.* 1997;**770**(1–2):192–201.

6. Armitage R, Hoffmann R, Trivedi M, Rush AJ. Sleep macro- and microarchitecture in depression: age and gender effects. *Sleep Res.* 1997;**26**:283.

7. Armitage R, Hudson A, Trivedi M, Rush AJ. Sex differences in the distribution of EEG frequencies during sleep: unipolar depressed outpatients. *J Affect Disord.* 1995;**34**(2):121–9.

8. Buysse DJ, Nofzinger EA. Sleep in depression: longitudinal perspectives. In: Oldham JM, Riba MB, eds. *American Psychiatric Press Review of Psychiatry.* Washington, DC, American Psychiatric Press. 1994;29–75.

9. Giles DE, Kupfer DJ, Rush AJ, Roffwarg HP. Controlled comparison of electrophysiological sleep in families of probands with unipolar depression. *Am J Psychiatry.* 1998;**155**(2):192–9.

10. Borbely AA, Tobler I, Loepfe M, *et al.* All-night spectral analysis of the sleep EEG in untreated depressives and normal controls. *Psychiatry Res.* 1984;**12**(1):27–33.

11. Kupfer DJ, Frank E, McEachran AB, Grochocinski VJ. Delta sleep ratio. A biological correlate of early recurrence in unipolar affective disorder. *Arch Gen Psychiatry.* 1990;**47**(12):1100–5.

12. Kupfer DJ, Grochocinski VJ, McEachran AB. Relationship of awakening and delta sleep in depression. *Psychiatry Res.* 1986;**19**(4):297–304.

13. Kupfer DJ, Reynolds CF, III, Ulrich RF, Grochocinski VJ. Comparison of automated REM and slow-wave sleep analysis in young and middle-aged depressed subjects. *Biol Psychiatry.* 1986;**21**(2):189–200.

14. Kupfer DJ, Ulrich RF, Coble PA, *et al.* Application of automated REM and slow-wave sleep analysis: II. Testing the assumptions of the two-process model of sleep regulation in normal and depressed subjects. *Psychiatry Res.* 1984;**13**(4):335–43.

15. Buysse DJ, Reynolds CF, III, Hauri PJ, *et al.* Diagnostic concordance for DSM-IV sleep disorders: a report from the APA/NIMH DSM-IV field trial. *Am J Psychiatry.* 1994;**151**(9):1351–60.

16. Reynolds CF, III, Buysse DJ, Kupfer DJ, *et al.* Rapid eye movement sleep deprivation as a probe in elderly subjects. *Arch Gen Psychiatry.* 1990;**47**(12):1128–36.

17. Armitage R, Roffwarg HP, Rush AJ, *et al.* Digital period analysis of sleep EEG in depression. *Biol Psychiatry.* 1992;**31**(1):52–68.

18. Thase ME, Buysse DJ, Frank E, *et al.* Which depressed patients will respond to interpersonal psychotherapy? The role of abnormal EEG sleep profiles. *Am J Psychiatry.* 1997;**154**(4):502–9.

19. Thase ME, Greenhouse JB, Frank E, *et al.* Treatment of major depression with psychotherapy or psychotherapy-pharmacotherapy combinations. *Arch Gen Psychiatry.* 1997;**54**(11):1009–15.

20. Giles DE, Jarrett RB, Roffwarg HP, Rush AJ. Reduced rapid eye movement latency. A predictor of recurrence in depression. *Neuropsychopharmacology.* 1987;**1**(1):33–9.

21. Rush AJ, Giles DE, Jarrett RB, *et al.* Reduced REM latency predicts response to tricyclic medication in depressed outpatients. *Biol Psychiatry.* 1989;**26**(1):61–72.

22. Jarrett RB, Rush AJ, Khatami M, Roffwarg HP. Does the pretreatment polysomnogram predict response to cognitive therapy in depressed outpatients? A preliminary report. *Psychiatry Res.* 1990;**33**(3):285–99.

23. Jarrett RB. Psychosocial aspects of depression and the role of psychotherapy. *J Clin Psychiatry.* 1990;**51** Suppl:26–35; discussion 35–8.

24. Shiromani PJ, Gillin JC, Henriksen SJ. Acetylcholine and the regulation of REM sleep: basic mechanisms and clinical implications for affective illness and narcolepsy. *Annu Rev Pharmacol Toxicol.* 1987;**27**:137–56.

25. Datta S, Calvo JM, Quattrochi J, Hobson JA. Cholinergic microstimulation of the peribrachial nucleus in the cat. I. Immediate and prolonged increases in ponto-geniculo-occipital waves. *Arch Ital Biol.* 1992;**130**(4):263–84.

26. Hobson JA, Datta S, Calvo JM, Quattrochi J. Acetylcholine as a brain state modulator: triggering and long-term regulation of REM sleep. *Prog Brain Res.* 1993;**98**:389–404.

27. Hobson JA, Stenade M. In: Mountcastle VB, Bloom FE, eds. *Handbook of Physiology.* Bethesda, American Physiological Society. 1986; 701–823.

28. Kushida CA, Zoltoski RK, Gillin JC. Expression of m2 muscarinic receptor mRNA in rat brain with REM sleep deprivation. *Sleep Res.* 1995;**24**:37.

29. McCarley RW, Hobson JA. Neuronal excitability modulation over the sleep cycle: a structural and mathematical model. *Science.* 1975;**189**(4196):58–60.

30. McCarley RW, Massaquoi SG. A limit cycle mathematical model of the REM sleep oscillator system. *Am J Physiol.* 1986;**251**(6 Pt 2):R1011–29.

31. Massaquoi SG, McCarley RW. Extension of the Limit Cycle Reciprocal Interaction Model of REM cycle control. An integrated sleep control model. *J Sleep Res.* 1992;**1**(2):138–43.

32. Luebke JI, Greene RW, Semba K, *et al.* Serotonin hyperpolarizes cholinergic low-threshold burst neurons in the rat laterodorsal tegmental nucleus in vitro. *Proc Natl Acad Sci U S A.* 1992;**89**(2):743–7.

33. Williams JA, Reiner PB. Noradrenaline hyperpolarizes cholinergic neurons in rat laterodorsal tegmentun in vitro. *Soc Neurosci Abstr.* 1992;**18**:975.

34. Aston-Jones G, Bloom FE. Activity of norepinephrine-containing locus coeruleus neurons in behaving rats anticipates fluctuations in the sleep-waking cycle. *J Neurosci.* 1981;**1**(8):876–86.

35. Hobson JA, McCarley RW, Nelson JP. Location and spike-train characteristics of cells in anterodorsal pons having selective decreases in firing rate during desynchronized sleep. *J Neurophysiol.* 1983;**50**(4):770–83.

36. Jacobs BL, Heym J, Trulson ME. Behavioral and physiological correlates of brain serotoninergic unit activity. *J Physiol (Paris).* 1981;**77**(2–3):431–6.

37. McGinty DJ, Harper RM. Dorsal raphe neurons: depression of firing during sleep in cats. *Brain Res.* 1976;**101**(3):569–75.

38. Steriade M. The corticothalamic system in sleep. *Front Biosci.* 2003;**8**:d878–99.

39. Robbins TW, Everitt BJ. Neurobehavioural mechanisms of reward and motivation. *Curr Opin Neurobiol.* 1996;**6**(2):228–36.

40. Steriade M, McCarley RW. Brainstem mechanisms of dreaming and of disorders of sleep in man. *Brainstem Control of Wakefulness and Sleep.* New York, Plenum. 1990;395–482.

41. Saper CB, Sherin JE, Elmquist JK. Role of the ventrolateral preoptic area in sleep induction. In: Hayaishi O, Inoue S, eds. *Sleep and Sleep Disorders: From Molecule to Behavior.* New York, Academic Press. 1997.

42. Panula P, Pirvola U, Auvinen S, Airaksinen MS. Histamine-immunoreactive nerve fibers in the rat brain. *Neuroscience.* 1989;**28**(3):585–610.

43. Khateb A, Fort P, Pegna A, Jones BE, Muhlethaler M. Cholinergic nucleus basalis neurons are excited by histamine in vitro. *Neuroscience.* 1995;**69**(2):495–506.

44. Lin JS, Kitahama K, Fort P, *et al.* Histaminergic system in the cat hypothalamus with reference to type B monoamine oxidase. *J Comp Neurol.* 1993;**330**(3):405–20.

45. Lin JS, Luppi PH, Salvert D, Sakai K, Jouvet M. [Histamine-immunoreactive

neurons in the hypothalamus of cats]. *C R Acad Sci III*. 1986;**303**(9):371–6.

46. Lin JS, Sakai K, Jouvet M. Evidence for histaminergic arousal mechanisms in the hypothalamus of cat. *Neuropharmacology*. 1988;**27**(2):111–22.

47. Lin JS, Sakai K, Jouvet M. Hypothalamo-preoptic histaminergic projections in sleep-wake control in the cat. *Eur J Neurosci*. 1994;**6**(4):618–25.

48. McCormick DA, Williamson A. Modulation of neuronal firing mode in cat and guinea pig LGNd by histamine: possible cellular mechanisms of histaminergic control of arousal. *J Neurosci*. 1991;**11**(10):3188–99.

49. Monti JM. Involvement of histamine in the control of the waking state. *Life Sci*. 1993;**53**(17):1331–8.

50. Shiromani PJ, Scammell T, Sherin JE, Saper CB. Hypothalamic regulation of sleep. In: Lydic R, Baghdoyan HA, eds. *Handbook of Behavioral State Control: Cellular and Molecular Mechanisms*. Boca Raton, CRC Press. 1999; 311–26.

51. Szymusiak R. Magnocellular nuclei of the basal forebrain: substrates of sleep and arousal regulation. *Sleep*. 1995;**18**(6):478–500.

52. McCormick DA. Cellular mechanisms of cholinergic control of neocortical and thalamic neuronal excitability. In: Steriade M, Biesold D, eds. *Brain Cholinergic Systems*. Oxford, Oxford University Press. 1990; 236–64.

53. Wainer BH, Mesulum MM. Ascending cholinergic pathways in the rat brain. In: Steriade M, Biesold D, eds. *Brain Cholinergic Systems*. Oxford, Oxford University Press. 1990; 65–119.

54. Cape EG, Jones BE. Differential modulation of high-frequency gamma-electroencephalogram activity and sleep-wake state by noradrenaline and serotonin microinjections into the region of cholinergic basalis neurons. *J Neurosci*. 1998;**18**(7):2653–66.

55. Metherate R, Cox CL, Ashe JH. Cellular bases of neocortical activation: modulation of neural oscillations by the nucleus basalis and endogenous acetylcholine. *J Neurosci*. 1992;**12**(12):4701–11.

56. Moore RY, Weis R, Moga MM. Efferent projections of the intergeniculate leaflet and the ventral lateral geniculate nucleus in the rat. *J Comp Neurol*. 2000;**420**(3):398–418.

57. Chou TC, Bjorkum AA, Gaus SE, *et al.* Afferents to the ventrolateral preoptic nucleus. *J Neurosci*. 2002;**22**(3):977–90.

58. Saper CB, Chou TC, Scammell TE. The sleep switch: hypothalamic control of sleep and wakefulness. *Trends Neurosci*. 2001;**24**(12):726–31.

59. Borbely AA, Baumann F, Brandeis D, Strauch I, Lehmann D. Sleep deprivation: effect on sleep stages and EEG power density in man. *Electroencephalogr Clin Neurophysiol*. 1981;**51**(5):483–95.

60. Borbely AA. A two process model of sleep regulation. *Hum Neurobiol*. 1982;**1**(3):195–204.

61. Feinberg I. Changes in sleep cycle patterns with age. *J Psychiatr Res*. 1974;**10**(3–4):283–306.

62. Tobler II, Franken P, Trachsel L, Borbely AA. Models of sleep regulation in mammals. *J Sleep Res*. 1992;**1**(2):125–7.

63. Dijk DJ, Beersma DG, Daan S. EEG power density during nap sleep: reflection of an hourglass measuring the duration of prior wakefulness. *J Biol Rhythms*. 1987;**2**(3):207–19.

64. Benington JH, Heller HC. Monoaminergic and cholinergic modulation of REM-sleep timing in rats. *Brain Res*. 1995;**681**(1–2):141–6.

65. Petit JM, Tobler I, Allaman I, Borbely AA, Magistretti PJ. Sleep deprivation modulates brain mRNAs encoding genes of glycogen metabolism. *Eur J Neurosci*. 2002;**16**(6):1163–7.

66. Werth E, Achermann P, Borbely AA. Brain topography of the human sleep EEG: antero-posterior shifts of spectral power. *Neuroreport*. 1996;**8**(1):123–7.

67. Finelli LA, Borbely AA, Achermann P. Functional topography of the human nonREM sleep electroencephalogram. *Eur J Neurosci*. 2001;**13**(12):2282–90.

68. De Gennaro L, Ferrara M, Curcio G, Cristiani R. Antero-posterior EEG changes during the wakefulness-sleep transition. *Clin Neurophysiol*. 2001;**112**(10):1901–11.

69. Borbely AA. From slow-waves to sleep homeostasis: new perspectives. *Arch Ital Biol*. 2001;**139**(1–2):53–61.

70. Finelli LA, Baumann H, Borbely AA, Achermann P. Dual electroencephalogram markers of human sleep homeostasis: correlation between theta activity in waking and slow-wave activity in sleep. *Neuroscience*. 2000;**101**(3):523–9.

71. Cajochen C, Foy R, Dijk DJ. Frontal predominance of a relative increase in sleep delta and theta EEG activity after sleep loss in humans. *Sleep Res Online*. 1999;**2**(3):65–9.

72. Cajochen C, Khalsa SB, Wyatt JK, Czeisler CA, Dijk DJ. EEG and ocular correlates of circadian melatonin phase and human performance decrements during sleep loss. *Am J Physiol*. 1999;**277**(3 Pt 2):R640–9.

73. Cajochen C, Knoblauch V, Krauchi K, Renz C, Wirz-Justice A. Dynamics of frontal EEG activity, sleepiness and body temperature under high and low sleep pressure. *Neuroreport*. 2001;**12**(10):2277–81.

74. Kingshott RN, Cosway RJ, Deary IJ, Douglas NJ. The effect of sleep fragmentation on cognitive processing using computerized topographic brain mapping. *J Sleep Res*. 2000;**9**(4):353–7.

75. Horne JA. Human sleep, sleep loss and behaviour. Implications for the prefrontal cortex and psychiatric disorder. *Br J Psychiatry*. 1993;**162**:413–19.

76. Horne J. Neuroscience. Images of lost sleep. *Nature*. 2000;**403**(6770):605–6.

77. Harrison Y, Horne JA, Rothwell A. Prefrontal neuropsychological effects of sleep deprivation in young adults–a model for healthy aging? *Sleep*. 2000;**23**(8):1067–73.

78. Harrison Y, Horne JA. The impact of sleep deprivation on decision making: a review. *J Exp Psychol Appl*. 2000;**6**(3):236–49.

79. Thomas M, Sing H, Belenky G, *et al.* Neural basis of alertness and cognitive performance impairments during sleepiness. I. Effects of 24 h of sleep deprivation on waking human regional brain activity. *J Sleep Res*. 2000;**9**(4):335–52.

80. Madsen PL, Holm S, Vorstrup S, *et al.* Human regional cerebral blood flow during rapid eye-movement sleep. *J Cereb Blood Flow Metab*. 1991;**11**(3):502–7.

81. Madsen PL, Schmidt JF, Holm S, *et al.* Cerebral oxygen metabolism and cerebral blood flow in man during light

sleep (stage 2). *Brain Res.* 1991;**557** (1–2):217–20.

82. Sakai F, Meyer JS, Karacan I, Derman S, Yamamoto M. Normal human sleep: regional cerebral hemodynamics. *Ann Neurol.* 1980;**7**(5):471–8.

83. Lydic R, Baghdoyan HA, Hibbard L, *et al.* Regional brain glucose metabolism is altered during rapid eye movement sleep in the cat: a preliminary study. *J Comp Neurol.* 1991;**304**(4):517–29.

84. Braun AR, Balkin TJ, Wesenten NJ, *et al.* Regional cerebral blood flow throughout the sleep-wake cycle. An H2 (15)O PET study. *Brain.* 1997;**120**(Pt 7):1173–97.

85. Buchsbaum MS, Gillin JC, Wu J, *et al.* Regional cerebral glucose metabolic rate in human sleep assessed by positron emission tomography. *Life Sci.* 1989;**45** (15):1349–56.

86. Maquet P, Peters J, Aerts J, *et al.* Functional neuroanatomy of human rapid-eye-movement sleep and dreaming. *Nature.* 1996;**383** (6596):163–6.

87. Franck G, Salmon E, Poirrier R, Sadzot B, Franco G. Study of regional cerebral glucose metabolism, in man, while awake or asleep, by positron emission tomography. *Rev Electroencephalogr Neurophysiol Clin.* 1987;**17**(1):71–7.

88. Gozukirmizi E, Meyer JS, Okabe T, *et al.* Cerebral blood flow during paroxysmal EEG activation induced by sleep in patients with complex partial seizures. *Sleep.* 1982;**5**(4):329–42.

89. Heiss WD, Pawlik G, Herholz K, Wagner R, Wienhard K. Regional cerebral glucose metabolism in man during wakefulness, sleep, and dreaming. *Brain Res.* 1985;**327**(1–2):362–6.

90. Maquet P, Dive D, Salmon E, *et al.* Cerebral glucose utilization during sleep-wake cycle in man determined by positron emission tomography and [18F]2-fluoro-2-deoxy-D-glucose method. *Brain Res.* 1990;**513** (1):136–43.

91. Maquet P, Franck G. Cerebral glucose metabolism during the sleep-wake cycle in man as measured by positron emission tomography. In: Horne J, ed. *Sleep '88.* New York: Gustav Fischer verlag; 1989; 76–8.

92. Meyer JS, Ishikawa Y, Hata T, Karacan I. Cerebral blood flow in normal and abnormal sleep and dreaming. *Brain Cogn.* 1987;**6**(3):266–94.

93. Nofzinger EA, Buysse DJ, Miewald JM, *et al.* Human regional cerebral glucose metabolism during non-rapid eye movement sleep in relation to waking. *Brain.* 2002;**125** (Pt 5):1105–15.

94. Hetta J, Onoe H, Andersson J, *et al.* Cerebral blood flow during sleep: a positron emission tomographic (PET) study of regional changes. *Sleep Res.* 1995;**24**:87.

95. Maquet P, Degueldre C, Delfiore G, *et al.* Functional neuroanatomy of human slow-wave sleep. *J Neurosci.* 1997;**17**(8):2807–12.

96. Andersson JL, Onoe H, Hetta J, *et al.* Brain networks affected by synchronized sleep visualized by positron emission tomography. *J Cereb Blood Flow Metab.* 1998;**18** (7):701–15.

97. Hofle N, Paus T, Reutens D, *et al.* Regional cerebral blood flow changes as a function of delta and spindle activity during slow-wave sleep in humans. *J Neurosci.* 1997;**17**(12):4800–8.

98. Phillips ML, Drevets WC, Rauch SL, Lane R. Neurobiology of emotion perception II: implications for major psychiatric disorders. *Biol Psychiatry.* 2003;**54**(5):515–28.

99. Phillips ML, Drevets WC, Rauch SL, Lane R. Neurobiology of emotion perception I: the neural basis of normal emotion perception. *Biol Psychiatry.* 2003;**54**(5):504–14.

100. Nofzinger EA, Nichols TE, Meltzer CC, *et al.* Changes in forebrain function from waking to REM sleep in depression: preliminary analyses of [18F]FDG PET studies. *Psychiatry Res.* 1999;**91**(2):59–78.

101. Nofzinger EA, Berman S, Fasiczka A, *et al.* Effects of bupropion SR on anterior paralimbic function during waking and REM sleep in depression: preliminary findings using. *Psychiatry Res.* 2001;**106**(2):95–111.

102. Nofzinger EA, Buysse DJ, Germain A, *et al.* Increased activation of anterior paralimbic and executive cortex from waking to rapid eye movement sleep in depression. *Arch Gen Psychiatry.* 2004;**61**(7):695–702.

103. McCarley RW. REM sleep and depression: common neurobiological control mechanisms. *Am J Psychiatry.* 1982;**139**(5):565–70.

104. Ho AP, Gillin JC, Buchsbaum MS, *et al.* Brain glucose metabolism during non-rapid eye movement sleep in major depression. A positron emission tomography study. *Arch Gen Psychiatry.* 1996;**53**(7):645–52.

105. Germain A, Nofzinger EA, Kupfer DJ, Buysse DJ. Neurobiology of non-REM sleep in depression: further evidence for hypofrontality and thalamic dysregulation. *Am J Psychiatry.* 2004;**161**(10):1856–63.

106. Nofzinger EA, Buysse DJ, Germain A, et al. Alterations in regional cerebral glucose metabolism across waking and non-rapid eye movement sleep in depression. *Arch Gen Psychiatry.* 2005;**62**(4):387–96.

107. Smith MT, Perlis ML, Chengazi VU, *et al.* Neuroimaging of NREM sleep in primary insomnia: a Tc-99-HMPAO single photon emission computed tomography study. *Sleep.* 2002;**25** (3):325–35.

108. Ebert D, Feistel H, Barocka A. Effects of sleep deprivation on the limbic system and the frontal lobes in affective disorders: a study with Tc-99m-HMPAO SPECT. *Psychiatry Res.* 1991;**40**(4):247–51.

109. Wu JC, Gillin JC, Buchsbaum MS, *et al.* Effect of sleep deprivation on brain metabolism of depressed patients. *Am J Psychiatry.* 1992;**149**(4):538–43.

110. Ebert D, Feistel H, Kaschka W, Barocka A, Pirner A. Single photon emission computerized tomography assessment of cerebral dopamine D2 receptor blockade in depression before and after sleep deprivation–preliminary results. *Biol Psychiatry.* 1994;**35**(11):880–5.

111. Volk SA, Kaendler SH, Hertel A, *et al.* Can response to partial sleep deprivation in depressed patients be predicted by regional changes of cerebral blood flow? *Psychiatry Res.* 1997;**75**(2):67–74.

112. Smith GS, Reynolds CF, III, Pollock B, *et al.* Cerebral glucose metabolic response to combined total sleep deprivation and antidepressant treatment in geriatric depression. *Am J Psychiatry.* 1999;**156**(5):683–9.

113. Wu J, Buchsbaum MS, Gillin JC, *et al.* Prediction of antidepressant effects of

sleep deprivation by metabolic rates in the ventral anterior cingulate and medial prefrontal cortex. *Am J Psychiatry.* 1999;**156**(8):1149–58.

114. Keshavan MS, Anderson S, Pettegrew JW. Is schizophrenia due to excessive synaptic pruning in the prefrontal cortex? The Feinberg hypothesis revisited. *J Psychiatr Res.* 1994;**28**(3):239–65.

115. Werth E, Achermann P, Borbely AA. Fronto-occipital EEG power gradients in human sleep. *J Sleep Res.* 1997;**6**(2):102–12.

116. Weiler MA, Buchsbaum MS, Gillin JC, Tafalla R, Bunney WE, Jr., Explorations in the relationship of dream sleep to schizophrenia using positron emission tomography. *Neuropsychobiology.* 1990;**23**(3):109–18.

Structural neuroimaging of narcolepsy

Eun Yeon Joo and Seung Bong Hong

Introduction

Narcolepsy is characterized by excessive daytime sleepiness (EDS), a disruption of sleep/wake behavior, cataplexy (sudden loss of muscle tone provoked by emotional stimuli), and the other rapid eye movement (REM) sleep phenomena such as sleep paralysis and hypnagogic hallucination. Hypocretin-containing neuron numbers are reduced in the hypothalamus of the narcoleptic brain [1]. The neuropeptide hypocretin appears to play a critical role in the neurobiology of narcolepsy [2–4]. Narcolepsy patients suffer from cognitive or emotional features in addition to sleep/wake disturbances. The responsible neuroanatomical substrates for those features have been studied.

MRI visual inspection

For the past decade, numerous brain magnetic resonance imaging (MRI) studies have been performed to identify the structural brain abnormalities of narcolepsy, but results have been controversial. The pontine tegmentum was first proposed as a possible main site of anatomical or functional impairments in narcolepsy because it controls transitions between sleep states. While T2-weighted hyperintensity in the pontine tegmentum was reported in three patients with narcolepsy [5], another two MRI studies found no pontine abnormalities in narcolepsy patients [6, 7]. However, the MRI abnormalities [5] could reflect non-specific age-related pontine vascular changes rather than a narcolepsy-related phenomenon, as they were indistinguishable from ischemic changes [8].

Voxel-based morphometry (VBM)

Differences in brain morphology that are not identifiable by routine visual inspection of individual brain MRI can be investigated using voxel-based morphometry (VBM). VBM allows between-group, statistical comparisons of tissue composition (gray and white matter) across all brain regions, based on high-resolution scans. Previous VBM studies reported equivocal results in narcolepsy patients.

One study insisted that there were no structural changes in brains of patients with hypocretin-deficient narcolepsy [9], while all other studies reported significant regional decreases in gray matter volumes (GMV) or concentration (GMC) [10–14].

Two of these studies reported decreases of GMC [10] or GMV [11] in the hypothalamus of narcolepsy patients (Figure 26.1A). These findings suggest that neuronal losses may affect hypocretinergic structures (i.e., the hypothalamus) as well as some major sites of hypocretin projections (i.e., the nucleus accumbens). Two other studies found decreases of GMV in 12 narcolepsy patients respectively in inferior temporal/frontal [12] and right prefrontal/frontomesial regions (Figure 26.1B) [13], possibly contributing to the cognitive impairments such as attentional deficits experienced by narcolepsy patients [15]. Our recent VBM study showed that 29 narcolepsy patients had reduced GMC in bilateral thalami, left gyrus rectus, bilateral frontopolar gyri, bilateral short insular gyri, bilateral superior frontal gyri, and right superior temporal and left inferior temporal gyri compared with 29 normal controls and furthermore, small volume correction revealed GMC reduction in bilateral nuclei accumbens, hypothalamus, and thalami (Figure 26.2) [14]. In particular, reduced GMC in the hypothalamus and nucleus accumbens in our study may support the prior hypothesis that these reductions are associated with EDS and cataplexy in narcolepsy patients. Our result suggests that areas with decreased GMC may serve possible roles in wake-sleep control, attention, or memory. Discrepancies of the results among several VBM studies might be due to differences in the analyses used (e.g., the statistical parametric mapping [SPM] version, modulated or unmodulated, grand mean scaling, absolute or relative thresholding, and sample size) and clinical characteristics of study patients (hypocretin deficiency, disease duration, medical treatment, etc.). Patient characteristics are quite variable from one study to another. More than half of the patients were medicated for EDS in three studies [9, 12, 13], and in another two studies, medication history was not mentioned [10, 11]. Only our study included unmedicated, drug-naïve narcolepsy patients [14]. More studies are needed to know whether brain structures are changed by pharmacological treatment. Among six VBM studies, four showed GMV changes [11–13] and the other two [10, 14] reported GMC reductions in narcolepsy patients. Optimized VBM can quantify either gray matter differences between subjects: relative distribution of gray matter concentration differences (GMC; no correction for non-linear normalization) or absolute gray matter volume differences (GMV; correction for non-linear normalization) [16]. It is not

Neuroimaging of Sleep and Sleep Disorders, ed. Eric Nofzinger, Pierre Maquet, and Michael J. Thorpy. Published by Cambridge University Press. © Cambridge University Press 2013.

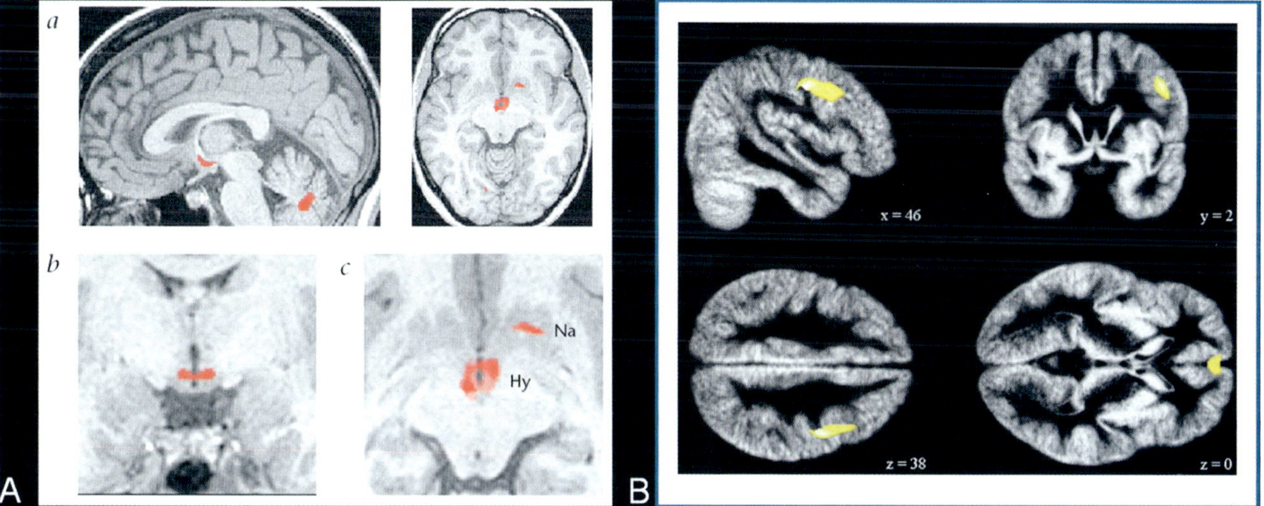

Figure 26.1 Brain regions showing reduced *gray matter volume* in patients with narcolepsy. (A) A significant decrease in gray matter was found in the hypothalamus (Hy) (a–c) and in the area of the right nucleus accumbens (Na). Significance levels for the one-tailed t-test were set at $P < 0.05$ and corrected for multiple comparisons. (Adapted from Draganski *et al.* [10].) (B) A cluster of gray matter loss was observed in the middle frontal gyrus of the right prefrontal (sagittal, coronal, and axial view) and in the frontomesial region (axial view) in narcolepsy patients. x,y,z refer to Talairach coordinates. (Adapted from Brenneis *et al.* [13].)

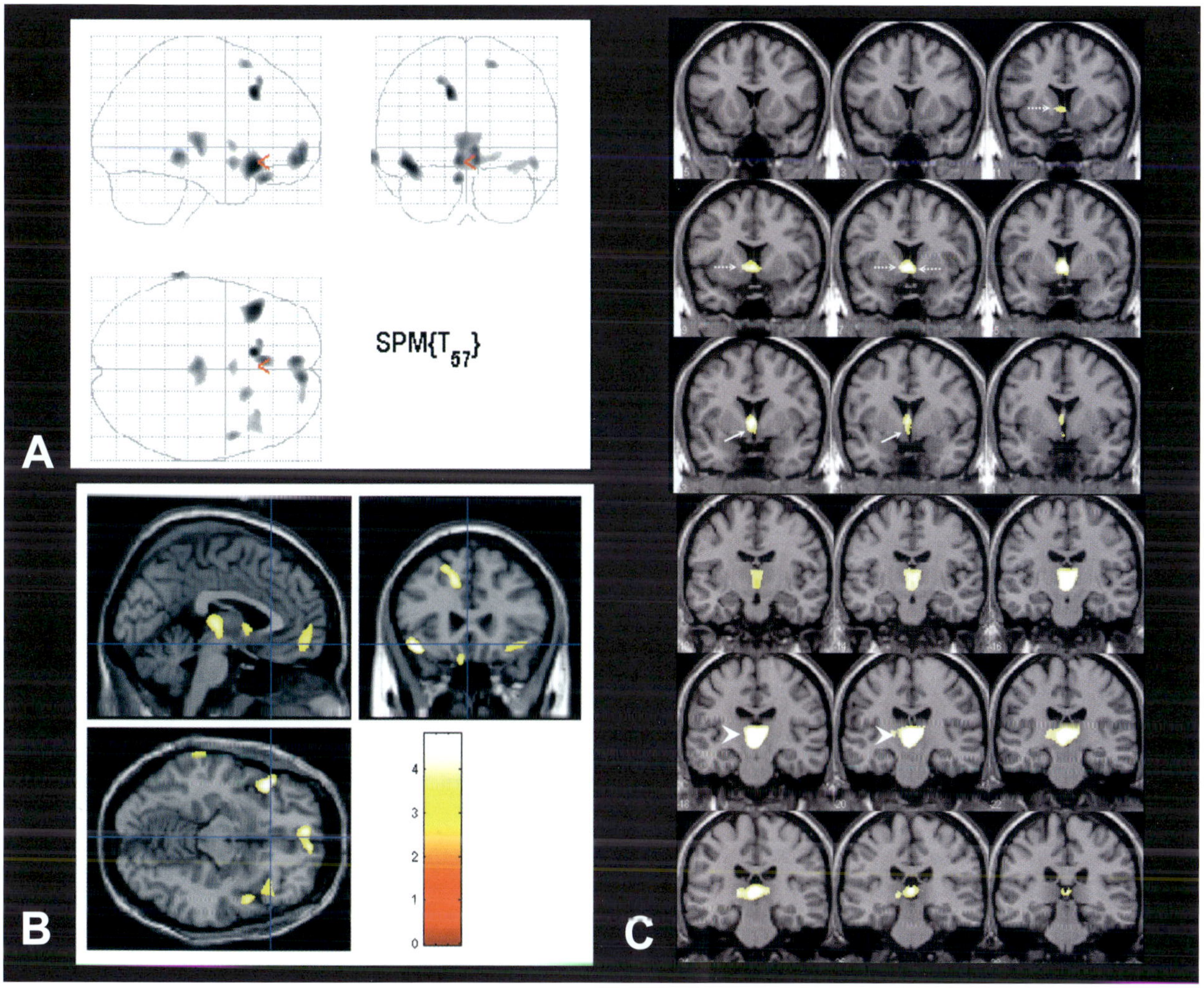

Figure 26.2 Brain regions showing reduced *gray matter concentrations* in patients with narcolepsy and cataplexy. (A) Overall areas showing reduced gray matter concentrations as a whole are shown in glass brain view. (B) Decreased gray matter concentrations in narcoleptics with cataplexy in: left gyrus rectus, bilateral thalami, bilateral frontopolar gyri, bilateral short insula gyri, bilateral superior frontal gyri, right superior temporal gyrus, and left inferior temporal gyrus are shown as T1 template overlaid MR image. Uncorrected $p < 0.001$ (extent threshold $kE < 100$ voxels). (C) Bilateral nuclei accumbens (dotted arrows), bilateral hypothalamus (solid arrows), and bilateral thalami (arrowhead) showed reduced gray matter concentrations at the level of false discovery rate corrected $p < 0.05$ with small volume correction. Superior to inferior panels are arranged in anterior to posterior direction in coronal images. (Adapted from Joo *et al.* [14].)

clear which one is more sensitive for detecting structural abnormalities of the brain.

Magnetic resonance spectroscopy (MRS) studies

As an advanced quantitative MR technique, proton magnetic resonance spectroscopy (^{1}H-MRS) has been used to assess the regional brain content of different compounds such as *N*-acetylaspartate (NAA), creatine (Cr), and phosphocreatine (PCr). Reduced NAA/Cr + PCr ratio indicates reduced neuronal function which could reflect neuronal loss (i.e., fewer neurons), but could also be due to reduced activity of existing neurons [17]. An earlier study found similar NAA/Cr + PCr ratios in the ventral pontine areas of 12 narcolepsy patients compared with 12 normal controls [18]. Other works showed that the spectral peak area ratios revealed a decrease in the NAA/Cr + PCr ratio in the hypothalamus of 23 and 16 narcolepsy patients [19, 20]. However, a subsequent MRS study did not find any changes in the hypothalamus or pontomesencephalic junction in 16 narcolepsy patients, but it found that myo-inositol was significantly lower in the right amygdala of narcolepsy patients, which suggested a possible hypothalamo-amygdala dysfunction in narcolepsy [21].

Analysis of cortical thickness

The VBM method has some limitations in representing gray matter morphology, and localization in the sulcal regions where the fine details of the anatomy are often obscured by a partial volume effect. On the other hand, the thickness of the cerebral cortex (ranging from 1.5 to 4.5 mm) reflects the density and arrangement of cells (neurons, neuroglia, and nerve fibers) [22]. Measuring cortical thickness using the cortical surface method has been suggested in studies of gray matter morphometry as a strategy for overcoming the limitation of volumetric analyses [23, 24]. It is known that the estimation of cortical thickness based on T1-weighted images represents a viable methodologic alternative to volumetric measurements for the assessment of subtle cortical changes in the human brain [25]. A cortical-thickness analysis performed at the nodes of a 3-dimensional polygonal mesh has the advantage of providing a direct quantitative index of cortical morphology [26]. In contrast with GMC or GMV analyses, cortical thickness measured from the cortical

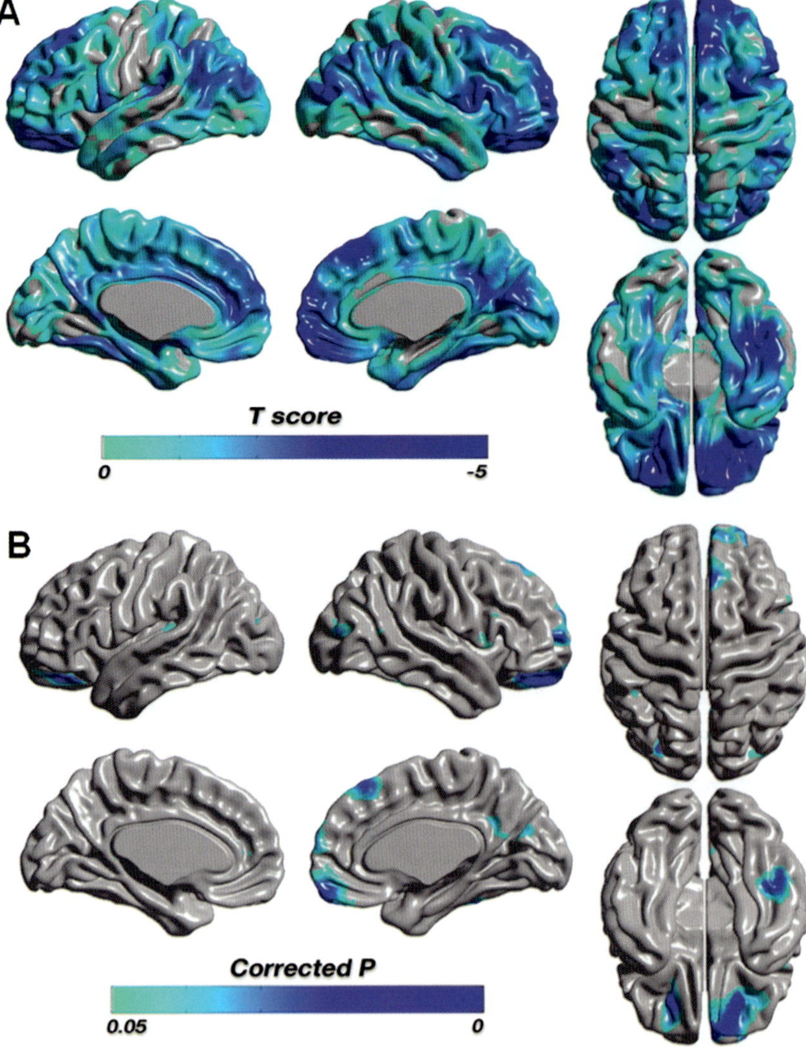

Figure 26.3 Statistical maps of differences in cortical thickness between narcolepsy patients with cataplexy and control subjects. (A) Statistical t-map with t-value range of −4.607 to 2.239 and positive values truncated. Most of the cortical area was thinner than in healthy control subjects. (B) A significant localized thinning of cortical thickness in patients was found in the orbitorectal gyri, the dorsolateral frontal gyri, the medial frontal gyrus, the cingulate gyrus, the middle and inferior temporal gyri, and the precuneus in the right hemisphere and the dorsolateral frontal gyri, the insular cortex, the posterior parietal lobule, and the middle occipital gyrus in left hemisphere at the level of false discovery rate corrected P < 0.05. (Adapted from Joo *et al.* [27].)

surfaces differentiates between cortices of opposing sulcal walls within the same sulcal bed, enabling more precise measurement in deep sulci and analysis of the morphology as a cortical sheet [26]. We measured the cortical thickness in 28 narcolepsy patients and 33 normal controls. Our result showed localized cortical thinning in the orbitofrontal gyri, dorsolateral and medial prefrontal cortices, insula, cingulate gyri, middle and inferior temporal gyri, and inferior parietal lobule of the right and left hemispheres in narcolepsy patients compared with normal controls (Figure 26.3) [27]. Moreover, significant negative correlation was observed between cortical thickness in the left supramarginal gyrus and the score on the Epworth Sleepiness Scale and between the cortical thickness in the left parahippocampal gyrus and the scores of general depressive symptoms on the Beck Depression Inventory. We proposed that cortical thinning of the prefrontal and limbic cortices, and parietal cortex in narcoleptic brains may provide a possible neuroanatomical explanation of the disturbances in attention, memory, emotion, and sleepiness of narcolepsy patients [27]. The results of a cortical-thickness analysis may be less subject to variation between laboratories compared to VBM analyses because thickness-measurement procedures are quite consistent [28]. Interestingly, the spatial distributions of cortical thinning [27] and of the reduced GMCs in the VBM study [14] in our laboratory were very similar even though the population of narcolepsy patients and the study periods were different. Cortical thinning of the dorsolateral prefrontal, orbitofrontal, and temporal cortices is consistent with the areas in which we observed significant reduced GMCs in narcolepsy patients [14].

Our VBM study also showed GMC reduction in the bilateral nuclei accumbens, hypothalamus, and thalami, which were not involved in the measurement of cortical thickness study because they are subcortical structures. Our previous studies about cerebral glucose metabolism and cerebral blood flow in narcolepsy showed decreased metabolism and cerebral perfusion in the hypothalamus and other brain regions [29, 30]. Similarities among neuroimaging studies in narcolepsy patients suggest that those findings are more reliable for revealing the neural substrates of the clinical symptoms and the pathophysiology of narcolepsy.

Conclusion

The neuroimaging studies have provided new information about brain abnormalities in narcolepsy patients. The computer-aided analysis of brain MRI in narcoleptic patients revealed structural abnormalities located in the hypothalamus, in agreement with a loss of hypocretinergic neurons in narcolepsy, as well as in various brain structures, possibly in relation with cataplexy and the cognitive and mood disturbances observed in narcolepsy patients. Higher tesla MRI scanners and further development of analysis software of brain MR images will be able to better characterize the structural changes in narcoleptic brains.

References

1. Thannickal TC, Moore RY, Nienhuis R, *et al.* Reduced number of hypocretin neurons in human narcolepsy. *Neuron.* 2000;**27**:469–74.

2. Taheri S, Zeitzer JM, Mignot E. The role of hypocretins (orexins) in sleep regulation and narcolepsy. *Annu Rev Neurosci.* 2002;**25**:283–313.

3. Sakurai T, Amemiya A, Ishii M, *et al.* Orexins and orexin receptors: a family of hypothalamic neuropeptides and G protein-coupled receptors that regulate feeding behavior. *Cell.* 1998;**92**:573–85

4. Nishino S, Ripley B, Overeem S, *et al.* Hypocretin (orexin) deficiency in human narcolepsy. *Lancet.* 2000;**355**:39–40.

5. Plazzi G, Montagna P, Provini F, *et al.* Pontine lesions in idiopathic narcolepsy. *Neurology.* 1996;**46**:1250–4

6. Bassetti C, Aldrich MS, Quint DJ. MRI findings in narcolepsy. *Sleep.* 1997;**20**:630–1.

7. Frey JL, Heiserman JE. Absence of pontine lesions in narcolepsy. *Neurology.* 1997;**48**:1097–9.

8. Desseilles M, Dang-Vu TD, Schabus M, *et al.* Neuroimaging insights into the pathophysiology of sleep disorders. *Sleep.* 2008;**31**:777–94.

9. Overeem S, Steens SC, Good CD, *et al.* Voxel-based morphometry in hypocretin-deficient narcolepsy. *Sleep.* 2003;**26**:44–6.

10. Draganski B, Geisler P, Hajak G, *et al.* Hypothalamic gray matter changes in narcoleptic patients. *Nat Med.* 2002;**8**:1186–8.

11. Buskova J, Vaneckova M, Sonka K, *et al.* Reduced hypothalamic gray matter in narcolepsy with cataplexy. *Neuroendocrinol Lett.* 2006;**27**:769–72.

12. Kaufmann C, Schuld A, Pollmacher T, Auer DP. Reduced cortical gray matter in narcolepsy: preliminary findings with voxel-based morphometry. *Neurology.* 2002;**58**:1852–5.

13. Brenneis C, Brandauer E, Frauscher B, *et al.* Voxel based morphometry in narcolepsy. *Sleep Med.* 2005;**6**:531–6.

14. Joo EY, Tae WS, Kim ST, *et al.* Gray matter concentration abnormality in brains of narcolepsy patients. *Korean J Radiol.* 2009;**10**:552–8.

15. Rieger M, Mayer G, Gauggel S. Attention deficits in patients with narcolepsy. *Sleep.* 2003;**26**:36–43.

16. Good CD, Johnsrude IS, Ashburner J, *et al.* A voxel-based morphometric study of ageing in 465 normal adult human brains. *Neuroimage.* 2001;**14**:21–36.

17. Rudkin TM, Arnold DL. Proton magnetic resonance spectroscopy for the diagnosis and management of cerebral disorders. *Arch Neurol.* 1999;**56**:919–26.

18. Ellis CM, Simmons A, Lemmens G, *et al.* Proton spectroscopy in the narcoleptic syndrome. Is there evidence of a brainstem lesion? *Neurology.* 1998;**50**:S23–6

19. Lodi R, Tonon C, Vignatelli L, *et al.* In vivo evidence of neuronal loss in the hypothalamus of narcoleptic patients. *Neurology.* 2004;**63**:1513–15.

20. Tonon C, Franceschini C, Testa C, *et al.* Distribution of neurochemical abnormalities in patients with narcolepsy with cataplexy: an in vivo brain proton MR spectroscopy study. *Brain Res Bull.* 2009;**80**:147–50.

21. Poryazova R, Schnepf B, Werth E, *et al.* Evidence for metabolic hypothalamo-amygdala dysfunction in narcolepsy. *Sleep.* 2009;**32**:607–13.

22. Parent A, Carpenter MB. *Human Neuroanatomy.* Baltimore, MD, Williams & Wilkins, 1995.

23. Fischl B, Dale AM. Measuring the thickness of the human cerebral cortex from magnetic resonance images. *Proc Natl Acad Sci U S A.* 2000;**97**:11050–5.

24. Kabani N, Le Goualher G, MacDonald D, Evans AC. Measurement of cortical thickness using an automated 3-D algorithm: a validation study. *Neuroimage.* 2001;**13**:375–80.

25. Hutton C, Draganski B, Ashburner J, Weiskopf N. A comparison between voxel-based cortical thickness and voxel-based morphometry in normal aging. *Neuroimage.* 2009;**48**:371–80.

26. Im K, Lee JM, Lee J, *et al.* Gender difference analysis of cortical thickness in healthy young adults with surface-based methods. *Neuroimage.* 2006;**31**:31–8.

27. Joo EY, Jeon S, Lee M, *et al.* Analysis of cortical thickness in narcolepsy patients with cataplexy. *Sleep.* 2011;**34**:1357–64.

28. Lin JJ, Salamon N, Lee AD, *et al.* Reduced neocortical thickness and complexity mapped in mesial temporal lobe epilepsy with hippocampal sclerosis. *Cereb Cortex.* 2007;**17**:2007–18.

29. Joo EY, Tae WS, Kim JH, *et al.* Glucose metabolism of hypothalamus and thalamus in narcolepsy. *Ann Neurol.* 2004;**56**:437–40.

30. Joo EY, Hong SB, Tae WS, *et al.* Cerebral perfusion abnormality in narcolepsy with cataplexy. *Neuroimage.* 2005;**28**:410–16.

Functional neuroimaging of narcolepsy

Thien Thanh Dang-Vu and Sophie Schwartz

Introduction

Functional neuroimaging techniques used to study narcolepsy include single-photon emission computed tomography (SPECT), positron emission tomography (PET), and functional magnetic resonance imaging (fMRI). SPECT shows the distribution of radioactive isotopes, the decay of which is associated with the emission of detectable single gamma photons. Examples of SPECT isotopes are ^{99m}technetium-hexamethylpropylene amine oxime (^{99m}Tc-HMPAO) and ^{99m}technetium-ethyl cysteinate dimer (^{99m}Tc-ECD), both indirect markers of regional cerebral blood flow (rCBF). PET shows the distribution of compounds labeled with positron-emitting isotopes, such as [^{15}O]-labeled water (H$_2$^{15}O), an indirect marker of rCBF, and ^{18}F-fluorodeoxyglucose (^{18}F-FDG), a marker of glucose metabolism (CMRglu). Functional MRI measures the variations in brain perfusion related to neural activity, using a method based on the assessment of the BOLD (blood oxygen level-dependent) signal. SPECT and PET can also be coupled with synthetic ligands to specific receptors of interest, in order to investigate neuromodulatory changes associated with a condition.

In this chapter, we will review functional brain imaging studies conducted in narcoleptic patients and evaluating different pathophysiological aspects of the disorder : (1) neurotransmission studies targeting the cholinergic, serotonergic, and dopaminergic systems (PET/SPECT); (2) the distribution of brain activity across the sleep-wake cycle (PET/SPECT); (3) the neural circuits involved in emotional and reward processing (fMRI).

Neurotransmission in narcolepsy

The role of various neurotransmitters in the pathophysiology of narcolepsy has been explored using PET or SPECT coupled with specific ligands: acetylcholine (ACh), serotonin (5-HT), and dopamine (DA). Results are summarized in Table 27.1.

Only one study evaluated ACh function in narcolepsy. PET coupled with [11C]N-methyl-4-piperidyl-benzilate (^{11}C-NMPB) was used to target muscarinic ACh receptors. No difference in muscarinic ACh binding was found in the pons, thalamus, striatum, and cerebral cortex of 11 patients compared with 21 controls [1].

Likewise there is a single work assessing 5-HT neurotransmission in narcolepsy. PET with 2′-methoxyphenyl-(N-2′-pyridinyl)-p-^{18}F-fluoro-benzamidoethylpiperazine (^{18}F-MPPF)

was employed to study 5-HT$_{1A}$ receptors. This study conducted on 14 patients showed an increase of 5-HT$_{1A}$ binding – particularly in the anterior cingulate, temporal, and mesio-temporal cortices – during sleep compared with wakefulness [2]. However, no control group was recruited, which prevents from confirming the specificity of this result to narcolepsy.

More interest was devoted to DA neurotransmission in narcolepsy. Several studies are available with either PET or SPECT. Studies of presynaptic DA transporter binding converge to demonstrate no significant modification in narcoleptic patients, either with [^{123}I](N)-(3-iodopropene-2-yl)-2β-carbomethoxy-3β-(4-chlorophenyl) tropane (^{123}I-IPT) SPECT [3] or ^{11}C-2β-carbomethoxy-3β-(4-fluorophenyl) tropane (^{11}C-CFT) PET [4]. As for postsynaptic D$_2$-receptor binding, only one study found a significant change between patients and controls: SPECT using ^{123}I-iodo benzamide (^{123}I-IBZM) demonstrated a D$_2$ binding increase in the striatum of seven narcoleptic patients [3]. In addition, a positive correlation was observed between striatal D$_2$ binding and the incidence of sleep attacks and cataplexy. However, other SPECT studies with IBZM [5, 6], as well as PET studies with [^{11}C]raclopride [7, 8] or N-(3-[^{18}F]fluoropropyl)-spiperone (FPSP) [9] did not confirm striatal changes in D$_2$ binding.

Altogether, available neuroimaging data do not consistently support the involvement of a neuromodulatory deficit in ACh, 5-HT, or DA systems for the pathophysiology of narcolepsy.

Brain perfusion and glucose metabolism in narcolepsy

Several functional neuroimaging studies were conducted to evaluate the distribution of brain activity during wakefulness and sleep in narcolepsy. Three of them described CMRglu [10, 11] and rCBF [12] patterns during resting wakefulness. Only preliminary reports compared rCBF values between sleep and waking [13, 14].

In a first PET study with ^{18}F-FDG PET, CMRglu during baseline wakefulness was compared between 24 narcoleptic patients and 24 healthy subjects [10]. Significant decreases were observed in the posterior hypothalamus and medio-dorsal thalamus of patients. In this study, three patients had narcolepsy without cataplexy, and four were treated with medications (stimulants, antidepressants). In addition, no electroencephalographic (EEG) recording was carried out to objectively monitor

Neuroimaging of Sleep and Sleep Disorders, ed. Eric Nofzinger, Pierre Maquet, and Michael J. Thorpy. Published by Cambridge University Press. © Cambridge University Press 2013.

Table 27.1. SPECT- and PET-ligand studies in narcolepsy

Study	Imaging	Target	Number of pat./ctrl.	Treatment	Results
Sudo *et al.* [1]	PET ^{11}C-NMPB	ACh (muscarinic)	11/21	None	No change
Derry *et al.* [2]	PET ^{18}F-MPPF	5HT$_{1A}$	14/0	12/14	N/A (no control group)
Eisensehr *et al.* [3]	SPECT IPT	DA (transporter)	7/7	None	No change
Rinne *et al.* [4]	PET ^{11}C-CFT	DA (transporter)	10/15	None	No change
Eisensehr *et al.* [3]	SPECT ^{123}I-IBZM	DA (D$_2$)	7/7	None	Increase in striatum
Hublin *et al.* [5]	SPECT ^{123}I-IBZM	DA (D$_2$)	6/8	None	No change
Staedt *et al.* [6]	SPECT ^{123}I-IBZM	DA (D$_2$)	10/10	None	No change
Khan *et al* [7]	PET [^{11}C]raclopride	DA (D$_2$)	17/32	12/17	No change
Rinne *et al.* [8]	PET [^{11}C]raclopride	DA (D$_2$)	7/7	6/7	No change
MacFarlane *et al.* [9]	PET FPSP	DA (D$_2$)	6/6	None	No change

N/A = not available.

the subjects' vigilance state during the study. To address these limitations, the same group then conducted a ^{99m}Tc-ECD SPECT study during wakefulness in 25 patients and the same number of controls: this time, all patients had a history of cataplexy and no history of pharmacological treatment (for sleepiness or cataplexy) [12]. Moreover, EEG was available during the study to ensure that the subjects were fully awake during the procedure. The study found decreased rCBF in the hypothalamus and thalamus, in line with the ^{18}F-FDG PET study. Additional significant decreases were also observed in the caudate, superior/middle frontal gyri, postcentral gyrus, parahippocampal gyrus, and cingulate cortex (Figure 27.1). A more recent study by another group used PET with ^{18}F-FDG during wakefulness in 21 patients with narcolepsy and cataplexy, and 21 matched controls. In contrast with the two previous studies, no significant CMRglu decrease was found. Instead, increases were observed in the anterior and mid cingulate cortex, and in the right visual association cortex. As in the earlier ^{18}F-FDG PET study, the two major limitations of these results are the inclusion of patients treated with psychostimulants and/or anticataplectic drugs (14 out of 21), and the absence of objective (EEG) monitoring of vigilance state.

In brief, with the exception of one ^{18}F-FDG PET study that found increased CMRglu particularly in the cingulate cortex [11], other functional neuroimaging studies during wakefulness confirmed a hypothalamic dysfunction in narcoleptic patients, in agreement with a deficit in the hypocretin system [10, 12]. Other hypoperfusions (thalamus, caudate, prefrontal, and postcentral cortices, limbic areas) might relate to clinical features associated with narcolepsy, such as altered emotional processing (see below) and attentional deficits.

As for the study of brain activity during sleep, early studies using ^{133}Xe inhalation showed that narcoleptics compared with controls had a lower rCBF during wakefulness mostly in the brainstem-cerebellum region, while at sleep onset compared to wakefulness rCBF decreased in controls but increased in narcoleptic patients in the same region [13, 15]. In contrast, a ^{99m}Tc-HMPAO SPECT study did not find any rCBF difference between wakefulness and rapic eye movement (REM) sleep in

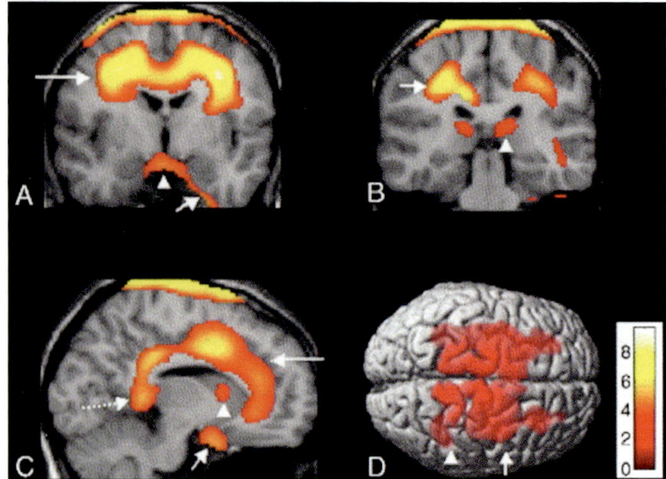

Figure 27.1 Brain perfusion decreases during wakefulness in narcolepsy. Brain mapping of the regions where cerebral perfusion is decreased in narcoleptic patients compared to normal subjects (^{99m}Tc-ECD SPECT). Results are overlaid on T1 MRI, and are significant at FDR-corrected $P < 0.05$. (A) Significant hypoperfusion was observed in bilateral anterior hypothalami (arrowhead) and in the right parahippocampal gyrus (short arrow). Bilateral cingulate gyri and white matters in bilateral middle frontal gyri (long arrow) showed decreased cerebral perfusion. (B) Hypoperfusion was evident in bilateral posterior thalami (arrowhead) and in the white matters of the bilateral postcentral and supramarginal gyri (short arrow). (C) In the sagittal view of right hemisphere, significant hypoperfusion was observed in the caudate nucleus (arrowhead), in the subcallosal gyrus (short arrow), the cingulate gyrus extending along corpus callosum (long arrow), and in the parahippocampal gyrus (dotted arrow). (D) 3-dimensional rendering view showing decreased cerebral perfusion in bilateral paracentral areas (arrowhead) and superior/middle frontal gyri (short arrow). The frontal lobe is on the right and the occipital lobe on the left. (Reprinted from *Neuroimage*; Vol. 28(2); Yeon Joo E, Hong SB, Tae WS, Kim JH, Han SJ, Cho YW, Yoon CH, Lee SI, Lee MH, Lee KH, Kim MH, Kim BT, Kim L. "Cerebral perfusion abnormality in narcolepsy with cataplexy"; pp 410–16; Copyright 2005, with permission from Elsevier.)

narcoleptic patients [14]. As this last study did not include a control group, the specificity of this result to narcolepsy could not be established. Future studies, using state-of-the-art functional neuroimaging techniques, should reevaluate brain activity patterns during the different stages of sleep in narcoleptic patients compared with controls.

Neural correlates of emotional processing in narcolepsy

Processing of emotional information potentially plays an important role in narcolepsy–cataplexy. Indeed it is well known that emotions, particularly those with a positive component (jokes, laughter, etc.), can trigger cataplectic episodes. Functional MRI studies therefore assessed brain responses to humorous stimuli in narcoleptic patients. In a first study, 12 narcoleptics with cataplexy and 12 controls were scanned during presentation of humorous and neutral pictures [16]. In patients, pharmacological treatment was discontinued for at least 14 days before the fMRI session. Humorous pictures (compared to neutral pictures) were associated with an increased amygdala response together with a decreased response in the hypothalamus of patients compared to controls (Figure 27.2). In a second fMRI study, a similar paradigm was used in 10 narcoleptic patients with cataplexy compared to 12 healthy controls [17]. Medications were stopped for at least five days prior to the experiment. In agreement with the previous study, higher brain response to humorous cartoons were observed in several areas including the amygdala (as well as the inferior frontal gyrus, superior temporal gyrus, insula, nucleus accumbens) in narcoleptics compared to controls. However, fMRI response in the hypothalamus to humorous stimulation was not found decreased in this study, but rather increased

Not only positive emotional stimulation was assessed with fMRI in narcolepsy. Brain responses to unpleasant stimuli were also investigated in nine unmedicated narcoleptic patients with cataplexy and nine matched controls [18]. The task consisted in an aversive conditioning paradigm (visual conditioning stimuli

and painful electrical stimulation). Results showed increased neural responses to conditioned stimuli in the amygdala and increased functional connectivity between the amygdala and medial prefrontal cortex in the control group but not in the narcolepsy group.

Altogether these studies suggest a dysfunction of amygdalo-hypothalamic and amygdalo-neocortical interactions during the processing of emotional information in narcoleptic patients, possibly underlying central mechanisms of cataplexy.

Neural correlates of reward processing in narcolepsy

Anticipation of reward (e.g., when playing games) constitutes a particular emotional experience prone to trigger cataplexy in humans [19], which suggests a potential involvement of the hypocretin system in reward brain circuits, and possible alterations of these circuits in narcolepsy with cataplexy. Accordingly, data in rodents show a close interplay between hypocretin neurons and reward-related brain regions, such as the nucleus accumbens and the DA ventral tegmental area [20–22]. In order to further evaluate a potential dysfunction of reward-related neural processes, an fMRI study was conducted in 12 unmedicated narcoleptic patients with clear-cut cataplexy and 12 matched healthy controls, while performing a task involving the mesolimbic and midbrain reward system [23]. This task consisted of a modifed version of a monetary incentive delay task. Brain responses to high motivational cues included the ventral tegmental area in the control group, but not in the narcolepsy group. Responses to successful trials (compared to failed trials) revealed increased activity in the ventromedial prefrontal cortex and nucleus accumbens in the control group but not in the patients group. Likewise, increased

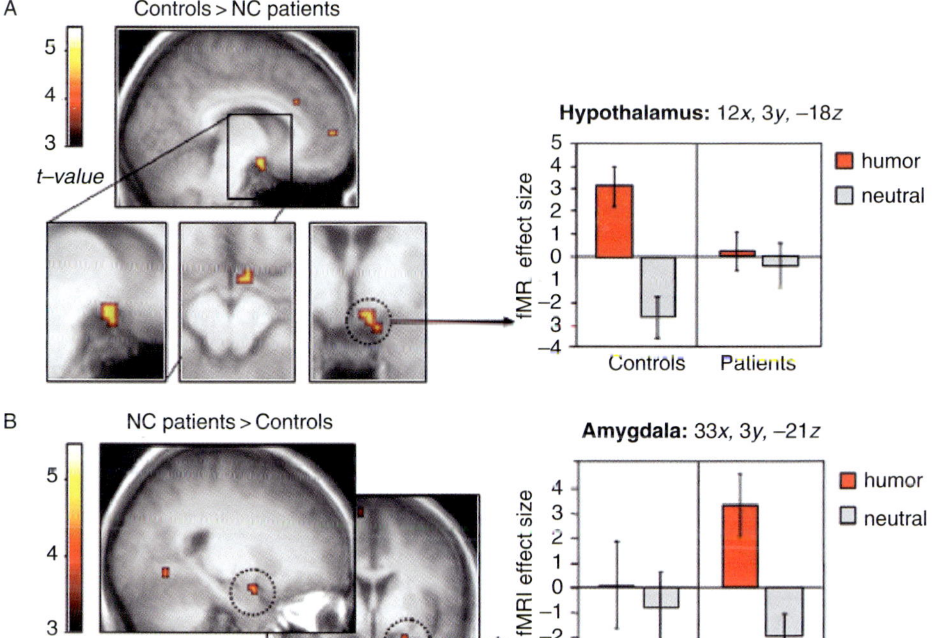

Figure 27.2 Neural correlates of emotional processing in narcolepsy. Functional MRI response is decreased in the hypothalamus (A) and increased in the amygdala (B) during presentation of humorous pictures compared to neutral pictures, and more so in narcoleptic patients than in healthy controls (p < 0.001). (Adapted from *Brain*; Vol. 131(Pt2); S. Schwartz *et al.*, "Abnormal activity in hypothalamus and amygdala during humour processing in human narcolepsy with cataplexy" ; pp 514–522; Copyright 2008, with permission from Oxford University Press.)

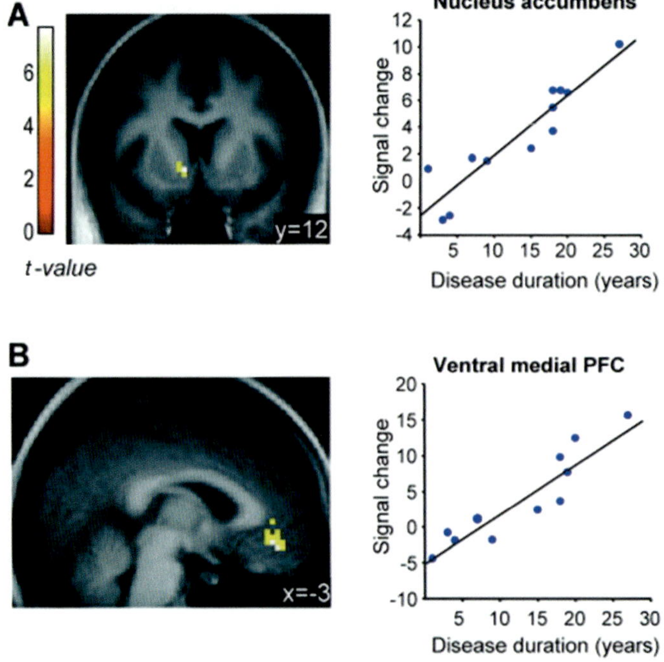

Figure 27.3 Neural correlates of reward processing in narcolepsy. Functional MRI responses to a monetary incentive delay task in narcoleptic patients. Brain responses to high motivational cues in the nucleus accumbens (A) and ventromedial prefrontal cortex (ventromedial PFC; B) are positively correlated with disease duration ($r^2 = 0.85$ and 0.82, respectively; $p < 0.001$). (Adapted from Annals of Neurology; Vol. 67(2); A. Ponz *et al.*, "Abnormal activity in reward brain circuits in human narcolepsy with cataplexy"; pp 190–200; Copyright 2010, with permission from John Wiley and Sons.)

brain responses to successful positively cued trials were found in the nucleus accumbens and lateral prefrontal cortex in controls; in narcoleptics increased responses to these trials were found in the amygdala, consistent with reports of increased amygdala response to stimuli associated with highly positive emotions (see above). Finally, in the narcolepsy group, significant positive correlations were found between disease duration and fMRI responses to high motivational cues in the nucleus accumbens and ventromedial prefrontal cortex (Figure 27.3). Altogether these findings show evidence for a disruption of neural circuits involved in reward processing in narcolepsy. Furthermore, these data suggest a progressive functional recovery of reward-related brain structures in narcoleptic patients with longer disease duration.

Conclusion

Functional brain imaging studies in narcolepsy can be summarized as follows:

1. Narcolepsy is not associated with a specific alteration of the central cholinergic or dopaminergic activity.
2. Functional brain activity patterns of narcoleptic patients during resting wakefulness are characterized by abnormalities located in the hypothalamus – in agreement with a loss of hypocretinergic neurons in this disease – as well as in various cortical areas, possibly in relation with cognitive and attentional deficits encountered by these patients.
3. Altered emotional processing associated with cataplexy also involves a dysfunction of the hypothalamus, in addition to neural changes within limbic structures, in particular the amygdala.
4. Narcolepsy with cataplexy finally involves a dysfunction of neural circuits implicated in reward processing and encompassing the nucleus accumbens and the midbrain ventral tegmental area.

Further studies should investigate more closely brain activity changes across the sleep/wake cycle in narcoleptic patients. Indeed narcolepsy not only induces severe daytime symptoms, but is also frequently associated with sleep disruption, including changes in sleep microarchitecture [24, 25].

Acknowledgements

This research was supported by the Fonds National de la Recherche Scientifique (Belgium), the Swiss National Science Foundation, the Fonds Léon Frédéricq (Belgium), the Belgian College of Neuropsychopharmacology and Biological Psychiatry, and the Canadian Institutes of Health Research.

References

1. Sudo Y, Suhara T, Honda Y, *et al.* Muscarinic cholinergic receptors in human narcolepsy: a PET study. *Neurology.* 1998;**51**(5):1297–302.

2. Derry C, Benjamin C, Bladin P, *et al.* Increased serotonin receptor availability in human sleep: evidence from an [18F]MPPF PET study in narcolepsy. *Neuroimage.* 2006;**30**(2):341–8.

3. Eisensehr I, Linke R, Tatsch K, *et al.* Alteration of the striatal dopaminergic system in human narcolepsy. *Neurology.* 2003;**60**(11):1817–19.

4. Rinne JO, Hublin C, Nagren K, Helenius H, Partinen M. Unchanged striatal dopamine transporter availability in narcolepsy: a PET study with [11C]-CFT. *Acta Neurol Scand.* 2004;**109**(1):52–5.

5. Hublin C, Launes J, Nikkinen P, Partinen M. Dopamine D2-receptors in human narcolepsy: a SPECT study with 123I-IBZM. *Acta Neurol Scand.* 1994;**90**(3):186–9.

6. Staedt J, Stoppe G, Kogler A, *et al.* [123I] IBZM SPET analysis of dopamine D2 receptor occupancy in narcoleptic patients in the course of treatment. *Biol Psychiatry.* 1996;**39**(2):107–11.

7. Khan N, Antonini A, Parkes D, *et al.* Striatal dopamine D2 receptors in patients with narcolepsy measured with PET and 11C-raclopride. *Neurology.* 1994;**44**(11):2102–4.

8. Rinne JO, Hublin C, Partinen M, *et al.* Positron emission tomography study of human narcolepsy: no increase in striatal dopamine D2 receptors. *Neurology.* 1995;**45**(9):1735–8.

9. MacFarlane JG, List SJ, Moldofsky H, *et al.* Dopamine D2 receptors quantified

in vivo in human narcolepsy. *Biol Psychiatry*. 1997;**41**(3):305–10.

10. Joo EY, Tae WS, Kim JH, Kim BT, Hong SB. Glucose hypometabolism of hypothalamus and thalamus in narcolepsy. *Ann Neurol*. 2004;**56** (3):437–40.

11. Dauvilliers Y, Comte F, Bayard S, *et al.* A brain PET study in patients with narcolepsy-cataplexy. *J Neurol Neurosurg Psychiatry*. 2010;**81**(3):344–8.

12. Yeon Joo E, Hong SB, Tae WS, *et al.* Cerebral perfusion abnormality in narcolepsy with cataplexy. *Neuroimage*. 2005;**28**(2):410–16.

13. Meyer JS, Sakai F, Karacan I, Derman S, Yamamoto M. Sleep apnea, narcolepsy, and dreaming: regional cerebral hemodynamics. *Ann Neurol*. 1980;**7** (5):479–85.

14. Asenbaum S, Zeithofer J, Saletu B, *et al.* Technetium-99m-HMPAO SPECT imaging of cerebral blood flow during REM sleep in narcoleptics. *J Nucl Med*. 1995;**36**(7):1150–5.

15. Sakai F, Meyer JS, Karacan I, Yamaguchi F, Yamamoto M. Narcolepsy: regional cerebral blood flow during sleep and wakefulness. *Neurology*. 1979;**29**(1):61–7.

16. Schwartz S, Ponz A, Poryazova R, *et al.* Abnormal activity in hypothalamus and amygdala during humour processing in human narcolepsy with cataplexy. *Brain*. 2008;**131**(Pt 2):514–22.

17. Reiss AL, Hoeft F, Tenforde AS, *et al.* Anomalous hypothalamic responses to humor in cataplexy. *PLoS One*. 2008;**3** (5):e2225.

18. Ponz A, Khatami R, Poryazova R, *et al.* Reduced amygdala activity during aversive conditioning in human narcolepsy. *Ann Neurol*. 2010;**67** (3):394–8.

19. Anic-Labat S, Guilleminault C, Kraemer HC, *et. al.* Validation of a cataplexy questionnaire in 983 sleep-disorders patients. *Sleep*. 1999;**22**(1):77–87.

20. Fadel J, Deutch AY. Anatomical substrates of orexin-dopamine interactions: lateral hypothalamic projections to the ventral tegmental area. *Neuroscience*. 2002;**111**(2):379–87.

21. Narita M, Nagumo Y, Hashimoto S, *et al.* Direct involvement of orexinergic systems in the activation of the mesolimbic dopamine pathway and related behaviors induced by morphine. *J Neurosci*. 2006;**26**(2):398–405.

22. Korotkova TM, Sergeeva OA, Eriksson KS, Haas HL, Brown RE. Excitation of ventral tegmental area dopaminergic and nondopaminergic neurons by orexins/ hypocretins. *J Neurosci*. 2003;**23**(1):7–11.

23. Ponz A, Khatami R, Poryazova R, *et al.* Abnormal activity in reward brain circuits in human narcolepsy with cataplexy. *Ann Neurol*. 2010;**67**(2):190–200.

24. Bove A, Culebras A, Moore JT, Westlake RE. Relationship between sleep spindles and hypersomnia. *Sleep*. 1994;**17** (5):449–55.

25. Khatami R, Landolt HP, Achermann P, *et al.* Insufficient non-REM sleep intensity in narcolepsy-cataplexy. *Sleep*. 2007;**30**(8):980–9.

Neuroimaging of treatment response in narcolepsy

Thien Thanh Dang-Vu

Introduction

Pharmacological management of narcolepsy–cataplexy is a symptomatic treatment, mainly focusing on the improvement of daytime sleepiness and the prevention of sleep attacks [1]. Therefore, the core of the treatment consists of psychostimulants. Amphetamines were among the earliest stimulant medications used to prevent sleep attacks in narcoleptic patients. Because of their side effects, they have now been largely replaced by non-amphetaminic stimulant medications, such as modafinil. Other medications are employed to prevent the occurrence of cataplectic episodes. Antidepressants such as venlafaxine for instance are commonly used in this perspective. Sodium oxybate is also now used in narcolepsy with cataplexy, and is particularly effective in improving sleep quality and reducing the number of cataplectic attacks [2].

This chapter will briefly review the neuroimaging findings dedicated to the effects of treatment in narcolepsy. These studies involved functional neuroimaging methods such as single-photon emission computed tomography (SPECT), positron emission tomography (PET), and functional magnetic resonance imaging (fMRI). The majority of them focused on modafinil, with also early reports on amphetamines and methylphenidate.

These studies are summarized in Table 28.1.

Amphetamines

The neural effects of a single dose of amphetamine in narcoleptic patients were studied in a preliminary fMRI report. This study resorted to an auditory and visual stimulation paradigm in two narcoleptic patients and three controls [3]. Drug administration in narcoleptics induced larger fMRI responses in primary and association sensory cortices, but paradoxically reduced responses in controls. This finding needs replication on larger samples.

Methylphenidate

Although commonly used to treat attention-deficit hyperactivity disorder, this amphetamine derivative is also frequently prescribed in narcoleptic patients to reduce daytime sleepiness. One study in five patients with narcolepsy used ^{133}Xe inhalation to assess regional cerebral blood flow (rCBF) changes before and after at least two weeks of treatment with methylphenidate [4].

Compared to baseline, treatment increased rCBF globally during wakefulness, and predominantly in the brainstem-cerebellum region. While increases in rCBF were seen from wake to sleep at baseline in the same region, treatment with methylphenidate attenuated these increases at sleep onset. Since the effects of medication were not evaluated in controls, the reported findings might not be specifically related to narcolepsy.

Modafinil

The effects of modafinil on brain function in narcoleptic patients were studied with SPECT, PET, and fMRI.

Modafinil effects were also studied in healthy populations. Brain perfusion changes induced by a single dose of modafinil (400 mg) in healthy subjects were investigated with ^{99m}Tc-ethyl eysteinate dimer (^{99m}Tc-ECD) SPECT [5]. During electroencephalographic (EEG) monitored wakefulness, modafinil (compared to placebo) induced higher rCBF in the pons, prefrontal gyrus, insula, cingulate gyrus, and left temporal and parahippocampal gyri. The study thus demonstrates that modafinil affects neural structures involved in arousal, emotions, and executive functions. This result is in agreement with an earlier fMRI study showing that a single dose of modafinil (200 mg) can counteract the negative effects of a single night of sleep deprivation on working memory while recruiting larger responses in prefrontal and parietal executive areas [6].

In narcoleptic patients single-dose treatment effects were also studied with fMRI. Brain responses to visual and auditory stimulation were assessed in eight patients and eight controls both before and after a single dose of modafinil (400 mg) [7]. No significant change was observed between pre- and post-modafinil conditions in either controls or narcoleptics. There was, however, a negative correlation between pre- and post-modafinil activation levels, in both groups. The effects of modafinil withdrawal were studied in a single-case fMRI study of a 20-year-old narcoleptic patient treated with modafinil (200 mg/day) for 24 months [8]. The patient and 38 control participants were submitted to an episodic memory task during fMRI acquisition. This task consisted of a face-encoding paradigm. The patient was scanned in two conditions: a first session after not taking modafinil for 32 h (acute withdrawal), and a second session 4 hours after her usual dose of modafinil. Acute withdrawal resulted in reduced behavioral performance, along with increased activation of the

Table 28.1. Functional brain imaging of pharmacological treatment in narcolepsy

Study	Imaging	Drug	Dose (daily)	Duration	Placebo	Paradigm	Number of pat./ctrl.	Results
Howard et al. [3]	fMRI	Dexamphetamine	10 mg	Single dose	No	Visual and auditory stimulation	2/3	Larger activation in sensory cortex of patients
Meyer et al. [4]	^{133}Xe inhalation	Methylphenidate	0.4–0.9 mg/kg	> 2 weeks	No	Resting wakefulness/ sleep onset	5/0	Global rCBF increases at wake, and attenuated increases at sleep onset, compared to before treatment
Ellis et al. [7]	fMRI	Modafinil	400 mg	Single dose	Yes	Visual and auditory stimulation	8/8	No significant change
Allen et al. [8]	fMRI	Modafinil	200 mg	> 24 months	No	Visual stimulation (memorization of faces)	1/38	Activation increase in hippocampus and decrease in prefrontal cortex after 32 hours off treatment ; normalization if only 4 hours off treatment
Kim et al. [9]	PET ^{18}F-FDG	Modafinil	100–400 mg	2 weeks	No	Resting wakefulness	7/8	Increased CMRglu in left hippocampus of patients
Joo et al. [10]	SPECT [^{99m}Tc]-ECD	Modafinil	100–400 mg	4 weeks	Yes	Resting wakefulness	32/0	Increased rCBF in prefrontal cortex and decreased rCBF in precentral cortex hippocampus, fusiform cortex, and cerebellum of patients
Dauvilliers et al. [11]	PET ^{18}F-FDG	Modafinil, mazindol, venlafaxine	Variable	?	No	Resting wakefulness	14/0	Increased CMRglu in cerebellum, pre- and postcentral gyri, compared to unmedicated patients

hippocampus and decreased responses in the prefrontal cortex compared to controls. On the other hand, usual modafinil intake during the second session increased performance and normalized brain responses compared to controls.

PET and SPECT were used to investigate brain activity changes induced by a prolonged administration of modafinil in narcoleptic patients. An ^{18}F-fluorodeoxyglucose (^{18}F-FDG) PET study evaluated brain glucose metabolism (CMRglu) during baseline wakefulness in eight patients and eight controls before and after two weeks of treatment with modafinil [9]. Decreased CMRglu was observed in the brainstem, hypothalamus, thalamus, and mesio temporal areas in narcoleptics compared to controls, both before and after treatment. Comparison of pre- and post-treatment conditions in patients showed a significant CMRglu increase in the left hippocampus with modafinil. As previously reported, treatment with modafinil also increases rCBF in mesio-temporal areas in healthy volunteers [5]. Therefore, the post-treatment hippocampal CMRglu increase might not be specific to narcolepsy. In a ^{99m}Tc-ECD SPECT study, rCBF during wakefulness was assessed in a sample of 32 narcoleptic patients treated with modafinil during four weeks compared with 21 placebo-treated patients [10]. EEG was recorded during the SPECT procedure to objectively monitor the subjects' alertness. The modafinil group (compared to the placebo group) displayed increased rCBF in dorsolateral and medial aspects of the prefrontal cortex, and decreased rCBF in precentral, hippocampal, fusiform, and cerebellar regions. No comparison with a group of healthy subjects was carried out in this study, which once again raises the question of the specificity of these results to narcolepsy. Finally, a more recent ^{18}F-FDG PET study compared CMRglu during wakefulness in 14 patients with narcolepsy–cataplexy treated with various psychostimulants and/ or anticataplectics compared with seven newly diagnosed patients in which treatment was not started yet [11]. Out of these 14 patients, 11 were treated with modafinil (100–500 mg/day), combined with an antidepressant used to treat cataplexy in seven of them (venlafaxine or paroxetine). Two were treated with another psychostimulant (mazindol) combined with venlafaxine, and one with venlafaxine alone. Compared with drug-naïve patients, treated narcoleptics had a higher CMRglu in the cerebellum and primary sensorimotor cortex. Given the heterogeneity of the treated group, these results are difficult to interpret, and contrast with the SPECT study that found decreased rCBF in the cerebellum and precentral gyrus with modafinil [10].

Conclusion

Functional neuroimaging has described the immediate effects of acute modafinil administration, but no well-defined neural changes could be demonstrated with a single dose of treatment in narcoleptic patients. Results obtained after weeks or months of administration of modafinil were quite divergent, and involved functional changes in several cortical areas (prefrontal, hippocampal, primary sensorimotor) as well as in the cerebellum. The significance of these changes remains unclear.

Further neuroimaging studies are needed to confirm these results using placebo-controlled protocols comparing patients and healthy volunteers. Future studies shall also use other technical modalities (e.g., structural imaging) and explore the effects of more recent medications (e.g., sodium oxybate) in narcolepsy. The development of new pharmacological targets, in particular in the hypocretinergic system, will eventually create the need for dedicated neuroimaging studies.

Acknowledgements

This research was supported by the Fonds National de la Recherche Scientifique (Belgium), the Fonds Léon Frédéricq (Belgium), the Belgian College of Neuropsychopharmacology and Biological Psychiatry, and the Canadian Institutes of Health Research.

References

1. Dauvilliers Y, Arnulf I, Mignot E. Narcolepsy with cataplexy. *Lancet.* 2007;**369**(9560):499–511.

2. Poryazova R, Tartarotti S, Khatami R, *et al.* Sodium oxybate in narcolepsy with cataplexy: Zurich sleep center experience. *Eur Neurol.* 2011;**65**(3):175–82.

3. Howard RJ, Ellis C, Bullmore ET, *et al.* Functional echoplanar brain imaging correlates of amphetamine administration to normal subjects and subjects with the narcoleptic syndrome. *Magn Reson Imaging.* 1996;**14**(9):1013–16.

4. Meyer JS, Sakai F, Karacan I, Derman S, Yamamoto M. Sleep apnea, narcolepsy, and dreaming: regional cerebral hemodynamics. *Ann Neurol.* 1980;**7**(5):479–85.

5. Joo EY, Tae WS, Jung KY, Hong SB. Cerebral blood flow changes in man by wake-promoting drug, modafinil: a randomized double blind study. *J Sleep Res.* 2008;**17**(1):82–8.

6. Thomas RJ, Kwong K. Modafinil activates cortical and subcortical sites in the sleep-deprived state. *Sleep.* 2006;**29**(11):1471–81.

7. Ellis CM, Monk C, Simmons A, *et al.* Functional magnetic resonance imaging neuroactivation studies in normal subjects and subjects with the narcoleptic syndrome. Actions of modafinil. *J Sleep Res.* 1999;**8**(2):85–93.

8. Allen MD, Hedges DW, Farrer TJ, Larson MJ. Assessment of brain activity during memory encoding in a narcolepsy patient on and off modafinil using normative fMRI data. *Neurocase.* 2012;**18**(1):13–25.

9. Kim YK, Yoon IY, Shin YK, Cho SS, Kim SE. Modafinil-induced hippocampal activation in narcolepsy. *Neurosci Lett.* 2007;**422**(2):91–6.

10. Joo EY, Seo DW, Tae WS, Hong SB. Effect of modafinil on cerebral blood flow in narcolepsy patients. *Sleep.* 2008;**31**(6):868–73.

11. Dauvilliers Y, Comte F, Bayard S, *et al.* A brain PET study in patients with narcolepsy-cataplexy. *J Neurol Neurosurg Psychiatry.* 2010;**81**(3):344–8.

Modafinil effects in narcolepsy

Michael T. Saletu and Gerda Saletu-Zyhlarz

Introduction

Neuroanatomy of wakefulness and cognition in narcolepsy

Wakefulness and cortical arousal are mediated by several ascending pathways with distinct neuronal components that project from the upper brainstem [1]. One pathway innervates the thalamus. The second branch projects into the lateral hypothalamus, basal forebrain, and cerebral cortex.

Lesions along this second branch are associated with narcolepsy, with the loss of hypocretin cells, in particular, contributing to the difficulty in maintaining arousal [1].

Functional neuroimaging studies of executive functioning have consistently demonstrated activation in an interconnected and distributed network of cortical areas. This network includes the dorsolateral prefrontal cortex, the cognitive division of the anterior cingulate, and the posterior parietal cortex [2]. There is evidence of a vulnerability of prefrontal cortical mechanisms in states of inadequate or disrupted sleep [3, 4].

The general pattern of cognitive dysfunction in narcolepsy is consistent with a reduction or limitation of cognitive processing resources in prefrontal areas. The hypothesized mechanism may be related to the above changes in the hypocretin system. A disruption of this system is associated with a deficient regulation of cortical activity and deficient vigilance.

Vigilance decrements may therefore be another treatment target of modafinil.

Modafinil increases subcortical and cortical monoaminergic neurotransmission

Modafinil is a unique wake-promoting compound that is pharmacologically and chemically distinct from other central nervous system stimulants [5]. The drug appears to have multiple effects on the ascending arousal pathway, promoting cholinergic, noradrenergic, serotoninergic, dopaminergic, and histaminergic arousal neurotransmission [5].

Varied findings suggest that modafinil may especially potentiate both dopamine (DA) and norepinephrine (NE) neurotransmission [5]. The drug has been demonstrated to bind directly to the dopamine transporter (DAT) and norepinephrine transporter (NET), which it inhibits at modest potency [5].

These effects are particularly prominent in the neocortex, and generally less potent or minimal in various subcortical areas [5]. Parenteral administration of modafinil leads to significantly increased (measured by microdialysis) extracellular DA and NE levels in the prefrontal cortex (PFC) of rats [6]. In post-mortem human brains, DAT is found not only in the striatum, but also throughout the neocortex, including the PFC, albeit at relatively lower concentrations [7].

In healthy humans (with or without sleep deprivation), working memory, recognition memory, sustained attention, and other tasks dependent on cognitive control are enhanced with modafinil [5, 8].

In a recent study, healthy volunteers underwent blood oxygen level-dependent (BOLD) functional magnetic resonance imaging (fMRI) while performing an emotional information processing task that activates the amygdala and two prefrontally dependent cognitive tasks – a working memory (WM) task and a variable attentional control (VAC) task [9]. BOLD fMRI revealed significantly decreased amygdala reactivity to fearful stimuli on modafinil compared with the placebo condition. During executive cognition tasks, a WM task and a VAC task, modafinil reduced the BOLD signal in the PFC and anterior cingulate. The authors concluded that modafinil enhances the efficiency of prefrontal cortical cognitive information processing, while dampening reactivity to threatening stimuli in the amygdala, a brain region implicated in anxiety.

Among adult psychiatric patients, there is evidence that modafinil improves several PFC-dependent cognitive functions in schizophrenia, major depression, adult attention-deficit hyperactivity disorder and detoxified alcohol-dependent patients [5, 10].

Modafinil in narcolepsy

The efficacy, safety, and tolerance of modafinil in narcolepsy patients have been demonstrated in two large nine-week, multicenter, placebo-controlled, fixed-dose trials in the USA [11, 12]. Daily treatment with 200 or 400 mg of modafinil resulted in significant improvements of the Multiple Sleep Latency Test (MSLT), Multiple Wakefulness Test (MWT), Epworth Sleepiness Scale (ESS), and Clinical Global Impression of Change (CGI-C) scores.

Neuroimaging of Sleep and Sleep Disorders, ed. Eric Nofzinger, Pierre Maquet, and Michael J. Thorpy. Published by Cambridge University Press. © Cambridge University Press 2013.

According to a recent meta analysis involving 1054 patients, modafinil – in comparison with placebo – showed significant benefits in terms of elimination of excessive daytime sleepiness assessed by the ESS – weighted mean difference (WMD) –2.73 points (95% CI –3.39, –2.08), MSLT – WMD 1.11 min (95% CI 0.55, 1.66), and MWT – WMD 2.82 min (95% CI 2.40, 3.24), as well as the number and duration of attacks of somnolence or sleep and naps per day, but did not differ from placebo in the number of attacks of cataplexy per day [13]. Compared with placebo, modafinil improved the quality of life of narcoleptic patients according to the SF-36 questionnaire, but was associated with more common nausea. It had similar effects on excessive daytime sleepiness as sodium oxybate and was associated with less common nausea.

Armodafinil, the longer-lasting isomer formulation of modafinil, is a wakefulness-promoting medication [5]. A multi-center randomized, double-blind, placebo-controlled 12-week study in narcolepsy found armodafinil to have various effects on cognition, as revealed by reaction time, episodic recall, and recognition tasks [14]. In a long-term study, armodafinil consistently improved subjective wakefulness and reduced fatigue of patients with sleepiness associated with narcolepsy [15]. Studies in animal models and neuroimaging in humans suggest that these effects may be related to specific actions of modafinil in the frontal cortex [5].

Unfortunately, there is a paucity of empirical studies objectively assessing and localizing the cognitive effects of modafinil in narcolepsy. Functional MRI has been used to detect regional brain responses to changes in sensory stimuli [16]. Mean cortical activation levels during the presentation of periodic visual and auditory stimulation showed no appreciable differences with either age or sex. Modafinil caused an increase in self-reported levels of alertness in seven of eight narcoleptic subjects, but there was no significant difference between mean pre- and post-treatment activation levels, as determined by fMRI for either normal or narcoleptic syndrome subjects receiving modafinil.

In another fMRI study with three drug-free narcoleptics, cerebral activation was mapped during the performance of a 2-back verbal working memory task [17]. In all subjects, during the first scan a bilateral and widespread activation in known nodes of the executive network was seen, including the lateral prefrontal, posterior parietal, and anterior cingulate cortices. There was a reduction in cerebral activation, especially but not exclusively in the PFC, associated with a slowing of performance from the first to the last tolerated scan. On stimulants, subjective alertness, activation, and objective performance were readily maintained.

A recent double-blind, placebo-controlled study investigated the effect of modafinil on cortical excitability in narcolepsy by means of transcranial magnetic stimulation (TMS) and explored the relation between these TMS measures and conventional measures of sleepiness [18]. Short-latency intracortical inhibition (SICI) was significantly increased in patients with narcolepsy. Modafinil induced oppositional changes and decreased SICI. Spearman rank correlation showed the highest correlation between SICI and the MSLT.

The authors concluded that a decrease in gamma-aminobutyric acid (GABA)ergic intracortical mechanisms reflected by TMS cortical excitability plays an important role in the wakefulness-promoting action of modafinil in narcolepsy.

Functional neuroimaging of therapeutic effects with LORETA

Neuroimaging of brain areas involved in wakefulness and attention can be performed by means of positron emission tomography (PET) and fMRI, but also by electrophysiological neuroimaging techniques [19, 20].

Electroencephalographic (EEG) low-resolution brain electromagnetic tomography (LORETA) was developed in order to identify brain regions that are involved in neuropsychiatric disorders and are the targets of therapeutic drug action [21–26].

LORETA computes a unique 3-dimensional electrical source distribution. It solves the non-unique "inverse" problem (i.e., the computation of the electric sources from surface data) by assuming that the smoothest of all possible source distributions is most plausible [21].

This assumption is consistent with electrophysiological findings showing highly correlated activity in neighboring neuronal populations. The LORETA version applied introduced, in addition to the smoothness constraint, a neuroanatomical constraint by restricting the solution space to cortical gray matter volume, as determined by the digitized Probability Atlas (Brain Imaging Centre, Montreal Neurological Institute) in the Talairach domain [27]. A voxel was labeled as gray matter if its probability of being gray matter was higher than 33% and higher than its probability of being white matter or cerebrospinal fluid.

EEG tomography (LORETA) in narcolepsy

Aim of the study

The aim of the study was (1) to investigate and localize brain regions responsible for vigilance decrements in narcolepsy patients as compared with age- and sex-matched normal controls by means of EEG tomography (LORETA) and (2) to identify target regions of modafinil in narcolepsy patients by means of LORETA (in addition to objectifying vigilance improvements by means of the conventional methods such as MSLT and ESS at the subjective behavioral level) [23].

Methods and findings

Sixteen drug-free narcoleptics and 16 normal controls were included in the baseline investigation.

The quantitative EEG differences observed were characterized by a significant decrease in alpha-2 power, mainly in the frontal, temporal, and parietal cortices of the right hemisphere, along with a global decrease in beta power, also accentuated over the right cortical brain areas, which demonstrates a deterioration of the frontotemporoparietal network of the "right hemisphere vigilance system" in narcolepsy [28].

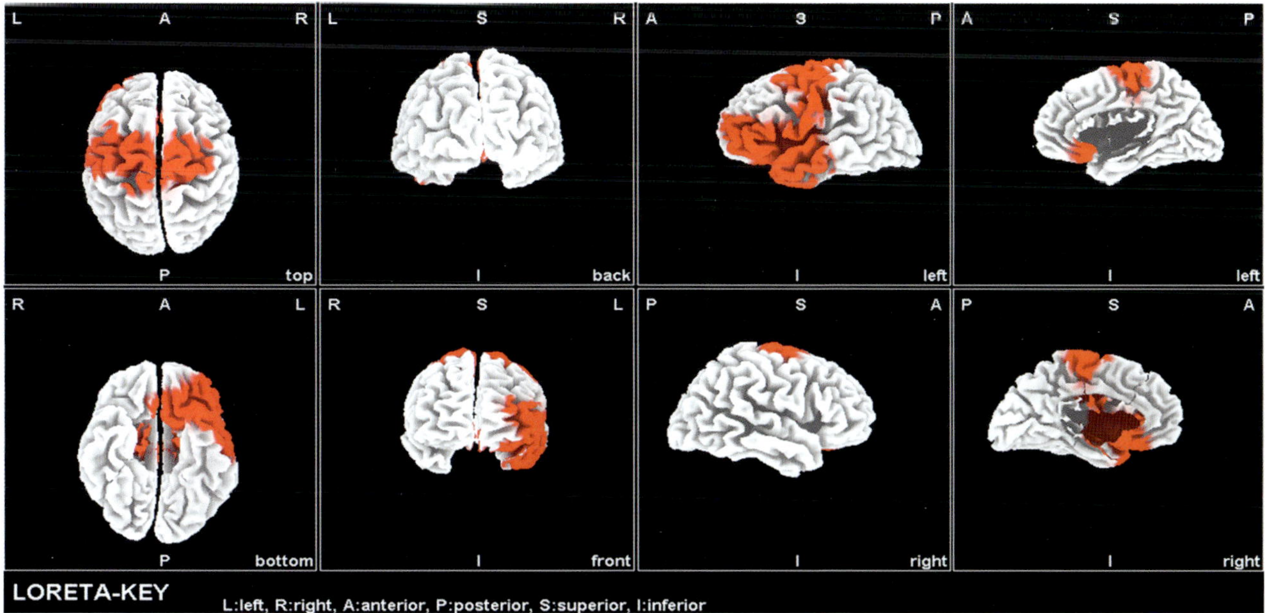

Figure 29.1 LORETA differences between modafinil (400 mg) and placebo during the resting recording after three-week therapy in narcoleptic patients (n = 15). Images depicting statistical parametric maps (SPMs) seen from different perspectives are based on voxel-by-voxel t-values of differences between modafinil and placebo for alpha-2 (10–12 Hz). Red colors indicate increases, blue colors decreases as compared to placebo. Structural anatomy is shown in gray scale. Modafinil induces an increase in fast alpha-2 power in the frontotemporal and sublobar cortical regions of the left hemisphere.

Subsequently, patients participated in a double-blind, placebo-controlled crossover study receiving a three-week fixed titration of modafinil (200, 300, 400 mg) and placebo.

Modafinil significantly improved daytime sleepiness, measured at the behavioral level by the ESS and at the neurophysiological level by the MSLT and LORETA tomography.

LORETA made it possible to identify and visualize target brain regions of modafinil for vigilance improvement. In the resting EEG, modafinil induced an increase in fast alpha-2 power in the frontotemporal and sublobar cortical regions of the left hemisphere, with the maximum in BA 11 of the inferior frontal gyrus (Figure 29.1). Beta 1–3 power increased in many brain regions, and predominantly in the left hemispheric temporoparietal and limbic cortices. In delta and theta power modafinil induced a decrease in frontal lobes, along with an increase in theta power in the left temporoparietal regions. Delta power increased in the left parietal cortex and in the right more than the left occipital and limbic lobes.

Conclusion

Thus, modafinil generally seems to exert its therapeutic mode of action more in the left than in the right hemisphere, which in narcolepsy seems to be the less affected part of the brain.

The decrease in alpha-2 power in narcolepsy patients as compared with normal controls and the increase in alpha-2 power under modafinil as compared with placebo confirm a "key–lock principle" in the diagnosis and therapy of neuropsychiatric disorders [22] and were both seen in the PFC. The latter has principal connections to the thalamus, hypothalamus, and basal forebrain, regions known to be involved in the neurological control of sleep and wakefulness. In general, our findings of a promotion of vigilance induced by modafinil are in line with the first human pharmaco-EEG data obtained in normal elderly subjects [29], as well as with findings in patients with vigilance decrements [10].

LORETA identifies brain regions linked to psychometric performance under modafinil in narcolepsy

Introduction

Since the early 1980s, several studies have attempted to demonstrate the relationship between sleepiness and cognitive performance in narcoleptic subjects [30–33]. The findings obtained generally failed to demonstrate significant performance differences to controls and remained inconclusive in the question of whether performance decrements in narcolepsy are explained by attentional or organic cognitive mechanisms.

Rieger *et al.* also found deficits in divided and flexible attention in narcolepsy [34]. Naumann *et al.* described deficits in some attention and all executive function tests, whereas memory and routine alertness tasks were only mildly impaired in narcolepsy, indicating a reduced capacity to maintain a sufficient level of alertness across longer periods of time when concentrating on a demanding task [35].

Aim of the study

In an additional analysis to the above study [23], we examined the effects of modafinil compared with placebo on cognitive performance and thymopsychic variables in narcoleptic patients [24]. Moreover, we correlated significant and clinically relevant psychometric changes in midmorning hours with neurophysiological alterations measured by EEG-LORETA at the same time. Finally, we explored the relation between these EEG-LORETA findings and MSLT results, which reflect objective sleepiness over one day, as well as ESS data, which indicate subjective sleepiness over one week.

Methods and findings

Mental performance was tested by means of a computerized version of the Pauli Test [36, 37]: within a time interval of 20 min, subjects had to add as many single-digit numbers as possible and react to two-digit solutions by pressing the last digit only. The test results reflect attention, concentration, mnestic aspects, and volition, which in turn depend on the individual's ability to keep activation at an adequate level over 20 min. Concerning the total number of calculations in the Pauli Test, patients performed significantly ($p < 0.01$) better under modafinil than under placebo (836 versus 790 calculations).

In the correlation analyses, we found a negative correlation between mental performance and EEG-LORETA power. The less theta and slow alpha-1 power in the midmorning EEG, the better arithmetic performance in the Pauli Test (Figure 29.2). In both frequency bands, the highest correlation coefficient as well as the highest percentage of voxels involved was seen in BA 10 of the medial frontal gyrus.

Thymopsychic variables included midmorning subjective well-being based on the von Zerssen BF-S Scale [38], the State-Trait Anxiety Inventory [39], the Beck Depression Inventory (BDI) [40], and the Symptom Checklist 90 (SCL-90) [41] as well as drive, mood, affectivity, and drowsiness in the morning, measured by means of 100-mm visual analog scales (VAS).

Compared with placebo, modafinil showed no significant group effect on thymopsychic variables, which sets it apart from the classical psychostimulants. This is of clinical relevance, as narcolepsy patients have a higher risk of developing psychiatric disorders (e.g., major depression, altered personality, or other psychiatric problems) than patients without narcolepsy [42, 43].

In the correlation analyses between subjective drowsiness and EEG-LORETA power, we demonstrated significant positive correlations in the delta, theta, and superimposed beta activity bands, reflecting vigilance changes in the sense of a drowsiness state.

Further analyses also showed significant correlations between midmorning EEG tomography and the widely used MSLT – although in a smaller number of voxels. However, the latter may be due to the fact that the EEG-LORETA data set obtained over a short period of time (3 min) was correlated with MSLT data averaged over a whole day. Finally, it seems understandable that the correlations between midmorning EEG-LORETA and subjective ESS data covering the last week did not reach the 1% level of statistical significance (as seen with all the other correlations), although at the 5% level, again significant correlations were found on the basis of these two very different data sets (objective versus subjective, short-term versus long-term sampling).

Conclusion

Modafinil did not influence thymopsychic variables in narcolepsy, but it significantly improved cognitive performance, which may be related to medial prefrontal activity processes identified by LORETA.

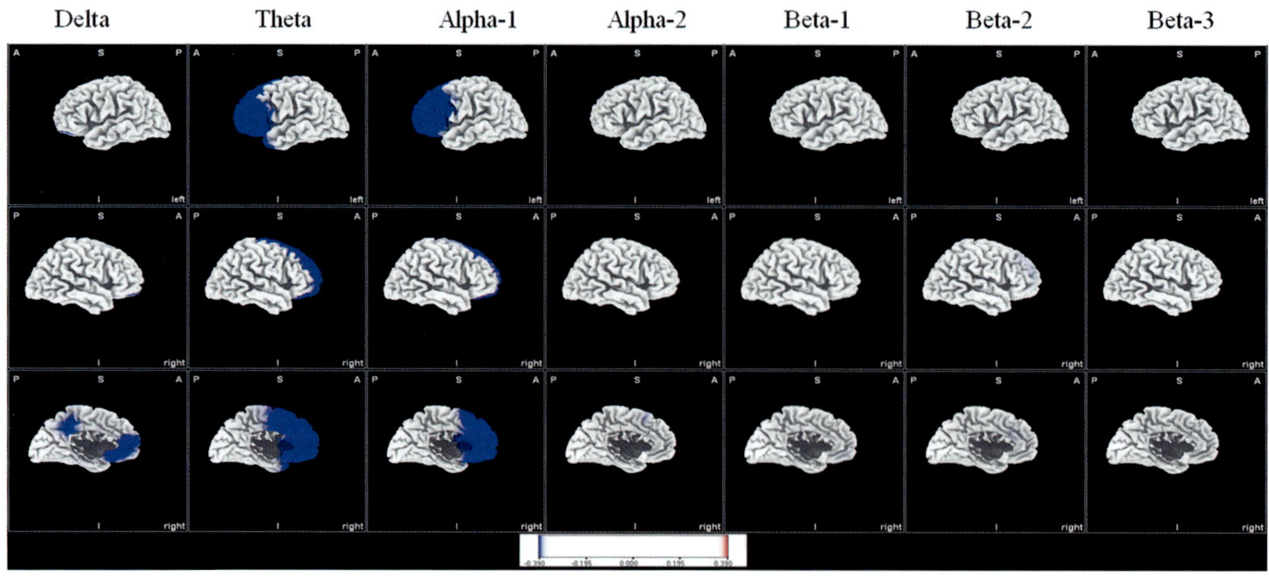

Figure 29.2 Correlations between mental performance and EEG-LORETA power based on surface-rendered LORETA images in narcolepsy. Images depicting SPMs seen from different perspectives are based on voxel-by-voxel Spearman rank correlation analysis between the total number of calculations in the Pauli Test and EEG-LORETA power in seven frequency bands (delta, theta, alpha-1, alpha-2, beta-1, beta-2, and beta-3 bands) in narcolepsy patients before and after treatment with placebo or modafinil (n: 3 × 15). Structural anatomy is shown in gray scale (A, anterior; I, inferior; P, posterior; S, superior). Significant negative correlations (blue color: $p < 0.01$) between EEG-LORETA power in the delta (1.5–6 Hz), theta (6–8 Hz), and slow alpha-1 (8–10 Hz), frequency range and the total score in the Pauli Test may be seen in different brain regions: the less the power in these slow frequency bands mainly over frontal regions, the better the performance in the arithmetic task.

Modafinil improves information processing speed and increases energetic resources for orientation of attention in narcoleptics: double-blind, placebo-controlled ERP studies with LORETA

Introduction

To bridge the currently wide gap between the neurotransmitter and the behavioral level and to improve temporal resolution up to the millisecond level, it may be useful to study the individual components of event-related brain potentials (ERPs). These include the N1 and P2 components, which reflect fundamental aspects of perception, such as initial orienting or attention-directing activity in the primary sensory projection areas [44, 45], and N2 and P300 components, which reflect fundamental aspects of cognition, such as the allocation of attentional resources for the evaluation of possible targets as well as the allocation of resources for stimulus encoding [46, 47].

Aim of the study

The aim of the study was to investigate cognition before and after modafinil as compared with placebo, utilizing LORETA to identify generators of ERP components in cortical regions [26].

Methods and findings

In a double-blind, placebo-controlled crossover design, 15 patients were treated with a three-week fixed titration scheme of modafinil and placebo. The ESS, MWT, and auditory ERPs (oddball paradigm) were obtained before and after the three weeks of therapy. Latencies, amplitudes, and LORETA sources were determined for standard (N1 and P2) and target (N2 and P300) ERP components.

ERP recordings were not performed on the same day as the MWT to avoid interference of the two vigilance test procedures.

Subjects were instructed to sit comfortably in a reclining chair situated in a constantly lit, sound-attenuated Faraday's cage, to open their eyes, and focus on a point 2.5 m straight ahead. A background noise (white noise of 45 dB SPL) was presented via earphones. The experiment started with a 1-min resting recording with eyes open. The two-tone oddball paradigm applied in this study was based on a design first reported by Squires *et al.* [48] and adapted for longitudinal studies by Semlitsch *et al.* [49]. Loud tone bursts (standard tone, probability 0.9, 1000 Hz, 50 ms duration, 5 ms rise/fall time, 90 dB SPL) were presented binaurally with a constant inter-stimulus interval of 1 s, randomly interrupted by soft tone bursts (target tone, probability 0.1, 1000 Hz, 50 ms duration, 5 ms rise/fall time, 70 dB SPL). The total number of tone bursts presented was 330. The subjects were asked to mentally count the soft tone bursts and report their number

at the end of the experiment. The error rate was calculated as the absolute difference between the number of target tones reported by the subject and the number of target tones actually presented.

Gold electrodes were attached to the scalp according to the international 10/20 system. Twenty-one channels, including 2 electro-oculography (EOG) and 19 EEG channels (Fp1, Fp2, F7, F3, Fz, F4, F8, T3, C3, Cz, C4, T4, T5, P3, Pz, P4, T6, O1, and O2 to averaged mastoids), were recorded by means of a Nihon Kohden 4421 G polygraph. Due to the high number of artifacts, the frontopolar electrodes were excluded from the analysis. The vertical EOG was recorded from an electrode at the mid-forehead to the average of one electrode below the left and one below the right eye. The horizontal EOG was recorded from the outer canthi (time constant: 1.0 s; high frequency response: 70 Hz; frequency range: 0.16–70 Hz; amplification: approximately 1:20 000 and 1:4000 for EEG and EOG, respectively). On-line data acquisition as well as data analyses were performed on a personal computer system using our software package [50]. The sampling frequency was 256 Hz, resulting in a time resolution of approximately 4 ms. After minimizing ocular artifacts based on regression analysis in the time domain [50, 51] and automatic artifact elimination [52], averaged ERP waveshapes were computed for target and standard tones. The analyzed time epoch was 1 s, including 100 ms pre-stimulus time. Waveforms were digitally filtered by means of a phase-linear, low-pass filter with a cutoff frequency of 20 Hz. Latencies and amplitudes of standard tone N1 and P2 as well as target tone N2 and P300 components were determined by the following procedure: peak latencies of the spatial average waveforms (i.e., average across 17 leads) were determined automatically and checked visually. If necessary, target tone N2 latency was determined with the aid of the difference waveform (target tone ERP – standard tone ERP). The amplitudes of the ERP components were measured at the defined latencies relative to pre-stimulus baseline (0–100 ms prior to stimulus onset). Thus, the component amplitudes measured at the different leads represent the topographic distribution at one single time point. Subsequently, on the basis of the scalp-recorded electric potential distribution, LORETA was used to estimate the 3-dimensional intracerebral current density distribution in 2394 voxels with a spatial resolution of 0.343 cm^3 [21]. The primary target was P300 latency. All p-values regarding intergroup differences are reported and displayed as graphs or images (statistical parametric maps, SPMs).

Modafinil normalizes cognitive ERP latencies

Our ERP study revealed significantly shortened N2 and P300 latencies under modafinil compared with placebo, which reflects an improvement of information processing speed. In a recent study we found prolonged latencies and reduced amplitudes in N2 and P300 components in the same drug-free patients as compared with normal controls, but no intergroup differences in N1 and P2 components [25]. This suggests impaired cognitive information processing in narcolepsy, while perception remains largely unaffected. Modafinil was

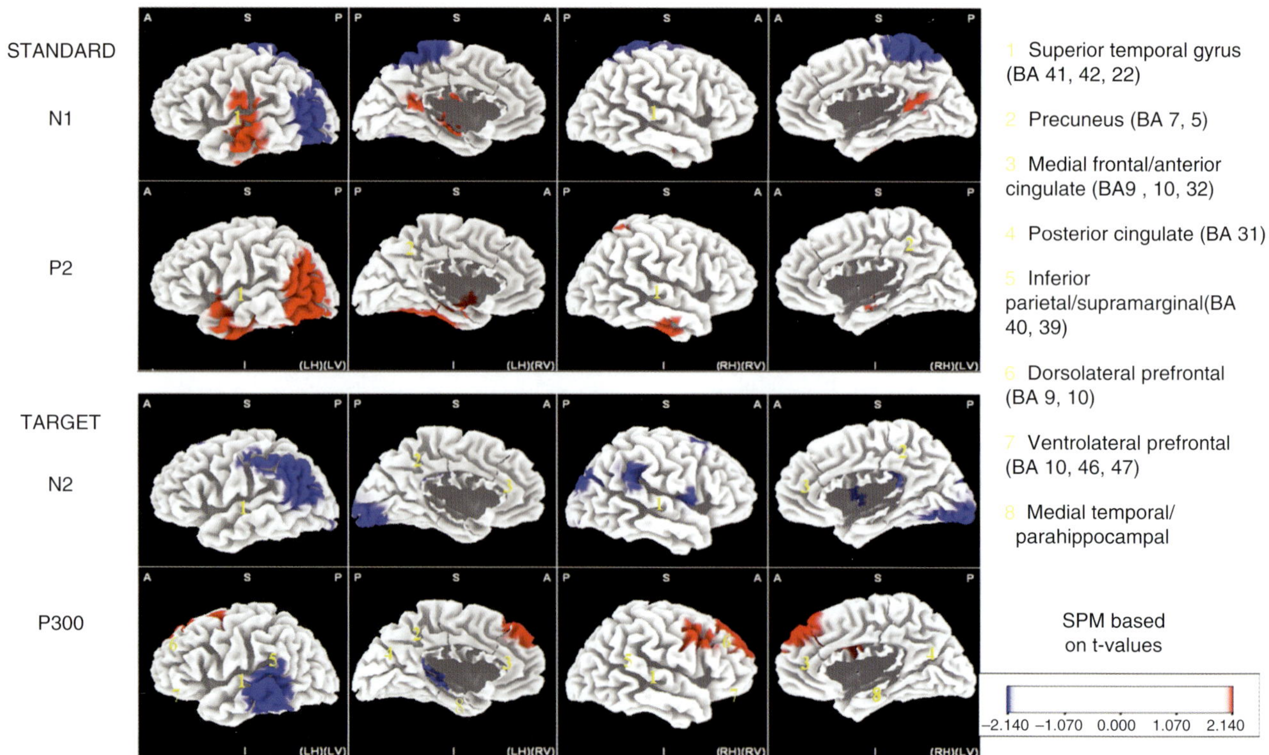

Figure 29.3 Differences between modafinil- and placebo-induced changes in standard N1 and P2 as well as target N2 and P300 LORETA source strength in 15 narcoleptic patients. Statistical differences based on t-values are projected to the left and right lateral and medial cortical surfaces (t > 2.06; p < 0.05; df = 28). Red colors represent significant increases, blue colors significant decreases after modafinil compared with placebo. The yellow numbers on the right side of the figure correspond to physiological standard N1 and P2 as well as target N2 and P300 generators. LORETA revealed increased source strength for N1 in the left auditory cortex. P300 source strength decreased in the left superior temporal gyrus and increased in the medial frontal regions and in the right dorsolateral prefrontal cortex.

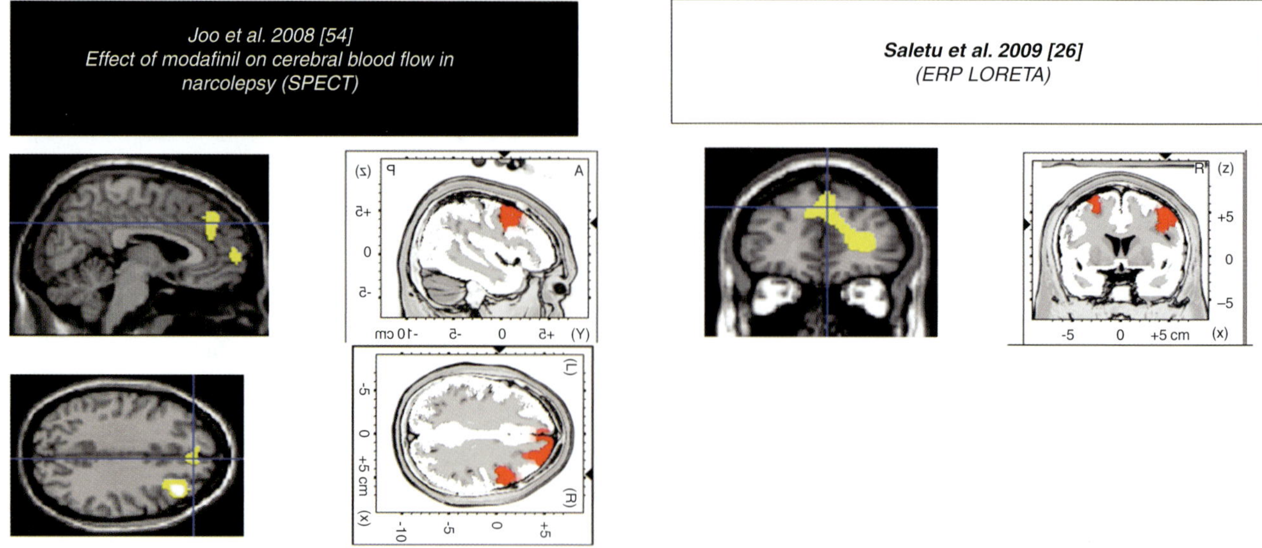

Figure 29.4 Comparison of brain SPECT and ERP LORETA showing similar modafinil-induced changes in narcolepsy. Brain SPECT (black background): SPM results demonstrating brain regions with rCBF increase or decrease after modafinil administration in narcolepsy patients. According to SPM overlaid on T1-weighted MR images, modafinil administration increases rCBF in bilateral medial prefrontal cortices and the right dorsolateral prefrontal cortex at an uncorrected p < 0.001. ERP LORETA (white background): regional differences in P300 LORETA source strength between modafinil-induced and placebo-induced changes in narcolepsy depicted in horizontal and vertical slices including all 2394 voxels. Modafinil increases source strength in the right dorsolateral prefrontal cortex for target P300 compared with placebo (p < 0.05; t > 2.05; df = 28).

shown to improve stimulus evaluation time, thereby tending to normalize cognitive information processing in narcoleptics, which confirms a "key–lock principle" in the diagnosis and therapy of impaired cognition in these patients.

Modafinil improves subjective sleepiness in narcolepsy

ESS scores improved significantly under modafinil as compared with placebo, which had been shown before [11, 12]. In the MWT, latency to sleep increased under modafinil, which, however, did not reach the level of statistical significance. The MWT was only used as an additional conventional method to objectify vigilance improvement.

LORETA identifies the medial and right dorsolateral prefrontal cortex as a target region of modafinil in regard to cognitive information processing

LORETA revealed increased source strength for N1 in the left auditory cortex and for P300 in the medial and right dorso-lateral prefrontal cortex (Figure 29.3).

A voxel-based morphometry (VBM) study in narcolepsy reported a significant gray matter loss in the right prefrontal and frontomesial cortices of patients, indicating a disease-related atrophy pattern, which may also be responsible for the reported prefrontal dysfunctions [53]. Comparing these findings with our study again reflects a "key–lock principle" in the diagnosis and therapy of the prefrontal dysfunction.

In a recent SPECT study before and after modafinil or placebo in narcolepsy, chronic modafinil treatment for four weeks increased regional cerebral blood flow (rCBF) in the right dorsolateral and anterior cingulate cortices, which confirms our results of this hot spot region for attention (Figure 29.4) [54]. The same group of scientists studied the effects of modafinil on rCBF in normal subjects and showed that a single dose of modafinil (400 mg at once) increased rCBF mainly in the thalamus and pons as well as in the prefrontal and cingulate cortices of healthy volunteers [55].

Functional imaging studies with sleep-deprived normal subjects, compared with narcolepsy patients, might clarify the question whether the increase in the medial and right dorso-lateral prefrontal cortices is specific for narcolepsy.

Conclusion

Our electrophysiological neuroimaging studies with LORETA identified the medial and right prefrontal cortices as a target region of modafinil in regard to cognitive information processing, as increased source density reflected increased energetic resources. Modafinil might work as a cognitive enhancer in narcolepsy, too.

Finally, our studies suggest that the same brain regions that have already been described as pathogenetically of interest in narcolepsy by morphological and functional MRI neuroimaging techniques may also be identified by electrophysiological neuroimaging.

References

1. Saper CB, Chou TC, Scammell TE. The sleep switch: hypothalamic control of sleep and wakefulness. *Trends Neurosci.* 2001;**24**:726–31.

2. Duncan J, Owen AM. Common regions of the human frontal lobe recruited by diverse cognitive demands. *Trends Neurosci.* 2000;**23**:475–83.

3. Muzur A, Pace-Schott EF, Hobson JA. The prefrontal cortex in sleep. *Trends Cogn Sci.* 2002;**6**:475–81.

4. Harrison Y, Horne JA, Rothwell A. Prefrontal neuropsychological effects of sleep deprivation in young adults – a model for healthy aging? *Sleep.* 2000;**23**:1067–73.

5. Minzenberg MJ, Carter CS. Modafinil: a review of neurochemical actions and effects on cognition. *Neuropsychopharmacology.* 2008;**33**:1477–502.

6. De Saint Hilaire Z, Orosco M, Rouch C, et al. Variations in extracellular monoamines in the prefrontal cortex and medial hypothalamus after modafinil administration: a microdialysis study in rats. *Neuroreport.* 2001;**12**:3533–7.

7. Ciliax BJ, Drash GW, Staley JK, et al. Immunocytochemical localization of the dopamine transporter in human brain. *J Comp Neurol.* 1999;**409**:38–56.

8. Saletu B, Grünberger J, Linzmayer L, et al. Pharmaco-EEG, psychometric and plasma level studies with two novel alpha-adrenergic stimulants CRL 40476 and 40028 (Adrafinil) in elderlies. *New Trends Exp Clin Psychiatry.* 1986;**2**:5–31.

9. Rasetti R, Mattay VS, Stankevich B, et al. Modulatory effects of modafinil on neural circuits regulating emotion and cognition. *Neuropsychopharmacology.* 2010;**35**:2101–9.

10. Saletu B, Saletu M, Grünberger J, et al. Treatment of the alcoholic organic brain syndrome: double-blind, placebo-controlled clinical, psychometric and electroencephalographic mapping studies with modafinil. *Neuropsychobiology.* 1993;**27**:26–39.

11. US Modafinil in Narcolepsy Multicenter Study Group (MiNMSG). Randomized trial of modafinil for the treatment of pathological somnolence in narcolepsy. *Ann Neurol.* 1998;**43**:88–97.

12. US MiNMSG. Randomized trial of modafinil as a treatment for the excessive daytime somnolence of narcolepsy. *Neurology.* 2000;**54**:1166–75.

13. Golicki D, Bala MM, Niewada M, et al. Modafinil for narcolepsy: systematic review and meta-analysis. *Med Sci Monit.* 2010;**16**:RA177–86.

14. Harsh JR, Hayduk R, Rosenberg R, et al. The efficacy and safety of armodafinil as treatment for adults with excessive sleepiness associated with narcolepsy. *Curr Med Res Opin* 2006;**22**:761–74.

15. Black JE, Hull SG, Tiller J, et al. The long-term tolerability and efficacy of armodafinil in patients with excessive sleepiness associated with treated obstructive sleep apnea, shift work disorder, or narcolepsy: an open-label extension study. *J Clin Sleep Med* 2010;**6**:458–66.

16. Ellis CM, Monk C, Simmons A, et al. Functional magnetic resonance imaging neuroactivation studies in normal subjects and subjects with the narcoleptic syndrome. Actions of modafinil. *J Sleep Res.* 1999;**8**:85–93.

17. Thomas RJ. Fatigue in the executive cortical network demonstrated in narcoleptics using functional magnetic resonance imaging – a preliminary study. *Sleep Med.* 2005;**6**:399–406.

18. Nardone R, Bergmann J, Lochner P, *et al.* Modafinil reverses hypoexcitability of the motor cortex in narcoleptic patients: a TMS study. *Sleep Med.* 2010;**11**:870–5.

19. Nofzinger EA. Functional neuroimaging of sleep. *Semin Neurol.* 2005;**25**:9–18.

20. Dang-Vu TT, Desseilles M, Petit D, *et al.* Neuroimaging in sleep medicine. *Sleep Med.* 2007;**8**:349–72.

21. Pascual-Marqui RD, Lehmann D, Koenig T, *et al.* Low resolution brain electromagnetic tomography (LORETA) functional imaging in acute, neuroleptic-naive, first-episode, productive schizophrenia. *Psychiatry Res.* 1999;**90**:169–79.

22. Saletu B, Anderer P, Saletu-Zyhlarz GM, *et al.* EEG topography and tomography in diagnosis and treatment of mental disorders: evidence for a key-lock principle. *Methods Find Exp Clin Pharmacol.* 2002;**24**(Suppl D):97–106.

23. Saletu M, Anderer P, Saletu-Zyhlarz GM, *et al.* EEG-tomographic studies with LORETA on vigilance differences between narcolepsy patients and controls and subsequent double-blind, placebo-controlled studies with modafinil. *J Neurol.* 2004;**251**:1354–63.

24. Saletu M, Anderer P, Semlitsch HV, *et al.* Low-resolution brain electromagnetic tomography (LORETA) identifies brain regions linked to psychometric performance under modafinil in narcolepsy. *Psychiatry Res.* 2007;**154**:69–84.

25. Saletu M, Anderer P, Saletu-Zyhlarz GM, *et al.* Event-related-potential low-resolution brain electromagnetic tomography (ERP-LORETA) suggests decreased energetic resources for cognitive processing in narcolepsy. *Clin Neurophysiol.* 2008;**119**:1782–94.

26. Saletu M, Anderer P, Saletu-Zyhlarz GM, *et al.* Modafinil improves information processing speed and increases energetic resources for orientation of attention in narcoleptics: double-blind, placebo-controlled ERP studies with low-resolution brain electromagnetic tomography (LORETA). *Sleep Med.* 2009;**10**:850–8.

27. Talairach J Tournaux P. *Co-Planar Stereotaxic Atlas of the Human Brain.* Stuttgart, Thieme, 1988.

28. Arruda JE, Walker KA, Weiler MD, *et al.* Validation of a right hemisphere vigilance system as measured by principal component and factor analyzed quantitative electroencephalogram. *Int J Psychophysiol.* 1999;**32**:119–28.

29. Saletu B, Frey R, Krupka M, *et al.* Differential effects of a new central adrenergic agonist – modafinil – and D-amphetamine on sleep and early morning behaviour in young healthy volunteers. *Int J Clin Pharmacol Res.* 1989;**9**:183–195.

30. Rogers AE, Rosenberg RS. Tests of memory in narcoleptics. *Sleep.* 1990;**13**:42–52.

31. Broughton R, Low R, Valley V, *et al.* Auditory evoked potentials compared to performance measures and EEG in assessing excessive daytime sleepiness in narcolepsy-cataplexy. *Electroencephalogr Clin Neurophysiol.* 1982;**54**:579–82.

32. Aguirre M, Broughton R, Stuss D. Does memory impairment exist in narcolepsy-cataplexy? *J Clin Exp Neuropsychol.* 1985;**7**:14–24.

33. Henry GK, Satz P, Heilbronner RL. Evidence of a perceptual-encoding deficit in narcolepsy? *Sleep.* 1993;**16**:123–127.

34. Rieger M, Mayer G, Gauggel S. Attention deficits in patients with narcolepsy. *Sleep.* 2003;**26**:36–43.

35. Naumann A, Bellebaum C, Daum I. Cognitive deficits in narcolepsy. *J Sleep Res.* 2006;**15**:329–38.

36. Pauli R, Arnold, W. *The Pauli Test; Its Correct Execution and Evaluation in BK.* Oxford, England, 1953.

37. Arnold W. *Der Pauli Test. Anweisung zur sachgemäßen Durchführung, Auswertung und Anwendung des Kraepelinschen Arbeitsversuchs*, Vol. 5. Springer-Verlag, Berlin, 1975.

38. Von Zerssen D, Koeller DM, Rey ER. Die Befindlichkeitsskala (B-S): Ein einfaches Instrument zur Objektivierung von Befindlichkeitsstörungen, insbesondere im Rahmen von Längsschnittuntersuchungen. *Arzneimittelforschung.* 1970;**20**:915–18.

39. Spielberger CD, Gorsuch R, Lushene RE. *STAI, Manual for the State-Trait Anxiety Inventory.* Palo Alto, CA, Consulting Psychologists Press, 1970.

40. Beck AT, Ward CH, Mendelson M, *et al.* An inventory for measuring depression. *Arch Gen Psychiatry.* 1961;**4**:561–71.

41. Derogatis LR, Rickels K, Rock AF. The SCL-90 and the MMPI: a step in the validation of a new self-report scale. *Br J Psychiatry.* 1976;**128**:280–9.

42. Roy A. Psychiatric aspects of narcolepsy. *Br J Psychiatry.* 1976;**128**:562–5.

43. Krishnan RR, Volow MR, Miller PP, *et al.* Narcolepsy: preliminary retrospective study of psychiatric and psychosocial aspects. *Am J Psychiatry.* 1984;**141**:428–31.

44. Näätänen R. Implications of event-related potentials data for psychological theories of attention. In: Renault M Kutas M, Coles MGH, Gailland AGM, eds. *Event-Related Potential Investigations of Cognition.* Amsterdam, North-Holland, 1989; 117–64.

45. Picton T, Hillyard S. Endogenous event-related potentials. In: Picton T, ed. *Human Event-Related Potentials. Handbook of Electroencephalography and Clinical Neurophysiology,* Vol. 3. *Amsterdam, Elsevier.* 1988; 361–426.

46. Polich J. P300 clinical utility and control of variability. *J Clin Neurophysiol.* 1998;**15**:14–33.

47. Halgren E, Marinkovic K, Chauvel P. Generators of the late cognitive potentials in auditory and visual oddball tasks. *Electroencephalogr Clin Neurophysiol.* 1998;**106**:156–64.

48. Squires NK, Squires KC, Hillyard SA. Two varieties of long-latency positive waves evoked by unpredictable auditory stimuli in man. *Electroencephalogr Clin Neurophysiol.* 1975;**38**:387–401.

49. Semlitsch HV, Anderer P, Saletu B, *et al.* Psychophysiological research in psychiatry and neuropsychopharmacology. I. Methodological aspects of the Viennese Psychophysiological Test-System (VPTS). *Methods Find Exp Clin Pharmacol.* 1989;**11**:25–41.

50. Anderer P, Semlitsch HV, Saletu B, *et al.* Artifact processing in topographic mapping of electroencephalographic activity in neuropsychopharmacology. *Psychiatry Res.* 1992;**45**:79–93.

51. Semlitsch HV, Anderer P, Schuster P, *et al.* A solution for reliable and valid reduction of ocular artifacts, applied to the P300 ERP. *Psychophysiology* 1986;**23**:695–703.

52. Anderer P, Saletu B, Semlitsch HV, *et al.* Perceptual and cognitive event-related potentials in neuropsychopharmacology: methodological aspects and clinical applications (pharmaco-ERP topography and tomography). *Methods Find Exp Clin Pharmacol.* 2002;**24**(Suppl C):121–37.

53. Brenneis C, Brandauer E, Frauscher B, *et al.* Voxel-based morphometry in narcolepsy. *Sleep Med* 2005;**6**:531–6.

54. Joo EY, Seo DW, Tae WS, *et al.* Effect of modafinil on cerebral blood flow in narcolepsy patients. *Sleep* 2008;**31**:868–73.

55. Joo EY, Tae WS, Jung KY, *et al.* Cerebral blood flow changes in man by wake-promoting drug, modafinil: a randomized double blind study. *J Sleep Res.* 2008;**17**:82–8.

Neuroimaging of Kleine–Levin syndrome

Maria Engström

Introduction

Recurrent hypersomnia was reported for the first time in multiple subjects by Kleine in 1925 [1]. Later Levin associated the syndrome with hyperphagia [2] and Critchley and Hoffman named the disease Kleine–Levin syndrome (KLS) [3]. KLS is characterized by periods of excessive sleep, cognitive impairment, altered perception, and behavioral disturbances. It is a relapsing disorder with mean duration of 14 years. The mean duration of sleep episodes is 12 days, but there is great individual variance ranging from 2 to 270 days. In mean, KLS patients have two episodes each year. However, some patients have sleep episodes as often as twice a month [4].

According to The International Classification of Sleep Disorders, revised by the American Academy of Sleep Medicine 2005, KLS patients should experience at least one of the following symptoms: hyperphagia, hypersexuality, odd behavior, or cognitive disturbances; in addition to recurrent episodes of hypersomnia. In a systematic study of 108 KLS patients, Arnulf *et al.* [4] showed that cognitive impairment (e.g., language and memory dysfunction, concentration difficulties, and temporal disorientation) and altered perception (e.g., dreamy state or derealization) occur in 100% of KLS patients, whereas hyperphagia and hypersexuality occur only in a KLS subset; 66% and 53%, respectively. KLS patients are asymptomatic between sleep periods; however, working memory deficits have been reported interictally and after relapse [5, 6].

The etiology of KLS is unknown and remains a challenge. Hypothalamic abnormality has been suggested due to the important function of the hypothalamus in sleep regulation. However, no consistent findings of hypothalamic pathology have been observed. Hormone and orexin levels are usually normal. So are routine blood tests as well as cerebrospinal fluid bacterial and viral serologies. Electroencephalogram (EEG) shows a non-specific slowing of background EEG activity during sleep periods in 70% of the cases, but no epileptic activity is reported. Birth difficulties are reported for a fourth of the patients, indicating possible perinatal brain injury. KLS onset is frequently associated with precipitating events, such as infections, alcohol intake, and sleep deprivation.

Finally, an overrepresentation in the Jewish population has been observed, pointing to a possible genetic component, eventually coupled to a genetic predisposition for infectious diseases [4, 7].

Neuroimaging in KLS

Different neuroimaging methods have been applied to further the knowledge of the neural concomitants of KLS. One objective with neuroimaging is to investigate whether KLS symptoms are caused primarily by structural (lesions or atrophy) or functional aberrations in the brain, for example functional connectivity disruption or neurotransmitter depletion. Another objective is to enhance the diagnosis by identifying imaging biomarkers of KLS. Due to the sparse occurrence of KLS, most neuroimaging reports are from case studies. However, a few authors report results from larger study groups. In the following sections the spectrum of neuroimaging in KLS are reviewed. A summary is found in Table 30.1.

Structural neuroimaging in KLS is made by standard magnetic resonance imaging (MRI) and computed tomography (CT). Brain tissue perfusion has most commonly been assessed by single-photon emission computed tomography (SPECT), which uses radioactive tracers to study cerebral blood flow. Cognitive function has been mapped by measuring the blood oxygen level-dependent (BOLD) response to stimuli or to spontaneous brain fluctuations in functional MRI (fMRI). Biochemical function in KLS has been assessed by means of proton magnetic resonance spectroscopy (^{1}H-MRS), which measures the concentration of proton containing metabolites in brain tissue. In addition, SPECT and positron emission tomography (PET) have been used to map metabolic and neurotransmitter distribution in a few KLS cases.

Morphology

Most structural imaging as assessed by MRI [5, 8–15] and/or CT [5, 10, 11, 13, 15–17] reveals no pathological findings. In four cases, lesions adjacent to the ventricular or cisternal system were reported. One patient had periventricular white matter lesions [18] and three patients had lipomas; either suprasellar lipomas [19] or lipoma at the posterior floor of the third ventricle [20]. Aberrations within the normal range in the pineal gland [21] and mamillary body [17] have been mentioned due to the anatomical location in areas that are associated with sleep regulation and amnesia.

Perfusion

Although structural neuroimaging in KLS is within the normal range in most cases, the vast majority of studies report

Neuroimaging of Sleep and Sleep Disorders, ed. Eric Nofzinger, Pierre Maquet, and Michael J. Thorpy. Published by Cambridge University Press. © Cambridge University Press 2013.

Table 30.1. Summary of structural and functional neuroimaging in KLS. When reporting number of cases (#), double counting has been avoided as far as possible

Method	# cases	Findings	Reference
Structural	**55**		
MRI	34	Normal	[5, 8–15]
CT	21	Normal	[5, 10, 11, 13, 15, 16, 17, 25]
MRI	1	Pineal gland aberration	[21]
MRI	1	Asymmetric mamillary body	[17]
MRI	1	Periventricular lesions	[18]
CT	3	Lipomas	[19, 20]
Perfusion	**19**		
MRI	1	Hypoperfusion thalamus	[18]
SPECT	6	Hypoperfusion thalamus	[11, 12]
SPECT	2	Hypoperfusion hypothalamus	[12, 21]
SPECT	6	Hypoperfusion basal ganglia	[11, 12, 21]
SPECT	7	Hypoperfusion frontal	[5, 8, 11, 12, 17, 21]
SPECT	8	Hypoperfusion temporal	[5, 9, 11, 12, 17, 21]
SPECT	1	Hyperperfusion thalamus	[14]
SPECT	1	Hyperperfusion basal ganglia	[14]
SPECT	3	Normal	[5, 15]
Cognitive	**10**		
fMRI (WM)	8	Hyperactivation thalamus	[6]
fMRI (WM)	8	Hypoactivation frontal	[6]
fMRI (TS)	1	Left/right dissociation	[18]
fMRI (RS)	9	Aberrant connectivity: Broca, Wernicke	[22]
Biochemistry	**8**		
^{1}H-MRS	1	Decreased NAA thalamus	[23]
^{1}H-MRS	4	Correlation BOLD NAA thalamus	[24]
^{1}H-MRS	2	Decreased glutamine thalamus	[18, 23]
PET	1	Normal glucose metabolism	[14]
SPECT	1	Reduced iomazenil frontotemporal	[14]
SPECT	1	Reduced dopamine function striatum	[25]

[WM = working memory; TS = tone stimuli; RS = resting state.]

hypoperfusion in several brain regions (see Table 30.1). Landtblom and coworkers [5, 17] were early in reporting frontotemporal hypoperfusion in KLS patients (Figure 30.1). Frontotemporal hypoperfusion in either the left or the right hemisphere or bilaterally is also observed in several case studies [8, 9, 11, 12, 21].

Huang *et al.* [11] investigated brain perfusion in seven KLS patients during an asymptomatic period and in five of those patients during hypersomnia. The main finding was hypoperfusion of bilateral thalami during hypersomnia, which was not observed during the asymptomatic period in any of the patients. These findings of thalamic hypoperfusion in the symptomatic state of KLS have been replicated in later case studies [12, 18] (however, see [14]).

Huang and coworkers [11] also observed significantly lower perfusion in all cortical areas as well as in the thalamus (as mentioned above) during the symptomatic period. However, they reported persistent frontotemporal hypoperfusion during the asymptomatic state in some subjects. Persistent hypoperfusion was most prominent in the subject with the longest clinical manifestation of KLS. Similar findings are reported in the case study by Hong *et al.* [12]. The authors observed lower perfusion in the symptomatic compared with the asymptomatic state in the bilateral thalami, the basal ganglia, the left hypothalamus, the medial frontal cortex (including the anterior cingulate cortex) as well as in the dorsolateral frontal and the left temporal cortices.

Additional SPECT findings show hypoperfusion in the hypothalamus [12, 21] and the basal ganglia [11, 12, 21]. However, a few patients were also found to have normal perfusion [5, 15].

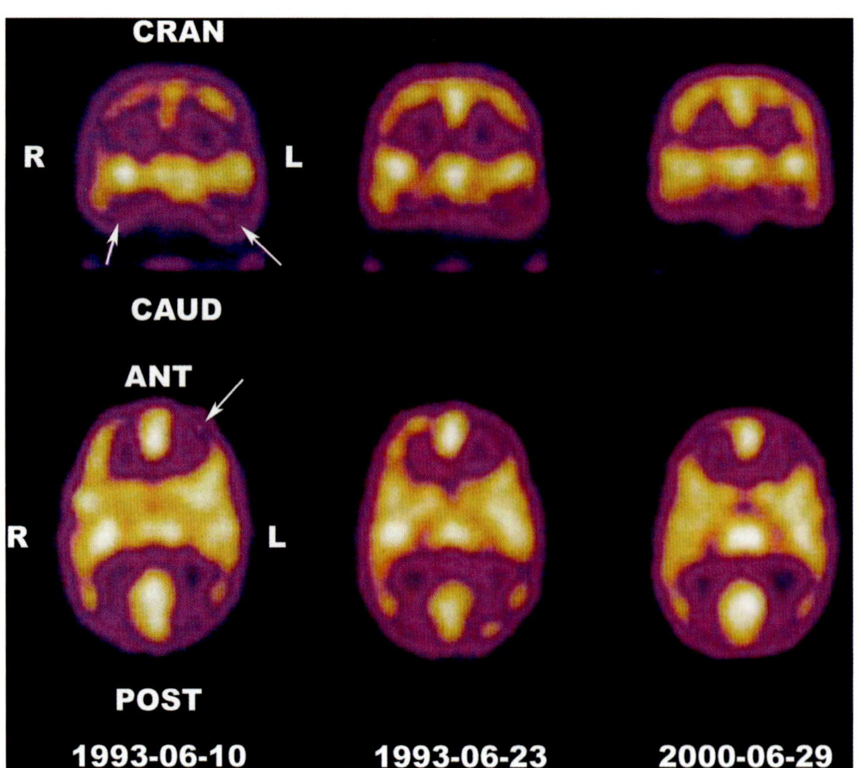

Figure 30.1 ^{99m}Tc-HMPAO-SPECT images with coronal and transaxial slices during a relapse with intense symptoms (10/06/1993) and after the disappearance of symptoms (23/06/1993) in a young male with Kleine–Levin syndrome showing marked hypoperfusion of the temporal and frontal regions, most prominent on the left side. Almost seven years after recovery (29/06/2000) there was a persisting slight hypoperfusion of the temporal lobes most prominent on the left side (Landtblom *et al. Acta Neurol Scand* 2002;**105**:318–21, printed with permission).

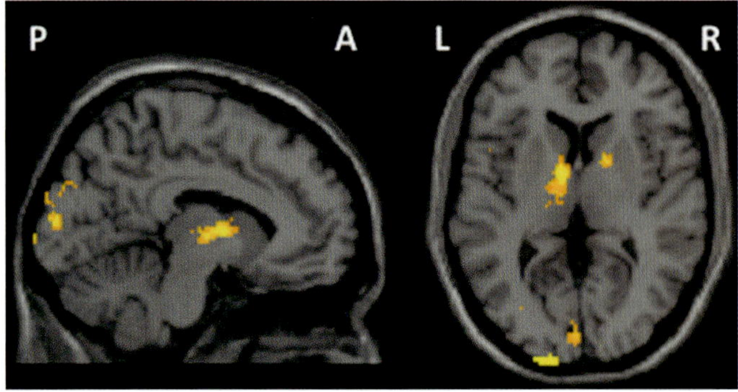

Figure 30.2 fMRI analyzed according to the general linear model showing BOLD hyperactivity in the thalamus and basal ganglia in KLS during performance of a verbal working memory task, which is tapping increasing task difficulty. The figure shows data, replicating earlier findings [6], from 18 KLS patients and 18 healthy controls for the contrast "KLS > controls." Cluster p-value: p < 0.001, Bonferroni corrected for multiple comparisons.

Cognition

Cognitive impairment and altered perception occur in all KLS patients during sleep episodes according to the review by Arnulf *et al.* [4]. It is thus pertinent to investigate the neural concomitants to cognitive function in KLS by functional neuroimaging. In fMRI, the BOLD response to localized neural events can be measured and visualized. Various cognitive tasks can be used to map the cerebral response to the function of interest, for example memory or language function. It is also possible to vary the difficulty of the task and in this way tap the cerebral response to task difficulty or effort.

Among different aspects of cognitive function, KLS patients were found to have persistent working memory problems [5, 6].

Engström *et al.* [6] showed interictal thalamic hyperactivation in eight KLS patients when they performed a verbal working memory task (reading span), which was analyzed for increasing task difficulty. These results have later been reproduced in a larger patient group (manuscript in preparation, Figure 30.2). In addition to the aberrant thalamic activation, the KLS patients also had reduced frontal activity, involving the anterior cingulate cortex and the adjacent prefrontal cortex, compared with healthy controls [6].

One drawback with fMRI in KLS is that most cognitive tasks require active participation. Thus, KLS patients have to be examined during the asymptomatic state. However, in order to image cognitive function during the symptomatic state it is possible either to use passive stimuli or investigate the spontaneous brain fluctuations during rest. One case study reported left-sided dominant cortical response to tone stimuli while the patient was in an asymptomatic state and right-sided response while in the symptomatic state [18]. Preliminary results on resting state fMRI of nine KLS patients indicate aberrant couplings within fronto temporo parietal networks, which are the cerebral representations of executive function [22]. KLS patients were found to have increased couplings to Broca's area and decreased couplings to Wernicke's area (Figure 30.3). In this study, however, the patients were examined during the asymptomatic state.

Biochemistry

N-Acetylasparate (NAA) is a biomarker for neuronal health, associated with either neuronal loss or neuronal dysfunction. One case study indicated decreased NAA/choline ratio in the thalamus during the symptomatic period compared with the

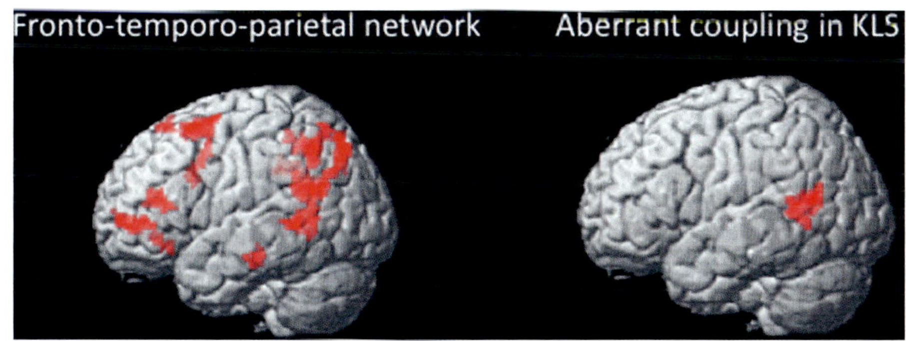

Figure 30.3 Resting state fMRI analyzed with independent component analysis (ICA). KLS patients had aberrant couplings to Wernicke's area (right) in a mainly left-lateralized fronto-temporo-parietal network (left). Cluster p-value: p = 0.009, Bonferroni corrected for multiple comparisons in region of interest.

asymptomatic period [23]. Tisell *et al.* have shown a negative correlation between NAA levels in the thalamus and the BOLD response to a verbal working memory task in a small group of KLS patients [24]. (The same task was used in [6].) These results have recently been reproduced in a larger group of 14 patients (manuscript in preparation). Two case studies reported increased glutamine metabolites in the thalamus during the symptomatic period compared with the asymptomatic period [18, 23].

Only two case studies have reported tracer active biochemistry imaging in KLS. Itokawa and coworkers [14] reported iomazenil hypoaccumulation in the left temporal lobe and the right frontal lobe suggesting reduced benzodiadepine binding to gamma-aminobutyric acid (GABA) receptors. Hoexter *et al.* [25] reported reduced striatal dopamine transporter potential in one KLS patient in the asymptomatic state.

Conclusions from neuroimaging in KLS

Hypothalamic pathology constitutes a main hypothesis for KLS etiology. This hypothesis is based on the important function of the hypothalmus in sleep and appetite regulation as well as regarding sexual activity. A minority (6%) of the structural imaging examinations reveal lesions in areas related to the hypothalamus (Table 30.1). Only two cases of hypothalamic hypoperfusion have been reported in the literature. Thus neuroimaging findings currently do not support the hypothalamic hypothesis, neither do the findings of normal hormone and orexin levels. However, three out of four post-mortem studies in primary and secondary KLS have reported autopsy findings in the hypothalamus [7]. Thus, the sparsity of neuroimaging findings in the hypothalamus might be a result of the detection limit for functional imaging in this region of the brain.

Another theory for the neural underpinnings of KLS is disturbed frontotemporal function. This theory is based on the frequent reports of hypoperfusion in frontotemporal regions and observations of memory and language problems in KLS [17]. The theory is also supported by the aberrant functional connectivity in frontal and temporal language areas and the dissociation of lateralization for auditory stimuli in the symptomatic and asymptomatic state [18, 22].

The most consistent finding in the neuroimaging literature is abnormalities in the thalamus. Hypoperfusion in the thalamus during the symptomatic state, which disappeared during the asymptomatic state, has been observed in three independent studies [11, 12, 18]. These findings indicate a recurrent aberration in the cerebral blood flow. However, the abnormal BOLD response, which is found in periods between sleep episodes, suggests an underlying thalamic involvement also in the asymptomatic state [6].

The theory of a thalamic involvement in KLS is supported by a couple of post-mortem investigations [7]. Both showed infiltration of inflammatory cells in the thalamus, indicating a regional encephalitis possibly caused by viral infection [16, 26]. KLS patients also manifest similar symptoms as patients with thalamic lesions [27, 28, 29, 30]. In a recent review on cognitive, affective, and behavioral disturbances following vascular thalamic lesions, it was reported that 90% of the patients with left or bilateral lesions had cognitive, behavioral, and/or mood alterations [31]. The majority of the patients exhibited moderate to severe memory impairments. Aphasia, with naming difficulties as the major problem, was commonly observed among patients with left-sided thalamic lesions. Apathy was the most commonly reported behavioral disturbance, which occurred in both unilateral and bilateral thalamic lesions, whereas hypersomnia was related to lesions in both thalami.

Thalamic nuclei project to widespread cortical and subcortical areas. The impact of thalamic lesions on a variety of functions might be explained by the crucial function of the thalamus in cerebral processing and/or a disconnection of the thalamo-striato-cortical loop. Lately, evidence for the so-called diaschisis hypothesis has evolved [31]. According to this hypothesis, dysfunction of the thalamus leads to metabolic and cerebral blood flow depression in functionally connected cortical regions. The hypothesis is supported by observations of thalamic lesions that are accompanied by frontotemporal hypometabolism [28, 30]. Together the neuroimaging findings in KLS indicate disruption of neural circuits involving frontotemporal regions as well as the thalamus and basal ganglia (Figure 30.4).

Future directions

Neuroimaging has identified plausible sources for hypersomnia as well as the cognitive, perceptive, and behavioral symptoms in KLS. However, more research is needed before the etiology of KLS is established and imaging methods that support the diagnosis are developed. Most of the previous neuroimaging reports are from case studies. It is therefore necessary to increase the study groups, but this could be a challenging issue since KLS is a rare disorder and most clinics do not encounter more than a handful of patients per decade. Thus, to enable sufficient patient

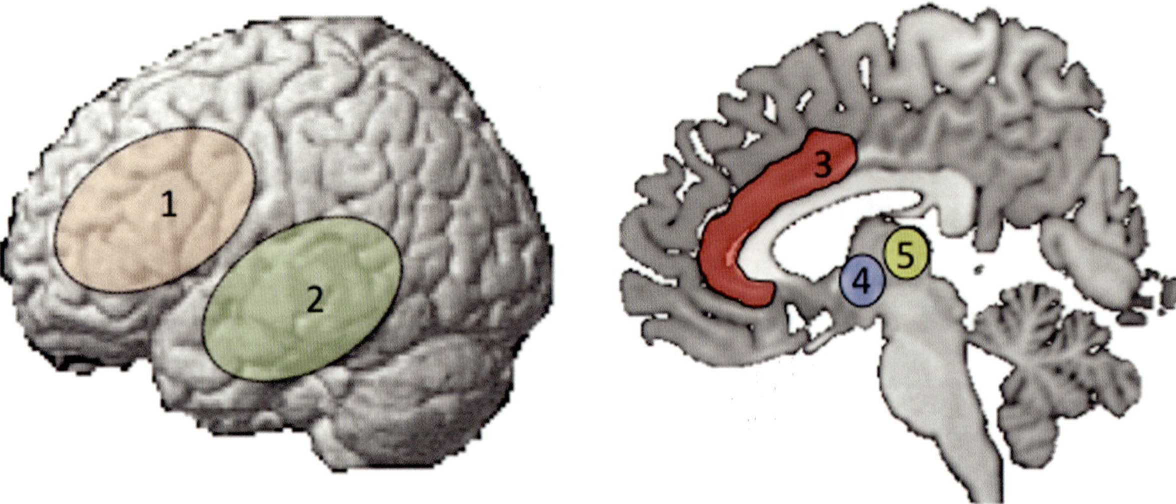

Figure 30.4 Brain regions affected in KLS. (1) Frontal lobe, (2) temporal lobe, (3) anterior cingulate cortex, (4) basal ganglia, (5) thalamus.

recruitment it is necessary to set up national centers for diagnosis and treatment and/or to apply a multicenter approach.

In neuroimaging it is important to evaluate which imaging modalities and/or protocols give necessary and sufficient information. In order to exclude secondary KLS caused by brain lesions, which are observable in standard MRI or CT, it is necessary to make structural imaging the first step in the examination chain. The second step is perhaps not so obvious to decide upon. Since cerebral blood flow is clearly indicative of dysfunction in KLS, assessment of brain perfusion is one attractive candidate. However, should perfusion preferentially be assessed with SPECT, as most centers have done so far, or is MRI perfusion a more appropriate method owing to its better spatial resolution? Further, fMRI gives valuable information about the functional networks of the brain. A verbal working memory task has been used to identify the thalamus as an important node of the (dys)functional network in KLS [6]. However, verbal tasks have the drawback of being language specific and could not easily be transferred to international protocols. It would therefore be interesting to study whether the same findings could be obtained from non-verbal tasks. Another problem with stimulus-driven fMRI is that it mostly requires active participation from the patients. This means that fMRI examinations using most cognitive tasks are not relevant for KLS in the symptomatic state. When examining KLS patients during sleep periods, resting state fMRI is an attractive alternative that has to be validated. In addition, the signal in MRI is dependent on the strength of the magnetic field. It is therefore relevant to investigate whether more information about the functional networks in KLS could be extracted at higher fields. This is certainly the case for MRS, where the possibility to quantify the levels of GABA and glutamate is substantially increased at higher fields. Finally, molecular imaging using PET could probably provide new information about KLS etiology as it could add knowledge about eventual neurotransmitter–receptor imbalance.

Summary

There are consistent findings across several studies pointing to malfunction of the thalamus and the frontotemporal cortex in KLS. There are also indications of functional aberration in the anterior cingulate cortex and the basal ganglia. However, most neuroimaging reports in KLS are from single cases. Clearly, more research is needed to ascertain the etiology and evolvement of KLS. Research is also needed to validate whether neuroimaging can support the diagnosis of KLS, in addition to clinical symptom assessment and neuropsychology.

References

1. Kleine W. Periodische schlafsucht. *Monats Psychiatr Neurol.* 1925;**57**:285–320.

2. Levin M. Periodic somnolence and morbid hunger: a new syndrome. *Brain.* 1936;**59**:494–504.

3. Critchley M, Hoffman H. The syndrome of periodic somnolence and morbic hunger (Kleine-Levin syndrome). *BMJ.* 1942;**1**:137–9.

4. Arnulf I, Lin L, Gadoth N, *et al.* Kleine-Levin syndrome: a systematic study of 108 patients. *Ann Neurol.* 2008;**63**:482–92.

5. Landtblom AM, Dige N, Schwerdt K, *et al.* Short-term memory dysfunction in Kleine-Levin syndrome. *Acta Neurol Scand.* 2003;**108**:363–7.

6. Engström M, Vigren P, Karlsson T, *et al.* Working memory in 8 Kleine-Levin syndrome patients: an fMRI study. *Sleep.* 2009;**32**:681–8.

7. Arnulf I, Zeitzer JM, File J, *et al.* Kleine-Levin syndrome: a systematic review of 186 cases in the literature. *Brain.* 2005;**128**:2763–76.

8. Arias M, Crespo-Iglesias JM, Perez J, *et al.* [Kleine-Levin syndrome: contribution of brain SPECT in diagrosis]. *Rev Neurol.* 2002;**35**:531–3.

9. Portilla P, Durand E, Chalvon A, *et al.* Hypoperfusion temporomesiale gauche en TEMP dans un syndrome de Kleine-Levin. *Rev Neurol (Paris).* 2002;**158**:593–6.

10. Dauvilliers Y, Mayer G, Lecendreux M, *et al.* Kleine-Levine syndrome. An autoimmune hypothesis based on clinical and genetic analysis. *Neurology.* 2002;**59**:1739–45.

11. Huang YS, Guilleminault C, Kao PF, *et al.* SPECT findings in Kleine-Levin syndrome. *Sleep.* 2005;**28**:955–60.

12. Hong SB, Yoo EY, Tae WS, *et al.* Episodic diencephalic hypoperfusion in Kleine-Levin syndrome. *Sleep.* 2006;**29**:1091–3.

13. Hirst J, Mignot E, Stein MT Episodic hypersomnia and unusual behaviors in a 14-year old adolescent. *J Dev Behav Pediatr.* 2007;**28**:475–7.

14. Itokawa K, Fukui M, Ninomiya M, *et al.* Gabapentin for Kleine-Levin syndrome. *Intern Med.* 2009;**48**:1183–5.

15. Lisk DR. Kleine-Levin syndrome. *Pract Neurol.* 2009;**9**:42–5.

16. Carpenter S, Yassa R, Ochs R. A pathologic basis for Kleine-Levin syndrome. *Arch Neurol.* 1982;**39**:25–8.

17. Landtblom AM, Dige N, Schwerdt K, *et al.* A case of Kleine-Levin syndrome examined with SPECT and neuropsychological testing. *Acta Neurol Scand.* 2002;**105**:318–21.

18. Billings ME, Watson NF, Keogh BP. Dynamic fMRI changes in Kleine-Levin syndrome. *Sleep Med.* 2011;**12**:531–2.

19. Servan J, Marchand F, Garma L, *et al.* Two new cases of Kleine-Levin syndrome associated with CT scan abnormalities. *Can J Neurol Sci.* 1993;**20**:S137.

20. Argenta G, Bozzao L, Petruzzellis MC. First CT finding in the Kleine-Levin-Critchley syndrome. *Ital J Neurol Sci.* 1981;**2**:77–9.

21. Lu ML, Liu HS, Chen CH, *et al.* Kleine-Levin syndrome and psychosis: observation from an unusual case. *Neuropsych Neuropsychol Behav Neurol.* 2000;**13**:140–2.

22. Engström M, Karlsson T, Landtblom AM. Resting state functional connectivity in patients with periodic hypersomnia. In: *Proceedings of the International Society for Magnetic Resonance in Medicine (ISMRM),* Stockholm, Sweden, 2010.

23. Poryazova R, Schnepf B, Boesiger P, *et al.* Magnetic resonance spectroscopy in a patient with Kleine-Levin syndrome. *J Neurol.* 2007;**254**:1445–6.

24. Tisell A, Engström M, Dahlqvist Leinhard O, *et al.* Combining fMRI with qMRS for under-standing the etiology of periodic hypersomnia. In: *Proceedings of the International Society for Magnetic Resonance in Medicine (ISMRM),* Hawaii, USA, 2009.

25. Hoexter MQ, Shih MC, Mendes DD, *et al.* Lower dopamine transporter density in an asymptomatic patient with Kleine-Levin syndrome. *Acta Neurol Scand.* 2008;**117**:370–3.

26. Fenzi F, Simonati A, Crosato F, *et al.* Clinical-features of Kleine-Levin syndrome with localized encephalitis. *Neuropediatrics.* 1993;**24**:292–5.

27. Guilleminault C, Qucra-Salva MA, Goldberg MP. Pseudo hypersomnia and pre-sleep behaviour with bilateral paramedian thalamic lesions. *Brain.* 1993;**116**:1549–63.

28. Stenset V, Grambaite R, Reinvang I, *et al.* Diaschisis after thalamic stroke: a comparison of metabolic and structural changes in a patient with amnesic syndrome. *Acta Neurol Scand.* 2007;**115**:67–71.

29. Bassetti C, Mathis J, Gugger M, *et al.* Hypersomnia following paramedian thalamic stroke: a report of 12 patients. *Ann Neurol.* 1996;**39**:471–80.

30. McGilchrist I, Goldstein LH, Jadresic D, *et al.* Thalamo-frontal psychosis. *Br J Psychiatry.* 1993;**163**:113–15.

31. De Witte L, Brouns R, Kavadias D, *et al.* Cognitive, affective and behavioural disturbances following vascular thalamic lesions: a review. *Cortex.* 2011;**27**:273–319.

Neuroimaging of cataplexy

Michael J. Thorpy

History

A 68-year-old woman had suffered from narcolepsy since she was 15 years old [1]. She had her first typical cataplectic episodes when she was 25 years old, while laughing, when surprised by meeting a known person in the street, or when speaking about emotionally challenging events of her past history. At age 68 years she abruptly stopped taking her clomipramine and had numerous cataplectic attacks, leading, over a two-month period, to full disabling status cataplecticus requiring inpatient care.

Polysomnographic findings

Her rapid eye movement (REM) sleep latency at night was 6 min. Her mean sleep latency during a multiple sleep latency test was 0.5 min, with three sleep onset REM periods among the four naps. She had undetectable hypocretin levels.

Imaging technique

The patient underwent two ^{99m}Tc-ethylcysteinate dimer brain single-photon emission computed tomography (SPECT) studies during symptomatic and asymptomatic periods of cataplexy on two non-consecutive days.

The perfusion brain tracer was administered within 10 s after the onset of cataplexy. After the cataplexy episodes the patient recovered full muscle tone within 2 min, and, when she could talk again, she accurately remembered all that she heard during the cataplectic episode.

The scan was performed in the half hour following the end of the clinical episode. Images (120 projections) were acquired using a three-headed gamma camera equipped with parallel high-resolution collimators (IRIX, Philips Medical Systems, Cleveland, USA) in a 128×128 matrix.

The asymptomatic study was performed three days after the initial study at the same time of day.

Symptomatic SPECT images were coregistered with asymptomatic images and both images were then coregistered with 3-dimensional magnetic resonance imaging (MRI). SPECT data were corrected for variable global cerebral blood flow after excluding voxels influenced by symptomatic-induced hyperperfusion in the symptomatic study, and a positive-difference image (symptomatic minus asymptomatic

SPECT) was calculated. The normalized subtracted SPECT and MRI volumes were merged for visual analysis.

Imaging findings

The positive-difference image (cataplexy minus rest) revealed hyperactivated areas corresponding anatomically to the cingular area (6-sd increase), the right and left orbitofrontal cortex (6-sd increase), the temporal cortex (4.5-sd increase), and the right putamen (6-sd increase) on brain MRI (Figure 31.1). The negative-difference image (rest minus cataplexy) did not identify any hypoperfused area.

Discussion

Neuroimaging of brain activity during intermittent short episodes of cataplexy, a transient and unpredictable neurological state, is difficult and it is easier to study cataplexy during status cataplecticus. There are, however, potential differences between routine cataplexy and the numerous cataplectic spells of status. During status, cataplexy is less often triggered by emotions and occurs more frequently. In addition, the abrupt clomipramine withdrawal that caused the rebound cataplexy in this patient, although it occurred two months previously, might have modulated the sensitivity of norepinephrine receptors in the brain. Although the patient did not have cataplexy during the asymptomatic brain SPECT, an asymptomatic period limited to 8 h does not guarantee normal baseline brain state. On the other hand, the state of the patient (complete atonia with full consciousness, lasting 1 to 2 min) during the cataplectic spells was not different from the usual cataplectic episodes.

This is the first imaging analysis comparing brain activation during a cataplectic episode with a non-symptomatic state in the same subject. While cingulate gyri and frontal white matter appear to be hypoperfused in narcoleptic patients outside any cataplectic event in this study, they were hyperperfused during cataplexy [2]. These data suggest that cataplexy is an overactive neuronal state, involving cortical and subcortical areas that are specific to the attacks and not activated between episodes.

Cataplexy appears as an intermediate stage between normal REM sleep and normal wakefulness Another striking

Neuroimaging of Sleep and Sleep Disorders, ed. Eric Nofzinger, Pierre Maquet, and Michael J. Thorpy. Published by Cambridge University Press. © Cambridge University Press 2013.

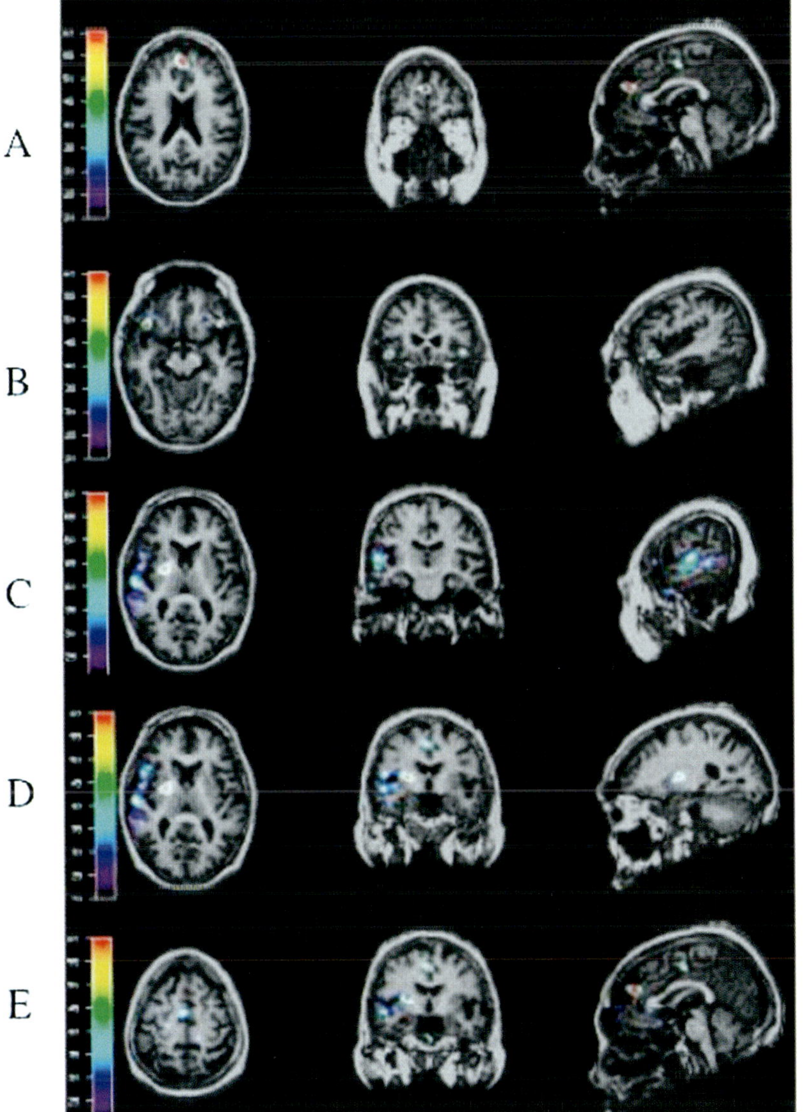

Figure 31.1 Brain functional imaging of cataplexy. Subtraction of cataplectic from non-cataplectic state single photon emission computed tomography coregistered to the magnetic resonance imaging study of the patient. The color scale indicates the intensity of changes expressed in standard deviations (sd) multiplied by a factor 10. Significant (sd > 2) perfusion increase was found in cingular (A, E), right and left orbitofrontal (B), right temporal (C), and right putamen (D) areas. No hypoperfusion could be detected with this technique.

characteristic of human REM sleep is right-hemisphere activation, as shown by SPECT imaging and spectral electroencephalographic (EEG) analysis [3, 4]. The right hemisphere is also more activated during cataplexy than is the left hemisphere.

Key points

- Neuroimaging shows cataplexy to be similar to REM sleep
- The right hemisphere is more activated during cataplexy than the left.

References

1. Chabas D, Habert MO, Maksud P, *et al.* Functional imaging of cataplexy during status cataplecticus. *Sleep.* 2007;**30**(2):153–6.

2. Yeon Joo E, Hong SB, Tae WS, *et al.* Cerebral perfusion abnormality in narcolepsy with cataplexy. *Neuroimage.* 2005;**28**:410–16.

3. Asenbaum S, Zeithofer J, Saletu B, *et al.* Technetium 99m HMPAO SPECT imaging of cerebral blood flow during REM sleep in narcoleptics. *J Nucl Med.* 1995;**36**:1150–5.

4. Bolduc C, Daoust AM, Limoges E, *et al.* Hemispheric lateralization of the EEG during wakefulness and REM sleep in young healthy adults. *Brain Cogn.* 2003;**53**:193–6.

Structural brain neuroimaging changes in obstructive sleep apnea

Paul M. Macey

Introduction

Obstructive sleep apnea (OSA) is accompanied by structural brain changes, as shown by neuroimaging findings from several groups. Changes in neural structure, reflected as gray matter loss, variations of metabolite levels, and alterations in water diffusion, appear in a variety of OSA populations, and likely reflect neural injury that contributes to the characteristics of the sleep disorder, including psychological and physiological comorbidities [1–10]. Complexities in identifying equivalent locations of brain structures across subjects and in the scanning and analysis techniques have resulted in a multitude of findings, with varying approaches used according to the particular research question being studied. Heterogeneity in OSA populations also contributes to variations in findings, since both apneic events and comorbidities of OSA are associated with neural changes. This chapter presents a summary of structural neuroimaging findings, including new data from our group. The chapter describes findings by technique, influences of factors other than the sleep disordered breathing on structural changes in OSA, and a summary of the brain regions shown across multiple studies to be affected in the disorder.

OSA neuroimaging findings by technique

Visual inspection

There is no evidence of clinically significant brain pathology in OSA [11], but subclinical changes in white matter were among the initial reports of magnetic resonance imaging (MRI) measurements in people with sleep disordered breathing. Visual inspection of brain images by an expert allows identification of white matter hyperintensities, which are a marker of accumulated vascular and other injury such as loss of fibers and demyelination, cell death, vessel damage, and silent infarcts [12]. Some OSA populations, especially severe OSA, show high levels of white matter hyperintensities [13–15], but others do not [16, 17], which may be due to confounding effects of aging and other factors contributing to the pathology, such as hypertension [12].

Magnetic resonance spectroscopy

Magnetic resonance spectroscopy (MRS) is a non-invasive MRI technique that allows quantification of metabolite levels, and

has been used to show alterations in brain regions of people with OSA indicative of reduced function and cell damage. Several studies report white matter differences in frontal occipital and parietal regions, especially in patients with severe OSA [5, 18–21]. Hippocampal changes in metabolite levels are also seen in adult and pediatric OSA populations [21–23]. Other brain areas may be affected, but the technique allows only selected, relatively large regions to be studied. Whole-brain approaches to MRS such as chemical-shift imaging remain problematic due to signal-to-noise issues, and suppression of signal from water in brain areas outside of medial forebrain areas ("outer volume" regions) [24].

Regional gray matter volume

In the past decade, available computing power, hard disk storage, and newly developed analytic techniques allowed the automatic analysis of anatomical T1-weighted images for the detection of regional gray matter changes in group comparisons over the whole brain, a process termed voxel-based morphometry (VBM) [25]. In 2002, our study demonstrated moderate reductions in gray matter volume across several cortical, limbic, and cerebellar areas [1]. Although these findings were initially only partially replicated [26–29],[1] more recent studies have confirmed the original phenomenon of reduced gray matter volume across multiple cortical and subcortical areas [6, 9, 30, 31], including secondary combined analysis of two OSA populations that individually showed no effect [8]. A related analysis of gray matter concentration also showed indications of injury in OSA [7].

Affected areas include diffuse frontal and parietal cortical regions, with the anterior cingulate showing some of the largest volume reductions. Limbic areas including the hippocampus and adjacent areas also show atrophy, as do cerebellar regions. The VBM approach has limited spatial resolution and sensitivity, but more targeted analyses allow certain brain structures to be assessed in more detail.

---

[1] Thomas *et al.* [28] reported "We performed voxel-based morphometric analysis on our data set (unpublished). The only positive result was a reduction in gray matter signal in the left hippocampus in the healthy subjects vs. hypoxic patients, which is similar to the conclusions of another report [Morrell]."

Neuroimaging of Sleep and Sleep Disorders, ed. Eric Nofzinger, Pierre Maquet, and Michael J. Thorpy. Published by Cambridge University Press. © Cambridge University Press 2013.

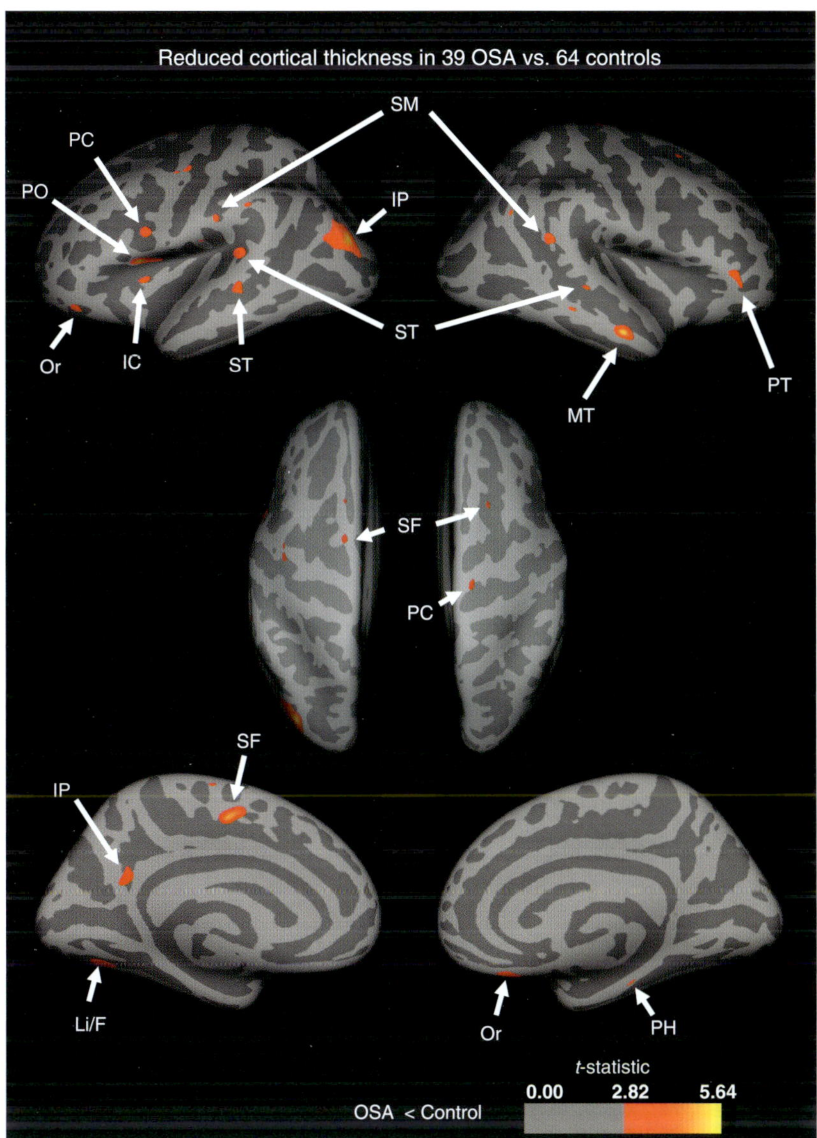

Figure 32.1 Reduced cortical thickness in OSA versus controls accounting for sex, with regions of significantly reduced thickness color-coded according to significance (t-statistic, scale bottom-right), and overlaid onto an inflated surface background (light gray, gyri; dark gray, sulci). IC = insular; IP = inferior parietal; Li/F = lingual/fusiform; MT = mid-temporal; Or = orbital; PC = precentral; PH = parahippocampal gyrus; PO = parsopercularis; PT = parstriangularis; SF = superior frontal; SM = supramarginal gyrus; ST = superior temporal.

Cortical thickness

The VBM analysis of regional gray matter volume is a whole-brain procedure, and can be influenced by partial volume effects[2] at the boundaries. An alternative approach to assessing cortical gray matter atrophy is assessing the thickness of the cortex, with software such as FreeSurfer or caret [32, 33]. Using FreeSurfer (http://surfer.nmr.mgh.harvard.edu/), we found cortical changes in a group of OSA patients [34], which we present here. We studied 39 recently diagnosed, untreated, moderate to severe OSA (apnea-hypopnea index [AHI] mean ± sd 35.8 ± 3.0 events/hour; age 46.1 ± 1.4 years; female: male 7:32) and 64 healthy control (age 47.5 ± 1.1; female:male 23:41) subjects. No subjects had any history of major medical illness or psychiatric condition. We calculated and analyzed cortical thickness using the FreeSurfer processing pipeline, and performed surface-based analysis using ANCOVA to compare cortical thickness between OSA and control groups (threshold: t-statistic > 2.5), with sex and total intracranial volume (to account for differences in skull size) as covariates. The software segments gray and white matter regions from a T1-weighted MRI scan, based on intensity differences and a-priori templates of tissue distributions [35]. Surface meshes are derived defining the pial and gray–white boundaries, and thickness is calculated based on the distance between these surfaces. After smoothing (10 mm kernel), surface-based statistics were performed using a linear model. Decreased cortical thickness in OSA versus controls appeared in multiple regions (Figure 32.1). Cortical thinning in OSA patients appeared in regions involved with cognition, verbal expression, and autonomic regulation. Neuropsychological and physiological characteristics of OSA likely derive in part from impaired function in these damaged brain structures. These findings, together with previously shown axonal deficits and gray matter loss, demonstrate the injurious consequences of OSA on neural tissue.

---

[2] Partial volume effect refers to the brain regions represented by one voxel containing more than one type of tissue. This phenomenon occurs at gray matter–white matter and gray matter–cerebrospinal fluid boundaries.

Diffusion tensor imaging (DTI)

Diffusion tensor imaging (DTI) is an MRI procedure sensitive to changes in structure, especially myelin and axonal alterations [36, 37]; OSA patients show extensive structural alterations, as measured by that technique [2]. There are several measurements that can be derived from DTI data, and we earlier assessed fractional anisotropy (FA), an index of directionality of water diffusion which is high in healthy white matter tracts. Changes to this index may represent different forms of pathology, not just cell death or atrophy. This measurement was especially sensitive to changes in OSA patients. In our study of 41 newly diagnosed, untreated OSA patients and 69 control subjects [2], we found that the cingulum bundle extending into the prefrontal cortex was affected (Figure 32.2), which is consistent with the gray matter alterations seen in the anterior cingulate cortex. Another group found similar, preliminary findings of reduced FA in OSA [38].

FA, the measure we and others used to demonstrate differences in newly diagnosed, untreated OSA subjects [2, 38], is an indirect measure of brain injury that varies with structural integrity, specifically the parallel organization of cellular objects within neural tissue [36]. The index is high in large axonal tracks, but low in gray matter (and zero in cerebrospinal fluid). Reductions in FA appear in the presence of fiber injury, including demyelination, shrinkage, and cell death [39]. Other pathologies that lead to reduced FA include fluid accumulation due to microvascular disease or larger lesions. Since the changes in the present study are primarily reflected in FA but are not visible, much of the injury is likely axonal or myelin damage, with more limited cellular death. Additional measures such as specialized MRI procedures which can partition myelin from axonal injury (e.g., magnetization transfer imaging [40], axial and radial diffusivity [41], axial and radial kurtosis [42]) need to be implemented to further refine our understanding of the pathology, and will be useful in determining whether the injury developed from hypoxia and other accompaniments of OSA, or preexisted the condition.

Volume reduction in specific structures

Due to the limitations of whole-brain analyses, we studied certain specific structures by manually tracing them, and analyzing volumes only of those structures. Certain structures such as the hippocampus can also be assessed for shape variations by group using morphometric techniques.

Hippocampus

The hippocampus is the most-studied distinct structure in OSA, and studies consistently show reduced hippocampal volumes associated with the disorder [9, 28, 29, 31]. We have also found reduced volumes of the hippocampus in OSA [43], as detailed below. We manually traced the left and right hippocampi in seven OSA patients (mean age = 48 ± 8, AHI = 32 ± 8) and 23 control subjects (age 53 ± 5) (Figure 32.3). We found that the hippocampal volume was lower in the OSA group, with the greatest differences on the left (2114 ± 400 vs. 2494 ± 382 mm^3, p = 0.03 raw volume, p < 0.01 scaled to head size), with the right also showing lower volumes (2309 ± 392 vs. 2571 ± 363 mm^3, p = 0.1 raw volume, p < 0.01 scaled to head size). A regional assessment using morphometric procedures [44] demonstrated that these changes were bilateral in the superior mid-hippocampal area and medial mid-to-posterior regions, with anterior reductions only on the left (Figure 32.3). The findings of atrophy in the hippocampus are consistent with the reduced metabolite levels found in MRS studies [22, 23].

Mammillary bodies

The mammillary bodies are small structures at the base of the anterior fornix which are part of the hippocampal/thalamic limbic circuitry associated with memory formation, amongst other roles, and are critical to normal functioning. Based on a preliminary visual inspection of anatomical scans, we hypothesized that OSA patients have reduced mammillary body volumes. Since these structures are too small for assessment with VBM, we implemented a new approach to test our hypothesis, which involved over-sampling the scans in order to accurately trace regions of interest, and demonstrated reduced volume in the mammillary bodies in untreated OSA patients [45]. These findings raise the question of whether nutrition deficiencies, of thiamine in particular, are contributing to the neural changes, as seen in other conditions [46, 47].

Cingulum bundle

Our whole-brain analysis indicated reduced axonal integrity in the region of the cingulum, but the area of change was diffuse

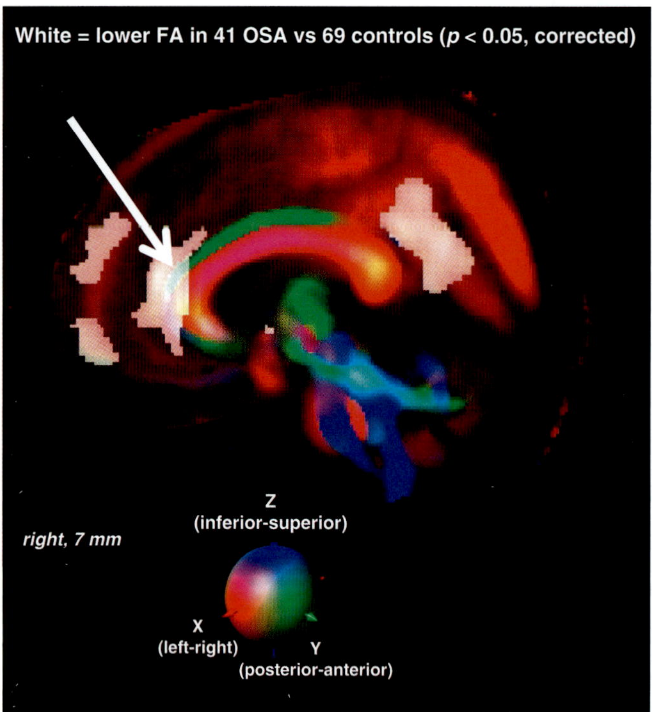

Figure 32.2 Reduced axonal integrity (lower FA) in OSA versus controls accounting for sex and age, with areas of significant difference shaded in white on a background illustrating the principal white matter tracks according to the key (bottom) [2]. The cingulum bundle shows reduced FA (arrow), and is colored green, with the underlying corpus callosum in red-orange. The background is the average of 110 subjects' spatially normalized images.

Table 32.1. Characteristics of the study population for comparison of brain injury in depressed versus non-depressed OSA subjects

	OSA		Control
	Depressed	Non-depressed	
N	11	15	38
BDI	18 ± 9 * †	5 ± 3 †	3 ± 3
Age (years)	50 ± 10	49 ± 8	49 ± 7
BMI (kg/m²)	30 ± 6 *	31 ± 3 *	24 ± 3
Handedness (left/both/right)	1/2/8	3/1/11	6/2/30
Gender (male/female)	5/6	3/12	14/24

Significant differences (p < 0.05): * vs. control; † OSA dep. vs. non-dep.
BMI = body mass index.

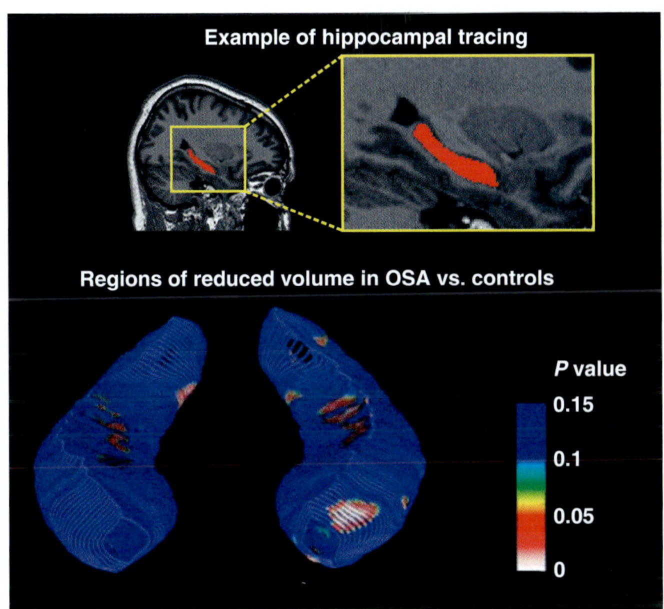

Figure 32.3 Top. Example of manually traced hippocampus on anatomical background. *Bottom*. Areas of reduced hippocampal volume in 7 OSA versus 23 control subjects, color-coded according to significance. The volume reductions were in the bilateral superior mid and medial mid-to-posterior hippocampus, with the left anterior hippocampus also showing atrophy.

across adjacent corpus callosum and cingulate cortex areas. We specifically assessed the cingulum bundle using fiber tracking based on DTI data, which allows anatomical localization of the cingulum, and quantification of size and other indices of structural integrity [48]. In a preliminary study, we found that OSA patients show reduced volume in the cingulum bundle [49]. This finding is consistent with the atrophy in anterior cingulate cortex and prefrontal regions, as well as altered structure throughout limbic regions.

Influences on OSA-related brain changes

Depression/anxiety symptoms

Psychological symptoms of depression and anxiety are associated with neural changes in non-OSA populations, so we hypothesized that the structural changes in OSA would be exacerbated in the presence of these symptoms. We found that both anxiety and depression in OSA are associated with indications of additional neural injury over that in the sleep disorder alone, most notably in limbic brain regions associated with these neuropsychological functions, including the insular cortex, anterior cingulate cortex, amygdala, and hippocampus [50, 51]. Additionally, thalamic, temporal, and brainstem areas were also affected.

We performed an additional study using DTI data looking at the differences in sites of injury in OSA patients with elevated depressive symptoms versus those with normal levels of such symptoms. From a sample of 26 moderate-to-severe OSA patients, 11 rated as "depressed" (elevated depressive symptoms as defined by a Beck Depression Inventory [BDI] > 9) and 15 as "non-depressed" (BDI < 9). We compared these against a group of 38 controls. Subject characteristics are shown in Table 32.1. We found that the depressed OSA subjects showed lower FA (reduced axonal integrity or myelin) in the sub-genu of the anterior cingulate cortex and in the posterior hippocampus, the two major areas associated with depression (Figure 32.4) [52, 53]. The non-depressed patients did not show such effects.

Male/female differences

The disorder is less prevalent in females than males, with women showing an incidence of OSA which is half or lower that found in men [54]. Furthermore, the characteristics of OSA differ between sexes [55]; women with OSA typically report different sleep-related complaints from males, and have a higher incidence of ankle edema and hypothyroidism [56]. However, male OSA patients typically present with more cardiovascular symptoms than females [57]. Other physiological differences appear in overnight blood pressure changes [58], upper airway muscle tone and arousal, and daytime fatigue [59–62]. Disease severity, as measured by apneic events per hour (AHI), tends to be lower in females, but women are symptomatic at lower AHI levels [55]. The incidence of certain neuropsychologic conditions, especially depression, is higher in women with OSA [56, 57, 63, 64]. The mechanisms underlying these differences are unknown, but may relate, in part, to

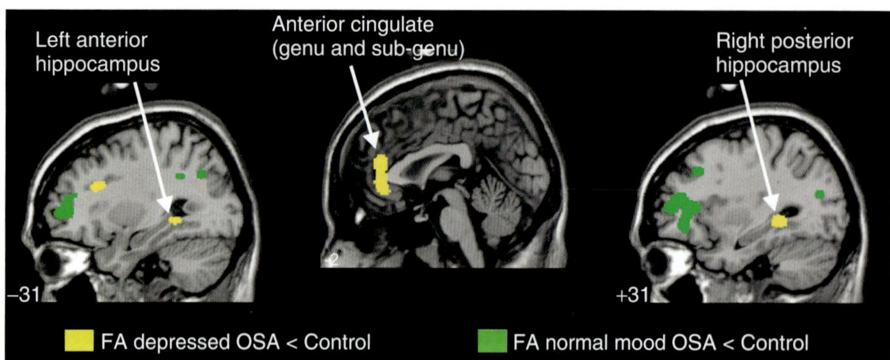

Figure 32.4 Areas of reduced FA (an indicator of axonal and myelin integrity) in depressed versus non-depressed OSA patients (see Table 32.1), highlighting the changes in depression-related regions.

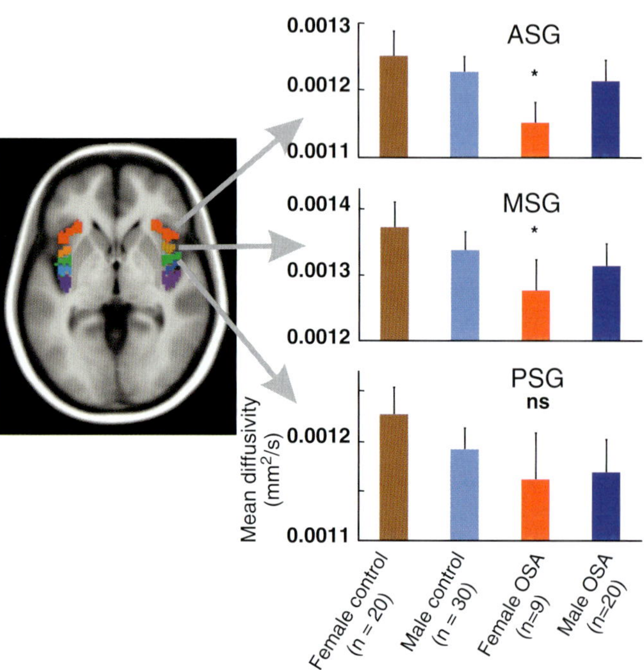

Figure 32.5 Altered structural integrity in OSA females relative to other groups in two right insular subregions (ASG = anterior short gyrus and MSG = mid short gyrus; p < 0.05, ANCOVA, age covariate). A third region (PSG = posterior short gyrus) showed no significant difference. The DTI index "mean diffusivity" shown here is sensitive to inflammatory conditions and cellular injury.

sex-based differences in brain function arising from differential injury of OSA-induced pathophysiology of brain tissue between genders [65].

We found a sex-by-OSA interaction on DTI measures including mean diffusivity, which is sensitive to various forms of neural injury, with OSA females showing lower values compared to all males and control females (Figure 32.5). The OSA males and females were matched for age and severity as measured with the AHI. The nature of the changes represented by these differences is unclear, but the findings emphasize the importance of considering sex differences in terms of impact of OSA on the brain.

Diabetes

In four diabetic OSA subjects, we found indications of much greater brain injury as compared with non-diabetic subjects

[66]. The affected brain areas include the mid and anterior cingulate cortices, together with adjacent corpus callosal regions. Other limbic areas affected were the insula and hippocampus. The measurement used was T2 relaxation time, which is sensitive to injury, especially cell death and vascular damage. The pilot study therefore suggests that the combination of diabetes and OSA may be especially harmful to the brain. However, this pilot study needs to be replicated in a larger sample to verify these findings.

Summary of affected brain regions

Many areas in the brain show structural impairments in OSA, including cortical, limbic, brainstem and cerebellar regions. Table 32.2 presents a synthesis of findings or OSA–control differences grouped by general brain area. Negative findings are not presented, and the findings should be considered liberal, as when other factors are accounted for, the OSA-specific differences sometimes become non-significant [9]. What is notable, however, is the consistency of differences appearing in certain regions, with limbic areas and in particular the hippocampus being especially affected. A common finding of impaired white matter by a variety of measures is also striking. An important point to note is that while white matter changes are usually interpreted as reflecting axonal and myelin alterations, glia are also very likely affected, and deserve further attention in future neuroimaging studies.

Summary

Numerous findings of brain structural changes in OSA give strong support to the notion that the disorder does cause brain injury. Animal studies of intermittent hypoxia support this interpretation. However, what remains unclear is the exact nature of these changes, including when they develop relative to disease progression. Neuroimaging methods give numerical measures that are associated with a variety of biological pathologies, and technical limitations due to scanning and analysis issues limit the interpretability of the data. A further critical confound is the influence on brain changes of co-occurring factors, including age, anxiety, BMI, depression, hypertension, sex, medication use, and other comorbidities, in addition to OSA-specific factors such as severity of occurrence and desaturation of apneas, and duration of

Table 32.2. Summary of published positive findings of affected brain structures in OSA. Note that some of these measures do not show a difference once covariates such as age, sex, BMI, and hypertension are controlled for (e.g., [9])

Area	Measure	Reference
Global		
Cortical gray matter volume	Volume (automatic segmentation)	[9]
White matter	White matter hyperintensities	[14, 15]
Surface cortical regions		
Frontal cortex	Regional gray matter concentration, VBM	[7]
	Regional gray matter volume, VBM	[1, 30]
Frontal white matter	Reduced FA	[2, 38]
	Metabolites	[20]
Lateral temporal cortex	Regional gray matter volume, VBM	[1, 8, 9, 30]
	Regional gray matter concentration, VBM	[7]
Parietal cortex	Regional gray matter concentration, VBM	[7]
	Regional gray matter volume, VBM	[1, 30]
	Reduced FA	[2]
	Metabolites	[5]
Parietal white matter	Reduced FA	[38]
	Metabolites (MRS)	[18, 19, 21]
Prefrontal cortex	Regional gray matter concentration, VBM	[7]
	Regional gray matter volume, VBM	[1, 30]
	Reduced FA	[2]
Temporal lobe white matter	Regional white matter volume, VBM	[9]
	Reduced FA	[2]
Ventral medial prefrontal/occipital cortex	Regional gray matter concentration, VBM	[7]
	Regional gray matter volume, VBM	[30]
	Reduced FA	[2]
Corpus callosum	Reduced FA	[2]
Limbic regions		
Amygdala	Regional gray matter concentration, VBM	[7]
Cingulate cortex, anterior	Regional gray matter concentration, VBM	[7]
	Regional gray matter volume, VBM	[1]
	Reduced FA	[2]
Cingulate cortex, mid	Regional gray matter concentration, VBM	[7]
Cingulate cortex, posterior	Reduced FA	[2]
Cingulum	Reduced FA	[2]
Fornix	Reduced FA	[2]
Hippocampus	Regional gray matter volume, VBM	[1, 9, 30]
	Regional gray matter concentration, VBM	[7]
	Volume (manual tracing)	[28, 29]
	Volume (automatic segmentation)	[9]
	Metabolites	[21–23]
Insula	Regional gray matter concentration, VBM	[7]
	Reduced FA	[2]
Mammillary bodies	Volume (manual tracing)	[45]
Parahippocampal gyrus	Regional gray matter volume, VBM	[1]
Basal ganglia		
Caudate	Volume (automatic segmentation)	[9]
	Regional gray matter concentration, VBM	[7]
Thalamus		
Dorsal/superior thalamus	Regional gray matter concentration, VBM	[7]
	Regional gray matter volume, VBM	[30]
	Reduced FA	[2]
Ventral thalamus	Reduced FA	[2]
Brainstem		
Ventral pons	Reduced FA	[2]
Cerebellar		
Deep nuclei	Reduced FA	[2]
Superior cerebellar cortex	Regional gray matter volume, VBM	[1, 8]
	Regional gray matter concentration, VBM	[7]
Interior cerebellar cortex	Regional gray matter volume, VBM	[0, 30]
	Regional gray matter concentration, VBM	[7]

disease. A need in the field is for carefully controlled, longitudinal studies (e.g., [21]), and multimodality measurements of brain structures to narrow down the underlying pathology. Simply put, we know that changes occur in the brain of people with OSA, but we do not know the causes, nature of pathology, or consequences of these changes, nor do we know how we should adapt treatment to account for central nervous system deficits.

Acknowledgements

This work was performed at the University of California at Los Angeles. No interventions were used in this study. Financial support was provided by the National Institutes of Health, HL-60296 (Ronald M. Harper) and NR-011230 (PMM). The author has no conflict of interest. The author thanks Dr. Ronald Harper for his support.

References

1. Macey PM, Henderson LA, Macey KE, *et al.* Brain morphology associated with obstructive sleep apnea. *Am J Respir Crit Care Med.* 2002;**166**(10):1382–7.

2. Macey PM, Kumar R, Woo MA, *et al.* Brain structural changes in obstructive sleep apnea. *Sleep.* 2008;**31**(7):967–77.

3. Henderson LA, Woo MA, Macey PM, *et al.* Neural responses during Valsalva maneuvers in obstructive sleep apnea syndrome. *J Appl Physiol.* 2003;**94**(3):1063–74.

4. Harper RM, Macey PM, Henderson LA, *et al.* fMRI responses to cold pressor challenges in control and obstructive sleep apnea subjects. *J Appl Physiol.* 2003;**94**(4):1583–95.

5. Tonon C, Vetrugno R, Lodi R, *et al.* Proton magnetic resonance spectroscopy study of brain metabolism in obstructive sleep apnoea syndrome before and after continuous positive airway pressure treatment. *Sleep.* 2007;**30**(3):305–11.

6. Canessa N, Castronovo V, Cappa SF, *et al.* Obstructive sleep apnea: brain structural changes and neurocognitive function before and after treatment. *Am J Respir Crit Care Med.* 2011;**183**(10):1419–26.

7. Joo EY, Tae WS, Lee MJ, *et al.* Reduced brain gray matter concentration in patients with obstructive sleep apnea syndrome. *Sleep.* 2010;**33**(2):235–41.

8. Morrell MJ, Jackson ML, Twigg GL, *et al.* Changes in brain morphology in patients with obstructive sleep apnoea. *Thorax.* 2010;**65**(10):908–14.

9. Torelli F, Moscufo N, Garreffa G, *et al.* Cognitive profile and brain morphological changes in obstructive sleep apnea. *Neuroimage.* 2011;**54**(2):787–93.

10. Ayalon L, Ancoli-Israel S, Klemfuss Z, Shalauta MD, Drummond SP. Increased brain activation during verbal learning in obstructive sleep apnea. *Neuroimage* 2006;**31**(4):1817–25.

11. Hentschel F, Schredl M, Dressing H. [Sleep apnea syndrome and cerebral lesions – a prospective MRI study]. *Fortschr Neurol Psychiatr* 1997;**65**(9):421–4.

12. Kapeller P, Schmidt R, Fazekas F. Qualitative MRI: evidence of usual aging in the brain. *Top Magn Reson Imaging.* 2004;**15**(6):343–7.

13. Aloia M, Arnedt J, Davis J, *et al.* MRI white matter hyperintensities in older adults with OSA. *Sleep.* 2001;**24**:A55.

14. Nishibayashi M, Miyamoto M, Miyamoto T, Suzuki K, Hirata K. Correlation between severity of obstructive sleep apnea and prevalence of silent cerebrovascular lesions. *J Clin Sleep Med.* 2008;**4**(3):242–7.

15. Minoguchi K, Yokoe T, Tazaki T, *et al.* Silent brain infarction and platelet activation in obstructive sleep apnea. *Am J Respir Crit Care Med.* 2007;**175**(6):612–17.

16. Davies CW, Crosby JH, Mullins RL, *et al.* Case control study of cerebrovascular damage defined by magnetic resonance imaging in patients with OSA and normal matched control subjects. *Sleep.* 2001;**24**(6):715–20.

17. Kiernan TE, Capampangan DJ, Hickey MG, Pearce LA, Aguilar MI. Sleep apnea and white matter disease in hypertensive patients: a case series. *Neurologist.* 2011;**17**(5):289–91.

18. Kamba M, Inoue Y, Higami S, *et al.* Cerebral metabolic impairment in patients with obstructive sleep apnoea: an independent association of obstructive sleep apnoea with white matter change. *J Neurol Neurosurg Psychiatry.* 2001;**71**(3):334–9.

19. Kamba M, Suto Y, Ohta Y, Inoue Y, Matsuda E. Cerebral metabolism in sleep apnea. Evaluation by magnetic resonance spectroscopy. *Am J Respir Crit Care Med.* 1997;**156**(1):296–8.

20. Alchanatis M, Deligiorgis N, Zias N, *et al.* Frontal brain lobe impairment in obstructive sleep apnoea: a proton MR spectroscopy study. *Eur Respir J.* 2004;**24**(6):980–6.

21. O'Donoghue FJ, Wellard RM, Rochford PD, *et al.* Magnetic resonance spectroscopy and neurocognitive dysfunction in obstructive sleep apnea before and after CPAP treatment. *Sleep.* 2012;**35**(1):41–8.

22. Bartlett DJ, Rae C, Thompson CH, *et al.* Hippocampal area metabolites relate to severity and cognitive function in obstructive sleep apnea. *Sleep Med.* 2004;**5**(6):593–6.

23. Halbower AC, Degaonkar M, Barker PB, *et al.* Childhood obstructive sleep apnea associates with neuropsychological deficits and neuronal brain injury. *PLoS Med.* 2006;**3**(8):e301.

24. Brown TR, Kincaid BM, Ugurbil K. NMR chemical shift imaging in three dimensions. *Proc Natl Acad Sci U S A.* 1982;**79**(11):3523–6.

25. Ashburner J, Friston KJ. Voxel-based morphometry – the methods. *Neuroimage.* 2000;**11**(6):805–21.

26. Macey PM, Harper RM. OSA brain morphology differences: magnitude of loss approximates age-related effects. *Am J Respir Crit Care Med.* 2005;**172**(8):1056–7; author reply 1057–8.

27. O'Donoghue FJ, Briellmann RS, Rochford PD, *et al.* Cerebral structural changes in severe obstructive sleep apnea. *Am J Respir Crit Care Med.* 2005;**171**(10):1185–90.

28. Thomas RJ, Rosen BR, Stern CE, Weiss JW, Kwong KK. Functional imaging of working memory in obstructive sleep-disordered breathing. *J Appl Physiol.* 2005;**98**(6):2226–34.

29. Morrell MJ, McRobbie DW, Quest RA, *et al.* Changes in brain morphology associated with obstructive sleep apnea. *Sleep Med.* 2003;**4**(5):451–4.

30. Yaouhi K, Bertran F, Clochon P, *et al.* A combined neuropsychological and brain imaging study of obstructive sleep apnea. *J Sleep Res.* 2009;**18**(1):36–48.

31. Canessa N, Castronovo V, Cappa SF, *et al.* Obstructive sleep apnea: brain structural changes and neurocognitive function before and after treatment. *Am J Respir Crit Care Med.* 2011;**183**(10):1419–26.

32. Fischl B, Sereno MI, Dale AM. Cortical surface-based analysis. II: Inflation, flattening, and a surface-based coordinate system. *Neuroimage.* 1999;**9**(2):195–207.

33. Van Essen DC. A Population-Average, Landmark- and Surface-based (PALS) atlas of human cerebral cortex. *Neuroimage.* 2005;**28**(3):635–62.

34. Macey PM, Kumar R, Woo MA, Harper RM. Reduced cortical thickness in obstructive sleep apnea patients. *Sleep.* 2009;**32**:A229.

35. Fischl B, Salat DH, Busa E, *et al.* Whole brain segmentation: automated labeling of neuroanatomical structures in the human brain. *Neuron.* 2002;**33**(3):341–55.

36. Le Bihan D, Mangin JF, Poupon C, *et al.* Diffusion tensor imaging: concepts and applications. *J Magn Reson Imaging.* 2001;**13**(4):534–46.

37. Kaufman JA, Ahrens ET, Laidlaw DH, Zhang S, Allman JM. Anatomical analysis of an aye-aye brain (*Daubentonia madagascariensis,* primates: Prosimii) combining histology, structural magnetic resonance imaging, and diffusion-tensor imaging. *Anat Rec A Discov Mol Cell Evol Biol.* 2005;**287**(1):1026–37.

38. Cappa S, Castronovo V, Scifo P, *et al.* Diffusion tensor imaging (DTI) in obstructive sleep apnea (OSA). *J Sleep Res.* 2008;**17**(Suppl 1):43.

39. Mac Donald CL, Dikranian K, Song SK, *et al.* Detection of traumatic axonal injury with diffusion tensor imaging in a mouse model of traumatic brain injury. *Exp Neurol.* 2007;**205**(1):116–31.

40. Koenig SH. Cholesterol of myelin is the determinant of gray-white contrast in MRI of brain. *Magn Reson in Med.* 1991;**20**(2):285–91.

41. Song SK, Sun SW, Ramsbottom MJ, *et al.* Dysmyelination revealed through MRI as increased radial (but unchanged axial) diffusion of water. *Neuroimage.* 2002;**17**(3):1429–36.

42. Poot DH, den Dekker AJ, Achten E, Verhoye M, Sijbers J. Optimal experimental design for diffusion kurtosis imaging. *IEEE Trans Med Imaging.* 2010;**29**(3):819–29.

43. Macey PM, Moiyadi AS, Kumar R, Woo MA, Harper RM. Reduced hippocampal volume in patients with obstructive sleep apnea. *Society for Neuroscience 2008 Abstracts.* 2008.

44. Thompson PM, Hayashi KM, de Zubicaray GI, *et al.* Mapping hippocampal and ventricular change in Alzheimer disease. *Neuroimage.* 2004;**22**(4):1754–66.

45. Kumar R, Birrer BV, Macey PM, *et al.* Reduced mammillary body volume in patients with obstructive sleep apnea. *Neurosci Lett.* 2008;**438**(3):330–4.

46. Harper C. The neuropathology of alcohol-related brain damage. *Alcohol Alcohol.* 2009;**44**(2):136–40.

47. Sullivan EV, Pfefferbaum A. Neuroimaging of the Wernicke-Korsakoff syndrome. *Alcohol Alcohol.* 2009;**44**(2):155–65.

48. Wang R, Benner T, Sorensen AG, Wedeen VJ. Diffusion Toolkit: a software package for diffusion imaging data processing and tractography. *Proc Intl Soc Mag Reson Med.* 2007;**15**:3720.

49. Richardson HL, Kumar R, Macey PM, *et al.* Cingulum bundle axonal integrity in obstructive sleep apnea. *Society for Neuroscience 2011 Abstract Viewer/Itineray Planner.* 2011.

50. Kumar R, Macey PM, Cross RL, *et al.* Neural alterations associated with anxiety symptoms in obstructive sleep apnea syndrome. *Depress Anxiety.* 2009;**26**(5):480–91.

51. Cross RL, Kumar R, Macey PM, *et al.* Neural alterations and depressive symptoms in obstructive sleep apnea patients. *Sleep.* 2008;**31**(8):1103–9.

52. Drevets WC, Price JL, Simpson JR, Jr., *et al.* Subgenual prefrontal cortex abnormalities in mood disorders. *Nature.* 1997;**386**(6627):824–7.

53. Neumeister A, Wood S, Bonne O, *et al.* Reduced hippocampal volume in unmedicated, remitted patients with major depression versus control subjects. *Biol Psychiatry.* 2005;**57**(8):935–7.

54. Young T, Evans L, Finn L, Palta M. Estimation of the clinically diagnosed proportion of sleep apnea syndrome in middle-aged men and women. *Sleep.* 1997;**20**(9):705–6.

55. Young T, Hutton R, Finn L, Badr S, Palta M. The gender bias in sleep apnea diagnosis. Are women missed because they have different symptoms? *Arch Intern Med.* 1996;**156**(21):2445–51.

56. Shepertycky MR, Banno K, Kryger MH. Differences between men and women in the clinical presentation of patients diagnosed with obstructive sleep apnea syndrome. *Sleep.* 2005;**28**(3):309–14.

57. Smith R, Ronald J, Delaive K, *et al.* What are obstructive sleep apnea patients being treated for prior to this diagnosis? *Chest.* 2002;**121**(1):164–72.

58. Lavie-Nevo K, Pillar G. Evening-morning differences in blood pressure in sleep apnea syndrome: effect of gender. *Am J Hypertens.* 2006;**19**(10):1064–9.

59. Jordan AS, McEvoy RD. Gender differences in sleep apnea: epidemiology, clinical presentation and pathogenic mechanisms. *Sleep Med Rev.* 2003;**7**(5):377–89.

60. Jordan AS, Wellman A, Edwards JK, *et al.* Respiratory control stability and upper airway collapsibility in men and women with obstructive sleep apnea. *J Appl Physiol.* 2005;**99**(5):2020–7.

61. Mohsenin V. Effects of gender on upper airway collapsibility and severity of obstructive sleep apnea. *Sleep Med.* 2003;**4**(6):523–9.

62. Pillar G, Lavie P. Psychiatric symptoms in sleep apnea syndrome: effects of gender and respiratory disturbance index. *Chest.* 1998;**114**(3):697–703.

63. Greenberg-Dotan S, Reuveni H, Simon-Tuval T, Oksenberg A, Tarasiuk A. Gender differences in morbidity and health care utilization among adult obstructive sleep apnea patients. *Sleep.* 2007;**30**(9):1173–80.

64. Quintana-Gallego E, Carmona-Bernal C, Capote F, *et al.* Gender differences in obstructive sleep apnea syndrome: a clinical study of 1166 patients *Respir Med.* 2004;**98**(10):984–9.

65. Hsu JL, Leemans A, Bai CH, *et al.* Gender differences and age-related white matter changes of the human brain: a diffusion tensor imaging study. *Neuroimage.* 2008;**39**(2):566–77.

66. Harper RM, Macey PM, Kumar R, Woo MA. Neural injury in diabetic versus non-diabetic obstructive sleep apnea patients: a pilot study. *Sleep.* 2009;**32**:A341.

Imaging the airway in obstructive sleep apnea

Joseph T. Daley and Richard J. Schwab

Introduction

Obstructive sleep apnea (OSA) is a common condition with significant morbidity and mortality. However, the pathogenesis of this condition remains incompletely understood. Imaging of the upper airway in subjects with and without OSA, during wake and sleep, has led to major advances in our knowledge of how upper airway anatomy and airway dynamics contribute to this disease. This chapter will focus on upper airway imaging and examine risk factors for OSA (both static and dynamic), and which of these anatomical factors are changed when successful treatment modalities are applied.

To discuss airway imaging, it is first necessary to establish the anatomical components and boundaries of the important upper airway regions. The upper airway, which extends from the nares to the larynx, can be divided into four anatomical regions: the nasopharynx, the retropalatal oropharynx, the retroglossal oropharynx, and the hypopharynx. The nasopharynx is defined as the region from the nasal turbinates to the hard palate. The retropalatal oropharynx begins at the hard palate, and has its inferior margin defined by the caudal margin of the uvula and soft palate. The retroglossal oropharynx extends from that point to the base of the epiglottis. The remaining portion of the pharynx from the base of the tongue to the larynx comprises the hypopharynx. Since the main sites of airway closure in OSA have been identified in the retropalatal and retroglossal oropharynx [1–3], the boundaries of these structures will be considered in greater detail.

The anterior oropharyngeal wall is formed mainly by the soft palate, tongue, and epiglottis. The posterior wall is bounded by the superior, middle, and inferior pharyngeal constrictor muscles, which lie anterior to the cervical spine. The lateral walls are complex structures that contain muscles (hyoglossus, styloglossus, stylohyoid, stylopharyngeus, palatoglossus, palatopharyngeus, and the pharyngeal constrictors), lymphoid tissue and the parapharyngeal fat pads. The lateral wall tissue is bounded by the parapharyngeal fat pads in the retropalatal region and by the mandibular rami in the retroglossal region [4–6]. Among these anatomical regions, no single critical area has been implicated in the pathogenesis of OSA. More likely, a combination of craniofacial and soft tissue variations in these upper airway regions converge in the individual patient to produce OSA pathology.

Studies of airway behavior during wake and sleep have used many modalities: endoscopy, cephalometry, and various modes of computed tomography (CT). Each of these upper airway imaging modalities has drawbacks. Endoscopy is invasive, requires local sedation, and can only simulate the conditions of apnea with manipulations such as the Mueller maneuver [7]. Cephalometry provides only 2-dimensional, static measurements. While CT is capable of volumetric and dynamic imaging, there are limitations in its ability to distinguish soft tissue structures (i.e., fat deposition), which may make it difficult to determine the role fat plays in the pathogenesis of OSA. In addition, the exposure to radiation, particularly over multiple scans, is problematic.

Magnetic resonance imaging (MRI) may be the best imaging modality for assessment of the upper airway and surrounding soft tissue and craniofacial structures. Advantages of MRI include that it can obtain high-resolution images of the upper airway and soft tissue in the axial, sagittal, and coronal planes. These data permit volumetric analysis, including 3-dimensional reconstruction of the upper airway and surrounding structures. MR images provide precise, accurate, and volumetric measurements of the upper airway and surrounding tissue (see Figure 33.1). In addition, MRI avoids radiation exposure, allowing for repeat measurements in subjects over time, which permits the capability of state-dependent imaging. However, there are limitations to MRI, including the inability to perform scans on morbidly obese or claustrophobia patients and those with metallic implants. Also, MRI is expensive and the noise of the machine may prevent or interrupt sleep. The advent of ultrafast MRI techniques has provided multiple images at multiple sites with sufficient image quality and temporal resolution to allow a dynamic assessment of the pharyngeal musculature. Recent work has reported attempted performance of MRI during natural sleep [8].

Structural and dynamic airway changes in normal breathing, sleep, and OSA

Examination of the airway during respiration provides insights into the dynamic behavior of the upper airway. Changes in the airway dimensions during respiration have been well characterized [30]. In inspiration upper airway area is relatively

Neuroimaging of Sleep and Sleep Disorders, ed. Eric Nofzinger, Pierre Maquet, and Michael J. Thorpy. Published by Cambridge University Press. © Cambridge University Press 2013.

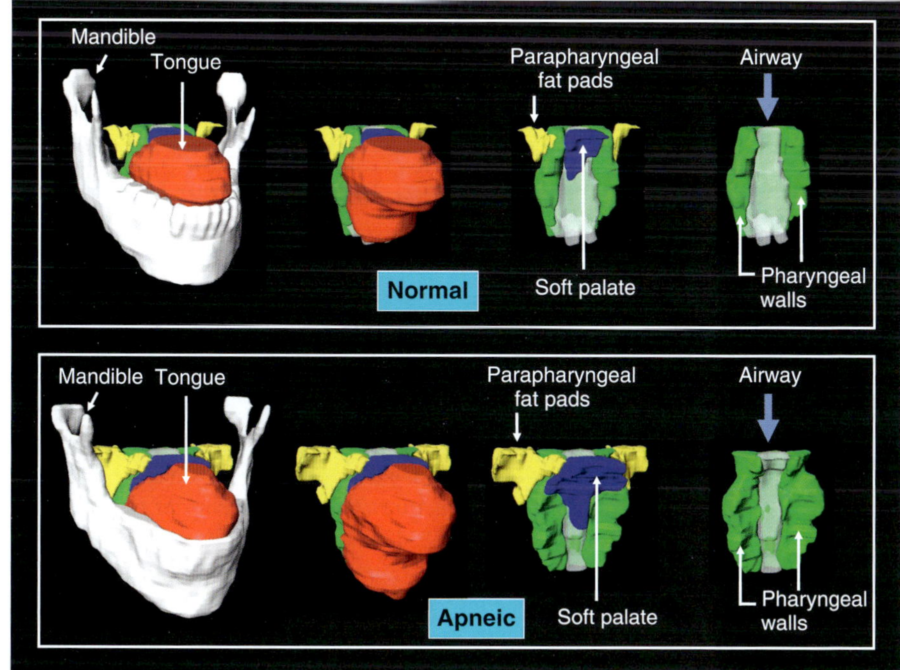

Figure 33.1 Volumetric reconstruction of axial MR images in a normal subject and a patient with sleep apnea. The mandible is depicted in white, the tongue in red, the soft palate in blue, the lateral parapharyngeal fat pads in yellow, and the lateral/posterior pharyngeal walls in green. The airway is depicted in gray/white. The normal subject has a larger airway than the patient with sleep apnea. The volume of the tongue, soft palate, parapharyngeal fat pads, and lateral pharyngeal walls of the patient with sleep apnea are all larger than in the normal subject.

constant, inferring a balance between airway dilator muscle activity and negative intraluminal pressure. During early expiration, increased intrathoracic pressure leads to maximal airway enlargement. Finally, in late expiration there is significant reduction in airway caliber to its smallest dimensions at end-expiration. These findings have also been replicated in patients with OSA [9]. Thus, the greatest susceptibility for airway collapse or narrowing is at the end of expiration or during inspiration. In addition, the respiratory-related changes in upper airway caliber demonstrated in CT studies [10, 11] were predominantly in the lateral dimension, suggesting that the lateral walls have an important role in modulating dynamic airway caliber. A study utilizing cine MRI also demonstrated an inverse relationship between airway caliber and the size of the lateral pharyngeal walls during normal respiration [12, 13]. The lateral pharyngeal walls remained relatively unchanged during inspiration, thinned in early expiration, and thickened towards the end of expiration. Thus, the lateral walls are likely to play an important role in mediating dynamic changes in upper airway area during respiration in patients with OSA.

Data from several studies have also shown that the airway can be characterized as a Starling resistor, where the balance of forces at one point along the tube may lead to local collapse, once the intraluminal pressure decreases below the surrounding tissue pressure [14, 15]. In order to further understand airway collapse MRI has been performed during sleeping and wake states in normal subjects [16]. The narrowest portion of the airway in sleeping subjects was in the retropalatal region. Retropalatal airway volume during sleep was reduced by 19%, while retroglossal airway volume was not significantly reduced [16]. In addition to confirming the regional collapsibility, this study identified the specific structures that directly reduced airway volume during sleep. Retropalatal airway narrowing was seen in both the

anterior-posterior and lateral dimensions. The decrease in anterior-posterior diameter was primarily due to posterior movement of the soft palate, while the lateral narrowing was mediated through thickening of the lateral pharyngeal walls.

The precise regions of airway compromise in OSA during wakefulness have been examined with various imaging techniques. The earliest studies observed that individuals with sleep apnea had decreased upper airway cross-sectional areas compared with controls, across all three major regions of the upper airway (naso-, oro-, and hypopharynx) using CT [17]. These findings have been replicated repeatedly using both CT and MRI [2, 6, 10, 11, 18–35], and have shown decreased airway cross-sectional area during wakefulness, regardless whether subjects were obese. Furthermore, using MRI, Cosentini and colleagues have demonstrated that minimal cross-sectional area of the airway correlates with apnea severity in a relatively linear fashion [33].

This decrease in upper airway cross-sectional area can be attributed to changes in configuration of the oropharynx in OSA. In normal patients, the airway is generally elliptical, with its widest diameter in the lateral dimension. In those with sleep apnea, the airway is generally narrowed laterally with its major axis shifted to the anterior-posterior plane [30, 32]. This lateral narrowing suggests that structures comprising the lateral walls of the airway are key in determining airway size and shape [6].

It is apparent that factors which influence the reduction in airway dimensions in OSA patients include both excessive soft tissue and altered bony structures. Craniofacial features which contribute to apnea severity include a small, posteriorly placed mandible (retro- or micrognathia), retroposition of the maxilla, and an inferiorly displaced hyoid [25, 36–44]. These structures may not be independent of one another, as one MRI study has shown that a large tongue volume may account for the differences seen with hyoid position [45]. Three-dimensional MR reconstructions have also been utilized to demonstrate soft tissue abnormalities in OSA patients, including increases in the volume of the tongue, soft palate, lateral parapharyngeal fat pads, and both the lateral and posterior pharyngeal walls (see Figure 33.1] [46]. Greater volume of the lateral pharyngeal walls, tongue, and total soft tissue correlates to increased likelihood of developing OSA. Although the lateral parapharyngeal fat pads are larger in OSA patients than controls [1, 30], they do not necessarily encroach on the airway lumen [6]. In addition, enlargement of the lateral peritonsillar walls has been shown to be a significant risk factor for the development of OSA (odds ratio 2.4), independent of body mass index (BMI) and neck circumference [47]. Other studies employing CT imaging have shown posterior displacement of the soft palate and tongue, in addition to lateral displacement of the pharyngeal walls, contributing to airway obstruction [23]. Finally, retropalatal airway closure in both normals and patients with OSA has been demonstrated during sleep utilizing sagittal ultrafast MRI [3].

Airway length is another important anatomical variable influencing airway collapsibility, as this may augment the chance of upper airway collapse by lengthening the "at-risk" portion of the airway. Using MRI and finite element analysis modeling, it has been shown that normal men have significantly increased pharyngeal airway length, greater soft palate cross-sectional area, and increased pharyngeal volume compared to females [48]. As a result of these factors, the male airway is more collapsible at any given negative airway pressure than the female airway [48].

Imaging findings underlying risk factors and exacerbators of OSA

Obesity

Obesity and increased neck circumference are the most studied contributors to OSA. Overall upper airway fat deposition appears to play a role in OSA. A strong correlation between apnea severity and the amount of fat encompassed between the mandibular rami has been described [29]. This overall fat deposition may exert its effects on the upper airway by increasing the surrounding tissue pressure, causing it to exceed the intraluminal pressure, leading to local collapse. Emerging data from imaging studies support the notion that regional adiposity of various structures in the upper airway has selective effects on airway dynamics and the risk of OSA. Greater adipose tissue deposition around the upper airway has been described in obese patients with sleep apnea [1, 6, 23, 29, 30, 49], even when compared with controls with the same BMI, neck circumference, and age [49]. This added fat mass may augment upper airway collapsibility either by directly decreasing airway cross-sectional area, or by providing an additional load to the posterior pharynx [50]. These imaging findings have been partially confirmed in studies directly examining tissue samples. The investigation of histological samples from patients who underwent soft palate resection

showed that patients with OSA had increased fat in the uvula and increased muscle tissue, when compared with those without OSA [51, 52]. Also, a recent post-mortem study demonstrated that the tongue has a high percentage of fat and that tongue weight and percentage of tongue fat are positively correlated with increasing obesity [53]. Apnea was not examined in this study, but these data suggest that tongue fat deposition and accumulation may be a physiological mechanism linking obesity and sleep apnea, particularly given the observation that increased tongue size is a risk factor for OSA.

Gender

Using a variety of imaging modalities, several studies have investigated gender-related anatomical upper airway differences. Women have a smaller upper airway, smaller neck size, smaller soft tissue structures/volume, and shorter upper airway length than men [20, 38, 48, 54–57]. As mentioned earlier, men have a longer upper airway, which appears to predispose it to collapse [48]. Gender differences in OSA may also be related to hormonal differences. Postmenopausal women have a higher prevalence of OSA compared to premenopausal women and postmenopausal women receiving hormone replacement therapy [58]. However, more research exploring gender differences in OSA pathogenesis is needed, particularly the specific role that hormones may play.

Age

Older patients with OSA tend to have more severe disease, suggesting that with age, changes occur within the airway predisposing it to regional collapse [59]. Potential mechanisms underlying these changes have been investigated using MRI. In a study of 38 elderly individuals, Malhotra and colleagues examined airway dimensions and physiological determinants of airway patency. Older patients had increased parapharyngeal fat pad size, even after correcting for BMI, and had posterior mandibles. In addition, older male subjects had diminished genioglossus muscle responses to negative pressure challenges, an activity which typically opposes collapse. Contrary to findings in younger women, elderly women had greater pharyngeal airway length, thus potentially predisposing older women to collapse on the basis of their airway configuration [60].

Upper airway edema

Edema may be an important contributor to enlargement of upper airway soft tissue structures in OSA. This may be especially critical in the soft palate, which experiences repetitive vibratory and negative pressure-related trauma during respiratory events. Research using MRI and quantitative magnetic resonance mapping examined T2 relaxation times of the lingual musculature in patients with sleep apnea and controls [61]. The T2 relaxation time is a physical property that varies with changes in tissue fluid content: short T2 relaxation times are typically associated with fibrosis while long T2 relaxation times are associated with tissue edema or increased fat content. Mean T2 relaxation times of lingual muscles in patients with OSA were significantly longer than those of the control group, suggesting the presence of increased edema or increased fat content of the tongue muscles in patients with OSA. Edema within the uvula in apneic patients has also been demonstrated histologically [62]. In addition to edema related to local trauma, recent studies postulate that large-scale fluid shifts occur from the legs to the neck when patients assume a recumbent position. This may have clinical significance in OSA, particularly in fluid-retaining states such as renal failure and congestive heart failure [63].

Body position

Body position changes also have an impact on the position of structures in the retropalatal region and clearly play a role in airway compromise in sleep apnea. The oropharynx is more susceptible to narrowing in the supine position. When measured using cephalometry, the oropharynx is significantly narrower in the supine position as opposed to when patients are upright, while the nasopharynx or hypopharynx show no significant change in diameter [64]. In addition, the soft palate and tongue are significantly thicker and the tongue becomes shorter in the supine position [64].

Genetics

OSA is known to have a significant familial component. Volumetric MRI has been employed to investigate whether or not oropharyngeal soft tissue structures segregate in a familial fashion [46]. These data demonstrated heritability for the size of tongue, lateral walls, and total soft tissue independent of obesity, craniofacial size, age, gender, and ethnicity. Further, it was demonstrated that the increased volume of the soft palate and lateral pharyngeal walls, and total soft tissue volume were associated with increased likelihood of having a sibling with OSA, after adjusting for potential confounders, including gender, age, ethnicity, craniofacial size, and visceral neck fat. These data suggest that heritable features of the upper airway soft tissue anatomy may underlie the genetic basis of OSA.

Taken together, these data implicate that changes in airway conformation and the size of structures surrounding the oropharynx are important identifiable risk factors for the development of OSA. As will be discussed below, interventions which successfully improve sleep disordered breathing often have positive impacts on these same factors, which may contribute to the reduction in airway collapsibility.

Imaging of treatment modalities and interventions to improve OSA

Continuous positive airway pressure (CPAP)

Several imaging modalities have been used to investigate the mechanism by which CPAP improves airway obstruction. Studies with CT and MRI have demonstrated increases in

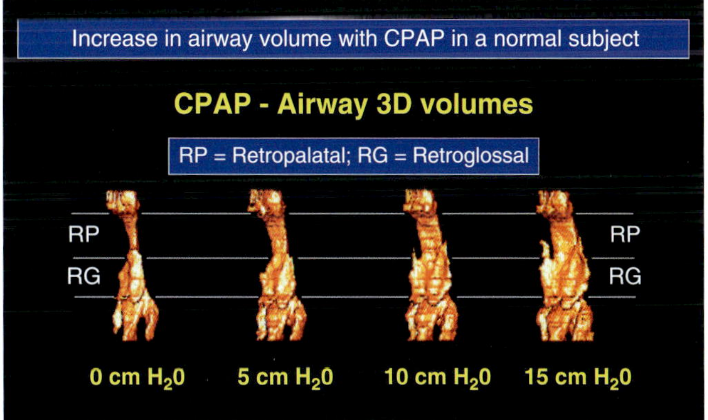

Figure 33.2 Volumetric reconstruction of axial MR images of the upper airway in a normal subject with progressively greater continuous positive airway pressure (CPAP) (0 to 15 cm H_2O) settings. The volume of the upper airway increases significantly in both the retropalatal (RP) and retroglossal (RG) regions with higher levels of CPAP. Note airway volume increases in the lateral dimension.

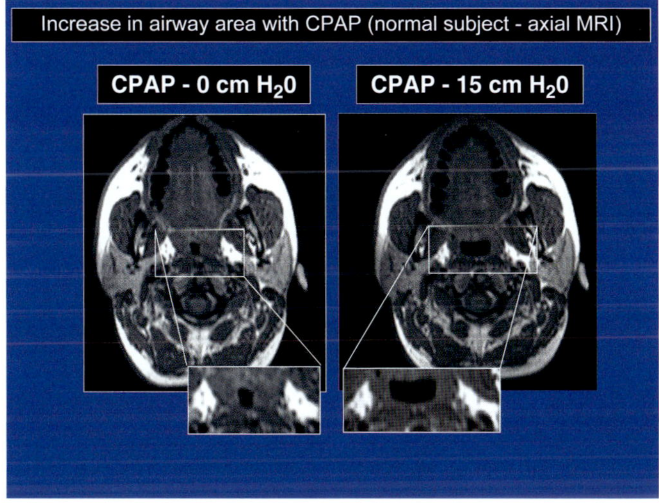

Figure 33.3 Comparison of axial retropalatal MR images in a normal subject at baseline and with continuous positive airway pressure (CPAP) at 15 cm H_2O. The retropalatal airway area is significantly greater at 15 cm H_2O than without CPAP. The enlargement in the retropalatal airway with CPAP is predominantly in the lateral dimension.

upper airway caliber during wakefulness with CPAP in subjects with and without OSA [2, 24, 65–67]. CPAP primarily increases the size of the upper airway in the lateral dimension (see Figures 33.2–33.4). Using CT, CPAP administration in both apneics and controls resulted in increases in total airway volume and lateral airway size [24]. There was a linear increase in airway cross-sectional area as "dosage" of CPAP was increased from 0 to 15 cm of water [24]. MRI studies, which are better able to describe soft tissue changes, have shown that the lateral pharyngeal walls also become compressed and thinner with increasing CPAP (see Figure 33.4) [2].

Weight loss

The significance of regional adiposity on the airway as described in the baseline state above is emphasized further

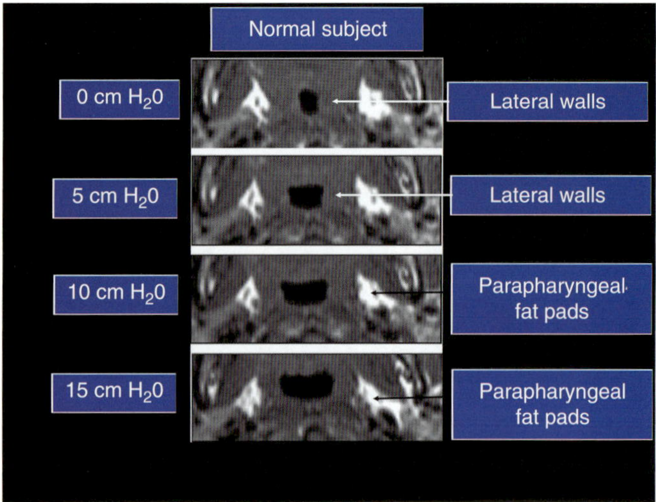

Figure 33.4 Comparison of axial retropalatal MR images in a normal subject (the same subject as in Figure 33.3) at baseline and with progressive increases in continuous positive airway pressure (CPAP) up to 15 cm H$_2$O. Increases in CPAP results in progressive thinning of the lateral pharyngeal walls but the parapharyngeal fat pads are not displaced. The increase in airway caliber with higher levels of CPAP is primarily in the lateral dimension; the anterior-posterior dimension of the airway does not increase significantly with CPAP.

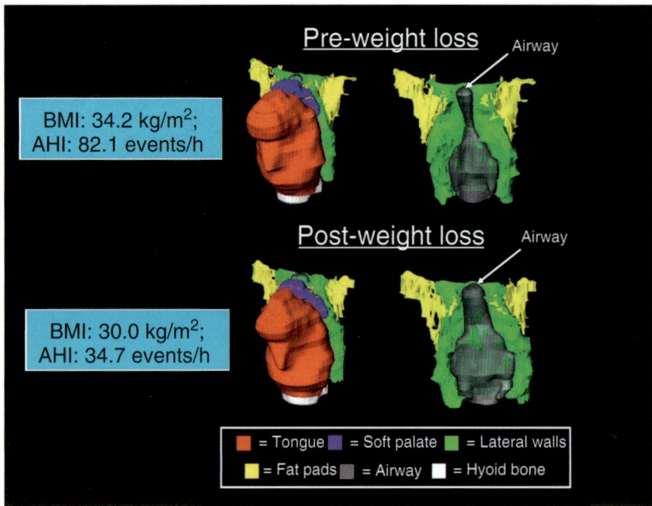

Figure 33.5 Volumetric reconstruction of axial MR images of the upper airway and surrounding soft tissue structures in a 50-year-old male before and after weight loss. The MR scans were performed five months apart: pre-weight loss (BMI: 34.2 kg/m^2; apnea-hypopnea index (AHI): 82.1 events/h) and post-weight loss (BMI: 30.3 kg/m^2; AHI: 34.7 events/h). The volume of the tongue, soft palate, parapharyngeal fat pads, and lateral walls all decreased with weight loss but the volume of the airway increased with weight loss. Percent differences in volume: tongue: (−8.7%); soft palate: (−7.4%); parapharyngeal fat pads: (−38.0%); pharyngeal lateral walls: (−4.5%); airway volume: (+35.0%).

by studies that have examined the effect of weight loss on airway caliber. Weight reduction in obese men with OSA increases the airway cross-sectional area [68] and decreases airway collapsibility [27] (see Figure 33.5). Similarly, weight loss in women has been shown to increase upper airway luminal volume, with a concomitant reduction in lateral pharyngeal wall and fat pad volume, as demonstrated by three-dimensional MRI [69].

Oral appliances

Oral appliances have been shown to increase posterior airway space [70, 71], airway cross-sectional area [72–74], and airway volume [75]. However, each of these changes may be device specific and the exact mechanism by which each device increases airway caliber remains elusive. While some investigators report increased retroglossal anterior-posterior airway diameter with oral appliances [71, 76], others have noted increases in the lateral dimension of the airway within the retropalatal region [70, 77]. Studies have confirmed that changes in the retropalatal and lateral dimensions with oral appliances are important in increasing airway caliber [77, 78]. Using volumetric MRI, Sutherland and coworkers [79] showed that two different types of oral appliances, the mandibular advancement splint and the tongue stabilizing device, shifted the parapharyngeal fat pads away from the airway. The mandibular advancement splint anteriorly displaced the muscles at the base of the tongue, while the tongue stabilizing device achieved a larger airway through anterior tongue displacement and an increase in lateral pharyngeal diameter. In addition, further analysis of the data from the tongue stabilizing device demonstrated that a greater increase in luminal volume with the oral appliance in place was associated with therapeutic effectiveness [79]. Further imaging studies with and without oral appliances may allow us to understand the complicated biomechanical interactions between the mandible, tongue, soft palate, and lateral walls when using these appliances. Such information may prove valuable in predicting which OSA patients will benefit most from oral appliances [78].

Surgery

Several surgical techniques have been developed with the intent of correcting the soft tissue and craniofacial abnormalities that predispose to OSA. Surgical techniques include uvulopalatopharyngoplasty (UPPP), uvulopalatopharyngoglossoplasty (UPPGP), transpalatal advancement pharyngoplasty (TPAP), sliding genioplasty or genioglossus advancement, hyoid advancement, maxillary-mandibular advancement, and many office-based procedures [80]. Given the complexity of OSA pathogenesis and the inter-individual variation in upper airway anatomy, selecting the appropriate procedure based on patient-specific factors is important. Nonetheless this is often difficult to achieve. No significant differences in upper airway dimensions were found for hyoid suspension surgery when comparing the patients before and after the procedure [81]. Cephalometry has not been shown to be useful in predicting outcome in nasal surgery for OSA [82]. Other studies have had inconsistent results in determining which patients are likely to respond to various surgical techniques, including UPPP [83, 84]. Despite their inconsistent results, these studies highlight a growing awareness of the need to evaluate patients preoperatively to help choose the appropriate procedure with the greatest likelihood of success.

One such procedure to examine the region of upper airway collapse in patients undergoing sleep apnea surgery is drug-induced sleep endoscopy. During drug-induced sleep endoscopy the airway is observed under pharmacologically (propofol) induced sleep. Drug-induced sleep endoscopy has been shown to identify patterns of upper airway obstruction in patients with OSA [85]. A recent review of the literature in patients undergoing drug-induced sleep endoscopy indicated that collapse occurs in different upper airway regions including the velopharynx, oropharynx, tongue base, and epiglottis and a multilevel collapse was often observed [86]. This suggests that regionally targeted surgical strategies could leave a patient with areas of residual collapse, and thus continued apnea. Moreover, evaluations of a particular surgical technique, or head-to-head comparisons, are difficult to perform because of the wide variety of surgical procedures and individual variation in the site of upper airway compromise. In addition to, or in conjunction with, structural measurements, computational modeling of the upper airway [87] may prove useful in predicting the response that a specific patient may have to different surgical interventions.

Conclusion

Over the previous several decades, imaging of the upper airway has successfully identified anatomical and physiological domains that underlie the pathogenesis of OSA. Imaging studies have identified clinical risk factors for OSA, including those related to obesity, age, gender, and genetics. Studies have shown that upper airway structure and function are important in the pathogenesis of OSA. Upper airway imaging has also begun to delineate the mechanisms of the different classes of therapies for OSA. We are beginning to identify the complex biomechanical interactions which occur between the anatomical factors that ultimately increase airway collapsibility and produce the pathological state. Routine imaging of the soft tissue and craniofacial structures of the head and neck are not a part of current clinical care. However, imaging can be used to classify patients for the purpose of targeting treatment modalities in order to enhance the success in treating sleep disordered breathing especially in patients undergoing upper airway surgery.

References

1. Horner RL, Mohiaddin RH, Lowell DG, *et al.* Sites and sizes of fat deposits around the pharynx in obese patients with obstructive sleep apnoea and weight matched controls. *Eur Respir J.* 1989;**2**:613–22.

2. Schwab RJ, Pack AI, Gupta KB, *et al.* Upper airway and soft tissue structural changes induced by cpap in normal subjects. *Am J Respir Crit Care Med.* 1996;**154**:1106–16.

3. Suto Y, Matsuo T, Kato T, *et al.* Evaluation of the pharyngeal airway in patients with sleep apnea: Value of ultrafast MR imaging. *AJR Am J Roentgenol.* 1993;**160**:311–14.

4. Kuna ST, Smickley JS, Vanoye CR. Respiratory-related pharyngeal constrictor muscle activity in normal human adults. *Am J Respir Crit Care Med.* 1997;**155**:1991–9.

5. Schwab RJ. Radiographic imaging in the diagnostic evaluation of sleep apnea. In: Weinberger SE, ed. *Uptodate (43) in Pulmonary and Critical Care Medicine;* 1996.

6. Schwab RJ, Gupta KB, Gefter WB, *et al.* Upper airway and soft tissue anatomy in normal subjects and patients with sleep-disordered breathing. Significance of the lateral pharyngeal walls. *Am J Respir Crit Care Med.* 1995;**152**:1673–89.

7. Ritter CT, Trudo FJ, Goldberg AN, *et al.* Quantitative evaluation of the upper airway during nasopharyngoscopy with the muller maneuver. *Laryngoscope.* 1999;**109**:954–63.

8. Barrera JE. Sleep magnetic resonance imaging: dynamic characteristics of the airway during sleep in obstructive sleep apnea syndrome. *Laryngoscope.* 2011;**121**:1327–35.

9. Yucel A, Unlu M, Haktanir A, Acar M, Fidan F. Evaluation of the upper airway cross-sectional area changes in different degrees of severity of obstructive sleep apnea syndrome: cephalometric and dynamic CT study. *AJNR Am J Neuroradiol.* 2005;**26**:2624–9.

10. Schwab RJ, Gefter WB, Hoffman EA, Gupta KB, Pack AI. Dynamic upper airway imaging during awake respiration in normal subjects and patients with sleep disordered breathing. *Am Rev Respir Dis.* 1993;**148**:1385–400.

11. Schwab RJ, Gefter WB, Pack AI, Hoffman EA. Dynamic imaging of the upper airway during respiration in normal subjects. *J Appl Physiol.* 1993;**74**:1504–14.

12. Schwab RJ. Properties of tissues surrounding the upper airway. *Sleep.* 1996;**19**:S170–4.

13. Welch KC, Ritter CT, Gefter WB, *et al.* Dynamic respiratory related upper airway imaging during wakefulness in normal subjects and patients with sleep-disordered breathing using MRI. *Am J Respir Crit Care Med.* 1998;**157**:A54.

14. Isono S, Remmers JE, Tanaka A, *et al.* Anatomy of pharynx in patients with obstructive sleep apnea and in normal subjects. *J Appl Physiol.* 1997;**82**:1319–26.

15. Morrell MJ, Arabi Y, Zahn B, Badr MS. Progressive retropalatal narrowing preceding obstructive apnea. *Am J Respir Crit Care Med.* 1998;**158**:1974–81.

16. Trudo FJ, Gefter WB, Welch KC, *et al.* State-related changes in upper airway caliber and surrounding soft-tissue structures in normal subjects. *Am J Respir Crit Care Med.* 1998;**158**:1259–70.

17. Haponik EF, Smith PL, Bohlman ME, *et al.* Computerized tomography in obstructive sleep apnea. Correlation of airway size with physiology during sleep and wakefulness. *Am Rev Respir Dis.* 1983;**127**:221–6.

18. Bradley TD, Brown IG, Grossman RF, *et al.* Pharyngeal size in snorers, nonsnorers, and patients with obstructive sleep apnea. *N Engl J Med.* 1986;**315**:1327–31.

19. Bohlman ME, Haponik EF, Smith PL, *et al.* CT demonstration of pharyngeal narrowing in adult obstructive sleep apnea. *AJR Am J Roentgenol.* 1983;**140**:543–8.

20. Brown IG, Zamel N, Hoffstein V. Pharyngeal cross-sectional area in normal men and women. *J Appl Physiol.* 1986;**61**:890–5.

21. Ell SR, Jolles H, Galvin JR. Cine CT demonstration of nonfixed upper airway obstruction. *AJR Am J Roentgenol.* 1986;**146**:669–77.

22. Hoffstein V, Zamel N, Phillipson EA. Lung volume dependence of pharyngeal cross-sectional area in patients with obstructive sleep apnea. *Am Rev Respir Dis.* 1984;**130**:175–8.

23. Horner RL, Shea SA, McIvor J, Guz A. Pharyngeal size and shape during wakefulness and sleep in patients with obstructive sleep apnoea. *Q J Med.* 1989;**72**:719–35.

24. Kuna ST, Bedi DG, Ryckman C. Effect of nasal airway positive pressure on upper airway size and configuration. *Am Rev Respir Dis.* 1988;**138**:969–75.

25. Rivlin J, Hoffstein V, Kalbfleisch J, *et al.* Upper airway morphology in patients with idiopathic obstructive sleep apnea. *Am Rev Respir Dis.* 1984;**129**:355–60.

26. Schwab RJ, Goldberg AN. Upper airway assessment: radiographic and other imaging techniques. *Otolaryngol Clin North Am.* 1998;**31**:931–68.

27. Schwartz AR, Gold AR, Schubert N, *et al.* Effect of weight loss on upper airway collapsibility in obstructive sleep apnea. *Am Rev Respir Dis.* 1991;**144**:494–8.

28. Series F, Cote C, Simoneau JA, *et al.* Physiologic, metabolic, and muscle fiber type characteristics of musculus uvulae in sleep apnea hypopnea syndrome and in snorers. *J Clin Invest.* 1995;**95**:20–5.

29. Shelton KE, Gay SB, Hollowell DE, Woodson H, Suratt PM. Mandible enclosure of upper airway and weight in obstructive sleep apnea. *Am Rev Respir Dis.* 1993;**148**:195–200.

30. Shelton KE, Woodson H, Gay S, Suratt PM. Pharyngeal fat in obstructive sleep apnea. *Am Rev Respir Dis.* 1993;**148**:462–6.

31. Shepard JW, Jr., Stanson AW, Sheedy PF, Westbrook PR. Fast-CT evaluation of the upper airway during wakefulness in patients with obstructive sleep apnea. *Prog Clin Biol Res.* 1990;**345**:273–9; discussion 280–2.

32. Shepard JW, Jr., Thawley SE. Evaluation of the upper airway by computerized tomography in patients undergoing uvulopalatopharyngoplasty for obstructive sleep apnea. *Am Rev Respir Dis.* 1989;**140**:711–16.

33. Cosentini T, Le Donne R, Mancini D, Colavita N. Magnetic resonance imaging of the upper airway in obstructive sleep apnea. *Radiol Med.* 2004;**108**:404–16.

34. Suratt PM, Dee P, Atkinson RL, Armstrong P, Wilhoit SC. Fluoroscopic and computed tomographic features of the pharyngeal airway in obstructive sleep apnea. *Am Rev Respir Dis.* 1983;**127**:487–92.

35. Stein MG, Gamsu G, de Geer G, *et al.* Cine CT in obstructive sleep apnea. *AJR Am J Roentgenol.* 1987;**148**:1069–74.

36. Bacon WH, Turlot JC, Krieger J, Stierle JL. Cephalometric evaluation of pharyngeal obstructive factors in patients with sleep apneas syndrome. *Angle Orthod* 1990;**60**:115–22.

37. deBerry-Borowiecki B, Kukwa A, Blanks RH. Cephalometric analysis for diagnosis and treatment of obstructive sleep apnea. *Laryngoscope.* 1988;**98**:226–34.

38. Guilleminault C, Partinen M, Hollman K, Powell N, Stoohs R. Familial aggregates in obstructive sleep apnea syndrome. *Chest.* 1995;**107**:1545–51.

39. Lyberg T, Krogstad O, Djupesland G. Cephalometric analysis in patients with obstructive sleep apnoea syndrome: II. Soft tissue morphology. *J Laryngol Otol.* 1989;**103**:293–7.

40. Lyberg T, Krogstad O, Djupesland G. Cephalometric analysis in patients with obstructive sleep apnoea syndrome. I. Skeletal morphology. *J Laryngol Otol.* 1989;**103**:287–92.

41. Lowe AA, Fleetham JA, Adachi S, Ryan CF. Cephalometric and computed tomographic predictors of obstructive sleep apnea severity. *Am J Orthod Dentofacial Orthop.* 1995;**107**:589–95.

42. Partinen M, Guilleminault C, Quera-Salva MA, Jamieson A. Obstructive sleep apnea and cephalometric roentgenograms. The role of anatomical upper airway abnormalities in the definition of abnormal breathing during sleep. *Chest.* 1988;**93**:1199–205.

43. Pracharktam N, Hans MG, Strohl KP, Redline S. Upright and supine cephalometric evaluation of obstructive sleep apnea syndrome and snoring subjects. *Angle Orthod.* 1994;**64**:63–73.

44. Riley R, Guilleminault C, Herran J, Powell N. Cephalometric analyses and flow-volume loops in obstructive sleep apnea patients. *Sleep.* 1983;**6**:303–11.

45. Chi L, Comyn FL, Mitra N, *et al.* Identification of craniofacial risk factors for obstructive sleep apnoea using three-dimensional MRI. *Eur Respir J.* 2011;**38**:348–58.

46. Schwab RJ, Pasirstein M, Pierson R, *et al.* Identification of upper airway anatomical risk factors for obstructive sleep apnea with volumetric magnetic resonance imaging. *Am J Respir Crit Care Med.* 2003;**168**:522–30.

47. Schellenberg JB, Maislin G, Schwab RJ. Physical findings and the risk for obstructive sleep apnea. The importance of oropharyngeal structures. *Am J Respir Crit Care Med.* 2000;**162**:740–8.

48. Malhotra A, Huang Y, Fogel RB, *et al.* The male predisposition to pharyngeal collapse: importance of airway length. *Am J Respir Crit Care Med.* 2002;**166**:1388–95.

49. Mortimore IL, Marshall I, Wraith PK, Sellar RJ, Douglas NJ. Neck and total body fat deposition in nonobese and obese patients with sleep apnea compared with that in control subjects. *Am J Respir Crit Care Med.* 1998;**157**:280–3.

50. Strobel RJ, Rosen RC. Obesity and weight loss in obstructive sleep apnea: a critical review. *Sleep.* 1996;**19**:104–15.

51. Stauffer JL, Buick MK, Bixler EO, *et al.* Morphology of the uvula in obstructive sleep apnea. *Am Rev Respir Dis.* 1989;**140**:724–8.

52. Zohar Y, Sabo R, Strauss M, *et al.* Oropharyngeal fatty infiltration in obstructive sleep apnea patients: a histological study. *Ann Otol Rhinol Laryngol.* 1998;**107**:170–4.

53. Nashi N, Kang S, Barkdull GC, Lucas J, Davidson TM. Lingual fat at autopsy. *Laryngoscope.* 2007;**117**:1467–73.

54. Mohsenin V. Gender differences in the expression of sleep-disordered breathing: role of upper airway dimensions. *Chest.* 2001;**120**:1442–7.

55. Whittle AT, Marshall I, Mortimore IL, *et al.* Neck soft tissue and fat distribution: comparison between normal men and women by magnetic resonance imaging. *Thorax.* 1999;**54**:323–8.

56. Brooks LJ, Strohl KP. Size and mechanical properties of the pharynx in healthy men and women. *Am Rev Respir Dis.* 1992;**146**:1394–7.

57. Dancey DR, Hanly PJ, Soong C, *et al.* Gender differences in sleep apnea: the role of neck circumference. *Chest.* 2003;**123**:1544–50.

58. Bixler EO, Vgontzas AN, Lin HM, *et al.* Prevalence of sleep-disordered breathing in women: effects of gender. *Am J Respir Crit Care Med.* 2001;**163**:608–13.

59. Young T, Shahar E, Nieto FJ, *et al.* Predictors of sleep-disordered breathing in community-dwelling adults: the sleep heart health study. *Arch Intern Med.* 2002;**162**:893–900.

60. Malhotra A, Huang Y, Fogel R, *et al.* Aging influences on pharyngeal anatomy and physiology: the predisposition to pharyngeal collapse. *Am J Med.* 2006;**119**:72 e79–14.

61. Schotland HM, Insko EK, Schwab RJ. Quantitative magnetic resonance imaging demonstrates alterations of the lingual musculature in obstructive sleep apnea. *Sleep.* 1999;**22**:605–13.

62. Launois SH, Feroah TR, Campbell WN, *et al.* Site of pharyngeal narrowing predicts outcome of surgery for obstructive sleep apnea. *Am Rev Respir Dis.* 1993;**147**:182–9.

63. Yumino D, Redolfi S, Ruttanaumpawan P, *et al.* Nocturnal rostral fluid shift: a unifying concept for the pathogenesis of obstructive and central sleep apnea in men with heart failure. *Circulation.* 2010;**121**:1598–605.

64. Ingman T, Nieminen T, Hurmerinta K. Cephalometric comparison of pharyngeal changes in subjects with upper airway resistance syndrome or obstructive sleep apnoea in upright and supine positions. *Eur J Orthod.* 2004;**26**:321–6.

65. Brown IB, McClean PA, Boucher R, Zamel N, Hoffstein V. Changes in pharyngeal cross-sectional area with posture and application of continuous positive airway pressure in patients with obstructive sleep apnea. *Am Rev Respir Dis.* 1987;**136**:628–32.

66. Collop NA, Block AJ, Hellard D. The effect of nightly nasal CPAP treatment on underlying obstructive sleep apnea and pharyngeal size. *Chest.* 1991;**99**:855–60.

67. Ryan CF, Lowe AA, Li D, Fleetham JA. Magnetic resonance imaging of the upper airway in obstructive sleep apnea

before and after chronic nasal continuous positive airway pressure therapy. *Am Rev Respir Dis.* 1991;**144**:939–44.

68. Rubinstein I, Colapinto N, Rotstein LE, Brown IG, Hoffstein V. Improvement in upper airway function after weight loss in patients with obstructive sleep apnea. *Am Rev Respir Dis.* 1988;**138**:1192–5.

69. Welch KC, Foster GD, Ritter CT, *et al.* A novel volumetric magnetic resonance imaging paradigm to study upper airway anatomy. *Sleep.* 2002;**25**:532–42.

70. Ishida M, Inoue Y, Suto Y, *et al.* Mechanism of action and therapeutic indication of prosthetic mandibular advancement in obstructive sleep apnea syndrome. *Psychiatry Clin Neurosci.* 1998;**52**:227–9.

71. Schmidt-Nowara WW, Meade TE, Hays MB. Treatment of snoring and obstructive sleep apnea with a dental orthosis. *Chest.* 1991;**99**:1378–85.

72. Gale DJ, Sawyer RH, Woodcock A, *et al.* Do oral appliances enlarge the airway in patients with obstructive sleep apnoea? A prospective computerized tomographic study. *Eur J Orthod.* 2000;**22**:159–68.

73. Liu Y, Park YC, Lowe AA, Fleetham JA. Supine cephalometric analyses of an adjustable oral appliance used in the treatment of obstructive sleep apnea. *Sleep Breath.* 2000;**4**:59–66.

74. Tsuiki S, Lowe AA, Almeida FR, Fleetham JA. Effects of an anteriorly titrated mandibular position on awake airway and obstructive sleep apnea severity. *Am J Orthod Dentofacial Orthop.* 2004;**125**:548–55.

75. Cobo J, Canut JA, Carlos F, Vijande M, Llamas JM. Changes in the upper airway of patients who wear a modified functional appliance to treat obstructive sleep apnea. *Int J Adult Orthodon Orthognath Surg.* 1995;**10**:53–7.

76. Bonham PE, Currier GF, Orr WC, Othman J, Nanda RS. The effect of a modified functional appliance on obstructive sleep apnea. *Am J Orthod Dentofacial Orthop.* 1988;**94**:384–92.

77. Ryan CF, Love LL, Peat D, Fleetham JA, Lowe AA. Mandibular advancement

oral appliance therapy for obstructive sleep apnoea: effect on awake calibre of the velopharynx. *Thorax.* 1999;**54**:972–7.

78. Johal A, Battagel JM, Kotecha BT. Sleep nasendoscopy: a diagnostic tool for predicting treatment success with mandibular advancement splints in obstructive sleep apnoea. *Eur J Orthod.* 2005;**27**:607–14.

79. Sutherland K, Deane SA, Chan AS, *et al.* Comparative effects of two oral appliances on upper airway structure in obstructive sleep apnea. *Sleep.* 2011;**34**:469–77.

80. Sher AE. Upper airway surgery for obstructive sleep apnea. *Sleep Med Rev.* 2002;**6**:195–212.

81. Stuck BA, Neff W, Hormann K, *et al.* Anatomic changes after hyoid suspension for obstructive sleep apnea: an MRI study. *Otolaryngol Head Neck Surg.* 2005;**133**:397–402.

82. Virkkula P, Bachour A, Hytonen M, *et al.* Snoring is not relieved by nasal surgery despite improvement in nasal resistance. *Chest.* 2006;**129**:81–7.

83. Isono S, Shimada A, Tanaka A, *et al.* Efficacy of endoscopic static pressure/area assessment of the passive pharynx in predicting uvulopalatopharyngoplasty outcomes. *Laryngoscope.* 1999;**109**:769–74.

84. Sher AE, Schechtman KB, Piccirillo JF. The efficacy of surgical modifications of the upper airway in adults with obstructive sleep apnea syndrome. *Sleep.* 1996;**19**:156–77.

85. Eric JK. Drug-induced sleep endoscopy. *Op Tech Otolaryngol Head Neck Surg.* 2006;**17**:230–2.

86. Ravesloot MJ, de Vries N. One hundred consecutive patients undergoing drug-induced sleep endoscopy: results and evaluation. *Laryngoscope.* 2011;**121**:2710–16.

87. Huang Y, White DP, Malhotra A. The impact of anatomical manipulations on pharyngeal collapse: results from a computational model of the normal human upper airway. *Chest.* 2005;**128**:1324–30

Neuroimaging of cognitive effects in obstructive sleep apnea

Robert Joseph Thomas and Suk-tak Chan

Introduction

The brain in sleep apnea has seen relatively less interest than the cardiovascular system, though symptoms related to abnormal brain function bring patients to the sleep clinic. This chapter will try to complement several others in this book, and make a case for the vulnerability of the brain to sleep pathology specifically in relation to cognition. A role for using advanced neuroimaging techniques to study brain function is more logical, and offers a large opportunity to answer clinically relevant questions.

Clinical and experimental evidence support a role for sleep pathology in brain health

Clinical and experimental evidence support a critical role for healthy sleep in normal brain function, vigilance, and cognition. Sleep apnea is probably the most important cause in sleep medicine for a direct sustained assault on the brain, and also indirectly through a range of mechanisms. Often epidemiological investigations point to clues supporting associations of a clinical state and target organ function. However, epidemiological investigation results linking sleep pathology and brain health, similar to those associating hypertension and brain structure and function, have been to date limited and inconclusive, but one recent exception linked sleep apnea and incident dementia risk [1]. Based on the variety of pathological processes induced by sleep apnea, it is a perfect storm to impair brain structure and function. Some of these mechanisms are summarized below, as they are all active in the obstructive sleep apnea (OSA) patient.

Sleep deprivation and fragmentation

The most consistent biological consequences of experimental sleep deprivation or restriction are attentional impairment and lapses, executive dysfunction, and affective change. Sleep duration is curtailed in modern day society, resulting in population-level sleep restriction. Chronic sleep restriction significantly increases amyloid beta (Aβ) plaque formation in amyloid precursor protein transgenic mice [2]. Stimuli that fragment sleep in controlled experimental situations, such as auditory stimuli, reliably induce sleepiness, executive dysfunction, and depressed mood. Experimental sleep fragmentation can induce insulin

resistance [3], a feature of the metabolic syndrome, which is associated with insulin resistance, silent brain infarction, periventricular hyperintensities, and subcortical white matter lesions [4, 5]. There are some recent data supporting an effect of sleep duration and prospective change in cognition [6].

Sleep hypoxia

Exposure to intermittent hypoxia in rodents results in impaired executive function, excessive sleepiness, and sensitivity to sleep deprivation [7–10]. There is evidence of neuronal injury in the hippocampus [11, 12] and basal forebrain [13], and neuronal loss in wake-promoting catecholaminergic systems [14]. Suggested mediating mechanisms include free radical-mediated injury, lipid peroxidation, induction of nitric oxide synthase, platelet activation factor, and apoptosis. Long-term potentiation mechanisms are impaired. Hypoxia upregulates beta-secretase activity, which can promote beta amyloid formation [15–18], and decreases neprilysin, important in beta amyloid clearance [19].

Using an oligemic model of cerebral hypoperfusion in the 3xTg-AD mouse model of Alzheimer's disease (AD), researchers transiently occluded both common carotid arteries and then examined the molecular and cellular pathways by which hypoperfusion influenced tau and Aβ proteins [20]. A single, mild, transient hypoperfusion insult acutely increased Aβ levels by enhancing beta-secretase protein expression. In contrast, transient hypoperfusion markedly decreased total tau levels, coincident with activation of macroautophagy and ubiquitin-proteosome pathways. Oligemia increased tau phosphorylated at serine and threonine, a tau epitope associated with paired helical filaments in AD patients. Despite the mild and transient nature of this hypoperfusion injury, the pattern of decreased total tau, altered phosphorylated tau, and increased Aβ persisted for several weeks post-oligemia. This study suggests that a single, mild, cerebral hypoperfusion event produces profound and long-lasting effects on both tau and Aβ [20].

Using a new technology (Single Molecule Arrays, SiMoA) capable of ultrasensitive protein measurements, a novel assay was developed to look for changes in serum Aβ42 concentrations in 25 resuscitated patients with severe hypoxia due to cardiac arrest [21]. After a lag period of ten or more hours, elevations in serum Aβ42 elevations were observed in all patients. Elevations ranged from approximately 80% to over 70-fold, with most elevations in the range of 3- to 10-fold (average approximately 7-fold). The magnitude of the increase correlated with clinical outcome. These data provide the first direct evidence in living humans that ischemia acutely increases $A\beta$ levels in blood. The results support the possibility that hypoxia may play a role in the amyloidogenic process of AD. The implications of these new exciting studies for hypoxic sleep states are obvious.

Hypoxia-cognition models in humans include exposure to altitude (although several studies have been inconclusive), patients with chronic obstructive airway disease, and sleep apnea. Executive dysfunction and some slowing in information processing are the primary domain impairments. A significant increase in amplitude and a delay in the evening decline in core body temperature raises the possibility of circadian effects [22]. Magnetic resonance spectroscopic assessments in adult with severe sleep apnea report reduced frontal white matter N-acetylaspartate and choline and poor post-treatment recovery. Hypoxia at altitude and in those with chronic obstructive lung disease is associated with alterations in cerebral phosphate metabolism and blood flow as assessed by magnetic resonance spectroscopy (MRS) and positron emission tomography (PET) [23–25].

Sleep and hemodynamic function

Sleep fragmentation is associated with daytime hypertension. Sleep deprivation causes mild blood pressure (BP) increases. Repetitive surges of BP are an invariant biological response to sleep fragmentation. Sleep apnea is a well-defined risk factor for secondary hypertension, and BP non-dipping [26–28]. Several studies have reported an associated between sleep fragmentation and BP non-dipping. Sleep with increased phasic electroencephalographic (EEG) activity called cyclic alternating pattern (CAP) is associated with non-dipping, while periods of sleep with paucity of such complexes (non-CAP) are associated with dipping of BP [29]. CAP is increased by a range of sleep fragmenting stimuli, including auditory stimulation, sleep apnea, epilepsy, and depression, and is more prevalent in patients with stroke and hypertension [30]. Sleep apnea is associated with an increased risk of strokes [31, 32].

A decrease in BP during sleep ("dipping") is a biomarker of health [33], and its absence ("non-dipping") is associated with a host of poor cardiac, neurological, metabolic, and renal outcomes. BP non-dipping is associated with an increased risk of stroke. Non-dipping is associated with brain atrophy and cognitive decline in elderly hypertensives. Abnormal circadian BP profiles are also common post-stroke. In one study of ischemic stroke patients, 46.2% were non-dippers and 36.9% were reverse dippers [34]. Dipping of lesser magnitude in systolic BP is associated with brain atrophy and worse functional status; and inadequate nocturnal BP dipping is associated with lower daytime cerebral blood flow. In acute stroke, loss of circadian BP variation occurs and may be associated with worse outcomes [35], and nocturnal BP dipping may be greater in patients with lacunar than non-lacunar infarcts.

Molecular medicine and sleep health

There are extensive changes in gene expression between behavioral states of sleep and wake and after sleep deprivation [36]. Functions of sleep may be to maintain synaptic homeostasis and promote macromolecule biosynthesis. There is also upregulation during sleep of genes involved in the synthesis of proteins and heme, maintenance of vesicle pools, and antioxidant enzymes, and genes encoding proteins of energy-regulating pathways. Wakefulness is an energetic challenge to the brain including the unfolded protein response, the electron transport chain, NPAS2, AMP-activated protein kinase, the astrocyte-neuron lactate shuttle, production of reactive oxygen species and uncoupling proteins [37, 38]. In all species studied to date, there is upregulation of the molecular chaperone BiP with extended wakefulness.

Sleep seems to have an important role for normal synaptic function and maintenance [39–42]. Wakefulness appears to be associated with net synaptic potentiation, whereas sleep may favor global synaptic depression, thereby preserving an overall balance of synaptic strength. In rat cortex and hippocampus, changes in the phosphorylation states of AMPARs, CamKII, and GSK3beta are consistent with synaptic potentiation during wakefulness and depression during sleep. Furthermore, the slope and amplitude of cortical-evoked responses increase after wakefulness, decrease after sleep, and correlate with changes in slow-wave activity, a marker of sleep pressure. Impairment of brain energetics and molecular mechanisms over prolonged periods of time has the capability to permanently alter brain structure and function.

Brain structure and function in sleep apnea syndromes

The published studies of brain neuroimaging in OSA are summarized in Table 34.1 [43, 44, 45–75], complemented by Figures 34.1 and 34.2, showing components of reversibility (or not) in OSA. Some of these studies are discussed in greater detail in other chapters in this book. For functional imaging and the associated cognition assessment, despite the use of different study protocols, different disease severities and durations, and variable scanner strengths, a common theme is reduced task-related network activation as assessed by blood oxygen level-dependent (BOLD) signals, with variable but incomplete post treatment recovery. The individual studies are too small to definitely answer a number of important clinical questions, and the protocols different enough that true pooling of data will not be possible, but the basic themes remain intact.

Morphological abnormalities in other disease states such as multiple sclerosis, stroke, and dementing illness correlate with cognition, and there is no reason to think that sleep apnea will be different. For example, in a study of 21 OSA patients vs. 21 control subjects, diminished regional and often unilateral gray matter loss was seen in multiple sites of the brain in patients, including the frontal and parietal cortex, temporal lobe, anterior cingulate, hippocampus, and cerebellum [63]. Reduced

Table 34.1. Summary of brain neuroimaging studies in OSA

Category	Study	Subjects	Results
MRS	Kamba *et al.* [53]	11 mild OSA patients (AI <20/h; 9M 2F; 48.3 ± 12.2 yrs); 12 moderate to severe OSA patients (AI ≥20/h, 10M 2F; 48.8 ± 14.1yrs), 15 controls	Significant decrease in NAA/Cho in periventricular white matter in moderate-severe OSA patients relative to healthy controls, and in moderate-severe OSA patients relative to mild OSA patients
MRS	Kamba *et al.* [57]	55 patients with habitual snoring and excessive daytime sleepiness (AHI = 43.78 ± 30/h; 49M 6F; 46.45 ± 12.64 yrs)	AHI had significant negative association with NAA/Cho for cerebral white matter
MRS	Kamba *et al.* [52]	25 OSAHS patients (AI ≥5/h; 6 patients with snoring but not OSA (AI <5/h) (26M 5F; 44.8 ± 12.8 yrs)	NAA/Cho, AI, AHI, and SpO$_2$min significantly interacted with age
MRS	Alchanatis *et al.* [43]	22 severe OSA (AHI = 70.6 ± 19.4/h; 22M; 49 ± 9.7 yrs), 10 healthy controls	OSA patients showed a significant reduction in the NAA, Cho, NAA/Cr and Cho/Cr, in frontal white matter relative to healthy controls
MRS	Bartlett *et al.* [54]	8 OSA patients (RDI >15; SaO$_2$ <90%; 8M; 48.7 yrs (41.1–56.4 yrs), 5 controls	Hippocampal NAA/Cr was significantly increased in OSA patients relative to healthy controls, and correlated with arousal index and BMI
MRS	Sarchielli *et al.* [55]	20 OSA patients (AHI = 16.65 ± 15.03/h; 20 controls	Significantly lower NAA/Cr was found in the frontal regions of OSA patients; negative correlation between AHI and NAA/Cr in the frontal regions of OSA patients
MRS	Sharma *et al.* [56]	18 apneic patients with OSA (AHI >5/h; 12M 6F; 48 ± 8.8 yrs), 32 controls	The NAA concentration was observed to be significantly lower in OSA in the left temporal and left frontal regions. The SpO$_2$min was significantly correlated with NAA in the left temporal region and left frontal gray region
MRS	Douglas *et al.* [105]	5 mice in chronic constant and intermittent hypoxia followed by normoxia	Chronic intermittent hypoxic mice had decreased NAA/Cr in hippocampus and thalamus relative to control mice
MRS	Rae *et al.* [67]	5 severe OSA patients with hypoxia (RDI = 68 ± 24; 8 severe OSA patients without hypoxia (RDI = 83 ± 20)	Oxygen desaturation >10% of sleeping baseline resulted in decreases in brain adenosine triphosphate levels, and increases in inorganic phosphate
MRS	O'Donoghue, *et al.* [44]	30 untreated OSA, 25-age matched controls. Mean AHI 71.5 ± 16.2, % SpO$_2$ below 90% 38.6 ± 19.3 % of total sleep time	Differences at baseline in frontal NAA/Cho and hippocampal Cho/Cr ratios. No longitudinal changes were seen with treatment. Significant negative correlations were seen between arousal index and frontal NAA/Cho and between % total sleep time at SpO$_2$ <90% and hippocampal Cho/Cr
fMRI	Thomas *et al.* [77]	16 patients with obstructive sleep-disordered breathing (OSDB) (RDI = 58.4 ± 15.7; 15M 1F; 40.3 ± 7.3 yrs) 16 healthy controls (11M 5F; 37.6 ± 6.3 yrs)	Working memory speed in OSDB was significantly slower than in healthy controls, and a group average map showed absence of dorsolateral prefrontal activation, regardless of nocturnal hypoxia; partial post-treatment recovery
fMRI	Ayalon *et al.* [51]	12 non-treated OSA patients (AHI = 35.1 ± 21.1/h; 11M 1F; 44.2 ± 11.9 yrs), 12 healthy controls (AHI = 1.9 ± 1.7/h; 11M 1F; 43 ± 9.1 yrs)	OSA patients showed increased brain activation in bilateral inferior frontal and middle frontal gyri, cingulate gyrus, areas at the junction of the inferior parietal and superior temporal lobes, thalamus, and cerebellum. OSA patients had decreased activation in the left postcentral and precentral gyri
fMRI	Henderson *et al.* [45]	2 severe OSA patients (RDI = 50 and 97; 2M; 47 yrs and 41 yrs)	Signal increases coincident with apneic periods emerged bilaterally in the cerebellar cortex, hippocampus, mediodorsal thalamus, frontal cortex and precentral gyrus. Signals declined bilaterally in the anterior cingulate cortex and postcentral gyrus
fMRI	Aloia *et al.* [46]	9 OSA patients (AHI = 42.4 ± 28.2/h; 5M 4F; 51.1 ± 9.3 yrs)	Treatment effects on 2-back-related brain activity: greater deactivation in the right posterior insula and over-activation in the right inferior parietal lobule
fMRI	Archbold *et al.* [58]	9 treatment-naïve moderate-severe OSA patients (AHI = 40.1 ± 28.1/h; 9M; 45.7 ± 6.6 yrs)	BOLD signal deactivations in posterior cingulate, retrosplenial, and inferior frontal regions during PASAT and 2-back. With increased disease severity, activation patterns were increased in the right parietal lobe, but decreased in the cerebellar vermis
fMRI	Ayalon *et al.* [48]	14 OSA patients (AHI = 34 ± 21/h; 13M 1F; 45.6 ± 11.7 yrs) 14 healthy controls (AHI <5/h; 13M 1F; 43.6 ± 8.6 yrs)	Patients with OSA showed decreased brain activation in cingulate, frontal, and parietal regions typically involved in attention tasks, compared with control subjects

Table 34.1. (cont.)

Category	Study	Subjects	Results
fMRI	Ayalon et al. [49]	14 OSA patients (AHI = 34 ± 21/h; 13M 1F; 45.6 ± 11.7 yrs), 14 healthy controls (AHI <5/h; 13M 1F; 43.6 ± 8.6 yrs)	Compared to controls, the OSA group showed more false positives during the No-Go trials, with decreased brain activation in the left postcentral gyrus, cingulate gyrus, and inferior parietal lobe, as well as right insula and putamen
fMRI	Castronovo et al. [59]	17 OSA patients (AHI = 50.14 ± 24.84/h; 43.93 ± 7.78 yrs) 15 age- and education-matched healthy controls (42.15 ± 6.64 yrs)	Compared to controls, never-treated OSA patients showed increased activations in the left frontal cortex, medial precuneus, and hippocampus, and decreased activations in the caudal pons. Neurocognitive domains showed improvement after treatment
fMRI	Ayalon et al. [50]	14 treatment-naïve young OSA patients, 14 treatment-naïve middle-aged OSA patients; controls: 14 young healthy controls, 14 middle-aged healthy	For both verbal learning and sustained attention tasks, decreased activation was detected for middle-aged sleep apnea relative to the other groups in task-related brain regions
fMRI	Sweet et al. [47]	10 OSA patients (AHI = 42.4 ± 28.2/h; 6M 4F; 51.1 ± 9.3 yrs)	The magnitude of deactivation during CPAP withdrawal was significantly associated with better working memory performance in the posterior cingulate and right postcentral gyrus, and greater sleepiness in the left and right medial frontal gyrus
fMRI	Prilipko et al. [69]	17 untreated OSA patients (AHI = 39.7 ± 22.8/h; 17M 43.2 ± 8.4 yrs), 7 age-matched healthy controls (AHI <5/h)	OSA patients demonstrated compensatory spatial recruitment of the task-positive network (maximal at 3-back) and of the default mode network (maximal at 2-back). AHI was positively correlated with BOLD signal in bilateral frontal regions
fMRI	Zhang et al. [70]	9 severe OSA patients (AI = 36.3 ± 4.5/h; 9M 38.4 ± 3.5 yrs) 9 age-matched healthy controls (9M, age 37.9 ± 3.1 yrs)	Patients with OSA showed reduced frontal activation in anterior cingulate, middle frontal gyrus, and inferior frontal gyrus and significantly increased activity in the right anterior prefrontal gyrus when being involved in mismatch tasks, when compared with healthy subjects; associated with oxygen desaturation duration and arousal index
Morphology	Macey et al. [63]	21 OSA patients (AHI = 34 ± 20/h; 21M; 49 ± 11 yrs) 21 healthy controls (21M; 47 ± 11 yrs)	Diminished regional and often unilateral gray matter loss in the frontal and parietal cortices, anterior cingulate, hippocampus, and cerebellum in OSA patients
Morphology	Morrell et al. [72]	7 OSA (AHI = 25–40/h; baseline nocturnal O_2 saturation = 92–97%), 7 healthy non-apneic controls	A significantly lower gray matter concentration within the left hippocampus in the apneic patients. No difference in total gray matter volumes
Morphology	O'Donoghue et al. [66]	27 untreated severe OSA patients before treatment (AHI = 71.7 ± 17/h; 27M; 45.7 ± 10.1 yrs), 24 controls	No areas of gray matter volume change were found in patients. Whole-brain volume decreases without focal changes after 6 months of CPAP.
Morphology	Kumar et al. [62]	16 OSA patients with anxiety symptoms, 7 controls with anxiety symptoms, 30 OSA patients without anxiety symptoms, 59 controls without anxiety symptoms	Significantly higher T2-relaxation values in anxious OSA, in subgenu, anterior, and mid-cingulate, ventral medial prefrontal and bilateral insular cortices, hippocampus extending to amygdala and temporal, and bilateral parietal cortices
Morphology/ PET	Yaouhi et al. [68]	16 OSA patients (AHI = 38.31 ± 14.33/h; 15M 1F; 54.75 ± 5.71 yrs), 14 healthy controls	Gray matter loss in the frontal and temporo-parieto-occipital cortices, the thalamus, hippocampal region, some basal ganglia and cerebellar regions, mainly in the right hemisphere. The decrease in brain metabolism was also right-lateralized, and involved the precuneus, the middle and posterior cingulate gyri, and the parieto-occipital cortex, as well as the prefrontal cortex
Morphology	Morrell et al. [71]	26 OSA patients in Australia (AHI = 71.5/h; 44.6 yrs), 25 healthy controls in Australia (AHI = 5.3/h; 42 yrs), 34 OSA patients in UK (AHI = 41.6/h; 49.3 yrs), 35 healthy controls in UK (AHI = 1.1/h; 48.9 yrs)	Patients with OSA had a reduction in gray matter volume in the right middle temporal gyrus compared with non-apneic controls. A reduction in gray matter was also seen within the cerebellum
Morphology	Joo et al. [74]	36 OSA patients (AHI = 52.5 ± 21.7/h; 36M; 44.7 ± 6.7 yrs) 31 non-apneic healthy controls (AHI = 2.8 ± 0.9/h; 31M; 44.8 ± 5.4 yrs)	Gray matter concentrations of OSA patients were significantly decreased in multiple locations including the left gyrus rectus, bilateral superior frontal gyri, right insula, bilateral caudate nuclei, bilateral thalami, and bilateral amygdalo-hippocampi.
Morphology	Torelli et al. [75]	16 OSA patients (12 patients, AHI = 31.6–106.3/h; 4 patients, AHI = 15.8–25.6/h; 13M 3F; 55.8 ± 6.7 yrs) 14 normal controls (9M 5F; 57.6 ± 5.1 yrs)	Volumes of cortical gray matter, right hippocampus, right and left caudate were smaller in patients compared to controls. VBM analysis showed regions of decreased gray matter volume in right and left hippocampus and within more lateral temporal areas in OSA patients

Table 34.1. (cont.)

Category	Study	Subjects	Results
Morphology	Canessa *et al.* [65]	17 OSA patients before treatment (AHI = 55.83 ± 19.08/h; 44.7 ± 7.63 yrs) 16 post-treatment, 15 controls	Cognitive impairments were associated with focal reductions of gray matter volume in the left hippocampus, left posterior parietal cortex, and right superior frontal gyrus. After treatment, cognitive improvements paralleled gray matter volume increases
PET	Antczak *et al.* [73]	7 OSA with excessive daytime sleepiness after >1 year CPAP, 7 OSA without persistent EDS	Glucose hypo-utilization in frontal areas in those with persistent sleepiness

AI = apnea index; AHI = apnea-hypopnea index; NAA = *N*-acetylaspartate; Cho = Choline; OSAHS = obstructive sleep apnea/hypopnea syndrome; Cr = Creatine; BMI = body mass index; RDI = respiratory distress index; PASAT = Paced Auditory Seinal Addition Task; CPAP = continuous positive airway pressure; VBM = voxel-based morphometry; EDS = excessive daytime sleepiness.

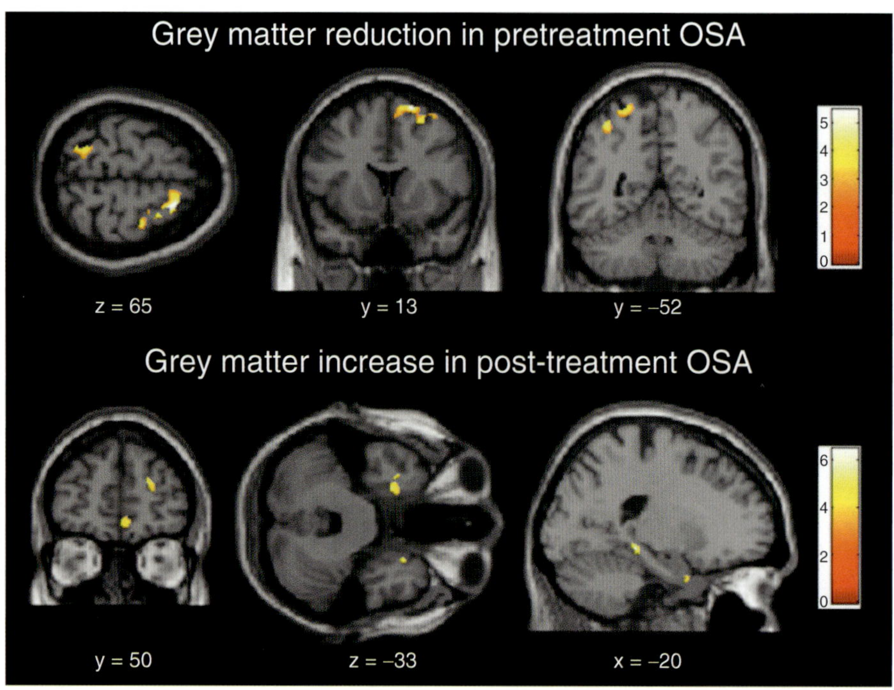

Figure 34.1 Structural imaging reversibility. A 17-subject study showing areas of "grey matter reduction" (using voxel-based morphometry) and the areas which showed post-treatment increases. Less important than the exact areas that are abnormal are reproducibility of such results, if the results are replicable in severe as well as milder disease, and what such studies may tell us about treatment efficacy. (From *Am J Respir Crit Care Med.* 2011;**183**:1419–26, with permission.)

mammillary body volume was reported by the same group [61]; they also used whole-brain maps of T2 relaxation time and showed apparent injury in depressed OSA subjects. The areas with abnormal signal included the mid- and anterior cingulate, anterior insular, medial prefrontal, parietal, and left ventro-lateral temporal cortices, left caudate nucleus, and bilateral hippocampus [60]. However, another group reported no impact of OSA on brain structure [66]. In a comparison of 39 severe sleep apnea patients vs. 64 controls, reduction in cortical thickness using FreeSurfer was noted in bilateral mid-parahippocampal gyrus, right amygdala, right medial prefrontal cortex, left posterior cingulate, and isolated areas in the right temporal cortex and left postcentral gyrus [76]. An assessment of white matter integrity using diffusion-weighted imaging in OSA patients showed multiple regions of lower fractional anisotropy in the anterior corpus callosum; anterior and posterior cingulate cortex and cingulum bundle; right column of the fornix; portions of the frontal, ventral prefrontal, parietal; and insular cortices; bilateral internal capsule; left cerebral peduncle; middle cerebellar peduncle and corticospinal tract; and deep cerebellar nuclei [64].

Neuroimaging abnormalities may be reversible [65]. In humans, sleep loss seems to disproportionately impair prefrontal-based cortical functions. Both increases and decreases in fMRI activation within the executive network (lateral and medial prefrontal, posterior parietal cortices), or lateral temporal cortex in a navigation task, have been reported. Our experience supports reductions rather than increases in activation in sleep apnea [77], narcolepsy [78], and following sleep deprivation [79]. Animal models support multiple mechanisms of neural injury in OSA [80]. However, traditional apnea-hypopnea index and sleep stages poorly predict cognition in clinical OSA.

Major confounders in functional magnetic resonance imaging (fMRI) studies of sleep apnea include obesity, resting O_2 and CO_2 levels, vascular function and hemodynamic reactivity, time from sleep, duration of task, type of task (executive function vs. encoding), and attention/vigilance (should the target

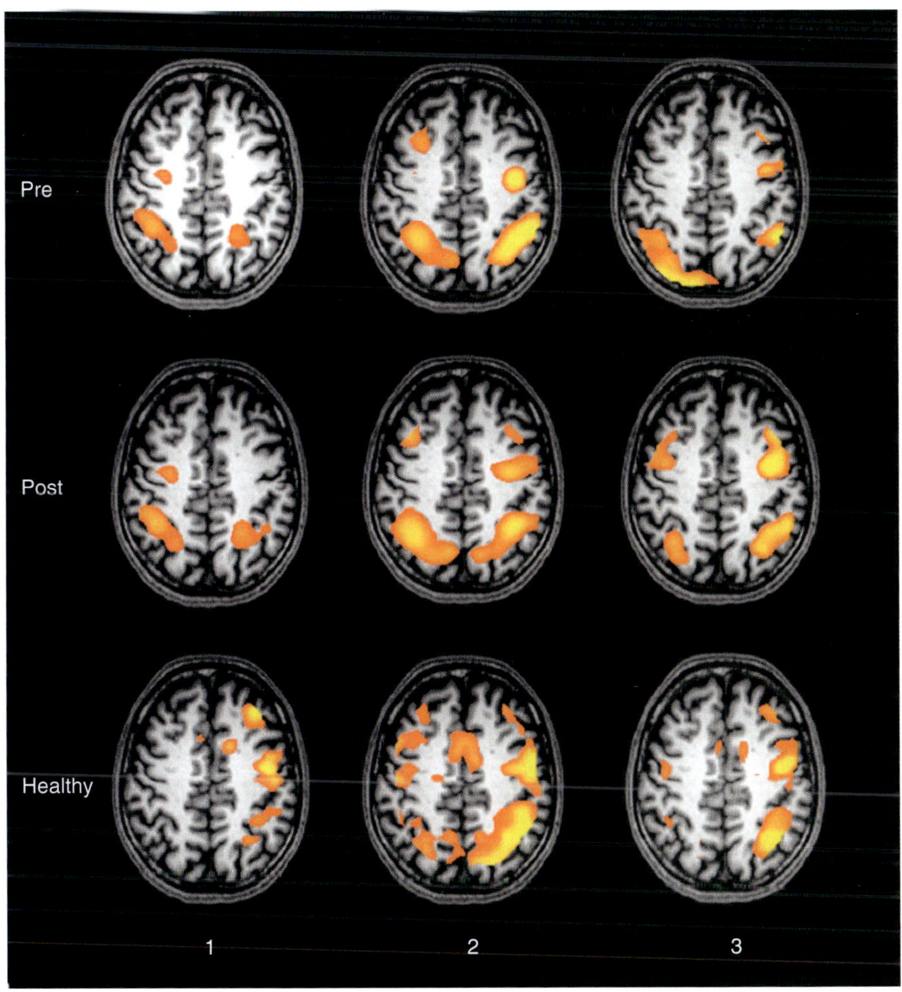

Figure 34.2 Functional imaging reversibility. At least partial reversibility of functional activation has been repeatedly demonstrated. In this figure, individual activation maps of 3 sleep apnea patients and 3 age-matched (within 5 years) healthy subjects. The well-documented individual differences in activation maps during functional imaging experiments are seen, but common themes can also be identified. Pretreatment (Pre) activation is seen in the posterior components of the executive network. Post-treatment (Post) activation in the anterior components of the network remains minimal. In contrast, the healthy subjects show activation in the lateral prefrontal and posterior parietal cortices. Larger number of subjects will be required to establish the true relationship of activation and performance; e.g., if activation remains less but performance normalizes, does that mean more efficient performance or lack of available reserve? How would such a system respond to stress (e.g., partial sleep deprivation) or a more difficult task? (From *J Appl Physiol.* 2005;**98**:2226–34, with permission.)

during scanning be speed or accuracy?). Of greatest relevance for sleep apnea is the possibility of altered hemodynamic responses to brain activation – perhaps future studies should use complementary procedures such as arterial spin labeling to obtain more direct blood flow information. Using multiple modalities such as PET, magnetoencephalography (MEG), structural MRI, and resting state/fMRI may offer complementary insights into brain health in sleep apnea patients.

Mechanisms by which pathological sleep may alter brain structure and function

Healthy aging is associated with changes in sleep architecture that suggest a weakening of the homeostatic sleep process. The resultant propensity to arousals makes sleep more vulnerable to disruptive influences. Polysomnographic changes with aging include reduced total sleep time, increased awakenings and lighter sleep, reduced slow-wave sleep and sleep apnea, changes amplified in conditions such as AD and Parkinson's disease. Treating sleep apnea in AD may result in improvements in cognition. Sleep is associated with a disproportionate reduction of metabolism in the high-order associative cortices. Sleep deprivation/fragmentation, and sleep apnea, alters task-related activation in the executive network. Transcranial magnetic stimulation has shown increased intracortical inhibition in severe untreated OSA patients.

Sleep and inflammation

Activation of innate systemic and nervous system inflammatory pathways occurs in sleep-deprived conditions [81]. Sleep apnea is associated with activation of a number of inflammatory pathways, possibly mediated by hypoxia [82]. Inflammation is also associated with the neuropathogenesis and clinical risk for cognitive decline and AD.

Vascular function

Sleep apnea is associated with carotid artery intimal thickening [83, 84]. Endothelial dysfunction, a known risk factor for vascular dysfunction, is a well-defined association of sleep apnea [85], and the mediator is probably nocturnal hypoxia. Desaturation–oxygenation cycles seen in sleep apnea result in significant oxidative stress [86] and generation of free radicals that can injure neurons.

Metabolic function

Diabetes is a risk factor for cognitive decline; a role in cognitive dysfunction and AD has been suggested and is still being explored. Sleep deprivation, sleep apnea, and experimental sleep fragmentation [3] are associated with impaired glucose tolerance and the metabolic syndrome. Hypoxia induces insulin resistance [87–89]. Oxidative stress may be important in AD and vascular dementia. Sleep apnea-related hypoxia induces a massive increase in sympathetic activation [90], with downstream vascular effects that could increase the risk of vascular dementia.

Hippocampal neurogenesis

The two sites for neurogenesis in the adult brain are the subventricular region and the dentate gyrus of the hippocampus. Hippocampal neurogenesis is reduced by sleep deprivation and fragmentation [91].

Electrophysiological and synaptic integrity

An additional mechanism through which OSA may impair brain health is through an adverse effect of synaptic downscaling effects of sleep. In the cerebral cortex, deep non-rapid eye movement (NREM) sleep manifests with low frequency variations in surface potentials that characterize EEG slow-wave activity. At the neuronal unit level, these events reflect synchronization (< 1 Hz) of cortical neuronal units between sustained firing (ON periods, which likely correspond to conditions of persistent membrane depolarization – "UP" states) and silent states (OFF periods, corresponding to membrane hyperpolarizations and "DOWN" states) [92]. During early NREM sleep after sustained wakefulness, periods of population activity (ON) are short, frequent, and associated with synchronous firing, while periods of neuronal silence are long and frequent. After sustained sleep, firing rates and synchrony decrease, while the duration of ON periods increases [93].

Delta power is a key homeostatic sleep drive marker. Cortical areas that have increased activity during the daytime, for example after daytime repetitive tasks, generate more slow waves locally. In the synaptic homeostasis model of NREM sleep, wake is associated with learning, leading to long-term potentiation (LTP) and strengthening of glutamatergic synapses, a process that eventually becomes unsustainable as the energy requirement for maintaining connections and associated firing increases. Sleep then occurs, leading to a proportional synaptic downscaling, leaving only the most robust connections intact. Synaptic downscaling during sleep would increase signal-to-noise ratio for the remaining connections, improving performance [40–42]. Sleep fragmenting stimuli inhibit the slow oscillation and the synaptic downscaling function, and could impair the coordinated interactions between hippocampal ripples and cortical spindles during slow-wave sleep. In rodents, sleep fragmentation impairs hippocampal LTP. Fragmenting stimuli may also have indirect effects, such as activation of glucocorticoid-related stress responses. Sleep-dependent learning could be inhibited by fragmented sleep, similar to that reported with motor learning in schizophrenia, cocaine users, and insomnia.

Gene–evironment interactions and the role of neuroimaging in sleep apnea

The apolipoprotein ε4 genotype is a risk factor for AD [94]. Apolipoprotein ε-deficient mice exhibit increased vulnerability to intermittent hypoxia-induced spatial learning deficits [95]. The apolipoprotein ε4 allele increases the risk of impaired cognition in OSA [96, 97]. Effects of hypoxia mediated through hypoxia-inducible factor 1alpha (HIF-1alpha), can contribute to the occurrence of AD by increasing beta-site amyloid precursor protein (APP) cleaving enzyme gene expression, protein level, and beta-secretase activity, resulting in a significant increase in the generation of Aβ [18, 98, 99]. An interaction of sleep hypoxia and the apolipoprotein ε4 allele in relation to neurocognitive performance or hippocampal structure/volume as determined by MRI can be determined in our proposed research. The presence of ε4 may also increase the risk of adverse effects of sleep apnea and hypoxia on cognition [95–97, 100].

Brain-derived neurotrophic factor (BDNF) may be a special link between sleep, cognition, and brain health. BDNF regulates neuronal survival and synaptic plasticity, including activity-dependent plasticity processes such as LTP, learning and memory [101]. A common sinde nucleotide polymorphism (rs6265) in the BDNF gene leads to a valine to methionine substitution at position 66 in the prodomain (Val66Met). The resulting trafficking defects include decreased variant BDNF distribution into neuronal dendrites, decreased secretory granule targeting, and impaired secretion. The variant participates in heterodimers less efficiently sorted into the regulated secretory pathway. This variant, which occurs naturally only in humans, influences regional brain volumes in the hippocampus (smaller) and hippocampal-dependent memory (impaired).

Supportive evidence of a central role for BDNF in sleep homeostasis has emerged, particularly providing a link between wake and use-dependent synaptic plasticity and subsequent slow-wave sleep [102–104]. BDNF enhances spontaneous sleep in rodents. Sleep deprivation impairs high-frequency stimulation-induced BDNF increases. Hippocampal BDNF is reduced by exposure to intermittent hypoxia, and exogenous administration prevents hypoxia-induced impairments in LTP.

Structural and functional imaging can help establish if genomic modifiers such as these modify the impact of sleep hypoxia or sleep fragmentation on the adult or pediatric brain structure and function, including cognition. Such "imaging genomics" has shown some utility in assessing the effects of stimulants in relation to catecholamine metabolizing pathway polymorphisms.

What neuroimaging can do to change "sleep apnea medicine"

For neuroimaging to impact the practice of clinical sleep medicine, specifically the diagnosis, treatment, and tracking of outcomes in sleep apnea syndromes, pretty pictures will not be enough. While neuroimaging being a part of the clinical evaluation and testing seems a remote possibility, research studies that ask specific questions and use the appropriate clinical cohorts, as well as large epidemiological studies, will be required. Examples of questions that may be better answered or at least significantly impacted by astute neuroimaging studies include: (1) Is there real brain injury or are these artifacts of technique, human variability, and vascular volume or reactivity changes? (2) Are the changes neuronal or glia? (3) What is the time course of development of pathological structural and functional imaging biomarkers, and what is the recovery time course? (4) Is full recovery possible, using as an analogy the resolution of cardiac ventricular hypertrophy after the treatment of hypertension? (5) What is the role of hypoxia? – this would need improved recognition of minimally hypoxic but symptomatic sleep apnea. (6) Why are some individuals with severe sleep apnea so minimally symptomatic, and vice versa? (7) What is the impact of pathological sleep on the developing brain? (8) Does the sleep apnea milieu increase the risk of vascular dementia (through hemodynamic stress) or AD (through hypoxia effects on beta amyloid metabolism and sleep fragmentation effects on cortical health)? (8) Does "residual sleepiness" in sleep apnea patients have a neuroimaging biomarker correlate? (9) Can neuroimaging provide more objective metrics of what is "biologically adequate compliance" than the now famous medical insurance-inspired "4 h average, 70% of the nights in a 4-week period, in the first 90 days" that is taking on a scientific glow?

References

1. Yaffe K, Laffan AM, Harrison SL, *et al.* Sleep-disordered breathing, hypoxia, and risk of mild cognitive impairment and dementia in older women. *JAMA.* 2011;**306**(6):613–19. Epub 2011/08/11.

2. Kang JE, Lim MM, Bateman RJ, *et al.* Amyloid-beta dynamics are regulated by orexin and the sleep-wake cycle. *Science.* 2009;**326**(5955):1005–7. Epub 2009/09/26.

3. Tasali E, Leproult R, Ehrmann DA, Van Cauter E. Slow-wave sleep and the risk of type 2 diabetes in humans. *Proc Natl Acad Sci U S A.* 2008;**105**(3):1044–9. Epub 2008/01/04.

4. Bokura H, Yamaguchi S, Iijima K, Nagai A, Oguro H. Metabolic syndrome is associated with silent ischemic brain lesions. *Stroke.* 2008;**39**(5):1607–9. Epub 2008/03/08.

5. Enzinger C, Fazekas F, Matthews PM, *et al.* Risk factors for progression of brain atrophy in aging: six-year follow-up of normal subjects. *Neurology.* 2005;**64**(10):1704–11. Epub 2005/05/25.

6. Ferrie JE, Shipley MJ, Akbaraly TN, *et al.* Change in sleep duration and cognitive function: findings from the Whitehall II Study. *Sleep.* 2011;**34**(5):565–73.

7. Sanfilippo-Cohn B, Lai S, Zhan G, *et al.* Sex differences in susceptibility to oxidative injury and sleepiness from intermittent hypoxia. *Sleep.* 2006;**29**(2):152–9.

8. Veasey SC, Davis CW, Fenik P, *et al.* Long-term intermittent hypoxia in mice: protracted hypersomnolence with oxidative injury to sleep-wake brain regions. *Sleep.* 2004;**27**(2):194–201.

9. Zhan G, Fenik P, Pratico D, Veasey SC. Inducible nitric oxide synthase in long-term intermittent hypoxia: hypersomnolence and brain injury. *Am J Respir Crit Care Med.* 2005;**171**(12):1414–20.

10. Morrell MJ. Residual sleepiness in patients with optimally treated sleep apnea: a case for hypoxia-induced oxidative brain injury. *Sleep.* 2004;**27**(2):186–7.

11. Gozal E, Gozal D, Pierce WM, *et al.* Proteomic analysis of CA1 and CA3 regions of rat hippocampus and differential susceptibility to intermittent hypoxia. *J Neurochem.* 2002;**83**(2):331–45. Epub 2002/11/09.

12. Hambrecht VS, Vlisides PE, Row BW, *et al.* Hypoxia modulates cholinergic but not opioid activation of G proteins in rat hippocampus. *Hippocampus.* 2007;**17**(10):934–42. Epub 2007/06/29.

13. Row BW, Kheirandish L, Cheng Y, Rowell PP, Gozal D. Impaired spatial working memory and altered choline acetyltransferase (CHAT) immunoreactivity and nicotinic receptor binding in rats exposed to intermittent hypoxia during sleep. *Behav Brain Res.* 2007;**177**(2):308–14. Epub 2007/01/16.

14. Zhu Y, Fenik P, Zhan G, *et al.* Selective loss of catecholaminergic wake active neurons in a murine sleep apnea model. *J Neurosci.* 2007;**27**(37):10060–71. Epub 2007/09/15.

15. Guglielmotto M, Tamagno E, Danni O. Oxidative stress and hypoxia contribute to Alzheimer's disease pathogenesis: two sides of the same coin. *ScientificWorldJournal.* 2009;**9**:781–91. Epub 2009/08/26.

16. Li L, Zhang X, Yang D, *et al.* Hypoxia increases Abeta generation by altering beta- and gamma-cleavage of APP. *Neurobiol Aging.* 2009;**30**(7):1091–8. Epub 2007/12/08.

17. Sun X, He G, Qing H, *et al.* Hypoxia facilitates Alzheimer's disease pathogenesis by up-regulating BACE1 gene expression. *Proc Natl Acad Sci USA.* 2006;**103**(49):18727–32. Epub 2006/11/24.

18. Zhang X, Zhou K, Wang R, *et al.* Hypoxia-inducible factor 1alpha (HIF-1alpha)-mediated hypoxia increases BACE1 expression and beta-amyloid generation. *J Biol Chem.* 2007;**282**(15):10873–80. Epub 2007/02/17.

19. Wang Z, Yang D, Zhang X, *et al.* Hypoxia-induced down-regulation of neprilysin by histone modification in mouse primary cortical and hippocampal neurons. *PLoS One.* 2011;**6**(4):e19229. Epub 2011/05/12.

20. Koike MA, Green KN, Blurton-Jones M, Laferla FM. Oligemic hypoperfusion differentially affects tau and amyloid-β. *Am J Pathol.* 2010;**177**(1):300–10. Epub 2010/05/18.

21. Zetterberg H, Mortberg E, Song L, *et al.* Hypoxia due to cardiac arrest induces a time-dependent increase in serum amyloid beta levels in humans. *PLoS One.* 2011;**6**(12):e28263. Epub 2011/12/24.

22. Coste O, Beaumont M, Batejat D, Beers PV, Touitou Y. Prolonged mild hypoxia modifies human circadian core body temperature and may be associated with sleep disturbances. *Chronobiol Int.* 2004;**21**(3):419–33.

23. Hochachka PW, Clark CM, Matheson GO, *et al*. Effects on regional brain metabolism of high-altitude hypoxia: a study of six US marines. *Am J Physiol*. 1999;**277**(1 Pt 2):R314–19.

24. Hamilton G, Mathur R, Allsop JM, *et al*. Changes in brain intracellular pH and membrane phospholipids on oxygen therapy in hypoxic patients with chronic obstructive pulmonary disease. *Metab Brain Dis*. 2003;**18**(1):95–109.

25. Shim TS, Lee JH, Kim SY, *et al*. Cerebral metabolic abnormalities in COPD patients detected by localized proton magnetic resonance spectroscopy. *Chest*. 2001;**120**(5):1506–13.

26. Suzuki M, Guilleminault C, Otsuka K, Shiomi T. Blood pressure "dipping" and "non-dipping" in obstructive sleep apnea syndrome patients. *Sleep*. 1996;**19**(5):382–7. Epub 1996/06/01.

27. Ziegler MG. Sleep disorders and the failure to lower nocturnal blood pressure. *Curr Opin Nephrol Hypertens*. 2003;**12**(1):97–102. Epub 2002/12/24.

28. Wolf J, Hering D, Narkiewicz K. Non-dipping pattern of hypertension and obstructive sleep apnea syndrome. *Hypertens Res*. **33**(9):867–71. Epub 2010/09/08.

29. Iellamo F, Placidi F, Marciani MG, *et al*. Baroreflex buffering of sympathetic activation during sleep: evidence from autonomic assessment of sleep macroarchitecture and microarchitecture. *Hypertension*. 2004;**43**(4):814–19.

30. Thomas RJ, Weiss MD, Mietus JE, *et al*. Prevalent hypertension and stroke in the Sleep Heart Health Study: association with an ECG-derived spectrographic marker of cardiopulmonary coupling. *Sleep*. 2009;**32**(7):897–904. Epub 2009/07/31.

31. Godoy J, Mellado P, Tapia J, Santin J. Obstructive sleep apnea as an independent stroke risk factor: possible mechanisms. *Curr Mol Med*. 2009;**9**(2):203–9. Epub 2009/03/12.

32. Yaggi HK, Concato J, Kernan WN, *et al*. Obstructive sleep apnea as a risk factor for stroke and death. *N Engl J Med*. 2005;**353**(19):2034–41. Epub 2005/11/12.

33. O'Brien E. Dipping comes of age: the importance of nocturnal blood pressure. *Hypertension*. 2009;**53**(3):446–7. Epub 2009/01/28.

34. Pandian JD, Wong AA, Lincoln DJ, *et al*. Circadian blood pressure variation after acute stroke. *J Clin Neurosci*. 2006;**13**(5):558–62. Epub 2006/05/09.

35. Ali K, Wei Leong KM, Houlder S, *et al*. The relationship between dipping profile in blood pressure and neurologic deficit in early acute ischemic stroke. *J Stroke Cerebrovasc Dis*. 2011;**20**(1):10–15. Epub 2010/06/12.

36. Cirelli C, Faraguna U, Tononi G. Changes in brain gene expression after long-term sleep deprivation. *J Neurochem*. 2006;**98**(5):1632–45.

37. Naidoo N. Cellular stress/the unfolded protein response: relevance to sleep and sleep disorders. *Sleep Med Rev*. 2009;**13**(3):195–204. Epub 2009/03/31.

38. Scharf MT, Naidoo N, Zimmerman JE, Pack AI. The energy hypothesis of sleep revisited. *Prog Neurobiol*. 2008;**86**(3):264–80. Epub 2008/09/24.

39. Vyazovskiy VV, Cirelli C, Pfister-Genskow M, Faraguna U, Tononi G. Molecular and electrophysiological evidence for net synaptic potentiation in wake and depression in sleep. *Nat Neurosci*. 2008;**11**(2):200–8. Epub 2008/01/22.

40. Esser SK, Hill SL, Tononi G. Sleep homeostasis and cortical synchronization: I. Modeling the effects of synaptic strength on sleep slow waves. *Sleep*. 2007;**30**(12):1617–30. Epub 2008/02/06.

41. Vyazovskiy VV, Riedner BA, Cirelli C, Tononi G. Sleep homeostasis and cortical synchronization: II. A local field potential study of sleep slow waves in the rat. *Sleep*. 2007;**30**(12):1631–42. Epub 2008/02/06.

42. Riedner BA, Vyazovskiy VV, Huber R, *et al*. Sleep homeostasis and cortical synchronization: III. A high-density EEG study of sleep slow waves in humans. *Sleep*. 2007;**30**(12):1643–57. Epub 2008/02/06.

43. Alchanatis M, Deligiorgis N, Zias N, *et al*. Frontal brain lobe impairment in obstructive sleep apnoea: a proton MR spectroscopy study. *Eur Respir J*. 2004;**24**(6):980–6.

44. O'Donoghue FJ, Wellard RM, Rochford PD, *et al*. Magnetic resonance spectroscopy and neurocognitive dysfunction in obstructive sleep apnea before and after CPAP treatment. *Sleep*. 2012;**35**(1):41–8. Epub 2012/01/05.

45. Henderson LA, Macey KE, Macey PM, *et al*. Regional brain response patterns to Cheyne-Stokes breathing. *Respir Physiol Neurobiol*. 2006;**150**(1):87–93. Epub 2005/12/13.

46. Aloia MS, Sweet LH, Jerskey BA, *et al*. Treatment effects on brain activity during a working memory task in obstructive sleep apnea. *J Sleep Res*. 2009;**18**(4):404–10. Epub 2009/09/22.

47. Sweet LH, Jerskey BA, Aloia MS. Default network response to a working memory challenge after withdrawal of continuous positive airway pressure treatment for obstructive sleep apnea. *Brain Imaging Behav*. 2010;**4**(2):155–63. Epub 2010/05/27.

48. Ayalon L, Ancoli-Israel S, Aka AA, McKenna BS, Drummond SP. Relationship between obstructive sleep apnea severity and brain activation during a sustained attention task. *Sleep*. 2009;**32**(3):373–81. Epub 2009/03/20.

49. Ayalon L, Ancoli-Israel S, Drummond SP. Altered brain activation during response inhibition in obstructive sleep apnea. *J Sleep Res*. 2009;**18**(2):204–8. Epub 2009/03/24.

50. Ayalon L, Ancoli-Israel S, Drummond SP. Obstructive sleep apnea and age: a double insult to brain function? *Am J Respir Crit Care Med*. 2010;**182**(3):413–19. Epub 2010/04/17.

51. Ayalon L, Ancoli-Israel S, Klemfuss Z, Shalauta MD, Drummond SP. Increased brain activation during verbal learning in obstructive sleep apnea. *Neuroimage*. 2006;**31**(4):1817–25. Epub 2006/04/22.

52. Kamba M, Inoue Y, Higami S, Suto Y. Age-related changes in cerebral lactate metabolism in sleep-disordered breathing. *Neurobiol Aging*. 2003;**24**(5):753–60. Epub 2003/07/30.

53. Kamba M, Suto Y, Ohta Y, Inoue Y, Matsuda E. Cerebral metabolism in sleep apnea. Evaluation by magnetic resonance spectroscopy. *Ame J Respir Crit Care Med*. 1997;**156**(1):296–8. Epub 1997/07/01.

54. Bartlett DJ, Rae C, Thompson CH, *et al*. Hippocampal area metabolites relate to severity and cognitive function in obstructive sleep apnea. *Sleep Med*. 2004;**5**(6):593–6. Epub 2004/10/30.

55. Sarchielli P, Presciutti O, Alberti A, *et al*. A 1H magnetic resonance spectroscopy study in patients with obstructive sleep apnea. *Eur J Neurol*. 2008;**15**(10):1058–64. Epub 2008/08/23.

56. Sharma SK, Sinha S, Danishad KA, *et al.* Proton magnetic resonance spectroscopy of brain in obstructive sleep apnoea in north Indian Asian subjects. *Indian J Med Res.* 2010;**132**:278–86. Epub 2010/09/18.

57. Kamba M, Inoue Y, Higami S, *et al.* Cerebral metabolic impairment in patients with obstructive sleep apnoea: an independent association of obstructive sleep apnoea with white matter change. *J Neurol Neurosurg Psychiatry.* 2001;**71**(3):334–9. Epub 2001/08/21.

58. Archbold KH, Borghesani PR, Mahurin RK, Kapur VK, Landis CA. Neural activation patterns during working memory tasks and OSA disease severity: preliminary findings. *J Clin Sleep Med.* 2009;**5**(1):21–7. Epub 2009/03/26.

59. Castronovo V, Canessa N, Strambi LF, *et al.* Brain activation changes before and after PAP treatment in obstructive sleep apnea. *Sleep.* 2009;**32**(9):1161–72. Epub 2009/09/16.

60. Cross RL, Kumar R, Macey PM, *et al.* Neural alterations and depressive symptoms in obstructive sleep apnea patients. *Sleep.* 2008;**31**(8):1103–9. Epub 2008/08/22.

61. Kumar R, Birrer BV, Macey PM, *et al.* Reduced mammillary body volume in patients with obstructive sleep apnea. *Neurosci Lett.* 2008;**438**(3):330–4. Epub 2008/05/20.

62. Kumar R, Macey PM, Cross RL, *et al.* Neural alterations associated with anxiety symptoms in obstructive sleep apnea syndrome. *Depress Anxiety.* 2009;**26**(5):480–91. Epub 2008/10/02.

63. Macey PM, Henderson LA, Macey KE, *et al.* Brain morphology associated with obstructive sleep apnea. *Am J Respir Crit Care Med.* 2002;**166**(10):1382–7. Epub 2002/11/08.

64. Macey PM, Kumar R, Woo MA, *et al.* Brain structural changes in obstructive sleep apnea. *Sleep.* 2008;**31**(7):967–77. Epub 2008/07/26.

65. Canessa N, Castronovo V, Cappa SF, *et al.* Obstructive sleep apnea: brain structural changes and neurocognitive function before and after treatment. *Am J Respir Crit Care Med.* 2011;**183**(10):1419–26. Epub 2010/11/03.

66. O'Donoghue FJ, Briellmann RS, Rochford PD, *et al.* Cerebral structural changes in severe obstructive sleep apnea. *Am J Respir Crit Care Med.* 2005;**171**(10):1185–90. Epub 2005/02/09.

67. Rae C, Bartlett DJ, Yang Q, *et al.* Dynamic changes in brain bioenergetics during obstructive sleep apnea. *J Cereb Blood Flow Metab.* 2009;**29**(8):1421–8. Epub 2009/05/14.

68. Yaouhi K, Bertran F, Clochon P, *et al.* A combined neuropsychological and brain imaging study of obstructive sleep apnea. *J Sleep Res.* 2009;**18**(1):36–48. Epub 2009/03/03.

69. Prilipko O, Huynh N, Schwartz S, *et al.* Task positive and default mode networks during a parametric working memory task in obstructive sleep apnea patients and healthy controls. *Sleep.* 2011;**34**(3):293–301A. Epub 2011/03/02.

70. Zhang X, Ma L, Li S, Wang Y, Wang L. A functional MRI evaluation of frontal dysfunction in patients with severe obstructive sleep apnea. *Sleep Med.* 2011;**12**(4):335–40. Epub 2011/03/15.

71. Morrell MJ, Jackson ML, Twigg GL, *et al.* Changes in brain morphology in patients with obstructive sleep apnoea. *Thorax.* 2010;**65**(10):908–14. Epub 2010/09/24.

72. Morrell MJ, McRobbie DW, Quest RA, *et al.* Changes in brain morphology associated with obstructive sleep apnea. *Sleep Med.* 2003;**4**(5):451–4. Epub 2003/11/01.

73. Antczak J, Popp R, Hajak G, *et al.* Positron emission tomography findings in obstructive sleep apnea patients with residual sleepiness treated with continuous positive airway pressure. *J Physiol Pharmacol.* 2007;58 Suppl **5** (Pt 1):25–35. Epub 2008/03/28.

74. Joo EY, Tae WS, Lee MJ, *et al.* Reduced brain gray matter concentration in patients with obstructive sleep apnea syndrome. *Sleep.* 2010;**33**(2):235–41. Epub 2010/02/24.

75. Torelli F, Moscufo N, Garreffa G, *et al.* Cognitive profile and brain morphological changes in obstructive sleep apnea. *Neuroimage.* 2011;**54** (2):787–93. Epub 2010/10/05.

76. Macey PM, Kumar R, Woo MA, Harper RM. Reduced cortical thickness in obstructive sleep apnea patients. *Sleep.* 2009;**32**:A229.

77. Thomas RJ, Rosen BR, Stern CE, Weiss JW, Kwong KK. Functional imaging of working memory in obstructive sleep-disordered breathing. *J Appl Physiol.* 2005;**98**(6):2226–34.

78. Thomas RJ. Fatigue in the executive cortical network demonstrated in narcoleptics using functional magnetic resonance imaging – a preliminary study. *Sleep Med.* 2005;**6**(5):399–406.

79. Thomas R, Kwong KK. Modafinil activates cortical and subcortical sites in the sleep deprived state. *Sleep.* 2006;**29**(11):1459–69.

80. Lim DC, Veasey SC. Neural injury in sleep apnea. *Curr Neurol Neurosci Rep.* **10**(1):47–52. Epub 2010/04/29.

81. Krueger JM. The role of cytokines in sleep regulation. *Curr Pharm Des.* 2008;**14**(32):3408–16. Epub 2008/12/17.

82. Kapsimalis F, Basta M, Varouchakis G, *et al.* Cytokines and pathological sleep. *Sleep Med.* 2008;**9**(6):603–14. Epub 2007/11/21.

83. Li C, Zhang XL, Liu H, Wang ZG, Yin KS. Association among plasma interleukin-18 levels, carotid intima-media thickness and severity of obstructive sleep apnea. *Chin Med J (Engl).* 2009;**122**(1):24–9. Epub 2009/02/04.

84. Minoguchi K, Yokoe T, Tazaki T, *et al.* Increased carotid intima-media thickness and serum inflammatory markers in obstructive sleep apnea. *Am J Respir Crit Care Med.* 2005;**172** (5):625–30. Epub 2005/08/27.

85. Budhiraja R, Parthasarathy S, Quan SF. Endothelial dysfunction in obstructive sleep apnea. *J Clin Sleep Med.* 2007;**3** (4):409–15. Epub 2007/08/19.

86. Lavie L. Oxidative stress–a unifying paradigm in obstructive sleep apnea and comorbidities. *Prog Cardiovasc Dis.* 2009;**51**(4):303–12. Epub 2008/12/27.

87. Iiyori N, Alonso LC, Li J, *et al.* Intermittent hypoxia causes insulin resistance in lean mice independent of autonomic activity. *Am J Respir Crit Care Med.* 2007;**175**(8):851–7. Epub 2007/02/03.

88. Polotsky VY, Li J, Punjabi NM, *et al.* Intermittent hypoxia increases insulin resistance in genetically obese mice. *J Physiol.* 2003;**552**(Pt 1):253–64. Epub 2003/07/25.

89. Ye J. Emerging role of adipose tissue hypoxia in obesity and insulin resistance. *Int J Obes (Lond).* 2009;**33** (1):54–66. Epub 2008/12/04.

90. Fletcher EC. Sympathetic over activity in the etiology of hypertension of obstructive sleep apnea. *Sleep*. 2003;**26**(1):15–19. Epub 2003/03/12.

91. Guzman-Marin R, Bashir T, Suntsova N, Szymusiak R, McGinty D. Hippocampal neurogenesis is reduced by sleep fragmentation in the adult rat. *Neuroscience*. 2007;**148**(1):325–33. Epub 2007/07/17.

92. Steriade M. Sleep oscillations and their blockage by activating systems. *J Psychiatry Neurosci*. 1994;**19**(5):354–8.

93. Vyazovskiy VV, Olcese U, Lazimy YM, *et al*. Cortical firing and sleep homeostasis. *Neuron*. 2009;**63**(6):865–78. Epub 2009/09/26.

94. Bu G. Apolipoprotein E and its receptors in Alzheimer's disease: pathways, pathogenesis and therapy. *Nat Rev Neurosci*. 2009;**10**(5):333–44. Epub 2009/04/03.

95. Kheirandish L, Row BW, Li RC, Brittian KR, Gozal D. Apolipoprotein E-deficient mice exhibit increased vulnerability to intermittent hypoxia-induced spatial learning deficits. *Sleep*. 2005;**28**(11):1412–17. Epub 2005/12/13.

96. Cosentino FI, Bosco P, Drago V, *et al*. The APOE epsilon4 allele increases the risk of impaired spatial working memory in obstructive sleep apnea. *Sleep Med*. 2008;**9**(8):831–9. Epub 2007/12/18.

97. Gozal D, Capdevila OS, Kheirandish-Gozal L, Crabtree VM. APOE epsilon 4 allele, cognitive dysfunction, and obstructive sleep apnea in children. *Neurology*. 2007;**69**(3):243–9. Epub 2007/07/20.

98. Li QY, Wang HM, Wang ZQ, *et al*. Salidroside attenuates hypoxia-induced abnormal processing of amyloid precursor protein by decreasing BACE1 expression in SH-SY5Y cells. *Neurosci Lett*. 2010;**481**(3):154–8. Epub 2010/07/06.

99. Guglielmotto M, Aragno M, Autelli R, *et al*. The up-regulation of BACE1 mediated by hypoxia and ischemic injury: role of oxidative stress and HIF1alpha. *J Neurochem*. 2009;**108**(4):1045–56. Epub 2009/02/07.

100. Spira AP, Blackwell T, Stone KL, *et al*. Sleep-disordered breathing and cognition in older women. *J Am Geriatr Soc*. 2008;**56**(1):45–50. Epub 2007/12/01.

101. Cowansage KK, LeDoux JE, Monfils MH. Brain-derived neurotrophic factor: a dynamic gatekeeper of neural plasticity. *Curr Mol Pharmacol*. 2010;**3**(1):12–29. Epub 2009/12/25.

102. Huber R, Tononi G, Cirelli C. Exploratory behavior, cortical BDNF expression, and sleep homeostasis. *Sleep*. 2007;**30**(2):129–39. Epub 2007/03/01.

103. Faraguna U, Nelson A, Vyazovskiy VV, Cirelli C, Tononi G. Unilateral cortical spreading depression affects sleep need and induces molecular and electrophysiological signs of synaptic potentiation in vivo. *Cereb Cortex*. 2010;**21**(12):2939–47. Epub 2010/03/30.

104. Faraguna U, Vyazovskiy VV, Nelson AB, Tononi G, Cirelli C. A causal role for brain-derived neurotrophic factor in the homeostatic regulation of sleep. *J Neurosci*. 2008;**28**(15):4088–95. Epub 2008/04/11.

105. Douglas RM, Miyasaka N, Takahashi K, *et al*. Chromic intermittent but not constant hypoxia decreases NAA/Cr ratios in neonatal mouse hippocampus and thalamus. *Am J Physiol Regul Integr Comp Physiol*. 2007;**293**(3):R1254–9. Epub 2006/11/02.

Neuroimaging of autonomic dysfunction and ventilatory control in obstructive sleep apnea

Paul M. Macey

Introduction

Autonomic function is disrupted in obstructive sleep apnea (OSA), which over time may contribute to the high incidence of cardiovascular comorbidities such as hypertension and its sequelae [1, 2]. Peripheral responses to various autonomic challenges highlight impaired reactivity in OSA, including muted and delayed heart rate responses [3, 4]. The source of the autonomic deficits likely includes altered neural regulation due to the structural brain changes that are present in OSA, as discussed in Chapter 32 [4–13]. Specifically, forebrain areas with regulatory roles for autonomic functions are injured in OSA, including the anterior and mid cingulate cortex, ventral medial prefrontal cortex, hippocampus, insular cortex, and thalamus. The set of both lower brainstem and hypothalamic and higher cortical and limbic regions involved in autonomic regulation has been termed the central autonomic network [14, 15], and structures within this network consistently show altered structure and function in people with OSA. This chapter summarizes functional neuroimaging findings from a variety of autonomic and respiratory challenges our group has performed in people with OSA. Previous findings and some new data are introduced.

OSA neuroimaging findings by challenge

Forehead cold pressor

A cold pressor challenge involves exposing a body region to a cold stimulus, which elicits a sympathetic activation that leads to a vasoconstriction and a blood pressure increase [16]. Additionally, when applied to the facial region, the "dive reflex" is triggered, which slows breathing rate in addition to the blood pressure increase and bradycardia [17]. We performed functional imaging during a forehead cold pressor challenge to assess the neural processes involved in mounting the cardio-respiratory responses in OSA and healthy control subjects [7]. We studied 10 OSA and 16 control subjects; this group of OSA subjects was heterogeneous, and included a combination of treated and untreated patients, and a range of comorbidities. Despite this variability, the OSA subjects showed distinct cardiovascular and respiratory responses, as well as significantly different neural patterns in multiple brain regions. The characteristic bradycardia was present in both OSA and control groups, but was more pronounced in controls. The normal reduction in breathing rate in controls was not present in OSA patients [7]. The regions of response are illustrated in the manuscript [7], but we also include a previously unpublished table listing affected regions (Table 35.1). Additionally, we recorded continuous blood pressure in a subset of subjects during a session outside of the scanner with the same cold pressor protocol. The blood pressure responses in the OSA patients were exaggerated, even when looking at only subjects without cardiovascular-influencing medications (Figure 35.1). The OSA subjects had a higher mean resting blood pressure, but this did not limit the rise in blood pressure, i.e., there was no ceiling effect. These combined findings demonstrate a failure of normal regulation of cardiovascular and respiratory responses to a standard autonomic challenge, likely due to impaired brain function in non-brainstem regions.

Valsalva maneuver

The Valsalva maneuver is an autonomic challenge involving straining by forceful expiration against a closed glottis, and the tasks elicit a sequence of blood pressure and heart rate responses mediated through a coordination of autonomic regulatory activity. The test is used to assess cardiovascular function in healthy and diseased populations. To assess OSA function, we collected functional magnetic resonance imaging (fMRI) and physiological signals while 8 OSA and 15 control subjects performed a sequence of three Valsalva maneuvers [4]. Both groups achieved the target expiratory pressure of 30 mmHg, but the heart rate responses were muted and delayed in the OSA group. Multiple brain regions were recruited during the challenge, with areas of differences including the anterior cingulate (an area of significant structural injury [5, 6]), the left and right insular cortices, the hippocampus, the cerebellar cortex, and the midbrain and pons [4]. These regions are recruited in healthy control subjects [18], but the patterns of response differed between groups, with both greater and lower magnitudes of fMRI signal changes in the OSA patients. A striking feature of the differences was the timing delay in the OSA subjects,

Neuroimaging of Sleep and Sleep Disorders, ed. Eric Nofzinger, Pierre Maquet, and Michael J. Thorpy. Published by Cambridge University Press. © Cambridge University Press 2013.

Table 35.1. Location of brain regions showing responses to a forehead cold pressor challenge in 10 OSA and 16 control subjects [7]. The statistical level (t-value), size of the region (number of $2 \times 2 \times 2$ mm voxels), and location of maximum of region in MNI co ordinates are shown

t-value	Voxels	X	Y	Z	t-value	Voxels	X	Y	Z
Control increase					Control & Δ OSA increase				
5.2	72	−36	8	12	5.3	476	40	0	14
4.7	199	56	2	−8	5.3	393	−40	−4	−14
4.6	229	42	−2	16	5.1	78	−8	34	18
4.4	29	36	−2	−14	4.7	127	−30	−72	−32
4.4	41	−28	26	−16	4.5	111	−18	−60	−26
4.1	87	−40	−4	−12	4.0	33	−58	−4	4
4.0	44	30	16	−14	3.7	60	28	−72	−30
3.9	21	6	−6	36	3.6	18	−54	6	−10
3.7	25	6	−4	−2	3.5	23	30	16	−14
3.7	37	−8	34	16	3.5	34	4	−6	42
3.6	22	−54	8	−18	3.3	12	4	0	0
3.5	57	−18	−52	−26	3.2	14	−4	−20	36
3.5	16	36	−24	−14	3.0	13	−36	−26	14
3.3	14	−12	−6	4	3.0	16	58	−28	−2
3.2	49	−34	−22	14	3.0	12	−14	−20	0
3.0	8	−30	−72	−32	3.0	14	−12	−66	−6
3.0	8	−58	−6	2	2.9	14	18	−22	8
					2.8	15	6	−46	42
Control decrease					Control & Δ OSA decrease				
4.1	41	8	−68	14	4.4	147	8	−70	12
3.8	12	8	−42	−30	3.3	15	6	−6	8
3.6	66	30	−64	−20	3.1	9	22	−18	−18
3.4	18	−14	−48	−56	3.1	29	−14	−60	4
3.2	7	58	−60	2	3.0	12	46	22	−2
3.2	9	−60	−52	16	2.9	15	32	−58	−22
3.1	29	−8	−52	4	2.8	7	−58	−52	14
OSA < Control					OSA > Control				
4.4	147	8	−70	12	4.7	14	−40	−74	−30
3.3	15	6	−6	8	3.3	6	36	26	−8
3.1	9	22	−18	−18	3.1	10	6	58	4
3.1	6	2	−38	−14	2.9	22	36	−62	−24
3.1	29	−14	−60	4	2.8	5	20	−76	−28
3.0	12	46	22	−2	2.7	6	−56	−14	10
2.9	15	32	−58	−22	2.7	3	8	−50	−26
2.9	3	18	0	−12	2.6	5	0	−54	20
2.8	7	−58	−52	14	2.6	4	4	54	12
2.6	6	−8	−70	14					

suggesting a slower responsiveness of the neural circuitry in responding to the challenge. This phase delay could also represent a lack of coordination of the rapidly changing afferent signals. The end result of a late and muted cardiovascular response presumably puts the patients at risk of acute periods of ischemia, and may contribute to further brain injury. The poor coordination of responses across multiple brain regions also suggests that other basic functions requiring central nervous system regulation would be impacted.

The earlier study suggested that timing differences were important, but the resolution of the fMRI signals at the time was low (6 s per volume), and the protocol was limited to 2:30

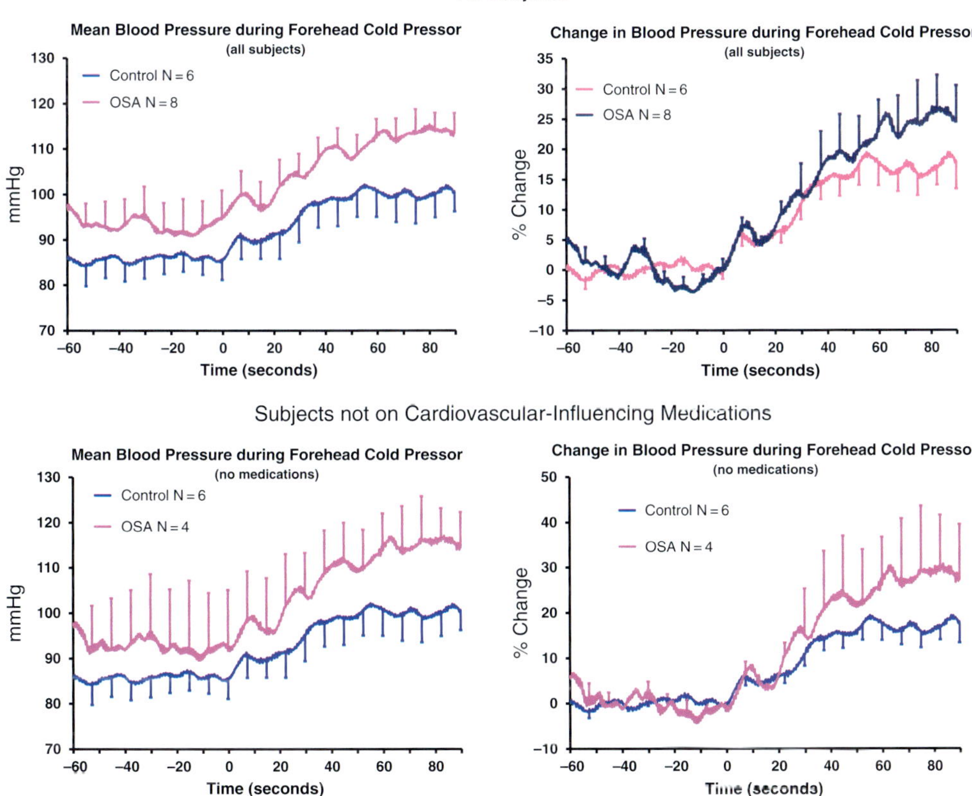

Figure 35.1 Continuous blood pressure responses to a forehead cold pressor challenge in OSA and control subjects (a subset of those assessed with fMRI [7]). The top row illustrates differential responses in all subjects, and the second row subjects who are not taking any potentially cardiovascular-altering medications. The left column shows raw values and the right percentage change.

minutes. In a more recent study, we repeated the Valsalva maneuver in a larger group of recently diagnosed OSA patients and controls using a higher-resolution paradigm, with longer recovery periods after the challenges. We studied 37 untreated moderate to severe OSA patients (age $46.3.0 \pm 8.8$ years, 24 males, apnea-hypopnea index (AHI) ≥ 15, mean $= 36.6 \pm 20.7$) and 58 healthy controls (age 46.9 ± 9.1 years, 38 males) while they performed a sequence of four 18 s Valsalva maneuvers at 1-min intervals. The fMRI scans were collected every 2 s, and pulse oximetry signals were recorded concurrently for measuring heart rate, in addition to load pressure. All subjects achieved the target pressure, but the heart rate responses were muted in the OSA group (Figure 35.2), as with the earlier study. To obtain more detailed understanding of the roles of a specific structure, we isolated the fMRI signals within subregions of the insular cortex by tracing the gyri on high-resolution anatomical images and extracting the functional signals from co-registered image volumes. The patterns of responses differed significantly between the OSA and control groups, with different timing of signal responses and different magnitudes across insular regions during the sympathetic phase of the challenge (Figure 35.2). The insular cortex, especially in

anterior regions, is considered as having modulatory roles during responses to autonomic stimuli, so the altered functional responses in this structure likely reflect a reduced capacity to respond at the central nervous system level to the demands of the stimulus.

Expiratory loading

Expiratory loading involves adding resistance to the expiratory phase of respiration, and simulates one aspect of the restricted breathing during obstructive apneic events. The challenge is relatively sustained but does not involve straining to the same degree as the Valsalva maneuver, and therefore does not result in blood pressure increasing to as great an extent as that challenge. However, a cardiovascular response should still be elicited. In a group of 9 OSA and 16 control medication-free subjects, we performed fMRI scanning during a 2 min expiratory loading task [3]. The OSA subjects failed to increase their heart rate in the normal manner, even though the breathing rate and average expiratory load pressure were similar in both groups. We assessed continuous blood pressure outside the scanner in a subset of subjects (8 OSA and 6 control), and found a greatly impaired blood

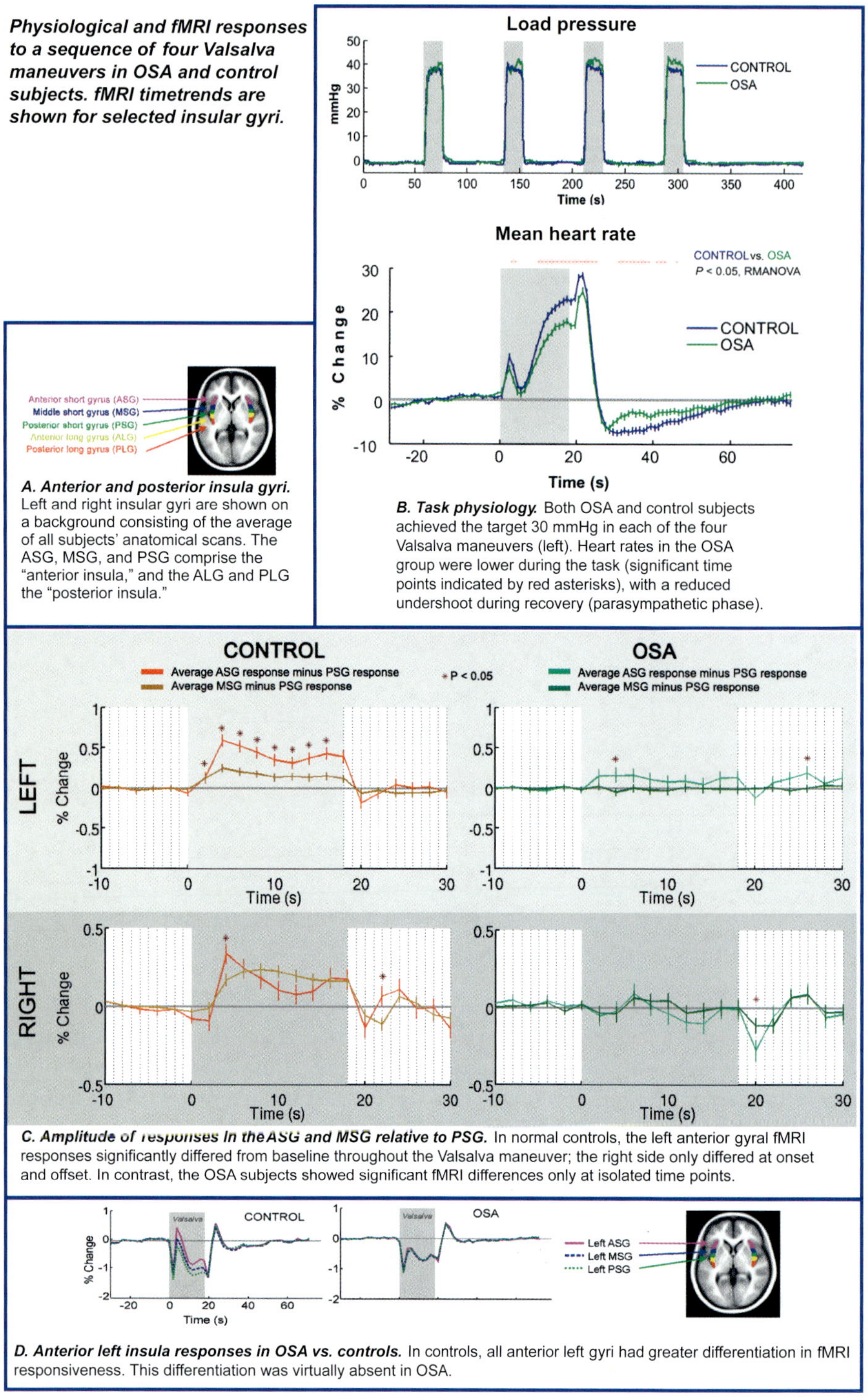
Physiological and fMRI responses to a sequence of four Valsalva maneuvers in OSA and control subjects. fMRI timetrends are shown for selected insular gyri.
Load pressure
mmHg
Time (s)
CONTROL
OSA
Mean heart rate
CONTROL vs. OSA
P < 0.05, RMANOVA
% Change
Anterior short gyrus (ASG)
Middle short gyrus (MSG)
Posterior short gyrus (PSG)
Anterior long gyrus (ALG)
Posterior long gyrus (PLG)
A. Anterior and posterior insula gyri. Left and right insular gyri are shown on a background consisting of the average of all subjects' anatomical scans. The ASG, MSG, and PSG comprise the "anterior insula," and the ALG and PLG the "posterior insula."
B. Task physiology. Both OSA and control subjects achieved the target 30 mmHg in each of the four Valsalva maneuvers (left). Heart rates in the OSA group were lower during the task (significant time points indicated by red asterisks), with a reduced undershoot during recovery (parasympathetic phase).
Average ASG response minus PSG response
Average MSG minus PSG response
* P < 0.05
LEFT
RIGHT
C. Amplitude of responses in the ASG and MSG relative to PSG. In normal controls, the left anterior gyral fMRI responses significantly differed from baseline throughout the Valsalva maneuver; the right side only differed at onset and offset. In contrast, the OSA subjects showed significant fMRI differences only at isolated time points.
Valsalva
Left ASG
Left MSG
Left PSG
D. Anterior left insula responses in OSA vs. controls. In controls, all anterior left gyri had greater differentiation in fMRI responsiveness. This differentiation was virtually absent in OSA.

Figure 35.2 Physiology and insular fMRI responses to the Valsalva maneuver in OSA and control subjects.

pressure response in OSA subjects, with the absence of the normal increase seen in controls (Figure 35.3A). These impaired cardiovascular responses in OSA are likely related to the altered functional responses in multiple brain regions. Examples of responses to the challenge are shown in Figure 35.3B, which illustrates the varying patterns across the two groups, with regions of similar responses, greater changes in controls over OSA, and areas of increase in OSA versus controls. These varied responses occurring in OSA despite a similar physiological challenge (in terms of respiratory rate and expiratory pressure) show that the sleep disorder is associated with altered function across a network of brain regions, and likely results in the poor coordination of cardiovascular responses.

Inspiratory loading

Inspiratory loading involves restricting the inspiratory phases of respiration, and mimics aspects of obstructive apneic events,

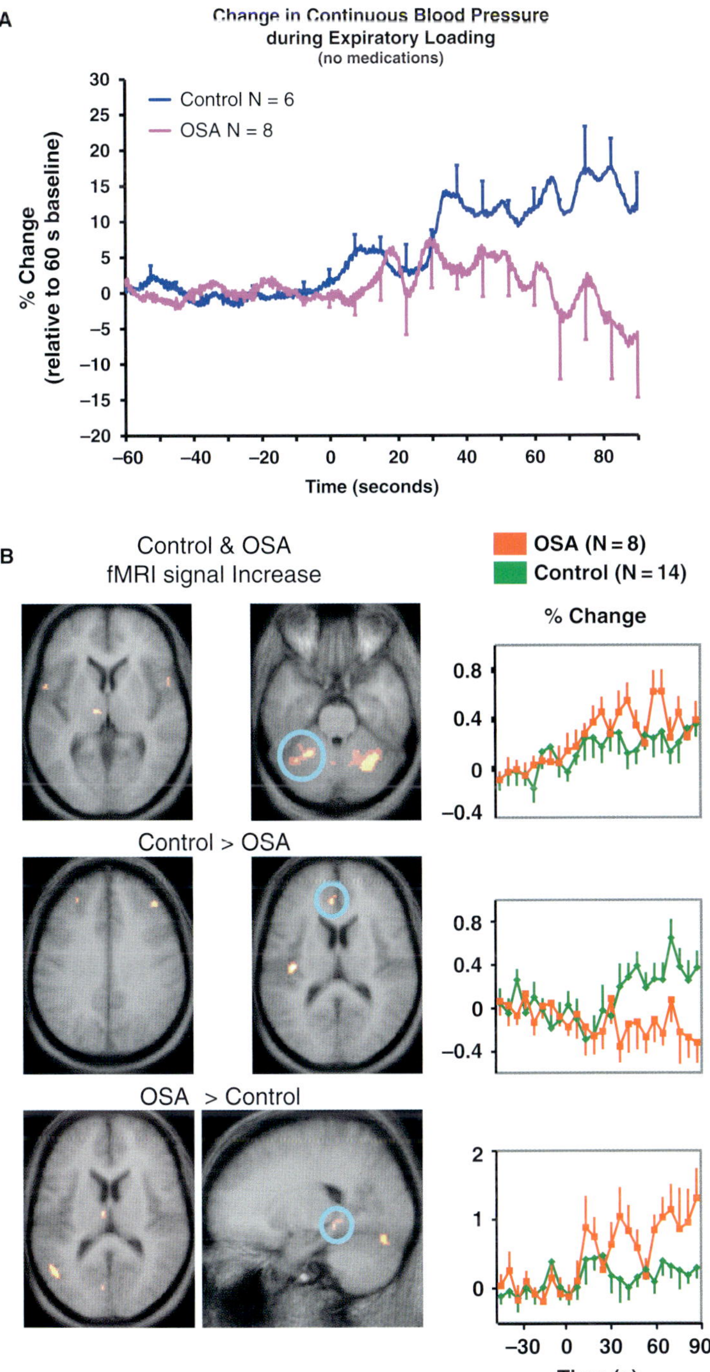

Figure 35.3 (A) Continuous blood pressure responses to an expiratory loading in eight OSA and six control subjects (a subset of those assessed with fMRI [3]). (B) fMRI responses to an expiratory loading in 8 OSA and 16 control subjects [3], illustrating areas of similar increases in both groups (superior cerebellar cortex, top row), an increase in control but not OSA (anterior cingulate, middle row), and greater increases in OSA vs. control (posterior right hippocampus, bottom row). The time-trends on the right show the group-mean response patterns.

with negative intrathoracic pressure in contrast with the positive intrathoracic pressure during expiratory loading or the Valsalva maneuver. We assessed fMRI responses in 7 OSA and 11 control subjects to a 2 min inspiratory loading challenge, while concurrently measuring heart rate and inspiratory pressure [19]. Both groups achieved similar negative pressures during the course of the challenge, with equivalent breathing rates [19]. However, heart rate responses in OSA lagged those in controls, and in a subset of subjects studied outside the scanner, continuous blood pressure rose rapidly and remained elevated in OSA versus controls [19]. The fMRI signal changes differed significantly in the two groups, especially in autonomically active regions including the anterior cingulate cortex, anterior insular cortex, cerebellar deep nuclei, and cerebellar cortices. Additional limbic regions including the hippocampus showed significantly different responses, as did medial midbrain and thalamic regions. While the inspiratory loading challenge involves respiratory and dyspneic as well as autonomic components, the impaired heart rate and blood pressure responses are consistent with inadequate regulation by the central autonomic network, including both higher cortical areas and thalamic and brainstem outflow regions.

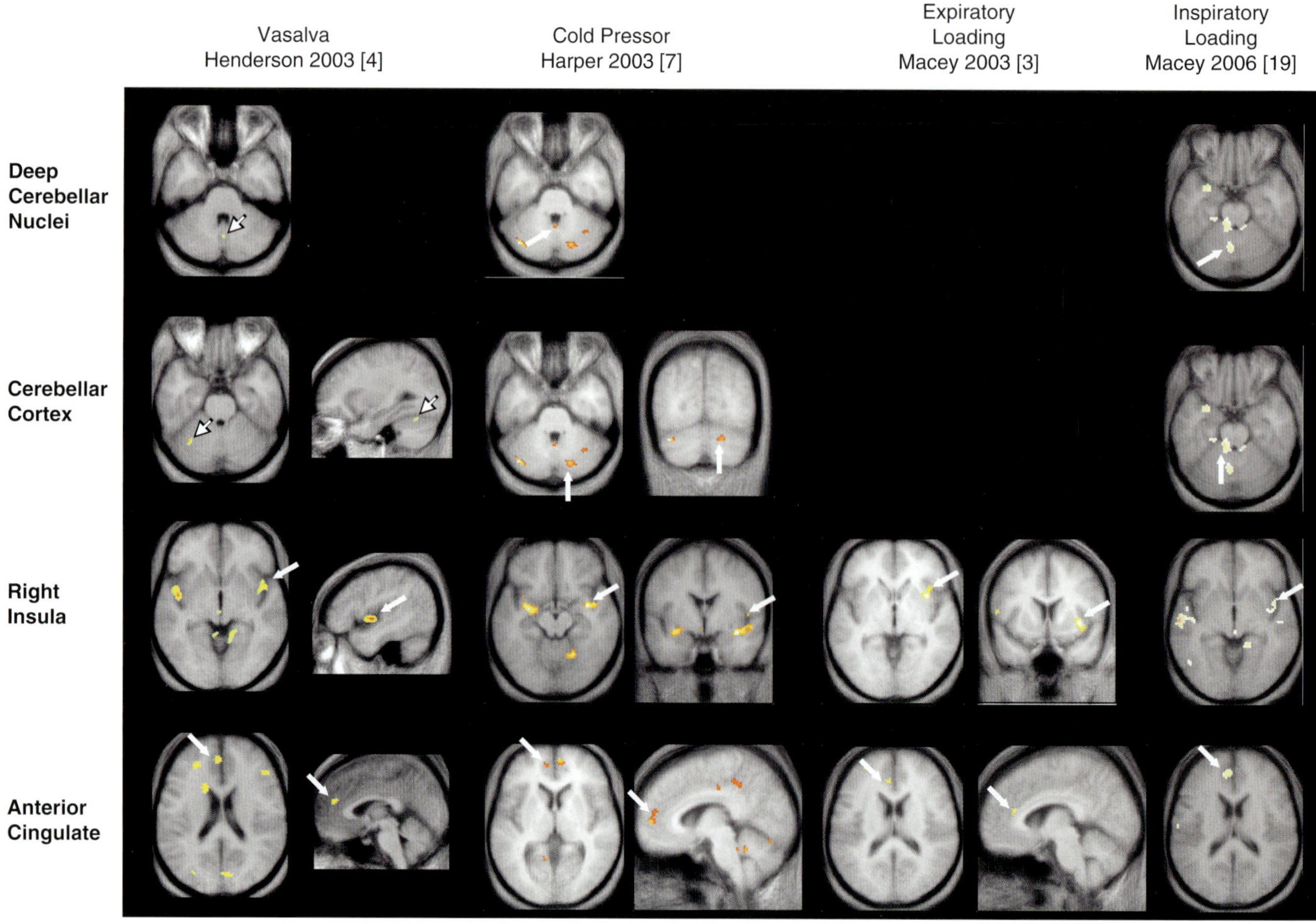

Figure 35.4 Summary of differences in fMRI signal changes between OSA and control subjects across four challenges [3, 4, 7, 19], illustrating areas of significantly altered neural patterns in similar brain regions including the cerebellar deep nuclei and cortex, anterior insula (especially on the right), and the anterior cingulate (especially on the left).

Summary of earlier studies

The four challenges performed in a group of subjects showing gray matter loss in multiple brain regions [5] demonstrate a remarkable consistency in structures showing altered function [3, 4, 7, 19]. A subset of such areas of difference across challenges is shown in Figure 35.4. These findings suggest that the gray matter loss leads to impaired function, with, for example, the left anterior insular being affected by all autonomic challenges as well as showing the greatest magnitude of gray matter volume reduction [5], and extensive axonal injury [6]. While the insular cortex did not show gray matter loss in the 2002 study, our later assessment of axonal integrity using diffusion tensor imaging (DTI) techniques did show impairments in white matter regions adjacent to and extending into the anterior insular cortices [6]. Whether the insular functional differences are due to damage just to the neighboring axons or to altered function across multiple brain regions is unknown, but worthy of further study. In particular, one of the limitations of the earlier studies was that the group of subjects who successfully performed the functional challenges without any technical issues was smaller than the group assessed for morphological changes, and a correlation between extent of structural change

and extent of functional differences in the same group could expand our understanding of the impact of neural damage.

One of the complexities with any autonomic challenge is isolating the intended stimulus. All the above tasks used to test function in OSA involve a combination of voluntary or passive actions related to respiration, blood pressure, motor control, temperature, as well as sensations of dysnea, pain, and other non-noxious experiences such as attention to visual cues. The inspiratory and expiratory loading tasks led to a degree of dyspnea in most subjects, as did the Valsalva maneuver to a lesser extent. The forehead cold pressor triggers the dive reflex, which elicits bradycardia and peripheral vasoconstriction as well as changes in cardio-respiratory coupling patterns [20]. Thus, the patterns of neural responses must reflect regulation of a combination of autonomic and other central nervous system-mediated functions.

Hand grip

In additional to the Valsalva maneuver performed with the newer protocols described above (i.e., Figure 35.2), we assessed neural and physiological responses to a brief static hand grip challenge, which elicits a rapid rise in heart rate and

A. Hand grip protocol

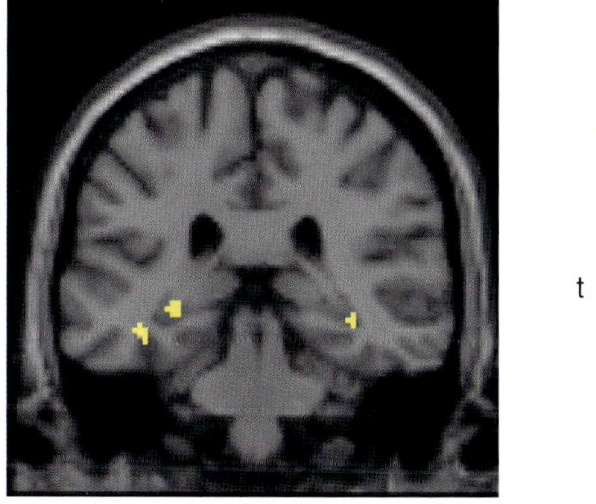
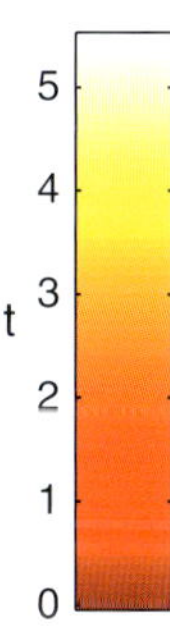

B. fMRI signal differences in 22 severe OSA vs. 47 matched control subjects (hippocampal areas)

Figure 35.5 (A) Hand grip protocol for fMRI assessment, illustrating the extended baseline and recovery periods needed to allow recovery to baseline. (B) Significant (p < 0.05, false discovery rate) fMRI signal differences between OSA and control subjects across four challenges, with the bilateral hippocampus and the parahippocampal gyrus showing differences in responses. The background is a single subject's T1-weighted anatomical image in standard space.

Patterns of differences

Most of the findings to date illustrate group differences in the magnitude of the signal responses during challenge periods, using the traditional "boxcar" method of fMRI analysis. Such differences included both higher and lower signals in the OSA patients, and responsiveness versus lack of responsiveness in some regions. Thus, despite the likely presence of neural injury, brain function in OSA is not uniformly affected, i.e., not all signals are lower or non-responsive in the sleep disorder. In many cases, a larger neural response is indicated by greater fMRI signal changes in the patient group, suggesting a greater demand on the regulatory system (a pattern seen in response to cognitive stimuli in OSA [13, 28]). Thus, the findings cannot be interpreted simplistically as neural injury resulting in reduced brain activity.

In addition to altered magnitude of fMRI signal changes, certain brain regions show delayed timing of responsiveness in OSA. The cerebellum, a region traditionally associated with coordination of motor control [29], shows both muted and phase-lagged responses to the Valsalva maneuver in OSA over control subjects, despite both groups performing the challenge in a similar fashion [4]. The blood pressure coordination roles for the cerebellar nuclei are well established [30–35], and these structures show activation in human neuroimaging studies to a variety of challenges that alter blood pressure [36–39]. The finding of delayed responsiveness even with the relatively coarse time resolution of 6 s demonstrates a significant impairment in the coordination of central responses. This impairment is presumably due to a combination of damage to the cerebellum itself, as well as to connecting axons from other regions, such as the cerebellar peduncles [5, 6].

Another abnormal pattern in OSA is altered insular functional neuroanatomy in response to autonomic stimuli, as seen with higher-resolution fMRI in response to the Valsalva maneuver (Figure 35.2). While timing differences also appear, what is remarkable is the lack of the normal functional differentiation across the anterior gyri of the insular cortex. In healthy controls, the anterior-most regions show the greatest signal increases during the sympathetic-dominant phases of the task, with more posterior areas showing significantly lower responses [40]. However, in OSA subjects, this anterior-posterior differential response is essentially absent (Figure 35.2), and may reflect a lack of capacity to adapt to the conditions elicited by the task (increased intrathoracic pressure and its sequelae). The muted heart rate increase in the OSA group is likely in part a reflection of this lack of normal neural function, although some of the difference in peripheral responses may relate to reduced cardiovascular reserve, given the higher heart rate of the OSA group. Nevertheless, the combination of muted heart rate responses and reduced functional differentiation in the insular cortex are of concern in the condition.

Summary

The findings of functional differences in similar brain regions across varying challenges in varying OSA

sympathetic outflow [21, 22]. This task does not involve significant changes in respiration. We used a brief (16 s) hand grip challenge to assess the responsiveness of 22 severe, untreated OSA patients (mean AHI 47 ± 17 events/hour; age 48 ± 9 years) and 46 control subjects (age 48 ± 8 years; normal Epworth Sleepiness Scale scores). Subjects squeezed to a subjective 80% of maximum for a total of four 16-s hand grip efforts, repeated every 76 s, and with a 58 s baseline (Figure 35.5A). The more extended scanning period enabled long enough recovery periods to allow for the subjects to return to baseline physiological conditions. Signals were detrended to remove global effects, and motion parameters were included as regressors, to exclude extraneous influences. Both groups showed signal increases in multiple motor, sensory, and autonomic areas, but significant differences appeared in the left and right hippocampi, extending into parahippocampal regions (Figure 35.5B; p < 0.05, false discovery rate). As with the left anterior cingulate, the impaired functional responses in the hippocampus are likely related to injury seen in this structure, as shown by our group and others [12, 23–27].

populations reinforce the importance of the central autonomic network in health and in a disordered state. We would add the cerebellum to the list of structures in that network, including both deep nuclei and cerebellar cortices. The combination of neural injury and dysfunction suggests a link between conditions such as intermittent hypoxia that damage brain structures and the chronic dysregulation of autonomic functions present in OSA. Several processes associated with OSA can lead to the development of hypertension, amongst which is endothelial dysfunction resulting from elevated sympathetic tone [41–44], oxidative stress [45, 46], and systemic inflammation [47, 48], but such phenomena are at least partially resolved by continuous positive airway pressure (CPAP), whereas hypertension is not [1, 49]. The question of whether treatment with CPAP restores neural function is unanswered, but the dysfunction is likely anchored at least in part to neural injury, which would be difficult to resolve with CPAP, at least in the short term. An unanswered question is whether acute inflammation in the brain impairs functional capacity; such pathology should resolve with CPAP [50, 51]. Perhaps the finding of difficult-to-treat hypertension in OSA, more so than hypertension in non-OSA populations [52], is related to the presence of more permanent neural impairments. Looking ahead, these neuroimaging findings confirm altered neural autonomic regulation in cross-sectional studies of OSA populations, but longitudinal assessment of autonomic function is required to determine the time course and potential reversibility of these changes.

Acknowledgements

This work was performed at the University of California at Los Angeles. No interventions were used in this study. Financial support was provided by the National Institutes of Health, HL-60296 (Ronald M. Harper) and NR-011230 (PMM). The author has no conflict of interest.

The author thanks Dr. Ronald Harper for his support.

References

1. Dudenbostel T, Calhoun DA. Resistant hypertension, obstructive sleep apnoea and aldosterone. *J Hum Hypertens.* 2012;**26**(5):281–7. doi: 10.1038/jhh.2011.47.

2. Grunstein R, Wilcox I, Yang TS, Gould Y, Hedner J. Snoring and sleep apnoea in men: association with central obesity and hypertension. *Int J Obes Relat Metab Disord.* 1993;**17**(9):533–40.

3. Macey PM, Macey KE, Henderson LA, *et al.* Functional magnetic resonance imaging responses to expiratory loading in obstructive sleep apnea. *Respir Physiol Neurobiol.* 2003;**138**(2–3):275–90.

4. Henderson LA, Woo MA, Macey PM, *et al.* Neural responses during Valsalva maneuvers in obstructive sleep apnea syndrome. *J Appl Physiol.* 2003;**94**(3):1063–74.

5. Macey PM, Henderson LA, Macey KE, *et al.* Brain morphology associated with obstructive sleep apnea. *Am J Respir Crit Care Med.* 2002;**166**(10):1382–7.

6. Macey PM, Kumar R, Woo MA, *et al.* Brain structural changes in obstructive sleep apnea. *Sleep.* 2008;**31**(7):967–77.

7. Harper RM, Macey PM, Henderson LA, *et al.* fMRI responses to cold pressor challenges in control and obstructive sleep apnea subjects. *J Appl Physiol.* 2003;**94**(4):1583–95.

8. Tonon C, Vetrugno R, Lodi R, *et al.* Proton magnetic resonance spectroscopy study of brain metabolism in obstructive sleep apnoea syndrome before and after continuous positive airway pressure treatment. *Sleep.* 2007;**30**(3):305–11.

9. Canessa N, Castronovo V, Cappa SF, *et al.* Obstructive sleep apnea: brain structural changes and neurocognitive function before and after treatment. *Am J Respir Crit Care Med.* 2010;**183**(10):1419–26.

10. Joo EY, Tae WS, Lee MJ, *et al.* Reduced brain gray matter concentration in patients with obstructive sleep apnea syndrome. *Sleep.* 2010;**33**(2):235–41.

11. Morrell MJ, Jackson ML, Twigg GL, *et al.* Changes in brain morphology in patients with obstructive sleep apnoea. *Thorax.* 2010;**65**(10):908–14.

12. Torelli F, Moscufo N, Garreffa G, *et al.* Cognitive profile and brain morphological changes in obstructive sleep apnea. *Neuroimage.* 2011;**54**(2):787–93.

13. Ayalon L, Ancoli-Israel S, Klemfuss Z, Shalauta MD, Drummond SP. Increased brain activation during verbal learning in obstructive sleep apnea. *Neuroimage.* 2006;**31**(4):1817–25.

14. Benarroch EE. The central autonomic network: functional organization, dysfunction, and perspective. *Mayo Clin Proc.* 1993;**68**(10):988–1001.

15. Loewy AD. Forebrain nuclei involved in autonomic control. *Prog Brain Res.* 1991;**87**:253–68.

16. Wirch JL, Wolfe LA, Weissgerber TL, Davies GA. Cold pressor test protocol to evaluate cardiac autonomic function. *Appl Physiol Nutr Metab.* 2006;**31**(3):235–43.

17. Khurana RK, Wu R. The cold face test: a non-baroreflex mediated test of cardiac vagal function. *Clin Auton Res.* 2006;**16**(3):202–7.

18. Fulbright RK, Troche CJ, Skudlarski P, Gore JC, Wexler BE. Functional MR imaging of regional brain activation associated with the affective experience of pain. *AJR Am J Roentgenol.* 2001;**177**(5):1205–10.

19. Macey KE, Macey PM, Woo MA, *et al.* Inspiratory loading elicits aberrant fMRI signal changes in obstructive sleep apnea. *Respir Physiol Neurobiol.* 2006;**151**(1):44–60.

20. Heath ME, Downey JA. The cold face test (diving reflex) in clinical autonomic assessment: methodological considerations and repeatability of responses. *Clin Sci.* 1990;**78**(2):139–47.

21. Mancia G, Iannos J, Jamieson GG, *et al.* Effect of isometric hand-grip exercise on the carotid sinus baroreceptor reflex in man. *Clin Sci Mol Med.* 1978;**54**(1):33–7.

22. Mark AL, Victor RG, Nerhed C, Wallin BG. Microneurographic studies of the mechanisms of sympathetic nerve responses to static exercise in humans. *Circ Res.* 1985;**57**(3):461–9.

23. Morrell MJ, McRobbie DW, Quest RA, *et al.* Changes in brain morphology associated with obstructive sleep apnea. *Sleep Med.* 2003;**4**(5):451–4.

24. Thomas RJ, Rosen BR, Stern CE, Weiss JW, Kwong KK. Functional imaging of working memory in obstructive sleep-disordered breathing. *J Appl Physiol.* 2005;**98**(6):2226–34.

25. Macey PM, Moiyadi AS, Kumar R, Woo MA, Harper RM. Reduced hippocampal volume in patients with obstructive sleep apnea. *Society for Neuroscience 2008 Abstracts.* 2008.

26. Bartlett DJ, Rae C, Thompson CH, *et al.* Hippocampal area metabolites relate to severity and cognitive function in obstructive sleep apnea. *Sleep Med.* 2004;**5**(6):593–6.

27. Halbower AC, Degaonkar M, Barker PB, *et al.* Childhood obstructive sleep apnea associates with neuropsychological deficits and neuronal brain injury. *PLoS Med.* 2006;**3**(8):e301.

28. Archbold KH, Borghesani PR, Mahurin RK, Kapur VK, Landis CA. Neural activation patterns during working memory tasks and OSA disease severity: preliminary findings. *J Clin Sleep Med.* 2009;**5**(1):21–7.

29. Thach WT, Goodkin HP, Keating JG. The cerebellum and the adaptive coordination of movement. *Annu Rev Neurosci.* 1992;**15**:403–42.

30. Zhang F, Iadecola C. Fastigial stimulation increases ischemic blood flow and reduces brain damage after focal ischemia. *J Cereb Blood Flow Metab.* 1993;**13**(6):1013–19.

31. Lutherer LO, Lutherer BC, Dormer KJ, Janssen HF, Barnes CD. Bilateral lesions of the fastigial nucleus prevent the recovery of blood pressure following hypotension induced by hemorrhage or administration of endotoxin. *Brain Res.* 1983 Jun 20;**269**(2):251–7.

32. Williams JL, Lutherer LO. Fastigial pressor response observed during an operation on a patient with cerebellar bleeding–anatomical review and clinical significance. *Neurosurgery.* 1994;**34**(2):379–80.

33. Hirano T, Kuchiwaki H, Yoshida K, *et al.* Fastigial pressor response observed during an operation on a patient with cerebellar bleeding–an anatomical review and clinical significance. *Neurosurgery.* 1993;**32**(4):675–7.

34. Achari NK, Downman CB. Autonomic effector responses to stimulation of nucleus fastigius. *J Physiol.* 1970;**210**(3):637–50.

35. Henderson LA, Richard CA, Macey PM, *et al.* Functional magnetic resonance signal changes in neural structures to baroreceptor reflex activation. *J Appl Physiol.* 2004;**96**(2):693–703.

36. Napadow V, Dhond R, Conti G, *et al.* Brain correlates of autonomic modulation: combining heart rate variability with fMRI. *Neuroimage.* 2008;**42**(1):169–77.

37. Henderson LA, Macey PM, Macey KE, *et al.* Brain responses associated with the Valsalva maneuver revealed by functional magnetic resonance imaging. *J Neurophysiol.* 2002;**88**(6):3477–86.

38. Kimmerly DS, O'Leary DD, Menon RS, Gati JS, Shoemaker JK. Cortical regions associated with autonomic cardiovascular regulation during lower body negative pressure in humans. *J Physiol.* 2005;**569**(Pt 1):331–45.

39. Critchley HD, Corfield DR, Chandler MP, Mathias CJ, Dolan RJ. Cerebral correlates of autonomic cardiovascular arousal: a functional neuroimaging investigation in humans. *J Physiol.* 2000;**523**(Pt 1):259–70.

40. Macey PM, Wu P, Kumar R, *et al.* Differential responses of the insular cortex gyin to autonomic challenges. *Auto Neurosin* 2012;**168**(1–2):72–81.

41. Narkiewicz K, van de Borne PJ, Montano N, *et al.* Contribution of tonic chemoreflex activation to sympathetic activity and blood pressure in patients with obstructive sleep apnea. *Circulation.* 1998;**97**(10):943–5.

42. Carlson JT, Hedner J, Elam M, *et al.* Augmented resting sympathetic activity in awake patients with obstructive sleep apnea. *Chest.* 1993;**103**(6):1763–8.

43. Hedner J, Ejnell H, Sellgren J, Hedner T, Wallin G. Is high and fluctuating muscle nerve sympathetic activity in the sleep apnoea syndrome of pathogenetic importance for the development of hypertension? *J Hypertens Suppl.* 1988;**6**(4):S529–31.

44. Fletcher EC. Sympathetic over activity in the etiology of hypertension of obstructive sleep apnea. *Sleep.* 2003;**26**(1):15–19.

45. Tamisier R, Pepin JL, Remy J, *et al.* 14 nights of intermittent hypoxia elevate daytime blood pressure and sympathetic activity in healthy humans. *Eur Respir J.* 2011;**37**(1):119–28.

46. Peled N, Greenberg A, Pillar G, *et al.* Contributions of hypoxia and respiratory disturbance index to sympathetic activation and blood pressure in obstructive sleep apnea syndrome. *Am J Hypertens.* 1998;**11**(11 Pt 1):1284–9.

47. Arnardottir ES, Mackiewicz M, Gislason T, Teff KL, Pack AI. Molecular signatures of obstructive sleep apnea in adults: a review and perspective. *Sleep.* 2009;**32**(4):447–70.

48. Kohler M, Stradling JR. Mechanisms of vascular damage in obstructive sleep apnea. *Nat Rev Cardiol.* 2010;**7**(12):677–85.

49. Barbe F, Duran-Cantolla J, Capote F, *et al.* Long-term effect of continuous positive airway pressure in hypertensive patients with sleep apnea. *Am J Respir Crit Care Med.* 2010;**181**(7):718–26.

50. O'Donoghue FJ, Wellard RM, Rochford PD, *et al.* Magnetic resonance spectroscopy and neurocognitive dysfunction in obstructive sleep apnea before and after CPAP treatment. *Sleep.* Jan 2012;**35**(1):41–8.

51. Macey PM. Is brain injury in obstructive sleep apnea reversible? *Sleep.* Jan 2012;**35**(1):9–10.

52. Pelttari LH, Hietanen EK, Salo TT, Kataja MJ, Kantola IM. Little effect of ordinary antihypertensive therapy on nocturnal high blood pressure in patients with sleep disordered breathing. *Am J Hypertens.* 1998;**11**(3 Pt 1):272–9.

Neuroimaging of treatment effects in obstructive sleep apnea

Mark S. Aloia and Vincenza Castronovo

Introduction

Obstructive sleep apnea (OSA) is a serious medical illness with significant comorbidities. OSA is characterized by repeated nocturnal disruptions of breathing. These disruptions involve either complete breathing cessations or partial cessations with accompanying oxygen desaturations. Events last at least 10 s to be characterized as significant and up to 7% of the general population has at least five of these events per hour of sleep. Many of these individuals have far more episodes than that, raising concern over the significant hypoxemia that can accumulate over the course of the night. Researchers have, for years, sought methods to quantify the consequences of OSA on the heart, the brain, and other key organ systems.

Neuroimaging studies have had broad scientific appeal in the study of OSA. Several studies have now been conducted on the neuroimaging consequences associated with OSA. These studies have taken the form of structural (e.g., voxel-based morphometry [VBM]) studies, functional (e.g., functional magnetic resonance imaging [fMRI]) studies, and chemical (magnetic resonance spectroscopy [MRS]) studies. The number of these studies is growing, but this area still fails to receive the attention from imaging researchers that has been given to other medical and psychiatric disorders. In general, structural neuroimaging studies have provided inconsistent evidence for generalized changes in gray matter, which may be related to differences in individual study samples. More consistent findings, however, have been reported regarding decreased hippocampal volume. This volumetric abnormality has been hypothesized to be associated with the effects of chronic, intermittent, nocturnal hypoxemia, although this model has not been formally tested. Epidemiological studies of structural white matter integrity generally have not found evidence of abnormalities in community-dwelling older adults with significant but undiagnosed breathing difficulties (Table 36.1).

OSA-associated dysfunction of the hippocampus is also supported from the findings from at least one MRS study [1]. Perhaps the most consistent finding of MRS studies, however, involves white matter dysfunction, particularly in the frontal lobes. The lack of convergence between MRS and structural MRI white matter findings should not be a primary concern given the variability in methodological approaches and sample characteristics. Specifically, negative structural white matter studies were often comprised of older adults from the general population, while spectroscopy samples contained middle-aged adults with clinically diagnosed OSA. In general, these results suggest that white matter abnormalities may be present in selected individuals who are at the greatest risk of vascular disease as a result of chronic apneic events. Existing models of central nervous system dysfunction have suggested that vascular compromise and endothelial dysfunction in OSA may preferentially damage small vessels in the brain, which could result in small vessel, white matter ischemia [2]. Some diffusion tensor imaging (DTI) studies have supported these findings.

Functional neuroimaging studies have also made vital contributions to the OSA literature. Functional MRI respiratory challenges provide support for OSA-related differences in neural function in multiple brain regions involved in respiratory and cardiovascular control, including regions in the motor, sensory, and autonomic integration brain areas. Although respiratory challenges conducted during wakefulness do not directly mimic the physiology of sleep disordered breathing, these studies nonetheless provide important insights into the neural mechanisms that may underlie the etiology or be involved in the physiological consequences associated with OSA. Results from the few fMRI studies in OSA individuals utilizing cognitive probes are mixed. Task-related results dependent upon the activation paradigm were evident in all studies. Some findings were consistent with fMRI studies of sleep deprivation, demonstrating compensatory recruitment of brain regions in untreated individuals.

Considered together, these neuroimaging findings provide support for the presence of OSA-associated neurofunctional and white matter impairments, particularly in the frontal lobes and hippocampus. Such impairment is consistent with proposed models of central nervous system and cognitive dysfunction in OSA implicating small vessel disease and prefrontal cortex [3, 4]. Given the relative paucity of experimental inquiry, however, additional studies are needed to more fully substantiate these models.

Several important limitations and considerations emerge from a review of the existing neuroimaging literature in OSA. Most notably, the vast majority of studies have included only male participants, thereby limiting generalizability of findings to men with OSA. Although the clinical presentation of OSA is

---

Neuroimaging of Sleep and Sleep Disorders, ed. Eric Nofzinger, Pierre Maquet, and Michael J. Thorpy. Published by Cambridge University Press. © Cambridge University Press 2013.

Table 36.1. Sample characteristics and major findings of reviewed OSA neuroimaging studies (BL + CPAP treatment)

Author, year published	Imaging modality	OSA subjects			Healthy subjects		Major findings	Comments
		N	Age	OSA severity	N	Age		
O'Donoghue et al., 2005 [7]	sMRI	27	46 (10)	AHI: 72 (17)	24	43 (9)	No group differences in gray matter in any regions of interest; slight decrease in whole-brain volume in OSA patients after 6 months PAP treatment	Only males. Threshold of $p < 0.05$ adjusted for multiple comparisons
Thomas et al., 2005 [14]	fMRI	16	40 (7)	RDI: 58 (16)	16	38 (6)	OSA: absence of activity in dorsolateral prefrontal cortex both before and after treatment; OSA patients performed more poorly on cognitive task compared with controls	15 male, 1 female
Canessa et al., 2011 [13]	VBM	17	44 (7.6)	AHI: 56 (19)	15	42 (6.6)	BL: impairments in most cognitive areas, mood and sleepiness associated with focal reductions of gray matter volume in the left hippocampus (entorhinal cortex), left posterior parietal cortex, and right superior frontal gyrus. After CPAP: significant improvements involving memory, attention, and executive-functioning that paralleled gray matter volume increases in hippocampal and frontal structures	Only males. No evaluation of controls after 3 months
Sweet et al., 2010 [16]	fMRI and 2-back	10	51.1 (9.3)	AHI: 42.4 (28)			Eleven clusters of significant 2-back-related deactivation identified. Significant further deactivation relative to the treatment adherent baseline was observed in the majority of these regions of interest during the withdrawal condition. The magnitude of deactivation during withdrawal was significantly associated with better working memory performance in the posterior cingulate and right postcentral gyrus, and greater sleepiness in the left and right medial frontal gyrus. Default mode network functions are further suspended as a result of a shifting of attention towards a more difficult active task in the context of lowered attentional capacity related to sleepiness	6 males, 4 females. 2 nights withdrawal. Limitation: lack of a resting control condition to confirm default mode network activity
Aloia et al., 2009 [17]	fMRI + 2-back verbal working memory paradigm under PAP (at least one week) or non-treatment (two consecutive nights)	9	51.1 (9.3)	AHI: 42.4 (28.2)			Treatment effects were significant, with greater deactivation in the right posterior insula and over-activation in the right inferior parietal lobule. The observed responses to PAP treatment withdrawal were more extreme in all regions of interest, such that 2-back-related activity increased and 2-back-related deactivation decreased further relative to the 0-back control task. The withdrawal of	5 males, 4 females

Table 36.1. (cont.)

Author, year published	Imaging modality	OSA subjects			Healthy subjects		Major findings	Comments
		N	Age	OSA severity	N	Age		
							PAP treatment in effectively treated individuals with OSA might result in the need to reallocate resources in order to perform at the same cognitive level	
Castronovo *et al.*, 2009 [15].	fMRI + 2-back working memory task	17	43.9 (7.8)	AHI: 50.1 (24.8)	15	42.1 (6.6)	OSA patients showed increased activations in the left frontal cortex, medial precuneus, and hippocampus, and decreased activations in the caudal pons without treatment. With treatment decreased activation in the left inferior frontal gyrus and anterior cingulate cortex, and bilaterally in the hippocampus. Neurocognitive tests mostly improved with treatment. Over-recruitment of brain regions (with the same level of performance on a working memory task) and decreases of activation in prefrontal and hippocampal structures after treatment→ possible neural compensation mechanism that is reduced by effective treatment.	Only males. No evaluation of controls at 3 months
Minoguchi *et al.*, 2007 [12]	MRI for silent brain infarction (SBI), levels of soluble CD40 ligand (sCD40L), soluble P-selectin (sP-selectin), PCR	50 OSA (24 after 3 months of CPAP)	Mild OSA 47.6 (1.9) Moderate to severe OSA 50.5 (1.7)	Mild OSA 10.9 (0.6) Moderate to severe OSA 44.9 (3.9)	15 obese	48.5 (3.1)	Percentage of patients with moderate to severe OSA with SBI (25.0%) higher than in obese control subjects (6.7%) or mild OSA (7.7%). Serum levels of sCD40L and sP-selectin higher in moderate-severe OSA than in obese ($p < 0.05$) or mild OSA ($p < 0.05$). CPAP significantly decreased serum levels of sCD40L ($p < 0.03$) and sP-selectin ($p < 0.01$) in moderate-severe OSA	Only males
Matsuo A *et al.*, 2011 [18]	Near-infrared spectrometry (NIRS) + hemoglobin indices	15 (9 with CPAP)	39.5 (7.1)	AHI: 66.3 (17.3)	12	31.9 (7.7)	Differential light absorbance of oxyhemoglobin (HbO) decreased during obstructive events; changes in total hemoglobin (HbT = HbO + HbD) and deoxyhemoglobin (HbD). HbD showed adverse increases, and the values of these hemoglobin indices returned to the baseline values at the end of each respiratory event in the OSAS group. The fluctuations in these cerebral hemoglobin indices during sleep were significantly larger in the OSAS group than in the control group. Moreover, in the OSAS group, these changes correlated strongly with the change in SpO_2. When using	14 male, 1 female

							CPAP, not only respiratory events but also the fluctuations in both the cerebral hemoglobin indices and SpO_2 were almost completely suppressed. Arterial oxygen desaturation is clearly related to cerebral oxygenation, and fluctuations of hemoglobin indices can be suppressed with CPAP	
Tonon et al., 2007 [19]	Single voxel H-MRS in parieto-occipital cortex + absolute concentrations of N-acetylaspartate (NAA), creatine, and choline were measured, acquiring spectra at multiple echo-times and using water as internal standard	14	48 (7)	RDI: 57 (24)	10		Normal global cognitive functioning before CPAP. Before CPAP: [NAA] in OSAS = 11.86 (0.8) significantly lower than in controls = 12.8 (0.93), p = 0.01. Positively correlated with minimum SpO_2 during sleep (r = 0.69; p = 0.006) and MSLT scores (= 0.62; p = 0.01). Cortical [NAA] reduction persisted after therapy 11.94 (1.3), p = 0.87 versus pre-CPAP. OSA patients have cortical metabolic changes consistent with neuronal loss even in the absence of vascular comorbidities. Metabolic changes persisted after CPAP in the absence of EDS, nocturnal arousals, and major cognitive deficits, likely related to hypoxic damage prior to CPAP treatment	Only males
Castronovo et al., 2010 [20]	DTI	15	43.7 (7.5)	AHI: 55.1 (19)	15	42.1 (6.6)	Extensive white matter alterations in OSA compared with controls. Patients after 12 months of CPAP treatment showed a decrease in FA localized in the superior-longitudinal fasciculus, bilaterally, in the fornix, in the fibers of the corpus callosum close to the anterior-frontal and prefrontal cingulated cortices. The comparison between controls and patients' FA maps along time revealed that the extension of the blobs decreases with time suggesting a possible role of the treatment	Only males. No evaluation of controls at 12 months

Age presented in mean (sd) for all studies.
OSA severity measures presented in mean (sd).
sMRI = Structural magnetic resonance imaging, MRS – magnetic resonance spectroscopy, fMRI – functional magnetic resonance imaging, VBM – voxel-based morphometry, DTI – diffusion tensor imaging, BL – baseline,
CPAP = continuous positive airway pressure;
AHI=Apnea Hypopnea Index; RDI=Respiratory Disturbance Index; OSAS = obstructive sleep apnea syndroms; EDS = excessive daytime sleeiness,

more common in men than in women [5, 6], the gender ratio of published studies does not generally reflect this prevalence. Consideration of the potential moderating effects of IQ and education is also important, particularly with respect to treatment adherence studies and performance on cognitive challenges. Age may also moderate the effect of OSA on brain structure and function. For instance, advanced age may mask the effects of OSA on cerebral integrity. Associations between sleep parameters and neuroimaging may be less robust among older adults given the myriad of age-related comorbid factors that could affect this relationship. Likewise, length of illness is a potentially confounding variable that is difficult to assess in the OSA patient and therefore difficult to investigate adequately. Several investigators have specifically focused on treatment-naive patients in an attempt to address this issue (e.g., [7–10]), but more direct assessment methods (e.g , bed partner questionnaire) may be necessary. Although examination of patients with a wide range of OSA severity is necessary to gain a thorough understanding of the clinical and physiological characteristics of the disorder, caution should be taken when comparing and interpreting results across studies. There may be a critical threshold associated with the clinical expression of OSA-related pathological insult to the brain. Similarly, very severe OSA patients may be more likely to have comorbid illness that may independently compromise the brain. In a study of hypertension in the Wisconsin Sleep Cohort, investigators suggested that the relationship between OSA and hypertension varied across OSA severity levels [11]. Clearly, continued examination of the complex relationship between disease severity and comorbid medical conditions is critical.

Perhaps one of the most significant problems associated with neuroimaging in OSA involves the sampling bias that exists when conducting MRI scans on obese OSA patients. Although body mass index is often reported in studies, the effect of body mass indices on observed findings is generally not explored nor discussed. In a practical sense, many OSA patients are unable to appropriately fit into the MRI scanner, which is limiting even further with functional scans, which often require participants to view a projection screen over their midsection. It is therefore likely that OSA samples included in neuroimaging studies represent only a subgroup of patients with the disorder. This limits interpretation regarding the interaction of OSA and obesity and/or any pathophysiological differences in OSA among obese and non-obese patients. There will likely be methods to remedy this problem as continued efforts increasingly focus on the utilization of these techniques in obesity, but investigators should be aware of this sampling bias until these issues are resolved.

A previous review of the neuroimaging studies in OSA called for specific attention to longitudinal studies of the treatment effects of OSA on neuroimaging.

This chapter focuses on those studies where treatment effects were considered. We will not reiterate baseline comparisons of imaging findings compared to normal, nor will we speak specifically of the various findings specific to certain cognitive challenges as there are other chapters devoted to

these concepts specifically. We will discuss these studies by combining them according to the imaging technique employed.

Structural imaging studies

There have been a total of three imaging studies in OSA examining the structural brain effects of treatment. All utilized continuous positive airway pressure (CPAP) as the treatment of choice. The first study, conducted by O'Donoghue *et al.*, examined structural brain changes associated with CPAP treatment over the course of six months [7]. Twenty-three patients were studied after six months of CPAP treatment with a mean of 5.8 ± 1.7 h of CPAP use per night. Six months of treatment resulted in slight, but rather insignificant, decreases in whole-brain volume (corresponding to a volume decrement of approximately 4%). These results stood up to more post hoc assessments applying different analyses to assess the degree to which findings were related to the analytical procedure itself. It was unclear as to whether or not this minimal effect was related to resolving edema or some indirect effect on the vasculature of the brain.

The second study examined MRI for silent brain infarction (SBI) in 24 treated OSA patients, longitudinally [12]. The patients were scanned prior to treatment and again after three months on CPAP. Adherence to CPAP was not reported. The percentage of patients with moderate to severe OSA who had SBI (25.0%) was higher than that of obese control subjects (6.7%) or patients with mild OSA (7.7%). SBI was located in subcortical white matter (54%), in the basal ganglia and thalamus (43%), and in the brainstem (3%) in patients with moderate to severe OSA. Levels of soluble CD40 ligand (sCD40L), soluble P-selectin (sP-selectin) and C-reactive protein (CRP) were also measured. Serum levels of sCD40L and sP-selectin were significantly higher in patients with moderate to severe OSA than in obese control subjects or patients with mild OSA. CPAP treatment in patients with moderate to severe OSA resulted in significant decrease of all variables: respectively, sCD40L 6.95 ± 0.79 to 4.62 ± 0.67 ng/ml, sP-selection 86.9 ± 6.4 to 67.2 ± 4.8 pg/ml, and CRP 0.28 ± 0.04 to 0.16 ± 0.03 mg/dl. These results suggest that platelet activation is increased in patients with moderate to severe OSA, and, in combination with an increased prevalence of SBI, may lead to an elevated risk of cerebrovascular morbidity. CRP is both a marker of inflammation and a factor in the pathogenesis of atherosclerosis as it works in part by activating endothelial cells and coronary artery smooth muscle cells. If OSA is the proximal mediator of increased systemic inflammation and platelet activation, these factors may play a potential role in the progression of atherosclerosis in patients with OSA. The hypoxic stress of OSA is potentially a proximal mediator of the systemic inflammation and platelet activation that lead to SBI in patients with OSA. If the hypoxic stress of OSA is a causal factor in promoting an inflammatory, platelet-activated state, then treatment with CPAP should act to decrease levels of CRP, sCD40L, and sP-selectin. Treatment of nocturnal hypoxic stress in patients with OSA can reduce serum levels of sCD40L and sP-selectin

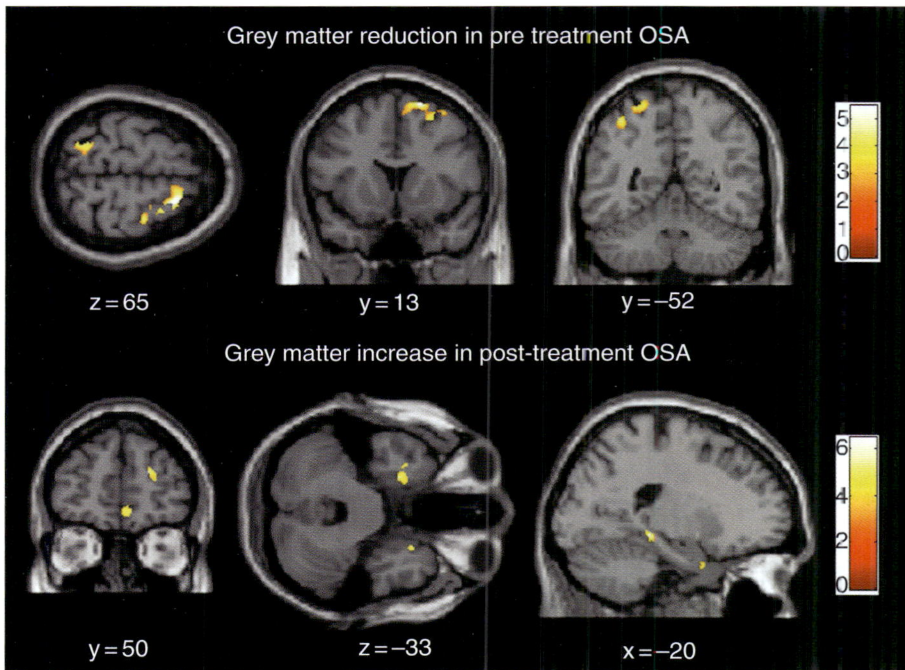

Figure 36.1 Structural brain changes in OSA before and after CPAP. *Top*: Regions showing a gray matter volume decrease in untreated OSA patients compared with control subjects (p , 0.05 corrected for multiple comparisons based on cluster-extent). *Bottom*: Regions showing a gray matter volume increase in post-treatment, compared with pretreatment (p , 0.05 corrected for multiple comparisons based on cluster-extent).

and, potentially, lower the risk for development of SBI. Thus, hypoxic stress in patients with moderate to severe OSA may be associated with activation of platelets and increased prevalence of SBI. CPAP was seen, in this study, to be an important treatment intervention for decreasing the cerebrovascular risk in this susceptible patient population.

The final study examined 17 patients after three months of CPAP treatment [13]. Focal reductions of gray matter volume were noted in the left hippocampus (entorhinal cortex), left posterior parietal cortex, and right superior frontal gyrus comparing patients with normal controls at baseline. Three months of CPAP treatment, however, resulted in increases in hippocampal and frontal volumes (Figure 36.1). What is even more interesting is that these brain changes correlated with changes on cognitive testing (improvements in memory, attention, and executive-functioning). All patients had documented adherence to treatment (5.8 ± 0.6 h/night; 82.5% of the nights). This is at least suggestive of the possibility that patients who use treatment consistently can have direct recovery on brain size that correlates well with functional changes.

Together, the structural studies suggest that there are some notable changes in the structure of the human brain when CPAP is used to correct OSA [7, 12, 13]. Some of these changes are even associated with cognitive changes in the expected cognitive domains and are seen with as little as only three months of treatment.

Functional studies

There are four functional imaging studies that examined treatment effects [14–17]. Again, all studies utilized CPAP as the treatment of choice. The first study was conducted by Thomas *et al.* [14]. This study made strong comparisons between OSA patients and normal controls, but only followed six participants after treatment. Treated patients continued to demonstrate a reduction in activity associated with a cognitive challenge compared with normal controls. This study suffered from a significant lack of power, but nonetheless started researchers thinking about the effects of CPAP on cognitive function during a cognitive challenge.

Castronovo *et al.* (2009) conducted a study following 17 patients over a three-month course of CPAP treatment [15]. These were the same patients reported in the structural study described above [13]. Baseline scanning noted over-recruitment of certain brain regions (left frontal cortex, medial precuneus and hippocampus) associated with a working memory task compared with normal controls. The authors reported that over-recruitment of brain regions was associated with the same level of performance, suggesting that patients required greater activation of brain networks to achieve the same levels of performance. Significant reductions of activation in both the prefrontal (left inferior frontal gyrus and anterior cingulated cortex) and hippocampal (bilateral hippocampus) regions of the brain were also reported when treatment imaging was compared to baseline imaging (Figure 36.2). These reductions were noted in areas of the brain that were noted to increase in size in the structural study described above. These results suggest that CPAP improves brain functioning in certain areas, but that it may not "normalize" function completely.

One study specifically examined the withdrawal of treatment employing functional neuroimaging methodology [16]. The study ran on the premise that patients often take a treatment holiday for a day or two without any assumed consequences. This study examined the changes in brain function associated with such a holiday. All patients had been strong users of CPAP for at least three months prior to entry into the study. Patients

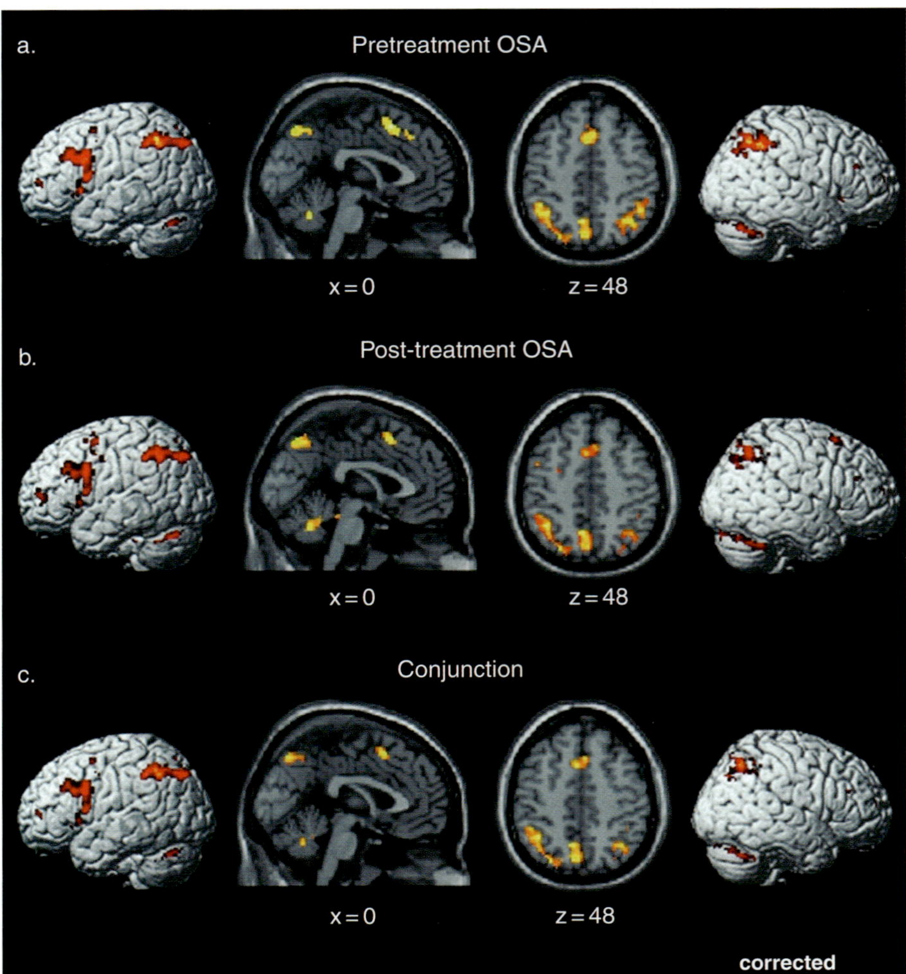

Figure 36.2 Common parametric effects of working memory load in pretreatment and post-treatment OSA patients. From top to bottom, the regions showing a significant linear increase of cerebral activation related to working memory load in pretreatment OSA patients (a), post-treatment OSA patients (b), and in both groups (c). P < 0.05 FWE (family-wise-error) corrected, based on cluster-extent.

were then examined after "treatment-on" and "treatment-off" conditions. Findings suggested specific over activation in the right inferior parietal lobe and deactivation in the right posterior insula associated with a working memory challenge under the treatment-off condition. It should also be noted that assumed brain effort (either to activate a region or deactivate a region) was stronger under the treatment-off condition. The authors concluded that resources required some reallocation and effort increased during the treatment holiday.

The same withdrawal study examined the effects of treatment holiday on the default mode network [17]. The authors demonstrated that the default mode network deactivates more when a cognitive challenge is administered under the treatment-off condition. This suggests that greater cognitive effort is required to perform the task as greater turning off of the default mode network is associated with treatment withdrawal and with relatively better cognitive performance. Although the two withdrawal studies had similar results, they need to be replicated as the methods and the participants were the same across studies.

The functional imaging studies together suggest that changes in brain function associated with working memory are evident when comparing treatment with no-treatment conditions in patients with OSA. Specifically, treatment often results in the recruitment of fewer cognitive resources to perform at the same level or better. Even treatment withdrawal for as few as two consecutive nights results in the over-recruitment of brain regions to perform a given cognitive task. These resource recruitments are sometimes related to sleepiness and other consequences of OSA, but they demonstrate functional brain changes, although sometimes subtle, associated with the effective use of CPAP.

Other imaging techniques

Matsuo *et al.* examined near-infrared spectroscopy (NIRS) during CPAP treatment in OSA patients [18]. The authors found that oxyhemoglobin (HbO) decreased during obstructive respiratory events, while total hemoglobin (HbT) and deoxy-hemoglobin (HbD) showed adverse increases and returned to the baseline values at the end of each respiratory event. These fluctuations correlated strongly with the change in peripheral O_2 saturation (SpO_2). During apnea or hypopnea events, cardiac output decreases, but cerebral arteries dilate mainly due to hypercapnia. These results support the idea that lowered cerebral resistance raises cerebral blood volume in spite of the reduction of cardiac output. With CPAP, not only respiratory events but also the fluctuations in both the cerebral hemoglobin indices and SpO_2 were almost completely suppressed (the maximum values of HbO, HbD, and HbT, as well as averaged values of HbD and HbT, were significantly smaller). These findings strongly support the fact that OSA treatment not only restores SpO_2 but also cerebral tissue oxygenation, leading to the stabilization of cerebral blood volume. This study partially explains the mechanism of the nocturnal occurrence of stroke in OSA and the effectiveness of CPAP for the prevention of stroke in these patients, although this requires further investigation. One significant limitation of this study is that measurements of NIRS were performed not during nocturnal sleep but during a short daytime nap mostly consistent of stage 1 and 2 non-rapid eye movement (NREM). The authors concluded that arterial oxygen desaturation is clearly related to cerebral oxygenation and that OSA-associated abnormalities in both Hbo and Hbd can be suppressed with CPAP treatment.

Another imaging and treatment-related study reviewed here employed MRS [19]. MRS is a technique that identifies metabolic changes in the brain using MRI. This study was suggestive of a loss of neurons in patients with OSA, replicating other MRS studies that compared OSA patients with normal controls. Moreover, this study examined changes in these brain metabolites after six months of CPAP treatment. Treatment did not normalize these metabolites. Metabolite changes were also not associated with sleepiness, cognitive dysfunction, or OSA severity. This suggests that there is a loss of neurons associated with the hypoxemia in OSA and that at least some of these changes are persistent even after six months of treatment. This final study is most striking in its report that metabolic changes to the brain that are associated with OSA are sometimes permanent. This is something many researchers and clinicians have suspected for years and calls into question the degree to which CPAP is needed or even effective at reducing the chance of further brain decline. The very supposition that OSA can lead to permanent brain damage and cell loss suggests that additional treatment studies and longitudinal non-adherence studies should be considered. Treatment providers can only advise patients as to the necessity of CPAP with significant investment in clinical research on the direct and indirect effects of CPAP on the brain.

The final imaging and treatment-related study employed the technique of DTI, which measures the flow of water through brain tissue [20]. This flow is relatively more focused and directed when tissue is compact, for example in intact white matter (axonal) tracts of the brain. Compromised white matter tracts can have functional consequences such as slowed information processing, impaired neurocognitive performance, and even aberrant emotional functioning, all of which have been reported in OSA. Macey *et al.*, in 2008, measured fractional anisotropy (FA), a measure of white matter integrity, among 41 patients with moderate to severe OSA and found a bilateral and nearly global white matter involvement in OSA compared with normal controls [21]. Castronovo *et al.*, in 2010, demonstrated the possible reversibility of white matter abnormalities with CPAP treatment [20] in the same 17 patients reported on above in the VBM and fMRI sections [13, 15]. They investigated white matter integrity in 17 male severe OSA patients after 3 and 12 months of CPAP treatment, confirming the hypothesis

of a "functional" sufferance of cellular tissue rather than a permanent tissue loss or cellular death. At baseline, OSA patients showed lower FA values in multiple supratentorial brain areas. In particular, in the right hemisphere, a significant decrease of FA values was observed at the level of subcortical white matter of the superior and inferior parietal lobes, including fibers of the superior longitudinal fasciculus, and at the level of deep frontal white matter, corresponding to a portion of the arcuate fasciculus. Also, another region showed lower FA corresponding to transcallosal connections from the medial prefrontal area. In the left hemisphere, a large area of subcortical white matter of the superior parietal lobe, containing fibers of the superior longitudinal fascicle, showed lower FA in the OSA group, as well as another region in the left inferior frontal gyrus including fibers of the frontal portion of uncinate fasciculus. After three months of treatment with CPAP only some of these areas showed a decrease of extension in OSA patients compared with controls. A full year of treatment with CPAP resulted in reductions of all areas, both with respect to baseline and with respect to the three-month follow-up. The clinical relevance of these findings is supported by the results of the correlation analysis that demonstrated a correlation between reduced FA and higher scores on the two sleepiness scales (Epworth Sleepiness Scale [ESS], Pittsburgh Sleep Quality Index [PSQI]). FA reductions were also related to increases of the time required to perform executive tasks, combined with more errors (Stroop, Paced Auditory Serial Addition Task [PASAT], Trial making A and B). In contrast, higher FA values were associated with better performance on short- and long-term memory tasks. This study is the first to demonstrate compromised DTI metrics among patients with OSA compared with normal controls across a number of white matter tracts. Moreover, the study found only some limited changes in DTI after three months of treatment but more notable changes were visible over the course of one year of treatment. It is important to note that despite the mechanism underlying these reported brain changes, both VBM and DTI demonstrate change with treatment in this sample. This may be the most important aspect of the three Italian studies (VBM, fMRI, and DTI [13, 15, 20]), regardless of the timing or extent of this change. Simply demonstrating changes with treatment is the first step in showing that at least some of the impairments seen in the brains of patients with OSA are remediable with treatment and are not due to permanent damage, suggesting the ability of OSA patients to recover from brain dysfunction.

Conclusions

Although fewer studies have been conducted to examine the effects of treatment for OSA on imaging outcomes, there are some compelling findings that merit further investigation. Several of these findings might be specific to the imaging technique employed. Others may simply be different views of the same recovery phenomenon. In either case, further investigation should be driven by specific theoretical models of the mechanisms of brain dysfunction in OSA. If these theorized mechanisms are predominantly cardiovascular, then measurements should take into account the cardiovascular comorbidity of patients and the degree to which the employed imaging technique may be affected by cardiovascular compromise. If the theorized effect is hypoxemia, then the methodology employed should make efforts to relate outcomes to levels of hypoxemia or to persistence of hypoxemia among patients. Data from CPAP devices themselves can also help identify non-responders to treatment to better explain the specific effects of CPAP on imaging outcomes. One must be careful, however, not to apply too much valence to imaging findings in this population, as imaging studies are limited in their ability to assess the effects of OSA for several reasons.

One involves the selection bias in imaging apneic obese patients. Scanners often accommodate only a portion of obese patients making a true representative sample of OSA patients difficult to scan. Also, hypertension can affect imaging outcomes and it is highly prevalent among OSA patients. Researchers should consider developing a working task force to determine common imaging techniques and parameters to apply to OSA studies, allowing better comparison between studies. Despite these limitations, the current cohort of studies offers promise to the imaging researcher that imaging can be utilized to detect important, and even clinically relevant, changes associated with treatment among OSA patients.

References

1. Bartlett DJ, Rae C, Thompson CH, *et al.* Hippocampal area metabolites relate to severity and cognitive function in obstructive sleep apnea. *Sleep Med.* 2004;**5**(6):593–6.

2. Lanfranchi P, Somers VK. Obstructive sleep apnea and vascular disease. *Respir Res.* 2001;**2**(6):315–19.

3. Aloia MS, Arnedt JT, Davis JD, *et al.* Neuropsychological sequelae of obstructive sleep apnea-hypopnea syndrome: a critical review. *J Int Neuropsychol Soc.* 2004;**10**(5):772–85.

4. Beebe DW, Gozal D. Obstructive sleep apnea and the prefrontal cortex: towards a comprehensive model linking nocturnal upper airway obstruction to daytime cognitive and behavioral deficits. *J Sleep Res.* 2002;**11**(1):1–16.

5. Young T, Palta M, Dempsey J, *et al.* The occurrence of sleep-disordered breathing among middle-aged adults. *N Engl J Med.* 1993;**328**(17):1230–5.

6. Shepertycky MR, Banno K, Kryger MH. Differences between men and women in the clinical presentation of patients diagnosed with obstructive sleep apnea syndrome. *Sleep.* 2005;**28**(3):309–14.

7. O'Donoghue FJ, Briellmann RS, Rochford PD, *et al.* Cerebral structural changes in severe obstructive sleep apnea. *Am J Respir Crit Care Med.* 2005;**171**(10):1185–90.

8. Morrell MJ, McRobbie DW, Quest RA, *et al.* Changes in brain morphology associated with obstructive sleep apnea. *Sleep Med.* 2003;**4**(5):451–4.

9. Alchanatis M, Deligiorgis N, Zias N, *et al.* Frontal brain lobe impairment in obstructive sleep apnoea: a proton MR spectroscopy study. *Eur Respir J.* 2004;**24**(6):980–6.

10. Ayalon L, Ancoli-Israel S, Klemfuss Z, *et al.* Increased brain activation during verbal learning in obstructive sleep apnea. *Neuroimage.* 2006;**31** (4):1817–25.

11. Lin L, Finn L, Zhang J, *et al.* Angiotensin-converting enzyme, sleep-disordered breathing, and hypertension. *Am J Respir Crit Care Med.* 2004;**170** (12):1349–53.

12. Minoguchi K, Yokoe T, Tazaki T, *et al.* Silent brain infarction and platelet activation in obstructive sleep apnea. *Am J Respir Crit Care Med.* 2007;**175**:612–617.

13. Canessa N, Castronovo V, Cappa SF, *et al.* Obstructive sleep apnea: brain structural changes and neurocognitive function before and after treatment. *Am J Respir Crit Care Med.* 2011;**183** (10):1419–26.

14. Thomas RJ, Rosen BR, Stern CE, *et al.* Functional imaging of working memory in obstructive sleep-disordered breathing. *J Appl Physiol.* 2005;**98** (6):2226–34.

15. Castronovo V, Canessa N, Ferini-Strambi L, *et al.* Brain activation changes before and after PAP treatment in obstructive sleep apnea. *Sleep.* 2009;**32**(9):1161–72.

16. Sweet LH, Jerskey BA, Aloia MS. Default network response to a working memory challenge after withdrawal of continuous positive airway pressure treatment for obstructive sleep apnea. *Brain Imaging Behav.* 2010;**4**(2):155–63.

17. Aloia MS, Sweet LH, Jerskey BA, *et al.* Treatment effects on brain activity during a working memory task in obstructive sleep apnea. *J Sleep Res.* 2009;**18**(4):404–10.

18. Matsuo A, Inoue Y, Namba K, Chiba H. Changes in cerebral hemoglobin indices in obstructive sleep apnea syndrome with nasal continuous positive airway pressure treatment. *Sleep Breath.* 2011;**15**:487–92.

19. Tonon C, Vetrugno R, Lodi R, *et al.* Proton magnetic resonance spectroscopy study of brain metabolism in obstructive sleep apnoea syndrome before and after continuous positive airway pressure treatment. *Sleep.* 2007;**30**(3):305–311.

20. Castronovo V, Scifo P, Aloia MS, *et al.* White matter integrity in obstructive sleep apnea (OSA): changes in diffusion tensor imaging (DTI) after CPAP treatment. *Sleep.* 2010;**33**: A115.

21. Macey PM, Kumar R, Woo MA, *et al.* Brain structural changes in obstructive sleep apnea. *Sleep.* 2008;**31**(7):967–77.

Structural and functional neuroimaging of congenital central hypoventilation syndrome

Ronald M. Harper and Rajesh Kumar

Introduction

Many insights into normal physiological processes are obtained by examining "Experiments of Nature," or disease processes which offer the opportunity to view mechanisms of loss of particular abilities. Congenital central hypoventilation syndrome (CCHS) is a condition with substantial potential to provide insights into normal breathing and autonomic control. The syndrome is rare, and results from defects in the paired-like homeobox 2B (*PHOX2B*) gene, which encodes a transcription factor that determines autonomic nervous system development [1–4]. The principal clinical concern is that breathing drive during sleep is lost, requiring mechanical nocturnal ventilation, and, with severe mutations, 24 h breathing support. In addition, ventilatory responses to CO_2 and O_2 are lost, and the sensitivity loss includes both automatic, unconscious changes in breathing patterns with alterations in chemical drive, as well as the perception of air hunger induced by hypercapnia or low O_2 [5–8]; for review, see [9]. The latter loss-of-emotion condition leads to failure to initiate breathing during otherwise innocuous behaviors, e.g., quiet, non-moving activities, and can result in damaging and potentially fatal scenarios. Remarkably, voluntary breathing efforts are retained, and ventilation increases to active or passive movement of the peripheral limbs [10, 11]. The loss of both integration of chemical drives to breathe, as well as disrupted emotional or affective drives provide a unique preparation to visualize with non-invasive imaging procedures the brain areas mediating those contributions to respiration.

Since autonomic nervous system development is targeted by *PHOX2B*, the consequences from mutations to parasympathetic and sympathetic functions are serious. Temperature control is severely affected, and both spontaneous blood pressure patterns, such as nocturnal "dipping," and evoked responses to challenges, including syncope with strain, heart rate acceleration to cold pressor stimulation, or patterns of heart rate to Valsalva maneuvers are altered [12, 13]. Other autonomic functions are modified; profuse sweating is common, and pupillary dilation is affected, often unilaterally, and visual focusing, as well as certain somatic eye movement coordination, is often difficult. The normal variation of heart rate with breathing is lost [14], and episodes of asystole are a constant threat in CCHS children with severe *PHOX2B* mutations [7]. Since sympathetic and parasympathetic regulation involves

brain structures located in such diverse areas as the prefrontal cortex, hypothalamus, midbrain, medulla, and cerebellum, and CCHS may modify structural integrity and function in any or all of those structures, as well as axons between structures, techniques which allow overall visualization of brain tissue injury and function are required. Structural and functional magnetic resonance imaging (MRI) procedures provide valuable tools to gain insights into these processes.

Although the greatest proportion of CCHS cases are detected in the newborn period, late-onset cases have also been found, even as late as adulthood, with the appearance of hypoventilation often accompanying a severe stress, such as brain meningeal infection, anesthesia, or severe respiratory illness [4, 7] Little is known of how these late-onset cases differ from traditional CCHS cases in brain structure and function, and this chapter focuses on classic CCHS cases in which symptoms appear early in life.

MRI tools for CCHS

The principal issues in CCHS are to determine what brain structures are damaged in CCHS to cause the loss of CO_2 and O_2 sensitivity, disturbances in autonomic function, and other affective and cognitive deficits. MRI procedures provide some of the few non-invasive means to assess the injured brain structures and function in this very rare syndrome. To evaluate gray matter injury, a variety of techniques have been used, including assessment of regional volume changes using high-resolution T1-weighted images, T2-relaxometry procedures, which assess free water within tissue, with altered values used as an index of injury, and mean diffusivity, which evaluates overall water diffusion within tissue, and also can assess tissue injury. In addition, it became apparent from both functional and structural studies of nuclear areas that white matter is also damaged in CCHS. Overall evaluation of white matter can be performed using a diffusion tensor imaging (DTI)-based technique, fractional anisotropy, which can examine fiber integrity. Specialized DTI-based techniques allow further examination of fiber injury; these techniques include axial and radial diffusivity, which assess water diffusion along the path of axons or at right angles to the axons, respectively, and can provide indications of axonal and myelin integrity, respectively. Fiber tractography

Neuroimaging of Sleep and Sleep Disorders, ed. Eric Nofzinger, Pierre Maquet, and Michael J. Thorpy. Published by Cambridge University Press. © Cambridge University Press 2013.

procedures are also useful for following the path and direction of fibers, as well as relative loss of fibers between particular structures over controls.

To demonstrate that the structural injury impacts function of affected brain structures, functional procedures (fMRI) using blood oxygen level-dependent (BOLD) contrast are implemented; since interactions between brain structures and timing of activation between areas are critical issues for physiological functions deficient in CCHS, data acquisition sequences are designed to be as rapid as possible to collect fMRI signals at appropriate temporal resolution.

Structural injury underlying autonomic deficits

Although the focus of scientific and clinical attention in CCHS has principally been on the loss of breathing drive during sleep, the autonomic ganglia are targeted by *PHOX2B* gene mutations, which, in addition to direct neural injury, or, possibly, surrounding glia, can then alter vascular supply to tissue. Additional injury may develop from hypoxic episodes as a consequence of ventilatory problems. T2-relaxometry procedures have revealed some of the injury contributing to the autonomic regulatory issues, as shown in Figure 37.1 (left). Thermoregulation, lost in CCHS, contributes to such symptoms as shivering in midsummer, inability to tolerate cold water immersion, and extreme difficulty to breathe with fever or high body temperature. Such temperature regulation depends on the integrity of the anterior hypothalamus, which is compromised in CCHS. A column of injury extends from the basal forebrain through the anterior hypothalamus, and continues to the posterior hypothalamus (Figure 37.1 [i]).

Blood pressure regulation is severely affected in CCHS; in addition to the hypothalamic injury, brain areas that dampen extremes of blood pressure elevation and lowering, important for understanding the nature of frequent syncope in CCHS, are damaged; these areas include the cerebellar cortex (Figure 37.1 [iv]). The ventral medial prefrontal cortex, genu of the cingulate, and mid- and posterior cingulate (Figure 37.1 [ii and iii]), essential structures for cardiovascular, and especially blood pressure, regulation also show injury. Impaired cerebral cardiovascular regulation is a major concern in CCHS, since a portion of the neural injury likely develops from early, compromised perfusion, induced by *PHOX2B* effects on autonomic

nuclei; the impaired cerebral vascular regulation in CCHS has been noted by arterial spin labeling imaging techniques [15].

Axial and radial diffusivity measures allow evaluation of fiber characteristics in affected brain areas. In particular, axial diffusivity has been valuable in demonstrating midbrain, medullary, and cerebellar injury [16]. Although cortical, cerebellar, and diencephalic areas which are involved in blood pressure control are severely affected, as shown by T2-relaxometry procedures, medullary regions are always a focus as regulatory sites for sympathetic action before projecting to the intermediolateral column of the spinal cord, and the ventro lateral medulla shows injury on the right side (Figure 37.1 [C, D]). Parasympathetic components of the autonomic nervous system are also affected, as shown by impaired pupillary dilation and secretory difficulties; the parasympathetic nuclei could not be isolated with the resolution of the technique used here, but are immediately adjacent to the periaqueductal gray, which shows significant injury (Figure 37.1 [A]). In addition, the midline raphe with its serotonergic neurons is damaged (Figure 37.1 [B]); serotonergic fibers play significant roles in chemoreception, as well as vascular dilation, temperature control, blood pressure, and pain [17, 18]. The damage to serotonergic fibers may play a critical role in dilation of the basilar arteries in CCHS [19].

As is the case for obstructive sleep apnea (OSA), the deep cerebellar nuclei, including the fastigial "autonomic" nuclei, are affected in CCHS [16, 20, 21], possibly a consequence of hypoxic episodes, or, as demonstrated in the Gensat *Phox2b* mouse atlases [22] (http://www.gensat.org/imagenavigator.jsp?imageID=62943), resulting from *PHOX2B* mutations affecting cerebellar glia or other tissue. The injury establishes a potential mechanism underlying the loss of coordination of blood pressure with breathing and movement in CCHS, paralleling serious consequences of fastigial damage in the animal literature [23].

The insular cortex, which plays essential roles in the baroreflex and in influencing hypothalamic action in a number of pain and other autonomic regulatory roles [24], is injured severely in CCHS (Figure 37.4). The cingulate cortex, portions of which are involved in sympathetic regulation, and other portions of which are implicated in initiation of urination and affect, such as perception of breathlessness, is injured, as is the principal fiber bundle within the cingulate cortex, the cingulum bundle (Figure 37.4 [c, d, g]). The ventral medial prefrontal

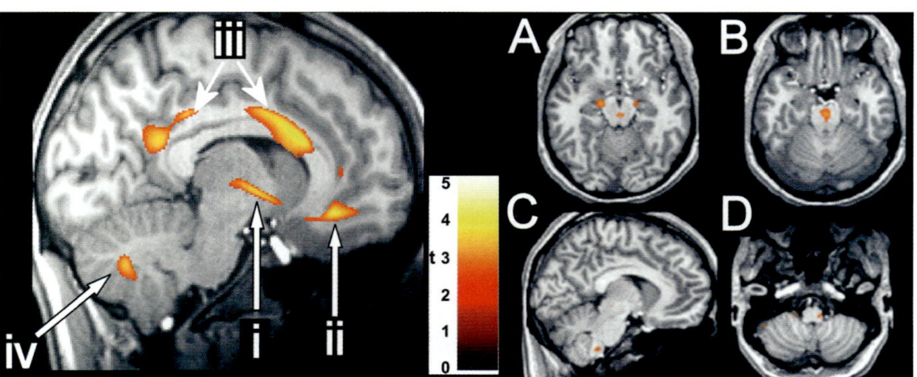

Figure 37.1 *Left*: T2-relaxometry procedures (free water within tissue) in 12 CCHS subjects relative to 28 age- and gender-matched controls, showing injury in hypothalamic (i) prefrontal and cingulate cortices (ii and iii), and cerebellar (iv) sites. *Right*: Axial diffusivity measures from 12 CCHS and 26 control subjects, showing injury in periaqueductal gray (PAG) and cerebral peduncles (A), PAG and raphe (B), and ventrolateral medulla (C, D). (Adapted from Kumar *et al.* [20] and Kumar *et al.* [16] with permission.)

cortex is affected (Figure 37.1 [ii]), as are areas within the temporal and parietal cortices. All of these structures with injury, and especially the ventrolateral medulla, caudal raphe, fastigial nuclei, insular, cingulate, and ventral medial prefrontal cortices likely contribute to the impaired cardiovascular and breathing responses to cold pressor, Valsalva, and respiratory challenges.

CO₂ and O₂ regulation

A principal issue in any examination of respiratory drive during sleep is to determine the nature of processes which mediate CO_2 drive, and the brain sites mediating responses to chemoreceptor processes. Studies to investigate the role of chemoreceptors role can obviously be assisted by conditions in which central chemoreception is lost, such as CCHS. The normal activation of brain sites to high CO_2 (5%) is remarkable, since fMRI signal responses to such a challenge reveal widespread involvement of brain structures, and that recruitment of brain structures is not confined to restricted medullary areas, as once believed, but includes cerebellar cortex and deep nuclei, midbrain, central pontine, and diencephalic areas [25]. Studies in CCHS subjects confirmed the widespread distribution of CO_2 regulatory structures, and indicate deficits in multiple sites in CCHS over controls, including dorsal medullary, raphe, locus coeruleus, ventral pons, cerebellar cortex, and medial hippocampus. A subset of fMRI signal responses to high CO_2 that differ from controls is shown in Figure 37.2.

Brain structures responding to hypoxia are also distributed in multiple areas, as would be expected from earlier evidence from animal studies showing hypothalamic, thalamic, medullary, and cerebellar roles in mediating low O_2 responses [26]. Functional MRI studies show participation of those multiple areas, as well as the basal ganglia, and limbic structures which project to the hypothalamus; CCHS subjects show various areas that significantly differ in amplitude from controls [26]. Widespread distribution of responses appears in reaction to hyperoxia (100% O_2) in CCHS [27]. Amelioration of the potentially serious consequences of hypoxemic involvement of limbic and other structures can be shown by addition of CO_2 [28].

In animal studies, intermittent hypoxic exposure, used to simulate apnea events in sleep disordered breathing, and thus alter brain structures accompanying OSA, is accompanied by significant injury in limbic and cerebellar areas [29–32]. Those brain areas affected by intermittent hypoxia may be especially at risk in children with CCHS, giving rise to the extensive injury found in limbic and cerebellar areas. Children with CCHS are exposed to multiple episodes of hypoxia from failure of ventilatory devices, unintended cessation of breathing during tranquil daytime waking periods from self-unrecognized hypoxia, or during periods of fever or overheating (temperature drive to breathing is lost in CCHS). These hypoxic episodes may add to existing genetic mutation-related injury in the condition.

The brain areas which fail to respond to high CO_2 in CCHS nearly overlay several regions of injury in CCHS, including traditional medullary areas involved both in chemosensation and in cardiovascular control. These structures include the locus coeruleus, which shows both significant injury, as indicated by DTI procedures, as well as failed responses to CO_2, assessed by fMRI. The caudal raphe, the source of serotonergic fibers which play a role in CO_2 detection and integration with arousal [17], shows substantial injury, as indicated by DTI-based axial diffusivity procedures, and impaired responses to CO_2, as shown by fMRI procedures (Figures 37.1, 37.2).

Injury to memory and other cognitive regulatory sites

Children with CCHS show a range of cognitive deficits, including memory problems, in addition to affect issues.

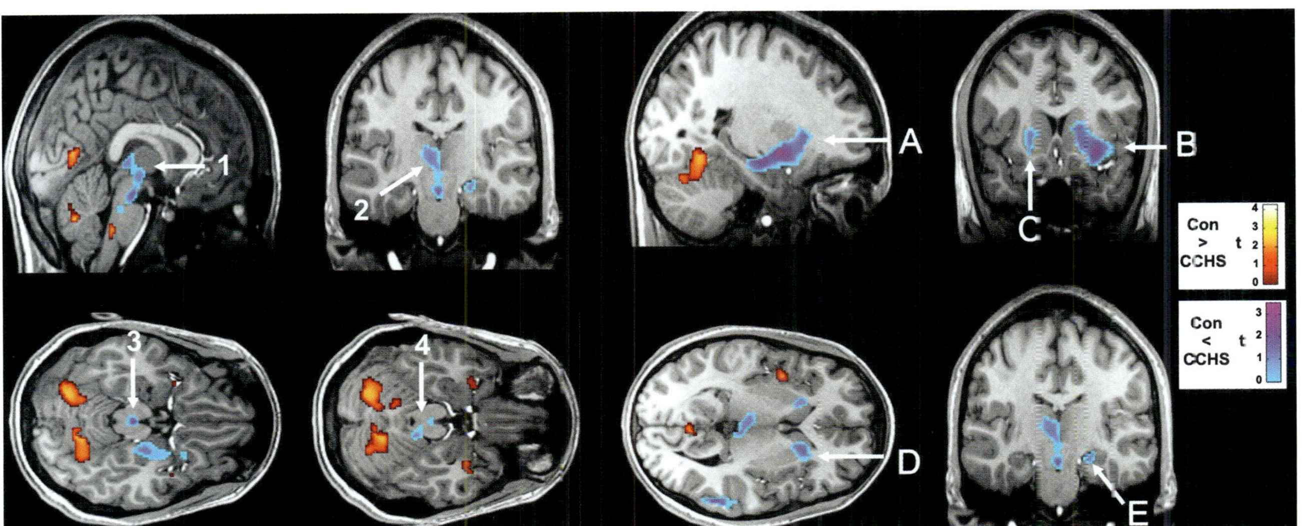

Figure 37.2 Differential fMRI signal responses to 5% CO_2, balance O_2, in CCHS relative to age- and gender-matched control subjects (adolescents) Widespread areas of the brain differed in CCHS, with larger signals in controls over CCHS indicated by the yellow-red clusters (dorsal medulla, cerebellar cortex, amygdala), and lower signals in controls (blue-green clusters) in the parabrachial pons/locus coeruleus (4), medial midbrain, raphe (3), ventral pons, extending to the dorsal thalamus, (1), caudate nucleus extending to the insular cortex and to the hippocampus (A, B, E), and caudate head, (D). (Derived from Harper *et al.* [25] with permission.)

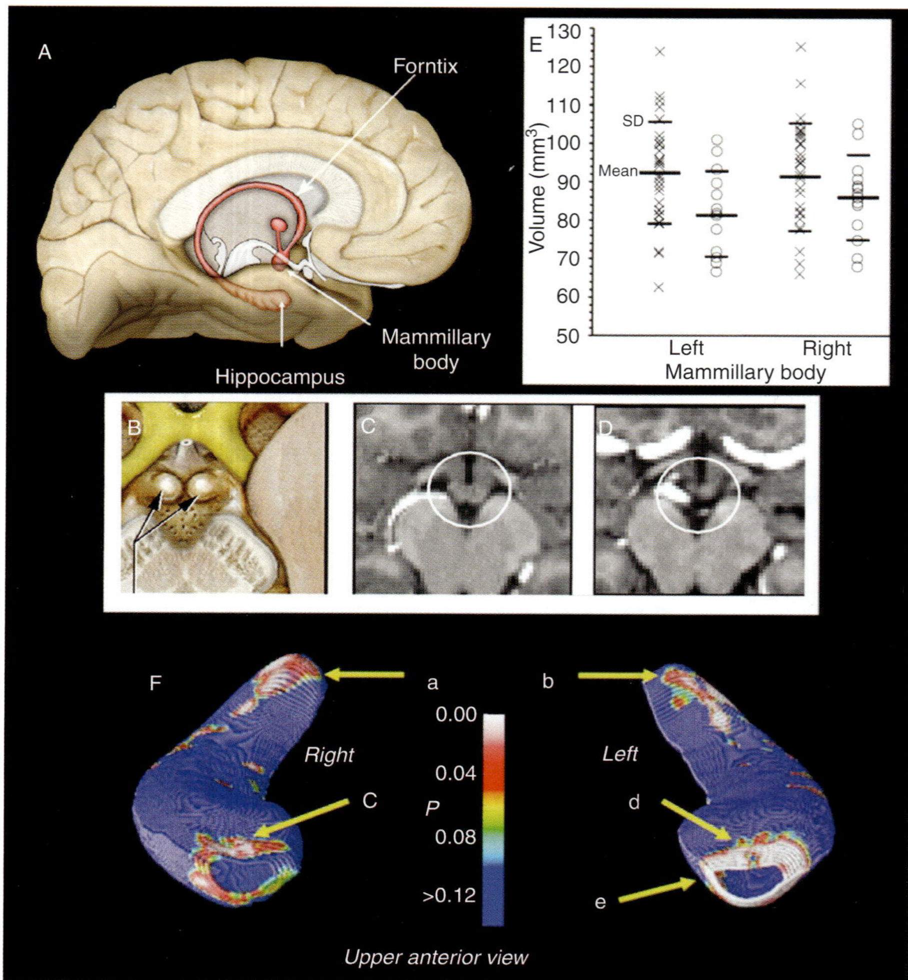

Figure 37.3 (A, B) Cartoons of hippocampus, fornix, and mammillary bodies (from Acerland International USA, with permission). (C, D) Mammillary bodies in a control (C), and an age- and gender-matched CCHS subject (D). (E) Scatterplots of left and right mammillary body volumes in control (x) and CCHS (o) subjects (from Kumar et al. [36]). (F) Regional hippocampal injury, reflected as surface deformations in CCHS subjects (a,b CA1/ CA2, near fimbria, c right rostral CA1–CA3, dentate gyrus, d left rostral CA1–CA3, e left ventral CA1, subiculum). (Redrawn from Macey et al. [35].)

Some of the cognitive deficits may stem from the cerebellar injury outlined earlier, and damage to cerebellar projections to the frontal cortex, as well as parietal, temporal, and frontal cortices and cingulate cortex injury found in T2-relaxation, mean diffusivity, and cortical thickness studies [20, 21, 33]. In addition, among the structures affected in CCHS is the hippocampal–fornix–mammillary body complex (Figure 37.3A). The hippocampus is injured in CCHS, as shown by mean diffusivity and DTI procedures, with regional shape deformations revealed by surface mapping techniques [21, 34, 35] (Figure 37.3F). Manual evaluation of high-resolution T1-weighted images shows substantially decreased volume in the mammillary bodies and cross-sectional areas of the fornix fibers [36]; (Figure 37.3 B–E). The hippocampal system, with its projections, is heavily used in memory processing and spatial orientation. Other fiber injury is apparent in the corpus callosum, especially in caudal and rostral areas [37]; the caudal areas may partially mediate issues of bilateral coordination of the ocular system and autonomic fibers which cross in that region of the corpus callosum in CCHS. The corpus callosum injury is paralleled by cortical injury, which appears as areas of thinning cortex, measured by FreeSurfer software [33, 38].

Temperature and affective contributions to breathing

An important, but seldom-considered, influence on breathing is from more-rostral brain areas including limbic projections to brainstem respiratory regulatory sites. The best known of these influences is from the hypothalamus, which exerts significant temperature drive to breathing, a drive that is lost in rapid eye movement sleep [39]. Other influences include signaling from the amygdala to respiratory phase-switching parabrachial pontine areas, influences that appear to be lost or modified during sleep [40], and have the potential to incorporate affective influences on breathing, such as inspiratory gasps on extreme fear, more-rapid pacing of breathing on excitement, and enhanced breathing efforts to the perception of breathlessness. This last sensation of dyspnea is notably lost in CCHS, with sometimes tragic results, since affected children will engage in breath-holding competitions with healthy playmates, not perceiving the extreme urge to breathe that normally accompanies high CO_2 or low O_2 levels. Brain areas implicated in serving that perception include the insular and cingulate cortices, as well as the amygdala and cerebellum [41, 42], all sites showing significant injury in CCHS, as indicated by T2-relaxometry, mean

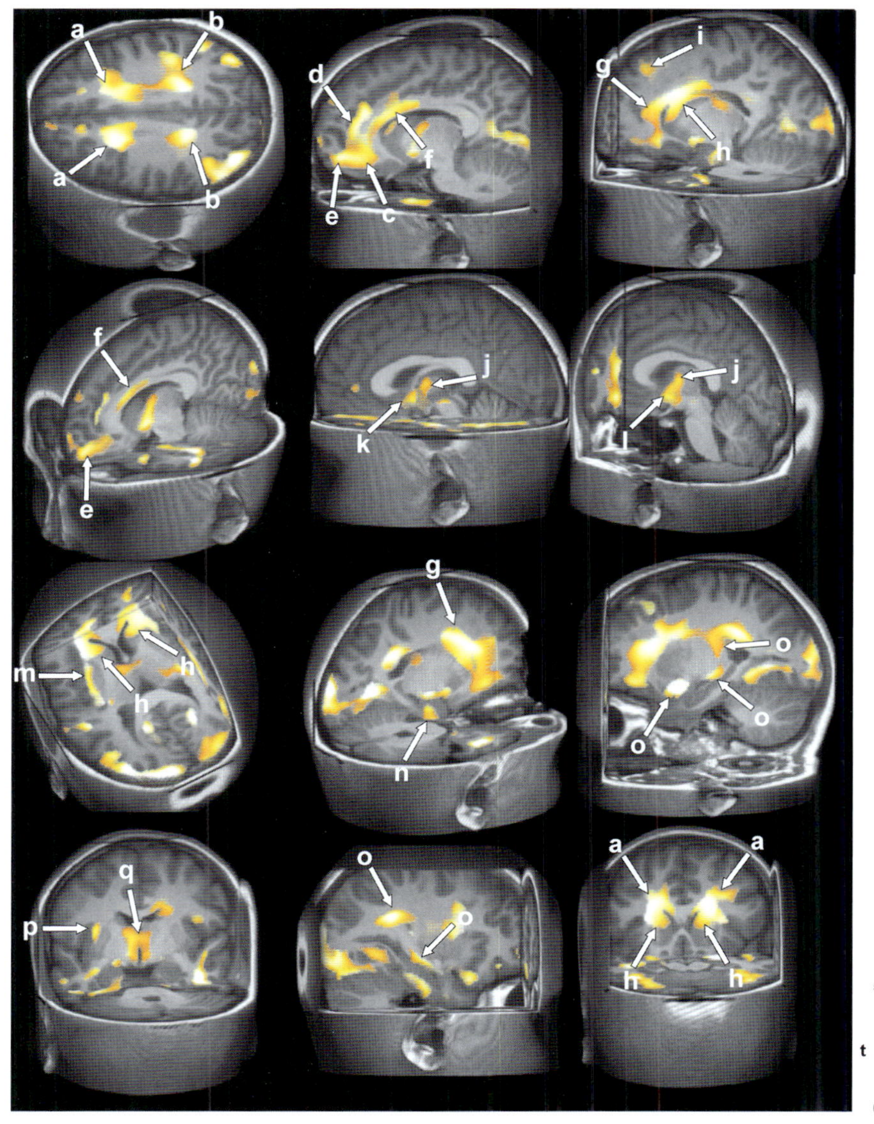

Figure 37.4 Three-dimensional views of brain structures showing both increased axial and radial diffusivity in CCHS relative to controls; deficient areas are represented as clusters with enhanced radial diffusivity values. Similar areas also show increased axial diffusivity values, but with differing significance levels. Areas associated with affect include the left genu and anterior cingulate cortices extending to the cingulum bundle (c,d,g); right prefrontal cortex (i); bilateral anterior fornix (k); bilateral hypothalamus extending to the anterior and midthalamus (j,); bilateral orbitofrontal cortex and nearby white matter; bilateral anterior hippocampus and amygdala (n); bilateral caudate nuclei (h); right anterior and left mid- and posterior insular cortices extending to the putamen (m,p); ventral medial prefrontal cortex and nearby white matter (e); bilateral nucleus accumbens; bed nucleus of the stria terminalis (BNST o,q), and bilateral inferior temporal lobes; bilateral temporal-occipital cortices. The bilateral superior, anterior, and posterior corona radiata (a,b), anterior and midbody of the corpus callosum (f) are also affected; further fiber injury in the corpus callosum (especially in the rostral and caudal fibers) are described elsewhere [37]. (From Kumar *et al.* [45].)

diffusivity, and axial and radial diffusivity procedures (Figures 37.1, 37.4) [16, 20, 21].

Motor areas

A remarkable aspect of the neural injury in CCHS is the distribution, with relative sparing of primary sensory and motor tracts, but significant injury to midline structures of the midbrain, limbic structures of the amygdala, hypothalamus, prefrontal, cingulate and insular cortices, and cerebellar regions. Except for bilateral isolated notches in the cerebral peduncles (Figure 37.1), the pyramidal tracts appear intact. Portions of the corpus callosum, the cingulum bundle, portions of the cerebellar peduncles, and fornix fibers are all affected.

Injury to sites mediating neurotransmitter action

Among the processes affected in CCHS appears to be the integrity of multiple neurotransmitter systems. The caudal raphe is affected (Figure 37.1), and presumably serotonergic fibers, which originate solely from the raphe system, are affected as well. The locus coeruleus, source of adrenergic fibers, is significantly injured, likely since *Phox2b* appears densely there in the adult mouse (http://www.gensat.org/imagenavigator.jsp?imageID=72012). Post-mortem human locus coeruleus material shows significant neuronal loss [43], and DTI and fMRI procedures show deficient structure and function (Figures 37.1 and 37.2). Structures which give rise to dopamine and cholinergic fibers are also modified; the ventral midbrain, incorporating the substantia nigra, as well as basal forebrain areas, which give rise to cholinergic neurons, show structural and functional deficits in CCHS (Figures 37.1 and 37.2); targets of dopamine fibers are also affected [44]. However, the effect on CCHS of specific neurotransmitter fiber injury has not yet been ascertained. Tracking of fibers from those structures is a difficult logistic task, since multiple fiber systems traverse those sites.

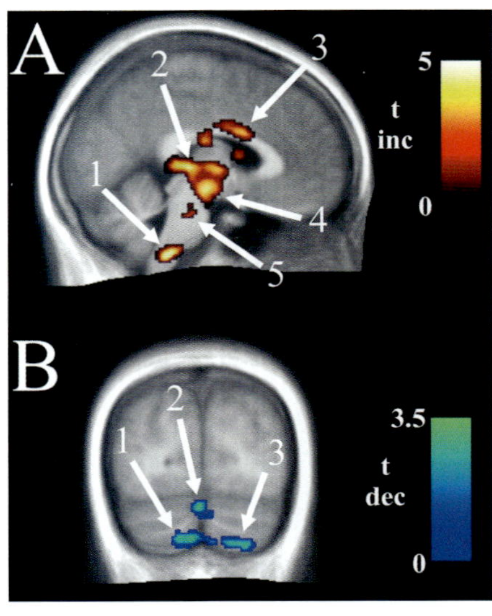

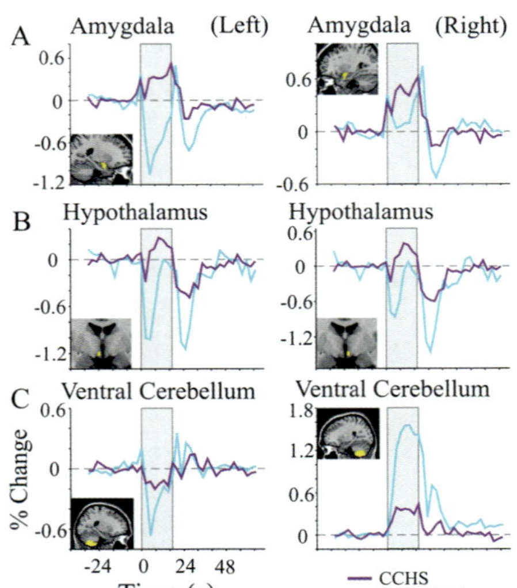

Figure 37.5 *Left*: (A) Clusters of fMRI signal differences in 9 CCHS from 25 controls, with larger CCHS signals in warm colors 1, ventral medulla; 2, midbrain; 3 cingulate cortex; 4, midbrain; 5, midline pons; (B) Clusters in which CCHS signals were lower than controls in cerebellar cortex 1–3, and deep cerebellar nuclei, 2. *Right*: Mean signal trends in CCHS and controls to a Valsalva challenge in left and right amygdala, hypothalamus, and ventral cerebellum, showing overall muting of signals, loss of asymmetry, i.e., normal difference in laterality, of signals in amygdala, significant time distortion in hypothalamus, and substantial muting in signals of cerebellum in CCHS patients. (From Ogren *et al.* [13], with permission.)

Functional MRI signal responses to ventilatory and autonomic challenges

Functional MRI responses to CO_2 and hypoxia in CCHS showed changes in amplitude or direction in sites mediating integration of those chemical senses. Such chemical challenges are difficult to precisely time to assess potential delays in interactions between areas. However, a range of ventilatory and pressor challenges can be closely timed with respect to onset of stimulation, and such challenges show remarkable timing distortion in addition to altered amplitude of responses. The signals are often delayed, or develop earlier in CCHS cases; such time shifts require assessment with rapid fMRI data sampling. The time-distorted signal development in autonomic areas are a concern with regards to integration of breathing and autonomic patterns; normally, substantial changes in breathing efforts are accompanied by large blood pressure changes, with syncope or other aberrant outcomes resulting if timing between the respiratory and cardiovascular systems is not well synchronized. If a precisely timed challenge, such as the Valsalva maneuver, which elicits both sympathetic and parasympathetic participation, is evaluated in CCHS with fMRI procedures, the distortions in both timing and amplitude of responses are especially apparent [13]. Figure 37.5 shows some of the areas that differ in the responses of CCHS individuals to the Valsalva maneuver from controls These include cingulate, hypothalamic, midbrain, and cerebellar sites (Figure 37.5, left, A, B; responses are larger in CCHS with warm-colored clusters, and lower in CCHS in cool-colored responses). Moreover, the potential for the condition to interfere with laterality of function, i.e., the representation of function on one side of the brain over the other, can be demonstrated. Figure 37.5 (right) shows mean fMRI signal trends (9 CCHS, 25 controls) in selected brain areas to the Valsalva maneuver that show amplitude or time differences, as well as laterality differences in CCHS subjects from controls. Signals are muted in all structures in CCHS, and time-altered in the hypothalamus; the cerebellum especially shows substantial muting. The amygdala shows a reversal of signals between left and right sides in controls, but that lateralization is lost in CCHS. Failure of lateralization of autonomic regulatory areas is of concern, since distortion of left–right organization can lead to a range of autonomic aberrations, including an enhanced risk for cardiac arrhythmia.

Summary

The rarity of CCHS cases places limits on determining brain mechanisms underlying the condition; post-mortem material is difficult to collect, and is usually obtained after many years of exposure to hypoxia, which imposes additional injury, confounding identification of initial injury induced by the genetic mutation. Structural and functional MRI procedures provide a valuable means to assess gray and white matter injury and impaired brain function in the syndrome, and, in the same fashion as numerous other disease processes, the descriptions have the potential to reveal normal mechanisms for serving breathing and autonomic functions. The evaluations have revealed the widespread distribution of brain areas responsive to CO_2 and O_2, unsuspected participation of sites involved in autonomic regulation, especially cardiovascular control and injury in sites that provide affective drive to breathe and temperature regulation, all functions that are defective in CCHS. Injury in cognitive and memory regulatory areas has also been revealed. In addition, DTI procedures have outlined the extent of white matter injury, information essential for describing functions in areas interconnected by those fibers. Additional DTI procedures have outlined separate myelin and axonal injury in the white matter of CCHS subjects. Many questions remain for the description of CCHS injury, such as when injury appears, to what extent injury develops from hypoxia, as opposed to initial damage from genetic mechanisms or defective perfusion induced by genetic processes, and the extent and nature of injury in late-onset forms of CCHS. As MRI technology improves, further differentiation of the nature of injury, especially finer discrimination of fiber injury, will be possible.

Acknowledgements

This research was supported by NICHD HD-22695. We thank Drs. P. M. Macey, M. A. Woo, H. L. Richardson and J. A. Ogren, and Ms. R. K. Harper.

References

1. Pattyn A, Morin X, Cremer H, *et al.* Expression and interactions of the two closely related homeobox genes *Phox2a* and *Phox2b* during neurogenesis. *Development*. 1997;**124**(20): 4065–75.

2. Pattyn A, Morin X, Cremer H, *et al.* The homeobox gene Phox2b is essential for the development of autonomic neural crest derivatives. *Nature*. 1999;**399** (6734):366–70.

3. Amiel J, Laudier B, Attie-Bitach T, *et al.* Polyalanine expansion and frameshift mutations of the paired-like homeobox gene PHOX2B in congenital central hypoventilation syndrome. *Nat Genet*. 2003;**33**(4):459–61.

4. Weese-Mayer DE, Rand CM, Berry-Kravis EM, *et al.* Congenital central hypoventilation syndrome from past to future: model for translational and transitional autonomic medicine. *Pediatr Pulmonol*. 2009;**44**(6):521–35.

5. Mellins RB, Balfour HH, Jr., Turino GM, *et al.* Failure of automatic control of ventilation (Ondine's curse). Report of an infant born with this syndrome and review of the literature. *Medicine (Baltimore)*. 1970;**49**(6):487–504.

6. Haddad GG, Mazza NM, Defendini R, *et al.* Congenital failure of automatic control of ventilation, gastrointestinal motility and heart rate. *Medicine (Baltimore)*. 1978;**57**(6):517–26.

7. Weese-Mayer DE, Berry-Kravis EM, Ceccherini I, *et al.* An official ATS clinical policy statement: congenital central hypoventilation syndrome: genetic basis, diagnosis, and management. *Am J Respir Crit Care Med*. 2010;**181**(6):626–44.

8. Shea SA. Life without ventilatory chemosensitivity. *Respir Physiol*. 1997;**110**(2–3):199–210.

9. Healy F, Marcus CL. Congenital central hypoventilation syndrome in children. *Paediatr Respir Rev*. 2011;**12**(4):253–63.

10. Gozal D, Marcus CL, Ward SL, *et al.* Ventilatory responses to passive leg motion in children with congenital central hypoventilation syndrome. *Am J Respir Crit Care Med*. 1996;**153** (2):761–8.

11. Gozal D, Simakajornboon N. Passive motion of the extremities modifies alveolar ventilation during sleep in patients with congenital central hypoventilation syndrome. *Am J Respir Crit Care Med*. 2000;**162**(5):1747–51.

12. Trang H, Girard A, Laude D, *et al.* Short-term blood pressure and heart rate variability in congenital central hypoventilation syndrome (Ondine's curse). *Clin Sci (Lond)*. 2005;**108** (3):225–30.

13. Ogren JA, Macey PM, Kumar R, *et al.* Central autonomic regulation in congenital central hypoventilation syndrome. *Neuroscience*. 2010;**167** (4):1249–56.

14. Woo MS, Woo MA, Gozal D, *et al.* Heart rate variability in congenital central hypoventilation syndrome. *Pediatr Res*. 1992;**31**(3):291–6.

15. Macey PM, Kumar R, Ogren JA, *et al.* Images in sleep medicine. Altered cerebral blood flow in a patient with congenital central hypoventilation syndrome. *Sleep Med*. 2010;**11** (6):589–90.

16. Kumar R, Macey PM, Woo MA, *et al.* Diffusion tensor imaging demonstrates brainstem and cerebellar abnormalities in congenital central hypoventilation syndrome. *Pediatr Res*. 2008;**64** (3):275–80.

17. Buchanan GF, Richerson GB. Central serotonin neurons are required for arousal to CO_2. *Proc Natl Acad Sci U S A*. 2010;**107**(37):16354–9.

18. Mason P. Contributions of the medullary raphe and ventromedial reticular region to pain modulation and other homeostatic functions. *Annu Rev Neurosci*. 2001;**24**:737–77.

19. Kumar R, Nguyen HD, Macey PM, *et al.* Dilated basilar arteries in patients with congenital central hypoventilation syndrome. *Neurosci Lett*. 2009;**467** (2):139–43.

20. Kumar R, Macey PM, Woo MA, *et al.* Neuroanatomic deficits in congenital central hypoventilation syndrome. *J Comp Neurol*. 2005;**487**(4) 361–71.

21. Kumar R, Macey PM, Woo MA, *et al.* Elevated mean diffusivity in widespread brain regions in congenital central hypoventilation syndrome. *J Magn Reson Imaging*. 2006;**24**(6):1252–8.

22. Gong S, Zheng C, Doughty ML *et al.* A gene expression atlas of the central nervous system based on bacterial artificial chromosomes. *Nature*. 2003;**425**(6961):917–25.

23. Chen CH, Williams JL, Lutherer LO. Cerebellar lesions alter autonomic responses to transient isovolaemic changes in arterial pressure in anaesthetized cats. *Clin Auton Res*. 1994;**4**(5):263–72.

24. Craig AD. Significance of the insula for the evolution of human awareness of feelings from the body. *Ann N Y Acad Sci*. 2011;**1225**:72–82.

25. Harper RM, Macey PM, Woo MA, *et al.* Hypercapnic exposure in congenital central hypoventilation syndrome reveals CNS respiratory control mechanisms. *J Neurophysiol*. 2005;**93** (3):1647–58.

26. Macey PM, Woo MA, Macey KE, *et al.* Hypoxia reveals posterior thalamic, cerebellar, midbrain, and limbic deficits in congenital central hypoventilation syndrome. *J Appl Physiol*. 2005;**98** (3):958–69

27. Woo MA, Macey PM, Macey KE, *et al.* FMRI responses to hyperoxia in congenital central hypoventilation syndrome. *Pediatr Res*. 2005;**57** (4):510–18.

28. Macey PM, Woo MA, Harper RM. Hyperoxic brain effects are normalized by addition of CO_2. *Plos Med*. 2007;**4** (5):823–35.

29. Gozal D, Daniel JM, Dohanich GP. Behavioral and anatomical correlates of chronic episodic hypoxia during sleep in the rat. *J Neurosci*. 2001;**21** (7):2442–50.

30. Veasey SC, Davis CW, Fenik P, *et al.* Long-term intermittent hypoxia in mice: protracted hypersomnolence with oxidative injury to sleep-wake brain regions. *Sleep*. 2004;**27**(2):194–201.

31. Pae EK, Chien P, Harper RM. Intermittent hypoxia damages cerebellar cortex and deep nuclei. *Neurosci Lett*. 2005;**375**(2):123–8.

32. Pae EK, Yoon AJ, Ahuja B, *et al.* Perinatal intermittent hypoxia alters gamma-aminobutyric acid: a receptor levels in rat cerebellum. *Int J Dev Neurosci*. 2011;**29**(8):819–26.

33. Macey PM, Moiyadi AS, Kumar R, *et al.* Decreased cortical thickness in central hypoventilation syndrome. *Cereb Cortex*. 2012;**22**(8):1728–37.

34. Kumar R, Nguyen HD, Macey PM, *et al.* Regional brain axial and radial diffusivity changes during development. *J Neurosci Res*. 2012;**90**(2):346–55.

35. Macey PM, Richard CA, Kumar R, *et al.* Hippocampal volume reduction in congenital central hypoventilation syndrome. *PLoS One*. 2009;**4**(7):e6436.

36. Kumar R, Lee K, Macey PM, *et al.* Mammillary body and fornix injury in congenital central hypoventilation syndrome. *Pediatr Res*. 2009;**66**(4):429–34.

37. Kumar R, Macey PM, Woo MA, *et al.* Selectively diminished corpus callosum fibers in congenital central hypoventilation syndrome. *Neuroscience*. 2011;**178**:261–9.

38. Dale AM, Fischl B, Sereno MI. Cortical surface-based analysis. I. Segmentation and surface reconstruction. *Neuroimage*. 1999;**9**(2):179–94.

39. Ni H, Zhang J, Glotzbach SF, *et al.* Dynamic respiratory responses to preoptic/anterior hypothalamic warming in the sleeping cat. *Sleep*. 1994;**17**(8):657–64.

40. Harper RM, Frysinger RC, Trelease RB, *et al.* State-dependent alteration of respiratory cycle timing by stimulation of the central nucleus of the amygdala. *Brain Res*. 1984;**306**(1–2):1–8.

41. Banzett RB, Mulnier HE, Murphy K, *et al.* Breathlessness in humans activates insular cortex. *Neuroreport*. 2000;**11**(10):2117–20.

42. Peiffer C, Poline JB, Thivard L, *et al.* Neural substrates for the perception of acutely induced dyspnea. *Am J Respir Crit Care Med*. 2001;**163**(4):951–7.

43. Tomycz ND, Haynes RL, Schmidt EF, *et al.* Novel neuropathologic findings in the Haddad syndrome. *Acta Neuropathol*. 2010;**119**(2):261–9.

44. Kumar R, Ahdout R, Macey PM, *et al.* Reduced caudate nuclei volumes in patients with congenital central hypoventilation syndrome. *Neuroscience*. 2009;**163**(4):1373–9.

45. Kumar R, Macey PM, Woo MA, Harper RM. Rostral brain axonal injury in congenital hypoventilation syndrome. *J Neurosci Res*. 2010;**88**:2146–54.

Neuroimaging of disorders of arousal and other parasomnias

Romy Hoque and Lourdes DelRosso

Introduction

For many years parasomnias, including disorders of arousal, have NOT been associated with known underlying pathology. With the development of new neuroimaging technologies in recent years sleep-related disorders can finally be associated with underlying neuroanatomical pathology. Case reports and other research studies are giving us greater insight into the underlying mechanisms of these disorders. This chapter reviews the current neuroimaging literature regarding disorders of arousal and parasomnias, particularly non-rapid eye movement (NREM) parasomnias. Rapid eye movement (REM) parasomnias including REM behavior disorder (RBD) are covered extensively in other chapters in this volume.

Disorders of arousal from NREM sleep

Sleepwalking

Bassetti *et al.* performed a ^{99m}Tc-ethyl cysteinate dimer (^{99m}Tc-ECD) single-photon emission computerized tomography (SPECT) study in a man (age not specified) with a 16-year history of sleepwalking [1]. Two separate ^{99m}Tc-ECD SPECT studies were performed. The first SPECT study was performed during normal slow-wave sleep. The second SPECT study was performed the following night with ^{99m}Tc-ECD injected 24 s after the onset of a sleepwalking episode while the patient was in electroencephalogram (EEG) verified slow-wave sleep. In comparison to wakefulness in healthy volunteers, the patient showed *increased* cerebral blood flow (CBF) in the posterior cingulate gyrus and the anterior cerebellum during sleepwalking. The authors noted an "absence of deactivation of the thalamus" during sleepwalking in contrast to "normal slow-wave sleep," and postulated sleepwalking may result in selective activation of thalamocingulate pathways. In comparison to wakefulness in healthy volunteers the patient showed *decreased* CBF during sleepwalking in the frontoparietal heteromodal association cortices. The decreased CBF in the frontoparietal heteromodal association cortices is postulated to be responsible for the lack of awareness and lack of recall during sleepwalking. (For more detail see Chapter 43.)

Hori *et al.* reported a 64-year-old man with an 8-month history of sleepwalking without recollection, an altered level of consciousness, and a left sixth cranial nerve palsy [2]. Cerebrospinal fluid (CSF) examination revealed an increased

opening pressure of 200 mmH$_2$O, 96 cells per cm^3 with 95 mononuclear cells, "increased protein" (amount not specified), and herpes simplex complement fixing antibody in the serum and CSF. Computerized tomography (CT) scan of the brain revealed a low density area in the right temporal lobe. EEG showed diffuse slowing; a more specific description was not provided in the article. Magnetic resonance imaging (MRI) showed increased T2-weighted image (WI) signal intensity in the right temporal lobe with extension into the right insular cortex. N-isopropyl-p-123-I-iodoamphetamine (123I-IMP) SPECT revealed increased accumulation of 123I-IMP in the right temporal lobe, and the authors postulated that the sleepwalking was due to the right temporal lesion.

Kushida *et al.* reported a 51-year-old man with Machado–Joseph disease and sleepwalking with occasional violent outbursts [3]. The episodes lasted from 5 to 20 minutes and occurred several times during the night. The patient would return to bed and awaken in the morning amnestic for the events, with only partial dream recall. Three polysomnograms (PSGs) revealed violent nocturnal behaviors arising primarily out of NREM sleep with kicking, thrashing about, and yelling. Given the complexity of the patient's behaviors the authors used the term "nocturnal wandering," which encompasses sleepwalking, RBD, and nocturnal seizures. Nocturnal seizures were less likely given the lack of: epileptiform activity on EEG, automatisms, prior seizure history, and improvement with carbamazepine or phenytoin. MRI of the brain showed the characteristic ponto cerebellar atrophy of Machado–Joseph disease. The authors noted they could not rule out the possibility that Machado–Joseph disease was involved in the nocturnal wandering; however, no cortical or thalamic lesions were noted that could directly explain the patient's behavior.

Hoque *et al.* reported a 51-year-old woman with zolpidem-induced sleepwalking, sleep-related eating disorder, and sleep-driving investigated using ^{18}F-fluorodeoxyglucose positron emission tomography (^{18}F-FDG PET) [4]. (For more detail see Chapter 53.)

Sleep terrors

DiGennaro *et al.* reported a 48-year-old woman with episodes of screaming during sleep [5]. PSG with full head 18-channel EEG showed one episode of screaming during slow-wave sleep with return to sleep in 10 minutes. PSG showed diffuse delta activity before and during the event, with tachycardia. No epileptiform activity was noted during the recording. MRI of the head showed a T2 WI hyper intense lesion in the right thalamus. Results of diffusion weighted imaging sequences, apparent diffusion coefficient imaging sequences, and administration of gadolinium contrast were not reported. Neurological examination was reported to be normal. The authors postulated that the right thalamic lesion might have altered the cortico-thalamic tract involved in sleep.

Mendez reported a 15-year-old boy with headaches and ataxia who underwent resection of a Grade I cerebellar astrocytoma arising near the fourth ventricle and adherent to the brainstem shown on CT [6]. Postoperatively his neurological examination showed dysarthria; ataxia; and bilateral fifth, sixth, and seventh cranial nerve palsies. He also developed postoperative sleep terrors consisting of screaming, and thrashing. After a few minutes he promptly returned to sleep, with partial recollection the next morning. At the age of 24 a diagnostic PSG showed arousals from slow-wave sleep, with vocalizations and looking around. Clonazepam 0.5 mg at bedtime decreased the episodes of sleep terrors. The author postulated that disruption of the nucleus tractus solitarius in the dorsum of the brainstem near the wall of the fourth ventricle may have been responsible for the patient's arousal from slow-wave sleep.

Disorders of arousal associated with REM sleep

Parasomnia overlap syndrome with RBD and sleepwalking

Limousin *et al.* reported a case of a 40-year-old woman with cerebellar ataxia (side unspecified); right third, fifth, seventh, eighth, nineth, and tenth cranial nerve palsies; and a right internuclear ophthalmoplegia (INO) [7]. MRI revealed T2 WI hyperintense/T1 WI hypo intense/gadolinium enhancing lesions in the right mesencephalic/pontine tegmentum, and the right medulla. CSF analysis did not show evidence of multiple sclerosis. She was treated with corticosteroids and all the cranial nerve palsies resolved with persistence of the cerebellar ataxia and the right INO. During the next two years the patient developed abnormal sleep behaviours, including violent behaviors (slapping) and sleepwalking. A diagnostic PSG revealed arousals from slow-wave sleep without abnormal movements, and REM sleep without atonia (RSWA). During REM sleep the patient exhibited RBD with mumbling, complex hand movements (e.g., writing, eating), and arm/leg jerks. A repeat MRI showed persistent increased T2 WI hyper intense/T1 WI hypo intense lesions in the right mesencephalic/pontine tegmentum and the right medulla. The authors postulated that the lesions of unknown etiology in the pontine tegmentum may have been responsible for the RBD/RSWA and the sleepwalking. (For more detail see Chapter 44.)

Nocturnal painful erections

Szucs *et al.* reported a 65-year-old man with a 10-year history of painful nocturnal erections that resolved upon awakening [8]. Diagnostic PSG with penile tumescence recording revealed three erections during REM sleep. Each erection lasted from 3 to 8 minutes followed by arousal from sleep and resolution of the erection. MRI of the spine was normal. MRI of the brain revealed compression of the left hypothalamus by the left posterior cerebral artery. The authors postulated that vascular compression of the anterior hypothalamus may have been responsible for the nocturnal painful erections given the role of the anterior hypothalamus' medial preoptic area in erection production in rat models.

Karsenty *et al.* reported a 45-year-old man with painful nocturnal erections starting two years after surgical resection of a thoracic T7 level spinal cord ependymoma seen on MRI [9]. The surgery resulted in amyotrophy of the left leg with normal muscle strength in the legs and normal gait. Sensation to light touch was reduced below the T5 level, with preservation of temperature and position sense. Diagnostic PSG with penile tumescence recording revealed three painful nocturnal erections during REM sleep. The authors noted that the association between the thoracic ependymoma and the nocturnal painful erections was unclear given the two-year event-free interval between the surgical resection and the onset of symptoms. Repeat MRI of the thoracic spinal cord five years after the surgical resection showed no recurrence of the ependymoma.

Other parasomnias

Sleep-related enuresis

Kikuchi *et al.* reported an 11-year-old girl with intractable nocturnal enuresis [10]. MRI of the brain revealed transection of the pituitary stalk with formation of an ectopic posterior pituitary lobe. The authors postulated that this finding was responsible for the nocturnal enuresis. Hunsballe, *et al.* reviewed the MRI of the pituitary gland in eight adults with primary enuresis [11]. MRI in seven patients was unremarkable and one patient had a Rathke's cleft cyst that was not considered clinically significant. The authors concluded that primary enuresis persisting into adulthood is not associated with detectable pathology of the pituitary gland.

Yu *et al.* studied 13 children with primary nocturnal enuresis and 15 healthy controls using intelligence tests and functional MRI (fMRI) [12]. The analysis between both groups revealed impairment in working memory in children and significant fMRI signal attenuation in the left posterior cerebellar lobes in children with primary nocturnal enuresis. The authors concluded that these two findings may potentially be associated with each other. Differences in pre frontal lobe function were not found between the two groups.

Lei *et al.* studied resting state fMRI in 16 children with primary nocturnal enuresis and 16 healthy controls [13]. Statistically significant differences in amplitude of low frequency fluctuation were noted in the left inferior frontal gyrus, the left medial frontal gyrus, and the left midbrain. The authors postulated that the abnormalities in the left inferior frontal gyrus and the left medial frontal gyrus may affect decision-making regarding voiding; and that abnormalities in the left midbrain may influence the internal signal transmission to the bladder control network.

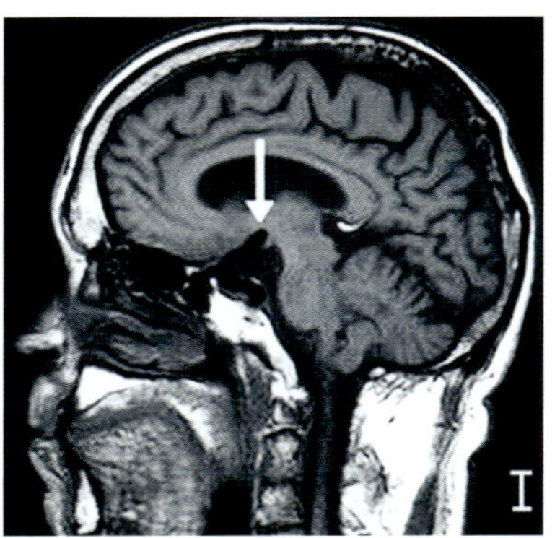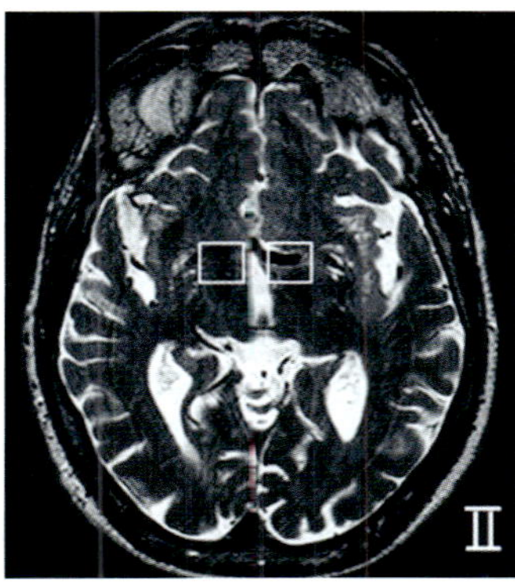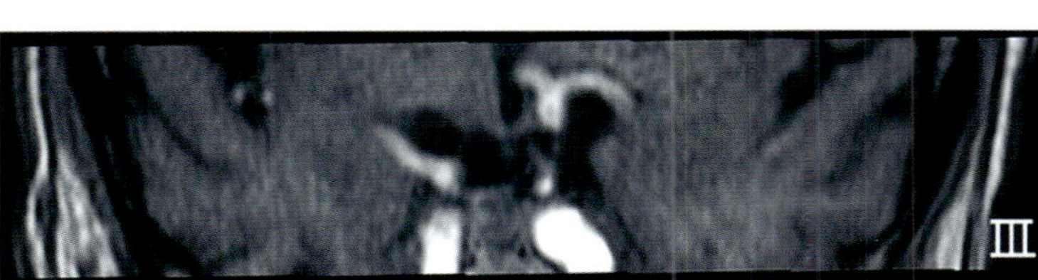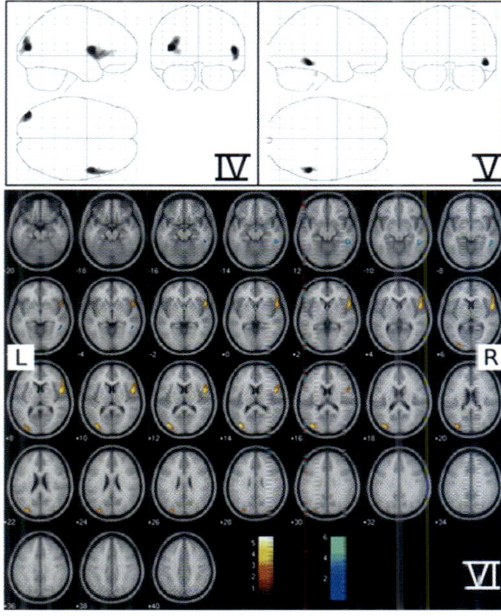

Figure 38.1 Neuroimaging in a case of peduncular hallucinosis. I: Brain magnetic resonance imaging (MRI) T1-weighted image (WI) with arrow showing impingement of the supraclinoid internal carotid artery in the left subthalamus. II: Brain MRI T2-WI with voxel placement for ^{1}H-magnetic resonance spectroscopy (MRS) in subthalami bilaterally. Distortion of left subthalamic region is evident compared to right. MRS showed decreased N-acetylaspartate (NAA) and choline (Cho) peaks in the left subthalamic region compared to the right subthalamic region. III: Magnetic resonance angiography (MRA) showing upward displacement of the left subthalamic region. IV–VI: Single Photon Emission Computerized Tomography (SPECT) of the brain displayed using glass brain (IV and V) and superimposed on T1-WI (VI). During visual hallucinations increased cerebral blood flow (CBF) is seen in the left middle occipital gyrus and right inferior frontal-rolandic opercular gyri (IV and V) and decreased CBF was seen in right middle temporal gyrus. (Reprinted with permission from Vetrugno, et al. [16].)

Exploding head syndrome

Salih et al. described exploding head syndrome that occurred at sleep onset in a 64-year-old woman with sarcoidosis and a normal neurological examination [14]. The patient reported sleep onset insomnia with the impression of a cracking sound shortly after losing consciousness. MRI of the head revealed a T2 WI hyper intense lesion at the pontomesencephalic lesion presumed to be neurosarcoidosis. Symptoms resolved with clonazepam 0.5 mg at bedtime. The authors postulated that the pontomesencephalic junction lesion was responsible for the exploding head syndrome symptoms.

Sleep-related hallucinations

The differential diagnosis of complex visual hallucinations in older adult patients includes peduncular hallucinosis associated with lesions in the midbrain, pons, or thalamus [15]. Vetrugno et al. reported a 72-year-old man with complex visual hallucinations of animals, people, and landscapes in the evening and when lying down to rest [16]. Neurological examination was normal. Routine daytime EEG was normal. Diagnostic PSG showed three episodes consistent with RBD. MRI showed non-specific T2 WI hyper intense lesions in the left subinsular cortex with normal diffusion-weighted imaging. Magnetic resonance angiography (MRA) showed an elongated and dilated left internal carotid artery, resulting in upward displacement of the left subthalamic region (Figure 38.1). ^{1}H-magnetic resonance spectroscopy (^{1}H-MRS) showed decreased N-acetylaspartate (NAA) and choline (Cho) peaks in the left subthalamic region compared to the right subthalamic region. SPECT during complex visual hallucinations showed increased CBF in the left middle occipital gyrus and the right inferior frontal-rolandic opercular gyri. An area of decreased CBF was noted in the right middle temporal gyrus. The authors postulated that the patient's symptoms may be attributable to vascular compression of the left subthalamus with subsequent release of motor (RBD) and hallucinatory (peduncular hallucinosis) phenomenon.

Sleep-related eating disorder/nocturnal eating syndrome

Lundgren et al. quantified serotonin transporter activity in nocturnal eating syndrome using the radiopharmaceutical ^{123}I-labeled 2-[2-(dimethylamino methyl phenyl thio]-5-iodophenylamine (^{123}I-ADAM) SPECT [17]. Uptake of ^{123}I-ADAM SPECT by the cerebellum was compared with ^{123}I-ADAM SPECT uptake in the midbrain, basal ganglia, and temporal lobes. Uptake ratios were generated for six patients with nocturnal eating syndrome and for six healthy controls. Patients with nocturnal eating syndrome had statistically significant increased ^{123}I-ADAM uptake in the midbrain compared to normal controls. The authors postulated that these findings may indicate a decrease in serotonin within the midbrain of patients with nocturnal eating syndrome.

Sleep-related headaches/hypnic headaches

Hypnic headaches are a form of sleep-related headaches that awakens the patient from sleep with a generalized or lateralized headache that usually lasts 5 to 30 min, with a frequency of at least 15 times per month for at least one month. Holle et al. studied 14 patients with hypnic headache and 14 age-matched and gender-matched healthy controls using MRI voxel-based morphometry [18]. Compared with healthy controls, patients with hypnic headaches showed statistically significant gray matter volume decrease in the left posterior hypothalamus. Smaller but still statistically significant gray matter volume loss was also noted in the operculum bilaterally, the right frontal lobe, the right cingulate cortex, and the left inferior temporal gyrus. The authors postulated that the gray matter volume decrease within the posterior hypothalamus may be a neuropathological indication of hypothalamic dysfunction in hypnic headaches given the role of the posterior hypothalamus in sleep and pain control.

Sleep-related groaning/catathrenia

Pevernagie *et al.* studied ten subjects aged 20 to 49 who presented with episodes of vocalization during prolonged expiration in REM sleep, the hallmark of catathrenia [19]. Seven patients underwent MRI scanning of the brain. No abnormalities were found in five of them. Parietal atrophy bilaterally with ventricular enlargement was reported in a 29-year-old man without any other medical or neurological conditions. A large left-sided frontal meningioma was reported in a 49-year-old woman. Resection of the meningioma did not improve or resolve the nocturnal groaning. The MRI findings in these two patients appeared unrelated to their catathrenia.

Conclusion

At the time of this review there were no MRI studies, SPECT studies, or PET studies of confusional arousals, recurrent isolated sleep paralysis, and sleep-related dissociative disorder. Future MRI, MRA, MRS, fMRI, SPECT, and PET studies into NREM and REM parasomnias may allow a better understanding of underlying pathophysiology. Individually each imaging modality has limitations. MRI, and MRA provide insights related to structure, but not underlying function. On the other hand MRS, SPECT, and PET provide insight into function, but spatial resolution is poor. These modalities when used in combination with clinical electrophysiology (e.g., EEG and PSG) may help provide better understanding into both structure and function of electrophysiologically verified parasomnias. Future studies combining both electrophysiology and multiple neuroimaging modalities may help in both the assessment of these disorders and the development of new treatment modalities.

References

1. Bassetti C, Vella S, Donati F, Wielepp P, Weder B. SPECT during sleepwalking. *Lancet*. 2000;**356**:484–5.

2. Hori T, Suzuki T, Terashima Y, *et al.* Chronic herpes simplex encephalitis with somnambulism: CT, MR and SPECT findings. *Jpn J Psychiatry Neurol*. 1990;**44**:735–9.

3. Kushida CA, Clerk AA, Kirsch CM, Hotson JR, Guilleminault C. Prolonged confusion with nocturnal wandering arising from NREM and REM sleep: a case report. *Sleep*. 1995;**18**:757–64.

4. Hoque R, Chesson AL, Jr. Zolpidem-induced sleepwalking, sleep related eating disorder, and sleep-driving: fluorine-18-flourodeoxyglucose positron emission tomography analysis, and a literature review of other unexpected clinical effects of zolpidem. *J Clin Sleep Med*. 2009;**5**:471–6.

5. Di Gennaro G, Autret A, Mascia A, *et al.* Night terrors associated with thalamic lesion. *Clin Neurophysiol*. 2004;**115**:2489–92.

6. Mendez MF. Pavor nocturnus from a brainstem glioma. *J Neurol Neurosurg Psychiatry*. 1992;**55**:860.

7. Limousin N, Dehais C, Gout O, *et al.* A brainstem inflammatory lesion causing REM sleep behavior disorder and sleepwalking (parasomnia overlap disorder). *Sleep Med*. 2009;**10**:1059–62.

8. Szucs A, Janszky J, Barsi P, *et al.* Sleep-related painful erection is associated with neurovascular compression of basal forebrain. *J Neurol*. 2002;**249**:486–7.

9. Karsenty G, Werth E, Knapp PA, *et al.* Sleep-related painful erections. *Nat Clin Pract Urol*. 2005;**2**:256–60; quiz 61.

10. Kikuchi K, Fujisawa I, Ohie T, *et al.* Ectopic posterior lobe of the pituitary gland and intractable nocturnal enuresis in a case with pituitary dwarfism. *Acta Paediatr Scand*. 1989;**78**:479–81.

11. Hunsballe JM, Lundorf E, Norgaard JP. The pituitary gland in nocturnal enuresis: MR findings. *Scand J Urol Nephrol*. 1996;**30**:85–7.

12. Yu B, Guo Q, Fan G, *et al.* Evaluation of working memory impairment in children with primary nocturnal enuresis: evidence from event-related functional magnetic resonance imaging. *J Paediatr Child Health*. 2011;**47**:429–35.

13. Lei D, Ma J, Du X, *et al.* Spontaneous brain activity changes in children with primary monosymptomatic nocturnal enuresis: a resting-state fMRI study. *Neurourol Urodyn*. 2012;**31**:99–104.

14. Salih F, Klingebiel R, Zschenderlein R, Grosse P. Acoustic sleep starts with sleep-onset insomnia related to a brainstem lesion. *Neurology*. 2008;**70**:1935–7.

15. Hoque R, Liendo C, Chesson AL, Jr. A girl who sees dead people. *J Clin Sleep Med*. 2009;**5**:277–9.

16. Vetrugno R, Vella A, Mascalchi M, *et al.* Peduncular hallucinosis: a polysomnographic and spect study of a patient and efficacy of serotonergic therapy. *Sleep Med*. 2009;**10**:1158–60.

17. Lundgren JD, Newberg AB, Allison KC, *et al.* 123I-ADAM SPECT imaging of serotonin transporter binding in patients with night eating syndrome: a preliminary report. *Psychiatry Res*. 2008;**162**:214–20.

18. Holle D, Naegel S, Krebs S, *et al.* Hypothalamic gray matter volume loss in hypnic headache. *Ann Neurol*. 2011;**69**:533–9.

19. Pevernagie DA, Boon PA, Mariman AN, Verhaeghen DB, Pauwels RA. Vocalization during episodes of prolonged expiration: a parasomnia related to REM sleep. *Sleep Med*. 2001;**2**:19–30.

Neuroimaging of Parkinson's disease and multiple system atrophy in patients with sleep disturbance

Jason Valerio and A. Jon Stoessl

Introduction

Sleep disturbances are common in patients with both multiple system atrophy (MSA) and Parkinson's disease (PD), where nearly all MSA patients [1] and an estimated 74–98% of PD patients [2] experience some form of sleep pathology. MSA and PD are both synucleinopathies, diseases characterized by abnormal aggregations of the protein alpha-synuclein in the central nervous sytem (CNS). The location of cellular deposition of the protein and neuronal networks affected leads to the clinical similarities as well as differences between these disorders. PD is clinically characterized by an asymmetric presentation of motor dysfunctions, specifically, bradykinesia, resting tremor, rigidity, and gait instability. MSA is a progressive neurodegenerative disease characterized by autonomic disturbances with varying degrees of cerebellar ataxia, parkinsonism, and pyramidal dysfunction. MSA patients are separated into MSA-P, if clinically predominant parkinsonian features are evident, and MSA-C, if a cerebellar syndrome predominates [3], despite pathology showing widespread alpha-synuclein oligodendroglial cytoplasmic inclusions. Given the widely distributed burden of pathology in PD and MSA, it comes as no surprise that significant non-motor complications of synucleinopathies have been increasingly appreciated and have garnered recent attention in the literature. Non-motor symptoms of PD and MSA, including mood disturbances, cognitive changes, pain, autonomic dysfunction, and sleep disturbances, represent a significant portion of the disability in each disease.

To better assess nocturnal disability, Chaudhari *et al.* developed a PD sleep scale (PDSS), an inventory of 15 commonly reported sleep disturbances. This scale has proven to be reliable and is employed in various countries [4]. Using tools such as the PDSS, a multitude of evidence suggests sleep dysfunction to be one of the most important determinants of quality of life (QOL) in PD [5]. Similar sleep rating scales and QOL questionnaires are being developed for MSA.

The focus of this chapter will be on primary sleep disorders in PD and MSA and insights provided by functional neuroimaging research. Specific disorders to be considered include excessive daytime sleepiness (EDS), sleep disordered breathing, restless legs syndrome/periodic limb movements in sleep (RLS/PLMS) and, rapid eye movement REM sleep behavior disorder (RBD). RBD is of particular interest and there are numerous neuroimaging studies investigating the relationship between synucleinopathies and RBD, but this will receive only limited attention here, as Chapter 40 is completely dedicated to this topic. Prior to delving into specific sleep disorders, the relevant neurochemical pathways in PD and MSA are reviewed.

Neuroimaging of common neurochemical pathways in PD, MSA, and sleep

Neurodegenerative disease manifests clinically when sufficient dysfunction occurs in vital neuronal networks. In PD and MSA, dopaminergic, serotonergic, noradrenergic, cholinergic, and hypocretin (orexin) systems are involved. The most important pathological process in PD is the degeneration of the nigrostriatal system; however, typical motor symptoms only appear once approximately 50% of nigral dopamine neurons and 80% of striatal dopamine is lost [6]. The Braak staging system for PD suggests that alpha-synuclein Lewy body deposition occurs in the vagal dorsal motor nucleus, magnocellular reticular nucleus, lower raphe nuclei (RN), and locus coeruleus (LC) prior to involvement of the substantia nigra (and hence prior to clinical manifestations of motor dysfunction). This is followed by involvement of the pedunculopontine nucleus (PPN), amygdala, basal nucleus of Meynert, thalamic nuclei, and olfactory, temporal and frontal cortices [7]. In MSA, alpha-synuclein oligodendroglial cytoplasmic inclusions affect similar nuclei, with additional degeneration affecting cerebellar Purkinje cells, the autonomic nuclei of the brainstem, the intermediolateral cell columns, and Onuf's nucleus of the spinal cord.

The aforementioned brainstem structures are intimately involved in the proposed physiology of REM sleep. These pathways are briefly summarized here, while a more comprehensive review is available elsewhere [8]. The cholinergic projections from the PPN and lateral dorsal tegmental nuclei (LDTN), along with serotonergic projections from the RN, noradrenergic input from the LC, and dopaminergic influence from the substantia nigra all influence "REM-off" regions, consisting of the ventrolateral part of the periaqueductal grey (vlPAG) and the lateral pontine tegmentum (LPT). Cortical and subcortical structures (thalamus, hypothalamus) directly and indirectly influence this pathway. The REM-off region is thought to have intimate connections with the sublaterodorsal nucleus

Neuroimaging of Sleep and Sleep Disorders, ed. Eric Nofzinger, Pierre Maquet, and Michael J. Thorpy. Published by Cambridge University Press. © Cambridge University Press 2013.

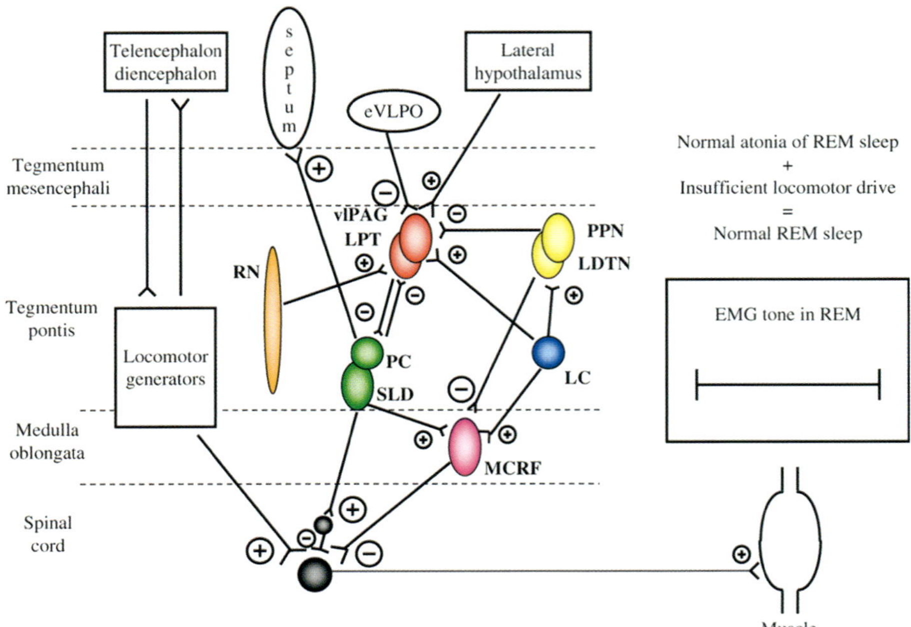

Figure 39.1 Important anatomical structures involved in REM sleep control and affected in PD and MSA. Based on the study of the rat with presumed corresponding human nuclei. The REM-off region, the vlPAG (in red) receives input from the serotonergic RN (orange), cholinergic PPN and LDTN (yellow), noradrenergic LC (blue), lateral hypothalamus, and eVLPO. There are also reciprocal connections with the REM-on region, SLD and PC (green). The REM-on region projects directly to spinal interneurons, and indirectly through the MCRF, causing active inhibition of anterior horn cells, which leads to atonia during REM sleep. Excitatory pathways are represented by encircled plus sign, inhibitory represented by encircled minus sign. PD = Parkinson's disease, MSA = multiple system atrophy, vlPAG = ventrolateral part of the periaqueductal grey matter, RN = raphe nucleus, PPN = pedunculopontine nucleus, LDTN = laterodorsal tegmental nucleus, LC = locus coeruleus, eVLPO = extended part of the ventrolateral preoptic nucleus, SLD = sublateral dorsal nucleus, PC = precoeruleus, MCRF = magnocellular reticular formation. (Boeve BF, Silber MH, Saper CB, Ferman TJ, Dickson DW, Parisi JE, *et al*. Pathophysiology of REM sleep behavior disorder and relevance to neurodegenerative disease. Brain. 2007 Nov;130 (Pt 11):2770–88. By permission of Oxford University Press.)

(SLD) or pre coereleus (PC), structures identified in animal models of RBD, but not as clearly delineated in humans. Direct and indirect gamma-aminobutyric acid (GABA)ergic and glycinergic neurons from this brainstem region project onto anterior horn cells of the spinal cord and their activity contributes to atonia during REM sleep (summarized in Figure 39.1 and Table 39.1). We will now explore each neurotransmitter in more detail, as it relates to PD, MSA, and sleep circuits.

Dopamine dysfunction

Traditional structural imaging, such as magnetic resonance imaging (MRI), provides limited information in PD, leading to a greater emphasis on functional neuroimaging for evaluating dopamine activity. Presynaptic dopamine function can be measured using three methods: [1] imaging the vesicular monoamine transporter type 2 (VMAT2) through [^{11}C]dihydrotetrabenazine ([^{11}C]DTBZ) labeling; [2] PET or SPECT imaging of dopamine transporter (DAT) binding using ligands such as (^{12}I-2-β-carbomethoxy-3 β-(4-iodophenyl)-N-(3-fluoropropyl) nortropane (^{123}I-FP-CIT) or [^{11}C]-D-threo-methylphenidate (^{11}C-MP); and [3] imaging of levodopa analogs, such as 6-[^{18}F]fluoro-levodopa (^{18}F-dopa), which are converted to [^{18}F]fluorodopamine (FDA) and taken up by dopamine neuron synaptic vesicles. Imaging of postsynaptic dopamine function relies on radiolabeled ligands that interact with dopamine receptors. Agonist and antagonist ligands include N-methylspiperone ([^{11}C] or [^{18}F]), [^{18}F]benperidol, [^{11}C]raclopride, [^{18}F]fallypride, [^{11}C]FLB 457, [^{11}C]N-propyl-nor-apomorphine and ^{11}C-labeled PHNO, and the older ligand ^{123}I-labeled (S)-2-hydroxy-3-iodo-6-methoxy-([1-ethyl-2-pyrrolidinyl]methyl) benzamide (^{123}I-IBZM). Each tracer has its advantages and disadvantages, and a description of each is beyond the scope of this chapter. An important consideration for the postsynaptic dopamine receptor tracers, however, is whether or not their binding is susceptible to competition from endogenous dopamine, as is the case for the agonist ligands and the lower antagonist ligands with lower affinity such as [^{11}C]raclopride and ^{123}I-IBZM. In contrast, high affinity ligands such as [^{18}F]fallypride or [^{11}C]FLB 457 can be used to label extra striatal dopamine receptors. The reader is referred to the review by Stoessl in 2011 [6] for further details.

Functional imaging has shown patterns that correspond to the clinical and neuropathological changes of PD. Neuroimaging of dopamine function has consistently shown a distinct rostral-caudal topographical distribution, with a preponderance of involvement in the posterior putamen and relative sparing of the caudate (Figure 39.2). Asymmetric involvement of the striatum, corresponding to the clinically asymmetric presentation of PD, is also recognized (Figure 39.2). As the disease progresses there is an overall decline in tracer uptake; the rostral-caudal gradient is maintained, but the asymmetry between the two sides becomes less prominent [9].

In MSA, in contrast to PD, conventional MRI may show atrophy of the putamen, middle cerebellar peduncles, pons, and cerebellum. Signal changes in these regions are also commonly reported [10]. The sensitivity and specificity of the structural changes visualized by MRI have been quite variable [11]; thus, for research purposes, there has been a greater reliance on functional imaging methods for evaluating MSA. In MSA-P, it is presumed that the majority of pathological change is in the nigrostriatal system, and similar to PD, a rostral-caudal gradient of putaminal degeneration has been reported [12]. While in MSA-C, the burden of the pathology is in the

Table 39.1. Neurochemical pathways in PD, MSA, and sleep with corresponding imaging modalities

Reference	Localization/ nuclei	Main neurotransmitters	Imaging modality/radiotracer	Sleep pathway	MSA or PD
[34, 59]	Raphe nucleus (RN)	Serotonin	[^{11}C]DASB (5-HT transporter), [^{11}C] WAY 100,635 (5-HT$_{1A}$ receptor) or α-[^{11}C]methyl-L-tryptophan (5-HT precursor)	Excitatory input to REM-"off" region Involved in arousal network Receives input from respiratory center nuclei	PD, MSA
[59]	Locus coerelus (LC)	Norepinephrine	^{11}C-RTI-32 (non-specific monoamine radioligand) [^{11}C] N-methylreboxetine (limited signal > age 50)	Excitatory input to LDTN and REM "off" region	PD, MSA
[34, 59]	Pedunculopontine nucleus (PPN)	Acetylcholine	Cholinesterase substrates: [^{11}C] PMP, [^{11}C]MP4A Presynaptic: [^{123}I] IBVM, Postsynaptic muscarinic ligands: ^{11}C-NMPB	Cholinergic input to thalamus, lateral hypothalamus, basal forebrain, and prefrontal cortex Involved in arousal network Inhibitory input to REM-off region Dysfunction of input to medullary nuclei contribute to OSA pathology	MSA > PD
[34, 59]	Lateral dorsal tegmentum (LDTN)	Acetylcholine	Cholinesterase substrates: [^{11}C] PMP, [^{11}C]MP4A Presynaptic: [^{123}I] IBVM, Postsynaptic muscarinic ligands: ^{11}C-NMPB	Thalamic cholinergic input Possible inhibitory input to MCRF Dysfunction of input to medullary nuclei contribute to OSA pathology	MSA > PD
[59]	Substantia nigra (SN)	Dopamine	Presynaptic: [^{11}C]DTBZ, [^{123}I-FP-CIT, ^{11}C-MP,^{18}F-Dopa Postsynaptic: N-methylspiperone ([^{11}C] or [^{18}F]), [^{18}F]benperidol, [^{11}C]raclopride, [^{18}F]fallypride, [^{11}C]FLB 457, [^{11}C] N-propyl-nor-apomorphine,^{11}C-labeled PHNO, and ^{123}I-labeled (S)-2-hydroxy-3-iodo-6-methoxy-([1-ethyl-2-pyrrolidinyl]methyl) benzamide (^{123}I-IBZM).	Not yet fully understood Possibly influences sleep wake states, and involved in arousal network Interacts with hypocretin secretion of the hypothalamus Possibly influences REM-off center	PD > MSA
[59]	Ventral periaqueductal gray matter (vlPAG)	Dopamine		REM "off" region Dual connection with REM "on" region	PD, MSA
[59]	Sublateral dorsal nucleus (or human equivalent)			REM "on" region Dual connection with REM "off" region Excitatory projections to spinal interneurons with inhibition of spinal motor neurons for REM atonia	?
[34, 59]	Tubero-mammillary nucleus (TMN)	Histamine		Receive input from the ventrolateral preoptic nucleus (VLPO) Projections to lateral hypothalamus Involved in arousal network	?
[34, 59]	Lateral hypothalamus	Hypocretin dopamine		Send input to cerebral cortex, and reciprocal connections to the LC and TMN Fire maximally during wake states Involved in hunger and foraging Excitatory input to REM "off" region	PD
[59]	Magnocellular reticular formation (MCRF)			Direct inhibitory input to spinal motor neurons	?
[34, 44]	Arcuate nucleus	Serotonin, acetylcholine, glutamate		Receives input from respiratory center nuclei	MSA

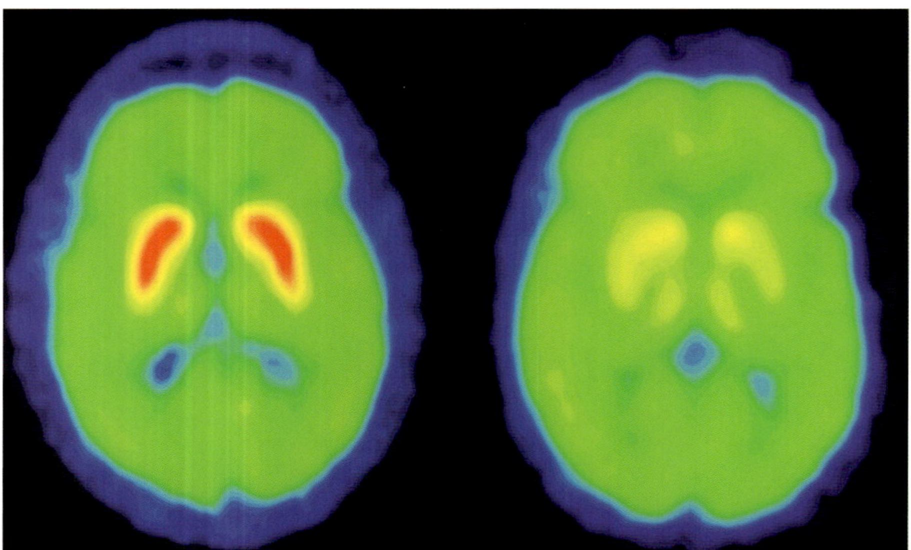

Figure 39.2 Dopamine transporter binding (VMAT2) in a healthy control (left) and a patient with moderate PD (right). There is an asymmetric and graded reduction of tracer uptake in the PD patient, affecting the putamen more than the caudate nucleus. VMAT = vesicular monamine transporter type 2; PD = Parkinson's disease.

olivopontocerebellar system, the neurodegenerative process is diffuse and the striatum and substantia nigra are still affected, albeit to a lesser extent. In fact, Munoz *et al.*, using ^{123}I-FP-CIT SPECT, recently demonstrated that 10/13 MSA-C patients without evidence of parkinsonism had subclinical presynaptic dopaminergic dysfunction of the putamen and caudate nuclei [13].

The neurotransmitter dopamine may play a role in REM sleep control, but there is limited direct evidence for this. There has been a clear relationship, however, with RBD and substantia nigra dysfunction (see RBD section). Dopamine may also play a role in regulation of the sleep/wake cycle with a wakefulness-promoting effect that is similar to histamine and hypocretin. There is also evidence that dopaminergic projections to the hypothalamus influence hypocretin release (see excessive day-time sleepiness section).

Cholinergic system

Along with the dopaminergic deficits, there is evidence supporting dysfunction in cholinergic neurotransmission in PD and MSA. Traditionally, cholinergic pathways to the cerebral cortex from the basal forebrain have been associated with higher cognitive function, including executive function, attention, learning, and memory. Cholinergic brainstem nuclei, however, play an important role in sleep physiology. The pedunculopontine tegmentum (PPT) and lateral dorsal tegmentum (LDT) have cholinergic neurons that project to the thalamus, lateral hypothalamus, basal forebrain, pontine and medullary reticular formation, cerebellum, and basal ganglia. The PPT/LDT cholinergic projections are felt to be involved in arousal, wakefulness, REM sleep dreaming, and immobility during REM sleep [8]. Neuropathological studies have shown loss of these cholinergic neurons in PD, MSA, and Lewy body dementia (LBD) [14–16]. Their involvement in the pathophysiology of RBD is still under debate [16], and is discussed in more detail below.

The cholinergic pathways can be labeled with cholinesterase substrates, such as N-[11C] methylpiperidyl propionate ([11C] PMP) or N-[11C]methylpiperidin-4-*yl* acetate ([11C]MP4A). These radioligands are acetylcholine analogs and are selective substrates for hydrolysis by acetylcholinesterase (AChE). Ligands binding to presynaptic vesicular acetylcholine transporters, such as ^{123}I-iodobenzovesamicol ([123I]IBVM), or postsynaptic muscarinic ligands, such as N-[11C] methyl-4-piperidyl benzilate (11C-NMPB), have been used to a lesser extent [6]. Using [11C]PMP with PET, Gilman *et al.* showed cholinergic dysfunction in the caudate nuclei, putamen, cerebellum, and mesencephalon of PD, MSA-P, and progressive supranuclear palsy (PSP) patients when compared to controls. A more substantial decrease in cholinergic activity was seen in MSA-P and PSP when compared to PD, including a significant change in [11C]PMP uptake in the pons. This study and others demonstrate that cholinergic function is lost throughout the cortex in PD and MSA-P, with evidence that the most severe reductions occur in PD with dementia [17].

Other neurochemical markers

Other monoaminergic pathways involved in sleep and affected in PD and MSA include the noradrenergic and serotonergic neurons. PET ligands that bind solely to norepinephrine plasma membrane transporters (NET) are not yet in widespread use. The best characterized, [11C]N-methylreboxetine, shows little specific binding beyond middle age [18] and may accordingly be of limited utility in the assessment of PD and related disorders. [11C]RT132 binds with similar affinity to DAT and NET, but in areas with minimal dopamine innervation this tracer can be used as a reasonable noradrenergic marker. Based on this, Remy *et al.* suggested a role of noradrenergic loss in the pathogenesis of depression in PD, and showed decreased [11C]RT132 binding in the LC and thalamus (as well as the anterior cingulate cortex (ACC), amygdala, and ventral striatum) in depressed PD patients compared with non-depressed PD patients [19]. In normal sleep, the LC is thought to act as an arousal system and influence REM and non-rapid eye movement (NREM) sleep circuits through connections with the vlPAG and LPT [8]. Corresponding with the Braak hypothesis, LC dysfunction likely occurs rapidly and early in PD. In one longitudinal study, the LC had the second most rapid annual decline in ^{18}F-dopa uptake (a non-specific monoaminergic marker) compared with other brainstem and subcortical structures, in early PD [20].

Not unlike the LC, the RN is thought to be part of the "REM-on" region through caudal projections to the LPT and vlPAG. Raphe serotonergic nuclei neurons can be divided into two groups: those that project to the forebrain, consisting of raphe dorsalis and nucleus centralis superior; and those that project caudally, consisting of nucleus raphe obscurus, raphe pallidus, and raphe magnus. Using a monoclonal antibody directed against tryptophan hydroxylase, a rate limiting enzyme of serotonin (5-HT) production, Kovacs *et al.* showed a paradoxical increase in the percentage of serotonium neurons with caudal projections in MSA, PD, and PSP tissue, compared to controls [21]. Imaging studies with the selective serotonin transporter ligand, ^{11}C-labeled 3-amino-4-(2-dimethylaminomethyl-phenylsulfamyl)benzonitinle ($[^{11}$C]DASB), have suggested preservation of caudal brainstem serotonergic neurons in early PD, even though forebrain serotonergic innervation may be affected [22]. Strecker *et al.* also demonstrated preserved $[^{11}$C]DASB binding in dorsal RN in early PD, accompanied by a significant negative correlation of serotonin transporter and DAT in the striatum. The authors proposed an up regulation of serotonin as a compensatory mechanism against dopamine loss [23]. Subsequent studies of PD with depression demonstrated increases in $[^{11}$C]DASB binding in depressed PD patients compared with controls in cortex [24], amygdala, hypothalamus, caudal RN, and posterior cingulate cortex [25], although non-depressed PD patients have widespread reductions in $[^{11}$C]DASB binding [26]. Thus, there are several sources of evidence suggesting varying serotonergic activity in subgroups of the RN, with possible upregulation in the caudal region. The impact this has on REM sleep is not yet known. An interesting observation consistently reported clinically is the manifestation of RBD in non-PD subjects using selective serotonin reuptake inhibitors (SSRIs). Future studies should focus on serotonin levels in the RN at differing stages of PD with and without RBD.

Hypocretin is a recently discovered lateral hypothalamic neurotransmitter whose loss of function leads to narcolepsy. Although cerebrospinal Fiuid levels of hypocretin are typically normal in PD, neuropathological studies of the hypothalamus have shown a reduction in hypocretin neurons in PD [2] and MSA [27]. PD patients can show similar clinical features to those with narcolepsy, albeit of lesser severity.

Sleep disorders in PD and MSA

Excessive daytime sleepiness

EDS is defined as a tendency towards drowsiness and sleep that interfere with normal daily functioning, commonly recognized by a score of 10 or greater on the Epworth Sleepiness Scale (ESS), although lower scores are associated with increased risk of falling asleep at the wheel in patients with PD [28]. An estimated 15–57% of PD patients and 29% of MSA patients suffer from EDS [29, 30]. EDS may be one of the most common non-motor symptoms in PD and MSA, although it has received the least attention in the literature. This is likely due to the multifactorial nature of EDS. A sleep survey comparing EDS in PD and MSA patients reported similar rates of EDS in each group but suggested distinct etiologies. Dopaminergic treatment and presence of RLS predicted EDS in PD, while sleep disordered breathing and sleep efficiency did so in MSA [30].

Dopamine has been implicated in the arousal system. On the one hand, dopamine antagonists, such as haloperidol or rispiridone, or dopamine depletion with reserpine or tetrabenazine are sedating, while drugs that increase extracellular levels of dopamine, such as methylphenidate, are wake promoting. However, all these drugs have effects on monoamines other than dopamine, in particular on norepinephrine and/or alpha adrenoceptors. In PD, dopamine agonists such as pramipexole or ropinirole are associated with EDS and sleep attacks in a dose-dependent pattern [31]. In the rat model, D_1 agonists increase hypocretin neuronal activity, while higher doses of D_2 agonists block this activity. Presumably, titrating D_2 agonists in a population with deficient hypocretin function, such as PD and MSA, would be sedating and have an effect similar to narcolepsy [31]. Indeed, PD patients can experience intrusive sleep events that resemble narcoleptic sleep attacks, which may have serious effects on daily activities, including driving [28].

An inverse correlation of ESS scores and presynaptic striatal dopamine activity, measured by ^{123}I-FP-CIT, was reported in patients with moderate PD (assessed by a Hoehn and Yahr score of 2). Despite similar levodopa doses, early PD patients did not show the same correlation, leading the authors to conclude that the primary neurodegenerative process is more important in EDS than dopaminergic replacement therapy [32]. Using $[^{11}$C]raclopride PET to assess hypothalamic dopamine receptors, Politis *et al.* demonstrated loss of D_2/D3 binding in the hypothalamus (Figure 39.3). This decrease in hypothalamic $[^{11}$C]raclopride binding was not correlated with levodopa dosage or disease duration [33]. The authors concluded that in PD, Lewy body pathology disrupts dopaminergic neurons and postsynaptic dopamine receptors in the hypothalamus [33]. EDS experienced by PD patients is likely partly due to neurodegeneration of dopaminergic, serotonergic, and noradrenergic neurons to arousal targets in the lateral hypothalamus, basal forebrain, and cerebral cortex [34], coupled with monoaminergic receptor alterations and loss of hypocretin neurons [2].

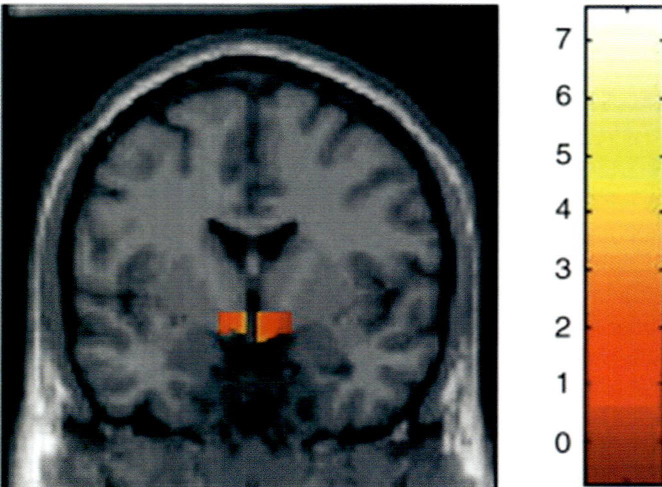

Figure 39.3 Coronal section of a statistical parametric map comparing PD patients (n = 14) with normal controls (n = 9). Yellow red areas represent hypothalamic areas with significant decreases in [^{11}C]raclopride uptake in PD patients compared to controls, with the bar on the right indicating z values. Correlation with EDS was not assessed in this study. PD = Parkinson's disease. (Reprinted from Experimental Neurology, 214, Politis M, Piccini P, Pavese N, Koh SB, Brooks DJ. Evidence of dopamine dysfunction in the hypothalamus of patients with Parkinson's disease: an in vivo 11C-raclopride PET study, 2008, with permission from Elsevier Ltd.)

Recent MRI studies have correlated alternate brain structures with EDS in PD. Kato *et al.* suggested a link between EDS in PD and widespread cortical and subcortical atrophy [35]. Matsui *et al.* demonstrated reduced fractional anisotropy in the fornix [36], implicating degeneration in this tract to be associated with EDS in PD.

Sleep disordered breathing

The reported frequency of sleep disordered breathing in PD varies from 40% to 50% [37, 38], while some authors have argued rates of obstructive sleep apnea (OSA) in PD are similar to the general population [39]. Conversely, sleep disordered breathing helps define the disease in MSA. It can manifest as central hypoventilation, OSA, and laryngeal stridor. Central hypoventilation consists of dysrhythmic breathing patterns, diminished hypoxic ventilator drive, Cheyne–Stokes respiration, and central sleep apnea. Central sleep apnea likely results from degeneration of brainstem respiratory center nuclei, including loss of serotonergic and cholinergic neurons in the arcuate nucleus of the ventral medulla, and serotonergic dysfunction in the RN [40, 41]. Central sleep apnea is more commonly reported in later stages of MSA.

OSA in MSA likely results from a combination of snoring and nocturnal laryngeal stridor. Laryngeal stridor may arise from paralysis of abductor laryngeal muscles or dystonia of adductor muscles [40, 41]. It is more common than central hypoventilation and is associated with sudden death during sleep [41]. Stridor during wake states is preceded by nocturnal stridor and may be indicative of disease progression. Iranzo *et al.* investigated continuous positive airway pressure (CPAP) in MSA patients with sleep dysfunction [42]. Of the 20 patients studied, 14 had vocal cord abduction dysfunction, and 5 had nocturnal stridor (complete laryngeal abduction dysfunction and OSA). Of the five patients with nocturnal stridor, four accepted CPAP, and in three of these patients CPAP completely abolished nocturnal stridor, OSA, and hemoglobin desaturation. CPAP is now used as a treatment strategy for nocturnal stridor and OSA. This therapeutic strategy improves sleep quality and improves median survival time in patients with nocturnal stridor [41]. Direct sleep video-laryngoscopy of a 57-year-old female with MSA confirmed inspiratory adduction of vocal cords and resolution with CPAP [43].

OSA is related to cholinergic activity in the thalamus, but not to dopaminergic activity in the striatum of MSA patients. In 15 patients with probable MSA, Gilman *et al.* demonstrated an inverse correlation between the density of [^{123}I]IBVM (iodobenzovesamicol, a ligand for the vesicular acetylcholine transporter) binding in the thalamus and the severity of the apnea-hypopnea index (AHI). As discussed above, the majority of cholinergic projections to the thalamus arise from PPT and LDT; thus, measuring radiotracer uptake in the thalamus serves as a surrogate for cholinergic dysfunction in these pontine nuclei. However, there was no relationship between striatal [^{11}C]DTBZ binding and AHI, suggesting that striatal dopaminergic dysfunction does not contribute to OSA [44]. Presumably, reduced caudal cholinergic projections of the PPT and LDT to medullary nuclei controlling upper airway tone contribute to the pathophysiology of OSA in MSA. Although central apnea was not measured in this study, disruption of cholinergic input to the medullary arcuate nucleus could, in theory, contribute to the increased rates of central sleep apnea events seen in MSA. MRI morphometry of MSA patients has shown a reduced area of the sagittal pons, but not midbrain, when compared to age-matched controls and PD patients. This group of MSA patients also showed a trend for higher risk of OSA [45]. Although this evidence on its own is not compelling, it does support the notion that pontine dysfunction is associated with OSA, and OSA is more prevalent in MSA as compared to PD.

Restless legs syndrome/periodic limb movements

Although controversial, a number of studies have supported an increased prevalence of RLS in PD patients, with some studies citing over double the prevalence compared with the general population [46]. RLS is defined by: [1] an urge to move the legs, which is usually accompanied or caused by unpleasant sensations; [2] symptoms occur during rest; [3] symptoms can be relieved by movement; [4] symptoms are worse in the evening or at night [47]. PLMS is a non-specific disorder, which occurs in association with various sleep pathologies including OSA, narcolepsy, RBD, and most importantly in 90% of patients with RLS. It is characterized by repetitive foot extension and dorsiflexion during sleep, and although these movements cause sleep disturbances, they are typically not recognized by the patient. PLMS in PD has not been investigated as thoroughly as RLS, but common dopaminergic neuronal pathways are suspected. There is no convincing association of RLS and PMLS in MSA patients [41].

Given the exacerbation of RLS symptoms with dopamine antagonists and treatment of RLS/PMLS symptoms with levodopa and dopamine agonists, an underlying central dopamine dysfunction has been suspected. Akathisia is a common side effect of dopamine antagonists, even in young healthy individuals, lending further support to a possible role for dopamine dysfunction in RLS. RLS symptoms also occur in PD patients as medication benefit wears off between doses [46].

Results from functional imaging studies of presynaptic dopamine function have been somewhat inconsistent. DAT imaging using ^{123}I-IPT and SPECT have shown significant differences in dopamine uptake in controls compared with RLS patients, but the findings may be technique dependent [48, 49]. One study examined ^{123}I-IPT striatal binding in 28 RLS patients compared with 29 patients with early PD and controls. PD patients had lower presynaptic ^{123}I-IPT binding, as would be expected, but there was no significant difference or dysfunction in ^{123}I-IPT binding in RLS [50]. This argues against a common pathophysiological presynaptic process and etiology between RLS and PD. Interestingly, Happe *et al.* in a separate study, showed that reduced striatal ^{123}I-FP-CIT was correlated with an increase in the number of PLMS events in patients diagnosed with PD [32]. The authors suggested that loss of dopaminergic cells in PD might be related to the intensity of PLMS, but the finding would of course also be consistent with PLMS occurring as a manifestation of more severe or more advanced PD. Most recently, Earley *et al.* demonstrated a significant decrease in DAT binding potential (using ^{11}C-d-*threo*-methylphenidate) in the putamen and caudate of patients with RLS. Finally, they suggested striatal SPECT DAT dysfunction in PD patients is easily visualized due to dopaminergic neuronal loss, but in RLS there is no neuronal loss, only decreased membrane-bound striatal DAT function due to iron deficiency and iron metabolism (discussed further below) [51].

Two studies by a single group, analyzing postsynaptic dopamine receptor binding have also shown an association between D_2 dysfunction and PLMS. Using ^{123}I-IBZM and SPECT, patients with PLMS again demonstrated decreased D_2 receptor binding [52, 53]. Interestingly, postsynaptic dopamine function in RLS patients has yielded inconsistent results. This poses the question of a distinct process occurring between PLMS and RLS.

Cervenka *et al.* used ^{11}C]raclopride and ^{11}C]FLB 457 to measure postsynaptic dopamine D_2 receptor binding in striatal and extrastriatal regions. Results demonstrated increased binding of radiotracers in the striatum, as well as the thalamus, insula, and ACC in RLS patients compared with controls. Increased binding would be in keeping with receptor upregulation or with reduced receptor occupancy due to lower levels of endogenous dopamine in the un-medicated state. The thalamus, insula, and ACC were chosen given their presumed involvement in medial nociceptive systems and in the affective motivational component of pain. This is one of the first studies using neuroimaging to explore the possible interaction between somatosensory processing and dopamine regulation in RLS, and supports the theory that RLS is a somato motor disorder. PET scans were performed twice in the same day, to assess for possible diurnal rhythm of dopamine variations; however, none was observed [54].

A dysfunction in iron metabolism has more recently been postulated as a mechanism for RLS/PMLS. Iron is a cofactor for tyrosine hydroxylase (TH), an enzyme involved in dopamine synthesis. Neuropathological studies have demonstrated that iron deficiency was associated with decreased D_2 receptors in the putamen of RLS brains, but normal D_1 and VMAT binding. This would offer an explanation for the normal dopaminergic presynaptic neuroimaging studies in RLS, but the abnormal ^{11}C]raclopride and ^{11}C]FLB 457 (D_2 receptor ligands) binding. Somewhat surprisingly, TH activity was in fact up regulated in the substantia nigra and the putamen of the same specimens. Whether iron deficiency produces an increase in TH and a dopaminergic abnormality, or paradoxically excess iron accumulation in PD is a response to dopaminergic cell degeneration, has yet to be elucidated.

MRI studies have revealed increased grey matter in the pulvinar of RLS patients [55] as well as widespread changes in fractional anisotropy in RLS, including subcortical white matter adjacent to primary and associate motor and somatosensory cortices, thalamus, motor projection fibers, and anterior cingulum [56]. Functional MRI studies have demonstrated activation of the thalamus and cerebellum during sensory leg discomfort; during combined sensory discomfort and PLMS, there was additional activation in the region of the red nucleus and the reticular formation [57].

Overall, the association between PD, RLS, and PMLS is complex, with inconsistent neuroimaging results. This may in part reflect the fact that RLS is likely to represent a sensorimotor disorder involving multiple circuits regulated by dopamine. The failure to consistently demonstrate presynaptic striatal dopaminergic dysfunction in RLS suggests that it is unlikely to have pathogenesis similar to PD, although the possibility of reduced activity in spinal dopamine projections in RLS (which would not be detected on radiotracer imaging) has been suggested (but not supported by autopsy studies [58]), and it is likely that PD predisposes to RLS.

REM sleep behavior disorder (RBD)

Unlike other sleep pathologies, RBD has been clearly associated with PD and MSA alike. Neuroimaging studies related to RBD and the synucleinopathies will be reviewed here; further discussion is provided in Chapter 40, which is dedicated to RBD. RBD is characterized by loss of normal motor atonia during REM sleep (REM sleep without atonia [RSWA]), and enactment of vivid dreams (dream enactment behavior [DEB]) [59]. RBD can be secondary to neurological diseases and has been commonly reported in synucleinopathies (MSA, LBD, PD, PD with dementia, pure autonomic failure) and more rarely in tauopathies (PSP, Alzheimer's disease), TDP-43opathy (amyotrophic lateral sclerosis), and genetic disease (spinocerebellar atrophy-3, Huntington's disease) [59]. In 1996, Schenck *et al.* were the first to describe the association between RBD and the future emergence of neurodegenerative disorders [60]. Later studies report a 10-year risk of 40% or higher of developing a

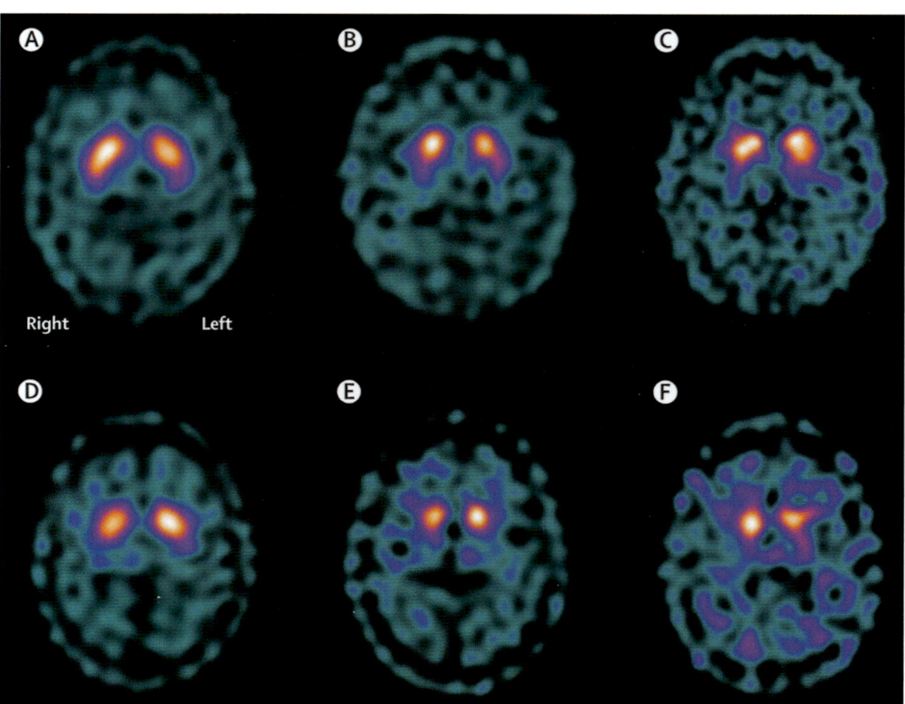

Figure 39.4 ^{123}I-FP-CIT SPECT imaging comparing a patient with idiopathic RBD who did not develop any evidence of parkinsonism (top row) and a patient with RBD who subsequently developed PD (bottom row). Patients compared at baseline (A,D), 1.5 years (B,E), and 3 year (C,F) follow up. ^{123}I-FP-CIT binding was reduced in the striatum (putamen > caudate nucleus) in the RBD patient who went on to develop PD. ^{123}I-FP-CIT = [123]I-2β-carbomethoxy-3β-(4-iodophenyl)-N-(3-fluoropropyl)-nortropane. RBD = rapid eye movement sleep behavior disorder. (Reprinted from Lancet Neurology, 10(9), Iranzo A, Valldeoriola F, Lomena F, Molinuevo JL, Serradell M, Salamero M, et al. Serial dopamine transporter imaging of nigrostriatal function in patients with idiopathic rapid-eye-movement sleep behavior disorder: a prospective study. 797–805., Sep 2011, with permission from Elsevier.)

synucleinopathy following a diagnosis of RBD [61]. However, the delay from RBD onset and motor symptoms of synucleinopathy can be as long as 50 years. A number of studies have now shown decreased presynaptic striatal dopamine function in idiopathic RBD, using [11C]DTBZ and PET [62], N-(3-iodopropen-2-yl)-2beta-carbomethocy-3beta-(4-chlorophemyl)tropane (^{123}I-IPT) SPECT [63, 64], and ^{123}I-FP-CIT SPECT [65]. Unlike in RLS, postsynaptic dopamine function has not proven to be abnormal in idiopathic RBD.

In a prospective study, Iranzo *et al.* tracked 43 patients with idiopathic RBD for up to five years following ^{123}I-FP-CIT SPECT imaging of striatal function and transcranial sonography of the substantia nigra. Of the 43 patients, 27 had either decreased radiotracer uptake or substantia nigra hyperechogenicity, and of these, 8 developed a synucleinopathy [66]. In a follow-up prospective study, Iranzo *et al.* performed serial ^{123}I-FP-CIT SPECT imaging, at baseline and 1.5 and 3 years, on 20 patients with idiopathic RBD. Patients with RBD demonstrated a more rapid rate of decline in DAT binding than healthy controls and the three patients who developed PD over the course of the study had the most striking dopaminergic dysfunction at baseline and the 3-year assessment (Figure 39.4) [67]. These studies demonstrate the tremendous potential of functional neuroimaging to predict and monitor the progression of disease patterns in idiopathic RBD.

This evidence supports an association between RBD and presynaptic dopaminergic dysfunction, but it is unclear whether the substantia nigra is directly involved in REM sleep control or whether abnormalities of DA imaging simply reflect premotor parkinsonism in those patients in whom RBD is an earlier manifestation of synucleinopathy. Brainstem nuclei believed to be involved in control of the REM sleep system

in humans include but are not limited to: LC, subcoeruleus complex, PPN, LDTN, magnocellular reticular formation (MCRF), SCD (or human equivalent), and substantive nigra (see Figure 39.1 and Table 39.1) [8], many of which are affected by Lewy body pathology. Theoretically, destruction in any of these pathways including cholinergic, noradrenergic or serotonergic projections could cause RBD and of these structures, the substantive nigra would be affected last, according to the Braak hypothesis. In patients with established early-stage PD, there is an inverse relationship between both absolute and percentage REM sleep duration and mesopontine uptake of ^{18}F-dopa [68]. This suggests increased monaminergic activity in those patients with reduced REM sleep, although it is not known whether this reflects compensatory increases in the activity of serotonergic neurons. A study comparing striatal VMAT binding of [11C]DTBZ, and thalamic presynaptic cholinergic terminals (^{123}I]IBVM) was performed on MSA patients with RBD and controls. Reduced radiotracer uptake in the thalamus and striatum was demonstrated in MSA patients, but only [11C]DTBZ binding in the striatum was inversely correlated with the severity of RBD. Recognizing the limitations of a correlational study, the authors concluded that cholinergic dysfunction in the PPT/LDT does not contribute to RBD [69].

Patients taking SSRIs and selective noradrenergic reuptake inhibitors (SNRIs) can develop RBD or aggravate RBD symptoms. Whether this is an unmasking of a future neurodegenerative process, or whether serotonin plays a key role in RBD pathogenesis is unknown. Future imaging with [11C]DASB in patients with idiopathic RBD may help solve some of these questions.

A number of structural MRI studies have appeared in the last year in patients with isolated RBD. Ellmore *et al.* [70]

demonstrated reduced putamen volume in RBD patients. Another study utilizing voxel-based morphometry found gray matter volume reduction in the cerebellum, pontine tegmentum, and parahippocampul gyrus [71]. Scherfler *et al.* [72] applied diffusion tensor techniques to demonstrate reduced fractional anisotropy in the midbrain and rostral pontine tegmentum as well as increased mean diffusivity (a measure of microstructural damage) in the pontine reticular formation.

Conclusions

Functional imaging and more recently MRI, particularly with measures of connectivity and microstructural damage, have provided tremendous insights into those neural networks involved in sleep physiology and their disruption in neurodegenerative disease. These studies have revealed dysfunction in dopaminergic, cholinergic, and serotonergic pathways in patients with PD and MSA. Coupled with our knowledge of sleep anatomy and sleep networks there is compelling evidence that degeneration of specific nuclei predispose to RBD and sleep disordered breathing. EDS is likely a multifactorial symptom in PD and MSA, with a primary disruption in arousal networks. RLS and PLMS coincide with PD, but a better understanding of their pathophysiology is still needed in order to clarify the significance of this association

In the future, a greater focus should be placed on non-dopaminergic pathways to evaluate sleep disorders in PD and MSA. Both current radiotracers and new radiotracers yet to be developed will provide further insights into the role of serotonin, acetylcholine, norepinephrine, histamine, and hypocretin in synucleinopathies. Preclinical detection of disease is one application of this technology that may come to fruition in the very near future. Ultimately, the development of therapeutics targeted towards preventing aggregation of proteins, or disease-modifying therapies in the premotor state will revolutionize the landscape of PD and MSA.

References

1. Colosimo C. Nonmotor presentations of multiple system atrophy. *Nat Rev Neurol.* 2011;7(5):295–8.

2. Thannickal TC, Lai YY, Siegel JM. Hypocretin (orexin) cell loss in Parkinson's disease. *Brain.* 2007;**130** (Pt 6):1586–95.

3. Halliday GM, Holton JL, Revesz T, Dickson DW. Neuropathology underlying clinical variability in patients with synucleinopathies. *Acta Neuropathol.* 2011;**122**(2):187–204.

4. Chaudhuri KR, Pal S, DiMarco A, *et al.* The Parkinson's disease sleep scale: a new instrument for assessing sleep and nocturnal disability in Parkinson's disease. *J Neurol Neurosurg Psychiatry.* 2002;73(6):629–35.

5. Scaravilli T, Gasparoli E, Rinaldi F, Polesello G, Bracco F. Health-related quality of life and sleep disorders in Parkinson's disease. *Neurol Sci.* 2003;**24**(3):209–10.

6. Stoessl AJ. Neuroimaging in Parkinson's disease. *Neurotherapeutics.* 2011;**8** (1):72–81.

7. Kingsbury AE, Bandopadhyay R, Silveira-Moriyama L, *et al.* Brain stem pathology in Parkinson's disease: an evaluation of the Braak staging model. *Mov Disord.* 2010;25(15):2508–15.

8. Boeve BF, Silber MH, Saper CB, *et al.* Pathophysiology of REM sleep behavior disorder and relevance to neurodegenerative disease. *Brain.* 2007;130(Pt 11):2770–88.

9. Nandhagopal R, Kuramoto L, Schulzer M, *et al.* Longitudinal progression of sporadic Parkinson's disease: a multi-tracer position emission tomography study. *Brain.* 2009;132(Pt 11):2970–9.

10. Watanabe H, Ito M, Fukatsu H, *et al.* Putaminal magnetic resonance imaging features at various magnetic field strengths in multiple system atrophy. *Mov Disord.* 2010;**25**(12):1916–23.

11. Brooks DJ, Seppi K. Proposed neuroimaging criteria for the diagnosis of multiple system atrophy. *Mov Disord.* 2009;24(7):949–64.

12. Wenning GK, Colosimo C, Geser F, Poewe W. Multiple system atrophy. *Lancet Neurol.* 2004;3(2):93–103.

13. Munoz E, Iranzo A, Rauek S, *et al.* Subclinical nigrostriatal dopaminergic denervation in the cerebellar subtype of multiple system atrophy (MSA-C). *J Neurol.* 2011;**258** (12):2248–53.

14. Hirsch EC, Graybiel AM, Duyckaerts C, Javoy-Agid F. Neuronal loss in the pedunculopontine tegmental nucleus in Parkinson disease and in progressive supranuclear palsy. *Proc Natl Acad Sci U S A.* 1987;**84**(16):5976–80.

15. Benarroch EE, Schmeichel AM, Parisi JE. Depletion of mesopontine cholinergic and sparing of raphe neurons in multiple system atrophy. *Neurology.* 2002;59(6):944–6.

16. Schmeichel AM, Buchhalter LC, Low PA, *et al.* Mesopontine cholinergic neuron involvement in Lewy body dementia and multiple system atrophy. *Neurology.* 2008;70(5):368–73.

17. Gilman S, Koeppe RA, Nan B, *et al.* Cerebral cortical and subcortical cholinergic deficits in parkinsonian syndromes. *Neurology.* 2010;74 (18):1416–23.

18. Ding YS, Singhal T, Planeta-Wilson B, *et al.* PET imaging of the effects of age and cocaine on the norepinephrine transporter in the human brain using (S, S)-[(11)C]O-methylreboxetine and HRRT. *Synapse.* 2010;64(1):30–8.

19. Remy P, Doder M, Lees A, Turjanski N, Brooks D. Depression in Parkinson's disease: loss of dopamine and noradrenaline innervation in the limbic system. *Brain.* 2005;128(Pt 6):1314–22.

20. Pavese N, Rivero-Bosch M, Lewis SJ, Whone AL, Brooks DJ. Progression of monoaminergic dysfunction in Parkinson's disease: a longitudinal 18F-dopa PET study. *Neuroimage.* 2011;**56**(3) 1463–8.

21. Kovacs GG, Kloppel S, Fischer I *et al.* Nucleus-specific alteration of raphe neurons in human neurodegenerative disorders. *Neuroreport.* 2003;14 (1):73–6.

22. Albin RL, Koeppe RA, Bohnen NI, *et al.* Spared caudal brainstem SERT binding in early Parkinson's disease. *J Cereb Blood Flow Metab.* 2008;28(3):441–4.

23. Strecker K, Wegner F, Hesse S, *et al.* Preserved serotonin transporter binding

in de novo Parkinson's disease: negative correlation with the dopamine transporter. *J Neurol.* 2011;**258** (1):19–26.

24. Boileau I, Warsh JJ, Guttman M, *et al.* Elevated serotonin transporter binding in depressed patients with Parkinson's disease: a preliminary PET study with [11C]DASB. *Mov Disord.* 2008;**23** (12):1776–80.

25. Politis M, Wu K, Loane C, *et al.* Depressive symptoms in PD correlate with higher 5-HTT binding in raphe and limbic structures. *Neurology.* 2010;**75** (21):1920–7.

26. Guttman M, Boileau I, Warsh J, *et al.* Brain serotonin transporter binding in non-depressed patients with Parkinson's disease. *Eur J Neurol.* 2007;**14**(5):523–8.

27. Benarroch EE, Schmeichel AM, Sandroni P, Low PA, Parisi JE. Involvement of hypocretin neurons in multiple system atrophy. *Acta Neuropathol.* 2007;**113**(1):75–80.

28. Hobson DE, Lang AE, Martin WR, *et al.* Excessive daytime sleepiness and sudden-onset sleep in Parkinson disease: a survey by the Canadian Movement Disorders Group. *JAMA.* 2002;**287**(4):455–63.

29. Schulte EC, Winkelmann J. When Parkinson's disease patients go to sleep: specific sleep disturbances related to Parkinson's disease. *J Neurol.* 2011;**258**(Suppl 2):S328–35.

30. Moreno-Lopez C, Santamaria J, Salamero M, *et al.* Excessive daytime sleepiness in multiple system atrophy (SLEEMSA study). *Arch Neurol.* 2011;**68** (2):223–30.

31. Arnulf I, Leu-Semenescu S. Sleepiness in Parkinson's disease. *Parkinsonism Relat Disord.* 2009;**15**(Suppl 3):S101–4.

32. Happe S, Baier PC, Helmschmied K, *et al.* Association of daytime sleepiness with nigrostriatal dopaminergic degeneration in early Parkinson's disease. *J Neurol.* 2007;**254**(8):1037–43.

33. Politis M, Piccini P, Pavese N, Koh SB, Brooks DJ. Evidence of dopamine dysfunction in the hypothalamus of patients with Parkinson's disease: an in vivo 11C-raclopride PET study. *Exp Neurol.* 2008;**214**(1):112–16.

34. Saper CB, Fuller PM, Pedersen NP, Lu J, Scammell TE. Sleep state switching. *Neuron.* 2010;**68**(6):1023–42.

35. Kato S, Watanabe H, Senda J, *et al.* Widespread cortical and subcortical brain atrophy in Parkinson's disease with excessive daytime sleepiness. *J Neurol.* 2012;**259**(2):318–26.

36. Matsui H, Nishinaka K, Oda M, *et al.* Disruptions of the fornix fiber in Parkinsonian patients with excessive daytime sleepiness. *Parkinsonism Relat Disord.* 2006;**12**(5):319–22.

37. Chotinaiwattarakul W, Dayalu P, Chervin RD, Albin RL. Risk of sleep-disordered breathing in Parkinson's disease. *Sleep Breath.* 2011;**15**(3):471–8.

38. Diederich NJ, Vaillant M, Leischen M, *et al.* Sleep apnea syndrome in Parkinson's disease. A case-control study in 49 patients. *Mov Disord.* 2005;**20**(11):1413–18.

39. Trotti LM, Bliwise DL. No increased risk of obstructive sleep apnea in Parkinson's disease. *Mov Disord.* 2010;**25**(13):2246–9.

40. Benarroch EE, Schmeichel AM, Low PA, Parisi JE. Depletion of putative chemosensitive respiratory neurons in the ventral medullary surface in multiple system atrophy. *Brain.* 2007;**130**(Pt 2):469–75.

41. Iranzo A. Sleep and breathing in multiple system atrophy. *Curr Treat Options Neurol.* 2007;**9**(5):347–53.

42. Iranzo A, Santamaria J, Tolosa E. Continuous positive air pressure eliminates nocturnal stridor in multiple system atrophy. Barcelona Multiple System Atrophy Study Group. *Lancet.* 2000;**356**(9238):1329–30.

43. Kuzniar TJ, Morgenthaler TI, Prakash UB, *et al.* Effects of continuous positive airway pressure on stridor in multiple system atrophy-sleep laryngoscopy. *J Clin Sleep Med.* 2009;**5**(1):65–7.

44. Gilman S, Chervin RD, Koeppe RA, *et al.* Obstructive sleep apnea is related to a thalamic cholinergic deficit in MSA. *Neurology.* 2003;**61**(1):35–9.

45. Gama RL, Tavora DG, Bomfim RC, *et al.* Sleep disturbances and brain MRI morphometry in Parkinson's disease, multiple system atrophy and progressive supranuclear palsy - a comparative study. *Parkinsonism Relat Disord.* 2010;**16**(4):275–9.

46. Peralta CM, Frauscher B, Seppi K, *et al.* Restless legs syndrome in Parkinson's disease. *Mov Disord.* 2009;**24** (14):2076–80.

47. Allen RP, Picchietti D, Hening WA, *et al.* Restless legs syndrome: diagnostic criteria, special considerations, and epidemiology. A report from the restless legs syndrome diagnosis and epidemiology workshop at the National Institutes of Health. *Sleep Med.* 2003;**4** (2):101–19.

48. Eisensehr I, Wetter TC, Linke R, *et al.* Normal IPT and IBZM SPECT in drug-naive and levodopa-treated idiopathic restless legs syndrome. *Neurology.* 2001;**57**(7):1307–9.

49. Michaud M, Soucy JP, Chabli A, Lavigne G, Montplaisir J. SPECT imaging of striatal pre- and postsynaptic dopaminergic status in restless legs syndrome with periodic leg movements in sleep. *J Neurol.* 2002;**249**(2):164–70.

50. Linke R, Eisensehr I, Wetter TC, *et al.* Presynaptic dopaminergic function in patients with restless legs syndrome: are there common features with early Parkinson's disease? *Mov Disord.* 2004;**19**(10):1158–62.

51. Earley CJ, Kuwabara H, Wong DF, *et al.* The dopamine transporter is decreased in the striatum of subjects with restless legs syndrome. *Sleep.* 2011;**34**(3):341–7.

52. Staedt J, Stoppe G, Kogler A, *et al.* Dopamine D2 receptor alteration in patients with periodic movements in sleep (nocturnal myoclonus). *J Neural Transm Gen Sect.* 1993;**93**(1):71–4.

53. Staedt J, Stoppe G, Kogler A, *et al.* Single photon emission tomography (SPET) imaging of dopamine D2 receptors in the course of dopamine replacement therapy in patients with nocturnal myoclonus syndrome (NMS). *J Neural Transm Gen Sect.* 1995;**99** (1–3):187–93.

54. Cervenka S, Palhagen SE, Comley RA, *et al.* Support for dopaminergic hypoactivity in restless legs syndrome: a PET study on D2-receptor binding. *Brain.* 2006;**129**(Pt 8):2017–28.

55. Etgen T, Draganski B, Ilg C, *et al.* Bilateral thalamic gray matter changes in patients with restless legs syndrome. *Neuroimage.* 2005;**24**(4):1242–7.

56. Unrath A, Muller HP, Ludolph AC, Riecker A, Kassubek J. Cerebral white matter alterations in idiopathic restless legs syndrome, as measured by diffusion tensor imaging. *Mov Disord.* 2008;**23** (9):1250–5.

57. Bucher SF, Seelos KC, Oertel WH, Reiser M, Trenkwalder C. Cerebral generators involved in the pathogenesis

of the restless legs syndrome. *Ann Neurol.* 1997;**41**(5):639–45.

58. Earley CJ, Allen RP, Connor JR, Ferrucci L, Troncoso J. The dopaminergic neurons of the A11 system in RLS autopsy brains appear normal. *Sleep Med.* 2009;**10**(10):1155–7.

59. Boeve BF. REM sleep behavior disorder: updated review of the core features, the REM sleep behavior disorder-neurodegenerative disease association, evolving concepts, controversies, and future directions. *Ann N Y Acad Sci.* 2010;**1184**:15–54.

60. Schenck CH, Bundlie SR, Mahowald MW. Delayed emergence of a parkinsonian disorder in 38% of 29 older men initially diagnosed with idiopathic rapid eye movement sleep behavior disorder. *Neurology.* 1996;**46**(2):388–93.

61. Postuma RB, Gagnon JF, Vendette M, *et al.* Quantifying the risk of neurodegenerative disease in idiopathic REM sleep behavior disorder. *Neurology.* 2009;**72**(15):1296–300.

62. Albin RL, Koeppe RA, Cherrin RD, *et al.* Decreased striatal dopaminergic innervation in REM sleep behavior disorder. *Neurology.* 2000;**55**(9):1410–12.

63. Eisensehr I, Linke R, Noachtar S, *et al.* Reduced striatal dopamine transporters in idiopathic rapid eye movement sleep behavior disorder. Comparison with Parkinson's disease and controls. *Brain.* 2000;**123**(Pt 6):1155–60.

64. Eisensehr I, Linke R, Tatsch K, *et al.* Increased muscle activity during rapid eye movement sleep correlates with decrease of striatal presynaptic dopamine transporters. IPT and IBZM SPECT imaging in subclinical and clinically manifest idiopathic REM sleep behavior disorder, Parkinson's disease, and controls. *Sleep.* 2003;**26**(5):507–12.

65. Stiasny-Kolster K, Doerr Y, Moller JC, *et al.* Combination of 'idiopathic' REM sleep behavior disorder and olfactory dysfunction as possible indicator for alpha-synucleinopathy demonstrated by dopamine transporter FP-CIT-SPECT. *Brain.* 2005;**128**(Pt 1):126–37.

66. Iranzo A, Lomena F, Stockner H, *et al.* Decreased striatal dopamine transporter uptake and substantia nigra hyperechogenicity as risk markers of synucleinopathy in patients with idiopathic rapid-eye-movement sleep behavior disorder: a prospective study [corrected]. *Lancet Neurol.* 2010 **9**(11):1070–7.

67. Iranzo A, Valldeoriola F, Lomena F, *et al.* Serial dopamine transporter imaging of nigrostriatal function in patients with idiopathic rapid-eye-

movement sleep behavior disorder: a prospective study. *Lancet Neurol.* 2011;**10**(9):797–805.

68. Hilker R, Razai N, Ghaemi M, *et al.* [18F]fluorodopa uptake in the upper brainstem measured with positron emission tomography correlates with decreased REM sleep duration in early Parkinson's disease. *Clin Neurol Neurosurg.* 2003;**105**(4):262–9.

69. Gilman S, Koeppe RA, Chervin RD, *et al.* REM sleep behavior disorder is related to striatal monoaminergic deficit in MSA. *Neurology.* 2003;**61**(1):29–34.

70. Ellmore TM, Hood AJ, Castriotta RJ, *et al.* Reduced volume of the putamen in REM sleep behavior disorder patients. *Parkinsonism Relat Disord.* 2010;**16**(10):645–9.

71. Hanyu H, Inoue Y, Sakurai H, *et al.* Voxel-based magnetic resonance imaging study of structural brain changes in patients with idiopathic REM sleep behavior disorder. *Parkinsonism Relat Disord.* 2012;**18**(2):136–9.

72. Scherfler C, Frauscher B, Schocke M, *et al.* White and gray matter abnormalities in idiopathic rapid eye movement sleep behavior disorder: a diffusion-tensor imaging and voxel-based morphometry study. *Ann Neurol.* 2011;**69**(2):400–7.

Neuroimaging of idiopathic REM sleep behavior disorder

Alex Iranzo

Introduction

Rapid eye movement (REM) sleep behavior disorder (RBD) is a parasomnia confined to REM sleep. It is characterized by abnormal motor and vocal behaviors (e.g., jerking, kicking, shouting, crying, laughing) and nightmares (e.g., being attacked or chased by people) linked to REM sleep without atonia. RBD is the result of the dysfunction of the brainstem structures that regulate muscle atonia during REM sleep. RBD can be idiopathic (iRBD) or secondary to neurological conditions [1, 2]. Longitudinal follow-up of individuals with iRBD showed that this parasomnia can precede the classical cognitive (mild cognitive impairment and dementia) and motor (parkinsonism and cerebellar syndrome) symptoms of three neurodegenerative diseases where brainstem damage is severe and common, namely Parkinson disease (PD), dementia with Lewy bodies (DLB), and multiple system atrophy (MSA) [3–5]. Neuroimaging has supported the concept that RBD can be considered an indicator of an underlying neurodegenerative disease. Neuroimaging can identify those iRBD individuals with higher risk for developing parkinsonism and dementia. This chapter summarizes findings from structural and functional neuroimaging studies in individuals with iRBD. If one aims to learn the neuroimaging abnormalities seen in iRBD, one must first attempt to understand (1) the mechanisms that generate REM sleep atonia in normal conditions, (2) the neuroimaging findings seen in normal REM sleep, and (3) the pathophysiology and clinical significance of RBD.

REM sleep physiology

REM sleep is characterized by rapid eye movements, skeletal muscle atonia, desynchronized electroencephalographic (EEG) activity, and dreams that usually have an emotional content. The core structures for REM sleep generation and REM sleep muscle atonia are located in the pontine tegmentum and the ventral medial medulla. In brief, these brainstem structures activate the cortex via the thalamus and basal forebrain, and inhibit the spinal cord motoneurons, resulting in muscle atonia. The limbic system and hypothalamus also modulate REM sleep [6–8].

Studies in rodents revealed the presence of REM-on and REM-off structures in the pontine tegmentum that form the base of a REM sleep generation model which is analogous to an electronic flip-flop switch. In this model, REM-on neurons inhibit REM-off neurons, and vice versa. REM-on neurons are gamma-aminobutyric acid (GABA)ergic in nature, are located in the subcoeruleus nucleus in the pons, and inhibit REM-off neurons. These REM-off cells are also GABAergic and are located in the lateral pontine tegmentum and ventrolateral periaqueductal gray matter in the pons.

The characteristic electroencephalographic activity of REM sleep is mediated by glutamatergic inputs from the precoeruleus area in the pons and parabrachial nucleus in the basal forebrain that reach the thalamus, hypothalamus, and prefrontal cortex. These structures send cholinergic, glutamatergic, and GABAergic projections to the cortex and hippocampus producing cortical activation.

REM sleep is also characterized by active inhibition of the motoneurons of the spinal cord, resulting in skeletal muscle atonia. This prevents self-injuries while the subject is dreaming. Neurons generating REM sleep atonia are glutamatergic cells localized in the ventral subcoeruleus nucleus that send their projections to the magnocellularis nucleus in the ventral medulla. The magnocellularis nucleus in turn inhibits the motoneurons of the spinal cord through GABAergic and glycinergic descending inputs. The glutamatergic descending neurons from the ventral subcoeruelus nucleus that decrease REM sleep electromyographic activity are modulated by direct and indirect projections from the brainstem and supratentorial structures. They include excitatory glutamatergic projections from the primary motor area of the frontal cortex, supplementary somatosensory area, central nucleus of the amygdale, and periaqueductal gray matter. The ventral subcoeruleus nucleus also receive afferents from cholinergic neurons of the pedunculopontine nucleus and laterodorsal tegmental nucleus, serotonergic neurons from the dorsal raphe, noradrenergic neurons from the locus coeruleus, and hypocretinergic neurons from the dorsolateral hypothalamus. Interestingly, the substantia nigra pars compacta, which contains dopaminergic neurons that innervate the putamen and caudate, does not seem to play a major role in the generation of REM sleep.

Neuroimaging of REM sleep

In humans, functional brain imaging has been used to evaluate the neural mechanisms and structures that regulate REM sleep.

Neuroimaging of Sleep and Sleep Disorders, ed. Eric Nofzinger, Pierre Maquet, and Michael J. Thorpy. Published by Cambridge University Press. © Cambridge University Press 2013.

Positron emission tomography (PET), evaluating metabolism or regional cerebral flow using ^{18}F-Fluorodeoxyglucose and radiolabed water ($H_2^{15}O$), and more recently functional magnetic resonance imaging (fMRI) have disclosed some areas that are activated and deactivated during REM sleep when compared with wakefulness and non-rapid eye movement (NREM sleep. Quantification of brain glucose metabolism in REM sleep shows a global level of activation which is similar to wakefulness. Compared with waking and NREM sleep, however, some brain structures in REM sleep enhance their activity while others decrease. Overall, neuroimaging of human REM sleep shows activation of the pons and limbic system including the amygdala, paralimbic structures, and visual occipital cortex, whereas the frontal cortex is deactivated [9–12] (Table 40.1). These structures mediate muscle tone (pons), emotions (limbic system), visual images (occipital cortex), and executive and memory functions (frontal cortex) [13]. Therefore, neuroimaging during REM sleep detects activation of the same brain areas that animal studies have shown to generate REM sleep [6–8].

Pathophysiology and clinical significance of RBD

Dysfunction of the REM sleep atonia network forms the neuropathological basis for RBD [1, 2, 6–8]. Available data in experimental cats and rodents, and in humans affected by neurodegenerative diseases and structural brain lesions indicate that RBD is the result of impairment of the brainstem nuclei that generate REM sleep atonia (the subcoeruleus nucleus in the pontine tegmentum and the magnocellularis

Table 40.1. Activated and deactivated brain structures during normal REM sleep detected by functional neuroimaging

Activated structures

Pons

Midbrain

Midbrain periaqueductal gray

Cerebellum hemispheres and vermis

Basal forebrain
– Caudal orbital
– Ventral striatum including the nucleus accumbens, substantia innominata, and olfactory tubercle

Basal ganglia
– Caudate
– Putamen

Thalamus
– Lateral geniculate bodies

Hypothalamus
– Anterior
– Lateral

Limbic system
– Amygdala
– Anterior cingulate gyrus
– Hippocampus

Paralimbic structures
– Parahippocampal gyrus including the entorhinal cortex, anterior cingulate cortex, and anterior insula

Medial prefrontal cortex

Mesial temporal cortex
– Auditory association cortex
– Inferior visual association cortex

Occipital cortex
– Primary visual cortex
– Lateral occipital

Deactivated structures

Frontal cortex
– Lateral orbital
– Dorsolateral prefrontal cortex (gyrus supramarginalis)
– Opercular cortex

Posterior insular cortex

Inferior parietal cortex
– Angular cortex
– Supramarginal cortex

Precuneus

Posterior cingulate gyrus

nucleus in the ventral medial medulla) and their anatomical connections, particularly with the amygdala. Experimental localized lesions in cats and rodents confined to the dorso-lateral pontine tegmentum (involving the subcoeruleus nucleus) and also to the medulla (impairing the magnocellularis nucleus) produce REM sleep without atonia associated with what looks like dream-enacting behaviors during unequivocal REM sleep. In addition, RBD is frequent in neurodegenerative diseases such as PD, DLB, and MSA probably because in these three conditions severe pathological changes are commonly found in the pons, medulla, and amygdala. Also, brainstem and limbic focal lesions (e.g., stroke, encephalitis) have been described in patients with acute or subacute RBD onset. Besides, the common occurrence of nightmares in human RBD can be explained by involvement of the emotional limbic system (e.g., central nucleus of the amygdala), whereas complex motor and vocal dream-enacting behaviors (e.g., gesturing, kissing, or giving long speeches) may result from an abnormal activation of the neocortex that reaches directly the spinal cord because its inhibition from the brainstem during REM sleep is lost [1, 2, 6–8].

In humans, iRBD is diagnosed when a patient with video-polysomnographic confirmation of REM sleep without atonia has no evidence of a neurological disease or other possible causes. Longitudinal follow-up of iRBD patients shows the frequent development of the classical motor and cognitive symptoms of PD, DLB, and MSA [3–5]. This is in line with post-mortem studies in PD showing that the pathological process in the subcoeruleus nucleus precedes substantia nigra damage. In some iRBD patients subclinical abnormalities can be detected, such as olfactory deficits [14], cognitive impairment on neuropsychological tests [15], dysautonomic abnormalities [16], and reduced cardiac ^{123}I-MBIG scintigraphy [17]. These features are common in patients with the established diagnosis of PD, DLB, and MSA. None of these features, though, are the cause or the consequence of RBD. They are epiphenomena caused by damage of several brain areas that are not associated with the regulation of REM sleep, like the olfactory system. Thus, available data indicate that RBD in humans can be considered part of the degenerative process damaging the structures that regulate REM sleep atonia in the lower brainstem.

Neuroimaging in idiopathic RBD

Overall, neuroimaging in RBD has detected the following findings:

1. Focal brain structural lesions (e.g., vascular malformations, tumors) in a few cases that were thought to be the direct cause of RBD.
2. Functional and morphological abnormalities in structures that regulate REM sleep in normal conditions such as the lower brainstem.
3. Functional abnormalities in areas that do not play a major role in the modulation of REM sleep but are frequently damaged in PD, DLB, and MSA such as the nigrostriatal dopaminergic pathway.

Neuroimaging studies in patients with RBD have mainly been performed in subjects with iRBD. Most studies are cross-sectional and included small samples of subjects. However, neuroimaging has increased our knowledge on the pathophysiology of RBD showing brainstem abnormalities. Neuroimaging has also supported the concept that this parasomnia can be the first manifestation of a neurodegenerative disease characterized by impairment of the nigrostriatal dopaminergic system. The main limitation of neuroimaging in RBD is its low spatial resolution to identify changes in the small, but important, nuclei located in the brainstem that regulate REM sleep. Proton magnetic resonance spectroscopy (^{1}H-MRS) in iRBD shows no abnormalities in the mesopontine tegmentum, whereas single-photon emission computed tomography (SPECT) demonstrates perfusion changes in the pons. However, SPECT is not able to depict which nuclei have or do not have perfusion changes within the pons due to its low spatial resolution. In contrast, diffusion tensor imaging (DTI) has higher spatial resolution and detects alterations in several pontine nuclei, including the subcoeruleus nucleus. The following sections cover the neuroimaging findings seen in iRBD. To better understand these findings, in each section the neuroimaging abnormalities that have been identified in PD, DLB, and MSA are summarized first.

Conventional brain magnetic resonance imaging (MRI) and computed tomography (CT)

Overall, visual assessment of brain magnetic resonance imaging (MRI) and computed tomography (CT) is unremarkable in subjects with iRBD. In a very few patients with RBD, status dissociatus (the most extreme form of RBD where wakefulness and sleep stages are not distinguishable) and parasomnia overlap syndrome (the combination of RBD and a NREM parasomnia in the same individual), MRI and CT have shown small ischemic lesions [18–23], hemorrhages from vascular malformations [24, 25], tumors [18, 26], demyelinating plaques [27–29], inflammatory lesions [30–35], and leukodystrophy [36] (Table 40.2). These lesions have mainly been found in the brainstem areas that regulate REM sleep atonia or in their anatomical connections. Most of them involved the mesopontine tegmentum or the medulla, where the subcoeruleus nucleus and the magnocellularis nucleus are located, respectively. RBD has also been described in subjects with mesopontine tegmentum plus amygdalar lesions [31]. Additionally, RBD has been reported in neurological conditions involving only either the limbic system [30] or the anterior thalamus [37] with no apparent primary brainstem damage.

One crucial question raised here is whether these structural lesions found in MRI and CT are the direct cause of RBD or are they simply incidental findings (Figure 40.1). We proposed the following criteria to determine when a focal brain lesion (e.g., vascular, inflammatory, tumoral, etc.) is the direct cause of RBD: (1) RBD onset should be temporally associated with the appearance of the brain lesion; (2) RBD onset should be coincident to the onset of other symptoms caused by the lesion if they do

Table 40.2. Lesions causing REM sleep behavior disorder, status dissociatus, and parasomnia overlap syndrome detected by MRI and CT

Author/ Reference	Lesion location	Lesion type	Sleep disorder
Schenck & Mahowald/ [18]	Mesopontine tegmentum	Ischemic infarct	Parasomnia overlap syndrome
Schenck & Mahowald/ [18]	Fourth ventricle	Astrocytoma	Parasomnia overlap syndrome
Kimura et al. / [19]	Left upper pons	Ischemic infarct	REM sleep behavior disorder
Condurso et al. / [20]	Medial pons	Ischemic infarct	Status dissociatus
Olson et al. / [21]	Pons	Ischemic infarct	REM sleep behavior disorder
Xi & Luning / [22]	Right paramedian pons	Ischemic infarct	REM sleep behavior disorder
Reynolds & Roy / [23]	Mesopontine tegmentum	Ischemic infarct	REM sleep behavior disorder
Provini et al. / [24]	Mesopontine tegmentum	Hemorrhage from cavernoma	Status dissociatus
Iranzo & Aparicio / [25]	Dorsolateral medulla	Hemorrhage from cavernoma	REM sleep behavior disorder
Zambelis et al. / [26]	Left pontocerebellar angle	Neurinoma	REM sleep behavior disorder
Plazzi & Montagna / [27]	Pons	Demyelinating plaque MS	REM sleep behavior disorder
Tippmann-Peikert et al. / [28]	Dorsal pons	Demyelinating plaque MS	REM sleep behavior disorder
Gómez-Choco et al. / [29]	Pons	Demyelinating plaque MS	REM sleep behavior disorder
Iranzo et al. / [30]	Bilateral amygdala	Potassium channel antibody-associated limbic encephalitis	REM sleep behavior disorder
Compta et al. / [31]	Bilateral dorsolateral midbrain and bilateral amygdala	Anti-Ma2-associated encephalitis	REM sleep behavior disorder
Mathis et al. / [32]	Dorsomedial pontine tegmentum	Encephalitis of unknown origin	REM sleep behavior disorder
Limousin et al. / [33]	Right pontine tegmentum and right dorsal medulla	Encephalitis of unknown origin	Parasomnia overlap syndrome
Blumenthal et al. / [34]	Thalamus, temporal lobe	Anti-Ma2-associated encephalitis	REM sleep behavior disorder
Flanagan et al. / [36]	Mesopontine tegmentum and anterior medulla	Adult autosomal dominant leukodystrophy	REM sleep behavior disorder
Perez-Diaz et al. / [35]	Pons and medulla	Clippers syndrome	REM sleep behavior disorder

MRI = magnetic resonance imaging; CT = computed tomography; MS = multiple sclerosis.

appear (e.g., oculomotor abnormalities, hypersomnia, limbic syndrome, etc.); (3) the lesion should be located in a brain area known to regulate REM sleep (e.g., mesopontine tegmentum, ventromedial medulla, amygdala, hypothalamus, etc.); (4) disappearance of the lesion when possible (e.g., by surgery in tumors or by immunotherapy in multiple sclerosis and autoimmune-mediated limbic encephalitis) is associated with remission or improvement of the RBD-related nocturnal symptoms and polysomnographic abnormalities; and (5) RBD is not better explained by another current disorder (e.g., PD) or medication use or withdrawal [25]. For example, in one patient from our series with isolated RBD of six years of duration and normal neurological examination, brain MRI showed mass effect on the left pons and medulla caused by vertebral artery dolicoectasy [25]. One would think that this finding was the cause of RBD, but the observations that the patient had hyposmia, neuropsychological tests showed marked visuospatial and memory impairment, and dopamine transporter (DAT) SPECT demonstrated reduced striatal tracer binding suggest that RBD in this case could represent an early marker of an underlying evolving neurodegenerative disease. Moreover, in another of our RBD patients, brain CT demonstrated a giant thalamic-parieto-occipital arteriovenous malformation in the left hemisphere [25]. We could only conclude that this lesion was not causing RBD after seven years of

clinical follow-up when we noticed that the patient gradually developed the classical symptoms of DLB (cognitive impairment, fluctuations, delusions, hallucinations, and parkinsonism responsive to levodopa). It should be noted, though, that some acute lesions in the pontine tegmentum may not cause RBD but other sleep abnormalities, including peduncular hallucinosis [38] or marked reduction of REM sleep time with physiological atonia [39]. On the other hand, we have seen one patient with iRBD and normal neurological examination in whom MRI disclosed marked atrophy of the pons and cerebellum. Two years later she developed urinary incontinence, orthostatic hypotension, and cerebellar syndrome fulfilling the diagnostic criteria for MSA (personal observation) (Figure 40.2).

Proton magnetic resonance spectroscopy

Proton magnetic resonance spectroscopy (^{1}H-MRS) is a non-invasive method which allows the detection of in vivo neuronal loss and metabolic alterations in localized brain areas. The main metabolic peaks detectable with ^{1}H-MRS are *N*-acetylaspartate (NAA), creatine-phosphocreatine (Cr), choline-containing compounds (Cho), and myo-inositol (mI). In brief, NAA is considered as a neuronal marker and its reduction reflects neuronal loss or damage, Cho increased or decreased concentrations suggest membrane turnover impairment, Cr changes

319

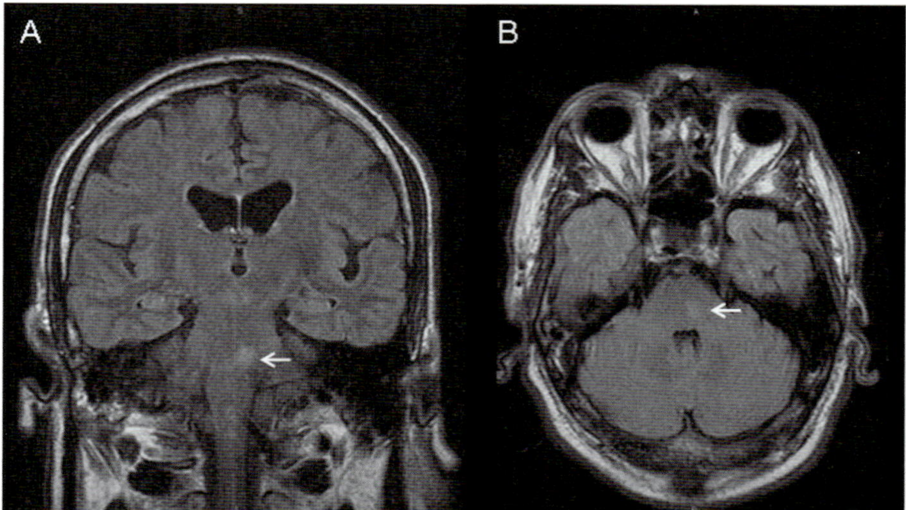

Figure 40.1 Coronal (A) and axial (B) T2 FLAIR-weighted brain MRI of a 72-year-old man with iRBD from our series. The patient reported an insidious onset of dream-enacting behaviors and nightmares that persisted for two years. Neurological examination was unremarkable and cranial MRI detected a lacunar ischemic infarction in the left pontine tegmentum (arrows).

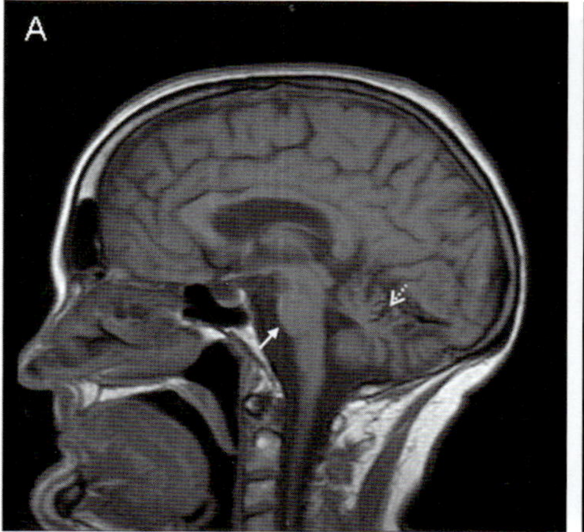
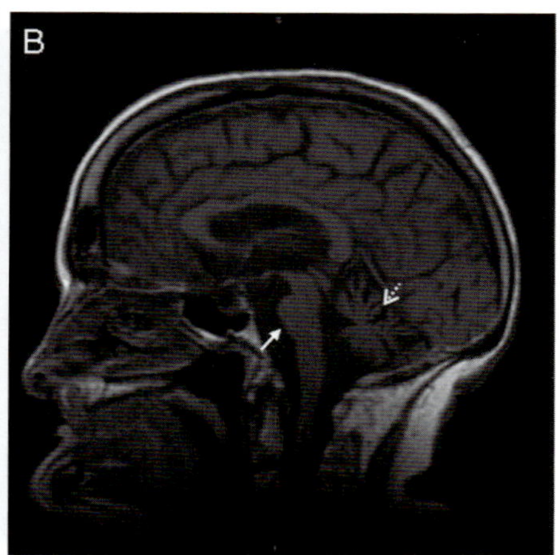

Figure 40.2 (A) Saggital T1-weighted brain MRI of a 64-year-old woman with iRBD, normal neurological examination, and absence of dysautonomic symptoms. MRI showed prominent pontine (continuous arrow) and cerebellar (dotted arrow) atrophy. (B) Two years later she developed dysautonomic symptoms and cerebellar syndrome and was diagnosed with multiple system atrophy. Repeated sagittal T1-weighted brain MRI disclosed more marked pontine (continuous arrow) and cerebellar (dotted arrow) atrophy than two years earlier.

indicate abnormality in energy metabolism, and mI provides information concerning the glial cells.

Most studies in PD have shown no ^{1}H-MRS abnormalities in the putamen, basal ganglia, and cortical areas. In contrast, ^{1}H-MRS shows reduced NAA in the putamen, medulla, and basal ganglia in MSA. ^{1}H-MRS in DLB shows lower NAA/Cr ratios in the bilateral hippocampus, indicating cell loss, and increased Cho/Cr ratio in cortical areas, reflecting increased membrane turnover.

Two studies have evaluated ^{1}H-MRS centered in the brainstem in subjects with iRBD (Table 40.3). They showed opposite results, probably due to methodological issues. Miyamoto et al. [40] were the first to investigate ^{1}H-MRS in iRBD. They reported the case of a 69-year-old man with iRBD in whom cranial MRI was normal and pontine ^{1}H-MRS (5.4 cm^3) presumably detected increased Cho/Cr ratio, suggesting functional impairment at the cell membrane level in the pons. The NAA/Cr ratio was normal suggesting the absence of neuronal loss. The validity of these findings is controversial since the authors compared a single 69-year-old patient with a previously published series of 26 healthy young subjects with a mean age of 25.5 (range, 21–32) years from another group of investigators, and were obtained with different acquisition parameters and echo-times [41].

Iranzo et al. evaluated ^{1}H-MRS centered on the mesopontine tegmentum in 15 untreated patients with iRBD and 15 healthy controls without RBD, matched for age and sex [42]. Cranial MRI was normal in all patients and controls. The first ^{1}H-MRS voxel covered the midbrain tegmentum from the posterior commissure to the isthmus rhombencephali and involved the mesopontine junction to ensure inclusion of the pedunculopontine nucleus. This voxel embraced the ventral tegmental area and a great extend of the substantia nigra pars compacta and periaqueductal gray matter. The second voxel covered the pontine tegmentum and included the subcoeruleus nucleus. Voxel volumes ranged from 3.4 to 4.3 cm^3 (Figure 40.3). There were no differences in NAA/Cr, Cho/Cr, and mI/Cr ratios between patients and controls. It was concluded that ^{1}H-MRS did not detect marked mesopontine neuronal loss or metabolic disturbances in iRBD. These results indicate that ^{1}H-MRS cannot detect the presence of small but important functional or anatomical abnormalities in iRBD in the two regions studied since this method can only detect few brain metabolites and may not be sensitive enough to detect damage in the brainstem structures that regulate REM sleep (e.g., subcoeruleus nucleus). These nuclei are too

Table 40.3. MRI studies in idiopathic REM sleep behavior disorder

Author/ Reference	Neuroimaging modality	Patients (number)	Age (years)	RBD duration (years)	UPDRS-III (score)	Findings
Iranzo et al. / [42]	^{1}H-MRS	15	65.7 ± 6.4	5.2 ± 3.0	NR	No abnormalities in the mesopontine tegmentum
Ellmore et al. / [43]	MRI-based volumetric measurement	5	52.6 ± 10.1	NR	4.6 ± 5.2	Reduced volumen of the putamen when compared with early PD and controls
Scherfler et al. / [44]	Voxel-based morphometry	26	67.4 ± 4.9	9.2 ± 6.4	2.1 ± 1.8	Increased gray matter density in both hippocampi
Hanyu et al. / [46]	Voxel-based morphometry	20	69.0 ± 7.0	6.0 ± 5.0	NR	Reduced gray matter density in pontine tegmentum, parahippocampal gyrus, and cerebellum
Unger et al. / [47]	Diffusion tensor imaging	12	59.9 ± 10.5	NR	NR	Increased FA in the olfactory tract. Decreased AD in the pontine tegmentum and right substantia nigra
Scherfler et al. / [44]	Diffusion tensor imaging	26	67.4 ± 4.9	9.2 ± 6.4	2.1 ± 1.8	Decreased FA and increased MD in the mesopontine tegmentum involving the LPT, vlPAG, FAG, SC, PC, LC, and PPN

[1] H-MRS = proton magnetic resonance spectroscopy; NR = no reported; FA = fractional anisotropy; AD = axial diffusivity; MD = mean diffusivity; LPT = lateral pontine tegmentum; vlPAG = ventrolateral periaqueductal gray matter; PAG = periaqueductal gray matter; SC = subcoeruleus nucleus; LC = locus coeruleus nucleus; PC = precoeruleus nucleus; PPN = pedunculopontine nucleus.

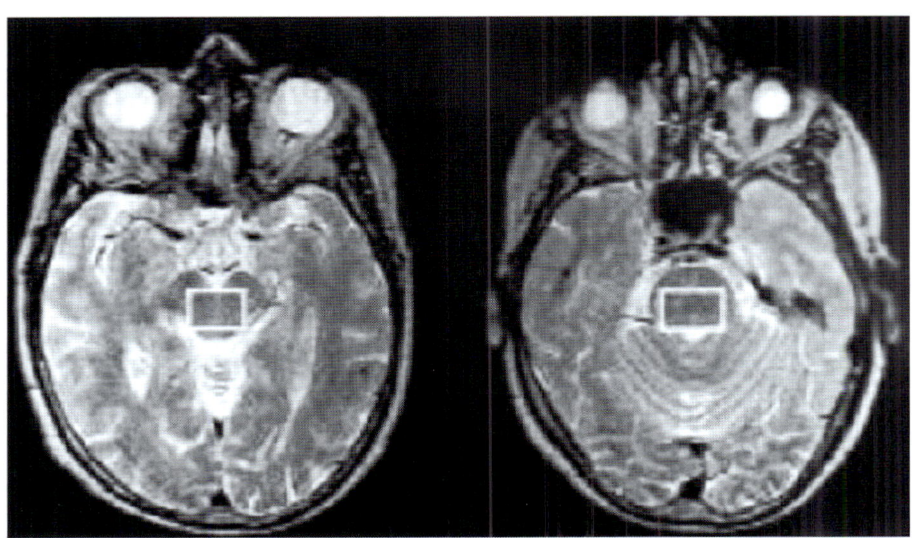

Figure 40.3 Axial T2-weighted MRI images of the volumes of interest in the midbrain (left) and pons (right) of iRBD patients who underwent a proton magnetic resonance spectroscopy study. (Reproduced, with permission, from [42].)

small to be individually studied with the spatial resolution of ^{1}H-MRS. Interestingly, ten years later, clinical follow-up showed that only 3 of the 15 iRBD patients evaluated with ^{1}H-MRS remained disease-free. During this interval of time, 12 patients were diagnosed with a neurodegenerative condition characterized by brainstem cell loss such as PD (n = 3), PD with associated dementia (n = 1), and DLB (n = 8) (unpublished observations). In two of the patients diagnosed with DLB, post-mortem examination showed severe cell loss and Lewy bodies in the mesopontine tegmentum including the subcoeruleus nucleus, the pedunculopontine nucleus, the substantia nigra pars compacta, the dorsal raphe, and the locus coeruleus.

Magnetic resonance imaging-based volumetric measurement

This method assesses morphological changes through volumetric quantification of different areas of the brain in vivo. In patients with the recent diagnosis of PD, this technique shows reduced volume of the putamen, whereas the volumes of the substantia nigra, caudate, pallidum, and total brain are normal. In early PD, reduced volume of the putamen may reflect decreased putaminal dopaminergic innervation from the substantia nigra. Patients with DLB also have reduced volumen of the putamen. In MSA, the volumes of the brainstem, putamen, thalamus, cerebellum, and hippocampus are significantly reduced.

There is only one publication that evaluated MRI-based volumetric measurement in iRBD, and only included five patients with this condition (Table 40.3). Ellmore *et al.* performed volumetric measurements of the putamen gray matter, caudate gray matter, and total brain (total gray matter plus total white matter) in five iRBD patients, seven early PD patients with RBD (Hoehn and Yahr scale of ≤2), and seven healthy controls [43]. Volumetric quantifications were derived from high-resolution T1-weighted 3 T MRI images. The total deep gray matter was measured in the putamen, caudate, amygdala, and hippocampus. The three groups were matched for sex and age. The mean age of the iRBD subjects was relatively low (mean age of 52.6 ± 10.1 years) for this population. Total brain volume and caudate volume were similar between the three groups. The iRBD group had smaller putamen volume when compared with the healthy group (about 20%). Unexpectedly, the putamen volume was bigger in the early PD-RBD group than in the iRBD group, and similar to the control group. The authors speculated that the normal putamen volume in the early PD-RBD group can be explained by a compensatory structural hypertrophy in the putamen as the result of decreased dopaminergic function in the early stages of PD. However, it may be argued that RBD can be considered a very early stage of PD and in this study the putamen volume was not increased, but reduced, in the iRBD group. As acknowledged by the authors, the main limitation of this study was the small number of patients included.

Voxel-based morphometry

Voxel-based morphometry (VBM) is a technique that measures gray and white matter volume from MRI using an automated technique throughout different voxels in the entire brain. VBM shows no marked gray matter volume reduction in early PD. In patients with later stages of PD, particularly when dementia is associated, VBM detects gray matter loss in all neocortical areas, the hippocampus, and limbic system. Studies with VBM T2-weighted MRI have not found increased white matter lesions in PD and PD with dementia. Reduced gray matter density in the cortex is more pronounced in DLB than in PD with dementia. In MSA, gray matter atrophy is seen in the striatum, midbrain, cerebellar hemispheres, and cortex.

Two studies have evaluated VBM in patients with iRBD (Table 40.3). These two studies reported different results that might reflect methodological issues. Scherfler *et al.* used VBM of 1.5 T T1-weighted MR images to assess for the presence of localized cortical gray matter and subcortical white matter changes in 26 iRBD subjects and 14 sex- and age-matched healthy controls [44]. VBM revealed neither decreased gray matter density nor white matter changes in the brain. In particular, no changes were found in the brainstem and in the amygdala. In contrast, VBM revealed increased gray matter density in both hippocampi and the adjacent parahippocampal gyrus. This was interpreted as an indicator of functional reorganization in this brain area. Cortical gray matter volume increases are likely to be related to sprouting of new connections, dendritic spine growth, and modification in the strength of existing connections. The increased gray matter volume in the

hippocampus as detected by VBM in this study is in line with a ^{99m}Tc-ethyl cysteinate dimer (^{99m}Tc-ECD) SPECT study reporting increased perfusion in the hippocampus of patients with iRBD [45]. The role of hippocampal activation in REM sleep is not entirely clear. A potential interaction in the consolidation of memory during sleep is suggested and impaired asymptomatic memory function occurs in iRBD patients [15].

In another study, Hanyu *et al.* applied VBM to 20 iRBD patients and 18 age-matched controls [46]. Patients and controls were not matched for sex. Compared with controls, patients with iRBD had significant gray matter volume reduction in the pontine tegmentum, anterior lobes of the right and left cerebellum, and left parahippocampal gyrus. Gray matter volume loss was not related to cognitive testing, polysomnographic variables, age, and RBD duration. The authors stated that this study provided in vivo evidence that structural lesions of the brainstem are responsible for the occurrence of RBD. The authors noted that the pattern of gray matter loss found in iRBD is consistent with morphological VBM changes commonly observed in patients with DLB and MSA.

Different results between the study by Scherfler *et al.* [44] and the study by Hanyu *et al.* [46] may reflect methodological and statistical issues. Scherfler *et al.* [44] excluded patients with structural MRI abnormalities (e.g., cortical atrophy, brainstem microangiopathy, and putaminal ring sign) and used linear regression analysis with the statistical threshold set to p = 0.001. In contrast, the study by Hanyu *et al.* [46] did not exclude patients with MRI abnormalities, used different statistical tests, and statistical threshold was set to p = 0.005.

Diffusion tensor imaging

DTI is a method which assesses microstructural brain tissue integrity in vivo. It is a unique form of MRI contrast that enables quantification of the direction of diffusing water molecules within the entire brain volume. Within fiber tracts, the motion of water molecules perpendicular to the main axonal direction is restricted to a greater extent than is the diffusion along the main axis, resulting in an anisotropically shaped space termed fractional anisotropy (FA). In addition, the mean diffusivity (MD) reflects the total magnitude of diffusion and hence provides information of alterations in the extracellular volume of both the gray and white matter compartments. MD is a parameter of brain tissue integrity and FA is a parameter of neuronal fiber integrity.

Both FA and MD were shown to be sensitive to brain tissue alterations in neurodegenerative conditions. In de novo untreated PD patients, DTI studies show reduced FA and increased MD in the substantia nigra, while no changes are observed in the pons, caudate, putamen, globus pallidus, and thalamus. PD patients with anosmia have reduced FA in the white matter surrounding primary olfactory areas, whereas those with associated dementia have decreased FA in the bilateral frontal, left temporal, and left parietal white matter. In patients with DLB, the pattern of FA reduction in the cortex is similar to that of patients with PD with dementia. However, white matter abnormalities are more severe and extend into occipital and visual association regions in DLB. Patients with DLB are characterized by elevated MD in the amygdala and decreased FA in the inferior longitudinal fasciculus. Abnormalities are also found in the caudate and the putamen of patients with DLB. In MSA, DTI shows increased MD and reduced FA in the pons, putamen, and cerebellum.

In iRBD, DTI has been assessed in two studies, which showed different results which may be related to different methodological issues (Table 40.3). Both have shown abnormalities in the pontine tegmentum where the nuclei that generate REM sleep are located. One of the studies found changes in the olfactory system and in the substantia nigra. This is in line with the frequent association of iRBD with olfactory defects and the later development of a neurodegenerative disease characterized by cell loss in the substantia nigra.

Unger *et al.* investigated FA as well as radial and axial diffusivity signal changes in 12 iRBD patients and 12 control subjects [47]. Controls were age matched but not sex matched (11 men versus 3 men). Surprisingly, one of the iRBD patients was only 38 years old. The authors reported decreases of axial diffusivity, a parameter assumed to indicate axonal loss, in the right substantia nigra in the midbrain and in the pontine tegmentum. The authors found no FA alterations in the brainstem, but detected FA decreases and radial diffusivity signal increases in cortical areas such as the fornix, the right visual stream, and the left superior temporal lobe. Increased FA was found in the thalamic radiation in the anterior limb of the internal capsule bilaterally and in the olfactory region. A decrease in radial diffusivity was also seen in the olfactory region. The fact that decreased FA was seen in the substantia nigra of only one side might reflect the typical asymmetric onset of PD and the potential transition state from RBD to PD in some of the patients evaluated. Interestingly, DTI detected abnormalities in the olfactory tract and most of the patients included in this study had olfactory deficits demonstrated by olfactory testing.

Scherfler *et al.* performed DTI to the same 26 iRBD subjects and 14 age- and sex-matched controls that also underwent VBM [44]. Statistical parametric mapping localized significant decreases of FA and increases of MD in the midbrain and pontine tegmentum. These brainstem abnormalities in FA and in MD were localized in some nuclei known to regulate REM sleep and REM sleep atonia, namely the subcoeruleus nucleus, lateral pontine tegmentum, ventrolateral periaqueductal gray matter, periaqueductal gray matter, locus coeruleus, precoeruleus nucleus, and pedunculopontine nucleus (Figure 40.4). These DTI findings suggest axonal and neuronal damage in the pontomesencephalic tegmentum, which appears to be subtle, as no marked gray or white matter atrophy was identified by VBM in the brainstem. The increased MD and decreased FA seen in the pons overlaps with areas of decreased axial diffusivity observed in the Unger *et al.* study [47]. Of note, in the study by Scherfler *et al.* [44] no FA and DM abnormalities were seen in the medulla, substantia nigra, basal ganglia, olfactory tract, and cortical areas. The different findings seen in these studies [44, 47] might be due to methodological differences, including number of patients evaluated, assessment of different diffusivity measures, measurements of diffusivity in 2D or 3D, different statistical methodology, and the distinct use of exclusion criteria for subjects with structural MRI abnormalities.

Perfusion and metabolism studies

SPECT and PET use intravenously injected radioactive tracers that are taken up by the brain. SPECT measures cerebral perfusion using a variety of ligands such as ^{99m}Tc-hexamethylpropylene amine oxime (^{99m}Tc-HMPAO SPECT), N-isopropyl-p-^{123}-I-iodoamphetamine (^{123}I-IMP SPECT), and ^{99m}Tc-ethyl cysteinate dimer (^{99m}Tc-ECD SPECT). PET evaluates glucose consumption using ^{18}F-fluorodeoxyglucose (^{18}F-FDG PET). A number of studies using SPECT and PET have found no major abnormalities in de novo PD patients with normal cognition. However, when mild cognitive impairment and dementia are associated in PD, then reduced perfusion and glucose hypometabolism are found in the cortex, whereas increased activity is seen in the brainstem, striatum, and cerebellum. As PD advances with time, metabolism shows a decline in the prefrontal and inferior parietal regions and an increase in the pons, subthalamic nucleus, internal globus pallidus, and primary motor cortex. In patients with DLB, ^{18}F-FDG PET studies show hypometabolism of all cortical areas with predominant damage in the occipital lobe. In MSA, ^{18}F-FDG PET shows reduced levels of metabolism in the brainstem, putamen, caudate, and cerebellum.

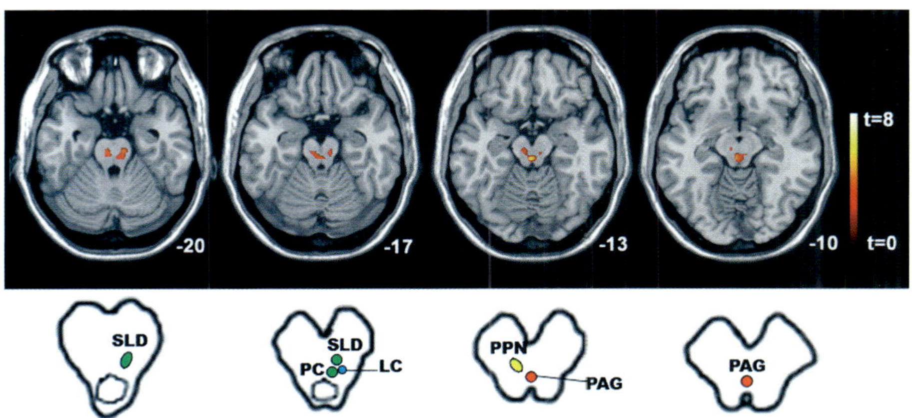

Figure 40.4 Statistical parametric mapping (t) axial intensity project on maps rendered onto a stereotactically normalized MRI scan, showing areas of significant increases of mean diffusivity values (color code, yellow to orange) in a cohort of patients with iRBD versus healthy control subjects. The number at the bottom right corner of each MRI scan corresponds to the z coordinate in Talairach space. Schematic drawings below correspond to the MRI and visualize proposed nuclei involved in REM sleep control. The REM-off region is represented by the periaqueductal gray matter (PAG) in red, and the REM-on region is represented by the precoeruleus (PC) and subcoeruleus (SLD) in green. Nuclei in yellow and blue are known to influence REM and non-REM sleep circuits. LC = locus coeruleus; PPN = pedunculopontine nucleus.

Table 40.4. Perfusion studies in idiopathic REM sleep behavior disorder

Author/Reference	Neuroimaging modality	Patients (number)	Age (years)	RBD duration (years)	UPDRS-III (score)	Findings
Shirawaka et al. / [48]	^{123}I-IMP SPECT	20	63.4 ± 8.5	NR	NR	Decreased cerebral perfusion in the pons and frontal lobe
Mazza et al. / [45]	^{99m}Tc-ECD SPECT	8	63.4 ± 8.5	7.5 ± 4.8	4.9 ± 2.8	Decreased cerebral perfusion in the frontal, temporal, and parietal lobes. Increased perfusion in the pons, right and left putamen, and right hippocampus
Vendette et al. / [49]	^{99m}Tc-ECD SPECT	20	64.9 ± 7.7	11 ± 8.6	4.2 ± 3.6	Decreased cerebral perfusion in the frontal, temporal, and parietal lobes. Increased perfusion in the pons, right and left putamen, and right hippocampus
Hanyu et al. / [52]	^{123}I-IMP SPECT	24	68.0 ± 7.0	6 ± 5	NR	Decreased cerebral perfusion in the parieto-occipital lobe, limbic lobe, and cerebellum

^{123}I-IMP = N-isopropyl-p-[123]-I-iodoamphetamine; SPECT = single-photon emission computed tomography; ^{99m}Tc-ECD = ^{99m}Tc-ethyl cysteinate dimer; NR = not reported.

In iRBD, publications evaluating cerebral perfusion with SPECT have reported controversial results, showing hypoperfusion, hyperperfusion, or normal perfusion in the pons (Table 40.4). These inconsistent results may be derived from methodological aspects. The low spatial resolution of SPECT, however, did not allow the identification of which structures are damaged or spared in the brainstem of the patients with iRBD. It should be noted that all these studies with SPECT were performed when individuals were awaken and not during REM sleep.

The first study that evaluated brain perfusion in iRBD was published by Shirawaka et al. who evaluated 20 male patients and 7 age-matched men as controls with ^{123}I-IMP SPECT [48]. This is a brief original publication where the authors found decreased blood flow in the upper portion of the frontal lobe and in the pons. No abnormalities were found in other cortical areas or in the striatum.

Mazza et al. investigated regional cerebral perfusion with ^{99m}Tc-ECD SPECT in eight untreated iRBD patients and nine sex- and age-matched controls [45]. Increased perfusion was detected in the pons and putamen bilaterally and in the right hippocampus. In addition, decreased perfusion was detected in frontal (including the primary cortex and supplementary motor areas) and temporoparietal cortices. The authors claimed that increased perfusion could reflect either compensatory mechanisms or disinhibition resulting from dysfunction of inhibitory structures. Conversely, decreased cortical perfusion was interpreted as the result of a deafferentation process due to dysfunction of the striato-thalamic network. Interestingly, quantitative EEG analysis and cognitive testing also point to cortical impairment in iRBD. The authors of this study stated that the metabolic pattern seen in their iRBD patients is similar to what is found in PD. The same group of investigators replicated their findings in 20 patients and 20 controls when they found the same pattern of decreased and increased cerebral flow also using ^{99m}Tc-ECD SPECT [49]. In addition, it was found that decreased perfusion in the frontal and occipital areas was associated with poorer performance in the color discrimination test. Also, there was a relationship between reduced hypoperfusion in the bilateral anterior parahippocampal gyrus and olfactory deficits. The ^{99m}Tc-ECD SPECT findings, however,

were not correlated with patients' age and RBD duration. Again the same group of investigators found that RBD patients with associated mild cognitive impairment had cortical hypoperfusion in the occipital, temporal, and parietal lobes when compared with iRBD without cognitive complaints [50]. The same authors found that when mild cognitive impairment is particularly linked to RBD, increased hippocampal perfusion at baseline may predict conversion to PD and DLB [51].

Hanyu et al. assessed regional cerebral blood flow using ^{123}I-IMP SPECT in 24 patients and 18 age-matched controls [52]. Patients and controls were not matched for sex (21 men versus 9 men). The authors found decreased regional cerebral blood flow in the parietal lobe, occipital lobe (precuneus), right limbic lobe, and cerebellum. These findings have been observed in patients with PD, DLB, and MSA. In this study, no abnormalities were detected in the brainstem, striatum, and frontal lobe.

Caselli et al. investigated ^{18}F-FDG PET in 17 patients with dream-enacting behaviors and 17 controls [53]. There was reduced glucose metabolism in the parietal, temporal, and posterior cingulated cortices. Of note, it is impossible to know if the patients with dream-enacting behaviors included in this study had RBD because they did not undergo nocturnal polysomnography to assess the electromyographic tone in REM sleep. Dream-enacting behaviors and nightmares can occur not only in RBD but also in a variety of conditions including severe obstructive sleep apnea, nocturnal frontal epilepsy, and sleepwalking.

Transcranial sonography and dopaminergic function imaging assessment of the nigrostriatal system

Braak et al. reported that the neurodegenerative process in PD begins in the olfactory bulb and in the lower brainstem where the nuclei responsible for REM sleep atonia are located. From there, the pathological process advances upwards through the substantia nigra in the midbrain, the amygdala, and finally reaches the cortex [54]. This temporal sequence is in agreement with the observation that RBD (as the result of brainstem dysfunction) and hyposmia (as the result of damage of the olfactory bulb) can both precede parkinsonism (as the result of dopaminergic cell loss in the substantia nigra) in some patients with PD. Thus, patients with PD have a premotor period characterized by the presence of non-motor symptomatology such as RBD and hyposmia. During this premotor period pathological changes in the nigrostriatal system develop several years before they reach a threshold (40–60% of dopaminergic cell loss in the substantia nigra and 70–80% reduction of dopamine content in the striatum) for the clinical appearance of parkinsonism.

As mentioned earlier, patients with iRBD commonly develop PD, DLB, and MSA, three diseases characterized by substantia nigra degeneration resulting in parkinsonism. Thus, assessment of the state of the nigrostriatal system could be helpful in identifying those patients with iRBD at a high risk for developing parkinsonism. Several neuroimaging studies have evaluated the morphological and functional state of the substantia nigra in iRBD. These studies have evaluated the echogenicity of the substantia nigra with transcranial sonography (TCS) and the nigrostriatal dopaminergic system with functional imaging. A cross-sectional study has shown that about 60% of the iRBD patients have subclinical reduced nigrostriatal dopaminergic innervation and/or hyperechogenicity of the substantia nigra [55]. A longitudinal study in iRBD showed that these two neuroimaging abnormalities are markers for the short-term conversion to PD, DLB, and MSA [55]. Another prospective study demonstrated that serial neuroimaging shows progressive nigrostriatal dopaminergic dysfunction with time [56]. Thus, available data indicate that it is possible imaging and monitoring the premotor stage of PD in subjects with iRBD.

Transcranial sonography

TCS is a non-invasive procedure which allows the measurement of the substantia nigra echogenic signal in the midbrain. In more than 90% of PD patients, TCS shows substantia nigra hyperechogenicity, a finding that is thought to reflect increased iron deposition. This is considered to be a marker for nigrostriatal vulnerability and early diagnosis of PD because it is identified in some healthy individuals who later developed PD, is frequently seen in PD

patients with early onset of parkinsonism, and is stable during the course of the disease. Midbrain hyperechogenicity is also observed in approximately 10% of healthy controls and has been proposed to be a potential risk marker for PD in these subjects. In PD the extent of midbrain hyperechogenicity does not correlate with the degree of nigrostriatal terminal dysfunction when assessed with DAT SPECT. This missing correlation suggests that dysfunction of presynaptic dopaminergic nerve terminals and substantia nigra hyperechogenicity are the result of different mechanisms and that dopaminergic dysfunction and increased iron content might be independent from each other. Midbrain hyperechogenicity occurs in the majority of patients with DLB and in up to 25% of the MSA subjects.

Hyperechogenicity of the substantia nigra has been found in about 40% of subjects with iRBD but not in subjects with RBD associated with narcolepsy, a disease where the state of the substantia nigra is normal (Table 40.5). Unger et al. evaluated five male iRBD subjects through a test battery comprising neurological examination, TCS, presynaptic dopaminergic nigrostriatal imaging with ^{123}I-N-3-fluoropropyl-2β-carbomethoxy-3β-(4-iodophenyl) nortropane (^{123}I-FP-CIT), and olfactory tests [57]. Substantia nigra echoginicity was considered enlarged when the area was greater than 0.20 cm^2. ^{123}I-FP-CIT uptake was considered reduced when the putamen or caudate ratios were lower than 2.6, but in this study the reference and control values were not reported to understand this 2.6 cut-off value in two distinct regions. This is the first study that evaluated combined dopaminergic imaging and TCS in iRBD, showing diverse patterns of abnormalities. Unilateral substantia nigra hyperechogenicity was seen in two patients, reduced ^{123}I-FP-CIT bilateral putamen uptake in one, and impaired sense of smell in all five. The patient with reduced ^{123}I-FP-CIT uptake had normal TCS. The two patients with substantia nigra hyperechogenicity had normal ^{123}I-FP-CIT striatal uptake.

Stockner et al. performed TCS in 55 individuals with iRBD and 165 age- and sex-matched controls [58]. Control subjects were recruited from a population-based cohort of 574 healthy individuals aged 50 and above, who were previously investigated by the same TCS examiner. The 90th percentile of the area of

Table 40.5. Transcranial sonography studies in idiopathic REM sleep behavior disorder

Author/Reference	Patients (number)	Age (years)	RBD duration (years)	UPDRS-III (score)	Findings
Unger et al. / [57]	5	66.0 ± 2.3	4.0 ± 2.5	2.6 ± 2.0	Unilateral substantia nigra hyperechogenicity in two (40%) patients
Stockner et al. / [58]	55	68.9 ± 7.8	8.9 ± 5.3	2.8 ± 3.1	Substantia nigra hyperechogenicity in 37% of the patients
Iwanami et al. / [59]	34	67.9 ± 6.1	5.3 ± 6.7	1.1 ± 2.1	Substantia nigra hyperechogenicity in 41% of the patients
Iranzo et al. / [55]	43	70.2 ± 6.9	9.5 ± 5.0	3.2 ± 3.4	Substantia nigra hyperechogenicity in 36% of the patients. Echogenicity of the substantia nigra did not correlate with ^{123}I-FP-CIT striatal uptake in DAT imaging
Miyamoto et al. / [70]	19	66.4 ± 4.9	3.5 ± 1.8	0.9 ± 1.0	Substantia nigra hyperechogenicity in 47% of the patients. Echogenicity of the substantia nigra did not correlate with FMT-PET striatal uptake in DAT imaging
Shin et al. / [60]	15	65.2 ± 8.7	5	1.7	Substantia nigra hyperechogenicity in 40% of the patients.

[1] FMT = 6-[^{18}F]Fluoro-meta-tyrosine.

echogenicity in the substantia nigra of the greater side was 0.20 cm^2 in control subjects. This was used as cut-off value to distinguish between normoechogenicity and hyperechogenicity. The echogenicity area was greater in the iRBD group than in the control group (0.20 ± 0.09 cm^2 versus 0.14 ± 0.05 cm^2). Substantia nigra hyperechogenicity occurred in 37% of the iRBD patients and in 11% of the controls. iRBD patients with midbrain hyperechogenicity had higher Unified Parkinson's Disease Rating Scale (UPDRS) motor score than those with normoechogenicity (3.7 ± 3.3 versus 2.1 ± 1.9), but this difference was not statistically significant. The authors concluded that the increased prevalence of midbrain hyperechogenicity in iRBD supports the potential role of this finding as a risk marker for PD.

Iwanami *et al.* performed TCS and olfactory testing in 34 patients with iRBD, 17 with PD, and 21 healthy controls [59]. All subjects in this study were male and groups were age matched. A cut off of greater than 0.20 cm^2 was used to define substantia nigra hyperechogenicity, which was found in 41% of the iRBD individuals, 53% of the PD patients, and 9.5% of the controls. The mean size of the echogenic area was 0.20 ± 0.13 cm^2 in iRBD, 0.22 ± 0.11 cm^2 in PD, and 0.06 ± 0.06 cm^2 in controls. Olfactory impairment was found in 79% of the patients with iRBD and in 100% with PD. Twelve percent of the iRBD subjects had abnormalities in both TCS and olfactory function. In the iRBD group there were no correlations between the size of the substantia nigra, olfactory testing, and RBD duration. The percentage of PD subjects with hyperechogenicity of the substantia nigra (53%) was much lower compared with previous reports that usually reach more than 90%. Shin *et al.* performed TCS in 15 iRBD individuals and found insufficient bone window in 3 (20%), hyperechogenicity (> 0.20 cm^2) in 6 (40%) and normoechogenicity in the remaining 6 (40%) [60].

Dopamine neuroimaging

One of the pathological hallmarks of PD, DLB, and MSA is the loss of dopamine neurons in the substantia nigra and the reduction of dopamine projections to the striatum leading to parkinsonism. Dopamine neuroimaging with SPECT and PET evaluates the presynaptic (substantia nigra) and postsynaptic (putamen and caudate) state of the nigrostriatal dopaminergic system. Its main application has been the visualization and quantification of the dopaminergic deficit in neurodegenerative diseases.

The postsynaptic dopaminergic function is evaluated by SPECT using ligands that bind to striatal D$_2$ dopamine receptors such as iodine-^{123} labeled 3-iodo-6methoxybenzamide (^{123}I-IBZM SPECT). For PET methods the tracer raclopride is used to evaluate the striatal dopamine D$_2$ binding.

The presynaptic nigrostriatal terminal function can be evaluated with 6-[^{18}F]-fluoro-L-dopa PET (^{18}F-dopa-PET), 6-[^{18}F]-fluoro-meta-tyrosine PET (FMT- PET), DAT SPECT, DAT-PET, and vesicular monoamine transporter PET (VMAT-SPECT).^{18}F-dopa-PET is a marker of presynaptic dopaminergic terminal function and reflects Dopa transport into the terminal, Dopa decarboxylase activity, and dopamine storage capacity. FMT-PET uses a radiotracer which is a substrate of the dopamine-synthesizing enzyme and is trapped in axon terminals without being released or further processed. DAT is a protein located in the presynaptic membrane on terminals of dopaminergic projections from the substantia nigra to the putamen and caudate and it provides a marker for dopamine terminal innervation. The brain vesicular monoamine transporter is the protein responsible for pumping neurotransmitters into synaptic vesicles. Several SPECT and PET radioligands for DAT are available. DAT SPECT radioligands include ^{123}I-FP-CIT (also referred to as ^{123}I-β-CIT-FP), (N)-(3-iodopropene-2-yl)-2β-carbomethoxy-3β-(4-chlorophenyl) tropane (^{123}I-IPT), ^{123}I-2β-carbomethoxy-3β-(4-iodophenyl) tropane (^{123}I-β-CIT), and ^{99m}Tc-TRODAT-1. PET radioligands for DAT include 2β-carbomethoxy-3-β-(4-fluorophenyl) tropane (^{11}C-β-CFT). Also, the density of the vesicular monoamine transporter type 2 (VMAT2) is measured with [^{11}C]dihydrotetrabenazine PET ([^{11}C]DTBZ-PET).

^{123}I-IBZM SPECT and PET using raclopride have shown that striatal D$_2$ binding is either normal or increased in PD patients. The striatal postsynaptic dopamine receptor density is intact in DLB. In contrast, striatal D$_2$ binding is reduced in MSA.

A number of studies showed reduced DAT uptake in PD, DLB, and MSA. DAT SPECT distinguishes DLB from Alzheimer's, disease. Low DAT uptake in basal ganglia demonstrated by SPECT or PET is considered a "suggestive feature" in the criteria for the diagnosis of DLB. Reduced DAT uptake also occurs in the parkinsonian and cerebellar subtypes of MSA. DAT imaging is also used to distinguish degenerative parkinsonism from esssential tremor and parkinsonism of vascular origin. PET and SPECT studies in PD have shown that an approximately 50% loss of dopamine terminals is required for the onset of motor symptoms. In hemiparkinsonian patients, the striatum contralateral to the more affected side shows about a 50% DAT loss, but the "asymptomatic" striatum shows about a 30% DAT loss. This finding led to the investigation of dopamine imaging in the premotor stage of PD, and subsequent studies were published for iRBD.

Overall, dopamine imaging studies in iRBD have shown normal striatal D$_2$ binding and reduced DAT striatal uptake in about 40% of the patients (Table 40.6). The reduction observed in iRBD is therefore less than the decrease required to cause manifest parkinsonism. In iRBD, neuroimaging has demonstrated that the dopaminergic deficit pattern is similar to the one that is seen in subjects with recent diagnosis of PD. The deficit is unilateral or asymmetrical, is more common and prominent in the putamen than in the caudate, and shows lack of correlation with age and echogenic size of the substania nigra.

The first two studies that showed reduced striatal dopaminergic innervation in iRBD were published in 2000. They represented the first evidence that subjects with RBD had nigrostriatal dopaminergic dysfunction. It was speculated if this finding was the cause of RBD or an epiphenomen of something that is occurring in the brain at the same time. Albin *et al.* determined the density of striatal dopaminergic terminals with [^{11}C]DTBZ-PET in 6 iRBD subjects and 19 controls [61]. Striatal [^{11}C]DTBZ-PET binding was reduced in all subjects with RBD in all striatal regions evaluated (posterior putamen, anterior putamen, and caudate). Reduced [^{11}C]DTBZ binding was seen in the posterior putamen in all six patients, in the anterior putamen in five, and in the caudate in four. [^{11}C]DTBZ binding reduction was 22% in the posterior putamen, 18% in the anterior putamen, and 11% in

Table 40.6. Dopamine imaging in idiopathic REM sleep behavior disorder

Author/Reference	Neuroimaging modality	Patients (n)	Age (years)	RBD duration (years)	UPDRS-III (score)	Findings
Albin et al. / [61]	[11C]DTBZ-PET	6	67.6 ± 6.4	10 ± 7.1	NR	Reduced [11C]DTBZ binding in all five patients, particularly in the posterior putamen
Eisensehr et al. / [62]	123I-IBZM SPECT 123I-IPT SPECT	5	58.5 ± 7.5	NR	NR	Normal 123I-IBZM SPECT. Reduced 123I-IPT SPECT uptake in all five patients, particularly in the putamen 123I-IPT SPECT uptake was higher in iRBD than in early PD
Eisensehr et al. / [63]	123I-IBZM SPECT 123I-IPT SPECT	8	62.3 ± 13.5	NR	NR	Normal 123I-IBZM SPECT. 123I-IPT SPECT uptake was reduced in patients with subclinical RBD and with clinical iRBD
Kim et al. / [65]	123I-FP-CIT SPECT	14	66.6 ± 4.5	4.1 ± NR	NR	Decreased entire striatal 123I-FP-CIT uptake in three patients Decreased 123I-FP-CIT uptake in putamen but not in caudate
Iranzo et al. / [55]	123I-FP-CIT SPECT	43	70.2 ± 6.9	9.5 ± 5.0	3.2 ± 3.4	Decreased striatal 123I-FP-CIT uptake in 40%, particularly in the putamen
Iranzo et al. / [56]	123I-FP-CIT SPECT	20	70.6 ± 6.0	9.6 ± 6.0	2.2 ± 1.7	Progressive reduction of 123I-FP-CIT uptake of 10–30%
Miyamoto et al. / [70]	FMT-PET	19	66.4 ± 4.9	3.5 ± 1.8	0.9 ± 1.0	Striatal FMT uptake did not correlate with substantia nigra echogenicity

the caudate. No interhemispheric differences were noted. The subject with the greatest reduction in [11C]DTBZ binding in the posterior putamen showed soft motor signs on clinical examination but not parkinsonism. The authors speculated that RBD could be the result of basal ganglia dysfunction leading to secondary dysfunction of the brainstem structures that modulate REM sleep atonia. Alternatively, the authors speculated that RBD also could result from primary dysfunction of the brainstem nuclei that regulate REM sleep, with temporally correlated pathology occurring within the basal ganglia.

Eisensehr et al. studied post- and presynaptic dopaminergic state with 123I-IBZM SPECT and 123I-IPT SPECT, respectively [62]. Subjects included were 5 iRBD subjects, 14 untreated PD patients with mild parkinsonism (Hoehn and Yahr stage I) and 7 controls. PD patients were younger than iRBD patients and controls. There was no information regarding whether PD patients had RBD or not. Controls and iRBD patients were matched. 123I-IBZM striatal uptake was similar between iRBD subjects and controls, indicating normal striatal dopamine D_2 density. All five iRBD patients had significantly reduced striatal 123I-IPT binding. In RBD patients, reduced 123I-IPT uptake was detected in the right and left putamen, and in the right and left caudate when compared with controls. In iRBD, decreased 123I-IPT uptake was more prominent in the putamen than in the caudate, but it was only statistically significant in the left side. iRBD patients had significantly higher right and left putamen 123I-IPT binding compared with the right and left putamen contralateral to the symptomatic body side of the PD patients. iRBD patients had similar right and left caudate 123I-IPT binding, compared with the right and left caudate contralateral to the symptomatic body side of the PD patients. In all striatal areas 123I-IPT uptake was similar between iRBD patients and ipsilateral areas to the symptomatic body side of the PD patients. The authors stated that reduction of striatal

dopaminergic neurons may play a role in the development of iRBD, or RBD may be the initial manifestation of an otherwise asymptomatic phase of PD.

Again, Eisensehr et al. studied neuroimaging in iRBD using 123I-IBZM and 123I-IPT SPECT [63]. Subjects were 8 with subclinical RBD, 8 with clinically manifest iRBD, 8 with untreated PD Hoehn and Yahr stage I, and 11 controls. All patients and controls reported by the same investigators in the previous study [62] were included in this study. The authors defined subclinical RBD as the incidental finding of REM sleep with increased electromyographic activity in subjects undergoing polysomnography plus absence of abnormal behaviors during video-polysomnography and no history of dream-enacting behaviors. They hypothesized that subclinical RBD shows a less severe reduced DAT viability than iRBD with clinical symptoms. 123I-IBZM uptake was normal in subclinical RBD and in iRBD. There was a significant decrease in 123I-IPT uptake from controls to patients with subclinical RBD, from patients with subclinical RBD to clinically manifest iRBD, and from patients with clinically manifest RBD to patients with PD contralateral to the clinically affected body side. Excessive long-lasting electromyographic activity during REM sleep was independently associated with 123I-IPT reduction of striatal dopamine transporters. The authors concluded that reduction in striatal dopamine content might cause increased electromyographic activity in RBD.

Stiasny-Kolster et al. reported 123I-FP-CIT SPECT and olfactory data in 30 patients with RBD of different origins [64]. Nineteen had clinical RBD (6 with "suspected" iRBD and 13 with symptomatic RBD, mostly associated with narcolepsy) and 11 had subclinical RBD associated with narcolepsy. Impaired olfactory function was seen in 97% of the patients. Among the six patients suspected to have iRBD, neurological examination at the time of the study showed that four fulfilled the UK Brain Bank criteria for the clinical diagnosis of PD, and one exhibited soft signs of parkinsonism but was considered to have iRBD. In this study only 11 subjects underwent ^{123}I-FP-CIT SPECT. None of the two subjects with true iRBD (when those who had PD instead were excluded) underwent DAT SPECT. Thus, this study does not provide data on neuroimaging in subjects with true iRBD. Three of the four patients with the new diagnosis of PD underwent DAT SPECT, and the result was abnormal in two. Striatal ^{123}I-FP-CIT binding was normal in the six patients with RBD linked to narcolepsy that underwent neuroimaging.

Kim *et al.* evaluated 14 patients with iRBD, 14 with early PD (Hoehn and Yahr stage I), and 12 normal controls with ^{123}I-FP-CIT SPECT [65]. iRBD patients showed a trend of lower ^{123}I-FP-CIT binding in the entire striatum than controls and the significance was revealed in the putamen, but not in the caudate. However, in 11 of the 14 iRBD patients, the ^{123}I-FP-CIT uptake in the putamen still remained within the normal range. ^{123}I-FP-CIT uptake in the caudate was similar between iRBD patients and controls. When compared with the PD group, the iRBD group had significantly higher ^{123}I-FP-CIT binding in the entire striatum, putamen, and caudate. ^{123}I-FP-CIT uptake in the putamen was decreased in most PD patients. In the iRBD group there was no correlation between phasic and tonic electromyographic activity in REM sleep and ^{123}I-FP-CIT binding in the basal ganglia. This finding suggested that another pathogenic process not related to nigrostriatal dopaminergic transmission may be implicated in the pathophysiology of RBD. Differences between the studies by Eisensehr *et al.* [63] and Kim *et al.* [65] regarding the relationship between reduced DAT striatal uptake and increased electromyographic activity in REM sleep may be related to methodological issues such as different methodology to quantify electromyographic activity in REM sleep (long-lasting activity versus tonic and phasic activity) and the use of different tracers (I-IPT versus ^{123}I-FP-CIT).

Paglionico *et al.* described the case of a 72-year-old woman with iRBD and normal neurological examination in whom ^{123}I-FP-CIT SPECT was normal and cardiac ^{123}I-MIBG scintigraphy showed reduced cardiac uptake [66]. This finding indicates that sympathetic cardiac terminals can be impaired in iRBD patients showing normal nigrostriatal dopaminergic function. Two years later, the same group of investigators reported two additional iRBD cases with the same imaging features plus normal autonomic tests [67]. Again, the same investigators described that in one of their patients ^{123}I-MIBG scintigraphy was abnormal at baseline and after 2 and 3 years without significant decline over time, while ^{123}I-FP-CIT SPECT was normal at baseline and after 2 years but turned to be abnormal at the 3-year assessment with the concomitant appearance of subtle clinical signs of parkinsonism [68]. Miyamoto *et al.* reported a 73-year-old man with iRBD where ^{123}I-MIBG scintigraphy showed reduced cardiac uptake and ^{11}C-β-CFT PET showed normal presynaptic nigrostriatal dopaminergic function [69]. Two and a half years later repeated ^{11}C-β-CFT PET showed reduced tracer uptake with a 4–6% decrease by year in the posterior putamen, anterior putamen, and caudate. This finding indicates that cardiac denervation may precede nigrostriatal dopaminergic deficit in iRBD.

Miyamoto *et al.* [70] evaluated FMT-PET and TCS in 19 male patients with iRBD. Nine (47%) patients had substantia nigra hyperechogenicity with a mean size of $0.31 \pm 0.12\,\mathrm{cm}^2$. Bilateral putamen and bilateral caudate FMT uptake was significantly lower in iRBD patients with substantia nigra hyperechogenicity compared with those with normoechogenicity. However, no correlation was found between substantia nigra echogenicity and striatal FMT uptake. Iranzo *et al.* in a similar approach involving 43 patients with iRBD found that (1) hyperechogenicity of the substantia nigra was seen in 36% of the subjects, (2) bilateral putamen and bilateral caudate ^{123}I-FP-CIT uptakes were similar in iRBD patients with substantia nigra hyperechogenicity and normoechogenicity, and (3) there was no correlation between substantia nigra echogenicity and ^{123}I-FP-CIT uptake [55].

In a prospective study conducted by Iranzo *et al.*, 43 iRBD subjects underwent ^{123}I-FP-CIT and TCS at baseline and were clinically assessed after 2.5 years of follow-up [55]. Seventeen (40%) patients had reduced ^{123}I-FP-CIT striatal binding that was more frequently found and was more severe in the putamen than in the caudate. Mean ^{123}I-FP-CIT binding was decreased by 8% in the putamen and by 7% in the caudate. Thirty-six percent had substantia nigra hyperechogenicity. Echogenic size of the substantia nigra did not correlate with striatal ^{123}I-FP-CIT uptake. Twenty-seven (63%) patients had reduced ^{123}I-FP-CIT uptake and/or substantia nigra hyperechogenicity. Four had reduced ^{123}I-FP-CIT uptake and substantia nigra hyperechogenicity, ten reduced ^{123}I-FP-CIT uptake and normal substantia nigra echogenicity, ten normal ^{123}I-FP-CIT uptake and substantia nigra hyperechogenicity, and three reduced ^{123}I-FP-CIT uptake and insufficient temporal bone windows on TCS. Fifteen subjects had both normal ^{123}I-FP-CIT uptake and substantia nigra echogenicity. The remaining patient had normal ^{123}I-FP-CIT uptake and insufficient temporal bone windows on TCS. After 2.5 years of clinical follow-up, eight (19%) subjects, all with reduced ^{123}I-FP-CIT uptake and/or substantia nigra hyperechogenicity at baseline, developed clinically defined PD (n = 5), DLB (n = 2), and MSA (n = 1). Patients with normal neuroimaging at baseline remained disease-free after the same follow-up period. The authors concluded that decreased striatal ^{123}I-FP-CIT binding and substantia nigra hyperechogenicity are useful markers to identify iRBD individuals at increased short-term risk for development of PD, DLB, and MSA. This suggested that iRBD subjects with these markers would be the ideal target population for entry into clinical trials to test disease-modifying agents.

In another prospective study, Iranzo *et al.* evaluated 20 iRBD patients that underwent serial ^{123}I-FP-CIT SPECT at baseline and again after 1.5 and 3 years [56]. Twenty matched controls underwent ^{123}I-FP-CIT SPECT at baseline and again after three years. All these individuals had participated in a previous study of DAT imaging and TCS [55]. Compared with controls, patients had reduced mean ^{123}I-FP-CIT binding in all four striatal regions at baseline and after three years. Striatal ^{123}I-FP-CIT uptake was reduced compared with that in controls in 10 (50%) patients at baseline and in 13 (65%) patients after three years. In patients, the mean reduction in ^{123}I-FP-CIT uptake from baseline to three years was 19% in the left putamen, 16% in the right putamen, 11% in the left caudate, and 7% in the right caudate. After adjustment for the

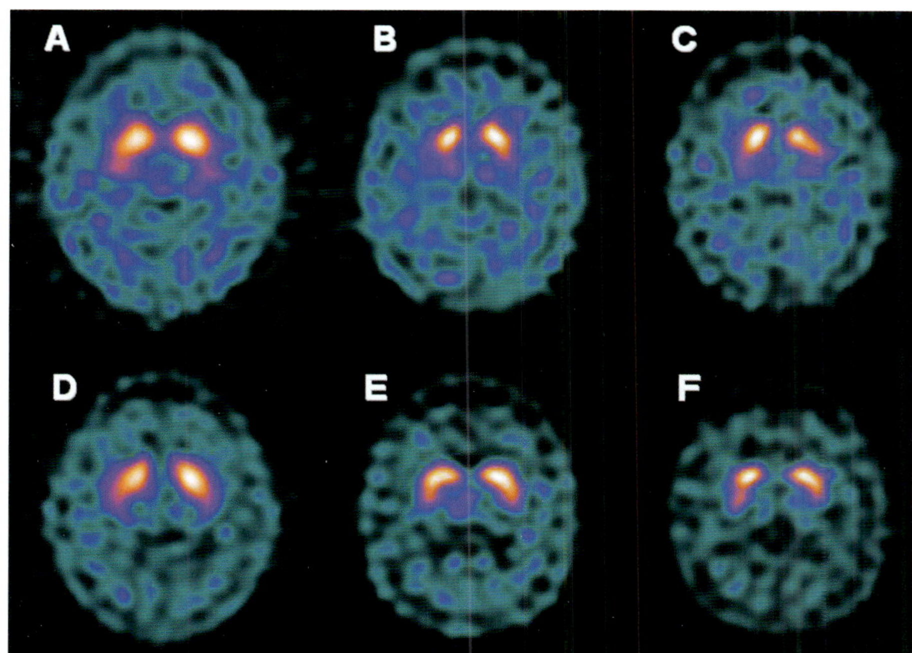

Figure 40.5 ^{123}I-FP-CIT SPECT images from a patient with iRBD who was diagnosed with PD (A, B, and C) and a patient with iRBD who remained disease-free (D, E, and F) at the three-year assessment. (A) Baseline UPDRS motor score of 3. (B) 1.5 years UPDRS motor score of 5. (C) 3 years UPDRS motor score of 14. (D) Baseline UPDRS motor score of 1. (E) 1.5 years UPDRS motor score of 1. (F) 3 years UPDRS motor score of 2.

baseline ^{123}I-FP-CIT uptake ratios, the decline in ^{123}I-FP-CIT binding at baseline to three years was greater in patients than in controls in the left putamen, right putamen, and left caudate, but not in the right caudate. At the three-year assessment, three patients were diagnosed with PD. These patients had the lowest ^{123}I-FP-CIT uptake at baseline and a mean reduction in ^{123}I-FP-CIT uptake at three years of 33% in the left putamen, 30% in the right putamen, 26% in the left caudate, and 24% in the right caudate (Figure 40.5). Thus, in RBD, serial ^{123}I-FP-CIT shows decline in striatal tracer uptake that reflects progressive nigrostriatal dopaminergic dysfunction with time. Longitudinal ^{123}I-FP-CIT SPECT can be used to monitor the progression of nigrostriatal deficits in patients with iRBD, and could be useful in studies of potential disease-modifying compounds in these patients. Thus, in iRBD there is a need to perform clinical trials with potential disease-modifying compounds where one of the end points could be evaluation of nigrostriatal dopaminergic function with ^{123}I-FP-CIT SPECT.

Summary

Neuroimaging has increased our knowledge on the physiopathology and clinical relevance of RBD. However, some of the studies showed conflicting results probably due to methodological issues (small samples, different technical aspects, and different statistical tests). Overall, neuroimaging has detected the following findings that have supported the hypothesis that RBD (1) is the result of the dysfunction of the brainstem structures that regulates REM sleep atonia and (2) may precede the onset of a neurodegenerative disease characterized by nigrostriatal damage, namely PD, DLB, and MSA.

1. In a few subjects with RBD, conventional MRI and CT have detected brainstem lesions (e.g., small lacunar infarcts, demyelinating plaques). Since the onset of the parasomnia was not always acute in all the cases reported, it is controversial whether the lesions detected were always the direct cause of RBD or they represent in some cases simple incidental findings.

2. In iRBD, abnormalities in the pons have been detected with VBM (gray matter volume reduction), DTI (reduced FA and increased mean diffusivity in the subcoeruleus nucleus, pedunculopontine nucleus, locus coeruleus, and substantia nigra), and perfusion studies with SPECT (decreased or increased cerebral perfusion).

3. In iRBD, MRI-based volumetric measurement shows a small putamen volume probably due to a presynaptic dopaminergic deficit. This is in line with dopaminergic imaging showing early decreased putaminal presynaptic dopaminergic deficit.

4. In about 40% of the subjects with iRBD, TCS demonstrates substantia nigra hyperechogenicity, a finding that suggests increased pathological iron deposition and is considered a marker for PD in the healthy population. In about 40% of the patients with iRBD, dopamine imaging shows reduced striatal dopaminergic innervation, while the postsynaptic dopaminergic state is normal. These findings indicate morphological and functional changes in the substantia nigra and nigrostriatal dopaminergic pathway.

5. Substantia nigra hyperechogenicity and reduced dopamine transporter uptake in the striatum are markers to identify iRBD individulas with a high risk for developing the classical symptoms of PD, DLB, and MSA

6. Serial DAT imaging shows progressive nigrostriatal dopaminergic dysfunction in iRBD. This finding can be used to monitor the response of putative disease-modifying agents in future trials in subjects with iRBD, particularly in those with abnormalities in TCS and dopamine imaging.

References

1. Iranzo A, Santamaria L, Tolosa E. The clinical and pathophysiological relevance of REM sleep behavior disorder in neurodegenerative diseases. *Sleep Med Rev.* 2009;**13**:385–401.

2. Boeve B. REM sleep behavior disorder. *Ann N Y Acad Sci.* 2010;**1184**:15–54.

3. Schenck CH, Bundlie SR, Mahowald MW. Delayed emergence of a parkinsonian disorder in 38% of 29 older men initially diagnosed with idiopathic rapid eye movement sleep behavior disorder: *Neurology.* 1996;**46**:388–92.

4. Iranzo A, Molinuevo JL, Santamaria J, *et al.* Rapid-eye-movement sleep behaviour disorder as an early marker for a neurodegenerative disease: a descriptive study. *Lancet Neurol.* 2006;**5**:572–7.

5. Postuma RB, Gagnon JF, Vendette M, *et al.* Quantifying the risk of neurodegenerative disease in idiopathic REM sleep behavior disorder. *Neurology.* 2009;**72**:1296–300.

6. Lu J, Sherman D, Devor M, Saper CB. A putative flip-flop switch for control of REM sleep. *Nature.* 2006;**441**:589–594.

7. Luppi PH, Clement O, Sapin E, *et al.* The neuronal network responsible for paradoxical sleep and its dysfunctions causing narcolepsy and rapid eye movement (REM) behavior disorder. *Sleep Med Rev.* 2011;**15**:153–63.

8. Saper CB, Fuller PM, Pedersen NP, Lu J, Scammell TE. Sleep state switching. *Neuron.* 2010;**68**:1023–42.

9. Maquet P, Péters JM, Aerts J, *et al.* Functional neuroanatomy of human rapid-eye-movement sleep dreaming. *Nature.* 1996;**383**:163–6.

10. Nofzinger EA, Mintum MA, Wiseman MB, Kupfer DJ, Moore RY. Forebrain activation in REM sleep: an FDG PET study. *Brain Res.* 1997;**770**:192–201.

11. Lövblad KO, Thomas R, Jakob PM, *et al.* Silent functional magnetic resonance imaging demonstrates focal activation in rapid eye movement sleep. *Neurology.* 1999;**53**:2193–5.

12. Dang-Vu TT, Schabus M, Desseilles M, *et al.* Functional neuroimaging insights into the physiology of human sleep. *Sleep.* 2010;**33**:589–603.

13. Hobson JA, Stickgold R, Pace-Schott EF. The neuropsychology of REM sleep dreaming. *Neuroreport.* 1998;**9**:R1–14.

14. Fantini ML, Postuma RB, Montplaisir J, Ferini-Strambi L. Olfactory deficit in idiopathic rapid eye movements sleep behavior disorder. *Brain Res Bull.* 2006;**70**:386–90.

15. Ferini-Strambi L, Di Gioia MR, Castronovo V, *et al.* Neuropsychological assessment in idiopathic REM sleep behavior disorder. *Neurology.* 2004;**62**:41–5.

16. Ferini-Strambi L, Oldani A, Zucconi M, Smirne S. Cardiac autonomic activity during wakefulness and sleep in REM sleep behavior disorder. *Sleep.* 1996;**19**:367–9.

17. Miyamoto T, Miyamoto M, Inoue Y, *et al.* Reduced cardiac ^{123}I-MBIG scintigraphy in idiopathic REM sleep behavior disorder. *Neurology.* 2006;**67**:2236–8.

18. Schenck C, Mahowald M. A polysomnographic, neurologic, psychiatric and clinical outcome report on 70 consecutive cases with REM sleep behavior disorder (RBD): sustained clonazepam efficacy in 89.5% of 57 treated patients. *Clev Clin J Med.* 1990;**57**(Suppl):9–23.

19. Kimura K, Tachibana N, Kohyama J, *et al.* A discrete pontine ischemic lesion could cause REM sleep behavior disorder. *Neurology.* 2000;**55**:894–5.

20. Condurso R, Aricò I, Romanello G, Gervasi G, Silvestri R. Status dissociatus in multilacunar encephalopathy with median pontine lesion: a video-polygraphic presentation. *J Sleep Res.* 2006;**15**(Suppl 1):212.

21. Olson EJ, Boeve BF, Silber MH. Rapid eye movement sleep behaviour disorder: demographic, clinical and laboratory findings in 93 cases. *Brain.* 2000;**123**:331–9.

22. Xi Z, Luning W. REM sleep behaviour disorder in a patient with pontine stroke. *Sleep Med.* 2009;**10**:143–6.

23. Reynolds TQ, Roy A. Isolated cataplexy and REM sleep behaviour disorder after pontine stroke. *J Clin Sleep Med.* 2011;**7**:211–13.

24. Provini F, Vertugno R, Pastorelli F, *et al.* Status dissociatus after surgery for tegmental ponto-mesencephalic cavernoma: a state dependent disorder of motor control during sleep. *Mov Disord.* 2004;**19**:719–23.

25. Iranzo A, Aparicio J. A lesson from anatomy: focal brain lesions causing REM sleep behaviour disorder. *Sleep Med.* 2009;**10**:9–12.

26. Zambelis T, Paparrigopoulos T, Soldatos CR. REM sleep behaviour disorder associated with a neurinoma of the left pontocerebellar angle. *J Neurol Neurosurg Psychiatry.* 2002;**72**:821–2.

27. Plazzi G, Montagna P. Remitting REM sleep behavior disorder as the initial sign of multiple sclerosis. *Sleep Med.* 2002;**3**:437–9.

28. Tippmann-Peikert M, Boeve BB, Keegan BM. REM sleep behavior disorder initiated by acute brainstem multiple sclerosis. *Neurology.* 2006;**66**:1277–9.

29. Gomez-Choco M, Iranzo A, Blanco Y, *et al.* Prevalence of restless legs syndrome and REM sleep behavior disorder in multiple sclerosis. *Multiple Sclerosis.* 2007;**13**:805–8.

30. Iranzo A, Graus F, Clover L. Rapid eye movement sleep behavior disorder and potassium channel antibody-associated limbic encephalitis. *Ann Neurol.* 2006;**59**:178–82.

31. Compta Y, Iranzo A, Santamaría J, Casamitjana R, Graus F. REM sleep behavior disorder and narcoleptic features in anti-Ma2-associated encephalitis. *Sleep.* 2007;**30**:767–9.

32. Mathis J, Hess CW, Bassetti C. Isolated mediotegmental lesion causing narcolepsy and rapid eye movement sleep behaviour disorder: a case evidencing a common pathway in narcolepsy and rapid eye movement sleep behavior disorder. *J Neurol Neurosurg Psychiatry.* 2007;**78**:427–9.

33. Limousin N, Dehais C, Gout O, *et al.* A brainstem inflammatory lesion causing REM sleep behaviour disorder and sleepwalking (parasomnia overlap disorder). *Sleep Med.* 2009;**10**:1059–62.

34. Blumenthal DT, Salzman KL, Digre KB, *et al.* Early pathological findings and long-term improvement in anti-Ma2-associated encephalitis. *Neurology.* 2006;**67**:146–9.

35. Perez-Diaz H, Rio Oliva C, Rodriguez Uranga JJ. Trastorno de conducta compleio de fases NREM v REM en un paciente con síndrome de Clippers. *Neurologia.* 2012;**27**(Espec Congr):136–7.

36. Flanagan EP, Gavrilova RH, Boeve BF, *et al.* Adult onset autosomal dominant leukodystrophy presenting with REM sleep behavior disorder. *Neurology.* 2012 (in press).

37. Lugaresi E, Provini F. Agypinia excitata: clinical features and pathophysiologic implications. *Sleep Med Rev.* 2001;5:313–32.

38. Cervera A, Sanchez-Valle R, Iranzo A, Blesa R, Santamaria J. Sleep studies in two patients with pontine haematomas and "peduncular" hallucinosis. *J Neurol.* 1999;246(Suppl 1):139.

39. Landau ME, Maldonado JY, Jabbari B. The effects of isolated brainstem lesions on human REM sleep. *Sleep Med.* 2005;6:37–40.

40. Miyamoto M, Miyamoto T, Kubo J, *et al.* Brainstem function in rapid eye movement sleep behavior disorder: the evaluation of brainstem function by MR spectroscopic (^{1}H-MRS). *Psychiatry Clin Neurosci.* 2000;54:350–1.

41. Michaelis T, Merboldt KD, Bruhn H, Hänicke, Frahm J. Absolute concentrations of metabolites in the adult human brain in vivo: quantification of localized proton MR spectra. *Radiology.* 1993;187:219–27.

42. Iranzo A, Santamaria J, Pujol J, *et al.* Brainstem proton spectroscopy in idiopathic REM sleep behavior disorder. *Sleep.* 2002;25:867–70.

43. Ellmore TE, Hood AJ, Castriotta RJ, *et al.* Reduced volume of the putamen in REM sleep behaviour disorder patients. *Parkinsonism Relat Disord.* 2010;16:645–9.

44. Scherfler C, Frauscher B, Schocet M, *et al.* White and gray matter abnormalities in idiopathic REM sleep behaviour disorder. A diffusion-tensor imaging and voxel-based morphometry study. *Ann Neurol.* 2011;69:400–7.

45. Mazza S, Soucy JP, *et al.* Assessing whole brain perfusion changes in patients with REM sleep behaviour disorder. *Neurology.* 2006;67:1618–22.

46. Hanyu H, Inoue Y, Sakurai H, *et al.* Voxel-based magnetic resonance imaging study of structural brain changes in patients with idiopathic REM sleep behavior disorder. *Parkinsonism Relat Disord.* 2012;18:136–9.

47. Unger MM, Belke M, Menzler K, *et al.* Diffusion tensor imaging in idiopathic REM sleep behavior disorder reveals microstructural changes in the brainstem, substantia nigra, olfactory region, and other brain regions. *Sleep.* 2010;33:767–73.

48. Shirakawa S, Takeuchi N, Uchimura N, *et al.* Study of image findings in rapid eye movement sleep behavioural disorder. *Psychiatry Clin Neurosci.* 2002;56:291–2.

49. Vendette M, Gagnon JF, Soucy JP, *et al.* Brain perfusion and markers of neurodegeneration in rapid eye movement sleep behavior disorder. *Mov Disord.* 2011;26:1717–24.

50. Vendette M, Montplaisir J, Gosselin N, *et al.* Brain perfusion anomalies in rapid eye movement sleep behaviour disorder with mild cognitive impairment. *Mov Disord.* 2012;27:1255–61.

51. Dang-Vu TT, Gagnon JF, Vendette M, *et al.* Hippocampal perfusion predicts impending neurodegeneration in REM sleep behaviour disorder. *Neurology.* 2012 (in press).

52. Hanyu H, Inoue H, *et al.* Regional blood flow changes in patients with idiopathic REM sleep behavior disorder. *Eur J Neurol.* 2011;18:784–8.

53. Caselli RJ, Chen K, Bandy D, *et al.* A preliminary fluorodeoxyglucose positron emission tomography study in healthy adults reporting dream-enactment behaviour. *Sleep.* 2006;29:927–33.

54. Braak H, Del Tredici K, Rub U, *et al.* Staging of brain pathology related to sporadic Parkinson's disease. *Neurobiol Aging.* 2003;24:197–211.

55. Iranzo A, Lomeña F, Stockner E, *et al.*, For the Sleep Innsbruck Barcelona (SINBAR) group. Decreased striatal dopamine transporter uptake and substantia nigra hyperechogenicity as risk markers of synucleinopathy in patients with idiopathic rapid-eye-movement sleep behaviour disorder: a prospective study. *Lancet Neurol.* 2010;9:1070–7.

56. Iranzo A, Valldeoriola F, *et al.* Progressive nigrostriatal dopaminergic dysfunction in idiopathic REM sleep behavior disorder: a prospective study. *Lancet Neurol.* 2011;10:797–805.

57. Unger MM, Möller JC, Stiasny-Kolster K, *et al.* Assesment of idiopathic rapid-eye-movement sleep behavior disorder by transcranial sonography, olfactory function test, and FP-CIT-SPECT. *Mov Disord.* 2008;23:596–9.

58. Stockner H, Iranzo A, Seppi K, *et al.* Midbrain hyperechogenicity in idiopathic REM sleep behavior disorder. *Mov Disord.* 2009;24:1906–9.

59. Iwanami M, Miyamoto T, Miyamoto M, Hirata K, Takada E. Relevance of substantia nigra hyperechogenicity and reduced odor identification in idiopathic REM sleep behavior disorder. *Sleep Med.* 2010;11:361–5.

60. Shin HY, Joo EY, Kim HY, Dhong HJ, Cho JW. Comparison study of olfactory function and substantia nigra hyperechogenicity in idiopathic REM sleep behaviour disorder. Parkinson's disease and normal control. *Neurol Sci.* 2012 (in press).

61. Albin RL, Koeppe RA, Chervin RD, *et al.* Decreased striatal dopaminergic innervation in REM sleep behavior disorder. *Neurology.* 2000;55:1410–12.

62. Eisensehr I, Linke S, Noachtar S, *et al.* Reduced striatal dopamine transporters in idiopathic rapid eye movement sleep behavior disorder. *Brain* 2000;123:1155–60.

63. Eisensehr I, Linke R, Tastch K, *et al.* Increased muscle activity during rapid eye movement sleep correlates with decrease of striatal presynaptic dopamine transporters. IPT and IBZM SPECT imaging in subclinical and clinically manifest idiopathic REM sleep behavior disorder, Parkinson's disease, and controls. *Sleep* 2003;26:507–12.

64. Stiasny-Kolster K, Doerr Y, Möller, *et al.* Combination of "idiopathic" REM sleep behavior disorder and olfactory dysfunction as possible indicator for α-synucleinopathy demonstrated by dopamine transporter FP-CIT-SPECT. *Brain* 2005;128:126–37.

65. Kim YK, Yoon IY, Kim JM, *et al.* The implication of nigrostriatal degeneration in the pathogenesis of REM sleep behavior disorder. *Eur J Neurol.* 2010;17:487–92.

66. Paglionico S, Labate A, Salsone M, *et al.* Involvement of cardiac sympathetic nerve endings in a patient with idiopathic RBD and intact nigrostriatal pathway. *Parkinsonism Relat Disord.* 2009;15:789–91.

67. Labate A, Salsone M, Novellino F, *et al.* Combined use of cardiac M-I123-iodobenzylguanidine scintigraphy and ^{123}I-FF-CIT single photon emission computed tomography in older adults with rapid eye movement sleep behavior

disorder. *J Am Geiatr Soc.* 2011;**59**:928–9.

68. Salsone M, Labate A, Quattrone A. Cardiac denervation precedes migrostinatal damage in idiopathic rapid eye movement sleep behaviour disorder. *Mov Disord.* 2012;**27**:1068–9.

69. Miyamoto T, Orimo S, Miyamoto M, *et al.* Follow-up PET studies in case of idiopathic REM sleep behaviour disorder. *Sleep Med.* 2010;**11**:100–1.

70. Miyamoto M, Miyamoto M, *et al.* Preclinical substantia nigra dysfunction in rapid eye movement sleep behaviour disorder. *Sleep Med.* 2012;**13**:102–6.

Cardiac ^{123}I-MIBG scintigraphic findings and REM sleep behavior disorder

Takashi Nomura and Yuichi Inoue

Introduction

Meta-iodobenzylguanidine (^{123}I-MIBG) is a radio-iodinated norepinephrine analog developed by Wieland *et al.* [1]. ^{123}I-MIBG scintigraphy has been widely used for the assessment of autonomic function in the field of cardiology [2]. Moreover, it is used for the assessment of autonomic dysfunction in neurodegenerative disorders and diabetic neuropathy. Cardiac uptake of ^{123}I-MIBG was reduced in patients with synucleinopathies including idiopathic Parkinson's disease (PD) and dementia with Lewy bodies (DLB) [3]. Based on this evidence, ^{123}I-MIBG imaging is considered a powerful tool to differentiate these two disorders from other parkinsonian syndromes including tauopathies [3, 4].

Rapid eye movement (REM) sleep behavior disorder (RBD) is characterized by vigorous and injurious behavior related to experiencing vivid, action-filled, and violent dreams in nocturnal REM sleep. REM sleep without atonia (RWA), in which phasic or tonic electromyography (EMG) appears mainly in the chin or legs on polysomonography (PSG), is an important physiological basis of RBD [5]. Notably, uptake on ^{123}I-MIBG scintigraphy is also reduced in patients with idiopathic RBD (iRBD) [6], and this finding is thought to support the close association between RBD and the above indicated synuclein pathology. In this section, we review the usefulness of ^{123}I-MIBG in neurology-specific sleep disorders with a particular focus on RBD.

The technique of ^{123}I-MIBG scintigraphy

The control center of the cardiac sympathetic nerve exists in the rostral venrolateral medulla [7]. The preganglionic sympathetic nerve descends to the anterior horn of the spine and synapses in the upper and lower cervical ganglia and upper thoracic ganglia [8]. Postganglionic noradrenergic sympathetic fibers enter the myocardium accompanying the blood vessels [4].

Meta-iodobenzylguanidine is a physiological noradrenergic analogue with guanidine-like constitution. It is transported actively into norepinephrine granules of sympathetic nerve terminals by the norepinephrine transporter, stored in these granules, and discharged by sympathetic activity (Figure 41.1). However, ^{123}I-MIBG does not bind to alpha and beta receptors of cardiac muscle.

Catecholaminergic innervation can be visualized in vivo by labeling of ^{123}I-MIBG with [123]iodine [9]. Active neuronal uptake of catecholamines is energy dependent and acts at low substrate concentrations. Thus, ^{123}I-MIEG scintigraphy displays not only the presence of noradrenergic innervation but also its functional capability [1].

Injection of ^{123}I-MIBG after approximately 20 minutes of rest in the supine position leads to a rapid early uptake, which may reflect sympathetic system integrity and cardiac sympathetic nerve terminal distribution (early phase of measurement) [4] Within several hours, ^{123}I-MIBG actively enters the sympathetic nerve terminals of the left ventricular wall mainly, and is washed out rapidly from non-neuronal tissues. The late phase after 3–4 h (late phase of measurement) reflects the active neuronal uptake of ^{123}I-MIBG without passive components, and is recommended for the diagnostic

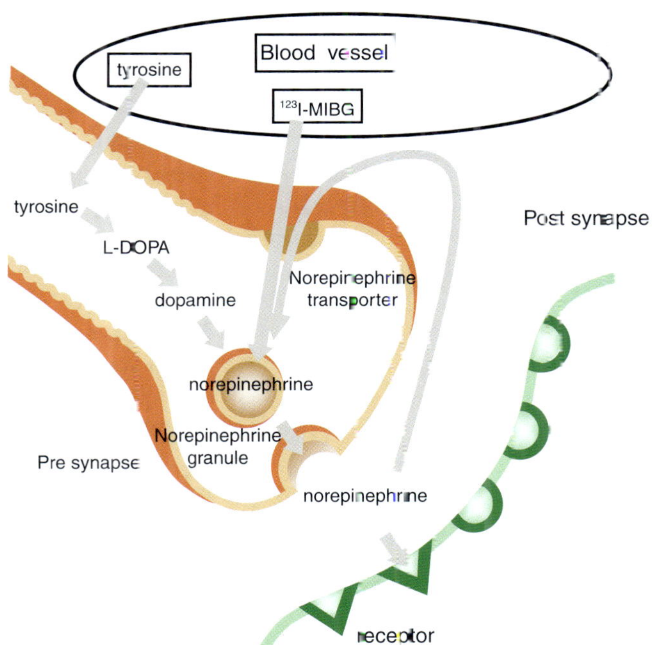

Figure 41.1 Norepinephrine and ^{123}I-MIBG kinetics in the sympathetic nerve terminal. ^{123}I-MIBG is a radio-iodinated analogue of norepinephrine. It is actively transported into norepinephrine granules of sympathetic nerve terminals by the norepinephrine transporter, stored in these granules, and discharged by sympathetic activity similar to norepinephrine.

Neuroimaging of Sleep and Sleep Disorders, ed. Eric Nofzinger, Pierre Maquet, and Michael J. Thorpy. Published by Cambridge University Press. © Cambridge University Press 2013.

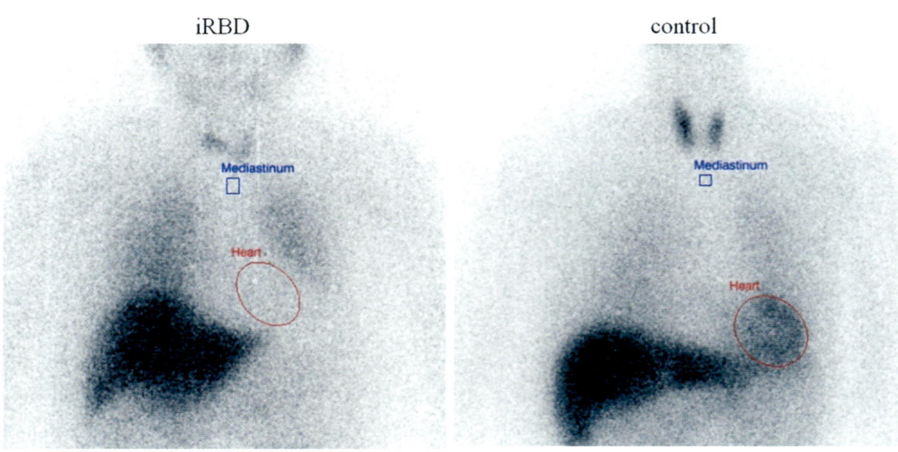

Figure 41.2 H/M ratio in the late phase of ^{123}I-MIBG scintigraphy in a patient with iRBD compared with controls. ^{123}I-MIBG myocardial scintigraphy indicated a reduced heart to mediastinum (H/M) ratio on images of the late phase in patients with iRBD compared with control (iRBD: 1.23 vs. control: 2.47).

examination of Lewy body disease [3, 4]. Cardiac uptake is quantified by comparing the ^{123}I-MIBG radiation emitted from regions of interest (ROI) placed over the heart and the mediastinum on planar images of the thoracic anterior view, and is expressed as the H/M ratio (Figure 41.2). Generally, the H/M ratio ranges from 2.0 to 2.6 by low energy collimators and from 2.6 to 3.4 by moderate energy collimators. The washout rate is calculated as [{(early phase counter in ROI on heart – early phase counter in ROI on background) – (late phase counter in ROI on heart – late phase counter in ROI on background)} / (early phase counter in ROI on heart – early phase counter in ROI on background)] because clearance of ^{123}I-MIBG in the heart is thought to be an index of sympathetic nerve activity or the capability of keeping norepinephrine in granules. A decreased value in the early phase indicates decreased density of sympathetic nervous terminals due to degeneration and/or denervation of the cardiac sympathetic nerve, impairment of norepinephrine transporter, impairment of vesicular monoamine transporter, and/or competition with norepinephrine. Alternatively, a decreased value in the late phase indicates a sympathetic nerve activity-dependent increase in norepinephrine and decreased ^{123}I-MIBG uptake due to impaired norepinephrine transporters and/or impaired retention of norepinephrine in sympathetic nerve terminals or granules. Thus, ^{123}I-MIBG scintigraphy is considered capable of detecting the impairment of postganglionic cardiac sympathetic nervous function.

This imaging modality has been confirmed as safe for humans. No serious adverse reactions have been noted. Mild adverse reactions, including burning at the injection site, nausea, palpitations, and non-specific ill-feeling were reported by only a few subjects [10].

Several commonly administered drugs including labetalol and reserpine competitively interact with the uptake of ^{123}I-MIBG into sympathetic nerve terminals. Moreover, tricyclic antidepressants impair norepinephrine transporters, resulting in decreased uptake. However, concurrent use of anti-parkinsonism drugs does not affect ^{123}I-MIBG uptake [11]. The only exception is monoamine oxidase B inhibitors, which reduce the H/M ratios of ^{123}I-MIBG. In order to obtain reliable results, these drugs should be avoided during the assessment of the temporal context for the cardiac sympathetic nervous system [9].

^{123}I-MIBG findings in Parkinson's disease

Hirayama *et al.* were the first to report a decrease in myocardial uptake of ^{123}I-MIBG in patients with PD [12]. Thereafter, several studies demonstrated the diagnostic reliability of reduced cardiac ^{123}I-MIBG uptake in PD patients. Patients with PD show not only decreased myocardial ^{123}I-MIBG uptake but also enhanced washout of ^{123}I-MIBG, which is a result of a reduced capability for retention of the substrate in the nerve terminals. This enhanced washout rate is observed even in patients with PD but without obvious reduction in H/M ratios in the early phase and may precede loss of nerve terminals [13].

The existence of a correlation between the severity of parkinsonian clinical features and ^{123}I-MIBG uptake remains controversial. Some investigators have reported no association between indices of PD severity and H/M uptake [14], while other studies found a greater decrease in H/M ratios in patients with higher disease severity, higher age, and longer disease duration [11]. Tremor-dominant PD patients were reported to have higher ^{123}I-MIBG uptake than those with postural instability and gait disorder, while reduced ^{123}I-MIBG uptake was linked to more severe bradykinesia, increased age at the onset of PD, and longer disease duration [14]. The existence of hallucinations was also reported to be closely linked to lower delayed H/M ratios than the disease duration or PD severity [15]. However, a clear consensus has not been reached yet in terms of the relationship between the clinical characteristics of PD and ^{123}I-MIBG uptake.

In general, ^{123}I-MIBG scintigraphy is regarded as an assessment of autonomic function. However, it is uncertain whether cardiac ^{123}I-MIBG uptake is correlated with clinical dysautonomic symptoms in patients with PD. Most clinical studies found no relationship between H/M ratios and dysautonomic symptoms or abnormal autonomic test results in PD patients [14, 16]. However, some investigators have reported a significantly higher ^{123}I-MIBG uptake in patients with PD without dysautonomia than in those presenting with dysautonomia [11, 17].

^{123}I-MIBG findings in α-synucleinopathies other than Parkinson's disease

Of note, early and late H/M ratios are significantly lower and washout rates are significantly higher in patients with DLB compared to those with Alzheimer's disease (AD), indicating a more severe postganglionic sympathetic denervation in the former group [13, 18]. Therefore, ^{123}I-MIBG scintigraphy may be useful for differentiating DLB from AD. However, additional parkinsonian features or orthostatic symptoms in DLB do not correlate with ^{123}I-MIBG findings [19].

Some studies dealt with ^{123}I-MIBG findings in pure autonomic failure (PAF) and found a reduced ^{123}I-MIBG uptake in patients with the disorder [13], but PD patients with dysautonomia cannot be distinguished from PAF patients by ^{123}I-MIBG scintigraphy [16].

Multiple system atrophy (MSA) presents as a poorly dopa-responsive parkinsonian syndrome with early autonomic dysfunction and cerebellar and/or pyramidal signs. In contrast to PD, autonomic dysfunction in MSA is caused by preganglionic rather than postganglionic denervation [20]. In agreement with this pathological characterization, the H/M ratio on ^{123}I-MIBG is usually normal with MSA despite severe autonomic symptoms. ^{123}I-MIBG scintigram has been reported to be more reliable for the differential diagnosis between PD and MSA than clinical autonomic testing with 80% sensitivity and 100% specificity [17]. However, a mild decrease in cardiac ^{123}I-MIBG uptake has been reported in patients with MSA [11]. With regard to this finding, measurement of tyrosine hydroxylase (TH)-immunoreactivity, which is a marker of sympathetic nerve function, showed a mild degeneration of the cardiac sympathetic nervous system possibly due to trans-synaptic degeneration in some MSA patients [21].

^{123}I-MIBG findings in atypical parkinsonian syndromes including tauopathies

Progressive supranuclear palsy (PSP) presents as a poorly dopa-responsive parkinsonian syndrome with ocular supranuclear palsy, gait disturbance at an early phase of the disease, and cognitive problems of subcortical origin. Patients with PSP show a significantly higher myocardial ^{123}I-MIBG uptake than those with PD [13, 20], but patients with PSP as a whole do not necessarily have normal ^{123}I-MIBG scintigraphic findings [3].

Few data are available for other tauopathy-related atypical parkinsonian syndromes. Among these, patients with corticobasal degeneration were reported to be distinguishable from PD in terms of an ^{123}I-MIBG scintigram in some studies [13].

^{123}I-MIBG findings in idiopathic REM sleep behavior disorder

Reports of ^{123}I-MIBG findings for iRBD are summarized in Table 41.1. Miyamoto *et al.* were the first to indicate markedly reduced ^{123}I-MIBG uptake in iRBD. They reported that all 13 patients with iRBD displayed clear reductions in cardiac

Table 41.1 Summary of ^{123}I-MIBG findings in idiopathic REM sleep behavior disorder

Author (year)	n	Results
Miyamoto (2006) [6]	13 (iRBD) 12 (PD) 8 (control)	The mean ratio of ^{123}I-MIBG uptake in the H/M ratio was reduced in patients with either iRBD or PD compared with controls.
Miyamoto (2008) [20]	13 (iRBD), 26 (PD) 6 (DLB), 10 (MSA) 13 (PSP), 9 (control)	Markedly reduced ^{123}I-MIBG uptake was shown in patients with iRBD, PD, and DLB
Miyamoto (2008) [40]	23 (iRBD with AHI <5) 9 (iRBD with 5< AHI <15) 15 (iRBD with AH >15) 16 (moderate to severe OSAS without RBD)	^{123}I-MIBG uptake was significantly decreased in all groups with iRBD compared with moderate to severe OSA without RBD
Oguri (2008) [22]	2 (iRBD)	Two patients with iRBD showed decreased ^{123}I-MIBG uptake
Kashihara (2010) [18]	13 (iRBD) 222 (PD) 50 (control)	^{123}I-MIBG uptake was significantly lower for patients with RBD than for those with early stage PD

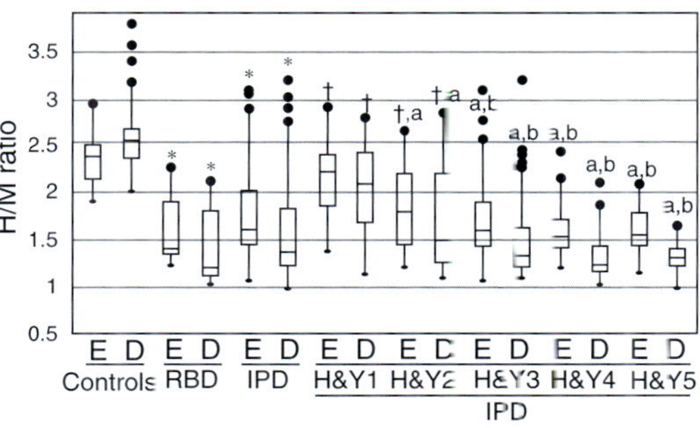

Figure 41.3 Box plots of the H/M ratio from patients with RBD and idiopathic PD (IPD) (total and each Hoehn and Yahr stage) and controls [23]. H&Y: Hoehn and Yahr, stage E: early image, D: delayed image. H/M ratios for delayed control images, for RBD, and for IPD in total and at each Hoehn and Yahr stage differ significantly from ratios for early images of the same group *: H/M ratios differ significantly from ratios of corresponding early or delayed images for the controls. †: H/M ratios differ significantly from ratios of corresponding early or delayed images for RBD. a: H/M ratios differ significantly from ratios of corresponding early or delayed images for IPD at Hoehn and Yahr stage 1. b: H/M ratios differ significantly from ratios of corresponding early or delayed images for IPD at Hoehn and Yahr stage 2.

^{123}I-MIBG uptake. The H/M ratios in the late phase were reduced comparably in patients with iRBD and in those with PD compared to controls [6]. In another report, mean values of the H/M ratio in both the early and late phase were significantly reduced in 31 patients with iRBD, 26 PD patients, and 6 patients with DLB compared to 10 MSA patients, 13 PSP patients, and 9 control subjects [20]. In that study, there was a significant correlation between the H/M ratio and duration of disease morbidity in iRBD patients [20]. Kashihara *et al.* also showed that H/M ratios in 13 iRBD patients and those in 220 PD patients were significantly reduced in both the early and late images as compared with 50 controls [18] (Figure 41.3). Oguri *et al.* reported two patients with RBD showing decreased ^{123}I-MIBG uptake [22], and the findings of those patients showed

that reduced ^{123}I-MIBG uptake in iRBD could not predict the development of PD.

In PD patients, RBD is frequently complicated [23], and RBD affected PD cases are likely to have a significantly lower H/M ratio in the late phase than non-affected cases [24].

Autonomic failure, ^{123}I-MIBG abnormality, and REM sleep behavior disorder

Autonomic dysfunction is common in α-synucleinopathies, and particularly marked in MSA [25]. Moreover, autonomic symptoms are likely to precede the development of motor symptoms in these disorders. Notably, autonomic dysfunction during wakefulness was reported to exist in up to 64% of iRBD cases by Ferini-Stambi et al. [26]. Fantini et al. also reported that cardiac and electroencephalographic activation associated with periodic leg movements during sleep is reduced in RBD [27]. On measures of beat-to-beat RR interval variability, there were clear differences between patients with iRBD and controls [28]. On the orthostatic standing test, iRBD patients were reported to show a larger blood pressure decrease than healthy controls [29]. These results indicate the existence of autonomic dysfunction in iRBD based on the pathological changes associated with synucleinopathy [14]. However, it has not been determined whether autonomic abnormalities can predict the development of neurodegenerative disease. In that regard, Postuma et al. reported that there were no differences in the level of autonomic dysfunction between iRBD patients who did or did not develop synucleinopathy [28].

It is widely accepted that not only clinical RBD symptoms but also clinically silent RWA on PSG (subclinical RBD) are frequently observed after the onset of synucleinopathies [23]. We reported that PD patients with clear RBD symptoms had reduced ^{123}I-MIBG uptake compared with those with subclinical RBD and those with normal REM sleep.

Moreover, multiple linear regression analysis revealed that only the existence of RBD symptoms was significantly associated with reduced ^{123}I-MIBG uptake among the subject PD patients [24]. In agreement with our result, Postuma et al. reported that a larger number of PD patients with RBD had orthostatic hypotension than PD patients without RBD [30]. Further studies investigating the association between the ^{123}I-MIBG findings and other autonomic measures in PD patients would be desirable.

Mechanism for reduced ^{123}I-MIBG uptake

Schenck et al. reported that 11 of 29 patients with previously diagnosed RBD developed PD during a period of approximately 13 years [31], and further longitudinal follow-up revealed that 17 of 26 patients with iRBD developed Parkinsonism and/or dementia over a period of 20.3 years [32]. Iranzo et al. reported that 20 of 44 patients with iRBD developed neurodegenerative disorders. In particular, nine patients developed PD within 11.5 years of follow-up [33]. Postuma et al. also conducted a follow-up study on 93 iRBD patients using life-table analysis to define disease risk over periods of 5, 10, and 12 years. The estimated 5-year, 10-year, and 12-year risk for developing neurodegenerative disease was 7.7%, 40.6%, and 52.4%, respectively, and the risk of the development in iRBD was substantial, with the majority of patients developing PD and DLB. [34]. Thus, iRBD can be hypothesized to occur in preclinical stages of PD. This phenomenon corroborates the proposed staging for the neuropathological process of PD outlined by Braak et al. [35] (Figure 41.4). According to this staging theory, the first stage of PD involves deposition of synuclein in the anterior olfactory nucleus and dorsal motor nucleus of the vagus. The degenerative changes in peripheral autonomic ganglia and unmyelinated lamina-1 spinal cord neurons are also involved in stage 1. Stage 2 is characterized by the changes in medullary and

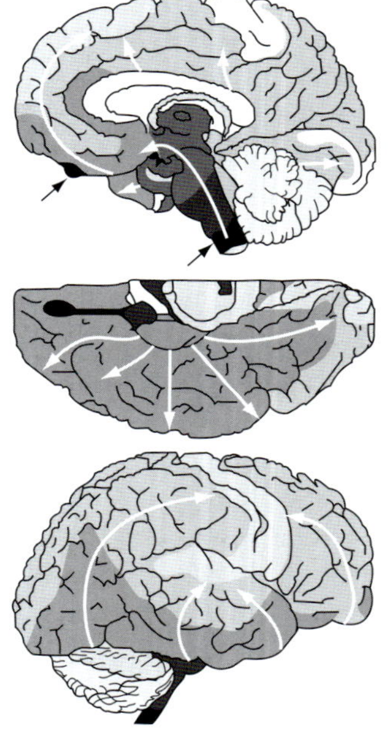

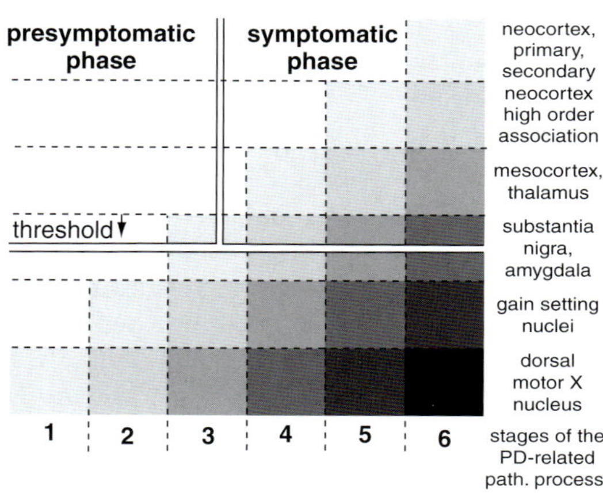

Figure 41.4 Proposed staging for the neuropathological process of Parkinson's disease [35]. Left image shows the upward progress of the PD-related brain pathology. It begins in the lower brainstem and ends in the cerebral cortex. Black arrows indicate the initial site of pathological changes. White arrows indicate the progressive direction of synuclein pathology. Right graphic indicates that the disease process begins at definite sites and progresses in a predictable manner with increasing severity. Changes in the topographical distribution pattern of the α-synuclein-immunoreactive inclusions in the brain can be used to define six neuropathological stages. The degenerative changes in Stage 1 include dorsal motor nucleus of the glossopharyngeal, vassal nerves, and anterior olfactory nucleus. Stage 2 is characterized by the changes in caudal raphe nuclei, gigantocellular reticular nucleus, and the coeruleus/subcoeruleus complex. Stage 3 affects pars compacta in the substantia nigra. Stage 4 involves the temporal neocortex and allocortex. Stages 5 and 6 severely affects the brain including neocortical areas.

pontine involvement affecting the lower raphae, the reticular formation, and the coeruleus/subcoeruleus complex. Stage 3 affects midbrain (including pars compacta of the substantia nigra), and in stages 4 to 6, cerebral cortical structures are affected.

The loss of sympathetic nerve fibers occurs very early in Lewy body disease [36]. TH-positive nerve fibers are also lost in the left ventricle early in the disease course of PD [37]. Some researchers have speculated that the initiation of neurodegeneration in the peripheral autonomic system occurs before synuclein pathology enters the central nervous system [38]. Thus, ^{123}I-MIBG uptake alterations may be the first subtle evidence of autonomic dysfunction in Lewy body diseases, which eventually become clinically manifest. Most patients with incidental Lewy bodies also have severe loss of TH-positive nerve fibers in the epimyocardial nerve, but the fibers are preserved in paraspinal and olfactory nerves [39]. Thus, iRBD might be a preclinical stage of PD or DLB. Further investigations in the evaluation of TH-positive cardiac postganglionic sympathetic nerves in patients with iRBD are necessary.

Clinical significance of ^{123}I-MIBG

Of note, the decrease in ^{123}I-MIBG uptake was present in almost 100% of iRBD patients. Thus, ^{123}I-MIBG scintigraphy has the potential to distinguish true RBD from pseudo RBD in which dream enactment behaviors occur in association with obstructive sleep apnea episodes [40]. However, considering that the H/M ratio is significantly lower for patients with iRBD than for those with early stage PD [18], the results of cardiac ^{123}I-MIBG uptake cannot necessarily predict the development of PD in iRBD patients. Therefore, investigation of this issue using multiple markers should be encouraged. There are a considerable number of potential clinical markers for the prediction of PD, including autonomic dysfunction, olfactory dysfunction, transcranial ultrasound of the substantia nigra, and radiological findings [41].

In PD, olfactory dysfunction is related to decreased ^{123}I-MIBG uptake, a fall in orthostatic blood pressure, and decreased heart rate variability [42]. As for iRBD, Stiasny-Kolster et al. reported that abnormal findings on single-photon emission computed tomography (SPECT) in combination with olfactory dysfunction could become an indicator of evolving α-synucleinopathies [43]. They found a lower threshold score, discrimination score, and identification score for olfactory function in RBD patients than controls. Patients with RBD have similar characteristics to patients with Lewy body disease in terms of olfactory dysfunction [43], cognitive impairment [44], reduction of striatal dopaminergic neurons [45], and increased echogenicity of transcranial ultrasound in the substantia nigra [46]. This supports the theory that the combination of ^{123}I-MIBG and other findings in iRBD might increase the sensitivity and specificity in predicting the future development of Lewy body disease.

In patients with PD, a pathological relationship between hallucinations and RBD has been reported [47, 48], and the occurrence of hallucinations in PD patients is regarded to be a risk factor for developing PD with dementia (PDD). Interestingly, the decrease in ^{123}I-MIBG uptake in PD patients with RBD was shown to be almost comparable with that of PDD [49]. This finding may indicate that ^{123}I-MIBG could be useful for predicting the development of PDD among PD patients.

Conclusion

Decreased ^{123}I-MIBG uptake is an important diagnostic tool for α-synucleinopathies. Moreover, most patients with iRBD have reduced ^{123}I-MIBG uptake, and an abnormal ^{123}I-MIBG finding supports the diagnosis of RBD. Although an abnormal ^{123}I-MIBG finding cannot predict the development of alpha-synucleinopathies among iRBD patients, the existence of RBD might be predictive of developing PDD in patients with PD. In the near future, ^{123}I-MIBG findings might help predict the development of PDD among PD patients affected with RBD.

References

1. Wieland DM, Wu JJ, Brown LE, *et al.* Radiolabeled adrenergic neuron-blocking agents: adrenomedullary imaging with [^{131}I] iodobenzylguanidine. *J Nucl Med.* 1980;21:349–53.

2. Merlet P, Valett H, Dubois-Rande JL, *et al.* Prognostic value of cardiac metaiodobenzyl-guanidine imaging in patients with heart failure. *J Nucl Med.* 1922;33:471–7.

3. Rascol O, Schelosky L. ^{123}I-Metaiodobenzylguanidine scintigraphy in Parkinson's disease and related disorders. *Mov Disord.* 2009;24: S732–41.

4. Taki J, Yoshita M, Yamada M, Tonami N. Significance of ^{123}I-MIBG scintigraphy as a pathophysiological indicator in the assessment of Parkinson's disease and related disorders: it can be a specific marker for Lewy body disease. *Ann Nucl Med.* 2004;18:453–61.

5. American Academy of Sleep Medicine. *International Classification of Sleep Disorders, 2nd edn: Diagnostic and Coding Manual.* Westchester, Illinois, American Academy of Sleep Medicine, 2005.

6. Miyamoto T, Miyamoto M, Inoue Y, *et al.* Reduced cardiac ^{123}I-MIBG scintigraphy in idiopathic REM sleep behavior disorder. *Neurology.* 2006;67:2236–8.

7. Dampney RA. Functional organization of central pathways regulating the cardiovascular system. *Physiol Rev.* 1994;74:323–64.

8. Owman C. Autonomic innervation of the cardiovascular system. In Bjorklund A, Hokfelt T, Owaman C, *et al.* eds. *Handbook of Chemical Neuroanatomy.* Elsevier, Amsterdam. 1988; 327–89.

9. Scisson JC, Shapiro B, Meyers L, *et al.* Metaiodobenzylguanidine to map scintigraphically the adrenergic nervous

system in man. *J Nucl Med.* 1987;**28**:1625–36.

10. Hirosawa K, Tanaka T, Hisada K, Bunko H. [Clinical evaluation of ^{123}I-MIBG for assessment of the sympathetic nervous system in the heart (multi-center clinical trial)]. *Kaku Igaku.* 1991;**28**:461–76.

11. Orimo S, Ozawa E, Nakade S, *et al.* ^{123}I-metaiodobenzylguanidine myocardial scintigraphy in Parkinson's disease. *J Neurol Neurosurg Psychiatry.* 1999;**67**:189–94.

12. Hirayama M, Hakusui S, Koike Y, *et al.* A scintigraphical qualitative analysis of peripheral vascular sympathetic function with meta-[123I] iodobenzylguanidine in neurological patients with autonomic failure. *J Auton Nerv Syst.* 1995;**53**:230–4.

13. Kashihara K, Ohno M, Kawada S, Okumura Y. Reduced cardiac uptake and enhanced washout of ^{123}I-MIBG in pure autonomic failure occurs conjointly with Parkinson's disease and dementia with Lewy bodies. *J Nucl Med.* 2006;**47**:1099–101.

14. Spiegel J, Hellwig D, Farmakis G, *et al.* Myocardial sympathetic degeneration correlates with clinical phenotype of Parkinson's disease. *Mov Disord.* 2007;**22**:1004–8.

15. Oka H, Yoshioka M, Onouchi K, *et al.* Impaired cardiovascular autonomic function in Parkinson's disease with visual hallucinations. *Mov Disord.* 2007;**22**:1510–14.

16. Reinhardt MJ, Jungling FD, Krause TM, Braune S. Scintigraphic differentiation between two forms of primary dysautonomia early after onset of autonomic dysfunction: value of cardiac and pulmonary iodine-123 ^{123}I-MIBG uptake. *Eur J Nucl Med.* 2000;**27**:595–600.

17. Courbon F, Brefel-Courbon C, Thalamas C, *et al.* Cardiac ^{123}I-MIBG scintigraphy is a sensitive tool for detecting cardiac sympathetic denervation in Parkinson's disease. *Mov Disord.* 2003;**18**:890–7.

18. Kashihara K, Imamura T, Shinya T. Cardiac ^{123}I-MIBG uptake is reduced more markedly in patients with REM sleep behavior disorder than in those with early stage Parkinson's disease. *Parkinsonism Relat Disord.* 2010;**16**:252–5.

19. Yoshita M, Taki J, Yokoyama K, *et al.* Value of ^{123}I-MIBG radioactivity in the differential diagnosis of DLB for AD. *Neurology.* 2006;**66**:1850–54.

20. Miyamoto T, Miyamoto M, Suzuki K, *et al.* ^{123}I-MIBG cardiac scintigraphy provides clues to the underlying neurodegenerative disorder in idiopathic REM sleep behavior disorder. *Sleep.* 2008;**31**:717–23.

21. Orimo S, Uchihara T, Nakamura A, *et al.* Axonal a-synuclein aggregates herald centripetal degeneration of cardiac sympathetic nerve in Parkinson's disease. *Brain.* 2008;**131**:642–50.

22. Oguri T, Tachibana N, Mitake S, *et al.* Decrease in myocardial ^{123}I-MIBG radioactivity in REM sleep behavior disorder: two patients with different clinical progression. *Sleep Med.* 2008;**9**:583–5.

23. Gagnon JF, Postuma RB, Mazza S, *et al.* Rapid-eye-movement sleep behaviour disorder and neurodegenerative diseases. *Lancet Neurol.* 2006;**5**:424–32.

24. Nomura T, Inoue Y, Hogl B, *et al.* Relationship between ^{123}I-MIBG scintigrams and REM sleep behavior disorder in Parkinson's disease. *Parkinsonism Relat Disord.* 2010;**16**:683–5.

25. Chaudhuri KR. Autonomic dysfunction in movement disorders. *Curr Opin Neurol.* 2001;**14**:505–11.

26. Ferini-Strambi L, Oldani A, Zucconi M, *et al.* Cardiac autonomic activity during wakefulness and sleep in REM sleep behavior disorder. *Sleep.* 1996;**19**:367–9.

27. Fantini ML, Michaud M, Gosselin N, *et al.* Periodic leg movements in REM sleep behavior disorder and related autonomic and EEG activation. *Neurology.* 2002;**59**:1889–94.

28. Postuma RB, Lanfranchi PA, Blais H, *et al.* Cardiac autonomic dysfunction in idiopathic REM sleep behavior disorder. *Mov Disord.* 2010;**25**:2304–10.

29. Frauscher B, Nomura T, Duerr S, *et al.* Investigation of autonomic function in idiopathic REM sleep behavior disorder. *J Neurol.* 2012;**259**:1056–61.

30. Postuma RB, Gagnon JF, Vendette M, *et al.* Manifestations of Parkinson disease differ in association with REM sleep behavior disorder. *Mov Disord.* 2008;**15**:1665–72.

31. Schenck CH, Bundlie SR, Mahowald MW. Delayed emergence of a parkinsonian disorder in 38% of 29 older men initially diagnosed with idiopathic rapid eye movement sleep behaviour disorder. *Neurology.* 1996;**46**:388–93.

32. Schenck C, Bundlie SR, Mahowald MW. REM behavior disorder (RBD): delayed emergence of parkinsonism and/or dementia in 65% of older men initially diagnosed with idiopathic RBD, and an analysis of the minimum & maximum tonic and/or phasic electromyographic abnormalities found during REM sleep. *Sleep.* 2003;**26**:A316.

33. Iranzo A, Molinuevo JL, Santamaria J, *et al.* Rapid-eye-movement sleep behaviour disorder as an early marker for a neurodegenerative disorder: a descriptive study. *Lancet Neurol.* 2006;**5**:527–7.

34. Postuma RB, Gagnon JF, Vendette M, *et al.* Quantifying the risk of neurodegenerative disease in idiopathic REM sleep behavior disorder. *Neurol.* 2009;**72**:1296–300.

35. Braak H, Bohl JR, Muller CM, *et al.* Stanley Fahn Lecture 2005: The staging procedure for the inclusion body pathology associated with sporadic Parkinson's disease reconsidered. *Mov Disord.* 2006;**21**:2042–51.

36. Merlet P, Valette H, Dubobis-Rande JL, *et al.* Prognostic value of cardiac metaiodobenzylguanidine imaging in patients with heart failure. *J Nucl Med.* 1992;**33**:471–7.

37. Fujishiro H, Frigerio R, Burnett M, *et al.* Cardiac sympathetic denervation correlates with clinical and pathologic stages of Parkinson's disease. *Mov Diord.* 2008;**23**:1085–92.

38. Orimo S, Amino T, ltoh Y, *et al.* Cardiac sympathetic denervation precedes neuronal loss in the sympathetic ganglia in Lewy body disease. *Acta Neuropathol* 2005;**109**:583–8.

39. Orimo S, Takahashi A, Uchihara T, *et al.* Degeneration of cardiac sympathetic nerve begins in the early disease process of Parkinson's disease. *Brain Pathol.* 2007;**17**:24–30.

40. Miyamoto T, Miyamoto M, Suzuki K, *et al.* Comparison of severity of obstructive sleep apnea and degree of accumulation of cardiac ^{123}I-MIBG radioactivity as a diagnostic marker for idiopathic REM sleep behavior disorder. *Sleep Med.* 2009;**10**:577–80.

41. Postuma RB, Montplaisir J. Predicting Parkinson's disease – why, when, and how? *Parkinsonism Relat Disord*. 2009;**15**:S105–9.

42. Oka H, Toyoda C, Yogo M, *et al*. Olfactory dysfunction and cardiovascular dysautonomia in Parkinson's disease. *J Neurol*. 2010;**257**:969–76.

43. Stiasny-Kolster K, Doerr Y, Moller JC, *et al*. Combination of 'idiopathic' REM sleep behaviour disorder and olfactory dysfunction as possible indicator for alpha-synucleinopathy demonstrated by dopamine transporter FP-CIT-SPECT. *Brain*. 2005;**128**:126–37.

44. Gagnon JF, Vendette M, Postuma RB, *et al*. Mild cognitive impairment in rapid eye movement sleep behavior disorder and Parkinson's disease. *Ann Neurol*. 2009;**66**:39–47.

45. Eisensehr I, Linke R, Noachtar S, *et al*. Reduced striatal dopamine transporters in idiopathic rapid eye movement sleep behaviour disorder. Comparison with Parkinson's disease and controls. *Brain*. 2000;**123**:1155–60.

46. Iwanami M, Miyamoto T, Miyamoto M, *et al*. Relevance of substantia nigra hyperechogenicity and reduced odor identification in idiopathic REM sleep behavior disorder. *Sleep Med*. 2010;**11**:361–5.

47. Arnulf I, Bonnet AM, Damier P, *et al*. Hallucinations, REM sleep, and Parkinson's disease: a medical hypothesis. *Neurology*. 2000 **55**: 281–8.

48. Nomura T, Inoue Y, Mitani H, *et al*. Visual hallucinations as REM sleep behavior disorders in patients with Parkinson's disease. *Mov Discrd*. 2003;**18**:812–17.

49. Nomura T, Nakashima K, Inoue Y, *et al*. Authors' reply to the comments of Miyamoto *et al*. regarding "Cardiac ^{123}I-MIBG accumulation in Parkinson's disease differ in association with REM sleep behavior disorder". *Parkinsonism Relat Disord*. 2011;**17**:654.

Neuroimaging and posttraumatic stress disorder

Ryan P. J. Stocker and Anne Germain

Introduction

Neuroimaging techniques have yielded significant advances in our understanding of the neural correlates of posttraumatic stress disorder (PTSD) during wakefulness in the last two decades. However, neuroimaging techniques remain underutilized to study sleep-related neural processes that may contribute to the pathophysiology and maintenance of PTSD. In this chapter, we first succinctly describe the current DSM-IV-TR diagnostic criteria for PTSD, as well as possible changes currently under consideration. We briefly review subjective and objective sleep findings in PTSD samples, and summarize neuroimaging findings from studies conducted during wakefulness in PTSD to highlight the potential of using neuroimaging in studying sleep. We conclude by discussing how well-established and novel neuroimaging methods may be applied to elucidate the neural underpinnings of PTSD during sleep, and how experimental paradigms can be used to probe sleep-specific neural circuits involved in PTSD. Finally, we offer a series of avenues for sleep neuroimaging research in trauma and PTSD research.

Definition of PTSD

While chronic, maladaptive stress reactions have been recognized under terms such as shell shock, combat neurosis, rape syndrome, railway spine, and many others, PTSD was first formally introduced in the third edition of the *Diagnostic and Statistical Manual of Mental Disorders* (DSM) in 1980. The latter was in recognition of chronic stress reactions experienced by combat veterans of the Vietnam War, and more generally, by survivors of extreme, stressful events including natural disasters, the Holocaust, and sexual assaults.

As summarized in Table 42.1 PTSD is an anxiety disorder that encompasses symptoms of re-experiencing (e.g., flashbacks, nightmares), avoidance (e.g., efforts to avoid thoughts or reminders of the trauma, emotional numbing), and hyperarousal (e.g., insomnia, hypervigilance), which are present for at least one month following the experience of a traumatic event, and are accompanied by significant distress and functional impairments. Potentially traumatic events include, but are not limited to, combat exposure, physical assaults, rape, and natural disasters.

A number of changes to the diagnosis of PTSD are currently under consideration for the fifth edition of the DSM. For instance, the definition of trauma (Criterion A) may be eliminated [1], restricted to include direct experiences of traumatic events [2], or expanded to include events when one gains knowledge that a violent or accidental event(s) happened to a close one, or prolonged exposure to negative aspects of a given event (e.g., recovery teams after natural disasters) [3]. The number of symptom clusters may be increased from three to four, to include specific manifestations of the persistent negative cognitive and affective responses that can result from trauma exposure. Finally, the number of required symptoms in each cluster is also under review [3].

Epidemiological studies indicate that between 50% and 90% of adults surveyed report having experienced at least one trauma over the course of their lives [4, 5]. However, rates of PTSD are significantly lower in the general population, with lifetime prevalence approximating 5% for men and 10% for women [6], but are often higher in survivors of interpersonal violence and combat-exposed military personnel. Recommended treatments for PTSD include selective serotonin reuptake inhibitors and exposure-based cognitive-behavioral techniques [7, 8]. Without treatment, PTSD tends to become chronic. Consequently, the direct and indirect societal costs associated with PTSD are astronomical (e.g., [9]).

A number of risk factors for the development of PTSD following trauma exposure have been identified: being a woman, prior trauma exposure, personal or family history of psychiatric disorders, poor social support, and peritraumatic dissociation (see [10] for review). As described below, sleep disturbances that precede or follow trauma exposure constitute significant risk factors for PTSD. Most importantly, sleep disturbances are one of the few modifiable PTSD risk factors, which offer a unique window to elucidate sleep-related neural mechanisms that may contribute to risk and psychological resilience, and to study brain circuits that are affected by PTSD across wakefulness and sleep states. However, neuroimaging studies in PTSD conducted to date have focused exclusively on structural and functional neural correlates of this pervasive disorder during wakefulness. In the reminder of this chapter, we review and discuss evidence in support of the hypothesis that sleep disturbances may reflect underlying neural processes that confer vulnerability or resistance to the potential adverse effects of traumatic stress, and that a better understanding of these sleep-related processes may provide

Neuroimaging of Sleep and Sleep Disorders, ed. Eric Nofzinger, Pierre Maquet, and Michael J. Thorpy. Published by Cambridge University Press. © Cambridge University Press 2013.

Table 42.1. DSM-IV-TR diagnostic criteria for posttraumatic stress disorder (PTSD)

Criterion A (both required)	Both required: • The person has experienced, witnessed, or been confronted with an event that involves actual or threatened death or serious injury, or a threat to the physical integrity of oneself or others • The person's response involved intense fear, helplessness, or horror
Criterion B: Intrusions	At least one of: • Distressing, recurrent, and intrusive recollections of the event • Distressing, recurrent nightmares • Flashbacks • Intense psychological distress to internal or external reminders of the event(s) • Intense physiological reactivity to internal or external reminders of the event(s)
Criterion C: Avoidance/ Numbing	At least three of: • Effortful avoidance of thoughts, feelings, or conversations about the event(s) • Effortful avoidance of activities, places. or people that trigger recollections of the event(s) • Partial or total amnesia of the event(s) • Loss of interest in significant activities • Feeling of detachment or alienation from others • Restricted affect • Sense of foreshortened future
Criteria D: Hyperarousal	At least two of: • Difficulty falling or staying asleep • Irritability or outbursts of anger • Concentration difficulties • Hypervigilance • Exaggerated startle response
Criterion E: Duration	• Symptoms persist for more than one month
Criterion F: Distress and Impairments	• Symptoms cause clinically significant distress or impairment in social, occupational, or other areas of functioning
Specifiers	• Acute: symptom duration is less than three months • Chronic: symptom duration is three months or more • Delayed onset: symptom onset is six months or more after the traumatic event(s)

insights to inform the development of effective prevention, detection, and intervention strategies.

Trauma exposure and sleep disturbances: an under-studied bidirectional relationship

Trauma exposure and chronic stress are often associated with the onset and persistence of sleep disturbances. However, sleep disturbances can persist long after acute or chronic stressors end, and in the absence of psychiatric comorbidities [11, 12]. Adverse childhood events, including abuse or neglect, are strongly associated with adult sleep disorders decades after adversity ended [11]. In turn, the persistence of sleep disturbances may contribute to later re-exposure to trauma [13]. Although a growing body of literature recognizes the long-term effects of early stress or trauma exposure on brain development and later brain functions (e.g., [14]), the potential neural mechanisms that underlie the relationship between early life stress/trauma exposure, sleep disturbances, and later psychiatric morbidities has not yet been directly and prospectively investigated. As detailed below, sleep neuroimaging methods are urgently needed to elucidate the neural circuits underlying trauma responses that can acutely and chronically affect regulatory brain sleep networks.

In adults, the onset of sleep disturbances following trauma exposure increases the risk of PTSD. In one study, subjective reports of insomnia occurring one month following a motor vehicle accident predicted the development of PTSD 12 months later [15], whereas actigraphic and polysomnographic measures of sleep disruption did not [16]. In survivors of traumatic injuries, another study observed that shorter rapid eye movement (REM) sleep duration characterized patients who later developed PTSD compared to those who did not [17], and that the duration of REM sleep was negatively correlated with insomnia severity as well as with PTSD symptom severity. Furthermore, non-rapid eye movement (NREM) sleep disruption also characterized trauma-exposed patients with and without PTSD compared to non-trauma-exposed subjects [18].

While the aforementioned studies highlight the impact of trauma exposure and sleep and subsequent development of PTSD, the presence of sleep disturbances *prior to trauma exposure* can also threaten psychological resilience, and heighten the risk of PTSD. Adults who reported bad dreams and other sleep disturbances prior to Hurricane Andrew were more likely to develop PTSD compared to individuals who did not report sleep disturbances prior to this natural disaster [19]. Preexisting sleep complaints also heightened the risk of PTSD and of other stress-related disorders three months after the occurrence of traumatic injuries [20]. These observations support a bidirectional relationship between trauma exposure and sleep disturbances, and subsequent development and/or persistence of PTSD. These observations also suggest that sleep monitoring and treatments early after trauma exposure may be a fruitful strategy to prevent the development of PTSD, and that screening for preexisting sleep disturbances and targeted treatments for sleep disturbances in populations at high risk for trauma exposure (e.g., emergency workers, firefighters fire, policemen and women, paramedics, military personnel) may enhance psychological resilience to trauma and reduce the risk for PTSD.

From a sleep neuroimaging perspective, elucidating the neural circuits that are affected by trauma exposure and that can contribute to sleep disruption may provide highly innovating and promising venues for prevention, early detection, and treatment of PTSD.

Sleep disturbances and PTSD

Nightmares and insomnia are PTSD symptoms of the re-experiencing and hyperarousal symptom clusters, respectively. Nightmares and insomnia are among the most common symptoms of PTSD. Although sleep avoidance is not a specific symptom of PTSD, it is also frequently endorsed by children and adults with PTSD. Other sleep disturbances are commonly endorsed by patients with PTSD, including bad dreams that are not related to traumatic events, sleep terrors and other arousal disorders, acting out dreams, and sleep paralysis [21–23]. The variety of sleep disturbances endorsed by individuals suffering from PTSD suggests that sleep-related regulatory mechanisms are globally disrupted in PTSD.

The severity of sleep complaints is significantly and positively correlated with daytime PTSD symptom severity [22], beyond the contributing effects of psychiatric comorbidity, age, sex, and PTSD chronicity. Sleep complaints contribute to symptoms of depression, suicidality, alcohol misuse, and poor perceived health in PTSD [24–26]. More recently, a five-year prospective study revealed that the presence of sleep disturbances prior to treatment initiation significantly reduced the likelihood of PTSD remission [27]. However, sleep-focused pharmacological or behavioral treatments can be used to effectively alleviate nightmares and insomnia in PTSD samples [28].

Despite the convergent observations that subjective sleep disturbances are a highly prevalent feature of PTSD, exacerbating the severity of the disorder, and adversely affecting treatment outcomes, objective indices of sleep disruption specific to PTSD have not be identified with polysomnography (PSG). PSG refers to the collection of physiological signals used to identify sleep stages and objective parameters of sleep disruption, such as wake time after sleep onset, nocturnal arousals, and sleep efficiency (or the ratio of time spent asleep to time spent in bed) below 85%. The absence of a specific objective profile of sleep anomalies may not be surprising, given the diversity of sleep complaints endorsed by patients with PTSD, which may be expected to arise from different underlying neural circuits. Nevertheless, a meta-analysis of PSG studies conducted in adults with PTSD detected modest effects suggesting an increased percentage of light sleep, decreased slow-wave sleep, and an increased rate of rapid eye movements during REM sleep in those with PTSD compared to those without PTSD [29]. An exploratory analysis revealed that age, sex, and comorbid depression or substance use disorders moderated the relationships between PTSD and sleep disturbances.

It is important to note that the presence of specific PSG-based anomalies is not required for the diagnosis of several sleep disorders that are endorse by patients with PTSD, including nightmares, insomnias, arousal disorders, and sleep-related movement disorders [30]. Rather, the diagnoses of these sleep disorders are all primarily based on the nature of presenting complaints, associated features, and functional consequences. Therefore, the presence of consistent and specific PSG findings in adults with PTSD should not be held as the gold standard to guide diagnostic and treatment plans for comorbid sleep disturbances. Inconsistent PSG findings may reflect PSG measurement limitations. A salient example in support of the latter comes from the observations that patients with insomnia show markedly different brain activity patterns during NREM sleep compared to healthy good sleepers, even in the absence of group differences on PSG sleep measures [31]. In a similar manner, changes in brain activity patterns during NREM sleep and REM sleep in PTSD may not be captured by PSG sleep measurement methods, but functional differences may be captured by sleep neuroimaging methods.

(Sleep) Neuroimaging in PTSD

While sleep neuroimaging techniques are the most promising approaches to uncover the neural circuits that underlie sleep disturbances and that are affected by trauma exposure, and, alternatively, to identify how sleep-related networks contribute to acute and chronic trauma responses, sleep neuroimaging in PTSD is in its infancy. In this section, we briefly review neuroimaging studies in PTSD, and highlight how they can inform much-needed sleep neuroimaging studies.

PTSD is conceptualized as a disorder of hyper-responsiveness to threat stimuli accompanied by dysfunctional inhibitory control of threat responses. As such, PTSD is thought to arise from a failure of recovery from trauma exposure, where behavioral, cognitive, emotional responses to the original threat(s) persist despite the termination of the threat. Animal studies have been instrumental in identifying the neurobiological underpinnings of fear responses, and have guided neuroimaging techniques used in PTSD, including positron emission tomography (PET), single photon emission computed tomography (SPECT), structural and functional magnetic resonance imaging (MRI), and magnetic resonance spectroscopy (MRS).

Consistent with animal models of fear learning and fear extinction, preclinical and clinical physiological and neuroimaging studies have implicated the amygdala, medial prefrontal cortex, and hippocampus in the neurobiology of normal and abnormal fear responses, including PTSD [32]. While these brain structures and regions are not regulatory sleep centers, they may nevertheless modulate sleep (see [33] for review).

Observations that chronic stress exposure was associated with smaller hippocampal volumes in animals [34] informed the initial structural MRI studies in adults with PTSD [35], and were corroborated by several (but not all) subsequent studies (see [36] for review). In animals, chronic sleep disruption reduces neurogenesis [37]. In humans, chronic primary insomnia has also been associated with reduced hippocampal volume [38]. One preliminary study suggested that insomnia severity is strongly and negatively correlated with volume of the CA3/dentate subfield, even when controlling for the effects of PTSD [39]. These findings raise the possibility that chronic sleep disruption may directly contribute to hippocampal anomalies in PTSD, which, in turn, may mediate daytime symptoms of PTSD. Whether structural changes can be detected in regulatory sleep centers in PTSD, or whether these alterations can be reversed using effective sleep-focused treatments in a manner analogous to changes observed in response to PTSD treatments, are areas of neuroimaging research that merit closer attention.

Functional neuroimaging studies have been the most common neuroimaging approach to study the neural correlates of PTSD during wakefulness. Resting state (waking) studies have been conducted with SPECT and PET. These have found alterations in the medial and dorsolateral prefrontal cortical regions, amygdala, and cerebellum in adults with PTSD compared to trauma-exposed subjects without PTSD (see [32] for review). Resting state functional MRI (fMRI) methods have been used to study the default mode network in PTSD. The default mode network refers to spontaneous, low frequency oscillations of the blood oxygen level-dependent (BOLD) signal that can be detected in the absence of processing demands [40]. This network including the medial prefrontal cortex, posterior cingulate, precuneus, and lateral parietal cortices, and reduced connectivity has been shown in the acute aftermath of natural disasters [41] and in chronic PTSD compared to non-PTSD samples [40]. Using similar methods to contrast activity of the default mode network during REM sleep and NREM sleep could be useful to elucidate how connectivity, and how daytime and sleep symptoms, may relate to these alterations.

Other commonly employed methods in studying the neural underpinnings of PTSD are activation and provocation paradigms combined with functional neuroimaging. In PET studies, the use of radiolabeled water ($H_2{}^{15}O$) was first combined with a symptom provocation study using script driven imagery to evaluate changes in regional cerebral blood flow (rCBF) in response to neutral or trauma-related scripts in trauma-exposed adults with and without PTSD [32]. This initial study reported increased rCBF in the right amygdala and rostral anterior cingulate cortex and reduced rCBF in Broca's area. Subsequent controlled neuroimaging studies using $H_2{}^{15}O$ or ^{18}F-fluorodeoxyglucose (^{18}F-FDG) PET imaging as well as fMRI paradigms have frequently replicated the findings that PTSD is associated with hyperactivation of the amygdala and hypoactivation of the ventromedial frontal regions in response to trauma- or threat-related scripts relative to control conditions compared to non-PTSD samples [32].

SPECT, PET, and fMRI neuroimaging methods have been used to study NREM and REM sleep in healthy subjects [42–45] and clinical samples of patients with major depression or insomnia (e.g., [31, 46–48]). We are currently using ^{18}F-FDG PET methods [43] to study the neurobiology of PTSD during sleep, and recently completed a pilot study to evaluate the neural correlates of PTSD in combat-exposed military veterans with and without PTSD during REM sleep relative to wakefulness (MH083035). As depicted in Figure 42.1, we found that combat-exposed veterans with PTSD showed significantly greater relative regional cerebral metabolic rate of glucose (rCMRglu) during wakefulness and REM sleep in large clusters that included the cerebellum, brainstem, precuneus, thalamus, dorsal striatum, and posterior, dorsal, anterior, and subgenual cingulate cortices, as well as amygdala, orbitofrontal cortex, and the occipitotemporal and parahippocampal gyri compared to veterans without PTSD [49]. These preliminary findings support the hypothesis that hyperactivation of brain regions involved in arousal regulation and fear responses can be detected across physiological states. However, the cross-sectional nature of this study does not provide information about the possible temporal relationship between the observed changes in relative rCMRglu during wakefulness and REM sleep. Specifically, increases in relative rCMRglu in PTSD during wakefulness may be a consequence of changes first occurring in REM sleep, or vice versa, or changes associated with PTSD may simultaneously affect wakefulness and REM sleep

In another pilot study, we explored the neural correlates of nightmare frequency estimates in combat-exposed veterans with and without PTSD. Analyses revealed a significant negative correlation between monthly nightmare frequency estimates and rCMRglu during REM in the amygdala and mPFC in the PTSD group (unpublished data). While these preliminary observations await replications in larger samples, they nevertheless support the

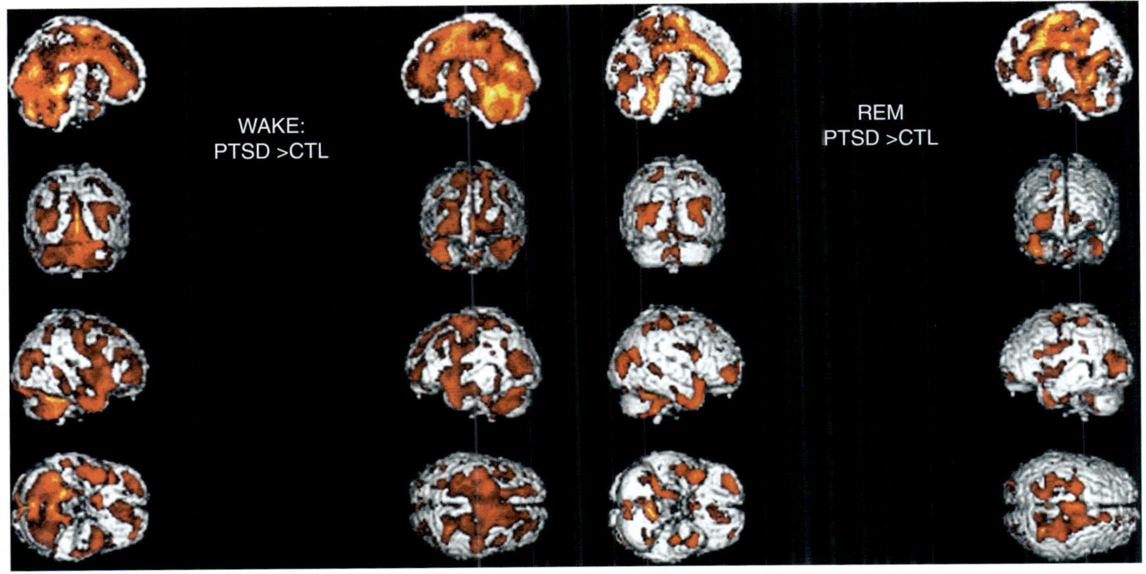

Figure 42.1 Brain regions where combat-exposed veterans with PTSD (n = 6) show greater relative rCMRglu than control veterans without PTSD (CTL; n = 6) during wakefulness (WAKE) and rapid eye movement (REM) sleep.

feasibility ^{18}F-FDG PET methodology to study the neural correlates of PTSD during REM sleep. A larger study that aims to replicate these findings, to expand our investigation to neural correlates of PTSD during NREM sleep, to study neural circuits that are normalized by effective treatment, and to explore neural predictors of sleep treatment response (PT073961; PI: Germain) is currently ongoing.

Summary and future directions

To date, neuroimaging methods have been scarcely applied to the field of sleep and PTSD research, despite burgeoning research highlighting the high potential for such methods for elucidating how sleep and sleep disturbances may contribute to heightened risk (or resilience) for poor psychiatric outcomes following trauma exposure. Specifically, a growing body of literature indicates that sleep disturbances are a predisposing and precipitating risk factor for PTSD (and other stress-related psychiatric disorders such as major depression and addictive disorders), and that sleep-focused treatments yield clinically meaningful improvements in daytime symptom severity and overall functioning. Thus, sleep neuroimaging methods are likely to provide novel insights to advance prevention, detection, and intervention strategies to prevent or accelerate recovery from trauma exposure and PTSD.

Studying and probing the neural correlates of PTSD during REM sleep and NREM sleep can significantly benefit research in both areas of sleep and in PTSD. For sleep researchers and clinicians, understanding the neural underpinnings of sleep disturbances in PTSD provides a unique clinical platform to test and translate innovative basic work on the functional role of sleep in emotion and memory processing (e.g., [50]). For PTSD researchers and clinicians, an integrated, 24-h approach to the evaluation and treatment of PTSD can inform efforts in developing effective prevention and treatment strategies aimed at enhancing psychological resilience to trauma and accelerating recovery from trauma reactions.

For instance, structural neuroimaging approaches have not been used to evaluate the acute or chronic stress exposure and/or PTSD on brain regions known to be involved in sleep regulation. Recent observations in adults with primary insomnia or PTSD that have shown smaller hippocampal volumes raise the possibility that structural changes in limbic regions may modulate regulatory sleep mechanisms. Additionally, in-depth assessments of trauma history in sleep disordered samples are also needed to clarify the relationships between trauma, sleep disturbances, and psychiatric outcomes.

Given the recent advances in sleep-guided fMRI studies, the use of fMRI methods appears to be ripe for dissemination of these methods to the study of sleep in PTSD (as well as other stress-related disorders). For instance, investigating the phasic activity in REM sleep and NREM sleep in relation to waking learning, memory, and affective processes could provide valuable knowledge to understand the mechanisms that underlie chronic hyper-responsiveness to threat stimuli in PTSD.

Finally, combining well-established sleep disruption paradigms with neuroimaging methods, in a way that parallels ongoing work in healthy samples may elucidate how sleep states contribute to emotional and cognitive deficits that are thought to maintain PTSD.

References

1. Kilpatrick DG, Resnick HS, Acierno R. Should PTSD Criterion A be retained? *J Trauma Stress*. 2009;**22**:374–83.

2. Spitzer RL, First MB, Wakefield JC. Saving PTSD from itself in DSM-V. *J Anxiety Disord*. 2007;**21**:233–41.

3. American Psychiatric Association. G 05 Posttraumatic Stress Disorder. DSM-V Development 2010 [cited 2011 Nov 1]; Available from: http://www.dsm5.org/ProposedRevisions/Pages/proposedrevision.aspx?rid=165

4. Seedat S, le Roux C, Stein DJ. Prevalence and characteristics of trauma and post-traumatic stress symptoms in operational members of the South African National Defence Force. *Mil Med*. 2003;**168**:71–5.

5. Breslau N, Kessler RC, Chilcoat HD, *et al*. Trauma and posttraumatic stress disorder in the community: the 1996 Detroit Area Survey of Trauma. *Arch Gen Psychiatry*. 1998;**55**:626–32.

6. Kessler RC, Sonnega A, Bromet E, Hughes M, Nelson CB. Posttraumatic stress disorder in the National Comorbidity Survey. *Arch Gen Psychiatry*. 1995;**52**:1048–60.

7. Stein DJ, Seedat S, van der Linden GJ, Zungu-Dirwayi N. Selective serotonin reuptake inhibitors in the treatment of post-traumatic stress disorder: a meta-analysis of randomized controlled trials. *Int Clin Psychopharmacol*. 2000;**15**(Suppl 2):S31–9.

8. Forbes D, Creamer M, Bisson JI, *et al*. A guide to guidelines for the treatment of PTSD and related conditions. *J Trauma Stress*. 2010;**23**:537–52.

9. Walker EA, Katon W, Russo J, *et al*. Health care costs associated with posttraumatic stress disorder symptoms in women. *Arch Gen Psychiatry*. 2003;**60**:369–74.

10. Ozer EJ, Best SR, Lipsey TL, Weiss DS. Predictors of posttraumatic stress disorder and symptoms in adults: a meta-analysis. *Psychol Bull*. 2003;**129**:52–73.

11. Bader K, Schafer V, Schenkel M, Nissen L, Schwander J. Adverse childhood experiences associated with sleep in primary insomnia. *J Sleep Res*. 2007;**16**:285–96.

12. Rosen J, Reynolds CF, III, Yeager AL, Houck PR, Hurwitz LF. Sleep disturbances in survivors of the Nazi Holocaust. *Am J Psychiatry*. 1991;**148**:62–6.

13. Noll JG, Horowitz LA, Bonanno GA, Trickett PK, Putnam FW. Revictimization and self-harm in females who experienced childhood sexual abuse: results from a prospective study. *J Interpers Violence*. 2003;**18**:1452–71.

14. Lupien SJ, McEwen BS, Gunnar MR, Heim C. Effects of stress throughout the lifespan on the brain, behaviour and cognition. *Nat Rev Neurosci*. 2009;**10**:434–45.

15. Koren D, Arnon I, Lavie P, Klein E. Sleep complaints as early predictors of posttraumatic stress disorder: a 1-year prospective study of injured survivors of motor vehicle accidents. *Am J Psychiatry.* 2002;**159**:855–7.

16. Klein E, Koren D, Arnon I, Lavie P. Sleep complaints are not corroborated by objective sleep measures in post-traumatic stress disorder: a 1-year prospective study in survivors of motor vehicle crashes. *J Sleep Res.* 2003;**12**:35–41.

17. Mellman TA, Pigeon WR, Nowell PD, Nolan B. Relationships between REM sleep findings and PTSD symptoms during the early aftermath of trauma. *J Trauma Stress.* 2007;**20**:893–901.

18. Mellman TA, Bustamante V, Fins AI, Pigeon WR, Nolan B. REM sleep and the early development of posttraumatic stress disorder. *Am J Psychiatry.* 2002;**159**:1696–701.

19. Mellman TA, David D, Kulick-Bell R, Hebding J, Nolan B. Sleep disturbance and its relationship to psychiatric morbidity after Hurricane Andrew. *Am J Psychiatry.* 1995;**152**:1659–63.

20. Bryant RA, Creamer M, O'Donnell M, Silove D, McFarlane AC. Sleep disturbance immediately prior to trauma predicts subsequent psychiatric disorder. *Sleep.* 2010;**33**:69–74.

21. Germain A, Hall M, Krakow B, Katherine Shear M, Buysse DJ. A brief sleep scale for Posttraumatic Stress Disorder: Pittsburgh Sleep Quality Index Addendum for PTSD. *J Anxiety Disord.* 2005;**19**:233–44.

22. Germain A, Buysse DJ, Shear MK, Fayyad R, Austin C. Clinical correlates of poor sleep quality in posttraumatic stress disorder. *J Trauma Stress.* 2004;**17**:477–84.

23. Lauterbach D, Behnke C, McSweeney LB. Sleep problems among persons with a lifetime history of posttraumatic stress disorder alone and in combination with a lifetime history of other psychiatric disorders: a replication and extension. *Compr Psychiatry.* 2011;**52**:580–6.

24. Ribeiro JD, Pease JL, Gutierrez PM, *et al.* Sleep problems outperform depression and hopelessness as cross-sectional and longitudinal predictors of suicidal ideation and behavior in young adults in the military. *J Affect Disord.* 2012;**136**:743–50.

25. Belleville G, Guay S, Marchand A. Impact of sleep disturbances on PTSD symptoms and perceived health. *J Nerv Ment Dis.* 2009;**197**:126–32.

26. Waldrop AE, Back SE, Sensenig A, Brady KT. Sleep disturbances associated with posttraumatic stress disorder and alcohol dependence. *Addict Behav.* 2008;**33**:328–35.

27. Marcks BA, Weisberg RB, Edelen MO, Keller MB. The relationship between sleep disturbance and the course of anxiety disorders in primary care patients. *Psychiatry Res.* 2010;**178**:487–92.

28. Maher MJ, Rego SA, Asnis GM. Sleep disturbances in patients with post-traumatic stress disorder: epidemiology, impact and approaches to management. *CNS Drugs.* 2006;**20**:567–90.

29. Kobayashi I, Boarts JM, Delahanty DL. Polysomnographically measured sleep abnormalities in PTSD: a meta-analytic review. *Psychophysiology.* 2007;**44**:660–9.

30. American Academy of Sleep Medicine. *International Classification of Sleep Disorders, Second Edition (ICSD-2): Diagnostic and Coding Manual.* Westchester, IL, American Academy of Sleep Medicine, 2005.

31. Nofzinger EA, Buysse DJ, Germain A, *et al.* Functional neuroimaging evidence for hyperarousal in insomnia. *Am J Psychiatry.* 2004;**161**:2126–8.

32. Liberzon I, Sripada CS. The functional neurocanatomy of PTSD: a critical review. *Prog Brain Res.* 2008;**167**:151–69.

33. Germain A, Buysse DJ, Nofzinger E. Sleep-specific mechanisms underlying posttraumatic stress disorder: integrative review and neurobiological hypotheses. *Sleep Med Rev.* 2008;**12**:185–95.

34. Watanabe Y, Gould E, McEwen BS. Stress induces atrophy of apical dendrites of hippocampal CA3 pyramidal neurons. *Brain Res.* 1992;**588**:341–5.

35. Bremner JD, Randall P, Scott TM, *et al.* MRI-based measurement of hippocampal volume in patients with combat-related posttraumatic stress disorder. *Am J Psychiatry.* 1995;**152**:973–81.

36. Woon FL, Sood S, Hedges DW. Hippocampal volume deficits associated with exposure to psychological trauma and posttraumatic stress disorder in adults: a meta-analysis. *Prog Neuropsychopharmacol Biol Psychiatry.* 2010;**34**:1181–8.

37. Guzman-Marin R, Bashir T, Suntsova N, Szymusiak R, McGinty D. Hippocampal neurogenesis is reduced by sleep fragmentation in the adult rat. *Neuroscience.* 2007;**148**:325–33.

38. Riemann D, Voderholzer U, Spiegelhalder K, *et al.* Chronic insomnia and MRI-measured hippocampal volumes: a pilot study. *Sleep.* 2007;**30**:955–8.

39. Neylan TC, Mueller SG, Wang Z, *et al.* Insomnia severity is associated with a decreased volume of the CA3/dentate gyrus hippocampal subfield. *Biol Psychiatry.* 2010;**68**:494–6.

40. Lanius RA, Bluhm RL, Coupland NJ, *et al.* Default mode network connectivity as a predictor of post-traumatic stress disorder symptom severity in acutely traumatized subjects. *Acta Psychiatr Scand.* 2010;**121**:33–40.

41. Lui S, Huang X, Chen L, *et al.* High-field MRI reveals an acute impact on brain function in survivors of the magnitude 8.0 earthquake in China. *Proc Natl Acad Sci U S A.* 2009;**106**:15412–7.

42. Maquet P, Peters J, Aerts J, *et al.* Functional neuroanatomy of human rapid-eye-movement sleep and dreaming. *Nature.* 1996;**383**:163–6.

43. Nofzinger EA, Mintun MA, Price J, *et al.* A method for the assessment of the functional neuroanatomy of human sleep using FDG PET. *Brain Res Brain Res Protoc.* 1998;**2**:191–8.

44. Braun AR, Balkin TJ, Wesensten NJ, *et al.* Regional cerebral blood flow throughout the sleep-wake cycle. An H2(15)O PET study. *Brain.* 1997;**120**:1173–97.

45. Wehrle R, Kaufmann C, Wetter TC, *et al.* Functional microstates within human REM sleep: first evidence from fMRI of a thalamocortical network specific for phasic REM periods. *Eur J Neurosci.* 2007;**25**:863–71.

46. Nofzinger EA, Buysse DJ, Germain A, *et al.* Increased activation of anterior paralimbic and executive cortex from waking to rapid eye movement sleep in depression. *Arch Gen Psychiatry.* 2004;**61**:695–702.

47. Smith MT, Perlis ML, Chengazi VU, *et al.* Neuroimaging of NREM sleep in primary insomnia: a Tc-99-HMPAO single photon emission computed tomography study. *Sleep.* 2002;**25**:325–35.

48. Bergmann TO, Molle M, Diedrichs J, Born J, Siebner HR. Sleep spindle-related reactivation of category-specific cortical regions after learning face-scene associations. *Neuroimage.* 2012;**59**:2733–42.

49. Germain A, James JA, Mammen O, Price J, Nofzinger EA. Functional neuroimaging of REM sleep in returning veterans with PTSD: an [18F]-FDG PET study. *Sleep.* 2011; A**242**:34(Suppl):A242.

50. Yoo SS, Gujar N, Hu P, Jolesz FA, Walker MP. The human emotional brain without sleep–a prefrontal amygdala disconnect. *Curr Biol.* 2007;**17**:R877–8.

Neuroimaging of sleepwalking

Michael J. Thorpy

History

A man aged 16 years reported one or two episodes of sleepwalking per night, usually within 2 hours of sleep onset [1]. He had a history of sleepwalking several times per week since childhood. There was a family history of sleepwalking. On examination he had drug-induced bilateral deafness. Awake electroencephalogram (EEG) and magnetic resonance imaging of the brain were normal.

Polysomnographic findings

During video-polysomnography an injection of ^{99m}Tc-ECD was given 24 seconds after the onset of sleepwalking. The episode of sleepwalking was seen during slow-wave sleep (Figure 43.1). The patient stood up with his eyes open and had a scared facial expression, then sat down. The EEG showed diffuse, high-voltage rhythmic delta activity.

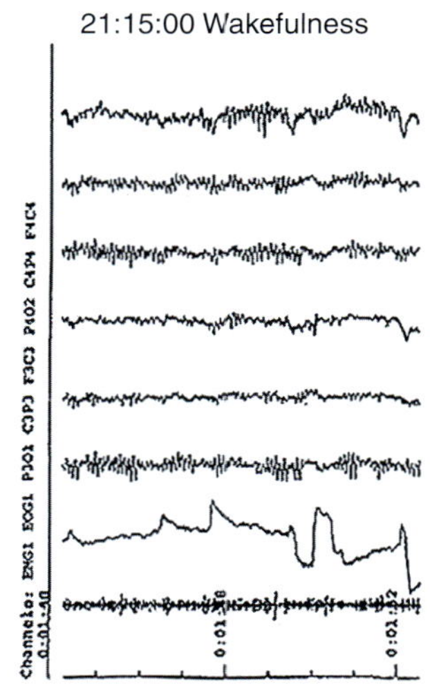

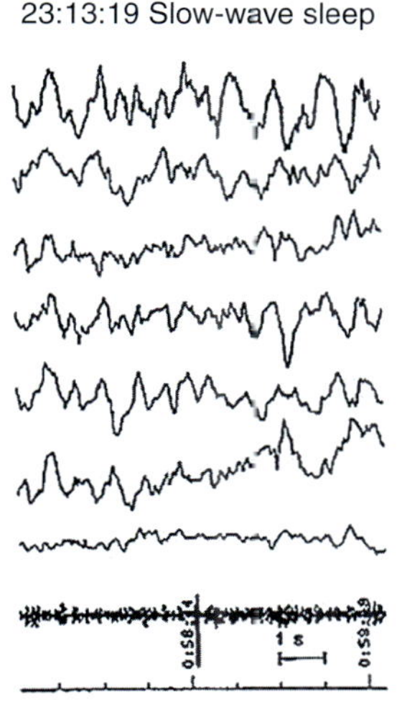

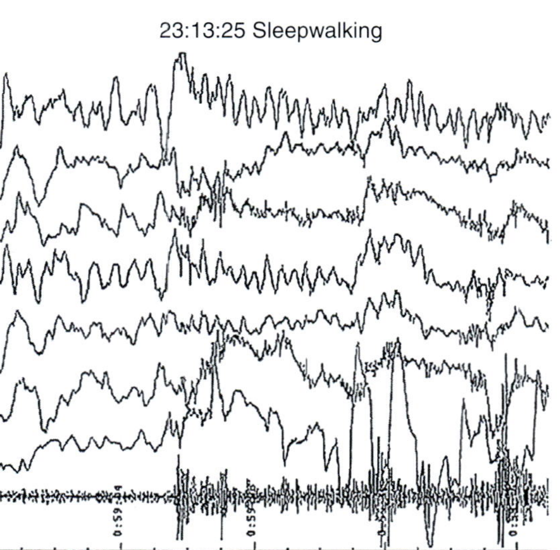

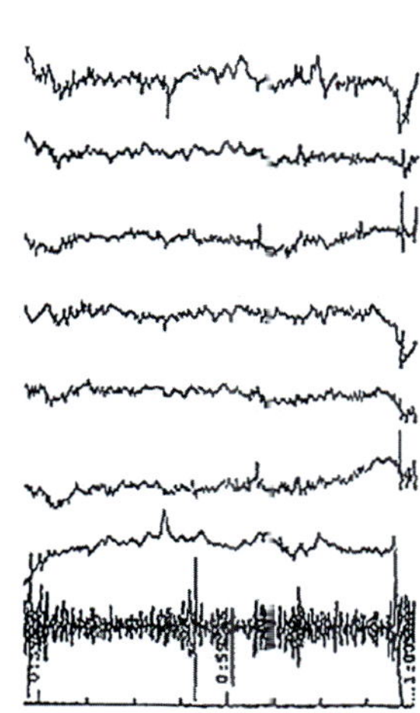

Figure 43.1 Video-polysomnography. Fifty minutes after sleep onset the patient is in stage 4 NREM sleep. Fifty-nine minutes after starting the recording, there is an episode of sleepwalking. There is sudden onset of a diffuse, high-voltage rhythmic delta activity. At the time of the injection of ^{99m}Tc-ECD the patient is sitting, but appears confused. There is diffuse theta activity with intermixed alpha, beta, and delta activities.

Neuroimaging of Sleep and Sleep Disorders, ed. Eric Nofzinger, Pierre Maquet, and Michael J. Thorpy. Published by Cambridge University Press. © Cambridge University Press 2013.

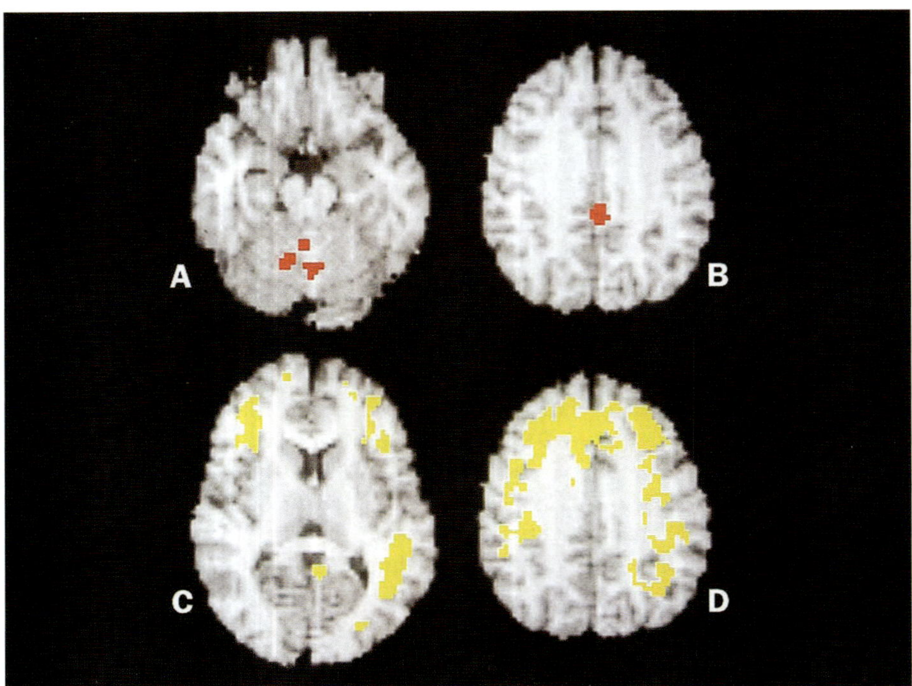

Figure 43.2 SPECT findings during sleepwalking after integration with the appropriate anatomical magnetic resonance image. During the sleepwalking, compared with quiet stage 3 to 4 NREM sleep, there was increased regional cerebral blood flow (>25%) in the anterior cerebellum, i.e., vermis (A), and in the posterior cingulate cortex (Brodmann area 23 [Tailarach coordinate x = −4, y = −40, z = 31], B). Large areas of frontal and parietal association cortices remain deactivated during sleepwalking, compared with data from normal volunteers during wakefulness (n = 24), as shown in the corresponding parametric maps (z-threshold = −3). The dorsolateral prefrontal cortex (C), medial frontal cortex (D), and left angular gyrus (C) are included within these areas.

Imaging technique

An injection of ^{99m}Tc-ECD was given 24 s after the onset of sleepwalking. Single-photon emission computerized tomography (SPECT) recordings were introduced into a computerized brain-atlas for analysis. First, the perfusion studies acquired during sleepwalking and slow-wave sleep (reference state) were normalized to the same global mean. Thereafter, subtraction images were calculated (sleepwalking minus slow-wave sleep). Regions of interest were delineated by the use of a threshold at a perfusion increase of more than 25% in relation to the reference state. Finally, z-scores were calculated by comparing findings in the patient during sleepwalking with the standard normal distribution in awake volunteers (n = 24).

Imaging findings

An increase of over 25% in regional cerebral blood flow during sleepwalking was related to the reference stage of slow-wave sleep, and was confined to the posterior cingulate cortex and to the anterior cerebellum (Figure 43.2, A, B).

Compared with awake normal volunteers (n = 24) a decrease in regional cerebral blood flow was found in the frontoparietal associative cortices during sleepwalking (Figure 43.2, C, D).

Discussion

During sleepwalking, the decreased regional cerebral blood flow in the frontoparietal cortices is consistent with a dissociated state consisting of both aroused motor activity and continuing sleep state. The deactivation of prefrontal cortices during normal sleep and sleepwalking is consistent with the lack of recall and the reduced self-awareness.

The activation of the cingulate cortex and the absence of a deactivation of the thalamus during sleepwalking differs from the profound deactivation seen during normal slow-wave sleep. This suggests that sleepwalking arises from activation of thalamocingulate pathways and persisting inhibition of other thalamocortical arousal systems.

The cingulate cortex modulates emotional behaviors and stimulation elicits motor, autonomic, and emotional responses similar to those seen in sleepwalking and sleep terrors. The activation of the posterior cingulate cortex in this patient may be related to the mental confusion and only transient motor activation of the sleepwalking episode. It suggests that the motor, vegetative, and emotional manifestations of sleepwalking and sleep terrors may be related to different activation patterns of the cingulate cortex.

Key points

- Sleepwalking is associated with reduced frontoparietal cerebral blood flow, activation of the cingulate cortex and absence of deactivation of the thalamus.
- The manifestations of sleepwalking may be associated with thalamocingulate pathway activation with the different clinical manifestations related to varied cingulate cortex activations.

Reference

1. Bassetti C, Vella S, Donati F, Wielepp P, Weder B. SPECT during sleepwalking. *Lancet*. 2000;**356**(9228):484–5.

Neuroimaging of the brainstem in parasomnia overlap disorder

Michael J. Thorpy

History

A 40-year-old woman developed acute rhombencephalitis with cerebellar ataxia, a facial palsy, diplopia, right hearing loss, dysphagia, and dysarthria [1]. She reported vivid dreams associated with vigorous movements while asleep. On examination, she had right third, fifth, sixth, seventh, eighth, ninth, and tenth nerve palsies plus a right internuclear ophthalmoplegia, and a static cerebellar ataxia.

Brain magnetic resonance imaging (MRI) suggested diffuse inflammatory lesions (Figure 44.1).

The patient was treated with high-dose corticosteroids and improved within five weeks, except for the cerebellar ataxia and the anterior internuclear ophthalmoplegia. Six months after the episode, she developed an acute C2–7 and D5–6 myelitis; the brain and spinal MRI were unchanged. Two years later she developed abnormal sleep behaviors.

Every night while asleep, and several times per night, she would speak, sing, have arm and leg jerks, and walk, open doors, walk into the kitchen or her son's room, but did not hurt herself and had no recall of any associated mental content. While dreaming of giving him a spanking she slapped her son. She was mainly amnestic for the episodes the next morning.

One year after the first neurological episode, she underwent video-polysomnography (Figure 44.2). Slow-wave sleep was interrupted by sudden arousals without any abnormal movement but she had nightly recurrent, quiet, sleep-associated walking episodes without dream recall suggestive of sleepwalking as an arousal disorder rather than as a rapid eye movement (REM) sleep behavior disorder (RBD).

Clonazepam was not beneficial but a 9 mg melatonin dose partially improved the frequency and severity of RBD and sleepwalking.

Polysomnographic findings

The video-polysomnography showed REM sleep that lasted 90 min (39% of total sleep time, when 17–23% was expected). There was enhanced chin muscle tone during 44% of REM sleep and increased phasic leg muscle activity (Figure 44.2). She spoke; mumbled; held up her neck; and displayed complex hand movements (looking like writing and eating), arm flailing, and leg jerking.

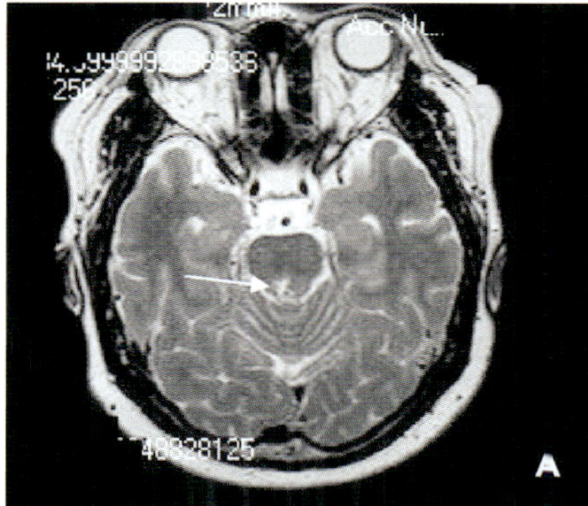
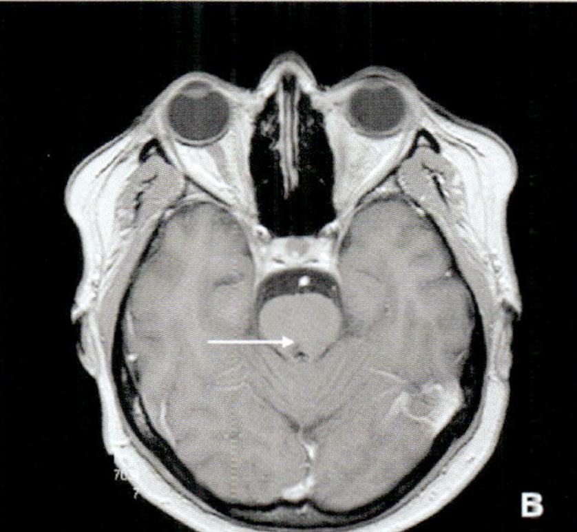
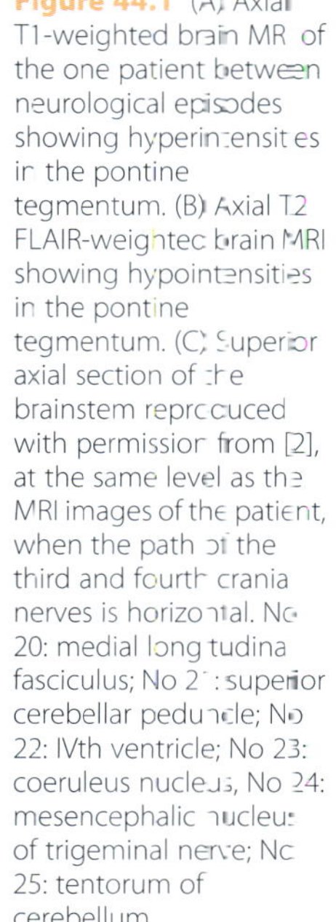
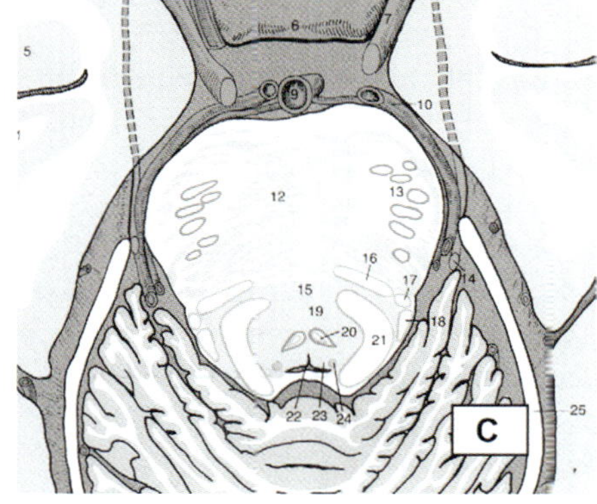

Figure 44.1 (A) Axial T1-weighted brain MRI of the one patient between neurological episodes showing hyperintensities in the pontine tegmentum. (B) Axial T2 FLAIR-weighted brain MRI showing hypointensities in the pontine tegmentum. (C) Superior axial section of the brainstem reproduced with permission from [2], at the same level as the MRI images of the patient, when the path of the third and fourth cranial nerves is horizontal. No 20: medial longitudinal fasciculus; No 21: superior cerebellar peduncle; No 22: IVth ventricle; No 23: coeruleus nucleus, No 24: mesencephalic nucleus of trigeminal nerve; No 25: tentorum of cerebellum.

The mean sleep latency during the multiple sleep latency test (MSLT) was 18.6 min with no sleep onset REM periods.

Neuroimaging of Sleep and Sleep Disorders, ed. Eric Nofzinger, Pierre Maquet, and Michael J. Thorpy. Published by Cambridge University Press. © Cambridge University Press 2013.

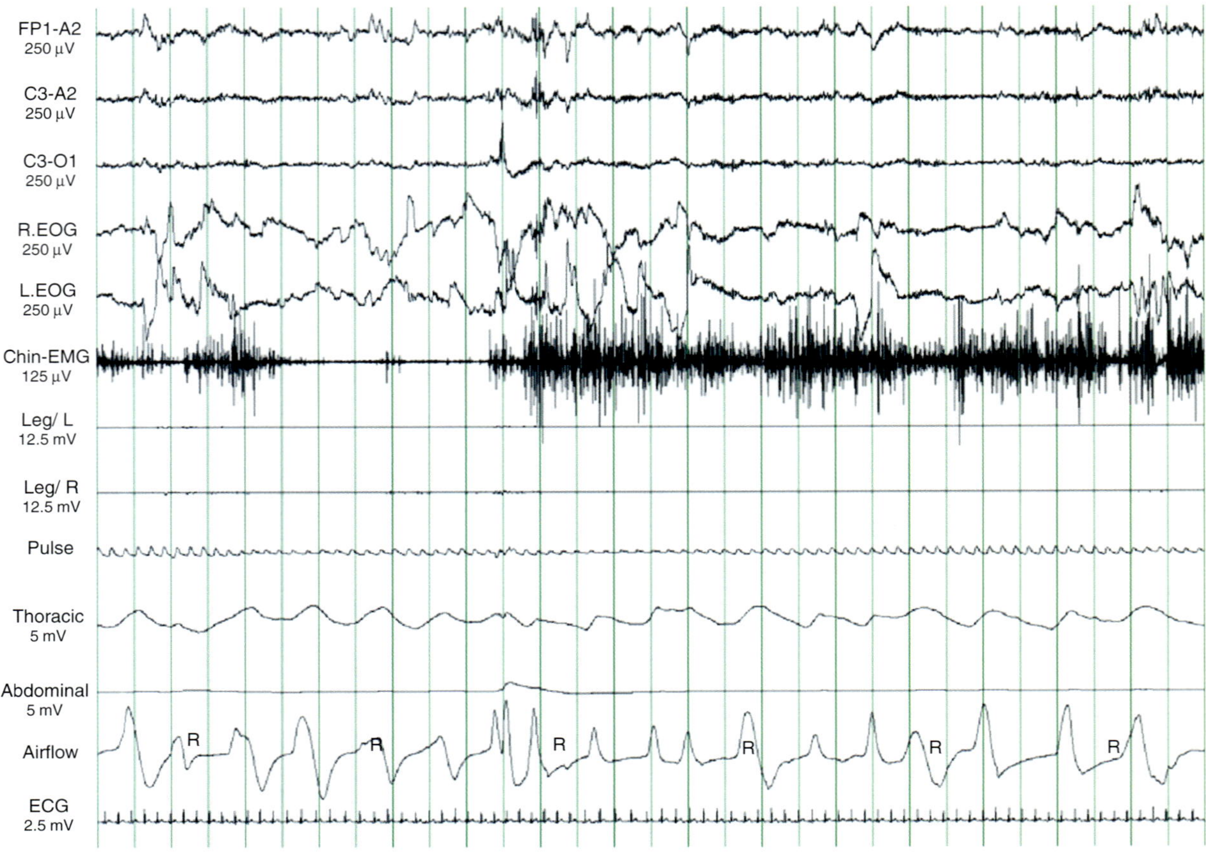

Figure 44.2 An example of a 1-min period of REM sleep without atonia in the patient, with enhanced tonic chin muscle tone during REM sleep. The montage includes, from top to bottom, electroencephalogram (EEG) (Fp1–A2, C3–A2, C3–01); right and left electro-oculograms; chin electromyogram; left and right tibialis anterior electromyogram; pulse, thoracic, and abdominal breathing efforts; airflow; and electrocardiogram (EKG).

Imaging technique

Axial T1-weighted brain MRI and gadolinium-enhanced T2-weighted and fluid-attenuated inversion recovery (FLAIR) sequences.

Imaging findings

On initial MRI, there were gadolinium-enhanced hyperintense signals on the T2-weighted and FLAIR sequences and hypointense signals on the T1-weighted sequences in the mesencephalic tegmentum, the fourth ventricle floor, and the right medulla, suggesting diffuse inflammatory lesions.

After one year the brain and spinal MRI were unchanged, with a small, persistent hyperintensity in the right pontine tegmentum (Figure 44.1A) and in the dorsal right medulla on T1 sequence and hypointensity on T2-FLAIR sequences (Figure 44.1B).

Discussion

This patient had a nightly recurring parasomnia overlap disorder, secondary to a recurrent inflammatory disease of the brainstem and spinal cord.

The parasomnia was attributed to small right lesions in the pontine tegmentum and in the medulla. The pontine lesion was small and included the medial longitudinal fasciculus and superior cerebellar peduncle, and probably the coeruleus and subcoeruleus nuclei. Lesions of the subcoeruleus nucleus can elicit RBD in animals. There is, however, no animal model of sleepwalking or parasomnia overlap disorder.

Nine previous RBD cases were associated with lesions of the brainstem of various causes (vascular disease, inflammation, tumor) that were mostly dorsal, median, and located from the mesencephalon to the lower/mid pontine tegmentum, and in one case in the medulla.

This patient had a unilateral lesion while the RBD movements were bilateral, suggesting that a unilateral lesion of the REM sleep atonia system is sufficient to increase the axial and bilateral limb muscle tone during REM sleep, and also to trigger sleepwalking.

Melatonin, which can improve RBD, also improved the parasomnia overlap disorder. Brainstem lesions have been reported previously in association with parasomnia overlap disorder.

This report provides evidence that lesions within or near the pontine tegmentum are associated with RBD and parasomnia overlap disorder and that a unilateral lesion by itself can cause RBD and sleepwalking.

Key points

- Neuroimaging showed a unilateral pontine tegmental lesion.
- Pontine tegmental lesions may be associated with both RBD and sleepwalking.

References

1. Limousin N, Dehais C, Gout O, *et al.* A brainstem inflammatory lesion causing REM sleep behavior disorder and sleepwalking (parasomnia overlap disorder). *Sleep Med.* 2009;**10** (9):1059–62. Epub 2009/04/02.

2. Kretschmann H-J, Weinrich W. *Cranial Neuroimaging and Clinical Neuroanatomy*, 3rd ed., revised and expanded. Stuttgart New York, Thieme. 2004;451.

Nocturnal wanderings and an arachnoid cyst

Alejandro Jiménez-Genchi and Yazmín de la Garza-Neme

History

The patient is a 15-year-old boy with a negative family and personal history for sleep, psychiatric, and epileptic disorders. When he was 14, he suddenly presented with episodes of sleepwalking-like behavior, characterized by walking into his parents' room, the bathroom, and the kitchen; he would also run and bang his head against objects while yelling obscene words. He did not remember any of the episodes and he reported no association with dream content. A few months after the first episode, he presented with urinary sphincter relaxation during an event, and also he experienced absence seizures.

Polysomnographic findings

An all-night polysomnographic (PSG) recording with audiovisual monitoring showed no abnormalities in sleep architecture parameters. However, he had eight paroxysmal episodes characterized by sudden hyperextension of the right hemibody, followed by the extension and the abduction of the right limb with the flexion of his fingers. During another episode, he suddenly sat up, put his legs out of bed, and then tried to get out of bed. This behavior was preceded by a spike discharge over the left frontocentral region with contralateral projection and secondary generalization during N2 stage of sleep (Figure 45.1).

Imaging technique

A brain MRI was performed in a 3-tesla scanner. T1-weighted image (T1WI), T2-weighted image (T2WI), fluid attenuated inversion recovery (FLAIR), and diffusion-weighted image (DWI) sequences were performed. In addition, a ^{99m}Tc-ECD SPECT (99m technetium ethyl cysteinated dimer single-photon emission computed tomography) was performed to evaluate any associated brain dysfunction.

Imaging findings

The MRI revealed a left temporal cyst (Figure 45.1). Axial T2WI showed an extra-axial cystic-appearing mass in the middle cranial fossa, isointense with cerebrospinal fluid (CSF). The temporal lobe appeared hypoplastic with dorsally displaced temporal horn. The coronal T1WI showed a sharply margined extra-axial fluid collection, also isointense with CSF. This cystic-appearing mass showed no restriction on DWI and suppressed completely on the FLAIR sequence. According to Galassi classification this is a type II cyst, with displacement of the temporal lobe and extension along the Sylvian fissure.

Interictal ^{99m}Tc-ECD (SPECT) scan showed impaired brain perfusion in the left temporal region (coronal view), corresponding with the arachnoid cyst (AC) found in MRI (Figure 45.1). There was an increased cerebral blood flow (rCBF) in the frontal region, more evident on the right side (axial and coronal views). These frontal changes were strongly correlated with the left frontocentral spike discharge with contralateral projection in the PSG recording.

Discussion

Episodic nocturnal wanderings, nocturnal paroxysmal dystonia, and paroxysmal arousals represent the clinical spectrum of nocturnal frontal lobe epilepsy (NFLE) [1].

Even when seizures are frequent manifestations of intracranial mass lesions, NFLE has rarely been associated to brain structure abnormalities [1]. Cystic lesions of the brain are easily recognized on both MRI and computed axial tomography by their morphological features (rounded shape, well-defined edges); nevertheless, MRI has a superior specificity for characterizing fluid collections in intracranial cysts on the basis of intensity patterns on cysts contents [2]. Particularly, ACs are sharply demarcated round/ovoid extra-axial masses that follow CSF attenuation/signal; FLAIR and DWI are considered the best sequences for distinguishing etiology of cystic-appearing intracranial masses [3]. Magnetic resonance spectroscopy (MRS) is also a useful technique because it can predict pathology in up to 90% of similar-appearing intracranial cystic lesions [4]. The use of MRS for the detection of abnormalities in the brain tissue adjacent to an AC has failed to show abnormalities suggestive of epileptogenic focus in epileptic patients with an incidental AC. This is consistent with reports of the absence of a relation between ACs and the location of the seizure focus [5] and the lack of superiority of surgical treatment over the conservative approach [6].

Distinguishing NFLE from arousal disorders on the basis of history presents a diagnostic challenge; therefore, PSG is highly recommended. During the PSG of the patient, we were able to document an episode of clear-cut epileptic activity with an origin in the frontal lobe. Moreover, the characteristics of the events also suggested an epileptic origin because the attacks were stereotypic, repetitive, and involved dystonic movements.

Neuroimaging of Sleep and Sleep Disorders, ed. Eric Nofzinger, Pierre Maquet, and Michael J. Thorpy. Published by Cambridge University Press. © Cambridge University Press 2013.

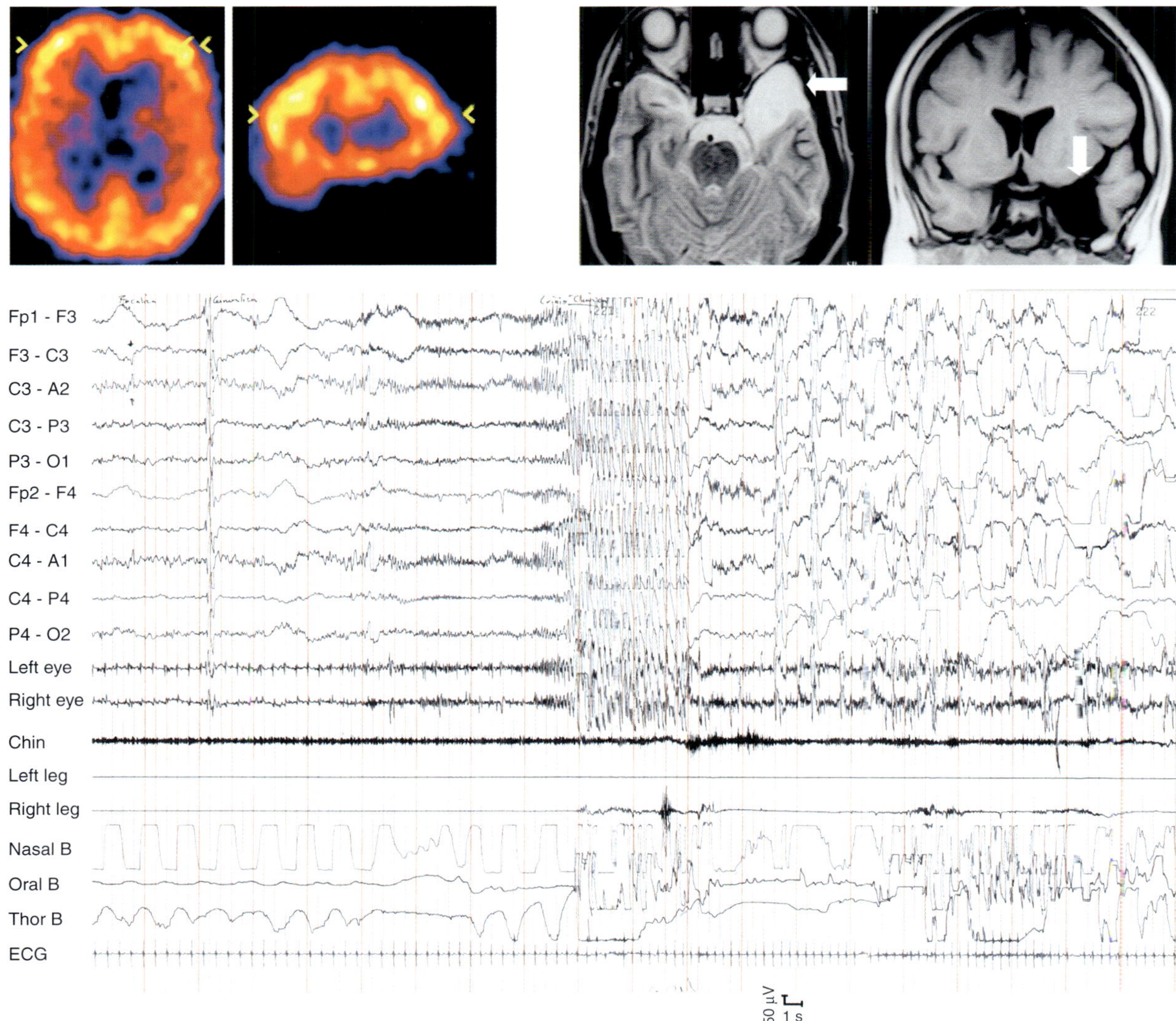

Figure 45.1 MRI images (upper right) show a large arachnoid cyst in the left temporal fossa. SPECT images (upper left) show a perfusion defect in cyst site (coronal slice) and hyperperfusion in bilateral frontal cortex (transverse slice). Before the beginning of a nocturnal wandering (bottom), EEG shows a spike discharge over the left frontocentral region with contralateral projection and secondary generalization after two seconds. The clinical attack begins during an arousal. Tachycardia and irregular breathing are also present. (Reprinted with permission from Jiménez-Genchi A, Díaz-Galvis J, García-Reyna JC, Avila-Ordoñez U. Coexistence of epileptic nocturnal wanderings and an arachnoid cyst. *J Clin Sleep Med* 2007;**4**:399–401.)

The frontal lobe involvement was supported by the hyperperfusion found in the interictal SPECT scan. In contrast to this finding, it has been reported that cerebral SPECTs of symptomatic patients with ACs show areas of decreased rCBF which correspond well with clinical symptoms and neuroimaging findings in 70% of cases [7].

Based on clinical findings and the results of MRI, SPECT, and PSG, we adopted a conservative approach. The patient was initially treated with magnesium valproate; however, a striking remission of attacks was observed when levetiracetam was added.

Key points

- Imaging techniques are valuable tools in the diagnostic assessment of sleep-related complex behavior.
- Imaging findings might be crucial for the therapeutic approach of sleep-related epilepsy.

References

1. Provini F, Plazzi G, Tinuper P, *et al.* Nocturnal frontal lobe epilepsy. A clinical and polygraphic overview of 100 consecutive cases. *Brain*, 1999;**122**:1017–31.

2. Kjos BO, Brant-Zawadzki M, Kucharczyk W, *et al.* Cystic intracranial lesions: magnetic resonance imaging. *Radiology.* 1985;**155**:363–9.

3. Mukherji SK, Chenvert TL, Castillo M. Diffusion-weighted magnetic resonance imaging. *J Neuroophthalmol.* 2002; **22**:118–22.

4. Ozisik HI, Sarac K, Ozcan C. Single-voxel magnetic resonance spectroscopy of brain tissue adjacent to arachnoid cysts of epileptic patients. *Neurologist.* 2008;**14**:382–9.

5. Arroyo S, Santamaria J. What is the relationship between arachnoid cysts and seizure foci? *Epilepsia.* 1997;**38**:1098–102.

6. Koch CA, Voth D, Kraemer G, Schwarz M. Arachnoid cysts: does surgery improve epileptic seizures and headaches? *Neurosurg Rev.* 1995;**18**:173–81.

7. Martínez-Lage JF, Valentí JA, Piqueras C, *et al.* Functional assessment of intracranial arachnoid cysts with TC99m-HMPAO SPECT: a preliminary report. *Childs Nerv Syst.* 2006;**22**:1091–7.

Structural and functional neuroimaging of restless legs syndrome and periodic limb movements in sleep

Thorleif Etgen

Definition, symptoms, and management

Restless legs syndrome (RLS) is a sensorimotor disorder of the sleep/wake cycle with the key feature being an urge to move the legs. [1]. Four essential criteria for RLS, as well as supportive and associated diagnostic features, have been established by the International RLS Study Group (Table 46.1) [2]. With an estimated prevalence of 7–9%, RLS is a very common sleep disorder [3].

Primary or idiopathic RLS is distinguished from secondary or symptomatic RLS which is associated with various conditions (e.g., iron deficiency, chronic kidney failure, and pregnancy) [4]. Two different phenotypes of RLS are defined on the basis of age at symptom onset: in patients with early-onset RLS, symptoms appear before the age of 45 years (possibly even before 30 years [5]) and they usually have a positive family history. Late-onset RLS starts after 45 years, often consists of a secondary form, shows a more rapid progression, and is often accompanied by neuropathy [2]. However, the two groups certainly overlap and are modified by genetic factors [4].

RLS as a sleep/wake cycle disorder has a circadian rhythm that mainly affects patients in the evening or at night. With increasing disease severity, however, the circadian rhythmicity changes and symptoms occur day and night. This phenomenon is particularly common in patients with augmentation, which is a paradoxical worsening of RLS symptoms and an earlier onset of symptoms during the day after initially successful treatment with dopaminergic agents [4].

Periodic limb movements in sleep (PLMS) are involuntary clonic-type movements of the lower extremities during sleep and typically involve bilateral ankle dorsiflexion, knee and hip flexion. PLMS occur in up to 85% of patients with RLS, are currently the only objective measure of RLS, and build a prominent cause of sleep disruption. PLMS are quantified by polysomnography and are defined as movements lasting > 0.5 s with an amplitude of at least 25% of the calibration amplitude, an intermovement interval of 4–90 s, occurring in a series of at least four consecutive movements. In adults, an index (number of PLMS per hour of sleep) of >15 for the entire night is considered pathological [1, 6]. However, PLMS are a non-specific motor phenomenon in sleep and can occur in many other conditions (e.g., narcolepsy, parkinsonian syndromes, rapid eye movement

sleep behavior disorder) [4]. In addition, periodic limb movements while awake (PLMW) are sometimes found in patients with RLS. In contrast, periodic limb movement disorder (PLMD) is defined as a clinically significant sleep disturbance with PLMS that cannot be accounted for by any other sleep disorder [1].

After exclusion and corresponding treatment of secondary RLS (iron supplementation in case of iron deficiency, for example), the first-line management of RLS consists of dopaminergic therapy. Either levodopa or non-ergot dopamine agonists (e.g., ropinirole, pramipexole, rotigotine) at night have proven to be an effective treatment. Opioids are widely used as second-line therapy if dopaminergic drugs fail or are insufficient. Anticonvulsants (like pregabalin or gabapentin) constitute an alternative, especially if RLS is accompanied by polyneuropathy or painful symptoms or if patients are resistant to dopaminergic drugs or opioids [4].

Pathophysiology and neuroanatomy

Revealing the pathophysiology of RLS requires explaining the four essential criteria. RLS cannot be attributed to one specific neuroanatomical location but is apparently a network disorder. Many regions of the nervous system, from the periphery to the cortex, contain structures that are involved in somatosensory perception as well as the generation of movement. This anatomical diversity is reflected in the many different topographical, genetic, and biochemical causes of RLS, either in isolation or in combination [4].

Dopamine

The dopamine system has been the focus of many studies as dopaminergic therapy is an outstanding effective treatment of RLS. Dopaminergic neurotransmission modulates neuronal interactions at very low doses; thus, a subtle receptor dysfunction or dopaminergic deficit may contribute to the pathophysiology of RLS. In addition, excitatory and inhibitory dopamine receptor systems seem to react differently depending on whether receptor stimulation is pulsed or continuous [4]. Metabolic neurotransmission studies of pre- and postsynaptic dopaminergic systems (see Chapter 47) revealed controversial results [7].

Neuroimaging of Sleep and Sleep Disorders, ed. Eric Nofzinger, Pierre Maquet, and Michael J. Thorpy. Published by Cambridge University Press. © Cambridge University Press 2013.

Table 46.1. Diagnostic criteria of RLS

Essential criteria	Description
1. Urge to move the legs	An urge to move the legs, usually accompanied or caused by uncomfortable and unpleasant sensations in the legs (sometimes the urge to move is present without the uncomfortable sensations and sometimes the arms or other body parts are involved in addition to the legs)
2. Worsening during rest	The urge to move or unpleasant sensations begin or worsen during periods of rest or inactivity such as lying or sitting
3. Relief by movement	The urge to move or unpleasant sensations are partially or totally relieved by movement, such as walking or stretching, at least as long as the activity continues
4. Worsening during night	The urge to move or unpleasant sensations are worse in the evening or night than during the day or only occur in the evening or night (when symptoms are very severe, the worsening at night may not be noticeable but must have been previously present)
Supportive clinical features	
1. Positive family history	RLS prevalence is 3–5 times greater among first-degree relatives of people with RLS than in first-degree relatives of people without RLS
2. Response to dopaminergic therapy	Nearly all people (>90%) with RLS show a positive therapeutic response – at least initially – to levodopa or a dopamine receptor agonist
3. Periodic limb movements	Periodic limb movements in sleep occur in at least 85% of cases
Associated features	
1. Natural clinical course	If age of symptom onset is >50 years, symptoms often occur abruptly and severely, whereas if age of onset is <50 years, onset is often more insidious
2. Sleep disturbance	Disturbed sleep is a common major morbidity
3. Normal physical examination	Physical examination is generally normal and does not contribute to the diagnosis, except for comorbid conditions or secondary causes of RLS

Allen *et al.* [2], Trenkwalder and Paulus [4]

Genetics

Linkage studies in families with RLS have so far identified eight loci that are associated with RLS, but no causally related sequence variant has yet been identified. In contrast to these linkage studies, genome-wide association studies detected gene variants conveying a differential risk of RLS in four chromosomal regions containing a total of five genes. The functions of the five genes that were identified are largely related to embryonic neuronal development and no functional relationship with RLS has so far been established [4].

Neurophysiology

Several electrophysiological studies suggest an increased hyperexcitability of spinal motor system and spinal sensory pathways which could result from dysfunction of descending control tracts [8].

Iron

Inadequate iron is a common cause of secondary RLS which resolves with iron supplementation. RLS severity is also associated with lower ferritin levels. Further clinical, laboratory, and neuroimaging evidence point to a regional iron deficiency in patients with RLS (see Chapter 47). As iron is a cofactor of tyrosine hydroxylase in dopamine production, this could serve as a link to the findings about the role of dopamine in RLS [3].

Conventional neuroimaging

Existing sparse data about conventional neuroimaging which encompasses computed tomography (CT) and magnetic resonance imaging (MRI) do not suggest any gross structural abnormalities being involved in the pathophysiology of idiopathic RLS or PLMS [9]. However, there are some reports in which the onset of RLS or PLMS coincided with a documented structural lesion (e.g., stroke). Though these cases have to be considered as symptomatic or secondary RLS or PLMS, nevertheless their neuroimaging results might help in discovering a possible neuroanatomical basis of RLS and PLMS.

The largest series of patients with poststroke RLS, with symptoms beginning within one week after stroke onset, found a prevalence of 12.4% stroke-related RLS (17 of 137 patients). The MRI-confirmed ischemic lesions were nearly all (94%) detected in subcortical structures such as the basal ganglia/corona radiata, internal capsule, lateral thalamus, and pons. Only one ischemic lesion (6%) was observed in the cortex (left temporo-occipital) [10]. Other case reports of RLS onset after stroke (Table 46.2) included also subcortical lesions such as the thalamus and lenticulostriate area [11, 12]. PLMS onset after stroke (Table 46.2) was observed in the internal capsule, cerebellum, corona radiata, and pons [13–17].

Other casuistics reported symptomatic PLMS in spinal cord lesions [18, 19]. Though a coincidental finding cannot be excluded, a close temporal association between the onset of the lesions and PLMS and, in some cases, improvement of PLMS after therapy support a cause–effect relationship.

Special neuroimaging

Voxel-based morphometry (VBM)

Voxel-based morphometry (VBM) is a modern neuroimaging analysis technique which is used to compare subtle focal differences in volume or density of gray (or occasionally white) matter. In VBM, high-resolution MRI scans are compared after segmentation, smoothing, and spatial normalization, using the statistical approach of statistical parametric mapping [20, 21]. This technique started in the mid 1990s and has since then increased tremendously in popularity [22].

The first VBM study in RLS was performed with 51 right-handed patients with an idiopathic RLS in two independent samples in two centers. The RLS group was compared with 51

Table 46.2. Casuistics of RLS and/or PLMS onset in patients after stroke

Author	Number of patients	Lesion localization	Latency from stroke to symptom onset	Symptoms
Lee et al. [10]	17	10 basal ganglia/corona radiata, 1 internal capsule, 1 thalamus, 1 temporo-occipital cortex 4 pons	7 days	RLS 12 both legs RLS 5 contralateral to lesion
Unrath & Kassubek [11]	1	Left thalamus	5 years	RLS unilaterally right leg
Sechi et al. [12]	1	Right lenticulostriate area	3 days	RLS + PLMS both legs
Kizilay et al. [13]	1	Right cerebellum	1 day	PLMS both legs
Lee et al. [14]	1	Left internal capsule	2 days	PLMS right leg
Anderson et al. [15]	1	Basal ganglia	No data	No data
Kang et al. [16]	1	Left corona radiata	7 days	PLMS right leg
Kim et al. [17]	2	1 left pons 1 left pons	1 day 2 days	PLMS right leg PLMS right leg

RLS = restless legs syndrome; PLMS = periodic limb movements in sleep

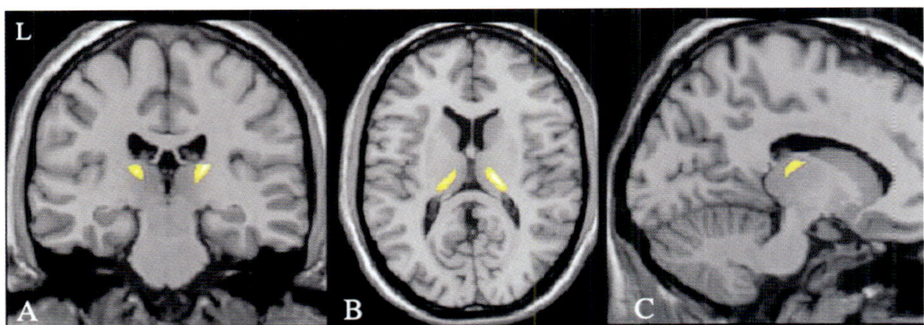

Figure 46.1 Result of VBM conjunction analysis showing bithalamic gray matter change in idiopathic RLS [23]. (Reprinted from *Neuroimage*, **24**(4), Etgen et al., Bilateral thalamic gray matter changes in patients with restless legs syndrome, 1242–7, Copyright (2005), with permission from Elsevier.)

sex- and age-matched healthy volunteers. Conjunction analysis was used to combine results from both centers. In patients with idiopathic RLS, both study centers observed independently a bilateral gray matter increase in the pulvinar. In the conjunction analysis including all patients and controls from both study centers, a significant gray matter increase in the pulvinar bilaterally was observed (Figure 46.1). This was the first demonstration of structural changes in the brain of patients with idiopathic RLS. According to the authors, these changes in thalamic structures either are involved in the pathogenesis of RLS or may reflect a consequence of chronic increase in afferent input of behaviorally relevant information [23]. As most patients of this study were on dopaminergic medication, this therapy might have an effect on the changes in thalamic gray matter. Therefore, the second VBM study focused on 14 RLS patients with no (n = 11) or minimal (n = 3) treatment. Using an optimized VBM protocol, no structural changes except for slightly increased gray matter density in the ventral hippocampus and in the middle orbitofrontal gyrus were detected [24]. Another VBM study of 63 mostly treated RLS patients revealed significant regional decreases of gray matter volume in the bihemispheric primary somatosensory cortex, which additionally extended into left-sided primary motor areas. All clusters correlated both with the severity of RLS symptoms and with disease duration [25]. Two

other recent VBM studies on small groups of RLS patients also failed to discover differences in gray matter. Celle et al. compared 17 untreated RLS patients with 54 controls and could not detect any significant structural changes in gray matter density [26]. Comley et al. examined 16 RLS patients naïve to dopaminergic drugs and 16 age- and sex-matched controls but found no significant differences [27].

One recent study detected a myelin decrease of approximately 25% in the frontal and temporal cortical brain tissue of RLS patients compared with controls. This was coupled with decreased ferritin and transferritin in the myelin fraction [28]. To expand these post-mortem findings, the authors additionally assessed white matter volume in RLS using VBM. Twenty-three RLS patients (mean age 55.6 years, mean severity score 24.4, average disease duration 12.6 years) were compared with 23 age- and gender-matched controls. Eighteen patients were treatment naïve, the remaining five RLS patients discontinued dopaminergic therapy at least one week prior to neuroimaging. VBM showed significant regional reduction of white matter volume among RLS patients in the corpus callosum, anterior cingulum, and white matter regions adjacent to the precentral gyrus [28].

Methodological and biological confounders might help to explain the striking differences between the studies (Table 46.3).

Table 46.3. Voxel-based morphometry studies of gray matter in RLS patients

Study	Patients (female/male)	Age (years)	Duration (years)	IRLSSG Score	Family history	Polysomnography	VBM protocol	Matched for age, sex, and handedness	Drugs	Result
Etgen[23]	Regensburg-28 (21/7)	53.3 (±8.0)	19.2 (±14.3)	29.5 (±13.4)	32%	No	Classical	A, S, H	Treated	Gray matter increase in pulvinar
	Munich-23 (17/6)	59.3 (±10.1)	11.4 (±11.1)	28.8 (±5.9)	52%	No		A, S, H		
Hornyak[24]	14 (9/5)	49.6 (±12.5)	16 (±12)	25.6 (±6.7)	64%	No	Optimized	A, S	Medication-free	NS
Unrath[25]	63 (45/18)	63.7 (±11.4)	22.3 (±18.2)	27.4 (±7.1)	46%	No	Optimized	A (40 controls)	Treated with dopaminergic drugs or opioids (except of 3)	Gray matter decrease in bihemispheric primary somatosensory cortex
Celle[26]	17 (16/1)	65.9 (±0.8)	No data	15.7 (±4.8)	No data	Yes	Optimized	A	No psychotropic or dopaminergic drugs	NS
Comley[27]	16 (8/8)	55 (±7)	27 (±12)	18.5 (±3.9)	56%	No	Optimized	A, S	No dopaminergic or opioid agonists	NS

VBM = voxel-based morphometry, IRLSSG = International Restless Legs Syndrome Study Group, A = age, S = sex, H = handedness, NS = not significant.

Initially, some unresolved methodological questions about VBM should be kept in mind. First, the relationship between gray matter concentration and MRI signal intensity is not clearly established [29]. Second, the problem of neuronal plasticity, including the mechanism and timing by which gray matter concentration changes with disease, is not understood; some recent papers suggest that cortical plasticity on a structural level in adult humans is already detectable after one week [30]. Third, practical aspects of the fidelity of VBM comparison data comprise the problem that many variables cause highly non-linear distortions in MR images, making them extremely difficult to register [29]. Any small registration error will lead to errors in VBM comparison data.

Most of the recent studies applied the optimized VBM protocol according to Good *et al.* [31], whereas the first study by Etgen *et al.* [23] used the standard or classical VBM protocol as the optimized version was not fully available in 2004. Optimized VBM includes incorporation of tissue-specific normalization parameters and automated removal of non-brain voxels from segmented images [31]. These advantages may allow a better detection of subtle changes compared with the standard VBM protocol [32]. In addition, thalamic areas might be more prone to partial volume effects causing problems in computational analysis [33]. The value of the results in the two studies reporting differences in gray matter between RLS patients and controls remains unclear as the results were only significant for uncorrected comparison and did not remain significant after multiple comparison [23, 25].

Several differences among the particular study populations may contribute to the divergent results. First, those studies with positive results employed group sizes > 20 patients [23, 25], whereas all three studies without differences in gray matter consisted of groups < 20 patients [24, 26, 27]. According to a recent analysis, larger group sizes allow optimal detection of volume loss in regions such as the hippocampus and thalamus [34]. Thus, the application of small control groups in VBM might hamper the detection of discrete, but significant, differences.

Second, some studies were not completely matched for age, gender, and handedness. Two studies were matched only for age [25, 26], two studies for age and gender [24, 27], and only one study for age, gender, and handedness [23]. However, several recent studies pointed out that age, gender, and handedness might influence the results of VBM studies. According to one study, a control group size of 70–90 subjects allowed optimal detection of volume loss in the hippocampus and thalamus and, at these group sizes, matched control groups did not consistently prove superior to deliberately "unmatched" groups of the same size [34]. Another VBM study revealed regional sex-specific differences of gray matter volume in middle-aged healthy individuals [35]. Correlations among gray matter volumes and age, gender, and hemisphere were partly described in a large VBM study of 1460 healthy young individuals [36]. Significant effects of handedness (especially in frontal regions) was found using group comparisons of left- and right-handed subjects' asymmetry maps [37].

Third, differences in age and percentage of RLS patients with a positive family history between the study groups may also account for divergent results as two potentially different phenotypes of RLS (early- vs. late-onset) are defined on the basis of age at symptom onset [3]. Differences in these phenotypes, including family history, suggest a variable etiology which may cause different results using VBM. Unfortunately, none of the studies explicitly incorporated the two different phenotypes or used a more homogenous group, for example, only RLS patients with early-onset as a group of late-onset RLS patients might have a mixture of primary and secondary RLS with symptoms exacerbated by other factors [3].

Fourth, though RLS is defined on pure clinical grounds, additional tests help to exclude secondary forms or RLS mimics. One common form of secondary RLS constitutes iron deficiency. Specific laboratory tests (e.g., iron, ferritin) to exclude iron deficiency were explicitly described only in the two studies with changes in gray matter [23, 25]. The other studies either performed a "routine blood test" (iron and ferritin do not belong to this group) [27] or mentioned only "secondary RLS as an exclusion criteria" (without details of laboratory testing) [24], or do not even differ between primary and secondary RLS [26]. In addition, polysomnographic findings like PLMS are supportive clinical features [1]. However, only one of all five VBM studies applied polysomnography as a selection criteria [26].

Finally, treatment with RLS-specific drugs presents another essential difference between the VBM studies with changes in gray matter and those without. Nearly all RLS patients in both studies with changes were treated with dopaminergic and/or opioidergic drugs [23, 25]. In the other three studies without changes most RLS patients were either medication-free [24] or had no treatment with dopaminergic, psychotropic, or opioidergic drugs [26, 27]. Therefore, the reported changes in gray matter could be drug-induced as antidopaminergic drugs lead to changes of basal ganglia volume [38, 39] and levodopa administration influences T1 MRI signal intensity in healthy subjects [40].

Diffusion tensor imaging (DTI)

Diffusion tensor imaging (DTI) mostly involves the characterization of white matter, and specifically, the directionality of white matter tracts. DTI generated maps may be used in the context of VBM but do not have to be, as a considerable amount of unique information resides in the maps themselves for individual subjects [29]. DTI involves the use of diffusion gradients sensitized to diffusion in multiple directions to determine the preferential directionality of diffusing spins [41]. With the understanding that spins diffuse more rapidly along white matter tracts as opposed to perpendicularly to them, this method can create voxel-wise maps of fractional anisotropy (FA) as well as computed maps of white matter tracts [29].

So far, DTI has been applied in two studies with RLS patients. Unrath *et al.* compared 45 idiopathic RLS patients with 30 healthy controls using quantitative whole brain-based DTI with computation of regional FA as a quantitative marker of white matter integrity. In the RLS group, multiple subcortical areas of significantly reduced FA were observed bihemispherically in close proximity to the primary and associate motor and somatosensory cortices, in the right-hemispheric thalamus (posterior ventral lateral nucleus), in motor projectional fibers, and adjacent to the left anterior cingulum [42]. Manconi *et al.* assessed 30 multiple sclerosis (MS) patients who suffered from secondary RLS. This group was compared with 52 MS patients without RLS. Neither whole brain, cerebellar, and brainstem T2-load nor mean diffusivity and FA showed any difference in MS patients with and without RLS. However, MS patients with RLS had significantly reduced average FA of the cervical cord compared with those MS patients without RLS [43].

Functional neuroimaging

Functional MRI (fMRI) assesses hemodynamic changes in the blood oxygen level-dependent (BOLD) signal, which is closely related to the electrical activity of nerve cells and allows analysis of cerebral activation [44]. Functional MRI has grown largely because of its non-invasiveness, relative ease of implementation, high spatial and temporal resolution, and, importantly, signal fidelity. The fMRI signal is robust and, for the most part, highly reproducible and consistent [29]. Despite many recent advancements in fMRI, it has only seldom be used in RLS patients.

The first landmark study questioning a possible central origin of sensory leg discomfort and PLMS was conducted by Bucher *et al.* in 1997 [45]. Nineteen idiopathic RLS patients (mean age 58 years) with polysomnographic features supporting RLS (all with PLMS and characteristic sleep profile) were matched with 15 right-handed controls without neurological disease. Eleven RLS patients were under levodopa treatment which was stopped at least seven days prior to fMRI. High-resolution proton density- and T2-weighted images of all 19 RLS patients excluded severe structural brain abnormalities. In all patients four conditions were examined: during a symptom-free period, during sensory leg discomfort, during combined PLMS and sensory leg discomfort, and during actively mimicking PLMS. Functional MRI with four to six slices revealed mainly bilateral activation of the cerebellum and contralateral activation of the thalamus during sensory leg discomfort. During the combined periodic limb movement and sensory leg discomfort conditions, patients also showed activity in the cerebellum and thalamus. In contrast to the sensory leg discomfort condition alone, the combined condition was associated with additional activation in the red nuclei and brainstem close to the reticular formation. Voluntary imitation of periodic limb movements by patients and control subjects was not associated with brainstem activity, but with additional activation in the globus pallidus and motor cortex [45].

In the second fMRI study seven right-handed untreated idiopathic RLS patients were investigated simultaneously with fMRI and electromyographic (EMG) recordings of the anterior tibial muscle [46]. Numerous clusters of positive correlation between fMRI signal and tonic EMG response were recorded in the contralateral and ipsilateral precentral and postcentral gyri, bilaterally in the precentral gyrus, the ipsilateral posterior cingulate, the contralateral cuneus, and ipsilateral lingual gyrus and the contralateral precuneus. Negative correlations were observed within the ipsilateral cingulate gyrus, the cerebellar vermis, and in the cerebellar hemispheres (ipsilateral and contralateral lobus

anterior) [46]. In addition, the study demonstrated that an increase of RLS-related sensory leg discomfort was significantly associated with a decrease of tonic muscle activity (as it happens at rest or during sleep) [46].

Astrakas *et al.* studied 25 idiopathic late-onset RLS patients and 12 sex- and age-matched controls. Beyond T2-relaxometry assessing brain iron content, whole-brain fMRI measured brain activation during active movement (dorsiflexion and plantarflexion of both feet) which is supposed to relieve lower limb symptoms in RLS. Between-group analysis detected significant differences with more activation in the RLS group in the dorsolateral prefrontal cortex of the left middle frontal gyrus, the left inferior frontal gyrus, and marginally in the cingulate gyrus [47].

Conclusion and practical approach

The results of the hitherto published conventional, special and functional neuroimaging studies underline the hypothesis of RLS being a network disorder (Figure 46.2).

The findings of conventional neuroimaging suggest that especially lesions of the subcortical brain areas (pyramidal tract and the basal ganglia–brainstem axis), which are involved in motor functions and sleep/wake cycles, may lead to RLS symptoms in patients after an ischemic stroke.

Special neuroimaging studies assessed the involvement of cortical and subcortical structures, respectively gray and white matter, in RLS. Two VBM studies revealed changes of gray matter of cortical (primary somatosensory cortex) and subcortical (thalamus) areas in patients with RLS, but these results could not be reproduced. Due to several methodological and biological confounders of the VBM studies, it remains therefore unclear whether these changes reflect a primary involvement in the pathophysiology of RLS or if they merely present an epiphenomenon of RLS (e.g., secondary change by RLS itself, effect

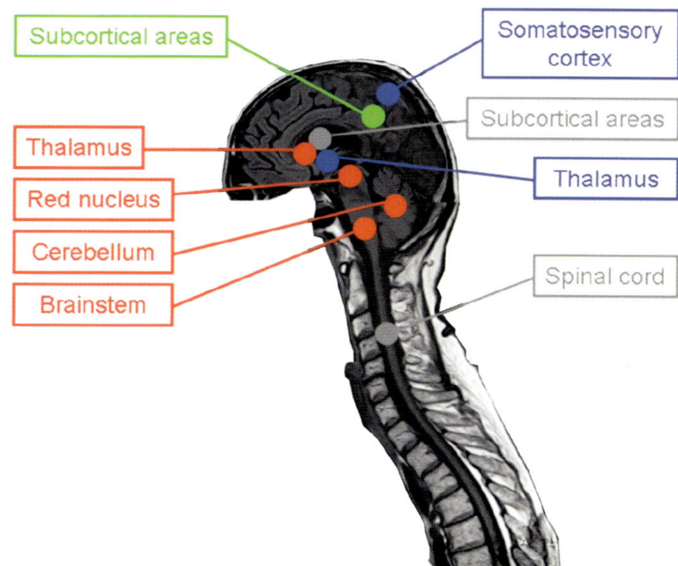

Figure 46.2 Synopsis of cerebral and spinal neuroimaging results in patients with RLS and/or PLMS (gray = lesion studies with conventional imaging, blue = voxel-based morphometry, green = diffusion-tensor imaging, red = functional MRI).

of RLS treatment). DTI and additional findings of a combined post-mortem and VBM study point to a possible wide-spread subcortical involvement of white matter areas; however, the relevance of these alterations is open as they may also mirror secondary changes in RLS.

Results from functional neuroimaging indicate an association of cerebellar and thalamic activation with sensory leg discomfort. Furthermore, participation of the red nucleus and brainstem in the generation of periodic limb movements in patients with RLS was observed.

Further neuroimaging studies would help in our limited understanding of RLS, for example a VBM study accounting for the problems of the current VBM studies or fMRI studies during sleep when symptoms of RLS occur.

From the practical point of view, currently there is no indication to perform any neuroimaging in patients with primary RLS or PLMS. In patients with secondary RLS or PLMS and further clinical evidence for a symptomatic lesion (e.g., ischemic stroke) neuroimaging (preferably MRI) is recommended.

References

1. Kushida CA. Clinical presentation, diagnosis, and quality of life issues in restless legs syndrome. *Am J Med.* 2007;**120**:S4–12.

2. Allen RP, Picchietti D, Hening WA, *et al.* Restless legs syndrome: diagnostic criteria, special considerations, and epidemiology. A report from the restless legs syndrome diagnosis and epidemiology workshop at the National Institutes of Health. *Sleep Med.* 2003;**4**:101–19.

3. Allen RP. Controversies and challenges in defining the etiology and pathophysiology of restless legs syndrome. *Am J Med.* 2007;**120**:S13–21.

4. Trenkwalder C, Paulus W. Restless legs syndrome: pathophysiology, clinical presentation and management. *Nat Rev Neurol.* 2010;**6**:337–46.

5. Winkelmann J, Muller-Myhsok B, Wittchen HU, *et al.* Complex segregation analysis of restless legs syndrome provides evidence for an autosomal dominant mode of inheritance in early age at onset families. *Ann Neurol.* 2002;**52**:297–302.

6. Zucconi M, Ferri R, Allen R, *et al.* The official World Association of Sleep Medicine (WASM) standards for recording and scoring periodic leg movements in sleep (PLMS) and wakefulness (PLMW) developed in collaboration with a task force from the International Restless Legs Syndrome Study Group (IRLSSG). *Sleep Med.* 2006;**7**:175–83.

7. Wetter TC, Eisensehr I, Trenkwalder C. Functional neuroimaging studies in restless legs syndrome. *Sleep Med.* 2004;**5**:401–6.

8. Paulus W, Dowling P, Rijsman R, *et al.* Pathophysiological concepts of restless legs syndrome. *Mov Disord.* 2007;**22**:1451–6.

9. Bucher SF, Trenkwalder C, Oertel WH. Reflex studies and MRI in the restless legs syndrome. *Acta Neurol Scand.* 1996;**94**:145–50.

10. Lee SJ, Kim JS, Song IU, *et al.* Poststroke restless legs syndrome and lesion location: anatomical considerations. *Mov Disord.* 2009;**24**:77–84.

11. Unrath A, Kassubek J. Symptomatic restless leg syndrome after lacunar stroke: a lesion study. *Mov Disord.* 2006;**21**:2027–8.

12. Sechi G, Agnetti V, Galistu P, *et al.* Restless legs syndrome and periodic limb movements after ischemic stroke in the right lenticulostriate region. *Parkinsonism Relat Disord.* 2008;**14**:157–60.

13. Kizilay F, Ozkaynak S, Hatipoglu E, *et al.* Periodic limb movement during sleep following cerebellar infarct. *Acta Neurol Belg.* 2010;**110**:284–6.

14. Lee JS, Lee PH, Huh K. Periodic limb movements in sleep after a small deep subcortical infarct. *Mov Disord.* 2005;**20**:260–1.

15. Anderson KN, Bhatia KP, Losseff NA. A case of restless legs syndrome in association with stroke. *Sleep.* 2005;**28**:147–8.

16. Kang SY, Sohn YH, Lee IK, Kim JS. Unilateral periodic limb movement in sleep after supratentorial cerebral infarction. *Parkinsonism Relat Disord.* 2004;**10**:429–31.

17. Kim JS, Lee SB, Park SK, *et al.* Periodic limb movement during sleep developed after pontine lesion. *Mov Disord.* 2003;**18**:1403–5.

18. Lee MS, Choi YC, Lee SH, Lee SB. Sleep-related periodic leg movements associated with spinal cord lesions. *Mov Disord.* 1996;**11**:719–22.

19. Yokota T, Hirose K, Tanabe H, Tsukagoshi H. Sleep-related periodic leg movements (nocturnal myoclonus) due to spinal cord lesion. *J Neurol Sci.* 1991;**104**:13–18.

20. Friston KJ, Holmes A, Poline J-B, Frith CD, Frackowiak RSJ. Statistic parametric maps in functional imaging: a general linear approach. *Hum Brain Mapp.* 1995;**2**:189–210.

21. Ashburner J, Friston KJ. Voxel-based morphometry – the methods. *Neuroimage.* 2000;**11**:805–21.

22. Wright IC, McGuire PK, Poline JB, *et al.* A voxel-based method for the statistical analysis of gray and white matter density applied to schizophrenia. *Neuroimage.* 1995;**2**:244–52.

23. Etgen T, Draganski B, Ilg C, *et al.* Bilateral thalamic gray matter changes in patients with restless legs syndrome. *Neuroimage.* 2005;**24**:1242–7.

24. Hornyak M, Ahrendts JC, Spiegelhalder K, *et al.* Voxel-based morphometry in unmedicated patients with restless legs syndrome. *Sleep Med.* 2007;**9**:22–6.

25. Unrath A, Juengling FD, Schork M, Kassubek J. Cortical grey matter alterations in idiopathic restless legs syndrome: an optimized voxel-based morphometry study. *Mov Disord.* 2007;**22**:1751–6.

26. Celle S, Roche F, Peyron R, *et al.* Lack of specific gray matter alterations in restless legs syndrome in elderly subjects. *J Neurol.* 2010;**257**:344–8.

27. Comley RA, Cervenka S, Palhagen SE, *et al.* A comparison of gray matter density in restless legs syndrome patients and matched controls using voxel-based morphometry. *J Neuroimaging.* 2012;**22**:28–32.

28. Connor JR, Ponnuru P, Lee BY, *et al.* Postmortem and imaging based analyses reveal CNS decreased myelination in restless legs syndrome. *Sleep Med.* 2011;**12**:614–19.

29. Bandettini PA. What's new in neuroimaging methods? *Ann N Y Acad Sci.* 2009;**1156**:260–93.

30. May A, Hajak G, Ganssbauer S, *et al.* Structural brain alterations following 5 days of intervention: dynamic aspects of neuroplasticity. *Cereb Cortex.* 2007;**17**:205–10.

31. Good CD, Johnsrude IS, Ashburner J, *et al.* A voxel-based morphometric study of ageing in 465 normal adult human brains. *Neuroimage.* 2001;**14**:21–36.

32. Keller SS, Wilke M, Wieshmann UC, Sluming VA, Roberts N. Comparison of standard and optimized voxel-based morphometry for analysis of brain changes associated with temporal lobe epilepsy. *Neuroimage.* 2004;**23**:860–8.

33. Karas GB, Burton EJ, Rombouts SA, *et al.* A comprehensive study of gray matter loss in patients with Alzheimer's disease using optimized voxel-based morphometry. *Neuroimage.* 2003;**18**:895–907.

34. Pell GS, Briellmann RS, Chan CH, *et al.* Selection of the control group for VBM analysis: influence of covariates, matching and sample size. *Neuroimage.* 2008;**41**:1324–35.

35. Chen X, Sachdev PS, Wen W, Anstey KJ. Sex differences in regional gray matter in healthy individuals aged 44–48 years: a voxel-based morphometric study. *Neuroimage.* 2007;**36**:691–9.

36. Taki Y, Thyreau B, Kinomura S, *et al.* Correlations among brain gray matter volumes, age, gender, and hemisphere in healthy individuals. *PLoS One.* 2011;**6**:e22734.

37. Herve PY, Crivello F, Perchey G, Mazoyer B, Tzourio-Mazoyer N. Handedness and cerebral anatomical asymmetries in young adult males. *Neuroimage.* 2006;**29**:1066–79.

38. Chakos MH, Lieberman JA, Bilder RM, *et al.* Increase in caudate nuclei volumes of first-episode schizophrenic patients taking antipsychotic drugs. *Am J Psychiatry.* 1994;**151**:1430–6.

39. Corson PW, Nopoulos P, Miller DD, Arndt S, Andreasen NC. Change in basal ganglia volume over 2 years in patients with schizophrenia: typical versus atypical neuroleptics. *Am J Psychiatry.* 1999;**156**:1200–4.

40. Salgado-Pineda P, Delaveau P, Falcon C, Blin O. Brain T1 intensity changes after levodopa administration in healthy subjects: a voxel-based morphometry study. *Br J Clin Pharmacol.* 2006;**62**:546–51.

41. Basser PJ, Jones DK. Diffusion-tensor MRI: theory, experimental design and data analysis - a technical review. *NMR Biomed.* 2002;**15**:456–67.

42. Unrath A, Muller HP, Ludolph AC, Riecker A, Kassubek J. Cerebral white matter alterations in idiopathic restless legs syndrome, as measured by diffusion tensor imaging. *Mov Disord.* 2008;**23**:1250–5.

43. Manconi M, Rocca MA, Ferini-Strambi L, *et al.* Restless legs syndrome is a common finding in multiple sclerosis and correlates with cervical cord damage. *Mult Scler.* 2008;**14**:86–93.

44. Norris DG. Principles of magnetic resonance assessment of brain function. *J Magn Reson Imaging.* 2006;**23**:794–807.

45. Bucher S, Seelos K, Oertel W, Reiser M, Trenkwalder C. Cerebral generators involved in the pathogenesis of the restless legs syndrome. *Ann Neurol.* 1997;**41**:639–45.

46. Spiegelhalder K, Feige B, Paul D, *et al.* Cerebral correlates of muscle tone fluctuations in restless legs syndrome: a pilot study with combined functional magnetic resonance imaging and anterior tibial muscle electromyography. *Sleep Med.* 2008;**9**:177–83.

47. Astrakas LG, Konitsiotis S, Margariti P, *et al.* T2 relaxometry and fMRI of the brain in late-onset restless legs syndrome. *Neurology.* 2008;**71**:911–16.

Functional neuroimaging of dopamine, iron, and opiates in restless legs syndrome

Thomas C. Wetter and Gerhard Klösch

Introduction

Restless legs syndrome (RLS) is a neurological sleep/wake disorder that is diagnosed according to clinical criteria proposed by the International RLS Study Group [1] (for the list of criteria see Chapter 46). RLS occurs frequently with an estimated prevalence of 2–10% in patients with a wide spectrum of complaints [2]. The essential criteria for RLS are found in both idiopathic (often familial) RLS with early onset and clinically similar secondary RLS associated with various conditions, including low serum ferritin levels, kidney failure, and pregnancy. In general, the course of this disorder is slowly progressive with age. In most patients with RLS, sleep disturbances and periodic limb movements (PLM) during sleep (PLMS) and wakefulness (PLMW) can be documented with overnight polysomnography. The first-line treatment for RLS includes dopaminergic agents, which are effective in low to moderate doses. Higher doses of dopaminergic drugs may induce augmentation – a paradoxical worsening of symptoms – which forces one to reduce the dose or to switch to another drug. Alternative treatments here include opioids and anticonvulsants [3].

Dopamine, opioids, and iron: pathophysiological aspects

Despite promising approaches in genetics and neurophysiology, the etiology of RLS remains unknown. Many regions of the central nervous system (CNS), from the periphery to the cortex, contain structures that may be involved in the pathophysiology of RLS [4] (see also Chapter 46). The rapid efficacy of dopaminergic drugs in RLS treatment can be taken as evidence for the role of dopaminergic neurotransmission. In controlled trials, dopaminergic agents have been shown to consistently provide complete or considerable relief from RLS symptoms and to lead to a significant decrease in PLM [5]. Indirect support for a role of the dopamine system in the pathophysiology of RLS is the observation that dopamine antagonists can worsen symptoms or even elicit RLS [6].

The dopaminergic system in the brain includes the nigrostriatal (A9), mesocortical and mesolimbic (A10), diencephalo-spinal (A11), and tuberoinfundibular hypothalamic (A12) pathways. There are two main groups of dopamine receptors, D_1-like (including D_1 and D_5) and D_2-like (including D_2, D_3,

and D_4) dopamine receptors. They are primarily found in the striatum, which is the region of interest of dopaminergic RLS imaging studies. The vast majority of striatal dopamine D_2 receptors are localized postsynaptically; therefore, imaging of dopamine D_2 receptors is frequently referred to as imaging of postsynaptic D_2 receptors [7]. The dopamine transporter (DAT) is a protein on the presynaptic dopaminergic nerve terminal, which controls dopamine levels by active reuptake after its interaction with the postsynaptic receptor [8] (Figure 47.1).

With regard to the opiate system, evidence for its involvement in RLS is also based on the known effects of opioid treatments. It has been shown that opiate antagonists like naloxone reactivated RLS in opiate pretreated patients, supporting the hypothesis of an endogenous opiate system dysfunction in RLS [9].

Iron deficiency in the brain has also been suggested to play a major role in the pathophysiology of RLS. Neuropathological data show reduced levels of iron in neuromelanin cells of RLS patients, suggesting that brain iron stores are decreased [10]. Iron is a cofactor for tyrosine hydroxylase; thus a deficiency in brain iron might result in a decrease in tyrosine hydroxylase, producing a dopaminergic abnormality [11].

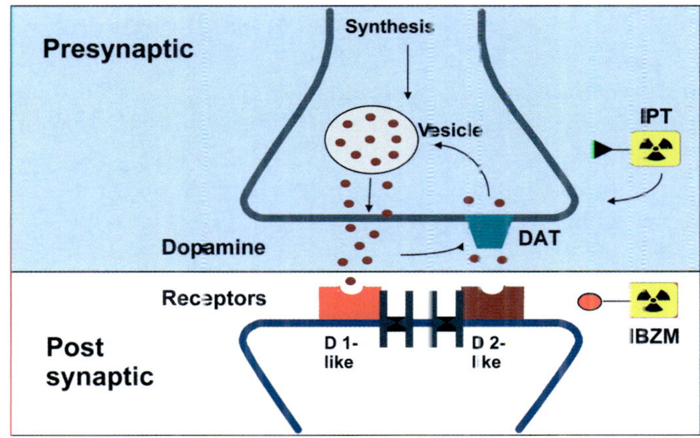

Figure 47.1 Simplified diagram of the terminal of a nigrostriatal dopaminergic cell and a postsynaptic cell in the striatum. Dopamine transporters are situated presynaptically in the membrane of the terminal. Dopamine D_2 receptors are shown only on the postsynaptic cell, whereas they are almost certainly also localized in low concentrations on presynaptic terminals.

Neuroimaging of Sleep and Sleep Disorders, ed. Eric Nofzinger, Pierre Maquet, and Michael J. Thorpy. Published by Cambridge University Press. © Cambridge University Press 2013.

Table 47.1. Radiolabeled ligands for SPECT and PET imaging of dopamine transporters and dopamine D_2 receptors used in RLS studies

Dopamine transporter	Dopamine D_2 receptor
^{123}I-IPT (SPECT)	^{123}I-IBZM (SPECT)
[^{123}I]β-CIT (SPECT)	[^{11}C]raclopride (PET)
[^{11}C]methylphenidate (PET)	[^{11}C]FLB 457 (extrastriatal brain regions) (PET)

Functional neuroimaging in restless legs syndrome

Functional neuroimaging techniques are powerful tools for investigating the complex patterns of functional neuroanatomy behind sleep and its disorders [12–14]. To evaluate the hypotheses that dysfunctional dopaminergic, opioidergic, or iron systems are involved in the pathophysiology of RLS, functional neuroimaging studies have been performed using single photon emission computed tomography (SPECT), positron emission tomography (PET), and, more recently, magnetic resonance imaging (MRI) [15].

Functional neuroimaging of the dopaminergic system

Radiolabeled ligands for SPECT and PET imaging of DAT and dopamine D_2 receptors in RLS are shown in Table 47.1.

SPECT studies

There are two different SPECT methods that are employed to document the regulation of both presynaptic dopamine neurons and postsynaptic dopamine D_2 receptors of the nigrostriatal dopaminergic pathway. Presynaptic dopaminergic systems can be measured by either iodine [^{123}I](N)-(3-iodopropene-2-yl)-2β-carbomethoxy-3β (4-chlorophenyl) tropane (^{123}I-IPT SPECT), [123]I-2β-carbomethoxy-3β-(4-iodophenyl) tropane (^{123}I-βCIT SPECT), or ^{99m}Tc-TRODAT-1. These compounds are cocaine analogs that bind with high affinity to DAT that are located in the presynaptic terminals of the neurons. In contrast, [123I]-iodobenzamide-SPECT (^{123}I-IBZM-SPECT) can provide information about postsynaptic striatal dopamine D_2 receptor binding (Figure 47.1).

Presynaptic dopamine receptor binding

A summary of presynaptic dopamine SPECT studies in patients with RLS is given in Table 47.2.

In an initial DAT imaging study, ^{123}I-IPT SPECT was used in drug-naïve patients with idiopathic RLS and long-term patients pretreated with L-Dopa monotherapy [16]. Because of a significant age difference between the drug-naïve and the pretreated RLS group, two age-matched control groups were investigated separately. The scans were performed between 11:00 and 16:00 h. The results showed that presynaptic striatal DAT binding in drug-naïve and L-Dopa-treated patients and controls was similar.

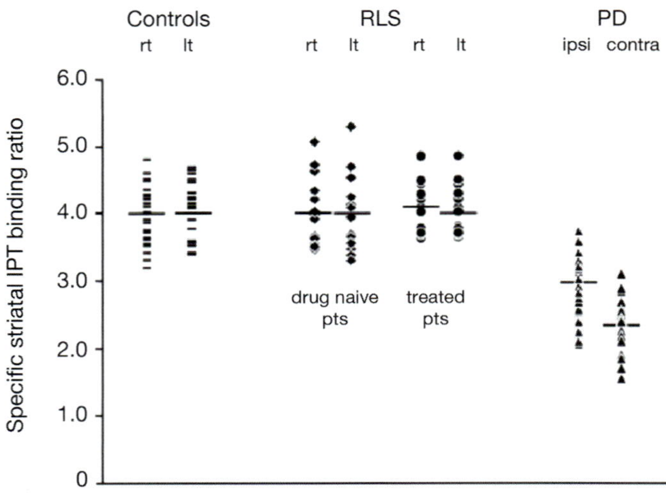

Figure 47.2 Specific striatal [123I]IPT binding in controls, RLS patients and patients with unilateral Parkinson's disease (PD) of Hoehn and Yahr stage I. (Figure and legend with permission from Linke R, Eisensehr I, Wetter TC, *et al.* Presynaptic dopaminergic function in patients with restless legs syndrome: Are there common features with early Parkinson´s disease? *Mov Disord* 2004; **19**: 1158–62.)

Michaud and colleagues [17] used [123]Iβ-CIT SPECT in patients with idiopathic RLS and healthy control subjects matched for age and gender. Scans were performed in the evening between 16:30 and 21:30 h the time of most pronounced symptomatology. In concordance with the previous study, no difference in striatal DAT binding between RLS patients and controls was detected. Similar results have been reported by Mrowka and coworkers [18].

To explore possible side-to-side asymmetry binding, Linke *et al.* [19] performed DAT imaging in idiopathic RLS patients using ^{123}I-IPT SPECT, and compared the results with patients with early Parkinson's disease (PD) and age-matched controls. In line with earlier studies, no differences in transporter binding between RLS patients and healthy controls were found. RLS and early PD showed no common characteristics, suggesting the involvement of different pathophysiologic pathways at the level of nigrostriatal presynaptic terminal function (Figure 47.2).

Postsynaptic dopamine receptor binding

An overview of postsynaptic dopamine SPECT studies is shown in Table 47.3.

Using the same study protocol as described above, Eisensehr *et al.* [16] studied postsynaptic dopamine receptor binding employing ^{123}I-IBZM SPECT. No differences between drug-naïve and L-Dopa-treated RLS patients and controls were detected. Similar to the IPT results, no between-group difference in the degree of striatal asymmetry of ^{123}I-IBZM binding and no correlation between various clinical parameters and ^{123}I-IBZM binding were reported. However, there was a significant negative correlation between age and postsynaptic D_2 receptor binding in patients and controls (Figure 47.3).

In accordance with these results, Tribl and coauthors [20] reported no differences between pretreated patients with idiopathic RLS and healthy controls in postsynaptic D_2 receptor

Table 47.2. SPECT studies of presynaptic dopamine receptor binding in RLS patients

Method	Patients/controls	Medication	Measure	Main results	Authors
^{123}I-IPT SPECT	Sample 1 14 patients 2 m, 12 f 67 ± 8 years 10 controls 7 m, 3 f 66 ± 7 years	Drug-naïve	ROI – background/background ROI: striatum, caudate, putamen; background: supratentorial brain regions excluding basal ganglia and thalamus	No differences between RLS and control groups in both samples; no correlation of IPT binding with duration of RLS symptoms, L-Dopa dosage, iron or ferritin levels, number of PLM, and sleep efficiency	Eisensehr et al. [16]
	Sample 2 11 patients 2 m, 12 f 67 ± 3 years 10 controls 7 m, 3 f 59 ± 18 years	Long-term L-Dopa pretreated; medication stopped two days prior to the scans			
[^{123}I]β-CIT SPECT	10 patients 6 m, 4 f 46 ± 8 years 10 controls 6 m, 4 f 46 ± 7 years	L-Dopa-naïve and free of other psychotropic drugs for at least three months	Basal ganglia – background/background	No differences between patients and controls. No associations between RLS severity, clinical parameters, and β-CIT binding	Michaud et al. [17]
^{123}I-IPT SPECT	Sample 1 14 patients 2 m, 12 f 67 ± 8 years	Drug-naïve	ROI – background/background ROI: striatum, caudate, putamen; background: supratentorial brain regions excluding basal ganglia and thalamus	No differences between RLS and healthy controls; no correlation of ^{123}I-IPT binding with duration of RLS symptoms and L-Dopa dosage. Significantly lower ^{123}I-IPT binding ipsi- and contralateral to the affected body side in PD patients compared to RLS patients or controls	Linke et al. [19]
	Sample 2 14 patients 6 m, 8 f 56 ± 10 years 29 patients with early PD 17 m, 12 f 53 ± 10 years 23 controls for both samples 19 m, 4 f 57 ± 15 years	Long-term L-Dopa pretreated; medication stopped two days prior to the scans			
[^{123}I]β-CIT SPECT	6 patients 2 m, 4 f 60 ± 4 years 7 controls 2 m, 5 f 55 ± 10 years	2 patients untreated, L-Dopa treatment stopped in 4 patients 12 h prior to the scans	Striatal region/background cortex	No differences between patients and controls in putamen or caudate nucleus	Mrowka et al. [18]

PD = Parkinson's disease; PLM = periodic leg movements; RLS = restless legs syndrome; ROI = region of interest.

binding using ^{123}I-IBZM SPECT. This was documented for ^{123}I-IBZM binding and several parameters including duration and severity of RLS.

Following the same DAT imaging study protocol, Michaud et al. [17] investigated postsynaptic dopaminergic receptors using ^{123}I-IBZM SPECT. The authors reported that the median striatal ^{123}I-IBZM binding was significantly reduced in patients compared to controls. In addition, nine of ten patients showed a mean striatal D_2 receptor binding below the mean value of the control group.

Table 47.3. SPECT studies of postsynaptic dopamine receptor binding in RLS patients

Method	Patients/controls	Medication	Measure	Main results	Authors
^{123}I-IBZM SPECT	12 patients (8 RLS, 4 PLMS only) 9 m, 3 f 56 years	No details at baseline reported. Treatment period included L-Dopa (375 mg, 5 patients) or bromocriptine (20 mg, 1 patient)	Specific uptake index: BG/brain contour (Cx) = BG (average)/Cx – BG	Significant reduction of BG/Cx ratio in the patient group compared with controls at baseline; after three months of L-Dopa or bromocriptine treatment ratios were unchanged in 4 patients; increase in 2 patients after medication was stopped two days before the study	Staedt et al. [21]
	4 controls 2 m (25; 59 years) 2 f (52; 57 years)				
^{123}I-IBZM SPECT	20 patients (14 RLS, 6 PLMS only) 14 m, 6 f 58 years	No details reported	BG/Cx	Lower ratio in patients; 2 patients had values within the control range; controls were significantly younger	Staedt et al. [22]
	10 controls 6 m, 4 f 42 years				
^{123}I-IBZM SPECT	4 patients (RLS/PLMS) 1 m: 54 years 3 f: 53; 61; 69 years	No details at baseline reported. Treatment period included L-Dopa (125, 200, 375 mg, 3 patients) or L-Dopa (200 mg) plus bromocriptine (10 mg, 1 patient)	Specific uptake index: BG/brain contour (Cx) = BG (average)/Cx – BG	Higher uptake in controls at baseline. Increase of binding after treatment for three months (3 patients) or eight months (1 patient)	Staedt et al. [23]
	10 controls No gender and age information reported				
^{123}I-IBZM SPECT	Sample 1 14 patients 2 m, 12 f 67 ± 8 years	Drug-naïve	ROI – background/background	No differences between RLS and control groups in both samples; no correlation of ^{123}I-IBZM binding with duration of RLS symptoms, L-Dopa dosage, iron or ferritin levels, number of PLM, and sleep efficiency. Significant negative correlation between age and receptor binding	Eisensehr et al. [16]
	10 controls 7 m, 3 f 66 ± 7 years		ROI: striatum, caudate, putamen; background: supratentorial brain regions excluding BG and thalamus		
	Sample 2 11 patients 2 m, 12 f 67 ± 8 years	Long-term L-Dopa monotherapy pretreated; medication stopped two days prior to the scans			
	10 controls 7 m, 3 f 59 ± 18 years				
^{123}I-IBZM SPECT	10 patients 6 m, 4 f 46 ± 8 years	L-Dopa-naïve and free of other psychotropic drugs for at least three months	BG – background/background	Significant reduction of striatal binding in RLS patients. No relation between RLS severity or PLMS indices and ^{123}I-IBZM binding	Michaud et al. [17]
	10 controls 6 m, 4 f 46 ± 7 years				
^{123}I-IBZM SPECT	14 patients 6 m, 8 f 57 ± 13 years	Ropinirol stopped one week or 60 h in 2 patients; L-Dopa, gabapentin, and zolpidem stopped 36 h prior to the scans (10 patients); 2 patients drug-free	Striatal/dorsolateral frontal cortex	No difference between patients and controls. No correlation of binding with gender, duration of RLS, severity of symptoms, sleep efficiency, PLM, PSQI	Tribl et al. [23]
	10 controls 8 m, 2 f 51 ± 20 years				

BG = basal ganglia; Cx = cortex; PLMS = periodic leg movments in sleep; PSQI = Pittsburgh Sleep Quality Index; RLS = restless legs syndrome; ROI = region of interest.

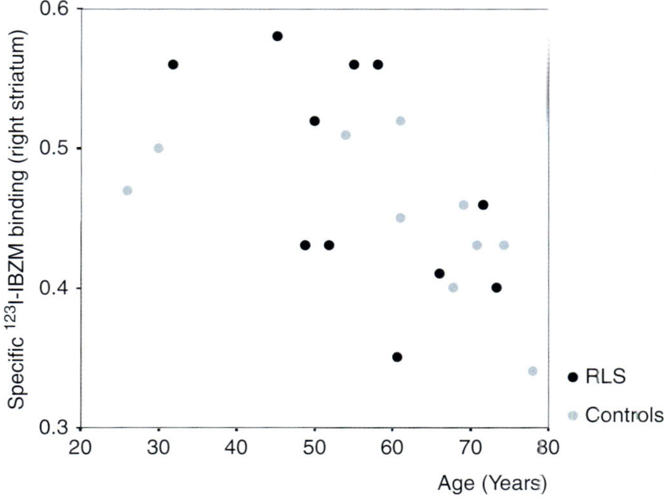

Figure 47.3 Significant inverse correlation (r = −0.60, p = 0.005) between age and right postsynaptic D$_2$ binding in patients and controls (T. C. Wetter, R. Linke, I. Eisensehr, et al, unpublished data, 2001).

In a series of earlier studies, Staedt *et al.* used ^{123}I-IBZM to investigate dopamine D$_2$ receptor alterations in patients with PLMS. In the initial study [21] 8 out of 12 patients with PLMS were diagnosed to have RLS. Six patients participated in a follow-up study subsequent to a three-month treatment period (for details see Table 47.3). At "baseline," the authors found a significant decrease in ^{123}I-IBZM binding in the basal ganglia of patients compared with controls. After treatment, the binding ratio increased in two patients, but remained unchanged in four patients. In a second study using a similar protocol [22] 14 out of 20 patients also were found to have RLS. Again, the authors reported a lower ^{123}I-IBZM binding in the striatum in the patient group. However, there was a significant age difference between patients and controls. In a third study, the ^{123}I-IBZM uptake and distribution was investigated before and during dopaminergic treatment in four PLMS/RLS patients. The main result was a higher ^{123}I-IBZM uptake in controls at baseline and an increase in striatal binding in all patients following treatment [23].

PET studies

PET is a reliable technique to measure the integrity of dopaminergic neurons, to visualize postsynaptic D$_2$ receptors, and to quantify presynaptic nigrostriatal dopaminergic neurons using the DAT as a neurochemical marker. To measure these targets, different PET ligands are available (Table 47.1). PET studies of the dopaminergic system are summarized in Table 47.4.

Integrity of dopaminergic neurons

^{18}F-dopa PET provides a measure of the structural and biochemical integrity of dopaminergic neurons: the uptake rate constant of ^{18}F-dopa is determined by the transfer of DOPA across the blood–brain barrier, its decarboxylation to fluorodopamine, and its retention in nerve terminals. In an initial PET study using ^{18}F-dopa in a small sample size, no abnormalities in presynaptic nigrostriatal dopaminergic projections were found among RLS subjects [24]. However, Turjanski and coworkers [25] detected a "mild" reduction of the mean ^{18}F-dopa uptake in the caudate and putamen. Subsequently, Ruottinen *et al.* [26] reported a significant reduction of ^{18}F-dopa uptake in the caudate nucleus and the putamen in drug-naïve patients with both RLS and periodic limb movement disorder (PLMD).

Dopamine D$_2$ receptor binding

Turjanski and coworkers [25] used [^{11}C]raclopride PET to image postsynaptic dopamine receptors in pretreated and drug-naïve RLS patients. Mean D$_2$ binding was reduced in both the caudate and the putamen. This study documented the lack of a relationship between striatal D$_2$ binding and clinical severity of RLS (Table 47.4). Červenka *et al.* used [^{11}C]raclopride and [^{11}C]FLB 457 to measure striatal and extrastriatal D$_2$ receptor availability both in the morning (between 10:00 and 12:00 h) and in the evening (starting at 18:00 h) [27]. Patients had significantly higher [^{11}C]raclopride and [^{11}C]FLB 457 binding potentials (BP) than controls in the striatum and extrastriatal regions such as the thalamus and anterior cingulated cortex. Images of [^{11}C]raclopride and [^{11}C]FLB 457 from a male control subject are shown in Figure 47.4.

Dopamine transporter (DAT)

To evaluate DAT binding potentials in the striatum of RLS subjects, [^{11}C]methylphenidate PET was used in a recent study [28]. PET scans were performed at two different time points of the day (starting at 08:30 and 19:30 h) in different groups of subjects. The results demonstrate that RLS patients had significantly lower DAT binding in the striatum compared with controls in both day and night scans. In line with the study by Červenka *et al.* [27] no diurnal differences for the total group or for controls and RLS separately were observed.

Summary

SPECT studies assessing presynaptic dopamine receptor binding (i.e., DAT imaging) with either IPT or β-CIT ligands reported no differences between idiopathic RLS patients and healthy age-matched controls [16–19]. These results were observed in drug-naïve and long-term L-Dopa pretreated patients, suggesting that striatal dopamine transporters are normal in RLS subjects. In contrast to these findings, one recent PET study assessing DAT imaging found a significant decrease in binding potentials in two independent samples, suggesting that membrane-bound striatal DAT, but not total cellular DAT, may be decreased in RLS [28]. PET studies of dopaminergic neurons integrity have, nonetheless, revealed mixed results with either unchanged [24] or reduced uptake of ^{18}F-dopa in the putamen and/or caudate [25, 26]. In the latter two studies, the reduced dopamine uptake was more

Table 47.4. PET studies of the dopaminergic system in RLS patients

Method	Patients/controls	Medication	Measure	Main results	Authors
^{18}F-dopa PET	4 patients 2 m, 2 f 59 ± 10 years 10 controls No gender information 58 ± 13 years	Medication stopped 36 h before the study	Caudate and putamen uptake	No difference in ^{18}F-dopa uptake for caudate and putamen between patients and controls	Trenkwalder et al. [24]
^{18}F-dopa PET	13 patients 6 m, 7 f 58 years 14 controls No gender information 59 years	Various RLS medication including L-Dopa stopped the night prior to the scans; 8 patients L-Dopa-naïve	Ki values: rate of uptake	All individual Ki values in the normal range. Significant reduction of mean ^{18}F-dopa uptake in the putamen. No correlation with RLS severity. No differences in mean uptake between drug-naïve and pretreated patients. Significant reduced Ki for putamen and caudate in L-Dopa-naïve patients	Turjanski et al. [25]
[^{11}C]raclopride PET	13 patients 6 m, 7 f 58 years 9 controls No gender information 57 years	Various RLS medication including L-Dopa stopped the night prior to the scans; 8 patients L-Dopa naïve	Bmax/Kd = BP	BP significantly reduced in caudate and putamen in patients. 6/13 patients below control range, 3 for putamen only. No correlation with RLS severity. Lower BP in putamen for L-Dopa-naïve patients vs. controls	
^{18}F-dopa PET	9 patients 6 m, 3 f 52 ± 10 years 27 controls 15 m, 12 f 53 ± 15 years	Drug-naïve with respect to RLS	Ki values: rate of uptake	Significant reduction of mean ^{18}F-dopa uptake in caudate (88%) and putamen (89%) in RLS patients compared with controls	Ruottinen et al. [26]
[^{11}C]raclopride PET and [^{11}C]FLB 457 (extrastriatal brain regions)	16 patients 8 m, 8 f 55 ± 7 years 16 controls 8 m, 8 f 56 ± 8 years 4 different PET examination sequences including morning and evening examinations	Naïve to dopaminergic drugs	Bmax/Kd = BP	Significantly higher BP values in the striatum in patients vs. controls. No differences in diurnal variability in BP Higher BP values in extrastriatal regions, significant for thalamus and ACC in patients vs. controls. No differences in diurnal variability in BP	Červenka et al. [27]
[^{11}C] methylphenidate PET	Day sample: 20 patients 6 m, 14 f 61 ± 9 years 20 controls 11 m, 9f 60 ± 8 years Night sample: 16 patients 5 m, 11 f 57 ± 10 years 14 controls 5 m, 9 f 58 ± 6 years	All CNS and RLS medication stopped at least 11 days prior to the scans	Total striatal DAT BP	Significantly lower striatal DAT binding in patients vs. controls on day and night scans. No diurnal differences in DAT for both groups. No correlation of DAT BP with clinical measures of RLS	Earley et al. [28]

ACC = anterior cingulated cortex; BP = binding potential; Bmax/Kd = ratio of receptor availability to the dissociation constant; CNS = central nervous system; DAT = dopamine transporter; Ki values = influx constants.

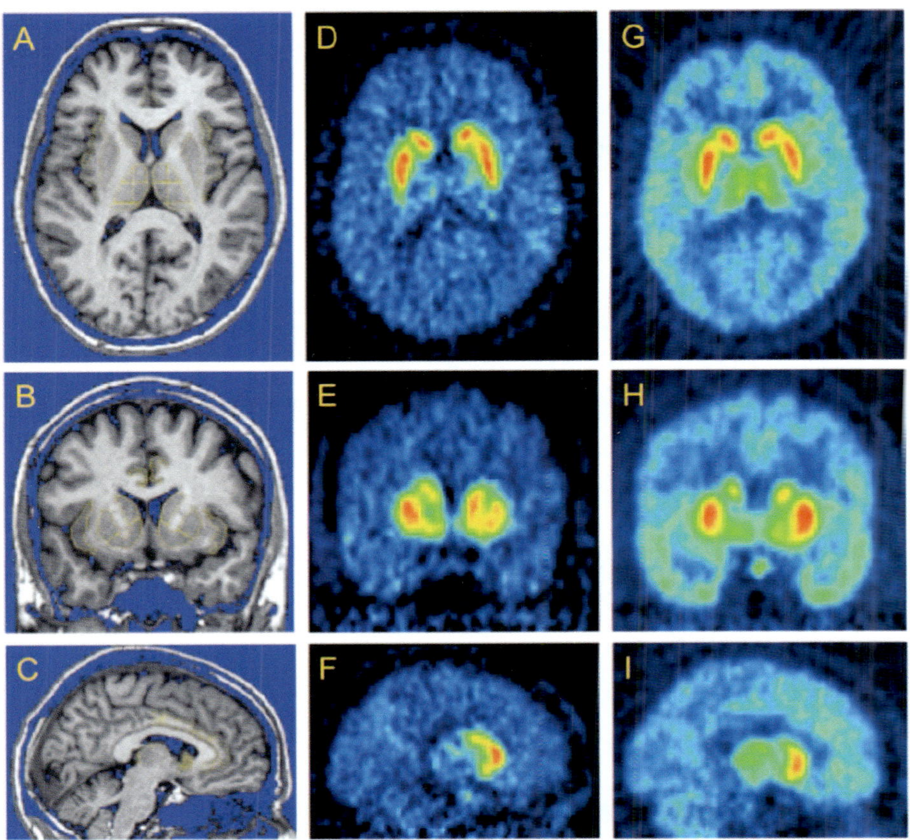

Figure 47.4 MR images showing ROIs (A–C) and PET images showing regional radioactivity after i.v. injections of [^{11}C]raclopride (D–F) and [^{11}C]FLB 457 (G–I). The projections are from top to bottom: horizontal, coronal, and sagittal. PET images shown are based on summed data from 9 min to the end of the examination. All images are from the same male control subject (Figure and legend with permission from Červenka S, Pålhagen SE, Comley RA, et al. Support for dopaminergic hypoactivity in restless legs syndrome: a PET study on D$_2$ receptor binding. *Brain* 2006;**129**:2017–28.)

pronounced than that seen in patients with PD or other neurodegenerative disorders.

With respect to postsynaptic D$_2$ receptor imaging studies, two SPECT studies [16, 20] found normal values either in drug-naïve or in pretreated patients, suggesting normal dopamine receptor bindings and receptor density in the nigrostriatal system. In contrast to these findings, Michaud *et al.* [17] and Staedt *et al.* [21–23] reported a reduced IBZM binding, suggesting a decreased number of D$_2$ receptors or a decreased affinity of D$_2$ receptors. An increased level of synaptic dopamine with attendant down regulation of D$_2$ would be a less likely explanation of the data, since presynaptic binding was normal. The studies by Staedt and coworkers, however, are limited by some methodological shortcomings. This makes conclusions more difficult as prior studies have shown an inverse correlation between striatal postsynaptic D$_2$ receptor binding and age (Figure 47.3). Two PET D$_2$ receptor studies have also yielded contradictory findings with either reduced [25] or increased [27] striatal and extrastriatal binding potentials. The latter study was consistent with the hypothesis of hypoactive dopaminergic neurotransmission in RLS.

The discrepancies among SPECT and PET studies may be due to different methodological issues (e.g., lower resolution with SPECT; medication, lack of age-matched controls; control of head movements during scanning). This makes it difficult to get a clear picture of how the dopaminergic neurotransmitter system may be involved in RLS. Given a central dopaminergic dysfunction, it has to be determined whether these alterations affect the nigrostriatal and/or other central dopaminergic systems (such as the diencephalospinal or mesolimbic pathways). Interestingly, studies that have included imaging of patients both in the morning and at night, when symptoms are more severe, have not found any differences in presynaptic [28] or postsynaptic [27] dopaminergic binding between both time points.

PET and SPECT studies on metabolism, pain, and the opioidergic system

A summary of the relevant studies is given in Table 47.5.

Global metabolic rate using PET

One study with ^{18}F-fluorodeoxyglucose (^{18}F-FDG PET) measured the overall cerebral metabolism by comparing RLS patients during a symptom-free period with healthy controls [24]. The global and regional metabolic uptake was normal in all six RLS patients. No association with severity or duration of the disease was found.

Regional cerebral blood flow using SPECT

One study investigated two family members with RLS during the state of pain induced by immobility, using semiquantitative regional cerebral blood flow (rCBF) SPECT using ^{99}Tc-HMPAO [29]. The authors found a 13% reduction in rCBF of

Table 47.5. PET and SPECT studies of metabolism, pain and the opioidergic system in RLS patients

Method	Patients/controls	Medication	Measure	Main results	Authors
^{18}F-FDG PET	6 patients 3 m, 3 f 55 ± 11 years	Medication likely to influence RLS stopped 36 h prior to the scans	Regional/global metabolic rate for glucose	Normal glucose metabolism in all patients. No difference in regional/global metabolic rate in various brain regions such as the pons, midbrain, cerebellum, caudate, putamen, thalamus, and cortical areas	Trenkwalder et al. [24]
	12 controls No gender information 56 ± 15 years				
^{99m}Tc-HMPAO SPECT	2 patients (familial RLS) 1 m (53 years) 1 f (36 years)	Scans were performed before and after treatment with L-Dopa	rCBF of caudate nucleus, thalamus, anterior cingulate cortex	13% reduction in rCBF of the caudate with increasing pain; 7% and 6.6% increase in rCBF in thalamus and anterior cingulated cortex with increasing pain	San Pedro et al. [29]
[11C] diprenorphine PET	15 patients 5 m, 10 f 45 ± 16 years	Dopaminergic medication stopped at least 48 h prior to PET scan; no treatment with opioids in both groups	Vd: volume of distribution quantifying ligand binding in various brain regions	No significant differences in opioid receptor binding between patients and controls. Negative correlation between ligand binding and RLS severity in specific brain areas involved in the medial pain system	von Spiczak et al. [31]
	12 controls 5 m, 7 f 46 ± 12 years				

rCBF = regional cerebral blood flow.

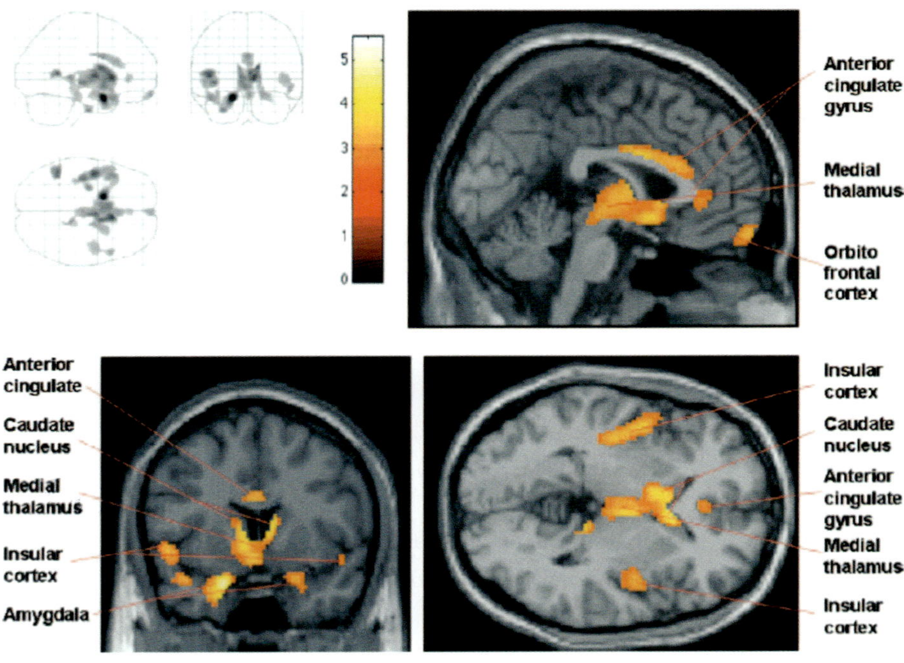

Figure 47.5 Localized clusters of negative correlations between [11C]diprenorphine Vd (n = 14) and RLS severity (IRLS) at p < 0.01 uncorrected threshold, cluster extent of 50 voxels. All clusters throughout the whole brain are demonstrated (top left) in the maximum intensity projection "glass brain" from SPM99. The top right and bottom two panels show significant clusters overlain on the Montreal Neurological Institute single subject representative brain from SPM99. The colour bar represents Z values of statistical significance. (Figure and legend with permission from Spiczak S, Whone AL, Hammers A, et al. The role of opioids in restless legs syndrome: an [11C] diprenorphine PET study. Brain 2005;**128**:906–17.)

the caudate nuclei with increasing pain. The rCBF reduction in the caudate may be associated with pain symptoms in RLS patients rather than with actual RL symptoms. Furthermore, a low caudate perfusion has been reported in chronic pain conditions [30].

PET studies of the opioid system

In a first study to measure opioid receptor binding in RLS patients, using [11C]diprenorphine PET, von Spiczak et al. [31] found no mean group differences between patients and controls. However, significant regional negative correlations between opioid receptor availability and the severity of RL symptoms were documented in areas serving the medial pain system such as the thalamus and amygdala (Figure 47.5).

Summary

In RLS patients, the endogenous opioid system appears to have redistributed binding that could compensate for unpleasant symptoms in direct correlation with the severity of RLS [32]. Existing data suggest that this effect may be modulated by dopamine and not by specific alterations of the endogenous opioid system [33]. Nevertheless, the findings of von Spiczak *et al.* [31] support the hypothesis that decreased opioid binding may lead to an increase in endogenous opioid release. The decrease in [^{11}C]diprenorphine binding may reflect the increased occupancy of opioid receptors by endogenous opioids, triggered by the severity of the RL symptoms. These patterns closely resembled changes seen in chronic pain conditions [29, 30].

Neuroimaging of iron

MRI studies

A summary of the studies is provided in Table 47.6.

In the 1980s MRI reports on T2-weighted MR images were published [34] showing decreased signal intensities in brain regions with high iron concentration. Since iron is known to vary between brain regions (e.g., [35]) and is substantially higher in dopaminergic brain areas such as the substantia nigra and striatum, MRI studies on brain iron have become an active area of research in RLS.

In 1999, Gelman *et al.* [36] introduced the R2* technique, a new way of calculating the relaxation rate, providing a more specific measure of regional brain iron. Applying this method, Allen and coworkers [37] conducted an MRI study in RLS patients and compared R2* relaxation rates with those of healthy subjects. In RLS subjects, reduced R2* rates were found in the putamen and substantia nigra, but not in the caudate nucleus. In addition, there was a correlation between the severity of RL symptoms and the reduction of R2* rates. It has also been shown that after a two-week infusion of iron dextran (for details see Table 47.6) brain iron concentrations as determined by MRI were increased in the substantia nigra and the prefrontal cortex [38]. In a subsequent study with a larger sample size, the mean "iron index" derived from the substantia nigra was significantly lower in early-onset RLS patients than in controls, whereas late-onset RLS patients and controls did not differ in distinct brain regions of interest (Table 47.6) [39]. Another 3 T MRI study [24] found that two patients with severe RLS and hemochromatosis had decreased R2* relaxation rates in the substantia nigra, red nucleus, and pallidum compared with healthy controls.

Godau and coauthors [40] used 1.5 T MRI and assessed substantia nigra echogenicity in RLS patients and healthy controls. For each subject, mean and standard deviation of T2 values were calculated. In all assessed brain regions (see Table 47.6) mean T2 values were higher in RLS patients than in controls, but statistical significances were only found in the head of the caudate nucleus, the thalamus, and the red nucleus.

No significant group differences were found in the substantia nigra, although this brain region is particularly rich in iron. In late-onset idiopatic RLS patients brain iron content was significantly higher only in the pars compacta of the substantia nigra, whereas other brain regions showed no differences compared with controls [41].

Summary

Imaging studies in RLS patients have detected changes in brain iron metabolism, which did not show a consistent association with reduced cerebrospinal fluid ferritin levels. Depending on the methods applied, reduced iron concentrations were found in the substantia nigra [37, 39, 41, 42] and putamen [37], prefrontal cortex [38], red nucleus [40, 41] and in the pallidum [42]. With respect to the caudate nucleus, results are ambiguous: Godau *et al.* [40] reported reduced iron concentrations, whereas other studies have failed to find any significant changes. Apart from methodological differences and physiological changes in local brain iron concentrations, other factors such as the severity and duration of RL symptoms may play a role in the discrepant findings. Iron deposits are substantially greater in dopaminergic brain areas such as the substantia nigra and striatum. There is evidence that iron is not only an important cofactor for tyrosine hydroxylase, the step-limiting enzyme in dopamine synthesis, but may also play a role in the functioning of postsynaptic D_2 receptors [43]. Moreover, MRI techniques are sensitive to iron bound to ferritin, but do not provide information on the relative amounts of H- and L-ferritin and the cellular compartment in which they are stored [41, 44].

Concluding remarks

Neuroimaging techniques provide new insights into the neurobiology of RLS. Consequently, SPECT, PET, and MR imaging of elements of the dopaminergic, opioid, and iron systems may contribute to the elucidation of pathophysiological mechanisms underlying this frequent sleep-related movement disorder. SPECT and PET studies of the nigrostriatal pre- and postsynaptic receptor binding potentials have produced controversial results, possibly reflecting a subtle receptor dysfunction of the central dopaminergic system. However, more refined investigations are necessary. Imaging studies of the opioidergic system are still limited, but available data point to an involvement of opioids in the pathophysiology of RLS. With regard to RL symptomatology, it is of particular interest that the dopamine system is involved in the modulation of nociceptive signals, which may contribute to the perception of pain and symptoms of restlessness. On the other hand, iron insufficiency may produce a dopaminergic abnormality contributing to the RLS pathology [11].

Table 47.6. MRI studies of the iron system in RLS patients

Method	Patients/controls	Medication	Measure	Main results	Authors
1.5 T scan (R2*)	5 patients 66.2 ± 10.5 years 5 age-matched controls 66.4 ± 16.8 years No gender information	Pevious treatment with dopaminergic drugs (no information about withdrawal of medication during fMRI investigation)	R2* rate of primary interest: substantia nigra, caudate, putamen Secondary interest: globus pallidus, cerebellum, thalamus, red nucleus, pons	Reduced R2* rate in patients in the putamen and substantia nigra but not in the caudate nucleus depending on the severity of the RL symptoms	Allen et al. [37]
1.5 T scan (R2*)	10 patients 62.4 ± 8.7 years 6 m, 4 f	MRI scans were performed within 48 h prior to treatment (single dose of 1000 mg iron dextran) and two weeks post treatment	R2* rate to estimate the local brain iron concentration in: dentate nucleus, pons, substantia nigra, red nucleus, globus pallidum, putamen, thalamus, caudate nucleus, frontal white matter, dorsolateral prefrontal cortex	Marginally non-significant increase of brain iron in the substantia nigra; significant increase in mean iron concentration in the prefrontal cortex in all patients; no significant group differences between responder/non-responder	Earley et al. [38]
	Patient group was divided into responder/non-responder (responder: 3 f/3 m)				
3 T scan (R2*)	2 patients 1 m (56 years) 1 f (40 years)	F: clonazepam M: no details reported	R2* values of substantia nigra, red nucleus, putamen, caudate, pallidum	Decreased R2* values in both patients in the substantia nigra, red nucleus, and pallidum compared with healthy controls	Haba-Rubio et al. [42]
	9 controls 5 m, 4 f 48 ± 9 years				
1.5 T scan (R2*)	41 patients 22 patients with early-onset RLS 57.1 ± 2.0 years 19 patients with late-onset RLS 67.4 ± 1.8 years	All psychoactive medication and any iron supplements were stopped two weeks prior to the investigation	Iron concentration ("iron index") was calculated from MRI measurements in 10 brain regions: substantia nigra (region of primary interest), dentate nucleus, pons, red nucleus, globus pallidus, putamen, caudate nucleus, thalamus, frontal white matter, and dorsolateral prefrontal cortex	Significantly lower R2* rate ("iron index") in the substantia nigra in early-onset RLS patients compared with controls; no differences between healthy controls and late-onset RLS patients	Earley et al. [39]
	39 controls 60.5 ± 1.7 years				
	Both groups were gender balanced				
1.5 T scan (T2)	6 patients 1 m, 5 f 60 ± 8 years	No details reported	Mean T2 values of various brain regions including substantia nigra, pallidum, putamen, head of caudate nucleus, red nucleus, thalamus, frontal and temporal white matter, hippocampus	Higher mean T2 values in RLS patients than in controls (2.9% vs. 7.8%), but statistically significant only in the head of the caudate nucleus, the thalamus, and the red nucleus	Godau et al. [40]
	19 controls 60 ± 12 years				
1.5 T scan (T2)	25 patients 11 m, 14 f 67 ± 9 years	No details reported	T2 relaxation time of various brain regions including substantia nigra, red nucleus, putamen, caudate nucleus, globus pallidus, thalamus, dentate nucleus	Significantly higher T2 relaxation time in patients in the substantia nigra pars compacta compared with controls	Astrakas et al. [41]
	12 controls 5 m, 7 f 66 ± 12 years				

R2* = relaxation rate; T = Tesla; T2 = spin-spin relaxation time.

References

1. Allen RP, Picchietti D, Hening WA, *et al.* Restless legs syndrome: diagnostic criteria, special considerations and epidemiology. a report from the restless legs syndrome diagnosis and epidemiology workshop at the National Institutes of Health. *Sleep Med.* 2003;**4**:101–19.

2. Ohayon MM, O´Hara R, Vitiello MV. Epidemiology of restless legs syndrome: a synthesis of the literature. *Sleep Med Rev.* 2012;**16**:283–95.

3. Montplaisir J, Allen RP, Walters A, *et al.* Restless legs syndrome and periodic limb movements during sleep. In: Kryger MH, Roth T, Dement WC, eds. *Principles and Practice of Sleep Medicine.* St. Louis, Missouri, Elsevier Saunders. 2011; 1026–37.

4. Trenkwalder C, Paulus W. Restless legs syndrome: pathophysiology, clinical presentation and management. *Nat Rev Neurol.* 2010;**6**:337–46.

5. Fulda S, Wetter TC. Where dopamine meets opioids: a meta-analysis of the placebo effect in RLS treatment studies. *Brain.* 2008;**131**:902–17.

6. Hoque R, Chesson AL. Pharmacologically induced/exacerbated restless legs syndrome, periodic limb movements of sleep, and REM behavior disorder/REM sleep without atonia: literature review, qualitative scoring, and comparative analysis. *J Clin Sleep Med.* 2010;**6**:79–83.

7. Booij J, Tissingh G, Winogrodzka A, *et al.* Imaging of the dopaminergic neurotransmission system using single-photon emission tomography and positron emission tomography in patients with parkinsonism. *Eur J Nucl Med.* 1999;**26**:171–82.

8. Marshall V, Grosset D. Role of dopamine transporter imaging in routine clinical practice. *Mov Disord.* 2003;**18**:1415–23.

9. Walters AS. Review of receptor agonist and antagonist studies relevant to the opiate system in restless legs syndrome. *Sleep Med.* 2002;**3**:301–4.

10. Allen RP, Earley CJ. Restless legs syndrome – a review of clinical and pathophysiologic features. *J Clin Neurophysiol.* 2001;**18**:128–47.

11. Connor JR, Xin-Shen W, Allen RP, *et al.* Altered dopaminergic profile in the putamen and substantia nigra in restless legs syndrome. *Brain.* 2009;**132**:2403–12.

12. Nofzinger EA. Neuroimaging and sleep medicine. *Sleep Med Rev.* 2005;**9**:157–72.

13. Dang-Vu TT, Desseilles M, Petit D, *et al.* Neuroimaging in sleep medicine. *Sleep Med.* 2007;**8**:349–72.

14. Desseilles M, Dang-Vu TT, Schabus M, *et al.* Neuroimaging insights into the pathophysiology of sleep disorders. *Sleep.* 2008;**31**:777–94.

15. Wetter TC, Eisensehr I, Trenkwalder C. Functional neuroimaging studies in restless legs syndrome. *Sleep Med.* 2004;**5**:401–6.

16. Eisensehr I, Wetter TC, Linke R, *et al.* Normal IPT and IBZM SPECT in drug-naive and levodopa-treated idiopathic restless legs syndrome. *Neurology.* 2001;**57**:1307–9.

17. Michaud M, Soucy JP, Chabli A, *et al.* SPECT imaging of striatal pre- and postsynaptic dopaminergic status in restless legs syndrome with periodic leg movements in sleep. *J Neurol.* 2002;**249**:164–70.

18. Mrowka M, Jöbges M, Berding G, *et al.* Computerized movement analysis and beta-CIT-SPECT in patients with restless legs syndrome. *J Neural Transm.* 2005;**112**:693–701.

19. Linke R, Eisensehr I, Wetter TC, *et al.* Presynaptic dopaminergic function in patients with restless legs syndrome: Are there common features with early Parkinson's disease? *Mov Disord.* 2004;**19**:1158–62.

20. Tribl GG, Asenbaum S, Happe S, *et al.* Normal striatal D_2 receptor bindings in idiopathic restless legs syndrome with periodic leg movements in sleep. *Nucl Med Commun.* 2004;**25**:55–60.

21. Staedt J, Stoppe G, Kogler A, *et al.* Dopamine D_2 receptor alteration in patients with periodic movements in sleep (nocturnal myoclonus). *J Neural Transm.* 1993;**93**:71–4.

22. Staedt J, Stoppe G, Kögler A, *et al.* Nocturnal myoclonus syndrome (periodic movements in sleep) related to central dopamine D_2 receptor alteration. *Eur Arch Psychiatry Clin Neurosci* 1995;**245**:8–10.

23. Staedt J, Stoppe G. Kögler A, *et al.* Single photon emission tomography (SPET) imaging of dopamine D_2 receptors in the course of dopamine replacement therapy in patients with nocturnal myoclonus syndrome (NMS). *J Neural Transm.* 1995;**99**:187–93.

24. Trenkwalder C, Walters AS, Hening WA, *et al.* Positron emission tomographic studies in restless legs syndrome. *Mov Disord.* 1999;**14**:141–5.

25. Turjanski N, Lees AJ, Brooks DJ. Striatal dopaminergic function in restless legs syndrome. 18F-dopa and [^{11}C]-raclopride PET studies. *Neurology.* 1999;**52**:932–7.

26. Ruottinen HM, Partinen M, Hublin C, *et al.* An FDOPA PET study in patients with periodic limb movement disorder and restless legs syndrome. *Neurology.* 2000;**54**:502–4.

27. Červenka S, Pålhagen SE, Comley RA, *et al.* Support for dopaminergic hypoactivity in restless legs syndrome: a PET study on D_2 receptor binding. *Brain.* 2006;**129**:2017–28.

28. Earley CJ, Kuwabara H, Wong DF, *et al.* The dopamine transporter is decreased in the striatum of subjects with restless legs syndrome. *Sleep.* 2011;**34**:341–7

29. San Pedro EC, Mountz JM, Mountz JD, *et al.* Familial painful restless legs syndrome correlates with pain dependent variation of blood flow to the caudate, thalamus, and anterior cingulate gyrus. *J Rheumatol.* 1998;**25**:2270–5.

30. Mountz JM, Bradley LA, Modell JG, *et al.* Fibromyalgia in women: abnormalities of regional blood flow in the thalamus and the caudate nucleus are associated with low pain threshold levels. *Arthritis Rheum.* 1995;**38**:926–38.

31. Von Spiczak S, Whone AL, Hammers A, *et al.* The role of opioids in restless legs syndrome: an [11C] diprenorphine PET study. *Brain.* 2005;**123**:906–17.

32. Walters AS, Ondo WG, Zhu W, Le W. Does the endogenous opiate system play a role in the restless legs syndrome? A pilot post-mortem study. *J Neurol Sci.* 2009;**279**:62–5.

33. Walters AS, Hening W, Cote L, *et al.* Dominantly inherited restless legs with

myoclonus and periodic movements of sleep: a syndrome related to the endogenous opiates? *Adv Neurol.* 1986;**43**:309–19.

34. Drayer B, Burger P, Darwin R, *et al.* Magnetic resonance imaging of brain iron. *AJR Am J Roentgenol.* 1986;**147**:103–10.

35. Bartzokis G, Aravagiri M, Oldendorfer WH, *et al.* Field dependent transverse relaxation rate increase may be specific measure of tissue iron stores. *Magn Reson Med.* 1993;**29**:459–64.

36. Gelman N, Gorell JM, Barker PB, *et al.* MR imaging of human brain at 3.0 T: preliminary report on transverse relaxation rates and relation to estimated iron content. *Radiology.* 1999;**201**:759–67.

37. Allen RP, Barker PB, Wehrl F, *et al.* MRI measurement of brain iron in patients with restless legs syndrome. *Neurology.* 2001;**56**:263–5.

38. Earley CJ, Heckler D, Allen RP. The treatment of restless legs syndrome with intravenous iron dextran. *Sleep Med.* 2004;**3**:231–5.

39. Earley CJ, Barker P, Horska A, *et al.* MRI-determined regional brain iron concentrations in early- and late-onset restless legs syndrome. *Sleep Med.* 2006;**7**:458–61.

40. Godau J, Klose U, Di Santo A, *et al.* Mulitregional brain iron deficiency in restless legs syndrome. *Mov Disord.* 2008;**8**:1184–7.

41. Astrakas G, Konitsiotis S, Margariti P, *et al.* T2 relaxometry and fMRI of the brain in late-onset restless legs syndrome. *Neurology.* 2008;**71**:911–16.

42. Haba-Rubio J, Staner L, Petiau C, *et al.* Restless legs syndrome and low brain iron level in patients with haemochromatosis. *J Neurol Neurosurg Psychiatry.* 2005;**76**:1009–10.

43. Unger EL, Wiesinger JA, Hao L, Beard JL. Dopamine D_2 receptor expression is altered by changes in cellular iron levels in PC12 cells and rat brain tissue. *J Nutr.* 2008;**12**:2487–94.

44. Connor JR, Boyer PJ, Menzies SL, *et al.* Neuropathological examination suggests impaired brain iron acquisition in restless legs syndrome. *Neurology.* 2003;**61**:304–9.

Neuroimaging and fatal familial insomnia

Daniela Perani and Pietro Cortelli

Introduction

The clinical and neuropathology features of fatal familial insomnia (FFI) were first reported in 1986 by Lugaresi *et al.* [1]. Subsequent reports from Lugaresi and his group examined in detail the alterations of the wake/sleep cycle, the dysautonomic and hormonal characteristics, and the neuropsychological traits that clinically typify FFI [2]. In the meantime, Gambetti and his collaborators demonstrated that FFI is a genetic prion disease characterized by a mutation in the prion protein (PrP) gene (*PRNP*), established the neuropathologic features, and defined the peculiar genotype linked to FFI, as well as the characteristics of the protease-resistant scrapie prion protein (PrPSc) present in FFI [3–5]. Additional studies showed that FFI can be transmitted to experimental animals, thus placing FFI within the group of transmissible prion diseases [6].

Currently, FFI has been definitely established as a distinct disease entity with worldwide distribution. It represents the third most frequent hereditary prion disease, and more than 40 apparently unrelated families are known to be affected. Although rare, FFI is an important disease on several accounts: it has widened the phenotypic spectrum of prion diseases, it has led to the discovery of a novel mechanism of phenotypic heterogeneity in human genetic diseases, and it has led to the identification of the two major forms of scrapie PrP in human prion diseases. Moreover, it is the first disease characterized by peculiar alterations in the wake/sleep cycle and other circadian rhythms that, together with the preferential pathological involvement of the dorsomedian and anterior thalamic nuclei, emphasize the role that the limbic portion of the thalamus plays in the regulation of sleep.

FFI therefore represents a disease model for the investigation of the integrative role of the limbic thalamus [7]. This chapter focuses on the neuroimaging alterations in FFI and their pathological correlates.

Genetic and clinical features

FFI is transmitted as an autosomal dominant trait and it is linked to a missense mutation at codon 178 of *PRNP* that results in the substitution of aspartic acid with asparagine in PrP (D178N) [3]. Allele-specific sequencing demonstrated that codon 129 of the PrP gene, the site of a common methionine/

valine polymorphism, is the determinant of the disease phenotypes linked to the D178N mutation. In patients affected by Creutzfeldt–Jakob disease (CJD) linked to the D178N mutation (CJD178), codon 129 located on the mutated allele is valine, whereas in patients with FFI, codon 129 is methionine [4].

Furthermore, because codon 129 located on the normal allele can be either methionine or valine, each of the FFI and CJD178 patient populations comprise patients that are homozygous and patients that are heterozygous at codon 129. The homozygous (Met/Met) FFI patients have on average a shorter disease duration than the heterozygous (Met/Val) patients, whereas the age at onset is not significantly different in the two patient populations [8]. Subsequent studies have shown that disease duration and clinical and pathological features differ in homozygous and heterozygous subjects [9].

FFI is a disorder with onset usually in mid life and it affects males and females equally; mean age of onset is 51 ± 7.1 years but with a range of 36 to 62 years in 14 pathologically verified patients. FFI leads to death within a mean disease course of 18 months (range 8–72 months). Two different disease courses are described, and attributed to the effect of the 129 PRNP codon polymorphism; homozygous subjects (Met/Met) have a short course of the disease (less than 11 months; mean 9.1 months) whereas heterozygous subjects (Met/Val) have a long (more than 11 months; mean 30.8 months) disease duration. Clinical symptoms and signs in FFI patients fall within three major categories: disturbances of wake and sleep, disturbances of autonomic functioning, and sensorimotor abnormalities. Insomnia is often the onset symptom, with patients complaining of unrefreshing sleep and frequent arousals during the night. In the course of the disease, falling asleep and maintaining nocturnal sleep or daytime naps become progressively harder, and sleep may be completely lost, resulting in complete agrypnia (organic insomnia). From disease onset patients also appear apathetic, indifferent to the surroundings, and as insomnia worsens, patients continuously try to sleep with the behavior of somnolence (close their eyes, drop their heads), but they cannot fall asleep. In the course of the disease, patients display additional peculiar oneiric disturbances (oneiric stupor), whereupon "wake" is abruptly interrupted by episodes of dreaming activity, during which patients perform automatic gestures mimicking daily-life activities (dressing, combing

Neuroimaging of Sleep and Sleep Disorders, ed. Eric Nofzinger, Pierre Maquet, and Michael J. Thorpy. Published by Cambridge University Press. © Cambridge University Press 2013.

their hair, drinking, eating, washing hands, manipulating non-existent objects) and are unresponsive to their environment. During the course of the disease, gesturing progressively becomes coarser and interspersed with tremor-like and spontaneous and evoked jerks and patients become confused and have increasing difficulties in reporting any dreaming content. Speech becomes increasingly slurred and weakens to the point of being incomprehensible. Gait becomes more and more uncertain and ultimately impossible unaided. Death is sudden, especially in 129 homozygous patients, or is preceded by an ever-increasing stupor state and an akinetic mutism.

Sleep disturbances are usually associated from the beginning with autonomic alterations, in the form of subtle pyrexia, especially in the evening; increased salivation and diaphoresis; and mild elevation of blood pressure, heart rate, and irregular breathing. Impotence may occur early in males, and sphincter control may be lost in the later stages of the disease, especially in the heterozygous patients. From disease onset there may be episodes of diplopia varying in duration.

Sporadic cases displaying clinical and pathological features indistinguishable from those of FFI have been reported under the term "sporadic fatal insomnia (sFI)." It is notable that little more than ten cases of proven sFI are methionine homozygous at codon 129 [10]. Furthermore, all sFI cases examined have PrPSc in very low amounts, as in FFI. In one case, sFI was transmitted to "humanized" transgenic mice that developed a disease characterized by a PrPSc of 19 kDa as in the human disease and histological lesions similar to those of sFI and FFI [11]. The co-occurrence of both sporadic and genetic forms of FI within the same family was recently described [12].

Laboratory findings

EEG and polysomnography

The electroencephalogram (EEG) background activity becomes progressively flattened and slow and then unreactive and monomorphic in the advanced stages. The periodic activity characteristic of CJD is usually absent throughout the course of FFI, even though bursts of repetitive diffuse 1- to 2-Hz sharp waves may appear in the advanced stages of long duration cases. These bursts are associated with diffuse and partial myoclonus.

The EEG 24-h recordings are characterized by a continuous oscillation between the EEG activity associated with normal, relaxed wakefulness and that associated with desynchronized theta activity. In more advanced stages, EEG patterns typical of synchronized sleep (spindling and delta activity) may be completely absent throughout the 24 h. Patients spend most of the recorded time in a non-wake/non-sleep-like state, characterized by a combination of alpha and theta EEG activity, similar to stage I sleep or better defined as "subwakefulness." Synchronized sleep progressively subsides and sleep spindles and K-complexes are altered and eventually disappear. Rapid eye movement (REM) sleep initially may remain normal or display a pathologically preserved muscle tone on antigravity muscles associated with increased myoclonic activity in limb muscles, similar to the patterns observed during REM sleep

behavior disorder (RBD). Notably, the cyclic organization of sleep is lost, with absence of the orderly transition between sleep stages and abrupt passages between wake and synchronized and REM sleep stages. Unlike synchronized sleep, REM sleep persists until the most advanced disease stages, appearing in isolated or clustered short-lasting (no longer than 20–30 s) episodes and is associated with oneiric behavior. Total sleep time is drastically reduced and sleep efficiency is severely impaired. Actigraphic recordings throughout 52 days in an FFI patient revealed an 80% increase in motor activity. Furthermore, indirect calorimetry in a closed respiratory chamber demonstrated that in this patient the 24-h energy expenditure was increased by an astonishing 60%, which may explain the wasting and emaciation typical of FFI [7].

Autonomic and hormonal findings

Autonomic studies in FFI have shown higher blood pressure and heart rate in the resting state with elevated levels of norepinephrine, which further increase on postural challenge or Valsalva maneuver. Baroreflex pathways remain unimpaired, indicating overall unbalanced autonomic control with preserved parasympathetic function but increased background and stimulated orthosympathetic activity [13]. Sympathetic skin response was abolished and muscle sympathetic nerve activity during resting wakefulness was found abnormally high in a AFFI patient [14]. Circadian rhythms of blood pressure and heart rate are present but with decreasing amplitude of the oscillations, until they disappear entirely in the late stages of the disease. Blood pressure mean values and body core temperature are persistently mildly elevated throughout the 24 h. Plasma cortisol is also persistently high in the presence of remarkably normal or even reduced corticotropin levels. Eventually secondary hypertension develops paralleled by increasing catecholamine levels and heart rate [2]. The nocturnal physiological elevation of somatotropin disappears in parallel with the loss of deep sleep, and prolactin maintains a normal circadian rhythmicity, which is lost only in the final stages of the disease [2]. Melatonin concentrations gradually decrease, showing a circadian oscillation in the early stages of the disease, which is subsequently lost [7]. Moreover, there is an increased sympathergic activation of central origin, associated with hypercortisolism and elevated catecholamine levels. The two- to three fold increases in serum norepinephrine level and the absence of the physiological nocturnal peak of melatonin secretion are the most prominent hormonal markers of the disease [7].

Neuropathology

The neuropathological hallmark of FFI is severe atrophy of the anterior ventral and mediodorsal thalamic nuclei with loss of 80–90% of the neurons and two- to threefold increase in astroglial cells, whereas spongiosis is conspicuously absent. The other thalamic nuclei are less and inconsistently affected. Atrophy of the inferior olives is also commonly found.

The involvement of other brain regions is a function of the disease duration, which, in turn, is largely related to the

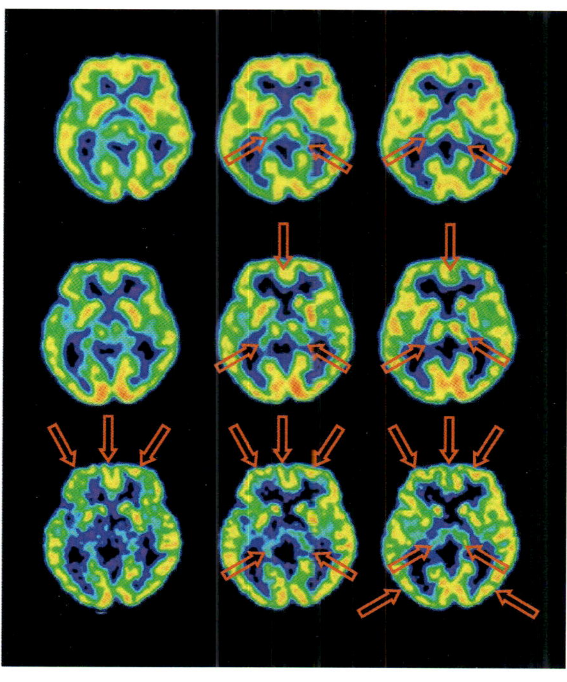

Figure 48.1 ^{18}F-FDG PET scans showing glucose hypometabolism in the thalamus and cingulate cortex as the typical marker in Met/Met homozygous FFI patients in the early phase of the disease, while the involvement of additional brain regions depends on disease duration and heterozygosis Met/Val. PET images represent regional cerebral metabolic rate of glucose consumption (rCMRglu), calculated using the kinetic constants and lumped constant reported by Reivich et al. [40]. (For details see [9].)

genotype at codon 129 of *PRNP*. Although the mesio-orbital frontal cortex and attendant substantia innominata (ventral pallidum and extended amygdala) may show spongiosis also in cases of short duration, the neocortex is affected by spongiosis, gliosis, and to a lesser extent by neuronal loss only in cases with more than 18 months' disease duration. Abundant apoptotic neurons have been found in the brains of FFI patients with a distribution that correlates closely with the distribution of the neuronal loss [15].

Neuroimaging

^{18}F-FDG PET

[18]F-fluorodeoxyglucose (^{18}F-FDG) positron emission tomography (PET) has consistently demonstrated the thalamic hypometabolism as a marker of FFI [9, 15–16, 17] (Figure 48.1). In particular, glucose hypometabolism in the thalamus and cingulate cortex is the typical pattern in Met/Met homozygous patients in the early phase of the disease, while the involvement of additional brain regions depends on disease duration [9].

Heterozygous subjects (Met/Val) with long disease duration usually present a more widespread hypometabolism that in addition to the thalamus involves frontal and other cortical regions (Figure 48.1). Comparison between neuropathological and ^{18}F-FDG PET findings in FFI patients showed that although hypometabolic areas and areas with neuronal loss co-distributed extensively, the hypometabolism was actually more widespread than neuronal loss and significantly correlated with the presence of protease resistant prion protein.

However, the relationship between the topography of PrPSc (prion protein) and neural dysfunction is unclear. First, the familial neurodegenerative diseases usually become symptomatic at mature age although the mutated protein thought to trigger the disease is present from the early stages of brain development. Second, prion diseases may differ from other neurodegenerative diseases in that the mutated protein probably maintains a normal conformation until some time in adulthood, when it changes conformation, converting adjacent PrPSc and ultimately leading to neuronal injury and loss. In FFI, PrPSc appears to be more widespread than suggested by lesions or even areas of hypometabolic function [9]. Furthermore, the magnitude of PrPSc is not correlated with clinical severity, nor does its distribution parallel that of cellular apoptosis [18]. Finally, structures that contain equal amounts of PrPSc (such as the thalamus and brainstem) are differentially vulnerable, the thalamus being much more so. In our published series, all FFI patients show similar amounts of PrPSc in the thalamus and brainstem. However, those whose disease runs a short duration show the least amount and most focal distribution of PrPSc, with the main accumulation being primarily in limbic areas (e.g., entorhinal cortex or the cingulate gyrus) and in subcortical structures (including the thalamus hypothalamus, and brainstem) [9]. With disease of longer duration, the abnormal protein becomes detectable in the cerebral cortex and eventually exceeds the amount observed in subcortical areas. Thus, two interpretations regarding the role of PrPSc are possible. Either PrPSc is not toxic and programmed cell death results from the loss of important signals from the normally protective PRNP, or PrPSc is toxic but different types of neural tissue are differentially vulnerable to it, in ways related to both tissue type and polymorphic status of codon 129.

A puzzling feature that FFI shares with other familial neurodegenerative diseases is that the clinical onset generally occurs at advanced age although the mutation is congenital, leaving an ample interval free of clinical signs during which the pathogenic effect of the mutation is unknown. Thus, two

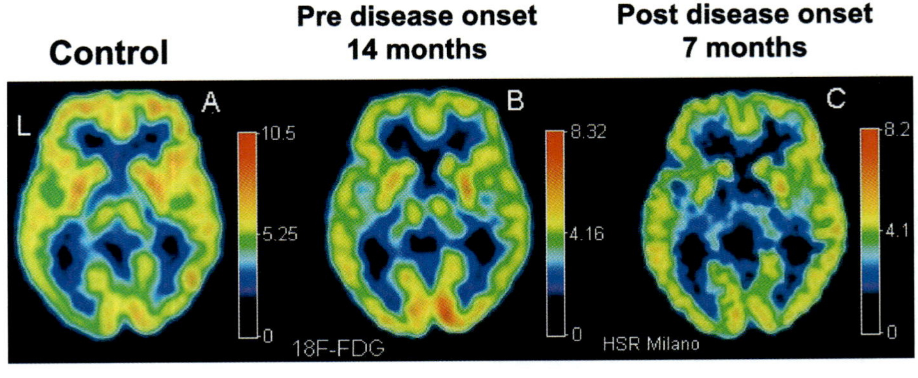

Figure 48.2 ^{18}F-FDG PET quantitative images of rCMRglu in a control and an FFI mutated subject. The ^{18}F-FDG PET findings indicated that the presence of the D178N-129M haplotype has no effect that can be detected even with functional neuroimaging before the disease becomes symptomatic. Only at a short time interval before clinical disease onset (14 months) when spectral analysis demonstrated a significant reduction of the sigma band with respect to the same examination performed 19 months earlier, brain metabolism was reduced in the thalamus (see [16]). OLC = occipital lateral cortex; rCRMglu = regional cerebral glucose consumption.

major unanswered questions concerning familial neurodegenerative diseases are when and where the degenerative process starts. A few serial ^{18}F-FDG PET studies carried out through the presymptomatic Alzheimer's disease, in individuals at risk for Alzheimer's disease because they were carriers of either an Alzheimer's disease pathogenic mutation or the Alzheimer's disease risk factor apolipoprotein E4 [19–23], showed significant changes in cerebral glucose metabolism (rCMRglu) when the carriers were still asymptomatic. Similar observations have been made in Huntington's disease and frontotemporal dementia [24, 25]. In long-lasting serial assessments of brain glucose metabolism with PET and sleep electrophysiology along with detailed clinical evaluations in carriers of the D178N-129M haplotype linked to FFI, who were clinically asymptomatic at the time of the initial evaluation, no abnormalities were detected [16]. The ^{18}F-FDG PET findings indicated that the presence of the D178N-129M haplotype has no effect that can be detected even with functional neuroimaging before the disease becomes symptomatic (Figure 48.2). Combined these findings indicate that tissue impairment, as revealed by impaired metabolism or atrophy, occurs long before the symptomatic onset in many neurodegenerative diseases but not in FFI. This discrepancy probably reflects the rapid course of FFI and other familial prion diseases [26] or the normal functioning of the mutated prion until it changes conformation to become PrPSc and accumulates in sufficient amount as a pathogenic isoform impairing neuronal metabolism and subsequently leading to the neuronal loss as found only at post-mortem examination. In a single case, however, the only detectable effect of the FFI-linked D178N-129M haplotype on brain metabolism was in the thalamus and at a short time interval (between 13 and 21 months) before

clinical disease onset. Noteworthy, at this time, none of the clinical, neurophysiological, and neuropsychological tests performed, including neurological examination, autonomic and neuropsychological evaluations, standard EEG, brain MR, and two night polysomnographic recordings, revealed abnormalities. However, while the macrostructure of sleep was normal, spectral analysis with calculation of the absolute and relative EEG power of the four main bands (delta [SWA 0.5–4.0 Hz], theta [TB. 4.5–8 Hz], alpha [AB 8.5–12 Hz], sigma [SA 12.5–16 Hz]) demonstrated a significant reduction of the sigma band with respect to the same examination performed 19 months earlier. On the other hand, the ^{18}F-FDG PET follow-ups performed in a few subjects after disease onset showed the progressive decrease of rCMRglu that affected specific brain regions: the thalamic metabolism had the worst decrease of 40 and 45% a few months after clinical onset; other patients showed metabolic reductions of 20% and 30% in the limbic cortex and the basal ganglia, respectively.

[11]C]-PK11195 PET

Microglia activation has a key role in the brain's immune response to neurodegeneration. Significant microglia activation was shown in vivo with ^{11}C]-PK11195 PET in patients with various neurodegenerative diseases. Neuroinflammation has been reported in prion disease, but only in post-mortem pathological assessment. In vivo microglia activation has never been investigated in human prion diseases, such as in FFI. It is possible that neuroinflammation has different roles and effects in these conditions.

The expression of the peripheral benzodiazepine receptor (PBR)/18-kDa translocator protein (TSPO) protein, linked to

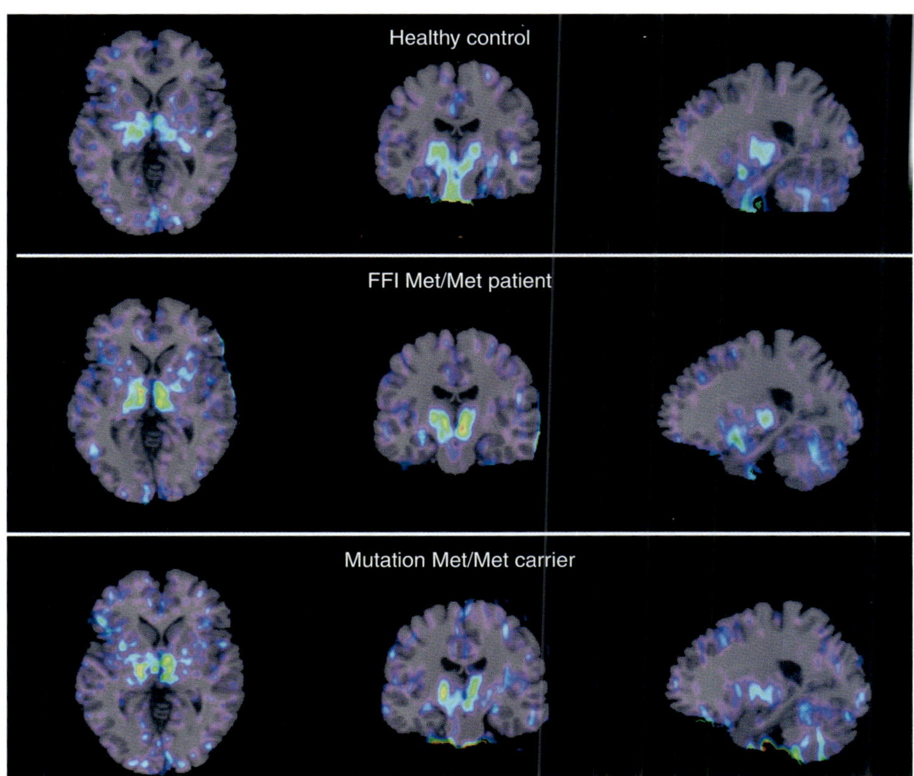

Figure 48.3 The figures show representative [^{11}C]-PK11195 PET slices: no significant changes in [^{11}C]-PK11195 uptake in the FFI patient and mutation carrier compared with the healthy control. Noteworthy, there were no significant increases in regions showing the major pathological changes in FFI (anterior and mediodorsal thalamus, anterior cingulate cortex).

microglia activation, was also assessed in unaffected carriers and one symptomatic case of FFI [27]. We obtained parametric images of [^{11}C]-PK11195 binding potential using simplified reference tissue model and cluster analysis to obtain the input function. There were no significant changes in [^{11}C]-PK11195 uptake in the FFI patient and mutation carriers, when compared with healthy controls (Figure 48.3). Noteworthy, there were no significant [^{11}C]-PK11195 binding potential increases in regions showing the major pathological changes in FFI (anterior and mediodorsal thalamus, anterior cingulate cortex). We suggest that microglia activation shown by post-mortem studies and correlated with the site of neuronal loss might be a late event in the FFI pathological course. The possibility that neuronal loss in prion diseases occurs through an apoptotic process has been postulated, and is consistent with the lack of inflammation in these disorders.

Apoptosis or programmed cell death is a dynamic process, the consequence of activating signals and specific protein synthesis in the dying cell. It differs from necrosis in that it is not accompanied by local inflammation. In FFI patients (but not controls), apoptotic tissue was observed in a distribution and abundance that closely correlated with neuronal loss [18]. The mechanism of apoptosis in FFI is unknown, although a possible cause is the differentiation of microglia into macrophages, which is known to occur following neural damage [28]. This transformation is accompanied by the release of cytotoxins including free oxygen radicals, cytokines, or nitric oxide (NO), which may contribute to both cell death and the gliosis observed in FFI.

[^{11}C] Flumazenil PET

Several PET studies have already successfully used the radioactive ligand [^{11}C] Flumazenil ([^{11}C] FMZ) for the evaluation of gamma-aminobutyric acid type A receptors (GABA$_A$)/benzodiazepine receptor density in the central nervous system. GABA$_A$ receptors imaging with [^{11}C] FMZ and PET has been applied to the study of neurodegenerative disorders for the evaluation of neuronal integrity in vivo. A PET study with [^{11}C] FMZ was employed to examine the density of benzodiazepine receptors in progressive supranuclear palsy, and found a global reduction of [^{11}C] FMZ binding of 13%, with a reduction of benzodiazepine receptor density in the anterior cingulate gyrus of 20%, although no significant changes in the density of receptors were found in the subcortical structures that exhibit the most pathological changes [29]. The density of GABA$_A$/benzodiazepine receptor was also studied in Huntington's disease, showing a significant decrease mainly in the caudate nucleus [30]. A PET study with [^{11}C] FMZ was used to investigate the degree of loss of GABAergic neurons in four types of cerebellar degenerations: multiple system atrophy of the ataxic type (MSAc), multiple system atrophy of the extrapyramidal/autonomic type (MSAp), sporadic olivopontocerebellar atrophy (sOPCA), and dominantly inherited olivopontocerebellar atrophy (dOPCA). This study found significantly decreased ligand influx in the cerebellum and brainstem of patients with MSAc and in patients with sOPCA, but not in patients with MSAp. Despite these differences in ligand influx, benzodiazepine binding was largely preserved in the cerebellar hemispheres, basal ganglia, thalamus, cerebellum,

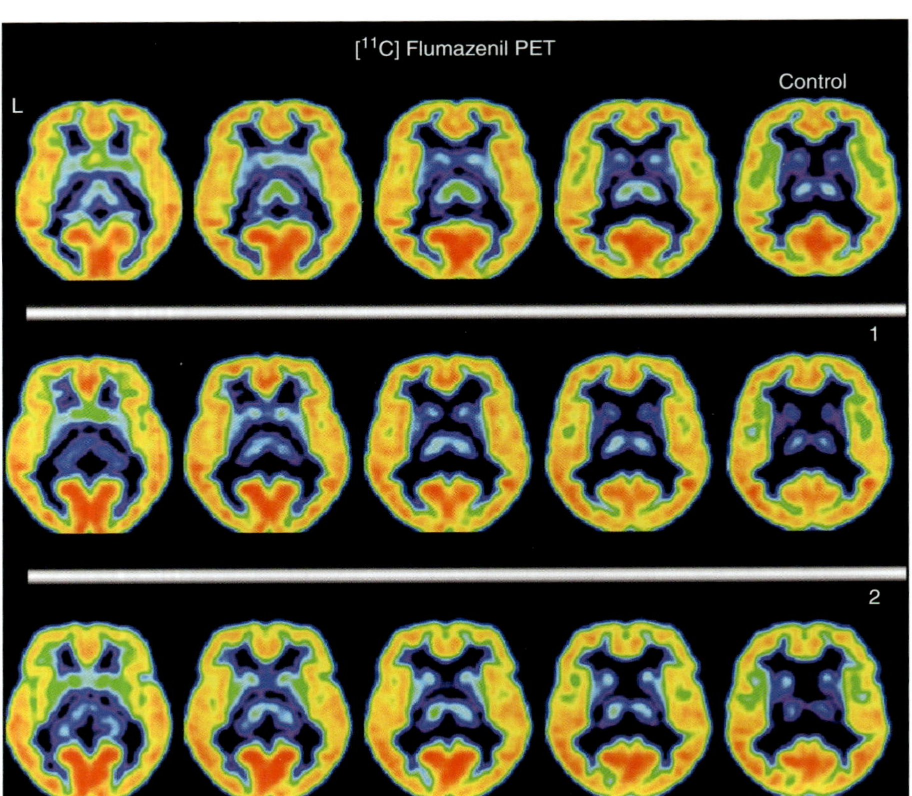

Figure 48.4 [¹¹C]FMZ PET quantitative images representing the GABA$_A$ receptor binding potentials in two twin patients (1 and 2) with very recent FFI diagnosis for evaluation of neuronal integrity in vivo. Consistent with the thalamic hypometabolism that is the typical disease hallmark, the most significant reduction of [¹¹C]FMZ binding potential is present in the thalamus bilaterally. No reductions are revealed in other cortical regions.

and brainstem of all patients [31]. As supportive features, cerebrovascular diseases are also associated with [¹¹C] FMZ binding potential reduction [32, 33].

Loss of the GABAergic neurons has been reported to be the first detectable neuropathological change in experimental models of prion diseases, which features the accumulation of an aberrant isoform of the prion protein [34].

To determine the timing of GABAergic system dysfunction and degeneration and its relationship to PrPSc accumulation during the course of prion disease in FFI, we used the central benzodiazepine receptor ligand [¹¹C] FMZ in two patients with very recent FFI diagnosis. Since coupling of central benzodiazepine receptors to GABA$_A$ receptors, which are widely expressed in cerebral cortical neurons, makes [¹¹C] FMZ a reliable marker of neuronal integrity, we also can obtain a measurement of neuronal loss.

The scenario of initial impairment of neuronal metabolism followed by neuronal death is supported by the present PET study employing [¹¹C] FMZ as a radioligand for the evaluation of neuronal integrity in vivo. Consistent with the thalamic hypometabolism that was the typical disease hallmark in both the cases in the very early phase of the disease, we also found the most significant reduction of [¹¹C] FMZ binding potential in the thalamus bilaterally, particularly in the anterior and dorsolateral thalamic nuclei. This reduction reflects the loss of intrinsic thalamic neurons that is also directly related to the metabolic functional defect confined to this area. No reductions were revealed in other cortical regions, apart from in the anterior cingulated cortex in one case (Figure 48.4).

Whereas CJD, Gerstmann–Sträussler–Scheinker syndrome, and kuru display overlapping clinical and neuropathological features, the clinical presentation and neuropathological hallmarks of FFI significantly differ from all other human prion diseases [35]. Previous studies demonstrated selective neuronal vulnerability of parvalbumin positive (PV1) GABAergic inhibitory interneurons in sporadic CJD and experimental transmissible spongiform encephalopathies (TSEs). In contrast, these neurons are mostly well preserved, or only moderately reduced, in FFI. Only PV1 neurons surrounded by isolectin-B4 positive perineuronal nets were severely affected in TSEs, suggesting a factor residing in this type of extracellular matrix around PV1 neurons as modulator for the selective neuronal vulnerability [34]. Clinically and neuropathologically, FFI clearly differs from all other human TSEs. Tissue pathology in FFI focuses on the thalamus, and there is little or no detectable tissue pathology in the cortex. Surprisingly, FFI shows only moderate (as compared to all other human TSEs in our series) loss of PV1 neurons and neuropil staining in the frontal cortex, which appears to be the only unequivocal diffuse pathological change in the FFI cortex [34, 35]. This moderate loss of cortical PV1 neurons likely accounts for the slight total neuronal cortical loss in FFI. However, this neuronal subset is well preserved in the temporal cortex and adjacent hippocampus, in striking contrast to all other TSE types. This adds another element to the exceptional position of FFI among human TSEs. It is possible that some differences in clinical presentation of FFI, as compared with other TSEs, might be due to the better preservation of PV1 cortical neurons.

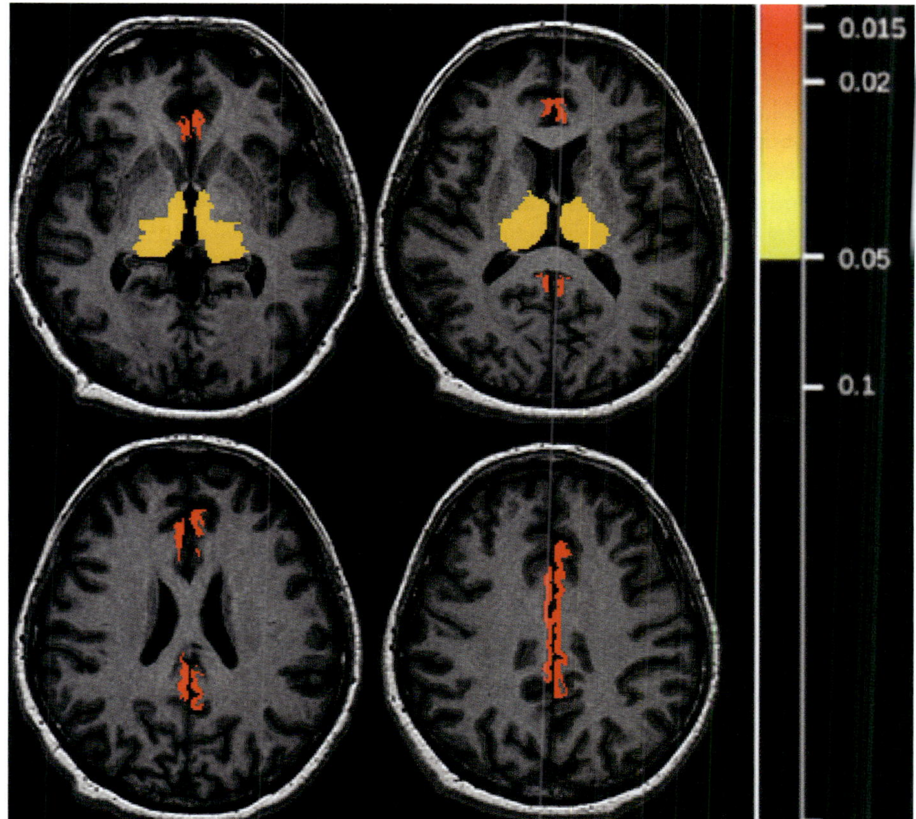

Figure 48.5 The regions of interest for which mean diffusivity value was significantly altered are shown in an FFI patient (D178N-129MM mutation) compared with controls and displayed as p-values (see color scale at right), back projected onto regions of interest selected by FreeSurfer, superimposed on T1 coronal images of the patient. The volumetric-DTI MRI studies were performed in the middle course of the disease (five months after the onset of insomnia disease duration: ten months). The figure highlights a bilateral involvement of the thalamus and cingulate cortex which were the only brain areas out of 14 selected regions of interest that demonstrated a mean diffusivity value significantly outside the distribution of the controls whereas the volume of these and all others structures selected was normal compared with those of the healthy controls. (Data unpublished, courtesy of Professor R. Lodi, University of Bologna, Italy.)

Our results are consistent with neuronal loss in selective brain regions in FFI. Neuropathological data report widespread neuronal loss post-mortem, with the most severe neuronal depletion in the thalamus (anterior and dorsolateral nuclei) [9, 18]. Neuronal loss in the thalamus and connected structures such as the anterior cingulate cortex is an early associated pathological event. We also suggest that both loss of intrinsic neurons containing benzodiazepine receptors and deafferentation of the cerebral cortex from distant brain regions contribute to cerebral cortical hypometabolism in FFI.

MRI diffusion and spectroscopy

FFI is probably the most challenging of TSEs to diagnose because brain lesions are mostly confined to the thalamus. Brain conventional magnetic resonance imaging (MRI) shows no specific changes in familial or sporadic forms of FI [36]. This is in contrast to the high value of brain MRI in the diagnosis of sporadic CJD, where, thanks to the use of FLAIR-T2 and diffusion imaging sequences, specific cortical or basal ganglia signal changes can be detected in 83–100% of definite cases [36, 37]. Considering FFI as a model of thalamic-restricted gliosis, a recent paper demonstrated that multisequences of magnetic resonance detected prion-induced gliosis in vivo that was confirmed by a neuropathologic examination performed only a few days after the radiological examination [38]. In particular, the patient's brain appeared normal on T2-weighted, FLAIR, and diffusion-weighted image sequences. Neither atrophy nor signal alterations were observed, notably not in the thalamus. When the apparent diffusion coefficient (ADC) of water was calculated from DWI data, an increased ADC value in the thalamus compared with at in the control group was revealed, suggesting gliosis. This finding was limited to the thalamus and not in other regions commonly involved in CJD, such as the caudate nucleus.

The proton MR spectroscopic (^{1}H-MRS) study showed a striking increase in the resonance of myo-inositol in the thalamus of the patient when compared with that of control cases, which also strongly indicates gliosis. The other brain regions of the patient evaluated with MRI were normal.

Another study reports a detailed clinical description of FFI in a large patient group, with respect to the M129V genotype [17]. Data on 41 German FFI patients were analyzed. Clinical features, proteins in the cerebrospinal fluid, MRI, ^{18}F-FDG PET, single-photon emission computed tomography (SPECT), polysomnography, and EEG were studied. Autopsy was performed for 21 of the FFI cases. As for the MRI data, general atrophy was found in 73% and thalamic changes in only 5% whereas on ^{18}F-FDG PET thalamic hypometabolism was present in 29%.

Recently, a combined volumetric and DTI MRI evaluation was carried out on a patient with FFI (D178N-129MM mutation) in the middle course of the disease (five months after the onset of insomnia disease duration: ten months). In comparison with healthy subjects, the only abnormality detected was a significant bilateral increase in ADC values in the thalamus and cingulate cortex (Figure 48.5, unpublished data courtesy of

Professor R. Lodi, University of Bologna, Italy) that, in turn, was associated with a normal volume of the same structures. These microstructural changes, similar to those detected in the thalamus of an FFI patient described by Haïk *et al.* [38] and reflecting glial activation and neuronal loss, show a distribution that parallels the findings obtained in FFI patients by ^{18}F-FDG PET studies [9, 15, 16] that found hypometabolic thalami and cingulated cortex as the most consistent metabolic alteration among FFI patients.

Within a large series of patients with clinically sporadic prion disease, a patient with definite FFI (D178N-129MV mutation) scanned 11 months after the onset of the inability to sleep was evaluated using conventional MRI and ^{1}H-MRS

[36]. On MRI, this case, as well as another patient with sFI, showed no brain signal intensity changes or atrophy. On the other hand ^{1}H-MRS performed in the thalamus found, as in other sporadic CJD patients, a severe reduction of the neuronal marker *N*-acetyl aspartate associated with a milder increase in the glial marker myo-inositol [36].

From the little MR data available in the literature [17, 36, 37] it can be concluded that in FFI severe thalamic neuronal loss and gliosis occur in the absence of thalamic or extra thalamic spongiosis which represents the pathological basis of the increased signal intensity in the cortex or basal ganglia detected, on FLAIR-T2 and diffusion-weighted images, in sporadic CJD [39].

References

1. Lugaresi E, Medori R, Montagna P, *et al.* Fatal familial insomnia and dysautonomia with selective degeneration of thalamic nuclei. *Engl J Med.* 1986;**315**(16):997–1003.

2. Montagna P. Fatal familial insomnia and the role of the thalamus in sleep regulation. In: Vinken PJ, Bruyn GW. *Handbook of Clinical Neurology*, Vol. 99. Amsterdam, Elsevier. 2011; 981–96.

3. Medori R, Tritschler HJ, LeBlanc A, *et al.* Fatal familial insomnia, a prion disease with a mutation at codon 178 of the prion protein gene. *Engl J Med.* 1992;**326**(7):444–9.

4. Goldfarb LG, Petersen RB, Tabaton M, *et al.* Fatal familial insomnia and familial Creutzfeldt-Jakob disease: disease phenotype determined by a DNA polymorphism. *Science.* 1992;**258** (5083):806–8.

5. Gambetti P, Petersen R, Monari L, *et al.* Fatal familial insomnia and the widening spectrum of prion diseases. *Br Med Bull.* 1993;**49**(4):980–94.

6. Telling GC, Parchi P, DeArmond SJ, *et al.* Evidence for the conformation of the pathologic isoform of the prion protein enciphering and propagating prion diversity. *Science.* 1996;**274** (5295):2079–82.

7. Montagna P. Fatal familial insomnia: a model disease in sleep physiopathology. *Sleep Med Rev.* 2005;**9**(5):339–53.

8. Montagna P, Cortelli P, Avoni P, *et al.* Clinical features of fatal familial insomnia: phenotypic variability in relation to a polymorphism at codon 129 of the prion protein gene. *Brain Pathol.* 1998;**8**(3):515–20.

9. Cortelli P, Perani D, Parchi P, *et al.* Cerebral metabolism in fatal familial insomnia: relation to duration, neuropathology, and distribution of protease-resistant prion protein. *Neurology.* 1997;**49**(1):126–33.

10. Capellari S, Strammiello R, Saverioni D, Kretzschmar H, Parchi P. Genetic Creutzfeldt-Jakob disease and fatal familial insomnia: insights into phenotypic variability and disease pathogenesis. *Acta Neuropathol.* 2011;**121**(1):21–37.

11. Mastrianni JA, Nixon R, Layzer R, *et al.* Prion protein conformation in a patient with sporadic fatal insomnia. *N Engl J Med.* 1999;**340**(21):1630–8.

12. Capellari S, Parchi P, Cortelli P, *et al.* Sporadic fatal insomnia in a fatal familial insomnia pedigree. *Neurology.* 2008;**70**(11):884–5.

13. Cortelli P, Parchi P, Contin M, *et al.* Cardiovascular dysautonomia in fatal familial insomnia. *Clin Auton Res.* 1991;**1**(1):15–21.

14. Donadio V, Montagna P, Pennisi M, *et al.* Agrypnia Excitata: a microneurographic study of muscle sympathetic nerve activity. *Clin Neurophysiol.* 2009;**120**(6):1139–42.

15. Perani D, Cortelli P, Lucignani G, *et al.* [18F]FDG PET in fatal familial insomnia: the functional effects of thalamic lesions. *Neurology.* 1993;**43** (12):2565–9.

16. Cortelli P, Perani D, Montagna P, *et al.* Pre-symptomatic diagnosis in fatal familial insomnia: serial neurophysiological and ^{18}F-FDG PET studies. *Brain.* 2006;**129**(3):668–75.

17. Krasnianski A, Bartl M, Sanchez Juan PJ, *et al.* Fatal familial insomnia: clinical features and early identification. *Ann Neurol.* 2008;**63**(5):658–61.

18. Gambetti P, Parchi P, Petersen RB, Chen SG, Lugaresi E. Fatal familial insomnia and familial Creutzfeldt-Jakob disease: clinical, pathological and molecular features. *Brain Pathol.* 1995;**5** (1):43–51.

19. Kennedy AM, Frackowiak RSJ, Newman SK, *et al.* Deficits in cerebral glucose metabolism demonstrated by positron emission tomography in individuals at risk of familial Alzheimer's disease. *Neurosci Lett.* 1995;**186**(1):17–20.

20. Fox NC, Warrington EK, Freeborough PA, *et al.* Presymptomatic hippocampal atrophy in Alzheimer's disease. A longitudinal MRI study. *Brain.* 1996;**119** (6):2001–7.

21. Reiman EM, Caselli RJ, Yun LS, *et al.* Preclinical evidence of Alzheimer's disease in persons homozygous for the ε4 allele for apolipoprotein E. *N Engl J Med.* 1996;**334**(12):752–8.

22. Perani D, Grassi F, Sorbi S, *et al.* PET study subjects from two italian FAD families with APP717 val to ileu mutation. *Eur J Neurol.* 1997;**4** (3):214–20.

23. Small GW, Ercoli LM, Silverman DHS, *et al.* Cerebral metabolic and cognitive decline in persons at genetic risk for Alzheimer's disease. *Proc Natl Acad Sci U S A.* 2000;**97**(11):6037–42.

24. Janssen JC, Schott JM, Cipolotti L, *et al.* Mapping the onset and progression of atrophy in familial frontotemporal lobar degeneration. *J Neurol Neurosurg Psychiatry.* 2005;**76**(2):162–8.

25. Kipps CM, Hodges JR. Cognitive assessment for clinicians. *J Neurol Neurosurg Psychiatry.* 2005;**76**(Suppl 1): i22–30.

26. Kong Q, Surewicz WK, Petersen RB, *et al.* Inherited prion diseases. In: Prusiner SB, ed. *Prion Biology and diseases.* New York, Cold Spring Harbor Laboratory Press. 2004; 673–775.

27. Perani D, Garibotto V, Florea I, *et al.* Lack of in vivo microglial activation in fatal familial insomnia as revealed by [11C]–PK11195 PET. *Abstract American Academy of Neurology 61st Annual Meeting,* 2009

28. Dorandeu A, Wingertsmann L, Chretien F, *et al.* Neuronal apoptosis in fatal familial insomnia. *Brain Pathol.* 1998;**8**(3):531–7.

29. Foster NL, Minoshima S, Johanns J, *et al.* PET measures of benzodiazepine receptors in progressive supranuclear palsy. *Neurology.* 2000;**54**(9):1768–73.

30. Künig G, Leenders KL, Sanchez-Pernaute R, *et al.* Benzodiazepine receptor binding in Huntington's disease: [11C]flumazenil uptake measured using positron emission tomography. *Ann Neurol.* 2000;**47** (5):644–8.

31. Gilman S, Koeppe RA, Junck L, *et al.* Benzodiazepine receptor binding in cerebellar degenerations studied with positron emission tomography. *Ann Neurol.* 1995;**38**(2):176–85.

32. Heiss WD, Grond M, Thiel A, *et al.* Permanent cortical damage detected by flumazenil positron emission tomography in acute stroke. *Stroke.* 1998;**29**(2):454–61.

33. Kuroda S, Shiga T, Houkin K, *et al.* Cerebral oxygen metabolism and neuronal integrity in patients with impaired vasoreactivity attributable to occlusive carotid artery disease. *Stroke.* 2006;**37**(2):393–8.

34. Guentchev M, Wanschitz J, Voigtländer T, Flicker H, Budka H. Selective neuronal vulnerability in human prion diseases: fatal familial insomnia differs from other types of prion diseases. *Am J Pathol.* 1999;**155**(5):1453–7.

35. Parchi P, Petersen RB, Chen SG, *et al.* Molecular pathology of fatal familial insomnia. *Brain Pathol.* 1998;**8** (3):539–48.

36. Lodi R, Parchi P, Tonon C, *et al.* Magnetic resonance diagnostic markers in clinically sporadic prion disease: a combined brain magnetic resonance imaging and spectroscopy study. *Brain.* 2009;**132** (10):2669–79.

37. Zerr I, Kallenberg K, Summers DM, *et al.* Updated clinical diagnostic criteria for sporadic Creutzfeldt-Jakob disease. *Brain.* 2009;**132** :2659–68.

38. Haïk S, Galanaud D, Linguraru MG, *et al.* In vivo detection of thalamic gliosis: a pathoradiologic demonstration in familial fatal insomnia. *Arch Neurol.* 2008;**65**(4):545–9.

39. Manners DN, Parchi P, Tonon C, *et al.* Pathological correlates of diffusion MRI changes in Creutzfeldt-Jakob disease. *Neurology* 2009;**72**:1425–31.

40. Reivich M, Alavi A, Wolf A, *et al.* Use of 2-deoxy-D[1–11C]glucose for the determination of local cerebral glucose metabolism in humans: variation within and between subjects. *J Cereb Blood Flow Metab.* 1982;**2**(3):307–19.

Neuroimaging of sleep-related epilepsies

Cheng Luo and Dezhong Yao

Introduction

Epilepsy is a brain disorder characterized by recurrent and unpredictable interruptions of normal brain function. Epileptic seizures result from abnormal paroxysmal brain activity and accompany the clinical manifestations [1]. Although the seizures are unpredictable, some regularity can be discovered in the epilepsy population. For example, some patients have seizures only in their sleep and sleep deprivation can trigger seizures.

The occurrence of seizures during sleep has been noted since antiquity. In 1885, Gowers reported that seizures occurred exclusively at night in one-fifth of patients [2]. Some recent reviews demonstrate that nearly one-third of all patients with epilepsy report a tendency to have seizures during sleep except their diurnal seizures [3, 4]. Nocturnal seizures are considered as a distinct subset of epilepsy, and include Rolandic epilepsy or benign epilepsy with centrotemporal spikes (BECTS), nocturnal frontal lobe epilepsy (NFLE), encephalopathy related to electrical status epilepticus during sleep (ESES), continuous spikes and waves during slow sleep etc. Extensive research reveals that sleep and epilepsy have a complicated interrelationship. Some patients report a higher rate of sleep problems, disturbed daytime behavior, poor-quality sleep, and anxieties about sleeping. Nocturnal seizures disrupt sleep structure, with consequent effects on daytime functioning of patients. On the contrary, the distinct states of sleep (i.e., non-rapid eye movement [NREM] sleep and rapid eye movement [REM] sleep) can influence epileptiform discharges on different levels. Recently, various advanced neuroimaging approaches have been adopted in epilepsy studies. In this chapter, we will focus on the application of neuroimaging approaches in sleep-related epilepsy, to help further understand the pathophysiological investigation of sleep and epilepsy.

These neuroimaging approaches, such as electroencephalography (EEG) and functional magnetic resonance imaging (fMRI), may provide not only a static representation of the patient, such as the structural imaging, but a highly dynamic or evolving entity related to the pathophysiology of illness or treatment interventions. On the other hand, the network of the interconnected brain regions is another issue of hot debate. The findings describe epilepsy on the overall view of brain, and challenge the concept of "localization-related" epilepsy. Furthermore, the brain connectivity may facilitate discovering the cognitive deficits in epilepsy.

Electroencephalography (EEG)

EEG is the most useful diagnostic procedure for epilepsy, and the most general method to diagnose and manage the epileptiform discharges. Likewise, EEG is also the essential element for investigation of the sleep structure. The interictal epileptiform discharge remains the hallmark of epilepsy, vividly demonstrating cortical hyperexcitability and hypersynchrony, and is present in the "normal" interictal state. The presence of an interictal spike helps to confirm a clinical diagnosis of epilepsy, aids in defining the epilepsy syndrome, provides information that assists in planning drug management, and helps to assess candidacy for epilepsy surgery.

In clinical practice, nocturnal seizures are rarely witnessed, and therefore a complete description is often lacking. The video-EEG is a powerful tool to determine when nocturnal seizures occur. Direct observation of epileptic events with video-EEG monitoring provides the ideal method of assessing the episodes. An early study using video-EEG recordings in 100 patients with NFLE showed that NFLE comprises a spectrum of distinct phenomena, different in intensity but representing a continuum of the same epileptic condition. And these clinical characterizations may contribute to understanding the pathogenic mechanisms and different clinical outcomes [5]. The video-EEG polysomnography combines video-EEG monitoring with standard polysomnographic recording, thus providing not only information to permit an accurate determination of sleep stage, but also more epileptic behavioral and discharge information. The approaches based on EEG play a critical role in discovering the relationship between sleep and epileptiform discharges.

Many authors have noted that generalized spike-wave discharges increase during sleep in humans as well as experimental animals [6]. The generalized epileptiform activity is wavelike in nature and may build up as oscillations, which are manifestations of the corticothalamic system. This system is also the main structure responsible for generating sleep oscillations. It comprises the cortical neurons, dorsal thalamic nuclei, and reticular nucleus of the thalamus. The slow oscillations (sleep spindles) in NREM have been found to be intimately associated with the formation of generalized spike-wave discharges. A recent review of the rat model of absence epilepsy suggests that the sleep spindles and the spike-wave discharges are considered as autonomous EEG phenomena and accompanied by different neuronal

Neuroimaging of Sleep and Sleep Disorders, ed. Eric Nofzinger, Pierre Maquet, and Michael J. Thorpy. Published by Cambridge University Press. © Cambridge University Press 2013.

processes and require different neurotransmitters [7]. However, the precise mechanism between the sleep and epileptic discharges is unclear.

Sleep may induce clinical seizures and interictal epileptiform discharges. Sleep activates both focal and generalized spikes in about one-third of all patients [6]. The occurrence of nocturnal seizures is influenced by sleep stage. These are most frequent in stage 2 NREM sleep, followed by stage 1 and stage 3 and 4 NREM sleep, and then REM sleep [6]. The common view of the influence of sleep on epileptiform discharges includes that NREM sleep activates interictal discharges and REM sleep inhibits interictal discharges. Shinnar et al. found that some patients had spike discharges that were only seen during sleep in 347 children with epilepsy [8]. Obtaining an EEG with adequate sleep improves the chances of detecting such discharges. Sleep may alter the morphology of epileptiform discharges. For example, Frost et al. found that compared with wakefulness, spikes seen in NREM sleep were of higher amplitude, longer duration, and less sharp, whereas spikes in REM sleep were of lower amplitude, shorter duration, and increased sharpness [9]. The typical 3 Hz per second spike and slow-wave complexes of children with absence epilepsy are replaced by either single spike-wave discharges or polyspike and wave configuration during sleep. On the other hand, sleep deprivation may increase cerebral irritability, which may result in epileptiform activity [10]. In clinical EEG practice, sleep deprivation becomes established as an activating method to elicit epileptiform activity.

Impairments of cognitive function are frequently reported in patients with epilepsy. Accumulated evidence indicates that specific sleep stages are involved in memory formation and cognitive performances [3]. For example, NREM may enhance and consolidate declarative memories, and REM sleep preferentially supports procedural and emotional memories. Memory disruption has been demonstrated in patients with nocturnal seizures, even in the benign form of epilepsy, such as BECTS. By using questionnaires, memory and phonological awareness difficulties are found in patients with BECTS [11]. Event-related potentials (ERP) were used to investigate cognitive function, and the smallest mismatch negativity to speech stimuli were found in individual patients with atypical BECTS and learning difficulties [12]. The other EEG character, the slope of slow waves during sleep, which is directly related to the degree of synchrony of the firing of cortical neurons [13], may be used to evaluate the cognitive impairment reduced by the epileptiform discharge during sleep. Bolsterli et al. found a significant difference of the slope of slow waves from the first to the last hour of sleep between the patients with ESES and the healthy controls, and speculated that the change in ESES may be associated with the cognitive regressions [14]. Although EEG is considered as the most useful diagnostic tool for epilepsy, it also is valuable to assess cognitive function in sleep-related epilepsy.

may localize abnormal neuronal activity at the origin of epileptiform discharges. Using simultaneous EEG and fMRI to study the human spontaneous NREM sleep, Kaufmann et al. described a specific pattern of decreased brain activity during sleep and suggested that this pattern must be synchronized for establishing and maintaining sleep [16].

EEG and fMRI are complementary imaging techniques, due to their respective strengths and weaknesses in terms of spatial and temporal resolution. Therefore, integrating EEG and fMRI may provide a combined imaging technique with a high level of dynamic temporal information and high spatial resolution [17]. There are three main methods to realize the fusion between EEG and fMRI. One proposed method is an "EEG-informed fMRI" algorithm, which requires the precise onset information of events or blocks such as the onset of epileptiform discharges and details of the actual hemodynamic response function (HRF). An alternative method, the "feature fusion" approach uses independent component analysis (ICA) to simultaneously analyze electromagnetic and hemodynamic data. A spatial pattern derived from fMRI can then be associated with a temporal waveform of EEG according to a common feature. The third approach is to use a statistical parametric map (SPM) obtained from fMRI to improve EEG source estimation. In this approach, SPM information can be used either to constrain the spatial locations of the likely sources of EEG, or to initially seed dipoles within the active regions found in the SPM for further dipole fittings. In addition, we proposed a new method for examining temporally coherent networks (TCNs) using scalp EEG in conjunction with data obtained by fMRI. In this approach, termed NEtwork based SOurce Imaging (NESOI), multiple TCNs derived from fMRI with ICA are used as the covariance priors of the EEG source reconstruction using parametric empirical Bayesian [18].

The potential of combined EEG and fMRI as a tool to explore mechanisms of epileptiform spike and seizure generation has been reviewed elsewhere [15]. One of the earliest studies to report on nocturnal seizures was based on spike triggered fMRI data in a girl with BECTS [19]. The finding showed that the fMRI activation in the ipsilateral face region of the somatosensory cortex in response to the epileptiform activity was consistent with facial sensorimotor involvement of BECTS seizures [19]. Recently, Masterton et al. reported similar localization with activation in association with centro-temporal spikes in BECTS by using EEG/fMRI [20]. A more recent study explored whether sleep-specific activity (sleep spindles, K-complexes, and vertex sharp waves) increase the sensitivity of EEG/fMRI of interictal epileptiform discharges in 11 patients with mono-focal epilepsy during sleep [21]. When considering the sleep-specific activity in SPM, it was possible to increase the statistical significance of the activated voxels inside the expected source of the interictal epileptiform discharge [21]. The sensitivity of EEG/fMRI increases by using the modified model; however, the findings implicate a complex relationship between sleep action and epileptiform discharges.

Simultaneous EEG and fMRI (EEG/fMRI)

Simultaneous EEG and fMRI scanning opens an opportunity to uncover the regions of the brain showing changes in the fMRI signal in response to epileptic spikes seen in the EEG [15]. It

Functional MRI (fMRI)

Functional MRI, which takes advantage of the observation that both blood flow and the ratio of oxy- to deoxyhemoglobin increase with neural activation (dynamic time course on each voxel), is another powerful and non-invasive tool to detect brain function. The main application of fMRI in epilepsy is the detection of cognitive function changes in patients, such as language and memory. Memory is considered to closely associate with the slow oscillations during sleep, i.e., memory consolidation. The epileptiform discharges interfere with the process, for example the nocturnal seizures, or directly relate with the structure related to memory, i.e., hippocampal in temporal lobe epilepsy (TLE).

The impairment of language, memory, or motor function after epileptic surgery, particularly memory impairment in temporal lobe resection, is a topic of great interest. Functional MRI could be used to determine the extent of these functions, and then give a prediction of the likely changes following surgery. In candidates for epilepsy surgery, the Wada test was used to determine language and memory dominance before fMRI. In the Wada test (intracarotid amobarbital test), the portions of one hemisphere supplied by the anterior circulation are transiently anesthetized using a bolus of short-acting amobarbital, allowing the contralateral hemisphere to be assessed independently [22]. The non-invasive fMRI is considered as a method to displace the Wada test. However, the Wada test provides more direct information about language and memory functions. The diagnostic value of fMRI and the Wada test seems to be rather complementary. Killgore *et al.* reported that the method of combined fMRI and the Wada test improved prediction of postoperative seizure control compared with either procedure alone [23].

In previous studies, task-related or resting state fMRI was commonly used to detect memory function in TLE patients. A lesion of the hippocampus, which is considered as a main structure related to memory function, may explain the abnormal findings in fMRI. Memory fMRI studies in mesial TLE have typically shown reduced activity in mesial TLE on the side of seizure onset [24]. Richardson *et al.* used event-related verbal encoding task fMRI to study memory function outcome after surgery in ten TLE patients with left hippocampal sclerosis [25]. Results revealed that fMRI provided the strongest independent predictor for evaluating memory outcome of surgery, and implicated the fMRI data in the high positive predictive value for memory decline individually [25]. Language fMRI is another application for patients with epilepsy. The language task may be relatively simpler than memory. Typically, participants will perform a task related to language in the fMRI scanner, such as a verb generation task, in which the participants are asked to generate an appropriate verb or noun as a response to the target displaying on the screen. In general, language function has left lateralization in normal subjects. However, using language fMRI, patients with left mesial TLE showed less left lateralization than other left-onset focal epilepsy patients [26] and also showed weaker functional connectivity between language network regions than normal individuals [27]. Abnormal lateralization of language function to the right in left mesial TLE patients correlated with the frequency of epileptiform discharges [28] and may correlate with mixed or left handedness [29].

Structural MRI

Structural MRI is widely adopted in clinical practice to detect lesions in brain and diagnose illness with MRI signs. Abnormalities in brain, including hippocampal sclerosis, malformation of cortical development, focal cortical dysplasia, tumors, brain trauma, etc., are associated with epilepsy. On the other hand, some patients with epilepsy are characterized by absence of structural, inflammatory, or metabolic brain lesions, and are designated "idiopathic." By using high-resolution T1 imaging or diffusion MRI, more and more reports have demonstrated the MRI abnormalities in patients with "idiopathic" or "benign" epilepsy, such as BECTS and idiopathic generalized epilepsy [30]. Although, these structural abnormalities are also found in some patients with sleep-related epilepsy, i.e. BECTS and ESES, no specific structural change was directly correlated to in the sleep-related epilepsy.

Even if structural MRI is unnecessary in BECTS, it is often performed before a specific diagnosis has been reached. Gelisse *et al.* reported that structural neuroimaging was abnormal in 14.8% of patients with BECTS in large samples (98 cases) [31]. In another group case (25 cases) study, Boxerman *et al.*, found that at least one abnormality was detected in 52% of BECTS patients by using brain structural MRI, suggesting that the routine brain MRI abnormalities were common in BECTS [32]. Recently, Sarkis *et al.* found that the prevalence of abnormalities in BECTS is 27% [33]. Additionally, hippocampal abnormalities were also found on the MRIs in BECTS, and they were almost ipsilateral to the main EEG findings [34]. Thus, it may be of interest to consider the function of an abnormal hippocampus in epileptogenesis, and especially its relation to epilepsy arising from the Sylvian cortex. A more recent study explored serial changes in frontal and prefrontal lobe volumes using three-dimensional MRI in patients with BECTS [35]. The findings suggest that longer active seizure periods, such as frequent spike waves coupled with the occurrence of frequent seizures in patients with BECTS, may be associated with prefrontal lobe growth disturbance, which relates to neuropsychological problems [35]. Although the prevalence and location of brain lesion in BECTS is variable in different studies, these abnormalities are non-specific for BECTS, and rarely Rolandic in location. The relationship between the lesion in the brain and the centro-temporal spikes requires additional study.

Diffusion tensor imaging (DTI), which quantifies the diffusion of water and characterizes the degree and direction of anisotropy, is another powerful tool of structural MRI. In epilepsy, DTI has been used to localize the epileptic foci and white matter tracts. Diffusion abnormalities have been found to lateralize in mesial TLE [36] and refractory partial epilepsy [37]; hence DTI may provide limited independent information beyond these more conventional measures. DTI data can be used to infer the presence, direction, and integrity of white matter tracts in the brain. Using DTI to tract white matter, we found that structural connectivity was significantly decreased between the posterior cingulate cortex/precuneus and bilateral medial temporal lobes in TLE patients [38]. Recently, Wang *et al.* used DTI to investigate the diffusion property in frontal lobe epilepsy, as characterized by brief, recurring seizures that arose in the frontal lobes of the brain while the patient was sleeping. Decreased fractional anisotropy (FA) was found in the frontal lobes and thalamus in patients with frontal lobe epilepsy compared with controls. The abnormalities in the frontal lobe white matter and the thalamus are considered to contribute to cognitive impairment in patients with frontal lobe epilepsy [39].

Brain networks

Human brain function is thought to rely on two principles of functional specialization and integration. Functional integration is implemented by the complex and reciprocal neural networks in the brain. Brain networks have been depicted in terms of functional connectivity by EEG, magnetoencephalography (MEG), and fMRI, and in terms of structural connectivity by DTI and morphological studies. The analysis of functional and structural connectivity networks provides new avenues for assessing complex network properties of healthy and diseased brain. Indeed, altered brain network topology has been shown in several psychiatric and neurological diseases.

For more than a decade, fMRI has been applied in the field of neuroscience to help us understand the brain network. Using correlation analysis, Biswal et al. first reported the correlated connectivity pattern of the spontaneous blood oxygen level-dependent (BOLD) signal in the motor system [40]. Since then, several analysis tools, such as independent component analysis, cluster analysis, etc., have been applied to fMRI data. Up to now, it has been suggested that at least 10 to 12 resting state functional networks (RSNs) can be detected from the brain cortex in fMRI. The fMRI data sets resulting from the task-related design or resting state are used to construct the brain network. Assessing functional connectivity in brain networks may allow for identification of more fundamental abnormalities underlying disease. Using resting state fMRI, Bettus et al. studied basal functional connectivity within the temporal lobes in eight patients with mesial TLE. The findings demonstrated decreased basal functional connectivity within epileptogenic networks but increased concomitant contralateral connectivity, possibly reflecting compensatory mechanisms [41]. This is the first resting state fMRI study to investigate the functional connectivity in epileptogenic networks in epilepsy [41]. Waites et al. evaluated the language functional network in TLE on the language task-related and resting state fMRI data, and found reduced connectivity at the language area in left TLE. These findings may reflect a disturbance of the language network during resting state in patients, which may be related to subtle language difficulties in the patient population [27]. Recently, using resting state fMRI on 18 mesial TLE patients, we built a functional brain network within 90 cortical and subcortical nodes. The findings suggested altered small-world properties in patients, along with a smaller degree of connectivity, smaller absolute clustering coefficients, and shorter absolute path length [42]. Recent network analyses have revealed that several distributed brain networks are involved in the genesis and manifestation of idiopathic generalized epilepsy based on the fMRI [43, 44].

An extension of functional connectivity, called functional network connectivity (FNC), has been developed. FNC is powerful in characterizing distributed changes in the brain by examining the interactions among different RSNs. Jafri and his colleagues conducted FNC analysis in schizophrenia, and found significant differences between patients and controls, suggesting deficiencies in cortical processing in patients [45]. Recently, in order to investigate the functional connectivity inter- and intra-RSNs in patients with partial epileptic seizures, we selected eight RSNs and conducted a systematical RSN analysis in a cohort of partial epilepsy patients and healthy controls. By dividing the eight RSNs into three subsystems, we found that intra-system connections were preserved for all the three subsystems, while the lost connections were confined to intersystem connections (Figure 49.1). These findings, in which the intra-system connections were preserved for all the three subsystems while the lost connections were confined to intersystem connections in patients with partial epilepsy, might suggest that decreased resting state functional connectivity and disconnection of FNC are two remarkable characteristics of partial epilepsy [46]. In our preliminary study, we also assessed the FNC among 10 RSNs in patients with BECTS with nocturnal seizures, 10 patients with BECTS (8 right, 2 left), and 12 controls. Then ten RSNs were selected to estimate the FNC in two subjects, among which some networks were related to primary perceptional function, including the lateral part of the visual network, the medial part of the visual network, the occipital visual network, the auditory network, and the sensorimotor network while others were higher level cognition networks, including the self-referential network, default mode network, dorsal attention network, and ventral attention network. The basal ganglia network appeared to be an important intermediary for modulation between sensory and higher level cognitive processing. The hierarchical disconnections of FNC (between the perceptional level and cognitive level) were also found in BECTS (Figure 49.2). The selective impairment of FNC had an important functional and theoretical implication in that it was unsuitable to understand the partial epilepsy only from a global or local view.

The brain network can be constructed on the structural MRI data. He et al. investigated large-scale anatomical connection patterns of the human cerebral cortex using cortical thickness measurements from MRI [47]. A recent study has derived whole-brain networks from volumetric data and obtained network measures (cortical thinning characteristic) in patients with TLE [48]. The network features were used to classify a given MRI scan into TLE or normal, and additional summary statistics related to the extent and spread of the disease were obtained. The proposed network approach improved classification accuracy (control and TLE) from 78% for non-network classifiers to 93% [48]. Meanwhile, the white matter tractography resulting from DTI was also used to describe the edge of the network. Hagmann et al. non-invasively mapped white matter pathways within and across cortical hemispheres in individual human participants and identified the core within the cortex with spatial and topological centrality [49]. Zhang et al. used the resting state fMRI signal correlations and DTI tractography to generate functional and structural connectivity networks in 26 idiopathic generalized epilepsy patients with tonic-clonic seizures [50]. Results showed that the patients

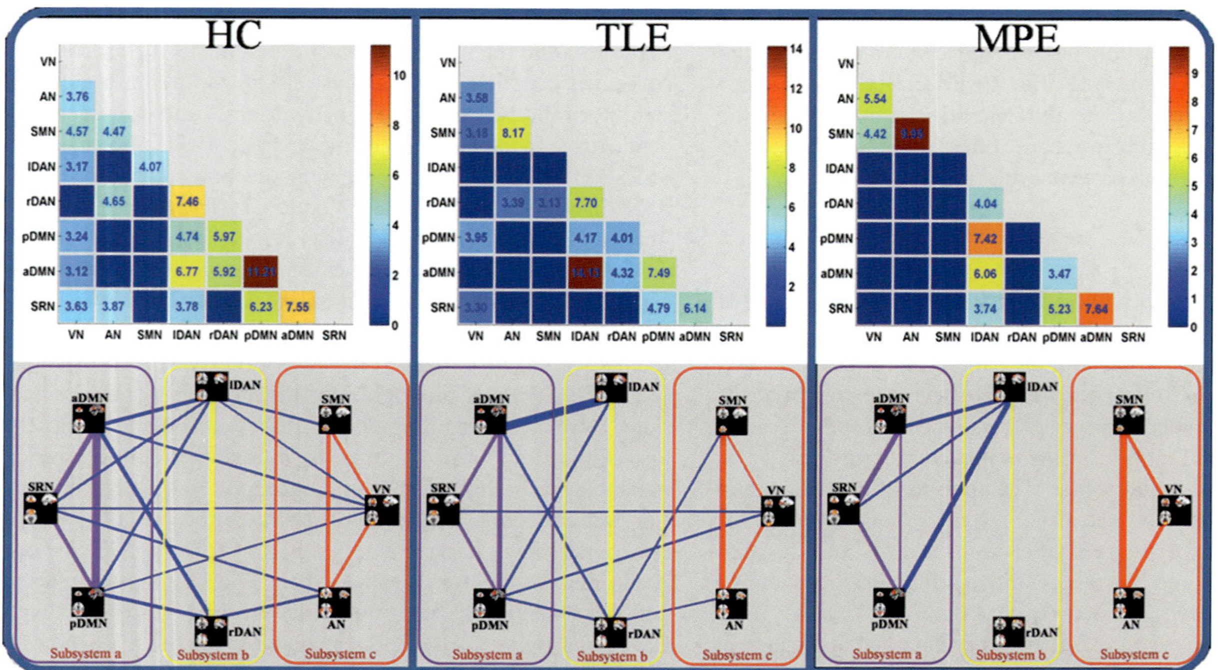

Figure 49.1 Correlation matrices representing results of FNC analysis for healthy control (HC, left), temporal lobe epilepsy (TLE, middle), and mixture partial epilepsy (MPE, right). Eight RSNs were identified by ICA, and used to assess the FNC in the three groups. Significant connections (P < 0.05 FDR-corrected) were marked by corresponding T values at upper of the figure. The network map was showed at the bottom of the figure. Three subsystems: (a) these RSNs (in the purple rectangle) related to information integration and modulation including the posterior part of the default mode network (pDMN), the anterior part of the default mode network (aDMN), and the self-referential network (SRN); (b) these RSNs (in the yellow rectangle) related to higher level cognition including the left dorsal attention network (lDAN) and right dorsal attention network (rDAN); (c) these RSNs (in the red rectangle) related to primary perceptual function including the sensorimotor network (SMN), visual network (VN), and auditory network (AN). The intensity of the temporal dependency between RSNs was indicated by the thickness of the corresponding line. (Reproduced from Luo *et al.* [46].) with permission.)

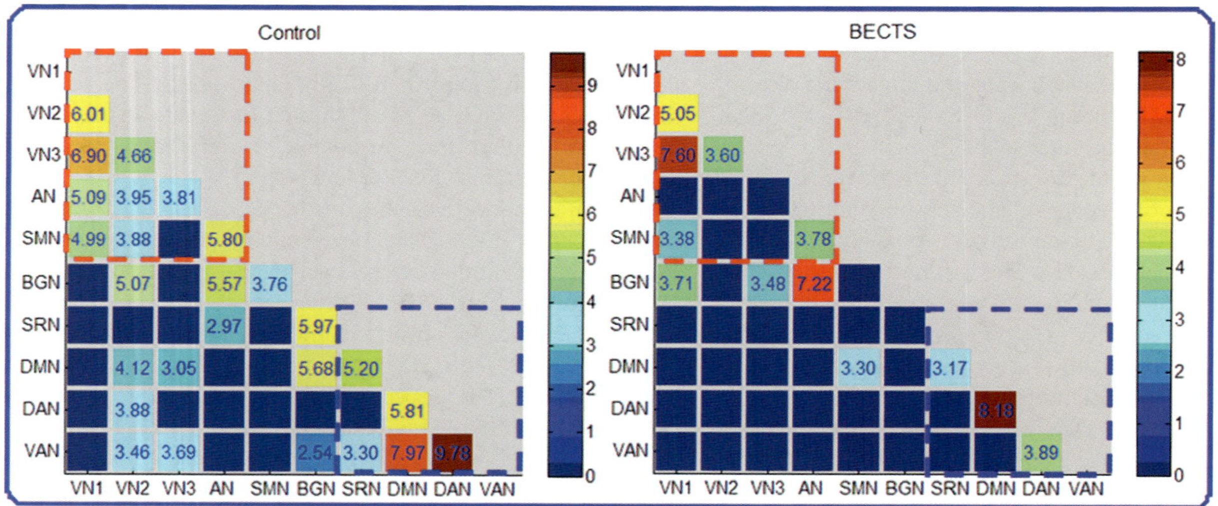

Figure 49.2 FNC (functional network connectivity) analysis for 12 controls (left) and 10 BECTS (right). Significant connections (p < 0.05 FDR-corrected) were marked by corresponding T-values (color bars). The networks (in the red dotted rectangle) related to primary function included the lateral part of the visual network (VN1), the medial part of the visual network (VN2), the occipital visual network (VN3), the auditory network (AN), and the sensorimotor network (SMN). The networks (in the blue dotted rectangle) related to higher level cognition included the self-referential network (SRN), default mode network (DMN), dorsal attention network (DAN), and ventral attention network (VAN). The basal ganglia network (BGN) was suggested as an important intermediary for modulation between sensory and higher level cognitive processing.

lost optimal topological organization in both functional and structural connectivity networks, and the degree of coupling between functional and structural connectivity networks was decreased [50].

Conclusion

Currently, neuroimaging research on epilepsy is vigorous and thriving, along with an eagerness to adopt new methods. However, there are relatively few studies focused on sleep and epilepsy. Obviously, the relationship between sleep and epilepsy is a complicated one. This complexity mainly lies in two aspects: one is the ambiguous electro-biological mechanism between the sleep activity and generalized epileptiform discharges, such as the relationship between spindle and generalized spike wave discharge; the other is the complex relationship between the nocturnal seizures and sleep structure. Simultaneous EEG and fMRI, and brain network approaches along with data acquisition during sleep in patients with epilepsy will be powerful means to evaluate these complicated relationships in the future.

Acknowledgement

This study was supported by the National Natural Science Foundation of China (Nos. 81071222, 81271547, 31170953), the 973 project 2011CB707803, and the PCSIRT and "111" project.

References

1. Engel J. A proposed diagnostic scheme for people with epileptic seizures and with epilepsy: report of the ILAE Task Force on Classification and Terminology. *Epilepsia*. 2001;**42**:796–803.

2. Gower WR. *Epilepsy and Other Chronic Convulsive Disease*, Vol. 1. London, William Wood, 1885.

3. Parisi P, Bruni O, Pia Villa M, *et al*. The relationship between sleep and epilepsy: the effect on cognitive functioning in children. *Dev Med Child Neurol*. 2010;**52**:805–10.

4. Sinha SR. Basic mechanisms of sleep and epilepsy. *J Clin Neurophysiol*. 2011;**28**:103–10.

5. Provini F, Plazzi G, Tinuper P, *et al*. Nocturnal frontal lobe epilepsy. A clinical and polygraphic overview of 100 consecutive cases. *Brain*. 1999;**122**(Pt 6):1017–31.

6. Kotagal P, Yardi N. The relationship between sleep and epilepsy. *Semin Pediatr Neurol*. 2008;**15**:42–9.

7. Sitnikova E. Thalamo-cortical mechanisms of sleep spindles and spike-wave discharges in rat model of absence epilepsy (a review). *Epilepsy Res*. 2010;**89**:17–26.

8. Shinnar S, Kang H, Berg AT, *et al*. EEG abnormalities in children with a first unprovoked seizure. *Epilepsia*. 1994;**35**:471–6.

9. Frost JD, Hrachovy RA, Glaze DG, *et al*. Sleep modulation of interictal spike configuration in untreated children with partial seizures. *Epilepsia*. 1991;**32**:341–6.

10. Rodin EA, Luby ED, Gottlieb JS. The electroencephalogram during prolonged experimental sleep deprivation. *Electroencephalogr Clin Neurophysiol*. 1962;**14**:544–51.

11. Northcott E, Connolly AM, Berroya A, *et al*. Memory and phonological awareness in children with Benign Rolandic Epilepsy compared to a matched control group. *Epilepsy Res*. 2007;**75**:57–62.

12. Metz-Lutz MN, Filippini M. Neuropsychological findings in Rolandic epilepsy and Landau-Kleffner syndrome. *Epilepsia*. 2006;**47**(Suppl 2): 71–5.

13. Vyazovskiy VV, Olcese U, Lazimy YM, *et al*. Cortical firing and sleep homeostasis. *Neuron*. 2009;**63**:865–78

14. Bolsterli BK, Schmitt B, Bast T, *et al*. Impaired slow wave sleep downscaling in encephalopathy with status epilepticus during sleep (ESES). *Clin Neurophysiol*. 2011;**122**:1779–87.

15. Gotman J, Kobayashi E, Bagshaw AP. *et al*. Combining EEG and fMRI: a multimodal tool for epilepsy research. *J Magn Reson Imaging*. 2006;**23**:906–20.

16. Kaufmann C, Wehrle R, Wetter TC, *et al*. Brain activation and hypothalamic functional connectivity during human non-rapid eye movement sleep: an EEG/fMRI study. *Brain*. 2006;**129**:655–67.

17. Laufs H, Daunizeau J, Carmichael DW, *et al*. Recent advances in recording electrophysiological data simultaneously with magnetic resonance imaging. *Neuroimage*. 2008;**40**:515–28.

18. Lei X, Xu P, Luo C, *et al*. fMRI functional networks for EEG source imaging. *Hum Brain Mapp*. 2011;**32**:1141–60.

19. Archer JS, Briellman RS, Abbott DF, *et al*. Benign epilepsy with centro-temporal spikes: spike triggered fMRI shows somato-sensory cortex activity. *Epilepsia*. 2003;**44**:200–4.

20. Masterton RA, Harvey AS, Archer JS, *et al*. Focal epileptiform spikes do not show a canonical BOLD response in patients with benign rolandic epilepsy (BECTS). *Neuroimage*. 2010;**51**:252–60.

21. Moehring J, Coropceanu D, Galka A, *et al*. Improving sensitivity of EEG-fMRI studies in epilepsy: the role of sleep-specific activity. *Neurosci Lett*. 2011;**505**:211–15.

22. Wada J, Rasmussen T. Intracarotid injection of sodium amytal for the lateralization of cerebral speech dominance. *J Neurosurg*. 1960;**17**:266–82.

23. Killgore WD, Glosser G, Casasanto DJ, *et al*. Functional MRI and the Wada test provide complementary information for predicting post-operative seizure control. *Seizure*. 1999;**8**:450–5.

24. Richardson MP. Strange BA, Duncan JS, *et al*. Preserved verbal memory function in left medial temporal pathology involves reorganisation of function to right medial temporal lobe. *Neuroimage*. 2003;**20**(Suppl 1):S112–19.

25. Richardson MP, Strange BA, Thompson PJ, *et al*. Pre-operative verbal memory fMRI predicts post-operative memory decline after left temporal lobe resection. *Brain*. 2004;**127**:2419–26.

26. Weber B, Wellmer J, Reuber M, *et al*. Left hippocampal pathology is associated with atypical language lateralization in patients with focal epilepsy. *Brain*. 2006;**129**:346–51.

27. Waites AB, Briellmann RS, Saling MM, *et al*. Functional connectivity networks are disrupted in left temporal lobe epilepsy. *Ann Neurol*. 2006;**59**:335–43.

28. Janszky J, Mertens M, Janszky I, *et al*. Left-sided Interictal Epileptic Activity Induces Shift of Language Lateralization in Temporal Lobe Epilepsy: An fMRI Study. *Epilepsia*. 2006;**47**:921–7.

29. Sveller C, Briellmann RS, Saling MM, *et al*. Relationship between language lateralization and handedness in left-hemispheric partial epilepsy. *Neurology*. 2006;**67**:1813–17.

30. Luo C, Xia Y, Li Q, *et al.* Diffusion and volumetry abnormalities in subcortical nuclei of patients with absence seizures. *Epilepsia.* 2011;**52**:1092–9.

31. Gelisse P, Corda D, Raybaud C, *et al.* Abnormal neuroimaging in patients with benign epilepsy with centrotemporal spikes. *Epilepsia.* 2003;**44**:372–8.

32. Boxerman JL, Hawash K, Bali B, *et al.* Is Rolandic epilepsy associated with abnormal findings on cranial MRI? *Epilepsy Res.* 2007;**75**:180–5.

33. Sarkis R, Wyllie E, Burgess RC, *et al.* Neuroimaging findings in children with benign focal epileptiform discharges. *Epilepsy Res.* 2010;**90**:91–8.

34. Lundberg S, Eeg-Olofsson O, Raininko R, *et al.* Hippocampal asymmetries and white matter abnormalities on MRI in benign childhood epilepsy with centrotemporal spikes. *Epilepsia.* 1999;**40**:1808–15.

35. Kanemura H, Hata S, Aoyagi K, *et al.* Serial changes of prefrontal lobe growth in the patients with benign childhood epilepsy with centrotemporal spikes presenting with cognitive impairments/behavioral problems. *Brain Dev.* 2010;**33**:106–13.

36. Goncalves Pereira PM, Oliveira E, Rosado P. Apparent diffusion coefficient mapping of the hippocampus and the amygdala in pharmaco-resistant temporal lobe epilepsy. *AJNR Am J Neuroradiol.* 2006;**27**:671–83.

37. Chen Q, Lui S, Li CX, *et al.* MRI-negative refractory partial epilepsy: role for diffusion tensor imaging in high field MRI. *Epilepsy Res.* 2008;**80**:83–9.

38. Liao W, Zhang Z, Pan Z, *et al.* Default mode network abnormalities in mesial temporal lobe epilepsy: a study combining fMRI and DTI. *Hum Brain Mapp.* 2011;**32**:883–95.

39. Wang XQ, Lang SY, Hong LU, *et al.* Changes in extrafrontal integrity and cognition in frontal lobe epilepsy: a diffusion tensor imaging study. *Epilepsy Behav.* 2011;**20**:471–7.

40. Biswal B, Yetkin FZ, Haughton VM, *et al.* Functional connectivity in the motor cortex of resting human brain using echo-planar MRI. *Magn Reson Med.* 1995;**34**:537–41.

41. Bettus G, Guedj E, Joyeux F, *et al.* Decreased basal fMRI functional connectivity in epileptogenic networks and contralateral compensatory mechanisms. *Hum Brain Mapp.* 2009;**30**:1580–91.

42. Liao W, Zhang Z, Pan Z, *et al.* Altered functional connectivity and small-world in mesial temporal lobe epilepsy. *PloS One* 2010;**5**:e8525.

43. Luo C, Li QF, Lai YX, *et al.* Altered functional connectivity in default mode network in absence epilepsy: a resting-state fMRI study. *Hum Brain Mapp.* 2011;**32**:438–49.

44. Luo C, Li QF, Xia Y, *et al.* Resting state Basal ganglia network in idiopathic generalized epilepsy. *Hum Brain Mapp.* 2012;**33**:1279–94.

45. Jafri MJ, Pearlson GD, Stevens M, *et al.* A method for functional network connectivity among spatially independent resting-state components in schizophrenia. *Neuroimage.* 2008;**39**:1666–81.

46. Luo C, Qiu C, Guo ZW, *et al.* Disrupted functional brain connectivity in partial epilepsy: a resting-state fMRI study. *PloS One.* 2011;**7**:e28196.

47. He Y, Chen ZJ, Evans AC. Small-world anatomical networks in the human brain revealed by cortical thickness from MRI. *Cereb Cortex.* 2007;**17**:2407–19.

48. Raj A, Mueller SG, Young K, *et al.* Network-level analysis of cortical thickness of the epileptic brain. *Neuroimage.* 2010;**52**:1302–13.

49. Hagmann P, Kurant M, Gigandet X, *et al.* Mapping human whole-brain structural networks with diffusion MRI. *PLoS One.* 2007;**2**:e597.

50. Zhang Z, Liao W, Chen H, *et al.* Altered functional-structural coupling of large-scale brain networks in idiopathic generalized epilepsy. *Brain.* 2011;**134**:2912–28.

Sleep, neuroimaging, and polysomnography of Wilson's disease

Sanjib Sinha and A. B. Taly

Introduction

Involuntary movements dominate the clinical profile in patients with Wilson's disease (WD) but nearly one-third of these patients also have psychiatric and behavioral abnormalities [1]. The pathological changes in the brain in WD are widespread and include areas involved in the regulation of sleep. Patients with WD have documented neuroanatomical, pathophysiological, and neurochemical basis for sleep disturbances [2–5]. In a questionnaire-based study, Portala *et al.* observed more frequent sleep abnormalities among patients of WD compared to the reference group [5].

Archana *et al.* [6, 7] evaluated the frequency and nature of sleep abnormalities using questionnaires and polysomnography (PSG) in 25 patients with WD (males: 18, age: 24.4 ± 9.25 years) compared with 25 healthy controls (all males; age 33.1 ± 9.7 years). Sleep questionnaires detected abnormalities in 16 patients and 8 controls. On the Pittsburgh Sleep Quality Index (PSQI), 15 patients had abnormal PSQI scores (>5) compared to 6 controls and mean PSQI score was significantly higher among patients ($p = 0.03$). Evaluation with the Epworth Sleepiness Scale (ESS) showed excessive daytime sleepiness (>10/24) in three patients and two controls. PSG detected sleep abnormalities in all the patients and 24 controls. However, patients had significantly reduced total sleep-time ($p = 0.001$), decreased sleep efficiency ($p = 0.001$), increased sleep onset latency ($p = 0.05$), and latency to stage 2 ($p = 0.02$), reduced deep sleep% – stage 3/4 ($p = 0.01$), and reduced rapid eye movement (REM) sleep% ($p = 0.04$). Correlation of PSG observations with phenotype revealed males had significantly more often bradycardia, both during awake ($p = 0.002$) and sleep ($p = 0.03$). Patients < 20 years had frequent tachycardia ($p = 0.01$), higher periodic limb movement (PLM) index ($p = 0.01$) and increased PLMs ($p = 0.01$) in non-rapid eye movement (NREM) sleep, and lesser REM sleep% ($p = 0.05$). Patients on de-coppering therapy had prolonged REM onset latency ($p = 0.03$) and mixed apnea events ($p = 0.04$). The isolated limb movement index in REM sleep was less in those with milder disease ($p = 0.05$) and without anticonvulsants ($p = 0.03$). We present the sleep profile in one of the patients with WD evaluated with MRI, sleep questionnaires, and PSG.

Patient description

Ms. K, an 18-year-old woman was first evaluated at our center at the age of 11 years for dystonia of limbs, bradykinesia, rigidity, seizures, and dysarthria of two-year duration. She had a history of brief-lasting jaundice (acute hepatitis) in the past. A diagnosis of WD was established based on the presence of Kayser–Fleischer (KF) ring, low serum ceruloplasmin (4 mg/dl) and serum total copper (12 µg/dl) levels, and elevated 24-h urinary excretion (250 mg/24 h). With de-coppering therapy (zinc and penicillamine), she had made substantial improvement. She did have brief periods of emotional disturbances during the course of the illness. There was no recurrence of seizures and she is currently off antiepileptic drugs. Liver function tests were normal and ultrasound examination did not reveal any evidence of cirrhosis. Currently, she has dysarthria and lower limb dystonia while walking. Magnetic resonance imaging (MRI) of the brain revealed diffuse cerebral atrophy, T2-weighted (T2 W) and FLAIR hyper intensity of putamen and thalami, and pallidal T2 W hypo intensity (Figure 50.1).

The ESS score was 9 while PSQI was 8, suggesting poor nighttime sleep quality. The PSG revealed decreased sleep efficiency. She exhibited increased REM sleep latency and overall reduction of REM sleep. Other parameters were within normal limits (Table 50.1). Figure 50.2 provides PSG records of four patients with WD.

Sleep profile in WD

While sleep abnormalities have been reported in a wide variety of extrapyramidal disorders, they are expected and reported in patients with WD; nevertheless further well-designed studies among patients with WD are important for a better understanding, and possible improvement with de-coppering therapy.

Questionnaires-based assessment

In our study significantly more patients with WD had higher scores when compared with controls (global PSQI index >5 in 15/25 patients and 5/25 controls, $p = 0.03$). Even though there was no significant difference between cases and controls in sleep quality and the onset latency, significantly more patients slept for less time (<6 h) (24% cases vs 0% control) and had poor

Neuroimaging of Sleep and Sleep Disorders, ed. Eric Nofzinger, Pierre Maquet, and Michael J. Thorpy. Published by Cambridge University Press. © Cambridge University Press 2013.

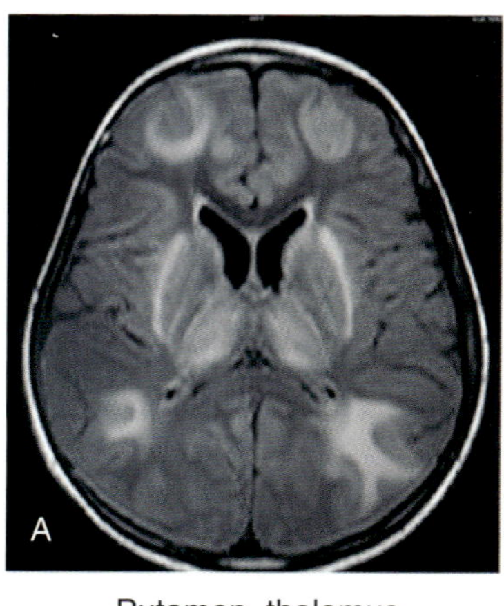

Putamen, thalamus,
subcortical white matter

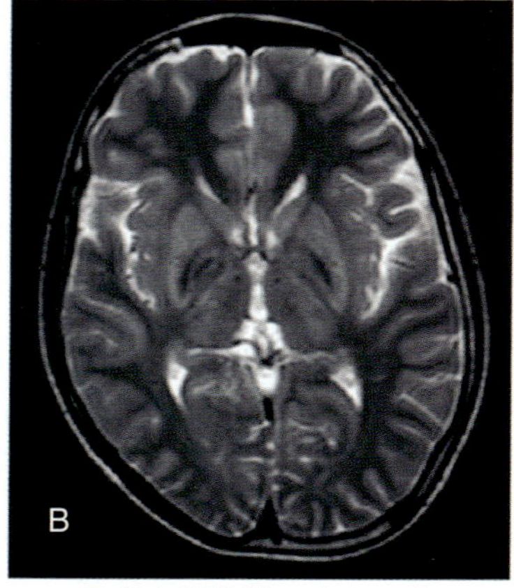

Pallidal T2 Hypointensity

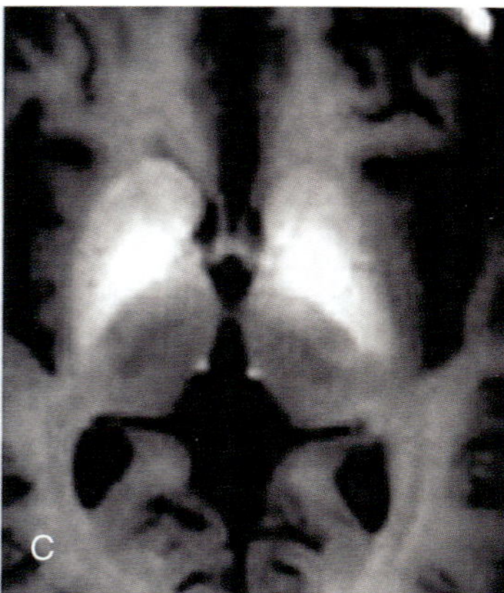

Pallidal T1 hyperintensity

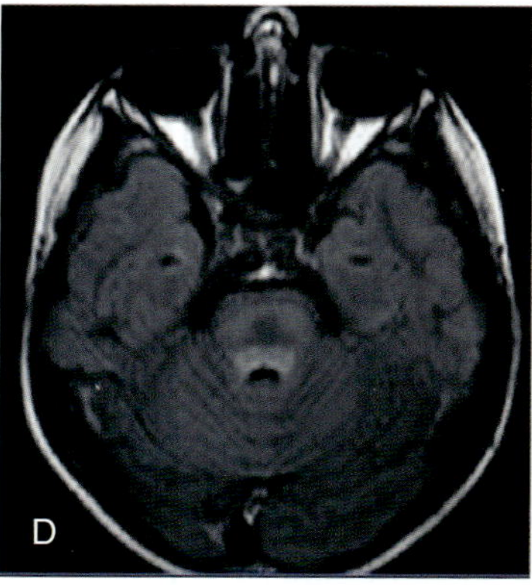

Pons: CPM-like (tripartite)

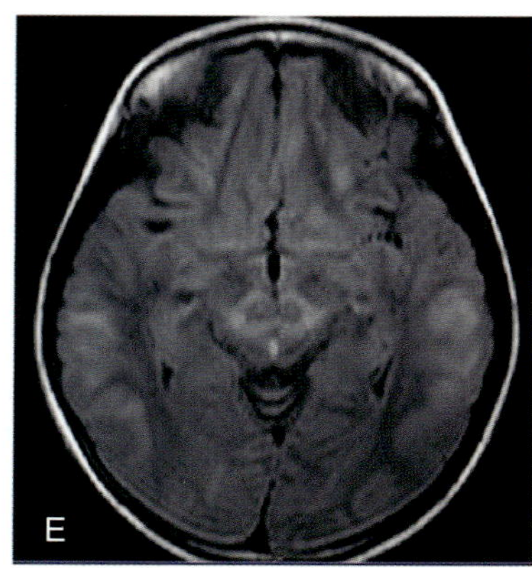

Midbrain: "Face of giant panda"

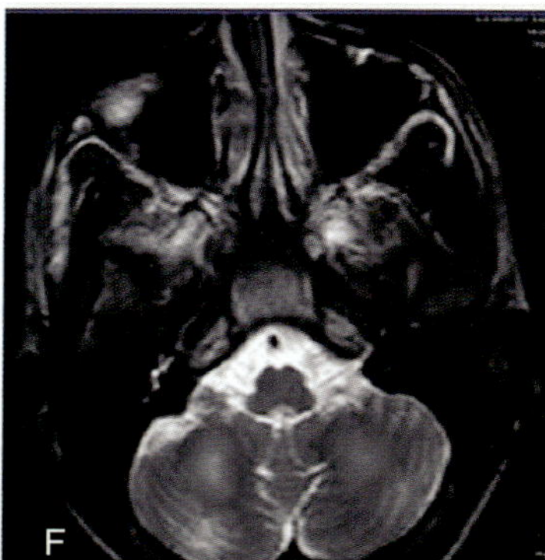

Cerebellar white matter

Figure 50.1 Various MRI features noted in patients with WD.

sleep efficiency (<75%; 28% of patients vs. 16.6% of controls) and frequent awakenings (50% of cases vs. 32 % controls), thus giving a higher global PSQI score in cases than controls. In the study by Portala *et al.*, there was no significant difference in sleep time during the night, but 59% of patients with WD had a significantly greater number of nocturnal awakenings than the reference group [5]. Patients with WD complained more frequently of not feeling rested after sleep, taking frequent naps, fatigue during the daytime, sleep paralysis, and cataplexy than the reference group [5]. In contrast, frequent daytime naps were not reported by the patients in our study. Excessive daytime somnolence (EDS >10) was noted in 12.5% of patients and 8.3% of controls and the difference was not significant. The study by Portala *et al.* used a different sleep inventory (Uppsala Sleep Inventory); hence direct comparison of the PSQI and ESS questionnaire used in our study is not possible [5, 7].

Polysomnography

In the study by Archana *et al.*, there were significant differences between WD and control groups [6]. Patients as a group had significantly reduced total sleep time (p = 0.001), decreased sleep efficiency (p = 0.001), increased sleep onset latency (p = 0.05) and latency to stage 2 (p = 0.02), reduced percentage of deep sleep i.e., stage 3 and 4 (p = 0.01), and less percentage of REM sleep (p = 0.04). Among the other PSG variables observed in this cohort, the control group had a significantly greater number of isolated movements in both REM and non-REM sleep. This meant that patients had fewer position changes and limb movements during sleep, probably due to the akinetic rigid state as part of the parkinsonian symptoms. Even though PLMs were found more often in WD than in the control group (6.24 vs. 3.21) this difference was not significant (p = 0.10). Patients on de-coppering therapy had a significantly prolonged REM sleep onset latency compared with controls (p = 0.03). Patients who were > 20 years of age had a greater percentage of REM sleep than younger patients, which is not in agreement with literature that cites reduced REM sleep with increasing age. The periodic limb movement index (number of PLMs/hour) and the number of PLMs in NREM sleep were significantly greater in younger patients. The isolated limb movement index in REM sleep was significantly less in patients with Chu stage 1 (mild disease) and in those patients who were not on anti epileptic drugs. Male patients had significantly lower heart rates (bradycardia) than female patients both during awake and in sleep state. Also, younger patients had tachycardia more often than older patients in sleep. Our study revealed that sleep abnormalities in WD varied as much as its clinical

Table 50.1. PSG parameters in one patient with Wilson's disease

Total study time (min)	400.00
Total sleep time (min)	234.00
Sleep efficiency (%)	58.6
Sleep onset latency (min)	11.90
Latency to N1	11.90
Latency to N 2	28.10
latency to N3	102.30
Latency to REM	235.00
N1%	17.70
N2%	68.70
N3%	7.00
REM%	6.60
NREM%	93.40
Apnea-hypopnea index (events/hour)	1.00
Apnea-hypopnea index (with arousal)	–
Central apnea/hypopnea	0.30
Obstructive apnea/hypopnea	0.80
Mixed apnea/hypopnea	–
Isolated index	1.30
Periodic limb movements(PLMs)/hour	1.50
Isolated index in REM	–
Isolated index NREM	5.00
Periodic index in REM	–
Periodic index in NREM	6.00
Isolated index with arousal	0.30
Periodic index with arousal	0.50
Arousal index/hour	4.90
No. of arousals	19.00
No. of awakenings	21.00
Minimum oxygenation awake (%)	96.00
Minimum oxygenation sleeping (%)	96.00
Minimum heart rate in awake (/min)	49.00
Maximum heart rate in awake (/min)	84.00
Minimum heart rate in sleep (/min)	49.00
Maximum heart rate in sleep (/min)	75.00

features. A number of other extrapyramidal disorders are known to have sleep abnormalities. PSG findings noted in various other extrapyramidal disorders published in the literature are shown in Table 50.2. Patients with WD have protean manifestations, MRI changes, multiple genetic mutations, and variable therapeutic response and course of illness, which might explain the variability.

MRI observations in WD

The topographic distribution and severity of changes caused by copper deposition, and/or encephalopathy due to hepatic dysfunction are variable. MRI is often recommended as a diagnostic tool for the neuropsychiatric form of WD because it is invariably abnormal and has a highly characteristic pattern. In a series of 100 MRIs in WD from our centre the salient findings were: atrophy of the cerebrum (70%), brainstem (66%), and cerebellum (52%) and T2 W and FLAIR signal changes in the putamen (72%), caudate (61%), thalami (58%), midbrain (49%), pons (20%), cerebral white matter (25%), cortex (9%), medulla (12%), and cerebellum (10%). The characteristic "face of giant panda" sign (12%) central pontine myelinosis-like changes (7%), and bright claustral sign (4%) were rather infrequent [11]. A sequential MRI study involving 50 patients during the course of therapy revealed variable imaging features: improvement (70%), status quo (20%), worsening (8%) and an admixture of improvement and worsening (2%). Hence, with treatment the majority of patients showed both clinical and MRI improvement [12]. It is important to recognize that the presence of central pontine myelinolysis-like changes and midbrain tectal plate signal changes can distinguish WD from other extrapyramidal disorders that involve basal ganglionic structures [13, 14]. Magnetic resonance spectroscopy (MRS) is a useful tool to look into the ongoing biochemical changes, in vivo. In a study of 40 patients and 30 controls who underwent in vivo 2-dimensional ^{31}P- and ^{1}H-MRS of basal ganglia using an image-selected technique, there was reduced breakdown and/or increased synthesis of membrane phospholipids and increased neuronal damage in basal ganglia in patients with WD [15].

Possible correlates of sleep abnormalities in WD

The imaging and pathological features of WD suggest that critical areas involved in the regulation of sleep are affected [11, 16]. As of now, there is no neuro anatomical correlation between PSG parameters and MRI abnormalities. Copper toxicity could be responsible for sleep abnormalities, but its role has not been substantiated. Activation of noradrenergic neurons of the locus coeruleus and serotoninergic neurons of dorsal raphe nuclei belonging to the monoaminergic system ("REM-off" cells) inhibits the cholinergic system. Patients with WD might have brainstem involvement and hence impairment in the monoaminergic system could occur. An abnormal metabolism of neurotransmitters, probably due to an increase in the activity of copper-containing enzymes like dopamine β-hydroxylase [3], with increased norepinephrine in the striatum, has been reported in WD [17, 18]. Nijeholt and Korf reported a decrease of both 5-hydroxyindole acetic acid (5-HIAA, a serotonin metabolite) and homovanillic acid (HVA, a metabolite of dopamine) in the lumbar cerebrospinal Fluid of patients of WD, before and during treatment with penicillamine [2]. This may require a larger cohort of patients with more specific anatomical sites of involvement.

Sleep studies among patients with WD are important for better understanding of underlying mechanisms. Recognition and treatment of sleep abnormalities in these patients may improve their quality of life.

Table 50.2. Comparative studies of PSG parameters in patients with extrapyramidal disorders

Parameters	PD–EDS	PSP	MSA	WD
	(Stevens *et al.*, 2004) [8]	(Arnulf *et al.*, 2005) [9]	(Wetter *et al.*, 2000) [10]	(Archana *et al.*, 2010) [6]
Number of subjects	$n = 10$	$n = 15$	$n = 10$	$n = 25$
Time in bed (min)	506.0 ± 66.0	541 ± 52	472.7 ± 15.7	473.9 ± 56.72
Total sleep time (min)	351.1 ± 53.7	347 ± 87	315.2 ± 51.6	306.6 ± 102.25
Sleep efficiency (%)	70.3 ± 15.1	64 ± 15	75.2 ± 8.9	64.6 ± 19.02
Sleep onset latency (min)	19.6 ± 19.7	22 ± 19	26.3 ± 17.8	49.7 ± 62.06
Stage 1%	10.8 ± 5.3	21 ± 12	12.6 ± 8.1	20.93 ± 14.18
Stage 2%	73.0 ± 6.8	44 ± 15	40.0 ± 12.5	56.83 ± 11.66
Stages 3 and 4%	4.6 ± 7.2	26 ± 13	5.6 ± 6.2	16.63 ± 10.22
REM%	11.6 ± 6.9	8 ± 6	9.2 ± 4.5	6.52 ± 5.75
Apnea hypopnea index (events/hour)	1.9 ± 2.5	25 ± 18	29.4 ± 14.3	0.32 ± 0.49
PLM index (events/hour)	4.2 ± 6.2	30 ± 27	25.8 ± 21.5	6.27 ± 7.84
Arousal index (events/hour)	10.7 ± 5.5	47 ± 28	–	21.2 ± 35.64
No. of awakenings	–	–	27.1 ± 9.1	25.20 ± 12.46

PD–EDS: Parkinson's disease–excessive daytime somnolence; PSP: progressive supranuclear palsy; MSA: multisystem atrophy; WD: Wilson's disease.

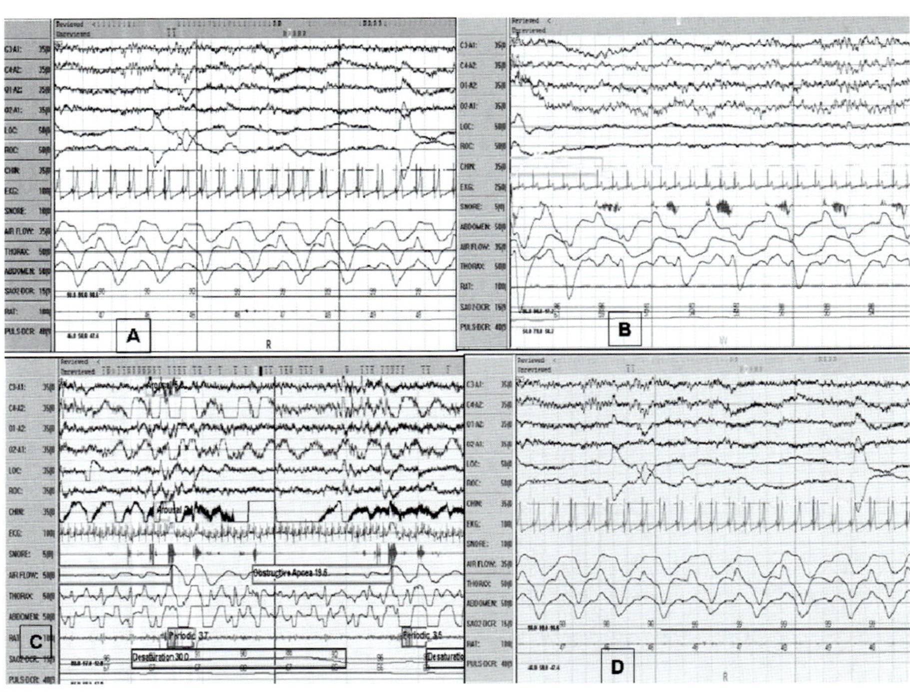

Figure 50.2 PSG observations in patients with WD. (A) REM sleep in a patient with WD who is 22 years old and presented with predominant symptoms of tremor. The left eye (LOC) and right eye (ROC) show REM and the chin electrode shows atonia (sweep speed 30 mm/s); (B) Snoring in a 26-year-old woman with WD observed in stage 2 sleep (sweep speed 30 mm/s); (C) Periodic limb movements in a 55-year-old gentleman who also has obstructive apnea, desaturation, and microarousals along with snoring (sweep speed 60 mm/s); (D) Bradycardia during REM sleep in an 18-year-old patient with WD (sweep speed: 30 mm/s).

References

1. Taly AB, Meenakshi-Sundaram S, Sinha S, Swamy HS, Arunodaya GR. Wilson disease: description of 282 patients evaluated over three decades. *Medicine*. 2007;**86**(2):112–21.

2. Nijeholt JL, Korf J. Wilson's disease and monoamines. *Arch Neurol*. 1978;**35**:617.

3. Barkhatova VP, Larsky G, Markova E, Ivanova-Smolenskaya IA, Demina EG. Changes in concentration of catecholamines in striatum of patients with hepatolenticular degeneration. In: Czlonkowska A, Van den Haner CJA, eds. *Proceeding of the 5 Symposium on Wilson's Disease*. Delft, Technical University. 1995;165–73.

4. Firneisz G, Szalay F, Halasz P, Komoly S. Hypersomnia in Wilson's disease: an unusual symptom in unusual case. *Acta Neurol Scand*. 2000;**101**:286–8.

5. Portala K, Westermark K, Ekselius L, Broaman JE. Sleep in patients with treated Wilson's disease. A questionnaire study. *Nord J Psychiatry*. 2002;**56**(4):291–7.

6. Archana NB, Sinha S, Taly AB, Panda S, Rao S. Sleep and Wilson's disease: polysomnography based study. *Neurol India*. 2010;**58**(6):933–938.

7. Archana NB, Sinha S, Taly AB, Panda S, Rao S. Sleep in Wilson's disease: questionnaire based study. *Ann Indian Acad Neurol*. 2011;**14**:31–4.

8. Stevens S, Comella CL, Stepanski EJ. Daytime sleepiness and alertness in patients with Parkinson's disease. *Sleep*. 2004;**27**(5):967–72.

9. Arnulf I, Merino-Andreu M, Bloch F, *et al*. REM sleep behavior disorder and REM sleep without atonia in patients with progressive supranuclear palsy. *Sleep*. 2005;**28**:349–54.

10. Wetter TC, Collado-Siedel V, Pollmacher T. Sleep and periodic leg movement patterns in drug free patients with Parkinson's disease and multiple system atrophy. *Sleep*. 2000;**23**:1–7.

11. Sinha S, Taly AB, Ravishankar S, *et al*. Wilson's disease: cranial MRI observations and clinical correlation. *Neuroradiology*. 2006;**48**(9):613–21.

12. Sinha S, Taly AB, Prashanth LK, *et al*. Sequential MRI changes in Wilson's disease with de-coppering therapy: a study of 50 patients. *Br J Radiol*. 2007;**80**:74–9.

13. Sinha S, Taly AB, Ravishankar S, Prashanth LK, Vasudev MK. Central pontine signal changes in Wilson disease: distinct MRI morphology and sequential changes with de-coppering therapy. *J Neuroimaging*. 2007;**17**:286–91.

14. Prashanth LK, Sinha S, Taly AB, Vasudev MK. Do MRI features distinguish Wilson's disease from other early onset extrapyramidal disorders? An analysis of 100 cases. *Mov Disord*. 2010;**25**(6):672–8

15. Sinha S, Taly AB, Ravishankar S, Prashanth LK, Vasudev MK. Wilson's disease: ^{31}P and ^{1}H MR spectroscopy and clinical correlation. *Neuroradiology*. 2010;**52**(11):977–85.

16. Meenakshi-Sundaram S, Mahadevan A, Taly AB, *et al*. Wilson's disease: a clinico-neuropathological autopsy study. *J Clin Neurosci*. 2008;**15**:409–17.

17. Nyberg P, Gottfries CG, Holmgren G, *et al*. Advanced catecholaminergic disturbances in the brain in a case of Wilson's disease. *Acta Neurol Scand*. 1982;**65**:71–5.

18. Kish S, Dozik S, Deck J, Shannak K, Hornykiewicz O. Brain adrenergic changes in a patients with Wilson's disease. *J Neuropathol Exp Neurol*. 1990;**49**:280

Functional neuroimaging: sedating medication effects

Hans-Peter Landolt and Emily Urry

Introduction

Healthy human sleep is characterized by the cyclic occurrence of non-rapid eye movement (NREM) sleep and rapid eye movement (REM) sleep, as well as a progressive decline of electroencephalographic (EEG) slow-wave activity (SWA, power within 0.75–4.5 Hz) in the course of a sleep episode. These characteristics reflect the influence of three basic processes that are assumed to underlie sleep/wake regulation [1]: (1) A sleep/wake-dependent, homeostatic process keeping track of "sleep need" accumulating during wakefulness and dissipating during sleep; (2) a sleep/wake-independent, circadian process determining the daily phases of high and low propensity for sleep, REM sleep, and wakefulness; and (3) an ultradian process reflecting the cyclic occurrence of NREM and REM sleep. According to the two-process model of sleep regulation (recently reviewed by [1]), the interaction between the homeostatic *Process S* and the circadian *Process C* regulates the variation of sleep propensity in waking, the alternation between wakefulness and sleep, NREM sleep intensity, and the timing of REM sleep. A high sleep efficiency reflecting a consolidated sleep episode without frequent arousals and state changes – but not necessarily a high proportion of deep slow-wave sleep – ensures the subjective perception of "good quality" sleep [2].

High prevalence of insomnia

Disturbed sleep as a consequence of acute and chronic insomnia is highly prevalent in society [3, 4]. Insomnia symptoms consist of difficulties of initiating or maintaining sleep, non-restorative or poor sleep quality, and reduced daytime functioning including emotional and cognitive impairments associated with the sleep problem. Non-pharmacological therapies (e.g., cognitive behavioral therapy) and/or sedative-hypnotic medications acting as allosteric agonistic modulators of gamma-amino butyric acid type A (GABA$_A$) receptors currently provide the most often used treatment options. These GABA$_A$ receptor modulators include the traditional benzodiazepines (BDZ) such as diazepam, midazolam, and triazolam, and the non-BDZ zolpidem, zaleplon, zopiclone, and eszopiclone, which are also known as "z-drugs." Because of concerns about unwanted effects of these GABAergic

agents (see below), recent research aimed to develop novel hypnotics targeting serotonin (5-HT), melatonin, hypocretin, or histamine receptors. These efforts have not yet led to major breakthroughs [5]. Thus, we will place the main focus of our review on neuroimaging studies investigating the effects of BDZ and z-drugs on regional glucose metabolism and brain perfusion as measured with ^{15}O-water (H$_2$^{15}O)-PET and blood oxygen level-dependent (BOLD) functional magnetic resonance imaging (fMRI) in wakefulness and NREM sleep. We will address the question whether the available studies can help us to better understand neurochemical and neuroanatomical mechanisms underlying physiological sleep and the neurobiological basis of insomnia. Selected findings from pharmacological studies in genetically modified mice, as well as neuroimaging results of the sedating antidepressant, mirtazapine, and of melatonin will also be included.

Most sedative-hypnotics target GABA$_A$ receptors

The GABA$_A$ receptors belong to the superfamily of ligand-gated ion channels, and mediate phasic and tonic inhibition in the central nervous system (CNS). These ubiquitous receptors form a chloride (Cl$^-$) ion pore, which is opened by GABA and structural analogs and inhibited by bicuculline and picrotoxin. They consist of various combinations of 19 different subunits (α, β, γ, δ, ε, θ, and ρ subunits). To form a Cl$^-$ ion channel in vitro with the full functional properties of native GABA$_A$ receptors, at least one α, one β, and one γ subunit are required [6]. Most GABA$_A$ receptors in the CNS are composed of two α subunits (α_1, α_2, α_3 or α_5), two β subunits, and one γ_2 subunit [7]. These receptors are present throughout the rodent brain, but have different regional and cellular distributions *in vivo*; α_1-, α_2-, α_3-, and α_5-containing receptor subtypes are attributed to largely distinct neuronal circuits [8] (Figure 51.1). In mice, α_1 is expressed in the cortex, thalamus, pallidum, and hippocampus; α_2 is expressed in the hippocampus, cortex, striatum, and nucleus accumbens; α_3 is expressed in the cortex and reticular nucleus of the thalamus; α_5 is expressed in the hippocampus and deep layers of the cortex.

Neuroimaging of Sleep and Sleep Disorders, ed. Eric Nofzinger, Pierre Maquet, and Michael J. Thorpy. Published by Cambridge University Press. © Cambridge University Press 2013.

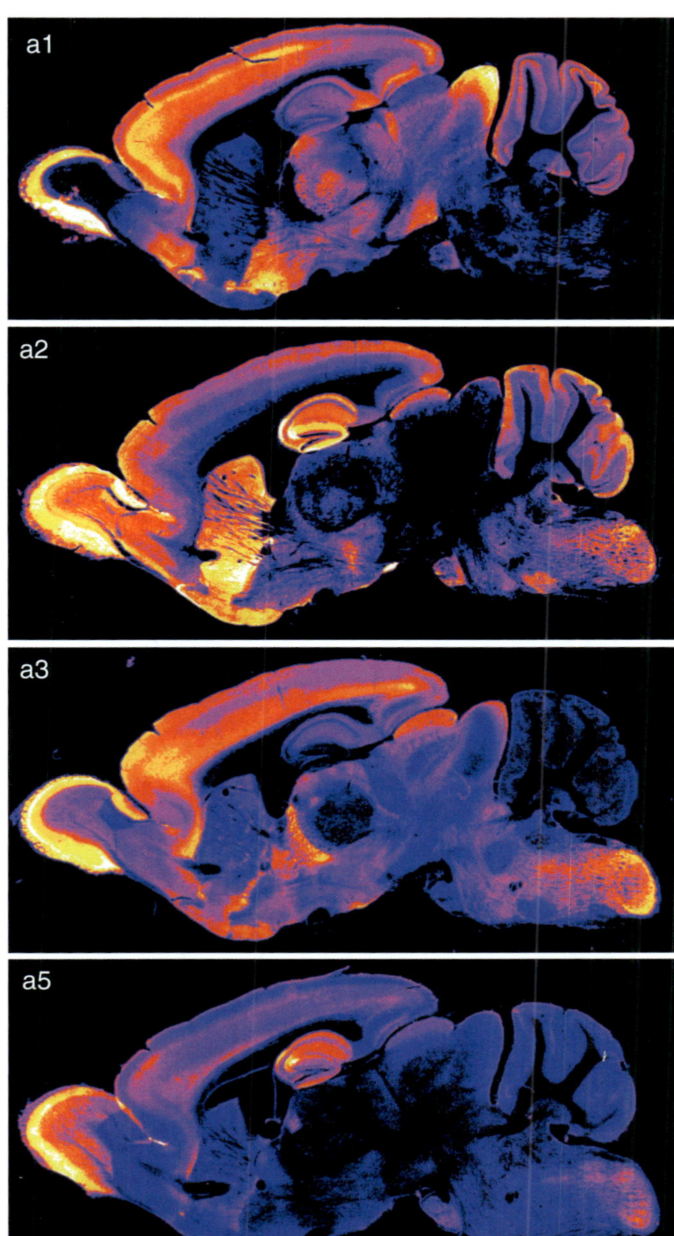

Figure 51.1 Immunohistochemical distribution of GABA$_A$ receptor subtypes in mouse brain. Color coding indicates different levels of α-subunit express on: white (high expression) > yellow > red > purple (low expression) > blue (no expression). (Reproduced, with permission, from [61].)

Flumazenil is a specific *antagonist* at the BDZ binding site of GABA$_A$ receptors containing α$_1$, α$_2$, α$_3$, or α$_5$ subunits. Position emission tomography (PET) studies with radio labeled flumazenil demonstrate that these receptors are widely expressed also in living human brain, particularly in the primary visual cortex and throughout frontal brain regions, especially in the lateral prefrontal and fronto basal cortices [9–11] (Figure 51.2). Lower receptor densities are found in the thalamus, caudate/putamen, pons, and cerebellum.

Complex role for GABA$_A$ receptor subunit(s) in hypnotic action of BDZ and z-drugs

Binding of BDZ and z-drugs at the interface between α and γ$_2$ subunits of GABA$_A$ receptors underlies their sedative-hypnotic properties (for reviews, see: [7, 12, 13]). The classical BDZ have similar binding affinities (i.e., probability to form a drug–receptor complex) to all GABA$_A$ receptors containing α$_1$, α$_2$, α$_3$, and α$_5$ subunits. By contrast, the z-drugs have different affinities, potencies (i.e., drug dose required to produce an effect of given intensity), and efficacies (i.e., maximum response achievable for a drug) at specific receptor subtypes that may result in specific, functionally discrete pharmacodynamics effects [14] (Table 51.1). For example, the imidazopyridine, zolpidem, has high affinity for α$_1$-containing receptors, ~ 20-fold reduced affinity for α$_2$- and α$_3$-containing receptors, and negligible affinity for α$_5$-containing receptors [15]. The pharmacodynamics of zolpidem suggests that α$_1$-containing GABA$_A$ receptors may be the important target for the sedative-hypnotic actions of BDZ and z-drugs. Studies in genetically modified mice indeed show that the α$_1$ subtype facilitates the sedative actions of these compounds [16]. Nevertheless, sedative and hypnotic properties appear to be mediated by different neuronal circuits. More specifically, enhancement of sleep continuity – as quantified by the number of brief awakenings in mice – occurs independently of α$_1$-containing GABA$_A$ receptors [17]. In accordance with these findings in transgenic animals, the effects of zolpidem and the physiological promotion of deep NREM sleep after sleep deprivation are separate also in humans, suggesting that they are mediated by different neurophysiological mechanisms [18]. It is possible that α$_2$-containing GABA$_A$ receptors are involved in the generation of deep NREM sleep [19, 20].

In conclusion, pharmacological studies in genetically engineered mice and healthy humans suggest complex roles for distinct GABA$_A$ receptors and their subunits in the physiology and pharmacology of sleep.

Functional neuroimaging of sedative-hypnotic medication effects during wakefulness

The clinical effects of ligands at BDZ binding sites not only consist of sedation and sleep induction, but also include anxiolysis, seizure suppression, and muscle relaxation. Moreover, they may also exert unwanted actions, including anterograde amnesia, addiction, dependence, and tolerance [7]. To better understand and eventually overcome the limitations of classical BDZ, research during the past two decades aimed to elucidate separable key functions of distinct GABA$_A$ receptor subtypes. Neuroimaging provides one promising approach to identify brain regions in which activity is affected by pharmacological agents. Localized effects of drugs may help to clarify their exact mechanisms of action in the brain, as well as to explain the clinical effects elicited in the patient.

At present, only a small number of placebo-controlled studies have examined the effects of sedative-hypnotics on brain activity in human subjects who are either awake or asleep. Experiments during wakefulness tend to use a combination of pharmacological and behavioral challenges during neuroimaging. This protocol enables researchers to clarify drug effects on regional brain activity during different states of cognitive activation. Behavioral tasks are selected to engage cognitive processes that are known to be influenced by the drug under investigation. For example, it is well established that acute BDZ administration in healthy volunteers produces dose-related decrements in episodic memory encoding, while leaving retrieval of previously encoded material intact (reviewed by [21]). As outlined above, GABA$_A$ receptors in the brain are known to be the initial sites of BDZ action. Nevertheless, the neural networks affected by BDZ administration during episodic encoding are yet to be clarified. It

is possible that they extend well beyond the sites of initial drug–receptor interactions.

Benzodiazepines

Different neuroimaging techniques including PET and fMRI were used to investigate the effects of diazepam, midazolam, triazolam, and lorazepam on brain activity during episodic memory encoding in healthy volunteers [22–28]. There is some discrepancy amongst the studies in regions showing BDZ-induced deactivation during performance of this task. This has been related to methodological differences in terms of experimental design (e.g., between- vs. within-subject manipulation of dose), type of stimuli (e.g., words vs. face-name pairs), modality of stimuli presentation (visual vs. auditory), and the nature of the control task to which the encoding task was compared. For example, Mintzer *et al.* [27] investigated memory encoding by comparing brain activity during more elaborate encoding (semantic categorization of words) with that during less elaborate encoding (orthographic categorization of words). By contrast, other research groups used "resting-wakefulness" as the control condition [23, 25]. These authors scanned blindfolded volunteers during the presentation of auditory tones, which they were instructed to ignore. Brain activation during resting wakefulness may reflect the "default mode network" consisting of precuneus, lateral parietal, ventromedial prefrontal, mid-dorsolateral prefrontal, and anterior temporal regions [29, 30]. This network has a high metabolic rate during resting wakefulness, which reduces following the introduction of specific tasks. It is thought to play an important role in the modulation of conscious processes, awareness, mental representations of the self, and inferential processing of context-related information.

Benzodiazepines (diazepam, midazolam, triazolam, lorazepam) induce deactivation of the prefrontal cortex and medial temporal lobe during episodic memory encoding

Despite the methodological differences, all but one study [24] revealed significant deactivation of the prefrontal cortex

Table 51.1. Relative functional effects of z-drugs at different GABA$_A$ receptors

z-drug	GABA$_A$ receptor subunit			
	α_1	α_2	α_3	α_5
Zolpidem				
Affinity	21x	1x	1x	Negligible
Potency	4–12x	2x	1x	Negligible
Efficacy	1x	1x	1x	Negligible
Zaleplon				
Affinity	4–17x	1–2x	1–2x	1x
Potency	3–33x	1–5x	1x	1–2x
Efficacy	1–2x	1x	2x	1x
Zopiclone				
Affinity	11x	7x	1x	2x
Potency	4–6x	1x	Conflicting data	4–6x
Efficacy	1x	1x	1x	1x
Eszopiclone				
Affinity	8x	5x	1x	8x
Potency	1x	4x	4–6x	10x
Efficacy	2x	4x	4x	1x

The lowest values for affinity, potency, and efficacy for each drug are assigned a reference value of 1x, and the other values for that drug characteristic are expressed relative to this.
Table adapted from [14].

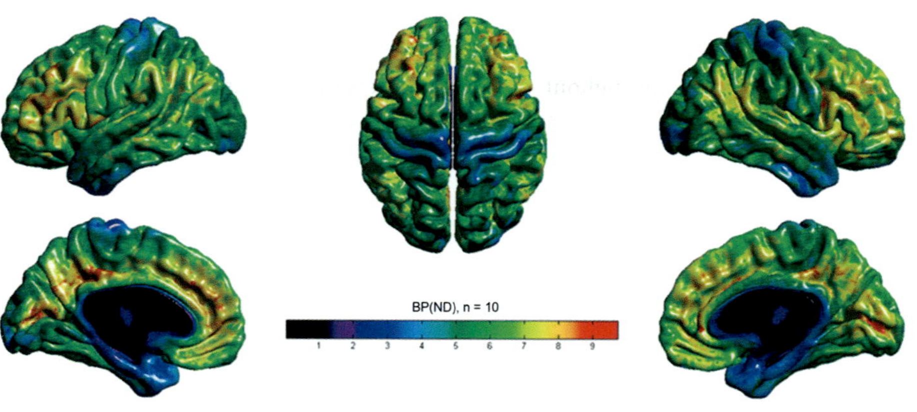

Figure 51.2 High-resolution, mean parametric maps of ^{18}F-flumazenil binding potential [BP(ND)] in healthy adults. (Reproduced, with permission, from [11].)

following BDZ administration during memory encoding. This region plays an important role in this step of episodic memory in humans (reviewed by [31]). It has been proposed that the prefrontal cortex is responsible for the initial control of reflective processes (e.g., selection and direction of processing resources, maintenance and manipulation of information) that ultimately lead to the transformation of sensory input into internal representations [31–33].

Another key region indicated in episodic memory is the medial temporal lobe (reviewed by [34]). There are large cortico-cortical direct reciprocal connections between the prefrontal cortex and the medial temporal lobe, passing through the uncinate fascicle, anterior temporal stem, and anterior corpus callosum [35]. Despite this, medial temporal structures have shown relative resistance to the effects of BDZ, with only two out of seven research papers revealing a significant deactivation within this region of interest during episodic memory encoding (hippocampus: [28]; parahippocampus: [27]). The medial temporal lobe is thought to bind together representations that were initially processed by the prefrontal cortex into a durable contextualized episodic memory trace [32, 33]. Thus, it is possible that the effects of BDZ on memory may be primarily mediated by impairment of encoding processes occurring in the prefrontal cortex, with relatively little effect on the integration or transfer of information to long-term memory [25].

Z-drugs

Zolpidem reduces visual cortex activation by flashing checkerboard

Functional MRI was recently used to investigate the effect of zolpidem on brain function during wakefulness [36]. Acute oral administration of the drug reduced the robust activation of the visual system produced by the presentation of a flashing checkerboard. These findings agree with previous fMRI studies which showed that other positive $GABA_A$ receptor modulators, such as alcohol [37], reduced activation during visual cortex stimulation. The observed effects may result from synaptic inhibitory activity. Developmental studies in rats suggest high expression of α_1 subunits in adult primary visual cortex [38]. Nevertheless, the functional significance of the imaging findings in humans remains unknown. It could be related to reported distortions in visual perception attributed to the drug, including blurred vision and hallucinatory experiences [39].

Sedating antidepressants and melatonin

Functional neuroimaging methods were also applied to the study of non-GABAergic agents, including sedating antidepressants and melatonin.

An fMRI study conducted in healthy volunteers examined the effects of mirtazapine on brain activation associated with behavioral inhibition and reinforcement processing [40]. This sedating antidepressant enhanced activation in the right lateral orbitofrontal cortex during behavioral inhibition and in both parietal cortices during reinforcement processing to monetary reward. Mirtazapine acts as an antagonist of $5\text{-}HT_{2A}$ receptors and as an agonist of $5\text{-}HT_{1A}$ receptors, suggesting that serotonin may play an important role in behavioral inhibition and reward processing. This effect may also underlie some of the therapeutic effects of serotonergic antidepressants [40].

Functional MRI was also used to investigate the effects of melatonin on brain activities during visual, auditory, and memory tasks, and their relation to the induction of sleepiness [41]. This study revealed that afternoon ingestion of melatonin, and not placebo, reduced task-related activity in the rostromedial aspect of the occipital cortex during a visual search task, and in the auditory cortex during a music task. The effects correlated with subjective measurements of fatigue. In addition, melatonin enhanced the activation in the left parahippocampus in an autobiographic memory task. These results demonstrate melatonin's ability to modulate brain activity in a manner resembling enhanced sleep pressure, despite participants being fully awake. Melatonin may induce sleep anticipation in the brain, so that sleep-related processes begin before actual sleep initiation [41].

Functional neuroimaging of sedative-hypnotic medication effects during sleep

The effects of pharmacological agents on regional brain activity during sleep can be investigated by employing neuroimaging and polysomnography simultaneously.

Benzodiazepines

Triazolam reduces blood flow in the prefrontal cortex and amygdala in NREM sleep

In an $H_2{}^{15}O\text{-}PET$ study in healthy volunteers, regional cerebral blood flow (rCBF) in NREM sleep was assessed in response to the BDZ triazolam [42]. Volunteers underwent two experimental nights – one placebo and one triazolam. Each night, two scans in wakefulness were obtained in a control condition with eyes closed, after which subjects took a treatment capsule. During sleep, three scans in superficial NREM sleep (stage 2) and three scans in slow-wave sleep were performed between 11:00 pm and 2:00 am. The EEG was recorded throughout the imaging session and used to determine the sleep states.

Compared with placebo, triazolam reduced blood flow in NREM sleep in the basal forebrain and amygdaloid complexes [42]. These findings indicate that triazolam has its main impact on the basal forebrain, rather than on other wake-promoting regions, including distinct nuclei of the brainstem, hypothalamus, and thalamus. The hypnotic effect of triazolam may thus result mainly from inhibition of the forebrain control system for wakefulness. Other imaging data show that the basal forebrain is deactivated in deep NREM sleep in healthy adults [43], possibly suggesting that deactivation of this region is involved in promoting physiological NREM sleep. The deactivation of the amygdaloid complexes, which contribute to emotional responses such as anxiety and fear, indicates that the anxiolytic effect of BDZ is also related to their hypnotic effect.

Z-drugs

Two studies employed PET imaging, in a double-blind, placebo-controlled manner, to assess the effects of zolpidem on brain function during sleep in healthy adults. These studies suggest that zolpidem has complex and varied influences on regional brain activity.

Studies in healthy volunteers

Zolpidem reduces regional cerebral glucose metabolic rate in the basal ganglia and limbic structures

Zolpidem induced changes in regional cerebral glucose metabolic rate as quantified with ^{18}F-fluorodeoxyglucose (^{18}FDG-PET) that varied directly with the plasma drug concentration [44]. These changes were unevenly distributed throughout the brain, and were greater in subcortical areas than lateral cortical areas. Specifically, compared with placebo, zolpidem elicited a reduction in absolute glucose metabolic rate in medial frontal cortical and cingulate regions, frontal white matter, putamen, thalamus, and hippocampus. Relative metabolic rate tended to decrease more on the left hemisphere than on the right hemisphere, and more in lateral temporal and occipital regions than in parietal and frontal regions. Within the right hemisphere, the paracentral lobule, medial frontal gyrus, frontal white matter, precuneus, posterior putamen, and midbrain showed relatively lower glucose metabolism. In the left hemisphere, lower glucose metabolism was seen in the posterior thalamus and anterior cingulate. Finally, zolpidem enhanced relative glucose metabolism in the right anterior thalamus, left frontal matter, and left superior colliculus.

The present findings indicate that zolpidem reduces absolute and relative metabolic rates in the cingulate cortex in proportion to its plasma concentration. In animals, this area is high in α_1-containing GABA$_A$ receptors [38]. On the other hand, several regions that are also high in α_1 subtype receptors (e.g., frontoparietal and sensorimotor cortices) are apparently unaffected, whereas areas such as the thalamus and putamen with relatively few α_1 subunits show lower metabolism after zolpidem when compared with placebo. Thus, arguably the present findings may not fully reflect the mechanisms of action and clinical effects of zolpidem. The unusually low plasma concentrations of the drug may be partly responsible for this.

Zolpidem reduces regional cerebral blood flow in the basal ganglia and insula

PET imaging during sleep was also used to investigate changes in rCBF following administration of zolpidem [45]. The study revealed that zolpidem induced distinct changes in rCBF in sleep-deprived, healthy volunteers in combined stages 2 and 4 and REM sleep. More specifically, relative rCBF was lower after zolpidem than after placebo in the basal ganglia (left putamen and caudate) and in the insula, yet it was higher in the parietal cortex (the superior and inferior parietal lobules of the neocortex) (Figure 51.3). Analyzing only NREM sleep, similar blood flow differences were apparent, but did not reach significance. In REM sleep, rCBF in the anterior cingulate was lower after zolpidem than after placebo, whereas rCBF in the occipital and parietal cortices, parahippocampal gyrus, and cerebellum was higher.

The generalizability of these findings is limited by the possible confounding effects of sleep deprivation. However, it is noteworthy that reduced rCBF in slow-wave sleep relative to waking or to all other sleep stages has been reported for the basal ganglia, insula, and anterior cingulate cortex (see [43] for recent review). Thus, the present evidence indicates that zolpidem promotes changes in rCBF that are typical for slow-wave sleep [45]. The observation that some effects of zolpidem are related to those of deep sleep is in agreement with the drug-induced shortening of sleep latency and the decrease in combined arousal variables [18]. Moreover, the reduced rCBF in the putamen and cingulate cortex could be related to the

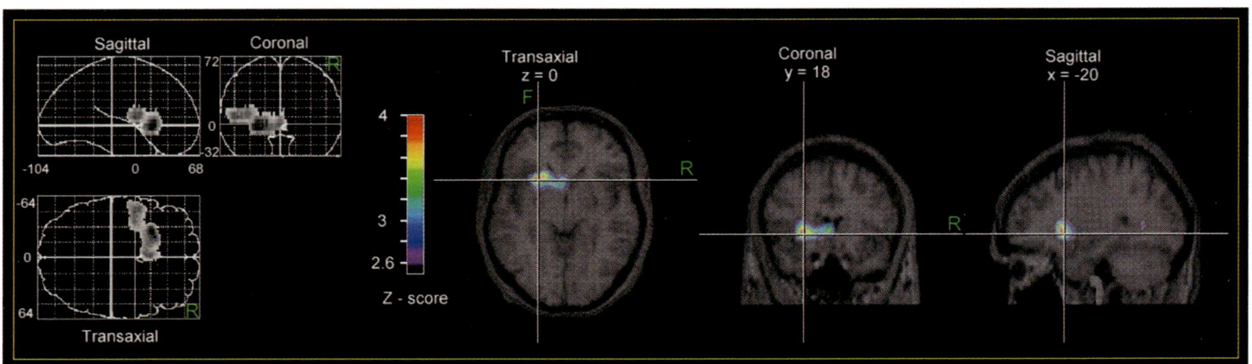

Figure 51.3 Brain regions showing lower rCBF during sleep after zolpidem compared with placebo assessed by statistical parametric mapping. Results are displayed above a threshold of Z = 2.58 (p < 0.005 uncorrected, n = 8). (Left) Statistical parametric map (SPM{Z}). The grey scale is arbitrary. (Right) Transaxial, coronal, and sagittal sections at a selected point of interest. The color scale for Z is indicated. (Reproduced, with permission, from [45].)

findings of Gillin *et al.* [44] who revealed that zolpidem decreased absolute glucose metabolic rate in these regions. Equally, the zolpidem-induced changes in absolute glucose metabolism tended to be larger in the midline than in the lateral cortical areas – an observation that is in accordance with the present study, in which the parietal cortex exhibited a relative increase in rCBF [45].

Studies in patients with neurological disorders

Zolpidem increases cerebral activity in patients suffering from neurological conditions

In the presence of brain injury, as opposed to healthy brain tissue, zolpidem has been shown to disproportionately enhance cerebral perfusion in areas that were hypoactive as a result of injury. This finding was demonstrated using single-photon emission computed tomography (SPECT) imaging in both neurologically diseased humans and baboons [46], and also using PET in a patient with postanoxic akinetic mutism [47]. Following zolpidem, the latter study revealed increased cerebral activity in the frontal cortex with both ^{18}F-FDG PET (at resting state) and $H_2^{15}O$-PET in an activating condition relative to resting state. During cognitive activation (object naming), zolpidem elicited increased activation in the anterior cingulate and orbitofrontal cortices. Interestingly, behavioral parameters were also affected, but in an apparently paradoxical manner. More specifically, despite being a "sedating hypnotic," zolpidem induced a transient improvement in motor and cognitive performance. Similar findings were reported in studies involving patients suffering from various neurological conditions, including brain injury [48–50], stroke [51], and Parkinson's disease [52], and in a patient in a vegetative state [53].

Given the small and specific nature of the patient samples in these studies, it is difficult to extrapolate the findings to other patients suffering from neurological disorders. Moreover, the neuronal mechanism underlying this paradoxical effect of zolpidem remains unknown. Nonetheless, some authors suggest that zolpidem may reverse the diaschisis phenomenon (i.e., loss of function in a portion of the brain that is at a distance from the site of injury, but neuronally connected), which prompts a recovery of cortical activity [48–50]. As proposed by Brefel-Courbon *et al.* [47], the stimulation of GABA function by zolpidem could interact with cortical-subcortical loops originating from the anterior cingulate and orbitofrontal cortices, which leads to disinhibition and thalamocortical over activity [54]. The improvement of function in the limbic loops could be related to both the reversal of a cortical-subcortical diaschisis, as well as to the improvement in motivational processes, which are necessary for speech and movement.

Eszopiclone may reduce glucose metabolism in the pontine and midbrain reticular activating system in patients with insomnia

Functional neuroimaging in patients with sleep disorders can provide clues to the underlying pathophysiology, as well as to the role of specific brain regions in generating and maintaining sleep. Imaging findings support the concept that persistent activity in distinct arousal networks, particularly continuous activation of the precuneus, is linked to impaired sleep quality in patients with insomnia [55, 56]. With regards to pharmacological interventions, sedative-hypnotics may provide an antidote to the proposed CNS hyperarousal seen in these patients during sleep. The current literature lacks placebo-controlled neuroimaging experiments that investigate the effects of hypnotics on brain activity in insomnia subjects. However, a preliminary, open-labeled study employed ^{18}F-FDG PET to assess the effects of eszopiclone, the S-enantiomer of the cyclopyrrolone, zopiclone, in eight individuals with primary insomnia [57]. Regarding its affinity, potency, and efficacy at different $GABA_A$ receptor subtypes (Table 51.1), this hypnotic can be considered to act preferentially at α_2/α_3 receptors [14]. Subjective measures of sleep, sleep quality, mood, and next-morning alertness improved from pre- to post-treatment. In addition, the reduction in relative regional glucose metabolism from waking to NREM sleep in an arousal network originating in the pontine reticular formation and ascending into the midbrain, subthalamic nucleus, thalamus, and cerebellum was more pronounced following eszopiclone than before. Related neocortical areas, including the orbitofrontal cortex, superior temporal lobe, right paracentral lobule of the posterior medial frontal lobe, right precuneus, dorsal cingulate gyrus, and parts of the frontal lobe showed a similar interaction with treatment. Reductions in relative metabolism after treatment were found in similar regions during sleep, but not in wakefulness. Thus, eszopiclone reverses a pattern of hyperarousal seen in insomnia patients in NREM sleep. The authors suggested that the inhibitory action of the drug focuses mainly on a CNS arousal neural network within sleep that includes the pontine and midbrain reticular activating system [57]. This research further validates the essential role of these structures in generating and maintaining sleep [55].

Conclusions and perspectives

Neuroimaging studies employing PET and fMRI have consistently found reduced brain activity in physiological slow-wave sleep when compared with wakefulness (see [43] for comprehensive recent review). The regional reductions in brain activity span cortical (prefrontal cortex, anterior cingulate cortex, and precuneus) and subcortical structures (brainstem, thalamus, basal ganglia, basal forebrain) (Table 51.2), including neuronal populations involved in awakening and arousal as well as areas that are highly active during wakefulness. Insomnia is characterized by difficulty initiating sleep, repeated awakenings with difficulty returning to sleep, or non-restorative/poor sleep quality [56]. Examining glucose metabolic rate with ^{18}F-FDG PET in wakefulness and NREM sleep revealed that patients with insomnia exhibit a smaller decrease than controls in relative glucose metabolism from waking to NREM sleep in the brainstem reticular core and hypothalamus [58]. These findings support the concept that

Table 51.2. Summary of regional changes in brain activity in slow-wave sleep when compared with wakefulness, and of effects of sedative-hypnotics in resting wakefulness and NREM sleep

	Brain structures (cortical regions, limbic and paralimbic structures, arousal centers)										References
	MPFC	Insula	Precuneus	BG	ACC	PHG	Amygdala	Hypothalamus	Thalamus	ARAS	
Slow wave sleep vs. wakefulness:											
rCBF ($H_2^{15}O$) in healthy volunteers	↓	↓	↓	↓	↓				↓	↓	[43, 55]
Glucose metabolism (^{18}F-FDG) in insomnia	↑	↑	↑		↑	↑	↑	↑	↑	↑	[56, 58]
Resting wakefulness:											
rCBF ($H_2^{15}O$) after midazolam	↓	↓		↓	↓				↓		[23, 25]
NREM sleep:											
rCBF ($H_2^{15}O$) after triazolam	↓	↓			↓					↓	[42]
Glucose metabolism (^{18}F-FDG) after zolpidem	↓		↓	↓	↓				↓		[44]
rCBF ($H_2^{15}O$) after zolpidem		↓		↓							[45]
Glucose metabolism (^{18}F-FDG) after eszopiclone in insomnia patients	↓		↓						↓	↓	[57]

↓ = decrease; ↑ = reduced decrease; some changes were only seen in one hemisphere. MPFC = medial prefrontal cortex; BG = basal ganglia; ACC = anterior cingulate cortex; PHG = parahippocampal gyrus; ARAS = ascending reticular arousal system (including brainstem and basal forebrain).

persistent activity in arousal networks may be linked to the impaired sleep quality in insomnia [55]. Drawing on human studies such as this, as well as on animal data, a neurobiological model of insomnia was recently proposed [56]. The authors postulate that insomnia is a disorder of sleep/wake regulation distinguished by ongoing wake-like activity in NREM sleep, which leads to simultaneous, and regionally specific, waking and sleeping neuronal activation. The model suggests that this persistent activity occurs in wake-active brain structures including distinct cortical regions, paralimbic cortex, thalamus, hypothalamus, and brainstem arousal centers.

The sedative-hypnotics midazolam, triazolam, and zolpidem reduce brain perfusion and/or glucose metabolism in healthy volunteers in restful wakefulness and NREM sleep in the medial prefrontal cortex, insula, basal ganglia, anterior cingulate cortex, and thalamus [23, 25, 42, 44, 45] (Table 51.2). These findings suggest that BDZ and z-drugs promote sleep by reducing arousal. Similar to their distinct changes in the sleep EEG referred to as "spectral BDZ signature" [12], these effects appear to be irrespective of chemical structure and differential affinity, potency, and efficacy at different subtypes of GABA$_A$ receptors. Moreover, sedative-hypnotic medication-induced changes in glucose metabolism and blood flow may not reflect the distribution patterns of different GABA$_A$ receptors in the brain. Apart from the thalamus, the most consistent deactivation in healthy volunteers occurs in limbic and paralimbic structures involved in emotional responses such as anxiety and fear. These observations indicate that anxiolysis is related to the hypnotic effects of both BDZ and zolpidem. Besides, augmenting the actions of endogenous GABA may be involved in sleep-promoting circuits. In support of this notion, a GABAergic deficit was linked to chronic insomnia in a patient with a mutation in the β_3 subunit of GABA$_A$ receptors [59]. It may be possible in the future, to design multi-modal imaging studies to investigate possible causal relationships among neurocircuitry, regional GABA concentrations, and distinct GABA$_A$ receptor dynamics.

A global reduction of GABA was also suggested in the brains of insomnia patients with proton magnetic resonance spectroscopy (^{1}H-MRS) [60]. Preliminary findings highlight the promising pharmacological intervention with eszopiclone for treating the regional cerebral disturbances seen in insomnia during sleep [56]. However, given the open-label protocol, the data should be interpreted with caution. Other research groups have investigated the effects of triazolam [41] and zolpidem [43, 44] on regional cerebral activity during sleep using blinded and placebo-controlled protocols. Their findings indicate that GABAergic hypnotics have the potential to ameliorate the cerebral over activity that is characteristic of insomnia. A caveat is that these studies were performed in healthy individuals with "good" sleep, and thus it is inappropriate to generalize the findings to patients. Indeed, zolpidem appears to increase cerebral activity in a region- and disease-specific manner in patients with neurological disorders rather than to decrease cerebral activity such as in healthy individuals. Going forward, in order to clarify the efficacy and mechanisms of action of sedating hypnotics in reducing CNS hyperarousal in insomnia, it is recommended that functional neuroimaging studies, of rigorous design, be employed to assess their effects on regional activity during sleep in insomniac samples.

Acknowledgements

We thank Dr. J.-M. Fritschy, Dr. C. La Fougère, and Dr. P. Achermann for providing us with their original figures.

References

1. Achermann P, Borbély AA. Sleep homeostasis and models of sleep regulation. In: Kryger MH, Roth T, Dement WC, eds. *Principles and Practice of Sleep Medicine*, 5th edn. St. Louis, MI, Elsevier Saunders. 2011; 431–44.

2. Akerstedt T, Hume K, Minors D, Waterhouse J. The meaning of good sleep – a longitudinal-study of polysomnography and subjective sleep quality. *J Sleep Res.* 1994;**3**(3):152–8.

3. Riemann D, Spiegelhalder K, Espie C, *et al.* Chronic insomnia: clinical and research challenges – an agenda. *Pharmacopsychiatry.* 2011;**44**(1):1–14.

4. Meyer G, Jennum P, Riemann D, Dauvilliers Y. Insomnia in central neurologic diseases – occurrence and management. *Sleep Med Rev.* 2011;**15**:369–78.

5. Wafford KA, Ebert B. Emerging anti-insomnia drugs: tackling sleeplessness and the quality of wake time. *Nat Rev Drug Discov.* 2008;**7**(6):530–40.

6. Pritchett DB, Luddens H, Seeburg PH. Type I and type II GABAA-benzodiazepine receptors produced in transfected cells. *Science.* 1989;**245**(4924):1389–92.

7. Rudolph U, Knoflach F. Beyond classical benzodiazepines: novel therapeutic potential of GABA(A) receptor subtypes. *Nat Rev Drug Discov.* 2011;**10**(9):685–97.

8. Fritschy JM, Möhler H. GABAA-receptor heterogeneity in the adult rat brain: differential regional and cellular distribution of seven major subunits. *J Comp Neurol.* 1995;**359**(1):154–94.

9. Frey KA, Holthoff VA, Koeppe RA, *et al.* Parametric in vivo imaging of benzodiazepine receptor distribution in human brain. *Ann Neurol.* 1991;**30**(5):663–72.

10. Salmi E, Aalto S, Hirvonen J, *et al.* Measurement of GABA(A) receptor binding in vivo with [C-11] flumazenil: a test-retest study in healthy subjects. *Neuroimage.* 2008;**41**(2):260–9.

11. la Fougere C, Grant S, Kostikov A, *et al.* Where in-vivo imaging meets cytoarchitectonics: the relationship between cortical thickness and neuronal density measured with high-resolution [(18)F] flumazenil-PET. *Neuroimage.* 2011;**56**(3):951–60.

12. Landolt HP, Gillin JC. GABA$_{A1a}$ receptors: involvement in sleep regulation and potential of selective agonists in the treatment of insomnia. *CNS Drugs.* 2000;**13**:185–99.

13. Mohler H. Review – GABA(A) receptors in central nervous system disease: anxiety, epilepsy, and insomnia. *J Recept Signal Transduct. Res.* 2006;**26**(5–6):731–40.

14. Nutt DJ, Stahl SM. Searching for perfect sleep: the continuing evolution of GABA(A) receptor modulators as hypnotics. *J Psychopharmacol.* 2010;**24**(11):1601–12.

15. Pritchett DB, Seeburg PH. Gamma-aminobutyric acid-A receptor a5-subunit creates novel type II benzodiazepine receptor pharmacology. *J Neurochem.* 1990;**54**:1802–4.

16. Crestani F, Martin JR, Mohler H, Rudolph U. Mechanism of action of the hypnotic zolpidem in vivo. *Br J Pharmacol.* 2000;**131**(7):1251–4.

17. Tobler I, Kopp C, Deboer T, Rudolph U. Diazepam-induced changes in sleep: role of the alpha 1 GABA(A) receptor subtype. *Proc Nat Acad Sci U S A.* 2001;**98**(11):6464–9.

18. Landolt HP, Finelli LA, Roth C, *et al.* Zolpidem and sleep deprivation: different effect on EEG power spectra. *J Sleep Res.* 2000;**9**(2):175–83.

19. Kopp C, Rudolph U, Tobler I. Sleep EEG changes after zolpidem in mice. *Neuroreport.* 2004;**15**(14):2299–302.

20. Kopp C, Rudolph U, Low K, Tobler I. Modulation of rhythmic brain activity by diazepam: GABA(A) receptor subtype and state specificity. *Proc Natl Acad Sci U S A.* 2004;**101**(10):3674–9.

21. Curran HV. Benzodiazepines, memory and mood – a review. *Psychopharmacology.* 1991;**105**(1):1–8.

22. Coull JT, Frith CD, Dolan RJ Dissociating neuromodulatory effects of diazepam on episodic memory encoding and executive function. *Psychopharmacology.* 1999;**145**(2):213–22.

23. Veselis RA, Reinsel RA, Beattie BJ, *et al.* Midazolam changes cerebral blood flow in discrete brain regions – an (H2O)-O-15 positron emission tomography study. *Anesthesiology.* 1997;**87**(5):1106–17

24. Bagary M, Fluck E, File SE, *et al.* Is benzodiazepine-induced amnesia due to deactivation of the left prefrontal cortex? *Psychopharmacology.* 2000;**150**(3):292–9.

25. Reinsel RA, Veselis RA, Dnistrian AM, *et al.* Midazolam decreases cerebral blood flow in the left prefrontal cortex in a dose-dependent fashion. *Int J Neuropsychopharmacol.* 2000;**3**(2):117–27.

26. Mintzer MZ, Griffiths RR, Contoreggi C, *et al.* Effects of triazolam on brain activity during episodic memory encoding: a PET study. *Neuropsychopharmacology.* 2001;**25**(5):744–56.

27. Mintzer MZ, Kuwabara H, Alexander M, *et al.* Dose effects of triazolam on brain activity during episodic memory encoding: a PET study. *Psychopharmacology.* 2006;**188**(4):445–61.

28. Sperling R, Greve D, Dale A, *et al.* Functional MRI detection of pharmacologically induced memory impairment. *Proc Natl Acad Sci U S A.* 2002;**99**(1):455–60.

29. Cavanna AE, Trimble MR. The precuneus: a review of its functional anatomy and behavioural correlates. *Brain.* 2006;**129**:564–83.

30. Legrand D, Ruby P. What Is self-specific? Theoretical investigation and critical review of neuroimaging results. *Psychol Rev.* 2009;**116**(1):252–82.

31. Fletcher PC, Henson RNA. Frontal lobes and human memory – insights from functional neuroimaging. *Brain.* 2001;**124**:849–81.

32. Otten LJ, Rugg MD. Task-dependency of the neural correlates of episodic encoding as measured by fMRI. *Cereb Cortex.* 2001;**11**(12):1150–60.

33. Paller KA, Wagner AD. Observing the transformation of experience into memory. *Trends Cogn Sci.* 2002;**6**(2):93–102.

34. Squire LR. Memory systems of the brain: a brief history and current perspective. *Neurobiol Learn Mem.* 2004;**82**(3):171–7.

35. Simons JS, Spiers HJ. Prefrontal and medial temporal lobe interactions in long-term memory. *Nat Rev Neurosci.* 2003;**4**(8):637–48.

36. Licata SC, Lowen SB, Trksak GH, MacLean RR, Lukas SE. Zolpidem reduces the blood oxygen level-dependent signal during visual system stimulation. *Prog Neuro psychopharmacol Biol Psychiatry.* 2011;**35**(7):1645–52.

37. Levin JM, Ross MH, Mendelson JH, *et al.* Reduction in BOLD fMRI response to primary visual stimulation following alcohol ingestion. *Psychiatry Res.* 1998;**82**(3):135–46.

38. Fritschy JM, Paysan J, Enna A, Mohler H. Switch in the expression of rat GABA(A)-receptor subtypes during postnatal-development – an immunohistochemical study. *J Neurosci.* 1994;**14**(9):5302–24.

39. Mintzer MZ, Frey JM, Griffiths RR. Zolpidem is differentiated from triazolam in humans using a three-response drug discrimination procedure. *Behav Pharmacol.* 1998;**9**(7):545–59.

40. Völlm B, Richardson P, McKie S, *et al.* Serotonergic modulation of neuronal responses to behavioural inhibition and reinforcing stimuli: an fMRI study in healthy volunteers. *Eur J Neurosci.* 2006;**23**(2):552–60.

41. Gorfine T, Assaf Y, Goshen-Gottstein Y, Yeshurun Y, Zisapel N. Sleep-anticipating effects of melatonin in the human brain. *Neuroimage.* 2006;**31**(1):410–18.

42. Kajimura N, Nishikawa M, Uchiyama M, *et al.* Deactivation by benzodiazepine of the basal forebrain and amygdala in normal humans during sleep: a placebo-controlled [O-15]H^{2}O PET study. *Am J Psychiatry.* 2004;**161**(4):748–51.

43. Dang-Vu TT, Schabus M, Desseilles M, *et al.* Functional neuroimaging insights into the physiology of human sleep. *Sleep.* 2010;**33**(12):1589–603.

44. Gillin JC, Buchsbaum MS, Valladares-Neto DC, *et al.* Effects of zolpidem on local cerebral glucose metabolism during non-REM sleep in normal volunteers: a positron emission tomography study. *Neuropsychopharmacology.* 1996;**15**(3):302–13.

45. Finelli LA, Landolt HP, Buck A, *et al.* Functional neuroanatomy of human sleep states after zolpidem and placebo: a H$_2$^{15}O-PET study. *J Sleep Res.* 2000;**9**(2):161–73.

46. Clauss RP, Dormehl IC, Oliver DW, *et al.* Measurement of cerebral perfusion after zolpidem administration in the baboon model. *Arzneim-Forsch Drug Res.* 2001;**51**(8):619–22.

47. Brefel-Courbon C, Payoux P, Ory F, *et al.* Clinical and imaging evidence of zolpidem effect in hypoxic encephalopathy. *Ann Neurol.* 2007;**62**(1):102–5.

48. Clauss RP, Nel WH. Effect of zolpidem on brain injury and diaschisis as detected by Tc-99m HMPAO brain SPECT in humans. *Arzneim-Forsch Drug Res.* 2004;**54**(10):641–6.

49. Clauss R, Sathekge M, Nel W. Transient improvement of spinocerebellar ataxia with zolpidem. *N Engl J Med.* 2004;**351**(5):511–12.

50. Cohen L, Chaaban B, Habert M. Transient improvement of aphasia with zolpidem. *N Engl J Med.* 2004;**350**(9):949–50.

51. Hall SD, Yamawaki N, Fisher AE, *et al.* GABA(A) alpha-1 subunit mediated desynchronization of elevated low frequency oscillations alleviates specific dysfunction in stroke – a case report. *Clin Neurophysiol.* 2010;**121**(4):549–55.

52. Daniele A, Albanese A, Gainotti G, Gregori B, Bartolomeo P. Zolpidem in Parkinson's disease. *Lancet.* 1997;**349**(9060):1222–3.

53. Clauss R, Nel W. Drug induced arousal from the permanent vegetative state. *Neurorehabilitation.* 2006;**21**(1):23–8.

54. Tekin S, Cummings JL. Frontal-subcortical neuronal circuits and clinical neuropsychiatry – an update. *J Psychosom Res.* 2002;**53**(2):647–54.

55. Nofzinger EA, Maquet P. What brain imaging reveals about sleep generation and maintenance. In: Kryger MH, Roth T, Dement WC, eds. *Principles and Practice of Sleep Medicine*, 5th edn. St. Louis, MI, Elsevier Saunders. 2011; 431–44.

56. Buysse DJ, Germain A, Hall M, Monk TH, Nofzinger EA. A neurobiological model of insomnia. *Drug Discov Today Dis Models.* 2011;**8**(4):129–37.

57. Nofzinger EA, Buysse D, Moul A, *et al.* Eszopiclone reverses brain hyperarousal in insomnia: evidence

from [18F]-FDG PET. *Sleep.* 2008;**31**: A232 (Abstract).

58. Nofzinger EA, Buysse DJ, Germain A, *et al.* Functional neuroimaging evidence for hyperarousal in insomnia. *Am J Psychiatry.* 2004;**161**(11):2126–9.

59. Buhr A, Bianchi MT, Baur R, *et al.* Functional characterization of the new human GABA(A) receptor mutation beta3(R192H). *Hum Genet.* 2002;**111**(2):154–60.

60. Winkelman JW, Buxton OM, Jensen JE, *et al.* Reduced brain GABA in primary insomnia: preliminary data from 4T proton magnetic resonance spectroscopy (¹H-MRS). *Sleep.* 2008;**31**(11):1499–506.

61. Rudolph U, Crestani F, Mohler H. GABA(A) receptor subtypes: dissecting their pharmacological functions. *Trends Pharmacol Sci.* 2001;**22**(4):188–94.

Functional neuroimaging of alerting medication effects

Robert Joseph Thomas

Introduction

Drugs that increase alertness can reduce subjective and objective sleepiness by mechanisms that may be probed using functional imaging. The term used is pharmacological magnetic resonance imaging (phMRI) when functional MRI techniques are used, though other imaging approaches are readily tagged with "ph." This review will provide a brief overview of some of the experimental challenges to obtain reliable phMRI data, summarize the published literature, and offer some plausible mechanistic insights into biological processes that mediate the effects of alerting medications, here generically termed "stimulants." As noted in Table 52.1, virtually all neurotransmitter systems that have alerting effects may be targeted by stimulant medications, though functional neuroimaging data are not yet available for some of them. Effects of drugs evaluated through cognitive event-related potentials are not covered here.

Pharmacological MRI (phMRI)

Positron emission tomography (PET) and functional MRI (fMRI) have been used for assessing stimulant effects, but with relevance to sleep and sleepiness, fMRI has been the dominant approach. Though blood oxygen level-dependent (BOLD) fMRI relies on a complex set of physiological processes, most phMRI studies performed tend to assume that the observed changes are predominantly due to activation of relevant neuronal circuits. The BOLD signal reflects signaling between neurons–glia–vascular entities, and the maintenance of a consistent level of vascular reactivity. Thus, the neurovascular coupling relationship has many opportunities to not reflect neural activity faithfully. These issues have been elegantly reviewed [1], and are pertinent to the functional imaging of stimulant effects.

A number of experimental measures have been proposed to improve the interpretability of BOLD fMRI studies [1]. These measures are: (a) the inclusion of one or more control tasks that explores a system not expected to be modulated (e.g., visual stimulation when investigating a cognitive task); (b) the recording of physiological parameters such as respiration during scanning and subsequent correction of possible between-group differences; (c) the assessment of baseline brain perfusion with methods such as arterial spin labeling, and vascular reactivity with CO_2 inhalation or acetazolamide; the inclusion of stimulus-related perfusion fMRI; (d) the recording of electrophysiological responses to the stimulus of interest; (e) simultaneous EEG-fMRI or combining fMRI with magnetoencephalography; (f) cerebral blood volume measurements; (g) rate of metabolic oxygen consumption measurements; and, when relevant, (h) animal studies investigating signaling between neural cells and blood vessels. Not all approaches would be relevant or even possible with each experiment.

Studies of alerting drugs/stimulants on functional brain activation have looked at regional BOLD changes or modulation of task-related activity. An important issue is a change in baseline neural activity from disease or drug, as the size of the task-related BOLD signal increase depends on the starting/resting neural activity. States of excessive sleepiness can be expected to have an effect on baseline neural activity, and be modified by top-down/motivational/volitional processes.

Table 52.1. Neurotransmitter system and stimulants drugs

Neurotransmitter	Example of clinical drug	Functional imaging data of class effect
Norepinephrine	Amphetamines, atomoxetine, selegiline	Yes
Dopamine	Amphetamines, methylphenidate, selegiline, modafinil, armodafinil	Yes
Hypocretin	Intranasal hypocretin	No
Acetylcholine	Donepezil	Yes
Glutamate	None for clinical use, but glutamate may be involved in the effects of amphetamine stimulants and modafinil	No
Adenosine	Caffeine	Yes
Neuropeptides (e.g., corticotropin-releasing hormone)	None for therapeutic use	No
Histamine	H_3 inverse-agonist tiprolisant	No

General functional imaging effects of amphetamines

Task-related brain activation modification by dextroamphetamine has been studied in healthy volunteers using O^{15} positron-emission to measure regional cerebral blood flow [2]. Dextroamphetamine (0.25 mg/kg) or placebo was administered in a double-blind, counterbalanced design 2 h before the study sessions separated by one to two weeks during performance of the Wisconsin Card Sorting Task, a neuropsychological test linked to a cortical network involving the dorsolateral prefrontal cortex and other association cortices, and Raven's Progressive Matrices, a non-verbal intelligence test linked to posterior cortical systems, and two corresponding sensorimotor control tasks. There were no significant drug or task effects on end-tidal CO_2 or on global blood flow. In the superior portion of the left inferior frontal gyrus, dextroamphetamine increased cerebral blood flow during the card sorting test but decreased it during the Ravens test. In the right hippocampus, blood flow decreased during the card sorting test but increased during the Ravens test.

Amphetamines have generally been reported to increase BOLD task-dependent activation in functional imaging studies [3, 4], though reductions have also been reported [5]. This effect is seen despite reductions in cortical blood flow by the drug [6, 7]. Experiments in rodents have investigated the functional connectivity structure underlying the widespread relative cerebral blood volume response to dextroamphetamine in the rat brain. Three distinct networks of brain regions exhibited closely coupled responses: one corresponding to primary dopamine projections from the midbrain to the striatum, a second consisting predominantly of forebrain cortical and basal ganglia regions, and a third including structures in the periventricular dopamine system [8]. Increased oxidative metabolism is a significant component of the cerebral metabolic response to acute cocaine challenge [9].

Cocaine induced focal signal increases in the nucleus accumbens/subcallosal cortex (NAc/SCC), caudate, putamen, basal forebrain, thalamus, insula, hippocampus, parahippocampal gyrus, cingulate, lateral prefrontal and temporal cortices, parietal cortex, striate/extrastriate cortices, ventral tegmentum, and pons and produced signal decreases in amygdala, temporal pole, and medial frontal cortex [10]. Brain regions that exhibited early and short duration signal maxima showed a higher correlation with rush ratings. These included the ventral tegmentum, pons, basal forebrain, caudate, cingulate, and most regions of the lateral prefrontal cortex. In contrast, regions that demonstrated early but sustained signal maxima were more correlated with craving than with rush ratings; such regions included the NAc/SCC, right parahippocampal gyrus, and some regions of the lateral prefrontal cortex. Sustained negative signal change was noted in the amygdala, which correlated with craving ratings. Similar results have been described in non-human primates, especially increased relative cerebral blood volume in the anterior cingulate, substantia nigra, ventral tegmental area, caudate (tail and head), putamen, and NAc [11]. In rodents, orexin antagonists inhibit

amphetamine responses [12]. Dextroamphetamine potentiates the response of the amygdala during the perceptual processing of angry and fearful facial expressions [13].

The effect of a functional polymorphism Val (158)-met in the catechol-O-methyltransferase gene, which has been shown to modulate prefrontal dopamine in animals and prefrontal cortical function in humans, on the modulatory actions of amphetamine on the prefrontal cortex were explored with phMRI [14]. Amphetamine enhanced the efficiency of prefrontal cortex function during a working memory task in subjects with the high enzyme activity Val/Val genotype, who have relatively less prefrontal synaptic dopamine, at all levels of task difficulty. In contrast, in subjects with the low activity Met/Met genotype, who tend to have superior baseline prefrontal function, the drug had no effect on cortical efficiency at low to moderate working memory load and caused deterioration at high working memory load. The results suggest an inverted-"U" functional-response curve to increasing dopamine signaling in the prefrontal cortex, and that individuals with genetic variants in catecholamine pathways may have differential responses.

Default mode network and stimulant drugs

The concept that the brain has a default or intrinsic mode of functioning has received increasing attention – a consistent network of brain regions, especially the posterior cingulate and precuneus, that shows high levels of activity when no explicit task is performed and participants are asked simply to rest [15, 16] remains controversial [17]. Assuming for now that default mode activity is a relevant component of brain biology, it is relevant to the understanding of sleepiness and stimulants effects [18]. The effect of sleep deprivation on functional connectivity within the default mode network and on brain regions typically activated during cognitive tasks were studied in 26 healthy participants [19]. A seed-based approach was used to examine pairwise correlations of low-frequency fMRI signal across different nodes in each state. Sleep deprivation was associated with significant selective reductions in default-mode functional connectivity and anti-correlated activity, meaning that the reciprocal activity differences were less pronounced or "blunted." Even a single night of sleep restriction reduces resting state functional connectivity [20].

Default mode network activity during working memory and visual attention tasks following the use of 20 mg of methylphenidate were evaluated in healthy subjects (16 each for drug and placebo) [21]. The group of subjects that received drug had higher activation in the parietal and prefrontal cortices, where there was increasing activation with increased cognitive load. There was also increased deactivation in the insula and posterior cingulate cortex, where regions were increasingly deactivated with increased cognitive load. In a study of children aged 9–15 years, when those with attention-deficit hyperactivity disorder (ADHD) were off-methylphenidate and task incentive was low, event-related default mode network deactivation was significantly attenuated compared to controls, but the two groups did not differ under high motivational incentives [22].

When children with ADHD were on-methylphenidate, motivational modulation of event-related default mode network deactivation was abolished, and no attenuation relative to their typically developing peers was apparent in either motivational condition. Treatment with methylphenidate normalized patterns to make them indistinguishable from that of typically developing children. This finding of methylphenidate improving suppression of default-mode activity in the ADHD patients has been replicated [23].

Caffeine

Caffeine is the most common stimulant used in the world. Adenosine antagonism is the core of its effect. This receptor-level antagonism is important in the context of function as adenosine likely plays a role in neurovascular coupling and this generation of the BOLD signal. PET has been used to quantify the effect of caffeine on whole brain and regional cerebral blood flow in humans [24]. A mean dose of 250 mg of caffeine produced approximately a 30% decrease in whole-brain cerebral blood flow; regional differences in caffeine effect were not observed. Pre-caffeine blood flow strongly influenced the magnitude of the caffeine-induced decrease. Caffeine decreased $PaCO_2$ and increased systolic blood pressure significantly; the change in $PaCO_2$ did not account for the change in cerebral blood flow.

Combined caffeine and glucose is associated with maintained performance but a decrease in activation in the bilateral parietal and left prefrontal cortices, which could suggest increased processing efficiency [25]. Caffeine reduces measures of resting state BOLD connectivity in the motor cortex, baseline cerebral blood flow, and the spectral energy in low-frequency BOLD fluctuations [26]. Caffeine increases the BOLD response [27] and can decrease cerebral blood flow [28]. The increase in BOLD response does not occur in all individuals [29], and it is unknown what role genetic modulation of adenosine metabolism may play. Sleep depth and response to sleep deprivation is modified by adenosine availability [30], and may in theory modify fMRI signals and the response to caffeine. In a study evaluating the difference between high and low users of caffeine, the BOLD signal change in the visual cortex was significantly greater in high users than in low users in the presence of caffeine, and the magnitude of the BOLD signal was significantly correlated with caffeine consumption [31]. Up regulation of adenosine receptors in high users may be involved.

Localized changes in oxygen consumption related to increased neural activity can result in a small and transient "initial dip" of the BOLD signal. The initial dip has been of great interest to the fMRI community because it may provide a more accurate and localized measure of neural activity than the conventional BOLD signal increase. Although potentially useful as a technique for human brain mapping, the initial dip is not always detected and has been a source of some controversy. The BOLD response to a 4-s long visual stimulus measured with a 3 T MRI system in five healthy volunteers both before and immediately after a 200-mg oral caffeine dose showed that caffeine reduced or eliminated the initial dip in all subjects [32]. Another study used both a 1-s long single trial stimulus and a 20-s long block stimulus in a 4 T magnet pre/post a 200-mg caffeine dose to assess BOLD signal kinetics and resting levels of cerebral blood flow using arterial spin labeling [33]. For both types of trials, the caffeine dose reduced the time to peak, the time after the peak at which the response returned to 50% of the peak amplitude, and the amplitude of the post-stimulus undershoot in all subjects. In some subjects, oscillations were observed in the post-stimulus portion of the response with median peak periods of 9.1 and 9.5 s for the single trial and block responses, respectively. Resting cerebral blood flow was reduced by an average of 24%.

Task-related functional activation studies of caffeine are few. In a study using a 2-back verbal working memory task, caffeine caused an increased response in the bilateral medial frontopolar cortex, extending to the right anterior cingulate cortex [34]. Caffeine can sustain regional brain activation patterns lost in acute hypoglycaemia [35].

Nicotine

Nicotine generally increases task-related activity in non-smokers and deprived smokers, but not active smokers [36–39]. Nicotine or nicotinic stimulation decreases the activity in the default mode network [40].

Atomoxetine

A selective norepinephrine reuptake inhibitor, the drug is licensed for use in ADHD but can be used in narcolepsy to inhibit cataplexy and also enhance alertness. The effect of 40 mg atomoxetine was evaluated using fMRI in 19 healthy volunteers. The drug improved inhibitory control and increased activation in the right inferior frontal gyrus when volunteers attempted to inhibit their responses (irrespective of success) [41].

Another study tested the effects of 80 mg atomoxetine on error monitoring in 12 healthy, male volunteers in a randomized double-blind, placebo-controlled, within-subjects design, during a combined Eriksen flanker–Go/No-Go task using fMRI [42]. At this dose, atomoxetine led to a significant increase in failed inhibition. There was an increase of the error signal (incorrect minus correct No-Go trials) under atomoxetine in bilateral inferior frontal cortex and pre-supplementary motor area. In this experiment, atomoxetine increased neural sensitivity for errors in healthy control subjects but this gain was accompanied by deterioration in inhibitory control, possibly reflecting a shift beyond the optimal working range of the norepinephrine system.

Cholinergic stimulation

The alerting effects of cholinergic stimulation are well recognized, but clinical use in conditions of excessive daytime sleepiness has not been readily possible or even well studied.

A comprehensive review of pharmacological imaging of cholinergic modulation of cognition has shown some consistent themes: (a) the direction of cholinergic modulation of sensory cortex activations depends upon top-down influences; (b) cholinergic hyperstimulation reduces top-down selective modulation of sensory cortices; (c) cholinergic hyperstimulation interacts with task-specific frontoparietal activations according to one of several patterns, including: suppression of parietal-mediated reorienting; decreasing "effort"-associated activations in prefrontal regions; and deactivation of a "resting state network" in medial cortex, with reciprocal recruitment of dorsolateral frontoparietal regions during performance-challenging conditions; (d) encoding-related activations in both neocortical and hippocampal regions are disrupted by cholinergic blockade, or enhanced with cholinergic stimulation, while the opposite profile is observed during retrieval; (e) many examples exist of an "inverted-U shaped" pattern of cholinergic influences by which the direction of functional neural activation (and performance) depends upon both task (e.g., relative difficulty) and subject (e.g., age) factors [43].

It is possible that low-dose cholinergic enhancement can augment the use of conventional stimulants. Opiate-induced sedation has been reportedly benefited by donepezil in a small case series of six subjects [44]. Thirty healthy volunteers were administered either a 5-mg daily dose of donepezil or placebo for 14–17 days, in a double-blind parallel group design prior to 24-h sleep deprivation [45]. A battery of cognitive tasks designed to measure different components of memory and executive function were administered. Despite partially reversing the decline in subjective alertness associated with sleep deprivation, treatment with donepezil failed to reverse significantly the decline in cognitive performance on any of the tasks [45]. An evaluation of donepezil effects following sleep deprivation used fMRI. The design was a double-blind, placebo-controlled, crossover study involving seven laboratory visits over two months in 26 healthy volunteers. Participants underwent four fMRI scans; two sessions (donepezil or placebo) followed a normal night's sleep, and two sessions followed a night of sleep deprivation [46]; 5 mg of donepezil was taken once daily for approximately 17 days. Subjects were scanned while performing a semantic judgment task and tested for word recognition outside the scanner 45 minutes later. Sleep deprivation increased the frequency of non-responses at encoding and impaired delayed recognition. No benefit of donepezil was evident when participants were well rested. When sleep deprived, individuals who showed greater performance decline from sleep deprivation improved with donepezil, whereas more resistant individuals did not benefit. Accompanying these behavioral effects, there was increased task-related activation in functionally relevant brain regions. The same research group also reported significant correlations between donepezil-induced increases in neural activation in the posterior cortical areas and improvement in accuracy during parametric task (perceptual and memory)-load manipulation of visual short-term memory [47] .

Modafinil

A phMRI study in the anesthetized rat mapped the circuitry activated by a single modafinil dose. Prominent and sustained activation was seen in the prefrontal and cingulate cortices, together with weaker but significant activation of the somatosensory cortex, medial thalamic domains, hippocampus, ventral striatum, and dorsal raphe [48]. Correlation analysis showed enhanced connectivity within a neural network including dopamine projections from the ventral tegmental area to the NAc.

To assess the effect of the wake-promoting drug modafinil on working memory and brain activation in the executive network, following a single night of sleep deprivation, a randomized, placebo-controlled, 4-arm, double-blind evaluation of a single 200-mg dose of modafinil on working memory (1-, 2-, and 3-back)-related functional brain activation and performance was done in eight medication-free men, aged 21 to 35 years. Performance in the deprived state was enhanced by modafinil only at an intermediate (2-back) level of task difficulty and was associated with the recruitment of increased cortical activation volumes [49]. Strong and consistent individual differences in performance were noted on the working memory tasks.

Metamphetamine-dependent individuals exhibit deficits in cognition and prefrontal cortical function. A randomized, double-blind, placebo-controlled, cross over study, using fMRI to examine the effects of a single dose of 200 mg modafinil on learning and neural activity related to cognitive function in abstinent, metamphetamine-dependent, and healthy control participants, has been reported [50]. Modafinil boosted learning in drug-dependent participants bringing them to the same performance level as control subjects; the control group did not show changes in performance with modafinil. After controlling for performance differences, drug-dependent participants showed a greater effect of modafinil on brain activation in the bilateral insula/ventrolateral prefrontal cortex and anterior cingulate cortices than control participants.

The acute effects of modafinil on prefrontal activation and cognitive control of motor activity in people with schizophrenia and prominent negative symptoms were examined using a crossover design in 12 subjects. Modafinil administration was associated with significantly greater activation of the dorsolateral prefrontal cortex during fMRI especifically in those with reduced baseline performance [51] A second report from the same group described an increase in anterior cingulate activation during a working memory task with a single 100 mg dose of modafinil [52].

Modafinil effects on neural circuits underlying affective processing and cognitive functions have been assessed in healthy volunteers in a double-blinded placebo-controlled trial (100 mg/day for seven days). Subjects underwent BOLD fMRI while performing an emotion information-processing task that activated the amygdala, and two prefrontal-dependent cognitive tasks – a working memory task and a variable attentional control task. BOLD fMRI revealed significantly decreased amygdala reactivity to fearful stimuli on modafinil compared with the placebo condition [53]. During the executive cognition tasks, modafinil reduced BOLD signal in the prefrontal cortex and anterior cingulate [53]. The study suggested that modafinil in low doses has a unique physiological profile compared with stimulant drugs: it enhances the efficiency of prefrontal cortical cognitive information processing, while dampening reactivity to threatening stimuli in the amygdala, a brain region implicated in anxiety.

Stimulants and disorders of excessive sleepiness

Functional imaging studies of stimulant effects in narcoleptics are limited (54–57), with results suggesting hypoactivation in executive areas that are more "normal" with the stimulant. Low-resolution brain electromagnetic tomography (LORETA) has reportedly shown a reduction in prefrontal delta with the use of modafinil, which correlated with cognitive performance [58]. Repetitive consecutive testing using fMRI has shown a progressive loss of functional activation, predominantly in the prefrontal cortex using a working memory 2-back task, that is prevented by modafinil and amphetamine treatment [55]. A study assessed the excitability of the motor cortex with transcranial magnetic stimulation (TMS) in 13 patients with narcolepsy and in 12 control subjects. Resting and active motor thresholds were higher in narcoleptic patients than in controls and intracortical inhibition was more pronounced in narcoleptic patients (59, 60). Activation during non-cognitive tasks are small, suggesting that task selection will be important in functional imaging studies of sleepiness in narcolepsy and related disorders.

Functional activation changes seen in narcoleptics need to be considered in light of reported structural differences, which could change network connectivity [61]. Anatomical differences between narcoleptics and controls are not visible on standard high-resolution MRI, but have been reported using voxel-based morphometry involving the hypothalamus, prefrontal and inferior temporal cortices, and insula (62–65). A completely negative study has also been reported [66]. Individual studies have had small sample sizes (often less than 20), and acquisition/analytic techniques have differences. Perhaps if investigators can pool all the available data a more definitive result may be obtained, and allow adjustment for possible disease durations. If indeed there are anatomical differences, and these differences reflect neuronal/synaptic loss or volumetric alterations, the possible reasons are open to speculation. These include trophic changes from changes in synaptic neurotransmission and autoimmune injury that occurred at the time of orexin neuronal loss. Any anatomical abnormality can impact functional activation.

The only randomized trial of stimulant use for residual sleepiness in treated sleep apnea patients using fMRI has been presented in abstract form. In a two-week, multicenter, randomized, double-blind, placebo-controlled study, 40 patients were randomized to armodafinil 200 mg/day or placebo [67]. The primary efficacy measure was change from baseline to final visit in activation volume of the dorsolateral

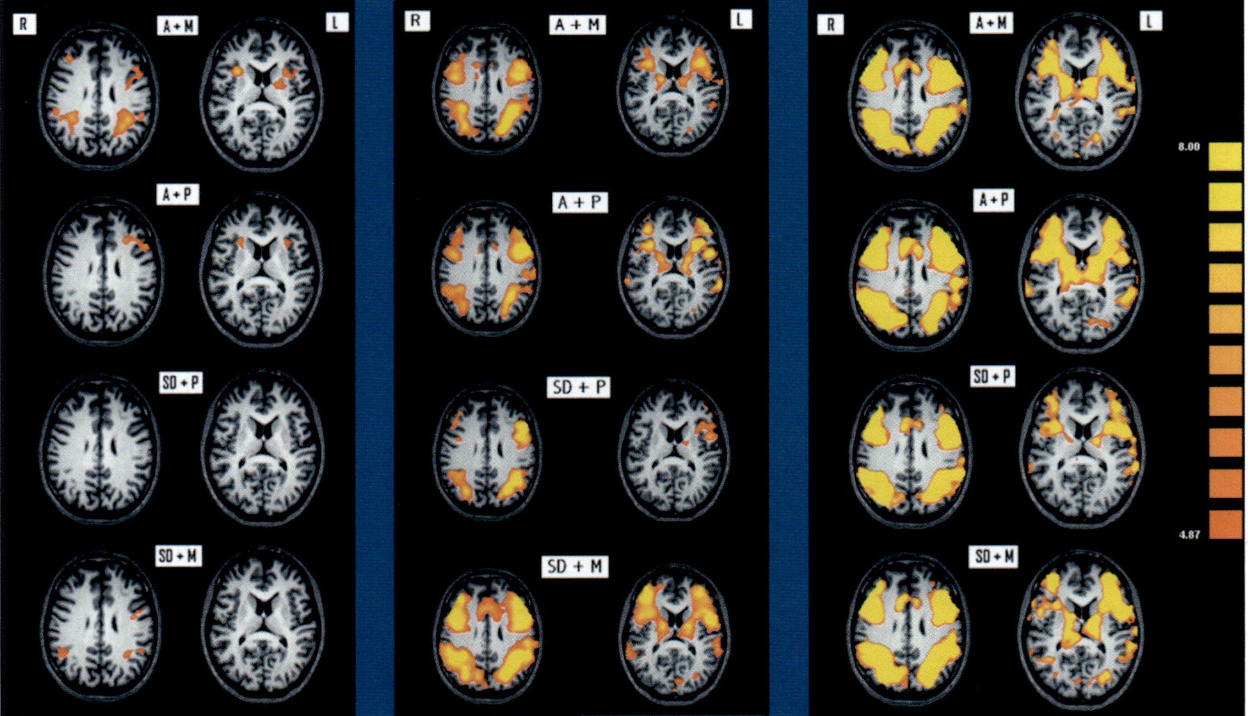

Figure 52.1 Sleep deprivation, drug (200 mg modafinil) and task-load effects assessed by fMRI at 3-tesla field strength. A: rested/alert, SD: 24-hours sleep deprivation, M: modafinil, P: placebo. Note that the greatest effect of the drug is in the 2-back condition, following sleep deprivation (middle panel, lowest figure set). When the task is easy, or the subject is able to perform a difficult (3-back) task, the drug has little effects on functional activation or performance. (From *Sleep* 2006;**29**:1471–81, with permission.)

prefrontal cortex (DLPFC) measured using fMRI. The key secondary measure was change in response latency on the 2-back working memory task performed during scanning. Other measures included activation volume in other predefined regions of interest (ROI), and % change in BOLD signal intensity and resting state activation in the ROI. Safety and tolerability were also assessed. Patients given armodafinil (n = 20) or placebo (n = 16) had similar demographic and baseline clinical characteristics. During the task, changes in activation volume in the DLPFC and other ROI and in 2-back response latency were not significantly different between groups, and changes in BOLD signal intensity in the ROI were inconsistent. While there are many interpretations of the results, they include the possibility that those with severe residual sleepiness despite perfect compliance with treatment have permanent injury to the relevant neural networks.

How can alerting drugs improve brain function?

Neuroanatomy, neurochemistry, and functional imaging offer some insights into how alerting drugs work. The simple explanation is that activity of specific alerting systems such as dopaminergic and noradrenergic systems occur. However, drugs show such precise specificity, and "promiscuity" is typical. Norepinephrine and cholinergic stimulation improve signal-to-noise ratios. Network connectivity may improve, and restoration of the correlated activity within the default mode network and anti-correlated activity within the default mode network and task-engaged network may occur. Drugs that increase motivation may enhance top-down influences. Adenosine antagonism may reduce effects of an endogenous sleep promoter and thus have multiple effects by modulating several neurotransmitter systems.

References

1. Iannetti GD, Wise RG. BOLD functional MRI in disease and pharmacological studies: room for improvement? *Magn Reson Imaging*. 2007;**25**(6):978–88. Epub 2007/05/15.

2. Mattay VS, Berman KF, Ostrem JL, *et al.* Dextroamphetamine enhances "neural network-specific" physiological signals: a positron-emission tomography rCBF study. *J Neurosci*. 1996;**16**(15):4816–22. Epub 1996/08/01.

3. Uftring SJ, Wachtel SR, Chu D, An fMRI study of the effect of amphetamine on brain activity. *Neuropsychopharmacology*. 2001;**25**(6):925–35. Epub 2001/12/26.

4. Knutson B, Bjork JM, Fong GW, *et al.* Amphetamine modulates human incentive processing. *Neuron*. 2004;**43**(2):261–9. Epub 2004/07/21.

5. Willson MC, Wilman AH, Bell EC, Asghar SJ, Silverstone PH. Dextroamphetamine causes a change in regional brain activity in vivo during cognitive tasks: a functional magnetic resonance imaging study of blood oxygen level-dependent response. *Biol Psychiatry*. 2004;**56**(4):284–91. Epub 2004/08/18.

6. Daniel DG, Weinberger DR, Jones DW, *et al.* The effect of amphetamine on regional cerebral blood flow during cognitive activation in schizophrenia. *J Neurosci*. 1991;**11**(7):1907–17. Epub 1991/07/01.

7. Gollub RL, Breiter HC, Kantor H, *et al.* Cocaine decreases cortical cerebral blood flow but does not obscure regional activation in functional magnetic resonance imaging in human subjects. *J Cereb Blood Flow Metab*. 1998;**18**(7):724–34. Epub 1998/07/15.

8. Schwarz AJ, Gozzi A, Reese T, Bifone A. Functional connectivity in the pharmacologically activated brain: resolving networks of correlated responses to d-amphetamine. *Magn Reson Med*. 2007;**57**(4):704–13. Epub 2007/03/29.

9. Ceolin L, Schwarz AJ, Gozzi A, Reese T, Bifone A. Effects of cocaine on blood flow and oxygen metabolism in the rat brain: implications for phMRI. *Magn Reson Imaging*. 2007;**25**(6):795–800. Epub 2007/04/20.

10. Breiter HC, Gollub RL, Weisskoff RM, *et al.* Acute effects of cocaine on human brain activity and emotion. *Neuron*. 1997;**19**(3):591–611. Epub 1997/10/23.

11. Jenkins BG, Sanchez-Pernaute R, Brownell AL, Chen YC, Isacson O. Mapping dopamine function in primates using pharmacologic magnetic resonance imaging. *J Neurosci*. 2004;**24**(43):9553–60. Epub 2004/10/29.

12. Gozzi A, Turrini G, Piccoli L, *et al.* Functional magnetic resonance imaging reveals different neural substrates for the effects of orexin-1 and orexin-2 receptor antagonists. *PLoS One*. 2011;**6**(1):e16406. Epub 2011/02/11.

13. Hariri AR, Mattay VS, Tessitore A, *et al.* Dextroamphetamine modulates the response of the human amygdala. *Neuropsychopharmacology*. 2002;**27**(6):1036–40. Epub 2002/12/05.

14. Mattay VS, Goldberg TE, Fera F, *et al.* Catechol O-methyltransferase val158-met genotype and individual variation in the brain response to amphetamine. *Proc Natl Acad Sci USA*. 2003;**100**(10):6186–91. Epub 2003/04/30.

15. Raichle ME, Snyder AZ. A default mode of brain function: a brief history of an evolving idea. *Neuroimage*. 2007;**37**(4):1083–90; discussion 1097–9. Epub 2007/08/28.

16. Cavanna AE, Trimble MR. The precuneus: a review of its functional anatomy and behavioural correlates. *Brain*. 2006;**129**(Pt 3):564–83. Epub 2006/02/10.

17. Morcom AM, Fletcher PC. Does the brain have a baseline? Why we should be resisting a rest. *Neuroimage*. 2007;**37**(4):1073–82. Epub 2007/08/08.

18. Gujar N, Yoo SS, Hu P, Walker MP. The unrested resting brain: sleep deprivation alters activity within the default-mode network. *J Cogn Neurosci*. 2010;**22**(8):1637–48. Epub 2009/03/26.

19. De Havas JA, Parimal S, Soon CS, Chee MW. Sleep deprivation reduces default mode network connectivity and anti-correlation during rest and task performance. *Neuroimage*. 2012;**59**(2):1745–51. Epub 2011/08/30.

20. Samann PG, Tully C, Spoormaker VI, *et al.* Increased sleep pressure reduces resting state functional connectivity. *MAGMA*. 2010;**23**(5–6):375–89. Epub 2010/05/18.

21. Tomasi D, Volkow ND, Wang GJ, *et al.* Methylphenidate enhances brain activation and deactivation responses to visual attention and working memory tasks in healthy controls. *Neuroimage.* 2011;**54**(4):3101–10. Epub 2010/10/30.

22. Liddle EB, Hollis C, Batty MJ, *et al.* Task-related default mode network modulation and inhibitory control in ADHD: effects of motivation and methylphenidate. *J Child Psychol Psychiatry.* 2011;**52**(7):761–71. Epub 2010/11/16.

23. Peterson BS, Potenza MN, Wang Z, *et al.* An FMRI study of the effects of psychostimulants on default-mode processing during Stroop task performance in youths with ADHD. *Am J Psychiatry.* 2009;**166**(11):1286–94. Epub 2009/09/17.

24. Cameron OG, Modell JG, Hariharan M. Caffeine and human cerebral blood flow: a positron emission tomography study. *Life Sci.* 1990;**47**(13):1141–6. Epub 1990/01/01.

25. Serra-Grabulosa JM, Adan A, Falcon C, Bargallo N. Glucose and caffeine effects on sustained attention: an exploratory fMRI study. *Hum Psychopharmacol.* 2010;**25**(7–8):543–52. Epub 2011/02/12.

26. Rack-Gomer AL, Liau J, Liu TT. Caffeine reduces resting-state BOLD functional connectivity in the motor cortex. *Neuroimage.* 2009;**46**(1):56–63. Epub 2009/05/22.

27. Chen Y, Parrish TB. Caffeine dose effect on activation-induced BOLD and CBF responses. *Neuroimage.* 2009;**46**(3):577–83. Epub 2009/03/18.

28. Perthen JE, Lansing AE, Liau J, Liu TT, Buxton RB. Caffeine-induced uncoupling of cerebral blood flow and oxygen metabolism: a calibrated BOLD fMRI study. *Neuroimage.* 2008;**40**(1):237–47. Epub 2008/01/15.

29. Laurienti PJ, Field AS, Burdette JH, *et al.* Relationship between caffeine-induced changes in resting cerebral perfusion and blood oxygenation level-dependent signal. *AJNR Am J Neuroradiol.* 2003;**24**(8):1607–11. Epub 2003/09/19.

30. Bachmann V, Klaus F, Bodenmann S, *et al.* Functional ADA polymorphism increases sleep depth and reduces vigilant attention in humans. *Cereb Cortex.* 2012;**22**(4):962–70. Epub 2011/07/08.

31. Laurienti PJ, Field AS, Burdette JH, *et al.* Dietary caffeine consumption modulates fMRI measures. *Neuroimage.* 2002;**17**(2):751–7. Epub 2002/10/16.

32. Behzadi Y, Liu TT. Caffeine reduces the initial dip in the visual BOLD response at 3 T. *Neuroimage.* 2006;**32**(1):9–15. Epub 2006/04/26.

33. Liu TT, Behzadi Y, Restom K, *et al.* Caffeine alters the temporal dynamics of the visual BOLD response. *Neuroimage.* 2004;**23**(4):1402–13. Epub 2004/12/14.

34. Koppelstaetter F, Poeppel TD, Siedentopf CM, *et al.* Does caffeine modulate verbal working memory processes? An fMRI study. *Neuroimage.* 2008;**39**(1):492–9. Epub 2007/10/16.

35. Rosenthal MJ, Smith D, Yaguez L, *et al.* Caffeine restores regional brain activation in acute hypoglycaemia in healthy volunteers. *Diabet Med.* 2007;**24**(7):720–7. Epub 2007/05/19.

36. Newhouse PA, Potter AS, Dumas JA, Thiel CM. Functional brain imaging of nicotinic effects on higher cognitive processes. *Biochem Pharmacol.* 2011;**82**(8):943–51. Epub 2011/06/21.

37. Azizian A, Monterosso J, O'Neill J, London ED. Magnetic resonance imaging studies of cigarette smoking. *Handb Exp Pharmacol.* 2009;(**192**):113–43. Epub 2009/02/03.

38. Kumari V, Gray JA, ffytche DH, *et al.* Cognitive effects of nicotine in humans: an fMRI study. *Neuroimage.* 2003;**19**(3):1002–13. Epub 2003/07/26.

39. Stein EA, Pankiewicz J, Harsch HH, *et al.* Nicotine-induced limbic cortical activation in the human brain: a functional MRI study. *Am J Psychiatry.* 1998;**155**(8):1009–15. Epub 1998/08/12.

40. Tanabe J, Nyberg E, Martin LF, *et al.* Nicotine effects on default mode network during resting state. *Psychopharmacology (Berl).* 2011;**216**(2):287–95. Epub 2011/02/19.

41. Chamberlain SR, Hampshire A, Muller U, *et al.* Atomoxetine modulates right inferior frontal activation during inhibitory control: a pharmacological functional magnetic resonance imaging study. *Biol Psychiatry.* 2009;**65**(7):550–5. Epub 2008/11/26.

42. Graf H, Abler B, Freudenmann R, *et al.* Neural correlates of error monitoring modulated by atomoxetine in healthy volunteers. *Biol Psychiatry.* 2011;**69**(9):890–7. Epub 2010/12/21.

43. Bentley P, Driver J, Dolan RJ. Cholinergic modulation of cognition: insights from human pharmacological functional neuroimaging. *Prog Neurobiol.* 2011;**94**(4):360–88. Epub 2011/06/29.

44. Slatkin NE, Rhiner M, Bolton TM. Donepezil in the treatment of opioid-induced sedation: report of six cases. *J Pain Symptom Manage.* 2001;**21**(5):425–38. Epub 2001/05/23.

45. Dodds CM, Bullmore ET, Henson RN, *et al.* Effects of donepezil on cognitive performance after sleep deprivation. *Hum Psychopharmacol.* 2011;**26**(8):578–87. Epub 2011/12/14.

46. Chuah LY, Chong DL, Chen AK, *et al.* Donepezil improves episodic memory in young individuals vulnerable to the effects of sleep deprivation. *Sleep.* 2009;**32**(8):999–1010. Epub 2009/09/04.

47. Chuah LY, Chee MW. Cholinergic augmentation modulates visual task performance in sleep-deprived young adults. *J Neurosci.* 2008;**28**(44):11369–77. Epub 2008/10/31.

48. Gozzi A, Colavito V, Seke Etet PF, *et al.* Modulation of fronto-cortical activity by modafinil: a functional imaging and Fos study in the rat. *Neuropsychopharmacology.* 2012;**37**(3):822–37. Epub 2011/11/04.

49. Thomas RJ, Kwong K. Modafinil activates cortical and subcortical sites in the sleep-deprived state. *Sleep.* 2006;**29**(11):1471–81. Epub 2006/12/14.

50. Ghahremani DG, Tabibnia G, Monterosso J, *et al.* Effect of modafinil on learning and task-related brain activity in metamphetamine-dependent and healthy individuals. *Neuropsychopharmacology.* 2011;**36**(5):950–9. Epub 2011/02/04.

51. Hunter MD, Ganesan V, Wilkinson ID, Spence SA. Impact of modafinil on prefrontal executive function in schizophrenia. *Am J Psychiatry.* 2006;**163**(12):2184–6. Epub 2006/12/08.

52. Spence SA, Green RD, Wilkinson ID, Hunter MD. Modafinil modulates anterior cingulate function in chronic schizophrenia. *Br J Psychiatry.* 2005;**187**:55–61. Epub 2005/07/05.

53. Rasetti R, Mattay VS, Stankevich B, *et al.* Modulatory effects of modafinil on neural circuits regulating emotion and cognition. *Neuropsychopharmacology.* 2010;**35**(10):2101–9. Epub 2010/06/18.

54. Allen MD, Hedges DW, Farrer TJ, Larson MJ. Assessment of brain activity during memory encoding in a

narcolepsy patient on and off modafinil using normative fMRI data. *Neurocase.* 2012;**18**(1):13–25. Epub 2011/10/12.

55. Thomas RJ. Fatigue in the executive cortical network demonstrated in narcoleptics using functional magnetic resonance imaging: a preliminary study. *Sleep Med.* 2005;**6**(5):399–406. Epub 2005/07/06.

56. Dang-Vu TT, Desseilles M, Schwartz S, Maquet P. Neuroimaging of narcolepsy. *CNS Neurol Disord Drug Targets.* 2009;**8**(4):254–63. Epub 2009/08/20.

57. Kim YK, Yoon IY, Shin YK, Cho SS, Kim SE. Modafinil-induced hippocampal activation in narcolepsy. *Neurosci Lett.* 2007;**422**(2):91–6. Epub 2007/06/30.

58. Saletu M, Anderer P, Semlitsch HV, *et al.* Low-resolution brain electromagnetic tomography (LORETA) identifies brain regions linked to psychometric performance under modafinil in narcolepsy. *Psychiatry Res.* 2007;**154**(1):69–84. Epub 2006/12/26.

59. Oliviero A, Della Marca G, Tonali PA, *et al.* Functional involvement of cerebral cortex in human narcolepsy. *J Neurol.* 2005;**252**(1):56–61. Epub 2005/01/18.

60. Howard RJ, Ellis C, Bullmore ET, *et al.* Functional echoplanar brain imaging correlates of amphetamine administration to normal subjects and subjects with the narcoleptic syndrome. *Magn Reson Imaging.* 1996;**14**(9):1013–16. Epub 1996/01/01.

61. Ellis CM, Monk C, Simmons A, *et al.* Functional magnetic resonance imaging neuroactivation studies in normal subjects and subjects with the narcoleptic syndrome. Actions of modafinil. *J Sleep Res.* 1999;**8**(2):85–93. Epub 1999/07/02.

62. Kaufmann C, Schuld A, Pollmacher T, Auer DP. Reduced cortical gray matter in narcolepsy: preliminary findings with voxel-based morphometry. *Neurology.* 2002;**58**(12):1852–5. Epub 2002/06/27.

63. Brenneis C, Brandauer E, Frauscher B, *et al.* Voxel-based morphometry in narcolepsy. *Sleep Med.* 2005;**6**(6):531–6. Epub 2005/07/05.

64. Buskova J, Vaneckova M, Sonka K, Seidl Z, Nevsimalova S. Reduced hypothalamic gray matter in narcolepsy with cataplexy. *Neuro Endocrinol Lett.* 2006;**27**(6):769–72. Epub 2006/12/26.

65. Joo EY, Tae WS, Kim ST, Hong SB. Gray matter concentration abnormality in brains of narcolepsy patients. *Korean J Radiol.* 2009;**10**(6):552–8. Epub 2009/11/04.

66. Overeem S, Steens SC, Good CD, *et al.* Voxel-based morphometry in hypocretin-deficient narcolepsy. *Sleep.* 2003;**26**(1):44–6. Epub 2003/03/12.

67. Rippon GA, Greve DN, Yang R, Dayno JM, Thomas RJ, Armodafinil fMRI Study Group. Effect of armodafinil on cortical activity and working memory in patients with residual excessive sleepiness associated with CPAP-treated OSA: an fMRI study. *Sleep.* 2010;**33**:A162.

Zolpidem-induced parasomnias

Romy Hoque

History

The patient is a 51-year-old African American woman with past medical history of hypertension, hyperlipidemia, depression, and mild obstructive sleep apnea with a previous diagnostic polysomnogram apnea-hypopnea index of ten events per hour. The patient had neither a personal nor family history of sleep-walking or other parasomnias. At age 44 the patient was started on non-extended release zolpidem 10 mg at bedtime for insomnia. A few weeks after starting zolpidem she began sleep-related walking, eating, and one episode of driving where she drove ten miles from home and was found asleep behind the wheel by local police. She had a vague recollection of this event and thought she was dreaming. After an evaluation by a sleep medicine physician the patient's zolpidem was gradually withdrawn. All sleep-related activities immediately ceased with discontinuation of zolpidem.

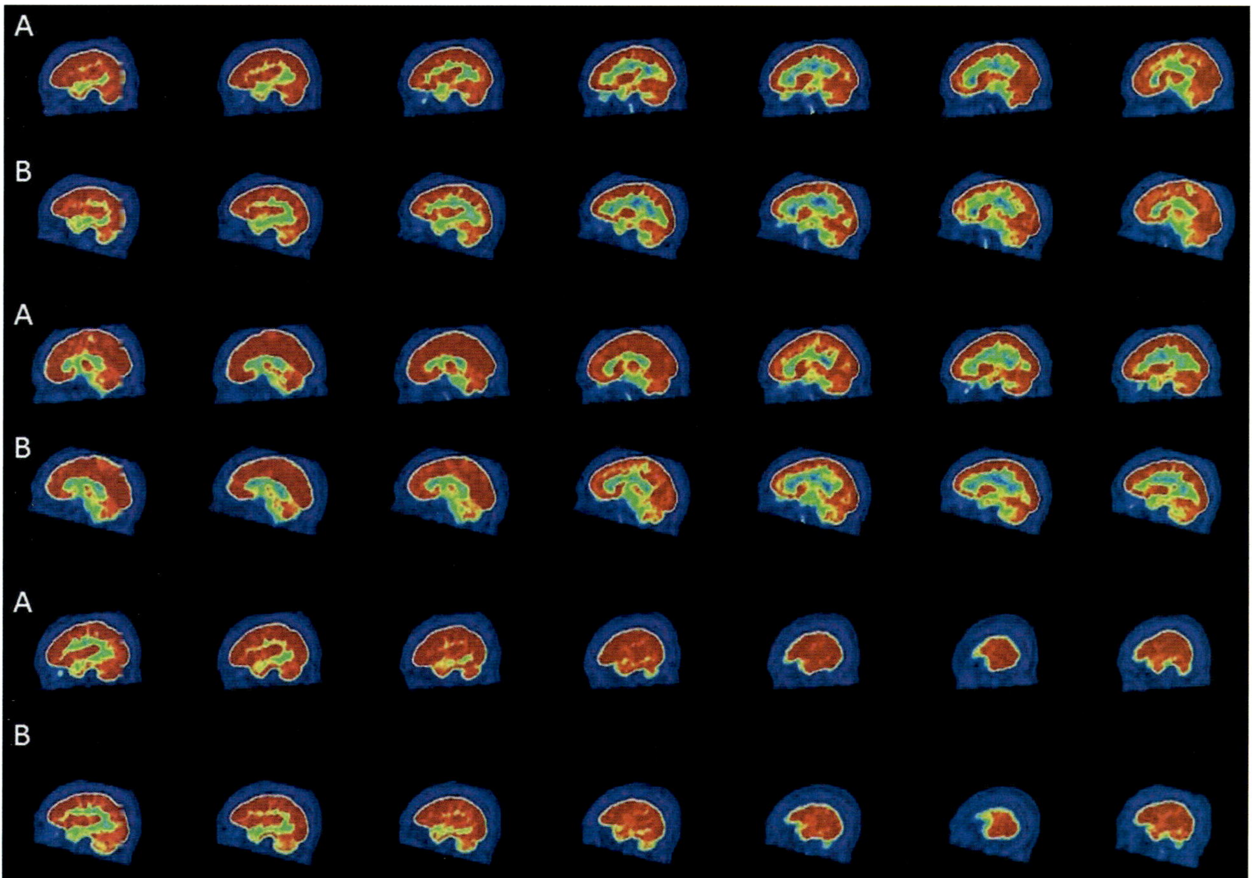

Figure 53.1 ¹⁸F-fluorodeoxyglucose positron emission tomography (¹⁸F-FDG PET) of a patient with zolpidem-induced sleepwalking, sleep-related eating disorder, and sleep-driving. (A) ¹⁸F-FDG PET off zolpidem. (B) ¹⁸F-FDG PET on zolpidem. FDG was administered to the patient 1 h after ingestion of 10 mg zolpidem. Statistical parametric mapping comparison of the two sequences shows no significant differences.

Neuroimaging of Sleep and Sleep Disorders, ed. Eric Nofzinger, Pierre Maquet, and Michael J. Thorpy. Published by Cambridge University Press. © Cambridge University Press 2013.

Imaging technique

Fluorine-18-fluorodeoxygluose positron emission tomography (^{18}F-FDG PET) was obtained one month after discontinuation of zolpidem. A second ^{18}F-FDG PET study was acquired the following day 1 h after oral administration of non-extended release zolpidem 10 mg with an expected zolpidem peak plasma concentration of 1.2 ± 0.2 h (Figure 53.1).

Imaging findings

Statistical parametric mapping of cerebral glucose metabolism showed no significant differences between the two ^{18}F-FDG PET studies [1].

Discussion

Zolpidem is an imidiazopyridine drug indicated for short-term insomnia at dosages ranging from 5 to 10 mg per day. Though considered a non-benzodiazepine since its imidiazopyridine structure differs from the typical benzodiazepine fusion of benzene and diazepine, zolpidem is a benzodiazepine receptor agonist with high affinity for the GABA$_A$ (gamma-aminobutyric acid type A) receptor expressing the α_1 subunit. This receptor corresponds to the ω_1 benzodiazepine receptor in the current benzodiazepine receptor nomenclature. Even though zolpidem is relatively specific for GABA$_A$ receptors with α_1 subunits, these receptors are expressed widely throughout the central nervous system. In addition zolpidem has a less recognized but limited binding affinity to ω_2 benzodiazepine receptors that are also widely expressed throughout the human brain.

In an attempt to identify focal zolpidem-induced changes in cerebral glucose metabolic rates ^{18}F-FDG PET studies were performed. Focal cortical changes in glucose metabolism associated with zolpidem use were not identified. Compared to wake, whole brain glucose cortical metabolic rates decrease in non-rapid eye movement (NREM) and REM sleep. One would expect a decline in glucose metabolic rate with the use of sleep-inducing hypnotics like zolpidem with its widespread cortical binding. However, the results show otherwise. The reasons for this are unknown. One possible explanation may be that PET is too insensitive a tool to detect subtle localized or generalized glucose metabolic rate differences on and off zolpidem in the normal brain.

Key points

- Zolpidem is a hypnotic indicated for short-term insomnia that acts at the GABA$_A$ receptor expressing the α_1 subunit.
- Sleep-related disorders including sleepwalking, sleep-related eating and even sleep-driving have been reported with zolpidem use.
- Pathophysiologic mechanisms underlying zolpidem's myriad effects have yet to be fully elucidated.

Reference

1. Hoque R, Chesson AL, Jr. Zolpidem-induced sleepwalking, sleep related eating disorder, and sleep-driving: fluorine-18-fluorodeoxyglucose positron emission tomography analysis, and a literature review of other unexpected clinical effects of zolpidem. *J Clin Sleep Med.* 2009;5:471–6.

Joint Commission International Accreditation:

Getting Started

SECOND EDITION

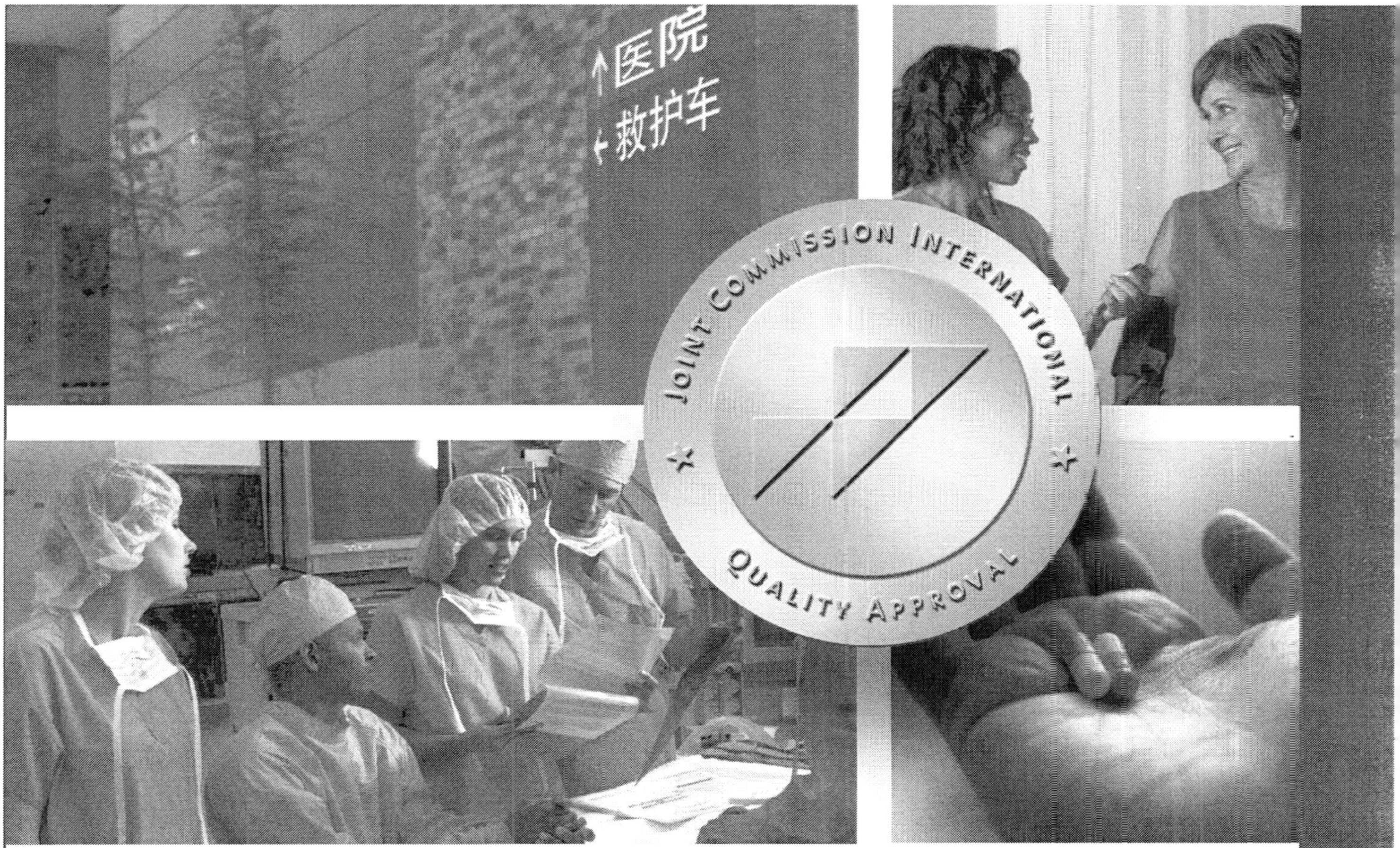

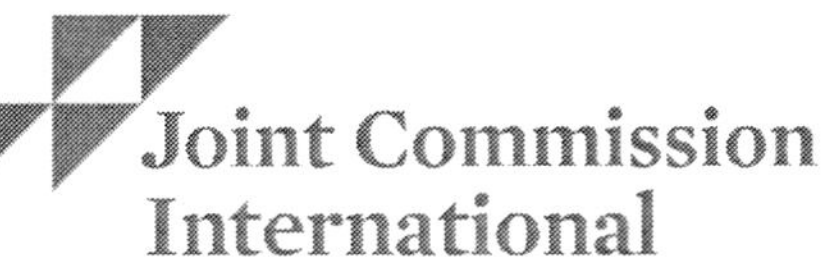

Joint Commission
International

Joint Commission International Accreditation: Getting Started, **Second Edition**

Manager, Publications: Paul Reis

Project Manager: Bridget Chambers

Production Manager: Johanna Harris

Executive Director: Catherine Chopp Hinckley, Ph.D.

Consulting Editor: Helen Hoesing, R.N., M.P.H., Ph.D.

Joint Commission International Reviewers: Siew Lee Cheng, R.N., M.S.N., C.C.N.S.; Bruce Frederick, R.N., M.N.; Catherine Chopp Hinckley, Ph.D.; Helen Hoesing, R.N., M.P.H., Ph.D.; Ann Jacobson, M.S.N., R.N., N.E.A.; Claudia Jorgenson, R.N., M.S.N.; Sherry Kaufield, M.A., F.A.C.H.E.; Paul vanOstenberg, D.D.S., M.S.

Joint Commission International Publications Advisory Board Reviewers: Malik Abdo Ali, M.D., M.P.H.; Ali Nasha`at Ali Sha`ar, M.D., M.Sc.; Kwong Ming Fock, M.B.B.S., M.Med., F.R.C.P., F.R.A.C.P., F.A.M.S.; Jorge César Martínez, M.D.; and Özlem Yildirim, Ph.D.

Joint Commission International

A division of Joint Commission Resources, Inc.

The mission of Joint Commission International (JCI) is to improve the safety and quality of care in the international community through the provision of education, publications, consultation, and evaluation services.

JCI educational programs and publications support, but are separate from, the accreditation activities of JCI. Attendees at JCI educational programs and purchasers of JCI publications receive no special consideration or treatment in, or confidential information about, the accreditation process.

Printed in the U.S.A. 5 4 3 2 1

Requests for permission to make copies of any part of this work should be mailed to
Permissions Editor
Department of Publications
Joint Commission Resources
One Renaissance Boulevard
Oakbrook Terrace, Illinois 60181, U.S.A.
permissions@jcrinc.com

ISBN: 978-1-59940-403-5
Library of Congress Control Number: 2010931662

For more information about Joint Commission International, please visit http://www.jointcommissioninternational.org.

For more information about Joint Commission Resources, please visit http://www.jcrinc.com.

CONTENTS

ACKNOWLEDGMENTS

Many thanks to everyone who gave time and energy to creating this book including consulting editor Helen Hoesing for going well beyond the expected in providing content and direction; Sherry Kaufield and Bruce Frederick for their content and reviews; reviewers Cathy Hinckley, Paul vanOstenberg, Claudia Jorgenson, Ann Jacobson, Siew Lee Cheng, Paul Chang, Ashraf Ismail, and Carlo Ramponi; and Joint Commission International Publications Advisory Board members Özlem Yildirim, Jorge César Martínez, Kwong Ming Fock, Malik Abdo Ali, and Ali Nasha`at Ali Sha`ar.

Thanks also to the many organizations whose generous donations of time and resources helped make this book a practical guide to JCI accreditation, including the following:

- Maria Grazia Allegretti, Santa Chiara Hospital, Trento, Italy
- Enrico Baldantoni, Azienda Provinciale per i Servizi Sanitari, Trento, Italy
- Angela Greco, Ospedale Regionale di Locarno, Locarno, Switzerland
- Jeff Guo, National Heart Centre Singapore
- Ann Higgins, Mater Private Hospital, Dublin, Ireland
- Grace Kim, Severance Hospital, Yonsei University College of Medicine, Seoul, Republic of Korea
- Dan Levinson, OCA Hospital, Monterrey, Nuevo León, Mexico
- Gaurav Loria, Apollo Hospitals Group, Chennai, India
- Virginia Maripolsky, Bangkok Hospital Medical Center, Bangkok, Thailand
- Mandy Seng, Institute of Mental Health, Singapore
- Diana Tan Yuen Lan, Changi General Hospital, Singapore
- Sharon Tay, Singapore General Hospital, Singapore
- Barbora Vaculíková, Na Homolce Hospital, Prague, Czech Republic
- John Wocher, Kameda Medical Center, Kamogawa, Chiba Prefecture, Japan
- Nellie Yeo, National Healthcare Group, Singapore

Finally, sincere thanks to Kathleen Vega for her excellent efforts in developing and writing this book.

HOW TO USE THIS BOOK

How do we get started? It's a question almost every health care organization asks when leaders first contact Joint Commission International (JCI) about accreditation. This newly updated edition of *Joint Commission International Accreditation: Getting Started* is intended to answer this question and provide tips, tools, and strategies to facilitate an organization's journey toward continuous standards compliance.

"How do *I* participate in the accreditation process?" This is a question posed by individual health care professionals throughout an organization seeking accreditation. The answer to this question depends on the health care professional who is asking it. Every individual health care provider can have an important role in the accreditation process.

If a hospital executive or leader poses the question, the answer starts with a commitment that sets the tone for safety and quality improvement. It requires a promise for adequate resource allocation, including financial, human, technology, and other resources. It requires that leaders accept the role of "champion" in the process of improving safety and quality in their organization. And it requires a commitment to actively participate in activities leading up to, during, and as a result of the accreditation survey.

If a hospital quality or accreditation expert asks how to participate, the answer focuses more on assessment, data analysis, implementation strategies, and overall survey preparation, although the quality improvement process eventually involves everyone from the executive suite to entry-level staff.

Finally, if an organization is fortunate enough to have other patient care staff members who ask about their role in accreditation, the answer is usually focused on activities such as contributing to quality and safety efforts, participating in improvement processes, and embracing change.

The Content of This Book

Fundamentally, *Joint Commission International Accreditation: Getting Started*, Second Edition, is a primer on the accreditation process that offers a wide range of information, answers the most basic questions, and discusses the purpose of quality and safety improvement efforts. It also introduces JCI's Clinical Care Program Certification (CCPC)—an assessment process that focuses on certifying a singular department or departments of an organization that provide specialized types of care.

Although many readers will want to research how all aspects of the accreditation process affect all health care professionals, the information in this book is segmented and targeted for maximum applicability to the groups described above: individual health care professionals, executives/leaders, quality improvement professionals, and patient care staff members. The four distinct sections of the book are designed to prevent each group from having to read the entire book in sequence to find out what its members want to know. Following is a brief description of the different sections:

- Section 1 provides an overview of accreditation and is important information for all individuals working in a health care organization to know. Everyone interested in the accreditation process should review this section.

- Section 2 provides valuable information for executives about establishing a foundation for accreditation, allocating resources, and participating in the on-site survey.

- Section 3 offers information for the quality/ accreditation specialist about the different activities involved in preparing for accreditation and how to structure performance improvement activities to achieve continuous standards compliance.

■ Section 4 targets all health care staff—specifically, the frontline workers—seeking information on their role in the accreditation process and how to effectively navigate the on-site survey.

The order of the sections is intentional: It is a logical progression of the accreditation process—establishing a basic foundation; identifying areas for improvement and implementing improvement initiatives; and encouraging staff participation in the preparation process.

New to This Edition

This is the second edition of *Joint Commission International Accreditation: Getting Started*. While keeping many of the effective elements of the first edition, this version offers several new items, including the following:

■ A comprehensive overview of JCI's accreditation process for, as well as other information on, Ambulatory Care, Care Continuum, Clinical Laboratory, Hospital, Medical Transport, and Primary Care, as well as Clinical Care Process certification. This overview reflects changes in JCI accreditation and certification policies, procedures, and standards, including the fourth edition of the JCI Hospital standards, published in July 2010 and effective starting 1 January 2011.

■ A stronger emphasis on tracer methodology, the key element in JCI's accreditation process, including forms and tools that can help organizations use tracer methodology to assess their performance on an ongoing basis

■ A greater focus on creating a culture of safety to support accreditation. A key element to a successful accreditation process is the framework that supports it. This book focuses on how organization leadership can establish this framework and support quality and safety efforts that contribute to accreditation.

■ Further details about using data to improve performance. This is a critical element in successful process and quality improvement. Without data driving the process, an organization cannot truly quantify the level and degree of its success. This new version discusses what types of data to use in assessing performance and provides data collection strategies to ensure appropriate, usable, and comparable data.

■ New tools, tips, and advice. Whether they relate to general quality improvement strategies or navigating the on-site survey, these resources can help an organization along its accreditation journey.

■ New and updated case studies. These vignettes come from accredited organizations and describe aspects of their preparation efforts.

■ A complete set of Online Extras. These resources and tools can help further an organization's efforts in seeking accreditation. Offered through the JCI Web site at www.jcrinc.com/JCIGS10/Extras, organizations can access these tools at any time. Within the text, readers are referred to these extras when they relate to a particular topic under discussion, using this logo: **Online Extras**

A full list of Online Extras is on page 147.

Recurring features in the book include the following:

■ **Notes from the Field.** These are brief narratives from JCI–accredited organizations that have successfully navigated the continuous accreditation journey. The notes describe organizations' processes for achieving accreditation, offer words of advice, or suggest specific strategies that proved effective in the organizations.

■ **Accreditation Strategies.** These are tips and suggestions organizations may want to consider when pursuing accreditation. Many of these are used in accredited organizations around the world.

■ **Expert Advice.** These are direct quotes from JCI leaders, consultants, and other experts in the field. They are meant to provide insight to the reader on the JCI accreditation process and how organizations can pursue high-quality and safe care through accreditation.

■ **Case Studies.** These longer features provide a detailed description of an accredited organization's efforts in seeking accreditation and continued standards compliance.

As this book demonstrates, JCI accreditation is a multifaceted experience that involves the entire organization. It takes commitment, focus, and a drive to succeed. This book can serve as an organization's guide to accreditation and offer ways to manage, expedite, and streamline the process.

And now, get started.

SECTION

1

ESSENTIAL KNOWLEDGE ABOUT JCI ACCREDITATION

This section provides general information on accreditation and, specifically, JCI's approach to accreditation and high-quality health care. Information in this section is useful for all individuals in a health care organization, including leaders, quality improvement experts, and staff.

Providing safe, high-quality care is a challenge for health care organizations around the world. Despite medical breakthroughs, an ever-expanding knowledge base, and enhanced technology, organizations still struggle to create systems that promote effective, safe, and high-quality care. Providing high-quality care helps organizations achieve desired patient outcomes while reducing the risks of unwanted events.

The Call for High-Quality Health Care

The Institute of Medicine (IOM) defines quality in health care as "the degree to which health care services for individuals and populations increase the likelihood of desired health outcomes and are consistent with current professional knowledge."[1] Other definitions of health care quality focus on not only the outcomes of care but also the management and support functions that are required to provide care effectively, efficiently, and safely.[2] Additional elements of quality care include patient and family involvement, accessibility to care, and timeliness of care.[3]

The pursuit of high-quality care is not a one-time event. Such activity must be ongoing and involve a solid infrastructure that supports change, adaptation, and improvement. It requires a system that collects and interprets information and identifies ways to improve.

Throughout the world, there is substantial variation in the development of health care quality improvement systems, with some health care organizations even lacking the basic infrastructure needed for quality improvement.[4] A recent survey by Shaw et al. showed that while a large majority of hospitals surveyed had formal, documented infrastructure to manage quality and safety, a minority had no designated mission, program, or coordination.[5]

The idea that health care organizations around the world must continue to improve the quality of health care they provide is not new, although it has received more attention in recent years. Currently, the call for improved health care quality and safety comes from many different sources. Political leaders around the globe, including presidents, prime ministers, ministers of health, and ministers of finance, are framing their arguments for reforming health care in terms of greater quality and the elimination or correction of practices that are deemed unsafe or wasteful. Several patient safety–focused organizations worldwide are also adding their voices to the quality and safety debate. For example, The Joint Commission, which is the United States–based arm of Joint Commission International (JCI), as well as the World Health Organization (WHO) and the International Society for Quality in Health Care (ISQua) are all promoting clearer accountability for the quality and safety of health care. These organizations are also encouraging health care organizations to adopt evidence-based practices to standardize the care they provide. At the same time, private and public insurance providers are seeking the best-quality care for their money. In some cases, insurance companies are refusing to pay for services of poor quality or services that involve a preventable error.

In addition to these voices, the Internet makes available a wealth of information regarding the science and practice of health care, and consequently the general public is becoming increasingly skilled in determining when care is not of sufficient quality. Patients and their families are also demanding that they play a greater role in their own care.[6]

To improve the quality and safety of care provided around the world, the international health care community must find ways to increase knowledge about high-quality care and patient safety and apply that information in a consistent manner so that patients benefit. To do this, organizations must go beyond previous quality improvement efforts and focus on doing the right things the right way the first time and embracing state-of-the-art quality concepts. One effective way to do this is through international accreditation.

What Is Accreditation?

Health care accreditation is a process in which a non-governmental entity, which is separate and distinct from the health care organization, assesses the organization to determine if it meets a set of standards. These standards are designed to improve quality of care and yield continuous improvement in structures, processes, and outcomes. Accreditation often involves some element of self-assessment, on-site evaluation, data and outcomes reporting, and follow-up.[7] Typically voluntary, participation in an accreditation process shows a proactive and visible commitment by an organization to continually ensure a safe environment for its patients and staff.

The heart of any accreditation program is the *standards* upon which all else is based—the evaluation methodology, decision process, evaluator training, and other operational elements. Such standards should be optimal, achievable, patient centered, and culturally adaptable in a way that stimulates continuous improvement. These standards should address both patient care and organization management activities and the integration between them. They should focus on proactive, systematic processes that help prevent error and ensure quality. Such standards can foster collaboration, joint planning, and a common vision about quality and safety that move organizations forward with a clear mission focus. In other words, the process of complying with well-crafted standards helps create an environment for change around a common set of expectations.[6]

While the standards on which accreditation is based are important, so is the other critical aspect of this process: the external, objective evaluation by an outside entity. This evaluation allows organizations to benchmark their success against the same standards many other organizations use in improving quality and safety and to identify opportunities for improvement.

The Changing Face of Accreditation

Accreditation began as a national concept. In other words, different countries had their own accreditation systems. The United States, Canada, and Australia have the oldest accreditation systems, while Germany, France, Ireland, and Spain have newer ones. In Asia, organizations in China, Thailand, India, and Malaysia are working to develop or expand national accreditation programs. Many other countries are in various stages of developing and implementing national standards and ultimately requiring compliance by their public or government-subsidized hospitals.

Since the concept of accreditation took shape, it has moved beyond national borders. International accreditation applies a common set of standards to any organization, regardless of where it is located. International standards are beneficial because they allow organizations across different countries to assess and compare quality and safety efforts. This type of accreditation, which JCI has pioneered, fosters a more standardized approach to improving quality and safety around the world.

Clarifying Terms

Accreditation is often confused with *licensure*, which is a different assessment process in which a government agency sets and requires compliance with minimum standards to protect public health and safety. Organizations must maintain their licensure in order to continue to operate and care for patients. In the licensure process, there are often many regulatory policies and procedures that must be met by health care organizations.

Accreditation also differs from *certification*, which evaluates an organization's special capabilities or unique skills to treat patients with chronic diseases such as diabetes and cardiac conditions, and for other specialty departments such as transplantation through the integration and coordination of care. Certification evaluates programs that are components of established hospitals. Although many aspects of preparing for certification are the same as preparing for accreditation, they are not the same. Accreditation recognizes an organization's complete commitment to quality and involves a comprehensive organizationwide survey, and certification demonstrates excellence in a certain aspect of operations, such as the treatment of a specific disease, condition, or clinical care service. (*See* "A Brief Look at JCI's Certification Program" on pages 15–16 for more information on certification.)

Accreditation should be considered a journey—not a destination. It is a process of continuously complying with standards that focus on key systems, patients, and performance improvement. This process creates a cultural shift toward quality that is almost impossible to reverse. Identification of quality indicators, measurement, analysis of data, monitoring, and continuous improvement become the norm. At all levels, staff feel empowered to make and sustain change.

Joint Commission International (JCI)

As mentioned earlier, JCI is the international arm of The Joint Commission, an independent, nonprofit, nongovernmental agency that has its headquarters near Chicago, Illinois, in the United States. The Joint Commission works to improve quality and safety of health care services through education and accreditation. For more than 55

years, The Joint Commission has surveyed health care programs in the United States through a voluntary accreditation process. Currently, the Joint Commission accredits nearly 20,000 organizations within the United States, including hospitals, ambulatory care clinics, behavioral health care centers, home care organizations, laboratories, and nursing homes.

Launched in 1999, JCI extends the Joint Commission mission worldwide. Through international accreditation, consultation, publications, and education JCI helps to improve the quality of patient care in many nations. JCI offers consulting services for both public and private health care organizations as well as local governments in nearly 90 countries. As of this printing, JCI accredits 333 and certifies 25 organizations in 42 countries.

In September 2007, JCI was awarded accreditation by ISQua. Accreditation by ISQua provides assurance that the standards, training, and processes used by JCI to survey the performance of health care organizations meet the highest international benchmarks for accreditation entities.

JCI provides accreditation for hospitals, ambulatory care facilities, clinical laboratories, care continuum services, medical transport organizations, and primary care centers, and provides clinical care program certification. (*See* "A Brief Look at JCI's Accreditation Programs" on pages 13–15 for more information on the different programs accredited by JCI.) JCI Consulting provides education, technical support, accreditation preparation, and other services to health care organizations in every region of the world. Educational areas include The International Essentials of Health Care Quality and Patient Safety™, a framework to help organizations begin the process of designing and implementing a risk reduction program that will lead to improved patient safety. It is important to note that the International Essentials framework is not the same as JCI accreditation, but it may eventually serve as a step toward accreditation. *See* Section 3 for more information.

The Mission of JCI

The mission of JCI is to improve the safety and quality of care in the international community through the provision of education, publications, consultation, evaluation, certification, and accreditation services. Fundamentally, JCI helps governments, hospitals, health care organizations, and health care–related organizations around the world evaluate, improve, and demonstrate the quality of patient care while respecting and accommodating specific legal, religious, and cultural factors that affect patients and their family members.

The Goals of JCI Accreditation

JCI was established to respond to a growing demand around the world for standards-based evaluation in health care. The purpose of JCI accreditation is to offer quantifiable benchmarks for patient care quality and an objective process for evaluating health care organizations that is based on international standards. Accreditation is designed to stimulate and demonstrate continuous, sustained improvement through a valid, reliable, and objective process while providing for cultural differences and needs across countries.

Within its accreditation process, JCI looks at important aspects of health care, such as how patients are assessed, the care of patients, medication safety, patient education, and patient rights. JCI also focuses on how organizations prevent and control infections and create an overall safe environment for patient care. Staff qualifications and education are also a part of the accreditation process. For example, a key question addressed within accreditation is: How does the organization ensure that physicians have and maintain the training and skills they need in order to do the procedures that they are performing?

What Makes JCI Accreditation Unique?

JCI accreditation addresses the same topics found in The Joint Commission's standards for health care organizations in the United States. However, JCI accreditation standards also reflect many of the quality control and quality leadership criteria found in the International Organization for Standardization (ISO) 9001 standards. In addition, JCI accreditation requirements address similar continuous improvement criteria to the European Foundation for Quality Management (EFQM) and the Malcolm Baldrige National Quality Award from the United States. For example, many of the concepts in the JCI standards, including quality management and improvement; leadership; staff education and training; and management of information, are similar to the Baldrige criteria. Likewise, there are linkages between JCI standards and the EFQM criteria regarding key processes in establishing organization policy and strategy and managing knowledge.

Although aspects of JCI accreditation are similar to aspects of accreditation by these other organizations, there are some significant differences. The most significant distinction is that the health care industry informs and participates in all aspects of JCI planning, development, and implementation of standards and other JCI resource materials. The JCI standards at the heart of the accreditation process are developed and agreed to by and for health care professionals from many parts of the world. This integration of the health care industry into JCI's activities distinguishes JCI accreditation from other forms of accreditation and certification, which are derived primarily from the domestic standards of an organization's home country or from industrial assessment models. The JCI standards thus provide a vehicle for incorporating rapidly emerging, globally relevant clinical science and technical advances into the accreditation process and also reflect multinational societal changes in health care. Consequently, the JCI standards are, to date, the only truly international consensus standards available that reflect the full scope of clinical and managerial functions found in contemporary health care around the world.

JCI strives to represent the needs and expectations of health care organizations throughout the world by maintaining an internationally based structure, including the following:

- International Board of Directors
- International Accreditation Committee
- International Standards Committee
- Regional advisory councils in the Middle East, Europe, Asia Pacific, Africa, and Latin America
- International offices in Europe, the Middle East, and Asia
- Collaborations with international agencies on research related to quality and safety
- International Publications Advisory Board

JCI also provides international translations of many products and participates in partnerships to provide culturally sensitive and local joint accreditation. (*See* Sidebar 1-1 on page 7; *see also* Sidebar 1-2 on pages 7–8 for frequently asked questions about JCI accreditation.)

What Does JCI Accreditation Involve?

JCI accreditation involves an on-site evaluation to ensure that standards are being met. However, before an on-site survey occurs, organizations are expected to take a critical look at their processes and procedures and embrace evidence-based practices and proactive risk reduction strategies. These practices and strategies can help the organization improve quality and safety and reduce the likelihood of an adverse event. (*See* Section 3, page 78, for more information on this self-evaluation, known as the baseline assessment.)

The on-site evaluation portion of accreditation involves an on-site survey that examines clinical and management systems and how patients receive services and treatment as they receive care. This survey evaluates the organization's compliance with standards based on interviews with staff and patients; on-site observations of patient care processes; and review of policies, procedures, and other documents provided by the organization. Compliance is scored through a consistent and transparent process, and all accreditation decisions are rule based. (*See* more specific information on the accreditation process in Section 3.)

Tracer methodology. One important element in the JCI on-site evaluation process is the use of tracer methodology. This methodology is a way to analyze a health care organization's systems of providing care, treatment, and services using actual patients as the framework for assessing standards compliance. Within this methodology, surveyors follow the experience of care for a number of patients through an organization's entire health care process. This allows the surveyors to accomplish many objectives, including the following:

■ Identify how an organization's systems function overall.
■ Pinpoint specific performance issues in one or more steps of a process or system.
■ Assess the interactions of processes or systems.
■ Determine if the organization's performance is consistent with JCI standards.

There are two types of tracers: *individual tracers* and *system tracers.* Individual or patient tracers follow the course of a patient's treatment within the organization, allowing surveyors to assess the health care organization's compliance with JCI standards in multiple departments by many caregivers offering a wide range of treatments and services. Surveyors can also determine if the organization is meeting the International Patient Safety Goals (*see* pages 18–19). Individual tracer activities allow surveyors to evaluate not only how an organization says it delivers services but also actual performance. For example, surveyors use individual tracers to understand the following:

■ The relationship among caregivers, disciplines, and departments involved in patient care
■ Integration and coordination of important processes
■ Opportunities for improvement

Individual tracer patients are generally selected from an active patient list. In other words, they are patients currently in the organization and receiving care. Typically, in order to provide the most effective opportunity for surveyors to understand organization performance, individuals selected for tracers are those who have received multiple or complex services.

During individual tracers, surveyors trace the care of patients by observing and talking to staff in the geographic area in which the individual received care. This may be the emergency room, radiology, surgery, recovery room, a long term care facility, a patient's home, or any other areas. Surveyors interact with staff members to discuss standards issues and how their performance directly relates to patient care. In this way, tracer methodology actively engages physicians, nurses, and other clinical and nonclinical staff in the survey process. This methodology allows all members of an organization to see directly how standards compliance issues can translate into potential vulnerabilities for patient quality and safety.

System tracers focus on important processes or functions that span an organization. Like individual tracers, system tracers may include visits to departments or areas directly involved in the process that is being discussed. JCI's current system tracers are medication management, infection control, and use of data. These tracers provide a forum for discussion of important topics related to the safety and quality of care at the organization level. Surveyors use system tracers to examine organization structure and how it impacts care and to understand how various health care systems are integrated with one another. For example, a medication management system tracer will provide information about how medications are selected, stored, prescribed, and dispensed; the pharmacy's role in verification and patient education; medication errors; and so on. Use of a data tracer will show how information is collected, safeguarded, and provided to caregivers when needed, and how data are used in many different decision and education processes.

At its core, tracer methodology moves the on-site survey away from high-level interviews and discussions with managers and leaders *about* policies and procedures. Instead, it focuses survey activities around those staff members actually delivering care. In short, it looks at policies and procedures in action. By using this methodology, surveyors can create an atmosphere that allows for an open exchange of information and ideas with staff. These discussions, combined with review of clinical charts and direct observations, make for a dynamic survey process that provides a complete picture of an organization's processes and services.

Tracer methodology is not only a tool for surveyors to

use during the on-site survey. When learned and used by staff members, it can be an excellent tool for an organization to use in ongoing self-assessment efforts. More information on how to use tracer methodology in preparing for accreditation can be found in Section 3.

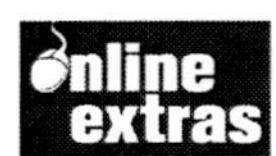

Several sample tracers and tracer tools are available in the Online Extras at www.jcrinc.com/JCIGS10/Extras.

Who Seeks JCI Accreditation?

JCI accreditation is used by different stakeholders for a variety of purposes. Stakeholders include the following:

- Health care organizations seeking to gain a competitive advantage in the marketplace by improving the quality and safety of care
- Public health agencies wishing to reduce risks to patients and strengthen community confidence in the quality and safety of care
- Health ministries seeking to improve health outcomes through recognized quality improvement activities, including professional advice and education on good practices that strengthen business operations and reduce wasted resources
- Others wishing to evaluate, improve, and demonstrate the quality of patient care in their country (for example, private insurance funds)

What Are the Benefits of JCI Accreditation?

As previously mentioned, JCI accreditation is a visible commitment by an organization to improve the quality of patient care the organization provides. By seeking accreditation, an organization opens its doors for an independent, top-to-bottom evaluation of patient-focused care activities, as well as organizational systems. JCI accreditation standards are widely published and publicly available, and JCI accreditation is known as the "gold standard" in accreditation around the world, making this external stamp of approval a valuable one. The following paragraphs take a brief look at some of the further benefits of JCI accreditation.

Ensures a Safe Environment That Reduces Risk

Every day people entrust their health or the health of their loved ones to health care organizations. In return, organizations have an obligation to provide the safest care possible. It is this obligation that inspires health care organizations to continuously improve services and processes to provide even better, safer care. As dedicated organizations know better, they do better. As they do better, patients have better outcomes. When patients have better outcomes, their confidence and satisfaction increase and an organization's reputation improves. An improved reputation can lead to an increase in patients and additional revenue to make further improvements.

The need for the health care industry to focus on patient safety is at the center of all JCI activities. (*See* Sidebar 1-3 on page 9.) Accreditation standards, International Patient Safety Goals, practica and other education events, Executive Briefings, books and other publications, electronic products, and on-site consulting all have the same intent—to contribute to JCI's commitment to patient safety and continuous improvement in the quality of care in health care organizations.

At its essence, accreditation can be defined as a risk reduction activity. Compliance with JCI accreditation standards is intended to reduce the risk of adverse outcomes and improve safety. For example, JCI standards emphasize the need to consider risks and to take action to reduce risks

(continued on page 9)

NOTES FROM THE FIELD

JCI–Accredited Organizations

As of July 2010, JCI has accredited 333 organizations and has certified 25 organizations in 42 countries, including Austria, Bangladesh, Barbados, Bermuda, Brazil, Chile, China, Costa Rica, Cyprus, Czech Republic, Denmark, Egypt, Ethiopia, Germany, Greece, India, Indonesia, Ireland, Israel, Italy, Jordan, Kingdom of Saudi Arabia, Korea, Lebanon, Malaysia, Mexico, Pakistan, Philippines, Portugal, Qatar, Singapore, Spain, Switzerland, Taiwan, Thailand, Turkey, United Arab Emirates, and Yemen.

Sidebar 1-1. Other JCI Activities

In addition to accreditation, JCI provides solutions to help health care organizations and agencies develop services, improve patient care, reduce costs, and comply with international standards and other goals. Since 1994, JCI has provided consultation services to governments, hospitals, insurance companies, and other health care organizations in more than 90 countries. Through its consulting operations, JCI offers the following services:

- Help with preparing for accreditation and improving operations. JCI offers consulting services related to standards compliance assessment and action planning. In addition, JCI offers customized education and training for leaders and staff on accreditation standards, the JCI survey process, quality improvement, and patient safety principles. JCI also provides education and train-the-trainer activities to help organizations train internal accreditation specialists.

- Opportunities for networking and education. JCI offers a variety of training and education tools to help enhance communication between JCI–accredited organizations and foster quality improvement. These include print publications and newsletters, e-learning products, online books, Web-based training, and subscription access to an online good-practices database. In addition, audio conferences, executive briefings, and multiday seminars help educate organizations on current and emerging patient safety and quality improvement topics. (*See* Section 3 for more information on these resources.)

- Assistance with developing a national or regional quality evaluation system. Starting with a foundation of evidence-based international standards and performance indicators, JCI works with key stakeholder groups to choose a model that meets the specific objectives for evaluating and improving health care quality and safety in a particular country or region. (*See* Section 3, page 89, for more about performance measures.) JCI assists national or regional governments or groups with the policy and infrastructure development required to build an effective and credible quality evaluation system. This process includes assistance with the development and implementation of the following system components:

- A set of standards and performance indicators that meet the unique needs of the country or region
- ♦ A standardized methodology for the evaluation of standards compliance
- ♦ Accreditation body policies and procedures
- ♦ Necessary governance and infrastructure supports for the national or regional accreditation body
- ♦ Surveyor selection, training, and management
- ♦ Information management planning

Although interaction with JCI's consultation services is not necessary for accreditation, it is a resource that can prove helpful in achieving continuous standards compliance. Further information on consultation services can be found at http://www.jointcommissioninternational.org/JCI-Advisory-Services/.

Sidebar 1-2. Frequently Asked Questions About JCI Accreditation

The following are some of the frequently asked questions about JCI accreditation, along with answers that may be useful in educating both leadership and staff.

Q: What is accreditation and how does it differ from the regulations that health care organizations must already follow?

A: Accreditation relies on state-of-the-art standards to evaluate a health care organization's demonstrated commitment to delivering effective, safe, and high-quality care. Health care accreditors such as JCI are private, not-for-profit

(continued on page 8)

Sidebar 1-2. Frequently Asked Questions About JCI Accreditation, *continued*

organizations that leverage optimal, ongoing improvements, as opposed to governmental regulators that mandate minimum standards for operation. Accredited organizations must continue to comply with all applicable regulations.

Q: Why do organizations seek accreditation if they are still subject to local and national regulations?
A: Organizations seek accreditation for the key reason that it is a way to provide better care. The by-products of better care are many—improved safety, increased patient satisfaction, cost efficiencies, physician and specialty staff recruitment and retention, private-payer requirements, distinction in a competitive health care marketplace, and so forth.

Q: Does accreditation mean that there is now only one way to do things? In other words, do all health care organizations accredited by JCI have to operate in the same way?
A: No. The goal of JCI accreditation will never be for all accredited organizations to operate in the same manner. Each organization must operate according to its defined mission, vision, and values, and the specific needs of the community and patient populations it serves. Accreditation provides a common framework of standards that can be used to provide safe, high-quality care. This standards framework, along with other established and published components that make up the accreditation process, provide a uniform method to evaluate health care organizations.

Q: Doesn't preparing for accreditation take up valuable time and resources that could be used for other activities?
A: Each organization must decide how to allocate its resources most wisely, but accreditation preparation does not necessarily have to add time to quality improvement efforts. Instead, some organizations might choose accreditation preparation as a new method for bolstering or even replacing current quality improvement activities. The accreditation preparation process helps organizations identify the things that are absolutely necessary in order to provide safe, high-quality care in a consistent manner. Ultimately, the amount of time and resources will depend on how different an organization's current performance is from the requirements in the standards. It is very important for an organization to understand the standards thoroughly before making any significant changes in order to focus efforts most effectively.

Q: What do surveyors hope to gain by talking with staff during the on-site survey?
A: The main open-ended question that surveyors ask is, "Why do you do it this way?" There is no right or wrong answer; instead, the surveyors' main interest is hearing from staff how they go about providing safe, high-quality care as part of their daily activities. Surveyors expect staff members to be able to describe *what* they do, *how they know* what to do, and *how to find out* what to do if they are not sure.

Q: Organization leaders have talked about the "business case for accreditation." What is this?
A: The "business case for accreditation" is the belief by many organizations that JCI accreditation makes good business sense. Accreditation incorporates accountability and quality improvement principles into daily operations in a way that benefits patients. By using JCI standards as the framework for doing the right things right the first time, health care organizations can improve quality of care in an efficient, cost-effective manner. Time and resources can be prioritized on those functions and activities that contribute to higher quality and safer care for patients. Organizations also use the distinction of JCI accreditation to attract patients and differentiate their operations. (*See* Sidebar 1-4 on page 11, for more about the business case for accreditation.)

before an unwanted event affects patients or staff. Through compliance with the standards, policies and procedures are standardized, and clinical pathways and other forms of evidence-based medicine are implemented to reduce unwanted variation. Adverse events are intensively analyzed to prevent their recurrence.

Several organizations that have pursued JCI accreditation have identified real benefits in terms of reduced risk and increased safety. For example, one hospital saw its mortality rate from health care–associated infections drop from 27% to 0% in one year.

Accreditation can help improve safety and quality throughout a health care organization. For example, health care organizations that are accredited have noted improvements in the following areas:

- Infection control, including fewer cases of ventilator-associated pneumonia, urinary tract infections, and central line–associated bloodstream infections (CLABSIs)
- Worker injury, such as needlestick injuries
- Hand hygiene
- Patient assessment, including assessment after transfer, emergency department triage, postsedation assessment, and allergy assessment
- Pain management
- Unscheduled readmissions
- Laboratory test turnaround
- Fall rates
- Pressure sores
- Security

Evaluates and Manages Quality Effectively

JCI's comprehensive patient care and operational standards provide a complete view of how an organization can go about delivering care to patients, no matter which services patients receive or where those services are delivered. Organizations that commit to using the standards as a

guide for developing, improving, implementing, and measuring their quality processes benefit from JCI's emphasis on safety and quality. The on-site accreditation survey process, as well as continued self-assessment of compliance with JCI standards, helps organizations identify and correct quality weaknesses and further improve strengths.

A recent study conducted in a 400-bed hospital in the Middle East showed a nearly 50% improvement in perceived quality after implementing JCI standards. Staff members, patients, and government entities all indicated the organization significantly improved the quality of care in areas such as leadership and management, patient safety, patient satisfaction, documentation, and ethical performance.[8]

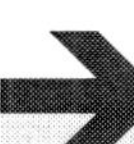

ACCREDITATION STRATEGY

Integrate Safety into Existing Processes

It is important to note that accredited organizations are not required to create new departments or structures or add staff to address the issue of patient safety. Rather, the standards require organizations to integrate safety into their existing processes. This includes making sure that the facility and the systems that keep it functioning are inspected, repaired, and improved when necessary and are monitored regularly. In addition, any identified risks to safety should be reduced or eliminated. (*See* Section 2, for more information about patient safety programs.)

Sidebar 1-3. **About the Terms *Safety* and *Security***

In many parts of the international health care community, the term *security* is used in place of the word *safety*. For the purposes of JCI and this book, *safety* refers to the degree to which the risks of treatment intervention and risks in the care environment are reduced for a patient and other persons, including health care providers. *Security* is protection from loss, destruction, tampering, or unauthorized access or use.

Builds Trust

When choosing a health care organization, patients prefer to go to an organization that provides safe, high-quality care. Accredited organizations can clearly illustrate their processes for providing such care and demonstrate that they are concerned for the patient and his or her health. Because the organization's quality and safety efforts are validated by an external, independent, and unbiased organization, accreditation can also raise community confidence in the health care organization, improve the reputation of that organization, and potentially attract new patients and payers.

Accreditation activities can also build trust between clinicians and organization leadership. By committing to working together to improve organization quality and safety, these two groups can open lines of communication and build trust where they may not have existed strongly before.

Creates a Learning Organization

A learning organization is one that is not satisfied with the status quo, but instead focuses on continuously improving and enhancing the way it conducts business. In learning organizations there is a culture of safety in which staff feel comfortable bringing up potential issues, and proactive risk reduction is the norm. JCI accreditation contributes to the development of a learning organization by encouraging a proactive approach in all aspects of patient care and management systems and processes. (*See* Section 2 for more information on establishing a culture that supports continuous learning.)

Participating in JCI accreditation also allows for benchmarking between organizations and can help standardize the level of, approach to, and quality of care provided across different organizations, systems, and countries. These international comparisons can promote learning and spread good practice.[9]

Improves Efficiency and Cost-Effectiveness

Fundamentally, it is more cost-effective to provide proactive care that reduces risk than to wait for adverse events to occur and address the consequences. As a result, organizations that focus on continuous compliance with JCI's proactive, evidence-based, risk reducing standards can provide the best possible care while maintaining efficiency and cost control. (*See* Sidebar 1-4 on page 11.)

Enhances Staff Recruitment, Retention, and Satisfaction

Organizations that value the contributions of staff and allow opportunities for professional development can better recruit and retain physicians, nurses, therapists, and other clinical and nonclinical staff. Seeking accreditation helps set the stage for a culture that emphasizes staff input and participation, enhances communication between disciplines, and offers education and training opportunities about quality improvement, risk reduction, and evidence-based care.

Involves Patients and Their Families in Care

Accreditation not only benefits an organization, it also benefits the patients that seek care within that organization. Patients in accredited organizations are involved in care decisions and care processes; have their rights respected and protected; receive education and communication in a way they can understand and can respond to; have their families involved—to the degree wanted—in care processes; and experience better care, shorter lengths of stay, and resultant lower medical bills.

Facilitates Medical Travel

Every year, people travel outside of their home country seeking medical care, and this number is increasing. Although it is difficult to project because of ever-changing environmental and political factors, it is estimated that the number of American patients traveling abroad for treatment will increase to 878,000 in 2010, reaching 1.6 million by 2012.[10] Such an increase could be worth US$20 billion per year to destination countries.[11] Medical travel is anything but an American phenomenon; patients from everywhere are seeking treatment everywhere. For example, statistics from the Tourism Authority of Thailand indicate that, of the 14 million visitors coming to Thailand each year primarily for medical reasons, more than 43.6% are from the United Arab Emirates.[12]

People engage in medical travel—traveling to another country for medical care—for a variety of reasons, including the following:

- To seek advanced technologies
- To look for better care than that provided in their own countries

Sidebar 1-4. Can Accreditation Save Money?

The quality of patient care is something every health organization must address. Poor-quality care can take many forms, including loss of records; delays of laboratory results, which yield delays in diagnoses and treatment; lack of chronic disease care, resulting in unnecessary hospitalization; patient falls; pressure ulcers; surgical site infections; and wrong-site surgery, to name a few. The results of poor quality can also vary and include wasted time and resources, negative patient outcomes, patient dissatisfaction, and significant expense. Sometimes, if poor-quality care is not addressed, it can lead to malpractice suits and legal action. One United States health system calculated that the cost of unresolved patient complaints was US$4 million a year for a service with 88,000 patient discharges.[1]

Proactively addressing quality issues in an organization can help avoid some of the costs associated with poor quality. For example, preventing a health care–associated surgical site infection through appropriate hand hygiene, site preparation, and other protocols can be much less expensive than treating such an infection after it occurs. There is considerable anecdotal evidence of the positive relationship between improved safety and enhanced financial performance. There is also quantitative evidence related to a specific set of interventions (such as a comprehensive fall reduction program) and decreased costs. All this evidence clearly demonstrates that reducing errors can decrease care costs and increase revenue.[2]

The process of accreditation helps organizations put systems and processes in place to proactively reduce the risk of poor quality. While there is a cost associated with accreditation, the costs of treating patients who fall victim to poor quality of care are often much more significant.

John Øvretveit, M.D.,* in his recent paper, "Does Improving Quality Save Money?" introduced a model that helps assign a cost value to quality improvement. This cost, spend, save/loss model can be used to assess the value added (or lost) by accreditation for patients or providers.

Three elements in this model help illustrate the cost-effectiveness of accreditation:

1. **Cost.** This is the cost to the organization of any adverse or poor quality that accreditation may reduce (in other words, potential savings).
2. **Intervention cost.** This is the cost to the organization of preparing for and undergoing accreditation.
3. **Savings or losses.** This is an estimate of the actual savings or losses as a result of accreditation.

By examining the costs of any adverse or poor-quality event; determining how much of those costs are reduced as a result of accreditation; and then comparing those figures with the costs of accreditation, organizations can determine whether accreditation is cost-effective for them.

Preliminary data from a study by JCI, in conjunction with Brandeis University and Jordan's Health Care Accreditation Council, indicate financial value of accreditation in the area of staff turnover. The study, performed from 2006 to 2008 and examining JCI–accredited hospitals versus a control group of nonaccredited hospitals, shows that the JCI–accredited organizations had a 3% decrease in staff turnover versus a 13% increase for the control group, resulting in a US$53,210 savings for accredited hospitals.

References

1. Øvretveit J.: *Does Improving Quality Save Money?* The Health Foundation, Sep. 2009.
   http://www.health.org.uk/publications/research_reports/does_quality_save.html (accessed 14 May 2010).
2. Healthcare Financial Management Association: *The Financial Manager's Role in Safety.* 19 Sep. 2008
   http://www.hfma.org/forums/healthcare/Healthcare_Compliance_Forum_Financial_Manager_Role_Safety.htm (accessed 14 May 2010).

---

* Dr. Øvretveit is a member of the Joint Commission Resources Board of Commissioners and the Joint Commission International Publications Advisory Board.

NOTES FROM THE FIELD

A Survey of Senior Leaders

A recent internal survey conducted by JCI asked senior leaders who have participated in the accreditation process for their thoughts about the benefits of accreditation. According to these leaders, accreditation is a way to achieve a standardized, quality-driven health care delivery system that helps organizations achieve a higher level of performance. Accreditation benefits patients by improving patient safety, patient rights, and coordination of care. It also reduces potential errors and allows for significant improvement in documentation to record the patient's chronological care experience. Achieving accreditation is also considered important for public image, political reasons, retention of existing staff, and the opportunity to become advisers for other health care organizations seeking to improve quality. Leaders further perceived accreditation as a useful marketing tool to recruit new staff, attracting top-performing physicians and nurses to their organizations.

- To obtain preventive or complex procedures at reduced costs
- To gain quicker access to medically necessary procedures

For example, Americans travel to India, Thailand, Singapore, Mexico, Costa Rica, and other countries for joint replacement, cosmetic surgery, dental treatments, or heart surgery to take advantage of costs that can be drastically lower than in the United States.

When seeking medical care in another country, patients look for organizations that offer high-quality care at a reasonable price. Individual patients are not alone in this quest. Multinational companies that have employees working abroad also need to know where their employees can receive high-quality health care. Because standards of care may vary widely from one health care facility to another and from one country to another, it is important that patients and employers look for assurances that a health care organization has publicly committed to safe, high-quality patient care.

To ensure that patients traveling abroad receive appropriate care, treatment, and services, many sources, including several safety-focused organizations, are recommending that individuals seek treatment in accredited organizations. For example, the International Medical Travel Association recently issued a position paper advocating that international health care organizations be held to high standards set by recognized accreditation authorities.[13] The American College of Surgeons also released a position statement encouraging patients seeking care abroad to search out high-quality care from board-certified physicians and to use accredited facilities.[14] The American Medical Association's position statement on medical tourism recommends that patients seek care only at institutions accredited by recognized international accrediting bodies and receive access to facility accreditation and outcomes data.[15] Deloitte's 2009 study of the state of medical tourism cites accreditation and oversight by neutral parties such as JCI as an important factor in maintaining quality of care across borders.[10]

JCI accreditation can help a health care organization respond to the recommendations of these safety-focused organizations and show patients, multinational companies, and international insurance providers that the organization values quality, works to ensure safe care, and proactively addresses risk. Accreditation can act as a symbol of quality that immediately communicates a certain standard of care. This can help draw patients to an organization and encourage new and expanded payer relationships.

JCI accreditation also ensures that organizations provide care that meets the needs of any patient. JCI standards require that patients and families be taught in a language they understand and that any cultural or other barriers to service are reduced. Other issues important to patients all over the world, such as patient rights, access to care, ethical admission practices, competency of staff, and quality of care, are also ensured through accreditation.

It is important to note that JCI takes no official position on the concept of medical travel, but does recommend JCI–accredited organizations as high-quality health care providers for all patients, local or distant, throughout the world.

A Brief Look at JCI's Accreditation Programs

JCI offers accreditation programs for the following types of organizations:

- Ambulatory care facilities
- Care continuum services
- Clinical laboratories
- Hospitals
- Medical transport organizations
- Primary care facilities

Each program is appropriate for a specific patient population within the continuum of health care services. In addition, there are specific eligibility criteria for each program. The following paragraphs provide a brief introduction to each of these different programs.

Ambulatory Care

This program is designed to support organizations providing care in ambulatory settings to strengthen patient safety efforts, improve risk management and risk reduction, and strengthen community confidence by demonstrating a commitment to quality and patient-centered care. The standards are organized around the important functions necessary for the provision of safe, high-quality care in a wide range of settings—from ambulatory dental and surgery centers to dialysis facilities and diagnostic radiology centers.

The standards are applicable to a variety of service models, including organizations that provide acute minor illness care, outpatient chronic care management, and even a broad array of medical and surgical services in freestanding facilities.

Specific areas addressed within the ambulatory care standards are the following:

- International Patient Safety Goals
- Patient access and assessment
- Patient care and continuity of care
- Patient rights and responsibilities
- Patient record and information flow
- Patient services and contracts
- Patient and family education
- Patient anesthesia and surgery
- Improvement in quality and patient safety
- Infection control and facility safety
- Human resource management
- Governance and leadership

The second edition of the JCI ambulatory care standards, published in October 2009, went into effect 1 April 2010. JCI standards are covered in more depth later in this chapter.

Care Continuum

The care continuum standards assess a variety of community-based care settings, such as home care, assisted living, long term care, and hospice care. The standards are equally applicable to social service models and medical care models of community-based care. They address community care as a continuum of services between acute and nonacute community settings, focusing on the integration of care and services in all phases of the patient's ongoing medical and social support.

For example, those standards that apply to private homes address complex medical care as well as social engagement and functional independence, which are major components of care in a home environment. Similarly, standards that relate to long term care and rehabilitation assess the quality of care and service delivery in settings ranging from short-term rehabilitation to long-term chronic care.

Standards within this program also measure and improve performance in meeting the unique needs of individuals at the end of life, including delivery of services for pain management and care within the context of an individual's spirituality and family.

Specific areas addressed within the care continuum standards are the following:

- Access and continuity of care and services
- Individual and family rights
- Assessment of needs
- Care, services, and support
- Pain management and end-of-life care and services
- Individual and family education
- Quality management and improvement
- Prevention and control of infections
- Organization management
- Environmental management and safety
- Staff management, qualifications, and education
- Management of information

As of the publication of this book, the first edition of the JCI care continuum standards, published in 2003, is still in effect. JCI standards are covered in more depth later in this chapter.

Clinical Laboratories

Clinical laboratories provide essential services for patient assessment and treatment. The clinical laboratory standards support a comprehensive, accurate, and objective standards-based assessment of laboratory processes and management practices for clinical laboratories of all types and complexities. The standards also offer benchmarks for individual laboratories wishing to evaluate their performance against established international industry standards. Reflecting the best practices of a number of recognized laboratory accreditation and quality certification agencies, these standards help laboratories demonstrate their efficiency, accuracy, and cost-effectiveness to multiple stakeholders.

Specific areas addressed within the clinical laboratory standards are the following:

- International Patient Safety Goals
- Management and leadership
- Development and control of policies and procedures
- Resource management and laboratory environment
- Quality control processes

The second edition of the JCI clinical laboratories standards, published in October 2009, went into effect 1 April 2010. JCI standards are covered in more depth later in this chapter.

Hospitals

Implemented in 1999, the hospital accreditation program is designed to evaluate all the functions of acute care hospitals, including both medical and psychiatric hospitals, as well as any related outpatient clinics and clinical laboratories. Equally applicable to both public and private hospitals, the hospital accreditation program assesses the quality of patient care from the time patients enter a facility until their discharge. The program also brings efficiency and best practices to all phases of management, from clarity of leadership's responsibility and accountability to critical facility-managed processes and board strategic planning. Fundamentally, the hospital standards focus on patient safety and risk reduction in clinical processes and help foster a culture of safety throughout an organization.

Specific areas addressed within the hospital standards are the following:

- International Patient Safety Goals

- Access to care and continuity of care
- Patient and family rights
- Assessment of patients
- Care of patients
- Anesthesia and surgical care
- Medication management and use
- Patient and family education
- Quality improvement and patient safety
- Prevention and control of infections
- Governance, leadership, and direction
- Facility management and safety
- Staff qualifications and education
- Management of communication and information

The fourth edition of the JCI hospital standards was published in July 2010; the effective date for compliance is 1 January 2011. JCI standards are covered in more depth later in this chapter.

Medical Transport

JCI created the medical transport standards to address a critical yet often overlooked component of quality care—emergency transport. These comprehensive standards are applicable to medical transport organizations associated with hospitals and those that are public and community based. They support multiple transport modes, including emergency treatment and transport services, nonemergency transport services, public and private ambulance services, air and water medical transport, and fire brigade emergency services. The standards offer a complete quality assessment of central dispatch, transport procedures, medical services provided during transport, infection control, and vehicle management and safety.

Specific areas addressed within the medical transport standards are the following:

- Governance, leadership, and direction
- Quality management and improvement
- Exposure to and transmission of biologic and chemical agents
- Facility, equipment, and vehicle management and safety
- Staff qualifications and education
- Management of information
- Access to services and coordination of services
- Patient and family rights
- Assessment of patients

■ Care of patients

■ Patient and family education

As of the publication of this book, the first edition of the JCI medical transport standards, published in 2002, is still in effect. JCI standards are covered in more depth later in this chapter.

Primary Care Centers

The primary care center program recognizes the important role of both public and private primary care centers in developed and developing countries and in both rural and urban settings. The primary care center standards are organized around the important functions common to all primary care centers. The standards focus on community integration, health promotion and disease prevention, first-contact medical services, and linkages to other parts of the health care delivery system. These functions apply to an entire primary care center as well as to each unit or service within the center. Standards that set expectations related to services that are not provided by the center (for example, an on-site pharmacy) are considered not applicable.

Specific areas addressed within the primary care center standards are the following:

■ International Patient Safety Goals

■ Community involvement and integration

■ Patient-centered services

■ Organization and delivery of services

■ Improvement in quality and safety

The first edition of JCI's primary care centers standards was published in July 2008 and became effective on publication. JCI standards are covered in more depth later in this chapter.

A Brief Look at JCI's Certification Program

In addition to accreditation programs, JCI offers certification in disease- or condition- specific care for a variety of health care programs. JCI's Clinical Care Program Certification (CCPC), formerly known as Disease- or Condition-Specific Care Certification, is different and distinct from accreditation. As previously mentioned, certification focuses on an organization's ability to integrate and coordinate care for treatment of a specific disease, condition, or clinical care service, such as diabetes, heart failure, and joint replacement.

CCPC is based on an assessment of compliance with consensus-based standards and criteria, the effective use of clinical guidelines, and an organized approach to performance measurement and improvement activities.

Certification standards apply in a variety of health care settings and address a wide range of programs:

■ Heart failure

■ Acute myocardial infarction

■ Primary stroke

■ Diabetes mellitus (Type 1) and/or diabetes mellitus (Type 2)

■ Chronic kidney disease (Stages I to IV)

■ End-stage renal disease

■ Palliative care (all types)

■ Traumatic brain injury

■ HIV/AIDS management

■ Cancer (all types)

■ Pain management

■ Asthma

■ Joint replacement (all types)

■ Transplantation (all types)

■ Chronic obstructive pulmonary disease (CCPD)

Areas evaluated for compliance are the following:

■ International Patient Safety Goals

■ Program leadership and management

■ Delivering or facilitating clinical care

■ Supporting self-management

■ Clinical information management

■ Performance, measurement, and improvement

The second edition of JCI's CCPC standards, published 1 January 2010, became effective 1 July 2010. JCI standards are covered in more depth in the next section of this chapter.

It is important to note that the path for CCPC is different than the path for accreditation. Although many of the topics discussed in this publication—for example, establishing a culture of safety (Section 2), allocating resources (Section 2), using data to improve performance (Section 3), conducting mock tracers (Section 3)—can be applied toward an organization's path to certification, accreditation is the main focus of this publication. Organizations pursuing certification should seek out supplemental resources to further help with that effort. More resources are available

from JCI at http://www.jointcommissioninternational
.org/CCPC-Certification/.

The JCI Standards: A Key Element in Accreditation

JCI standards are the fundamental building blocks on which JCI accreditation rests. The following paragraphs further define the JCI standards.

What Is a Standard?

Standards are statements of expectation that define the structures and processes that must be substantially in place in an organization to enhance the safety and quality of care. To be effective, a standard must withstand the test of time and be applicable not only on the day it is written, but on a continuing basis.

Standards can be developed from a variety of sources, from professional societies to panels of experts, and from research studies to government regulations. Standards might evolve from a consensus of what are "best practices," given the current state of knowledge and technology, or from common accepted practice.

Standards are generally classified as addressing a system's input (or structures), the processes the organization carries out, or the outcomes it expects from its care or services.[16]

- *Structure standards* look at the system's inputs (such as human resources), the design of a building, the availability of personal protective equipment for health care workers (such as soap, gloves, and masks), and the availability of equipment and supplies (such as microscopes and laboratory reagents).

- *Process standards* address the activities or interventions carried out within the organization in the care of patients or in the management of the organization or its staff. Process standards for a hospital or health care center might address such areas as patient assessment, patient education, medication administration, equipment maintenance, and staff supervision. Recently, professional bodies have developed explicit process standards called "clinical guidelines." Such guidelines are based on scientific medical evidence (evidence-based medicine). Governmental agencies, insurers, and professional bodies are promoting the use of clinical guidelines in the management of common or high-risk clinical conditions.

- *Outcome standards* look at the effect of the interventions used on a specific health problem and whether the

expected purpose of the activity was achieved. Examples of outcomes, both positive and negative, are patient mortality, wound healing, infection, delivery of a healthy infant without complications, and resolution of an infection through the appropriate use of antibiotic therapy.

The foundation of JCI standards is based on principles of quality management and continuous quality improvement. As a result, JCI standards include a balance of structure, process, and outcome standards and set optimal, achievable expectations. (*See* Sidebar 1-5 on page 17.)

For all programs, JCI standards are patient-focused and organized around the systems and functions of care in a health care organization. They are grouped by those functions related to providing patient care and those related to providing a safe, effective, and well-managed organization. These functions apply to the entire organization as well as to each department, unit, or service within the organization. (*See* "A Brief Look at JCI's Accreditation Programs" on pages 13–15, for a specific list of the areas the standards address.)

How Are JCI Standards Created?

A 16-member international task force, composed of experienced physicians, nurses, administrators, and public policy experts, guides the development and revision process of the JCI standards. The task force consists of members from six major world regions:

- Africa
- Asia and the Pacific Rim
- Central and Eastern Europe
- Latin America and the Caribbean
- Middle East
- Western Europe

When updating or creating new standards, the task force develops an initial draft based on scientific literature, evidence-based best practices, and feedback from surveyors, accredited organizations, staff, experts, and so forth. The work of the task force is refined based on an international, Internet-based field review of the standards; input from JCI Regional Advisory Councils in Asia Pacific, Europe, and the Middle East; and feedback from other experts and individuals with unique content expertise.

To further ensure that JCI standards apply worldwide and accommodate cultural differences, an international standards committee continues the work of the task force and makes recommendations about updates and modifications that keep the standards current and relevant.

Sidebar 1-5. Frequently Asked Questions About JCI Standards

Q: When there are national or local laws related to a standard, which applies?

A: When a standard is related to a law or regulation, whichever sets the higher or stricter requirement applies. This means that if a standard is stricter than a country's law, the standard must be met. If a law is higher or stricter than a standard, the law must always be followed.

Q: What if religious beliefs or cultural practices conflict with standards?

A: JCI is very respectful of this issue throughout the world. When religious beliefs or cultural practices appear inconsistent with the standards, organizations have the opportunity to demonstrate how they can meet the standards within their cultural or religious norms.

Q: Are JCI standards the same as United States standards?

A: Development of JCI's standards is actively overseen by an international task force whose members are drawn from each of the world's populated continents. Although many of the standards are similar, domestic standards reflect the many local, state, and national laws that govern health care in the United States and do not apply internationally. International standards are broader based in order to respect country and cultural differences. JCI standards are comparable to United States. standards n expectations and intensity, but different.

Q: How frequently are JCI standards updated?

A: JCI standards are usually updated every three years. Information and experience related to the standards are gathered on an ongoing basis. If a standard no longer reflects contemporary health care practice, commonly available technology, quality management practices, or patient-centered care, it is revised or deleted. It is currently anticipated that the standards will continue to be revised and republished as required and not on a scheduled basis. In addition, if information between formal updates is considered to be important enough, changes to the current edition are made and communicated to the field for immediate implementation. (*See* "A Brief Look at JCI's Accreditation Programs," on pages 13–15 for specific dates of standards updates.)

The Three Components of Every Standard

Each JCI standard is made up of three distinct components:

1. The standard. This is the written requirement with which organizations must comply.
2. The intent statement. This is a brief explanation of a standard's rationale, meaning, and significance. Intent statements often contain detailed expectations of the standards that are evaluated in the on-site survey process.
3. The measurable elements. These are the requirements of the standard and its intent statement that will be reviewed and assigned a score during the accreditation survey process. Each element is also reflected in the standard or intent statement. Listing the measurable elements is intended to provide greater clarity to the standards and help organizations educate staff about the standards and prepare for the accreditation survey.

Sidebar 1-6 on page 18 shows a sample of a JCI standard, intent statement, and measurable elements from the hospital accreditation program, specifically the "Assessment of Patients" (AOP) chapter. (**Note:** This standard is current as of the publication of this book, but organizations should consult their current comprehensive accreditation manual for actual standards, intents, and measurable elements.)

Complying with JCI Standards

Because the JCI standards have multiple dimensions, they require multiple sources of information in order to illustrate compliance. For example, document review can reveal whether organizations have specific policies in place. Likewise, staff training logs and interviews with staff can

Sidebar 1-6. Standard AOP.1

All patients cared for by the organization have their health care needs identified through an established assessment process.

Intent of AOP.1

When a patient is admitted to an organization for care (ACC.1), staff members then need to completely assess the patient to establish the reason the patient is there. The specific information the organization requires at this stage, and the procedures for getting it, depend on the patient's needs and the setting in which care is being provided—for example, inpatient or outpatient care. Organization policy and procedures define how this process functions and what information needs to be gathered and documented.

Measurable Elements of AOP.1

1. Organization policy and procedure define the assessment information to be obtained for inpatients.
2. Organization policy and procedure define the assessment information to be obtained for outpatients.
3. Organization policy identifies the information to be documented for the assessments.

This is one standard of the many applicable to health care organizations. A complete list of the standards can be found in the accreditation manual for each program.

illustrate staff knowledge, while clinical observation and patient interviews can highlight particular practices. JCI standards are designed to foster consistent evaluation, so all surveyors evaluating all types of evidence should reach one score. (More information about assessing compliance can be found in Section 3, on pages 81–83.)

Proactively Enhancing Safety Through the International Patient Safety Goals

Providing medical care to multiple patients is a complex endeavor, involving multiple disciplines, varying diseases, and limited time. Because of its complexity, the health care environment is at risk for serious errors. These errors are devastating for patients, their families, and the health care professionals involved. Yet, many of the same errors are repeated over and over again at health care organizations around the globe.

To help prevent the occurrence of serious errors, JCI created the International Patient Safety Goals (IPSG). Like the JCI standards, the IPSG are designed to help organizations enhance safety and yield more positive patient outcomes. The goals represent proactive strategies to reduce the risk of medical error. They reflect good practices proposed by leading patient safety experts and provide clear priorities and

solutions for improving patient safety. The IPSG have accompanying requirements that focus on well-defined, practical, and cost-effective actions that can be implemented in all organizations, no matter their size or location.

JCI introduced the concept of the IPSG in 2006. When developing the goals, a task force of JCI surveyors and consultants selected six goals from among those currently in place for health care organizations accredited by The Joint Commission in the United States. A survey was then distributed to 153 representatives of JCI–accredited organizations and 35 representatives from organizations preparing for JCI accreditation to evaluate the feasibility of the goals. Based on these survey results, JCI tested the goals within the accreditation process and began requiring compliance with the goals in 2007.

The IPSG help accredited organizations address specific areas of concern in some of the most problematic areas of patient safety. Following are the six current IPSG:

Goal 1: Identify Patients Correctly

Goal 2: Improve Effective Communication

Goal 3: Improve the Safety of High-Alert Medications

Goal 4: Ensure Correct-Site, Correct-Procedure, Correct-Patient Surgery

Goal 5: Reduce the Risk of Health Care–Associated Infections

Goal 6: Reduce the Risk of Patient Harm Resulting from Falls

The IPSG are structured in the same manner as JCI standards, including a requirement, an intent statement, and measurable elements. As with the standards, the requirement is the precise goal the organization is expected to meet. The intent statement further explains the requirement's intended achievements. The measurable elements are the components of the goal that are scored by the JCI surveyor during an on-site accreditation survey. (*See* Sidebar 1-7 on pages 20–22 for a complete listing of the goals and their intent statements.)

Complying with the goals requires daily vigilance in best practices. Although health care organizations must strive for continuous compliance, they do not need to create any extra documentation to prove compliance to JCI. Surveyors will review whatever documentation an organization has that is relevant, interview the organization's leaders and direct caregivers, and make direct observations of performance to determine whether the requirements have been implemented and how consistently they are being performed. With that said, organizations that choose to create extra documentation or other methods for measuring compliance with the goals are expected to comply with their own requirements.

Certain Goals May Present More Challenges Than Others

Data collected from JCI surveyors justify the existence of the IPSG as an initiative to highlight some of health care's most serious patient safety issues and illustrate which of these issues are more difficult to resolve than others.

The data, which were collected 1 January 2009 through 31 December 2009, show the following:

- Of 93 JCI surveys in 2009, only 28 organizations, 30% of those surveyed, were in full compliance with the IPSG.
- Goal 4, Ensure Correct-Site, Correct-Procedure, Correct-Patient Surgery, had the highest rate of noncompliance among hospitals at 44%.
- Goal 6, Reduce the Risk of Patient Harm Resulting from Falls (29% noncompliant), and Goal 3, Improve the Safety of High-Alert Medications (25% noncompliant), were also particularly difficult to meet.
- Goal 5, Reduce the Risk of Health Care–Associated Infections, had the highest rate of compliance—91% of organizations surveyed were compliant.

Making the Commitment

A health care organization that wishes to be accredited must complete and submit an application for survey. This document provides essential information about the health care organization. For example, a hospital seeking JCI accreditation will be asked to provide the number of inpatient beds, the average daily inpatient census, and the types of clinical medical services provided (obstetrics, surgical, oncology, and so forth). The hospital must also provide information about the top five patient diagnoses at discharge, the top five surgical procedures, hospital departments, and areas where anesthesia and sedation are administered. Other programs are required to submit similar information that, combined with basic information about ownership, allows JCI to better understand the type of organization seeking accreditation and develop a survey plan that meets the unique characteristics of that organization. For example, JCI requires organizations to submit a copy of any license from regulatory agencies or other bodies needed to provide care to patients with their application. Health care organizations should apply for survey by using the application forms found on the JCI Web site at http://www.jointcommissioninternational.org/Why-Become-Accredited/ (all applications are available by clicking on the program-specific button). (*See* Section 3, pages 116–117, for more information about submitting an application for survey.)

While the application process may be the initial interaction between JCI and the organization, an organization's preparation efforts for JCI accreditation should begin long before that time. For most organizations, the process of preparing for a JCI accreditation survey will take between 12 and 24 months. In some cases, although it is not a requirement of JCI, in order to achieve compliance with the standards, an organization may address its allocation of resources, which could include enhancements to the facility, recruiting and training staff, and redesigning care delivery processes and systems.

For an organization to be successful in achieving accreditation, the process of preparation must be a priority. Pursuing JCI accreditation requires a strong commitment from all members of an organization, including leadership, quality management, and frontline staff. The remainder of this book takes a closer look at what is required of different individuals in an organization and helps organizations get started on the rewarding pursuit of JCI accreditation.

Sidebar 1-7.   International Patient Safety Goals

Following is a list of the IPSG and their intent statements. An applicability grid follows the text. Please note: These goals have been updated for publication in *Joint Commission International Accreditation Standards for Hospitals*, Fourth Edition, which was published in July 2010 with requirements effective as of 1 January 2011. Consult your applicable comprehensive accreditation manual for current requirements.

Goal 1: Identify Patients Correctly (IPSG.1)

The organization develops an approach to improve accuracy of patient identifications.

Intent

Wrong-patient errors occur in virtually all aspects of diagnosis and treatment. Patients may be sedated, disoriented, or not fully alert; may change beds, rooms, or locations within the organization; may have sensory disabilities; or may be subject to other situations that may lead to errors in identification. The intent of this goal is twofold: first, to reliably identify the patient as the person for whom the service or treatment is intended; second, to match the service or treatment to that individual patient.

Policies and/or procedures are collaboratively developed to improve identification processes—in particular, the processes used to identify a patient when giving medications, blood, or blood products; taking blood or other specimens for clinical testing; or providing any other treatments or procedures. The policies and/or procedures require at least two ways to identify a patient, such as the patient's name, identification number, birth date, or other ways. The patient's room number or location cannot be used for identification. The policies and/or procedures clarify the use of two different identifiers in different locations within the organization, such as in ambulatory care or other outpatient services, the emergency department, or operating theatre. Identification of the comatose patient with no identification is also included. A collaborative process is used to develop the policies and/or procedures to ensure that they address all possible identification situations.

Goal 2: Improve Effective Communication (IPSG.2)

The organization develops an approach to improve the effectiveness of communication among caregivers.

Intent

Effective communication—which is timely, accurate, complete, unambiguous, and understood by the recipient—reduces errors and results in improved patient safety. Communication can be electronic, verbal, or written. The most error-prone communications are patient care orders given verbally and those given over the telephone, when permitted under local laws or regulations. Another error-prone communication is the reporting back of critical test results, such as the clinical laboratory telephoning the organization to report the results of a critical lab value.

The organization collaboratively develops a policy and/or procedure for verbal and telephone orders that includes the writing down, legibly (or entering into a computer), the complete order or test result by the receiver of the information; the receiver reading back the order or test result; and the confirmation that what has been written down and read back is accurate. The policy and/or procedure identifies permissible alternatives when the read-back process may not always be possible, such as in the operating theatre or in emergency situations in the emergency department or intensive care unit.

Goal 3: Improve the Safety of High-Alert Medications (IPSG.3)

The organization develops an approach to improve the safety of high-alert medications.

Intent

When medications are part of the patient treatment plan, appropriate management is critical to ensuring patient safety. High-alert medications are those medications involved in a high percentage of errors and/or sentinel events,

<table>
<tr><td>**Sidebar 1-7.**</td><td>**International Patient Safety Goals,** *continued*</td></tr>
</table>

medications that carry a higher risk for adverse outcomes, as well as look-alike, sound-alike medications. Lists of high-alert medications are available from organizations such as the World Health Organization or the Institute for Safe Medication Practices. A frequently cited medication safety issue is the unintentional administration of concentrated electrolytes (for example, potassium chloride [equal to or greater than 2 mEq/mL concentrated], potassium phosphate [equal to or greater than 3 mmol/mL], sodium chloride [greater than 0.9% concentrated], and magnesium sulfate [equal to or greater than 50% concentrated]). Errors can occur when staff are not properly oriented to the patient care unit, when contract nurses are used and not properly oriented, or during emergencies. The most effective means to reduce or eliminate these occurrences is to develop a process for managing high-alert medications that includes removing the concentrated electrolytes from the patient care unit to the pharmacy.

The organization collaboratively develops a policy and/or procedure that identifies the organization's list of high-alert medications based on its own data. The policy and/or procedure also identifies any areas where concentrated electrolytes are clinically necessary as determined by evidence and professional practice, such as the emergency department or operating theatre, and identifies how they are clearly labeled and how they are stored in those areas in a manner that restricts access to prevent inadvertent administration.

Goal 4: Ensure Correct-Site, Correct-Procedure, Correct-Patient Surgery (IPSG.4)
The organization develops an approach to ensuring correct-site, correct-procedure, and correct-patient surgery.
Intent
Wrong-site, wrong-procedure, wrong-patient surgery is an alarmingly common occurrence in health care organizations. These errors are the result of ineffective or inadequate communication between members of the surgical team, lack of patient involvement in site marking, and lack of procedures for verifying the operative site. In addition, inadequate patient assessment, inadequate medical record review, a culture that does not support open communication among surgical team members, problems related to illegible handwriting, and the use of abbreviations are frequent contributing factors.

Organizations need to collaboratively develop a policy and/or procedure that is effective in eliminating this alarming problem. The policy includes a definition of surgery that incorporates at least those procedures that investigate and/or treat diseases and disorders of the human body through cutting, removing, altering, or insertion of diagnostic/therapeutic scopes. The policy applies to any location in the organization where these procedures are performed.

Evidence-based practices are described in The (US) Joint Commission's Universal Protocol for Preventing Wrong Site, Wrong Procedure, Wrong Person Surgery™.

The essential processes found in the Universal Protocol are

■ marking the surgical site;

■ a preoperative verification process; and

■ a time-out that is held immediately before the start of a procedure.

Marking the surgical site involves the patient and is done with an instantly recognizable mark. The mark should be consistent throughout the organization, should be made by the person performing the procedure, should take place with the patient awake and aware, if possible, and must be visible after the patient is prepped and draped. The surgical site is marked in all cases involving laterality, multiple structures (fingers, toes, lesions), or multiple levels (spine).

The purpose of the preoperative verification process is to

■ verify the correct site, procedure, and patient;

■ ensure that all relevant documents, images, and studies are available, properly labeled, and displayed; and

■ verify any required special equipment and/or implants are present.

(continued on page 22)

Sidebar 1-7. International Patient Safety Goals, *continued*

The time-out permits any unanswered questions or confusion to be resolved. The time-out is conducted in the location the procedure will be done, just before starting the procedure, and involves the entire operative team. The organization determines how the time-out process is to be documented.

Goal 5: Reduce the Risk of Health Care–Associated Infections (IPSG.5)

The organization develops an approach to reduce the risk of health care–associated infections.

Intent

Infection prevention and control are challenging in most health care settings, and rising rates of health care–associated infections are a major concern for patients and health care practitioners. Infections common to many health care settings include catheter-associated urinary tract infections, bloodstream infections, and pneumonia (often associated with mechanical ventilation). Central to the elimination of these and other infections is proper hand hygiene. Internationally acceptable hand hygiene guidelines are available from the World Health Organization (WHO), the United States Centers for Disease Control and Prevention (US CDC), and various other national and international organizations. The organization has a collaborative process to develop policies and/or procedures that adapt or adopt currently published and generally accepted hand hygiene guidelines and for the implementation of those guidelines within the organization.

Goal 6: Reduce the Risk of Patient Harm Resulting from Falls (IPSG.6)

The organization develops an approach to reduce the risk of patient harm resulting from falls.

Intent

Falls account for a significant portion of injuries in hospitalized patients. In the context of the population it serves, the services it provides, and its facilities, the organization should evaluate its patients' risk for falls and take action to reduce the risk of falling and to reduce the risk of injury should a fall occur. The evaluation could include fall history, medications and alcohol consumption review, gait and balance screening, and walking aids used by the patient. The organization establishes a fall-risk reduction program based on appropriate policies and/or procedures. The program monitors both the intended and unintended consequences of measures taken to reduce falls. For example, the inappropriate use of physical restraints or fluid intake restriction may result in injury, impaired circulation, or compromised skin integrity. The program is implemented.

Applicability Grid

Setting	IPSG.1	IPSG.2	IPSG.3	IPSG.4	IPSG.5	IPSG.6
Ambulatory Care	X	X	X	X	X	X
Care Continuum*						
Clinical Laboratories	X	X		X	X	
Hospital	X	X	X	X	X	X
Medical Transport*						
Primary Care	X	X	X	X	X	X
Clinical Care Program (Certification)	X	X	X	X	X	X

*At the time of this publication, these programs' standards had not been updated since the institution of the IPSG. Although the IPSG are not included in a program's comprehensive accreditation manual and are not an official part of the JCI on-site accreditation survey, organizations accredited or seeking accreditation in these programs are strongly urged to consider the application of the goals to their everyday caregiving activities.

Case Study 1-1.   Changi General Hospital

Organization Name: Changi General Hospital (CGH)
Location: Singapore
Years accredited: 2005, 2008
About Changi General Hospital: CGH is a 788-bed, 26-ward hospital in Singapore. Opened in 1998, CGH includes 22 specialist clinics with nearly 100 consultation rooms to cater to the outpatient needs of the community.

The Decision to Pursue JCI Accreditation

CGH leadership, led by its Chairman Medical Board, and Chief Executive Officer, chose to pursue JCI accreditation for reasons applicable to leadership, staff, patients, and clinicians. Those reasons are detailed in the following paragraphs.

Leadership

JCI accreditation does the following for CGH leadership:

- Supports CGH's mission, vision, and strategic thrusts, which include the following:
  - Being dedicated to improving the health of the community in the region
  - Accomplishing goals through cooperation with other caregivers to provide high-quality health care that is integrated, accessible, affordable, and appropriate to the community's needs
  - Valuing and recognizing the contribution of every staff member and fostering a culture of innovation and lifelong learning
  - Maintaining core values that include integrity, compassion, commitment, teamwork, professionalism, openness, social responsibility, and CARE values (CARE = **C**onsistency and continuous improvement, **A**ttention to details, **R**espect for others, and **E**xcellence in medical care and service)
- Represents a continuation of the quality journey started with accreditation by the ISO and Occupation Health and Safety Assessment Series (OHSAS)
- Permits comparison and benchmarking with best health care practices
- Along with JCI standards, gives additional focus on continuous quality improvement and patient safety

Staff

The following points describe what JCI accreditation does for CGH staff:

- Provides an integrated structure for improving quality and patient safety
- Facilitates merging science with quality improvement (for example, practice guidelines, clinical pathways, research)
- Provides a framework for professional accountability
- Improves professional staff development
- Improves employee safety and security
- Promotes teamwork and values employee opinions

Patients

CGH patients benefit from JCI accreditation in the following ways:

- More and better patient and family involvement in care decisions and care processes
- Access to a quality-focused organization
- Respected and protected patient rights
- Understandable education and communication
- End-of-life care and pain management that are appropriate to patient needs
- Better care, shorter hospital stays, and lower hospital bills

Clinicians

CGH clinicians benefit from JCI accreditation in the following ways:

- Decreased infection rates
- Improved clinical outcomes
- Decreased risks of practice
- Increased staff safety
- Lower medico-legal and insurance costs
- Enhanced professional standing of hospital and staff

The Journey to Accreditation

First, CGH leadership and quality personnel devised a time line for their accreditation journey and carried out the following activities:

- **Sent a team to the JCI Practicum in Chicago in July 2004.** This team became the JCI

(continued on page 24)

Case Study 1-1. Changi General Hospital, *continued*

Steering Committee and included senior management, as well as leaders from the medical, nursing, allied health, and administration departments.

⮞ **Formed quality assurance teams known as JCI Work Groups and distributed tasks according to the chapters in the *JCI Accreditation Standards for Hospitals*.** Each JCI Work Group had a balanced composition of members—physicians, nurses, allied health staff, and administrators—as appropriate to the topic of the JCI chapter. The primary task of each JCI Work Group was to review its JCI chapter and write policies that would be aligned with the JCI standards and measurable elements.

⮞ **Established a JCI Secretariat Team.** This team was made up of executives in the Clinical Services Department to help coordinate all activities necessary for JCI accreditation.

⮞ **Held a one-day strategic planning session.** This occurred approximately 10 months before the expected date of the JCI accreditation survey, during which the hospital's senior management gathered to confirm and convey their commitment toward JCI accreditation to clinician leaders, nursing administrators, allied health leaders, and administrators. Management's plans for preparing for JCI accreditation were shared with all present.

⮞ **Rewrote and approved accreditation policies and plans.** Policies were written by the respective JCI Work Groups and subsequently discussed and approved at medical board meetings. The policies were then implemented and monitored for compliance, as well as for implementation problems. In cases where there were practical problems in implementing the policy, the policy was reviewed and sent through another round of revision and approval. All finalized policies were then uploaded to the JCI Web portal (*see* below) of the hospital's intranet.

⮞ **Produced educational and publicity materials for staff.** These included posters (*see* Figure 1 on page 26), internal JCI newsletters (*see* Figure 2 on page 27), a pocket guide (*see* Figure 3 on page 28), a pocket card, and computer log-on screens. The organization also created a motivational slogan, "JCIA: Mission Possible," which it used in many internal communications.

⮞ **Set up a JCI Web portal on the hospital's intranet.** All information pertaining to JCI accreditation was uploaded on this portal, including policies and plans, JCI newsletters, and teaching slides. This allowed staff to access the information readily.

⮞ **Conducted staff education sessions.** After CGH's Chief Executive Officer and Chairman Medical Board announced that the hospital was going for JCI accreditation, staff education took place on several levels. Large-scale sessions ("town hall meetings") for information sharing and teaching were held in the hospital's auditorium, where up to 350 staff could gather to listen and learn. Smaller-scale sessions were conducted by individual departments with their respective staff. Tailored teaching sessions were also held for specific groups, such as Infection Control, Pharmacy, and Information Technology.

⮞ **Started a JCI "countdown to the survey" date.** The number of days remaining until the JCI accreditation survey date was counted down on the JCI intranet portal and via a printed "JCI countdown calendar" in all major hospital areas. These initiatives created an appropriate sense of urgency as the survey date drew nearer.

⮞ **Conducted internal audits by an internal JCI accreditation team.** A pool of internal auditors was formed, co-opting members from the medical, nursing, allied health, and administration departments. The JCI Secretariat Team maintained the internal audit schedule. The internal audits covered all areas of the hospital. Each audit team ideally comprised a physician, a nurse, and an administrator. However, if that composition could not be achieved on the particular day, the team still went on its audit. The team members were each given a checklist for the place that they were auditing, and a "scribe" took notes for them. Upon completion of the audit, the scribe collated the auditors' findings and sent a consolidated report to the person in

Case Study 1-1. Changi General Hospital, *continued*

charge of the area audited (for example, the Ward Nurse Manager). A list of gaps and non-compliances were also sent to the person in charge of the audited area, with a request to write down the corrective actions taken to close the compliance gaps and make improvements. The corrective actions were then compiled and kept by the JCI Secretariat Team.

- An external assessment (also known as a mock audit) was conducted by JCI consultants nine months before the actual survey. All efforts were made to close the gaps identified by the consultants.
- The on-site survey was conducted, resulting in CGH being accredited by JCI on 11 June 2005. (Note: After its success with its initial JCI hospital accreditation, CGH was reaccredited on 26 April 2008 and achieved JCI certification in two disease-specific care areas—Heart Failure (25 January 2007 and 7 January 2010) and Acute Myocardial Infarction (25 January 2007 and 9 January 2010).

Quality Personnel and Other Staff

CGH already had a Clinical Quality section within its Clinical Services Department and a Quality Management Office before deciding to pursue accreditation with JCI. In addition, various departments such as Nursing, Allied Health, Human Resource Development, and Corporate Affairs had teams within them looking at quality issues.

The responsibilities of the Clinical Quality section include the following:

- Managing incidents, clinical complaints, and sentinel events
- Conducting analyses of adverse clinical events to determine the root causes and making recommendations for improvement and prevention of similar occurrences. Clinical Quality also monitors the implementation of the recommendations and checks if the process improvements have achieved the desired effects (CGH employs the Plan, Do, Check, Act methodology—*see* Section 3).
- Conducting patient safety walkabouts to garner feedback from staff regarding safety issues in their areas of work (*see* Section 2). The

feedback is collated and the relevant departments are asked to help with solutions for improvement.

- Collaborating with the Patient Safety Committee to teach performance improvement concepts, such as root cause analysis and crew resource management
- Monitoring clinical indicators and presenting the performance and trends to the Performance Improvement Committee
- Providing secretarial support for multiple committees, such as the Medical Audit Committee, Patient Safety Committee, Performance Improvement Committee, Medical Board, Tissue Audit Committee, and Medical Ethics Committee

After embarking on the path to JCI accreditation, the Clinical Quality section and Quality Management Office collaborated, and members from Clinical Quality formed the JCI Secretariat Team.

The responsibilities of the Quality Management Office include the following:

- Monitoring service quality indicators, such as appointment lead times and consultation waiting times
- Overall monitoring of the indicators in the Hospital Score Card
- Monitoring the hospital's workload statistics and presenting them on a quarterly basis to senior management
- Reporting data to the Ministry of Health and corporate parent SingHealth on a regular basis
- Arranging for service quality training for staff
- Organizing service quality awards and customer satisfaction surveys
- Coordinating the activities and preparation for audits, such as those for ISO, OHSAS, and JCI

Many leaders and staff were already in place at CGH before its path to accreditation started. Two executives were hired to be part of the JCI Secretariat Team to provide administrative support for the hospital's JCI preparation and accreditation survey.

(continued on page 26)

Case Study 1-1. Changi General Hospital, *continued*

Figure 1. Posters Promoting Patient-Safe Care

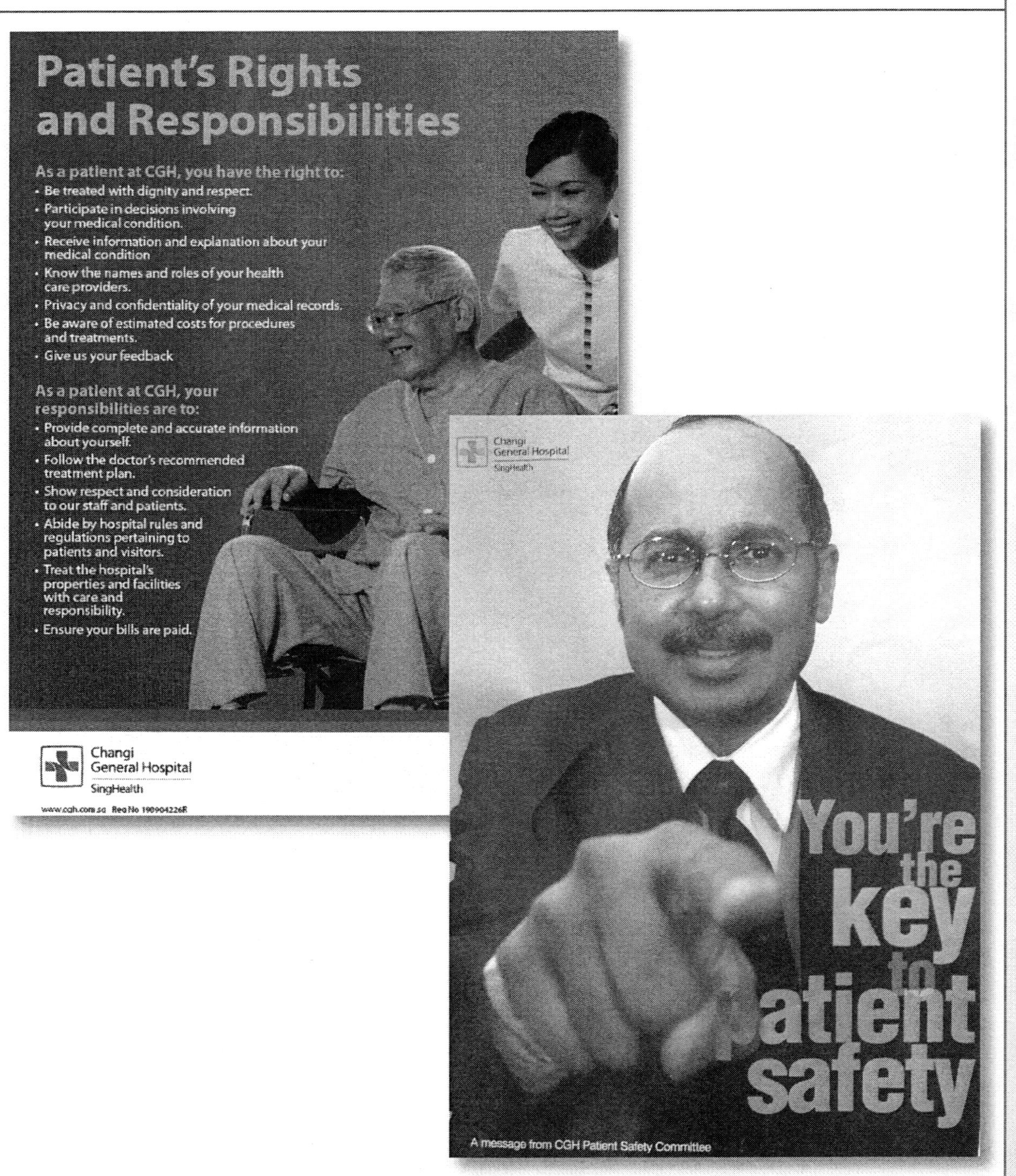

Source: Changi General Hospital, Singapore. Used with permission.

Case Study 1-1. Changi General Hospital, *continued*

Figure 2. Internal JCI Newsletter

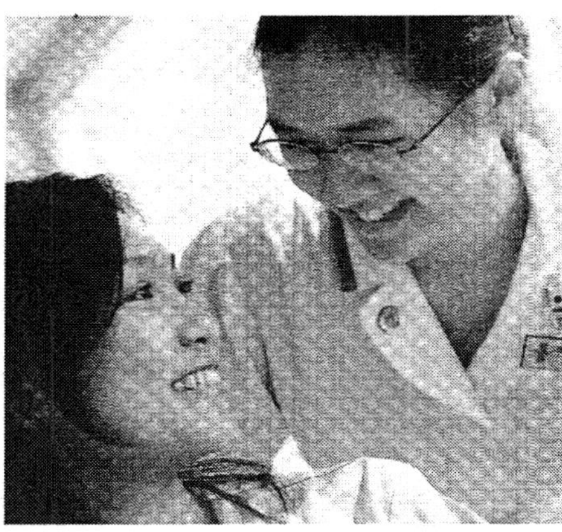

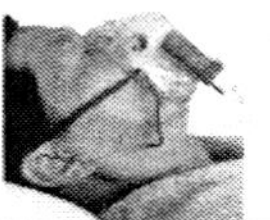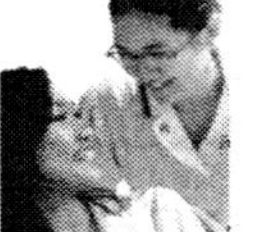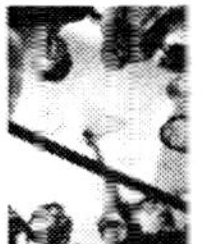

Patient
Safety
Patient care & safety
top priorities for CGH
PRIME

Upholding
Patient's Rights
Patient and family
involved in care decisions
PRIME

Continuous
Improvement
Working round the
clock to sustain
improvement
HOME

JCIA TIMES

4 PAGES IN ONE PART ■ MITA (P) 001/01/2005   TARGET APRIL 05 ■ FREE

JCIA Issue No. 3   20 JANUARY 2005

Patient Rights and Safety

A series of JCIA briefings were conducted for staff from 16 to 19 October 2004 as part of the JCIA Awareness Programme. 4 Modules were covered during each briefing.

We have covered Module 2 – General Safety and Fire Safety in the previous issue and we will be focusing on Module 3 – Patient Rights and Safety in this issue.

Patients have the right to:

- Privacy and Confidentiality
- Choose treatment
- Refuse treatment
- Second opinion
- Receive clear and concise information about their medical care
- Receive considerate, respectful and compassionate care

Protect patients' rights – Some simple Do's:

- Do log out after using computers in patient care areas
- Do close doors and curtains during treatment
- Do cover patients appropriately during treatment and transport
- Do lower your voice in areas where patient privacy and confidentiality could be compromised.

Common types of medical errors are:

- Diagnostic error
- Equipment failure
- Infection - nosocomial infection, post surgical wound infection
- Blood transfusion related injuries
- Misinterpretation of medical orders
- Medication error
- Wrong site surgery

To reduce medical errors, staff must:

- Identify patient - check ID tag (name, NRIC)
- Check for drug allergy
- Ensure correct patient for correct site operation
- Verify medical orders
- Document findings and management plan clearly

Source: Changi General Hospital, Singapore. Used with permission.

(continued on page 28)

Case Study 1-1.   Changi General Hospital, *continued*

Figure 3. Pocket Guide

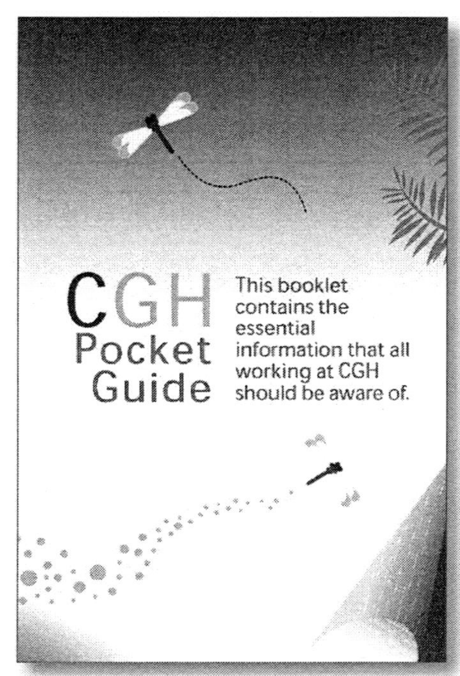

Patient's Rights and Responsibilities
All patients are provided with a booklet on CGH Patient's Rights and Responsibilities.

Our patients have a RIGHT to:
- Be treated with dignity and respect.
- Participate in decisions involving his/her medical condition.
- Receive information and explanation about his/her medical condition.
- Know the names and roles of his/her health care providers.
- Confidentiality and privacy of his/her medical records.
- Give us feedback.

Our patients have a RESPONSIBILITY to:
- Provide complete and accurate information about his/her health.
- Follow the doctor's prescribed treatment plan and to discuss if any changes are needed.
- Show respect and consideration to our staff and patients.
- Ensure that his/her hospital bills are paid.

Privacy and Confidentiality
Our patients have a right to privacy and confidentiality. Here are some simple Do's and Don'ts that we should practise:

DOs
- Log-out after using computers in patient care areas.
- Close doors and curtains during treatment and examination.
- Cover patients appropriately during treatment and transport.
- Modulate voice volume in areas where privacy could be compromised. THINK ABOUT WHAT YOU SAY AND WHERE YOU SAY IT.

DON'Ts
- Do not share computer passwords.
- Do not discuss patient-specific information in public areas like lifts, food courts and hallways.
- Do not display patient-specific information on noticeboards accessible to the public.
- Do not leave medical records or casenotes in public areas or unattended by staff.

Source: Changi General Hospital, Singapore. Used with permission.

Case Study 1-1. Changi General Hospital, *continued*

No other new staff were specifically hired for the purpose of helping with JCI accreditation, but some staff were redeployed to be part of the Steering Committee, Work Groups, and Secretariat Team.

A major challenge CGH faces for quality improvement is to bring together all the various initiatives of the various departments so that they form a well-coordinated effort to improve quality hospital-wide. In short, CGH leaders and staff need to guard against working in "silos."

Obstacles to JCI Accreditation

As mentioned earlier, a group of leaders was selected to attend the JCI Practicum in Chicago to start the JCI accreditation journey for CGH. This group then formed the JCI Steering Committee, which would lead and train the rest of the hospital staff. Despite this, CGH leaders found it challenging to find others to lead and champion the hospital's JCI efforts. CGH leaders needed to convince staff that JCI accreditation was a worthwhile effort that would help make the hospital safer for patients and staff and raise the quality of clinical care and service provided.

Resistance to JCI accreditation could be categorized three ways:
- There was a natural resistance to change from current practices.
- There was also skepticism, particularly among physicians, some of whom felt that JCI accreditation was merely an exercise to obtain a certificate. Some senior physicians remarked that they had been "practicing this way without JCI for more than 20 years," and nothing adverse had happened to their patients.
- Some physicians felt that the enormous expenditure of time and effort to obtain JCI accreditation would translate to only minimal gains in performance. In particular, this was viewed as additional work, over and above the demands of their daily duties.

The JCI Steering Committee met with CGH staff to explain the intent behind JCI accreditation. This core group helped to persuade other staff that the JCI standards would indeed help to improve patient safety and quality of care, and that because many of the core principles behind the standards were already being practiced routinely, JCI accreditation did not constitute a major change in the way CGH managed its patients.

Some additions and modifications in procedures were required in order to comply with the standards. CGH needed to approach all patient care and managerial activities in a more systematic way, backed up by written policies and more complete documentation. Thus physicians' clerking sheets and nurses' patient assessment forms were revamped, and many other new or revised forms were introduced. Staff felt that too much time was spent on filling in forms, and this paperwork took time away from actual patient care. The importance of good and complete documentation was emphasized to all staff. It was explained that this was good practice, and the information was necessary for the management of patients. Also, good documentation would stand the organization in good stead in the unfortunate event of a medico-legal case.

Writing good policies also proved to be a challenge. Enunciating the necessary practices in unambiguous language turned out to be harder than expected. CGH leaders realized that what initially appeared to be well-written policies sometimes proved difficult to implement. CGH overcame these problems by seeking further feedback from staff as to readability and relevance of the policies during implementation. The policies were then revised according to feedback and reviewed again. As mentioned previously, the plan-do-check-act method constituted CGH's policy development cycle.

To help win over other skeptics, particularly clinicians, data were collected and tracked to provide evidence of improvement in key areas—for example the reduction in infection rates. As the group of "believers" grew, the JCI effort gathered momentum, and more and more staff came on board to contribute.

(continued on page 30)

Case Study 1-1.   Changi General Hospital, *continued*

One way CGH staff could literally "sign on" to the commitment to quality was visible—a huge poster in a common area with the message "We Are the Key to Clinical Quality," which staff were invited to sign as a pledge.

Emphasis on Cooperation

CGH leaders report that the JCI accreditation experience helped to bring out an unprecedented level of cooperation among all categories of hospital staff, as everyone was working toward a common goal, that of improving patient safety and quality of care via compliance with JCI standards. As Professor Fock Kwong Ming, then Chairman Medical Board who headed CGH's decision to become accredited, once said, "There are people whom I've not spoken to in many years, but for the sake of JCI accreditation, I spoke with them to gain their collaboration."

Advice to Organizations Considering JCI Accreditation

CGH leaders want any organizations considering JCI accreditation to consider the following factors when making their decision:

- ⊃ JCI provides a comprehensive set of standards and an accreditation process that are designed to help the organization improve patient safety and quality of care.
- ⊃ Embarking on JCI accreditation requires a significant commitment of resources—people, time, effort, and finances.
- ⊃ It is critical to have good leaders who can engage the staff and drive the JCI efforts.
- ⊃ Be prepared to handle resistance, as inevitably there will be skeptics who do not believe in JCI accreditation.
- ⊃ Be prepared for an increase in data collection and data management tasks. Develop a mindset based on the use of data for concrete evaluations and improvement.

Finally, CGH's advice is, "Just do it."

Special thanks to Dr. Diana Tan Yuen Lan, Director of Clinical Services and Quality Management, for her contributions to this case study. Dr. Tan thanks the following colleagues for their contributions and support:

- *Professor Fock Kwong Ming, Senior Consultant, Gastroenterology*
- *Ms. Aileen Lim, Executive, Clinical Services*
- *Ms. Preetha Ramachandran, Executive, Clinical Services*
- *Mr. T. K. Udairam, Chief Executive Officer, Changi General Hospital*
- *Associate Professor Low Cheng Ooi, Chairman Medical Board, Changi General Hospital (from October 2007)*

SECTION 1

REFERENCES

1. Institute of Medicine: *Crossing the Quality Chasm: A New Health System for the 21st Century.* Washington, DC: National Academy Press, 2001.

2. Whittaker S.: Definitions of quality in health services. *Building Quality in Health Care* 1:5–8, 2007.

3. Timmons K.: An international approach to quality and patient safety. *Building Quality in Health Care* 1:15–18, 2007.

4. Spencer E., Walshe K.: National quality improvement policies and strategies in European healthcare systems. *Qual Saf Health Care* 18(suppl. 1):i22–i27, Feb. 2009.

5. Shaw C., et al.: Do European hospitals have quality and safety governance systems and structures in place? *Qual Saf Health Care* 18(suppl. 1):i51–i56, Feb. 2009.

6. VanOstenberg P.: Joint Commission International (JCI): A partner in quality and safety. *Jt Comm J Qual and Patient Saf* (Global Supplement) pp. 5–8, 2004.

7. Smits P., et al.: Conceptualizing performance in accreditation. *Int J Qual Health Care* 20: 47–52, 2008.

8. Hassan D.K., Goes J., Pasternak D.: Are Joint Commission International standards effective in improving quality performance? A longitudinal study. *JCInsight* 3, Jan. 2009. http://www.jointcommissioninternational.org/JCInsight/ JCIezine/Are-Joint-Commission-International-Standards-Effective-in-Improving-Quality-Performance (accessed 14 May 2010).

9. Lombarts M.J.M.H., et al.: Application of quality improvement strategies in 389 European hospitals: Results of the MARQuIS project. *Qual Saf Health Care* 18(suppl. 1):i29–i37, Feb. 2009.

10. Deloitte Center for Health Solutions: *Medical Tourism: Consumers in Search of Value.* 2008. http://www.deloitte .com/assets/Dcom-UnitedStates/Local%20Assets/Documents/ us_chs_MedicalTourismStudy(3).pdf (accessed 14 May 2010).

11. Ehrbeck T., Guevara C., Mango P.D.: Mapping the market for medical travel. *McKinsey Quarterly* May 2008.

12. Thailand: Health and medical tourism update. *International Medical Travel Journal* 15 Apr. 2010. http://www.imtj.com/ news/?EntryId82=195271 (accessed 14 May 2010).

13. Accreditation: IMTA issues position paper. *International Medical Travel Journal* Sep. 2008.

14. American College of Surgeons: Press Release: *Patient Safety Issues Prompt American College of Surgeons to Release Statement on Medical and Surgical Tourism.* 8 May 2009. http://www.facs.org/news/surgtourism.html (accessed 14 Jun. 2010).

15. American Medical Association Council on Medical Service: *Medical Care Outside the United States.* Report 1-A08. http://www.ama-assn.org/ama1/pub/upload/mm/372/a-08cms1.pdf (accessed 14 May 2010).

16. Rooney A.L., vanOstenberg P.R.: *Licensure, Accreditation, and Certification: Approaches to Health Services Quality.* Quality Assurance Project, 1999. http://www.qaproject.org/pubs/ pubsmonographs.html#licensure (accessed 14 May 2010).

SECTION 2

ACCREDITATION FOR THE HEALTH CARE EXECUTIVE

This section explores the role of leadership in accreditation and the commitments and decisions leaders must make to support accreditation. It is designed for use by an organization's leadership, including executives, members of the governing body, and clinical leaders.

Every health care organization has leaders. They are the people behind the organization's success or failure. They set the tone, create the vision, define the culture, identify the priorities, and monitor the organization's success and the way it conducts its business. They are responsible for governance, administration, and oversight of the quality and safety of care the organization provides. These leaders may include the organization's CEO, administrator, governing body leaders, senior managers, and other managerial and clinical leaders.

Although pursuing accreditation requires an organizationwide commitment, the support, participation, and involvement of organization leaders is vital toward the success of accreditation efforts. Organization leaders commit to the accreditation process, allocate resources to the process, support changes that come about as a result of the process, and act as visible champions of the accreditation effort.

To lay the groundwork for accreditation, organization leaders must define, emphasize, and nurture a culture based on safety, quality, and continuous performance improvement. Creating such a culture is an important leadership responsibility that contributes to an environment that supports accreditation and meets patient needs.

By making their expectations consistently clear throughout the organization, leaders can also influence the attitudes and behaviors of staff toward the accreditation process. Failure by the health care executive to emphasize the importance of improving organization performance through accreditation sends a message that other goals are more important. Indeed, leaders are the critical link between the concept of performance improvement and its implementation through employee participation.[1]

Choosing Accreditation

Before starting on the accreditation journey, organization leaders must decide whether accreditation is a worthwhile pursuit and appropriate for their particular organization. To establish this leadership commitment for accreditation, it is important for leaders to consider the process from different perspectives, including the following:

- How can accreditation benefit the organization? As discussed in Section 1, accreditation has been shown to help organizations assess, evaluate, and improve the quality of their services; recruit the most skilled clinical staff; fulfill public demand for high-quality health care; and meet regulatory and payment requirements.

- How does accreditation reflect the organization's values and support its mission and goals? Examining the unique needs of the organization and patients served can help leaders see directly how accreditation can support these critical organization elements. By doing this, leaders can identify tangible ways that accreditation supports current organization efforts on behalf of patients.

- How can accreditation improve clinical processes? Compliance with the standards can help an organization improve, standardize, and structure many different clinical processes, such as admission, assessment of patients, care planning, and facility management.

- How will accreditation help with quality and performance improvement efforts? Because accreditation is based on the concept of regular, proactive, and comprehensive performance improvement, leaders should be able to see how the pursuit of accreditation can support and enhance existing performance improvement efforts.

- How will accreditation fit into daily operations? Continued compliance with standards is possible only if organizations incorporate compliance efforts into the day-to-day operations of staff and leadership.

- How will accreditation meet the organization's needs related to competitiveness in the marketplace? Leaders should understand how accreditation will provide credibility and external validation of their organization. They should understand the needs of their customers and other stakeholders for such validation and consider how their stakeholders will view accreditation.

- How will accreditation activities mesh with strategic planning efforts? Accreditation is a significant undertaking and must be in line with an organization's overall strategic direction. It is through the strategic planning process that leaders commit vital resources to the accreditation process.

- Are organization leaders prepared to embark on this never-ending journey? When an organization starts the accreditation process, the process must become part of the very fabric of the organization. Leaders should assess their level of commitment and understanding of the time involved.

The comprehensive, demanding process of Joint Commission International (JCI) accreditation might not be right for all organizations. The difficulty is, in fact, part of its appeal. Only those organizations truly committed to

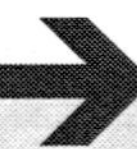

ACCREDITATION STRATEGY

Surveying the Board

To assess leadership's feelings toward and commitment to accreditation, organization leaders may want to survey boards of directors, senior leaders, clinical leaders, and other stakeholders to evaluate their commitment to the journey.

EXPERT ADVICE

Commitment

Committing to accreditation is no different than any other new undertaking within an organization. It requires additional resources initially but results in reduced costs and increased revenue if it is planned well. Commitment starts at the top. Leadership has to clearly identify their reasons for seeking accreditation, and if they are not clear and passionate, their board and other leaders will never agree to provide resources—people, financial, or other resources. But accreditation also should be looked upon as if it is an investment, because continued quality improvement will reduce costs. You learn to do your job better, with more efficiency and less waste.

—Helen Hoesing, R.N., M.P.H., Ph.D.,
JCI Senior Consultant

Why Pursue Accreditation?

Some (leaders) say they seek accreditation to become a world-class facility. A few will talk about the benefits of being able to compare data on core measures with other organizations in order to improve their care. Leaders don't usually refer to "marketing" as being a reason to pursue accreditation, but they say they want their organization to be identified as being as successful as and usually better than other hospitals in the area. These are all valid and important reasons, but in conversations with effective leaders they will inevitably get down to their bottom line—they truly want to improve quality and patient safety. The focus on improving quality and patient safety becomes like an umbrella that protects the whole organization from making decisions that ultimately harm patients.

—Helen Hoesing, R.N., M.P.H., Ph.D.,
JCI Senior Consultant

quality and safety in every aspect of operations will be successful in achieving accreditation. Leaders who understand this fact can make an informed decision to either wholeheartedly support accreditation or determine that their organization is not yet ready for the challenge.

The Roles of Different Leadership Groups

Every health care organization should have a leadership structure that supports operations and sets the tone for safety and quality across the organization. Depending on the type and size of the organization, this leadership structure may be complex, consisting of multiple groups—a governing board, senior leaders, and clinical leaders—or it may be simple, consisting of one or two individuals.

When an organization chooses to pursue accreditation, different leadership groups play different roles in the process. Each organization pursuing accreditation should identify its leaders and involve them in the process because who the leaders are and how they lead within an organization have a very real impact on the success and value of accreditation. The following paragraphs take a brief look at different leadership groups and discuss their critical roles in accreditation efforts.

Governing Board

This agency, group of individuals, or owner is responsible for overseeing the operations of an organization and is held accountable for the quality of services an organization provides. Governance is also responsible for the financial health and reputation of an organization. This group allocates resources for operation, ensures organizational management, and monitors compliance with laws and regulations. Governance is the highest level of decision making and responsibility for an organization.

Although governance duties associated with financial health and operations management are important, they should not eclipse or replace board responsibilities for quality and safety. The governance of an organization sets the framework for supporting safe and high-quality patient care. This framework includes the mission statement, policies and procedures, and resources necessary to improve performance. As a group, boards must promote quality improvement and patient safety efforts, as well as allocate resources to support these efforts.

So what does a board that is focused on quality and safety look like? Research shows that better outcomes are associated with governing boards that do the following[2]:

- Spend more than 25% of their time on quality issues.
- Receive a formal quality performance measurement report.
- Engage in a high level of interaction with physicians on quality strategies.
- Compensate senior executives, in part, based on quality improvement performance.
- Identify the chief executive as the person with the greatest impact on quality improvement.

In addition, boards should regularly engage in the following activities to communicate their commitment to quality and safety efforts[3]:

- Review data about organizational safety performance.
- Review adverse event reporting and root cause analysis (RCA). (*See* page 46 for information on RCA.)
- Provide resources for improving organizational infrastructure, education, and staffing.
- Hold leadership accountable for addressing safety issues.

To help engage a governing board in safety and quality, organizations may want to consider the following actions[4]:

- Structure board meeting agendas so that quality and safety are given the same amount of attention as financial issues.
- Engage the board in discussions regarding safety measures that should be used to gauge organization performance
- Discuss the organization's performance in relation to evidence-based best practices.
- Strengthen aspects of the organization's strategic plan that relate to quality of care and safety.
- Educate the board. As a group, board members must be knowledgeable and able to participate fully in discussions about quality improvement, safety issues, and accreditation. Many organizations urge trustees to attend conferences and lectures on quality and safety. Others arrange retreats where board members can talk with quality experts in health care and other fields, explore international and organizational trends, and look at key trouble spots within the organization in more depth than is possible at monthly or quarterly meetings.

The board's role in accreditation. Although the board will not be involved in the day-to-day work necessary for an organization to become accredited, its commitment to the process is essential. When governance pays attention to an issue, such as accreditation, that issue gets the attention of executive leadership, physician leadership, and ultimately the entire organization.[5] When the board sets priorities and reviews data, providers at every level know that their efforts to improve care are an organizational priority and that the organization's leadership pays attention to those efforts.[6]

It is important to realize that if the governing body sees accreditation as a process that could potentially reveal poor performance rather than opportunities for improvement, solid ongoing support from executive leadership, physician leadership, and organizational staff may be difficult to achieve. Conversely, if the governing board views accreditation as an organizational imperative, it will be more likely to make and implement decisions that support accreditation, allocate the resources necessary to achieve accreditation, and contribute in other ways that support improved organization performance.

Senior Leaders

The senior leaders of an organization—the chief executive officer, president, chief operating officer, chief financial

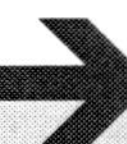

ACCREDITATION STRATEGY

Keeping the Governing Body Involved

To keep the governing body involved in and supportive of the accreditation process, it may be useful to ask a governing body representative to serve on high-level accreditation committees. (*See* page 40 for more information on accreditation committees.) Providing regular and frequent written and oral reports to the governing body also keeps these leaders informed as to the status and progress of accreditation initiatives. Effective communication helps make governing body members become interested and dedicated partners in the accreditation process.

officer, chief nursing officer, chief medical officer, and so on—are responsible for an organization's overall, day-to-day operations. This includes high-level work to develop plans and policies necessary to carry out the organization's mission, vision, and goals. In addition, senior leaders must oversee procurement of essential supplies, maintenance of the physical facility, financial management, and quality management. More than any other entity, these leaders are responsible for the administrative operations of the organization that support safe and high-quality care and ultimately foster an organization's ability to meet its mission, vision, and goals.

To be effective, executive leaders must place a priority on safety and quality efforts and ensure that policies, processes, and procedures in an organization reflect that priority. They must discuss safety and quality issues at senior executive meetings, regularly review data about safety and quality, follow up on issues at the senior level, discuss safety and quality issues with frontline staff, and respond to identified issues quickly and effectively to yield real change. Senior leaders should prioritize their calendars to be

Involving the Governing Board

Because governing boards generally do not meet very often, it can be difficult to keep members updated and enthusiastic about the accreditation effort. Leaders should spend some time at the beginning of the accreditation process strategizing how they will accomplish this. Some organizations make accreditation preparation a standing agenda item at every meeting. Others invite board members to participate on committees or to champion specific aspects of the work. One organization I am aware of asked board members to choose one standards category that interested them and pledge to attend at least one committee meeting related to that interest each month. Their presence had a motivating effect on everyone.

—Sherry Kaufield, M.A., F.A.C.H.E.,
Executive Director, International Services, JCI

available for data review sessions, meetings with project leaders, and other activities that support safety and quality.

Senior leaders' role in accreditation. A health care organization's senior leaders will be the ones to choose accreditation as a way to promote quality and safety. Their solid and visible championing of accreditation and their continuing involvement throughout the accreditation process are essential for quality to become and remain the organization's priority.

Senior leaders must serve as advocates for quality improvement, "marketers" of unified standards, and mentors for other leaders and organization staff. Committed leaders understand the benefits of accreditation, and they communicate excitement to staff about the ultimate goal—achieving and maintaining the highest possible levels of patient care. This attitude can help overcome any anxiety or resistance to accreditation. Leading by example on quality councils and task forces is important because clinical leaders and other staff within the organization will not focus on accreditation if it is not a visible priority of senior management.

Leaders can further demonstrate their commitment to accreditation by investing their time in the planning process. Health care executives likely will not personally develop accreditation-related quality improvement projects, but they should be involved in and aware of them, offering input on priorities and showing interest in the planning process. (*See* Sidebar 2-1 on page 38.) Completely delegating to others within the organization may send the wrong message about the importance of accreditation and quality improvement.

Before championing accreditation and cultivating an improvement culture for other leaders and staff, senior leaders should self-assess current quality improvement competencies and knowledge and augment existing capacity with new information and tools. Leaders may also want to seek out training to improve their communication skills because interactive, open communication is a hallmark of successfully accredited organizations.

Clinical Leaders

Although the governing body of an organization is ultimately accountable for the quality and safety of care the organization provides, the clinical staff—both physicians and nurses—directly provide and participate in the delivery of that care. Clinicians have a significant impact on resource utilization; the delivery, safety, and quality of health care; and the speed and effect of efforts designed to improve the safety and quality of health care. Consequently, organizations should leverage this unique

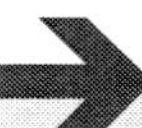

Opportunities for Communication

Throughout the accreditation process, leaders should remain sensitive to the heavy demands of the process on clinical leaders, department managers, and general staff. One way to do this is to provide opportunities for two-way communication about the accreditation process in which those affected by change can voice their concerns, confusion, and worries about the new ways of conducting business Allowing time for this type of interaction is crucial to keeping an organization on track.

Sidebar 2-1. Using Tracers as a Leadership Tool

As described in Section 1, tracer methodology is a key component of the survey process that allows JCI surveyors to follow the experiences of a patient throughout an organization. Organizations can integrate this same methodology into their own systems improvement activities.

The quality/accreditation specialist is likely to drive the majority of organizational efforts to conduct "mock" or practice tracers to improve organization performance (*see* Section 3, beginning on page 113). However, health care executives who view this process as a leadership tool will see their organizations reap the greatest benefits. Benefits include an improved focus on the systems that contribute to safety and quality of patient care. Benefits also include staff members who engage in systems thinking, gain a better understanding of their colleagues' duties, and work as effective members of a team.

To support these mock tracer efforts, leaders can do the following:

- Make an organizational commitment to using the tracer methodology.
- Allocate the resources necessary for education.
- Work with the individual who is leading tracer efforts to set a realistic time frame for conducting the initial and follow-up tracers.
- Request regular updates on the process.
- Realize that the process will not be perfect at first and communicate this fact to staff involved.
- Demonstrate a willingness to modify processes, tools, and focus as the tracers progress.
- Frame all communication about the tracer methodology as a means for improving patient safety and quality of care—the aim of all individuals at the organization.
- Reward improvements.

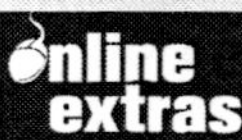 "Use of Tracers as a Leadership Tool," a helpful slide presentation, is available in the Online Extras at www.jcrinc.com/JCIGS10/Extras.

---

perspective and empower clinical leaders to become drivers in efforts to improve safety and quality.[7]

By focusing on improving quality and safety, increasing collaboration, and helping reduce risk, clinical leaders can become more engaged in the organization—to the benefit of themselves, patients, and the organization as a whole.

Gaining the support of clinical leaders. Support for accreditation by clinical leaders is crucial to an organization's success. To enlist this support and engage clinical leaders in the accreditation process, senior leaders and governing boards must outline why accreditation is worth the investment in time and talent. Clinical leaders must understand how the accreditation process will ultimately affect and improve patient care.

Clinical leaders may have limited time for performance improvement and accreditation activities. Senior leaders, including the chief medical officer and the chief nursing officer, who involve clinical leaders where their input can

EXPERT ADVICE

Finding a "Champion"

There has to be a "champion," and an organization's path to accreditation is normally much more successful if the champion comes from top leadership. When we don't see this commitment from top leadership, the organization not only has a difficult time understanding the benefits of accreditation; it often has a difficult time even becoming accredited. The leader helps to define and communicate the benefits of accreditation to staff. This is critical to success.

—Helen Hoesing, R.N., M.P.H., Ph.D.,
JCI Senior Consultant

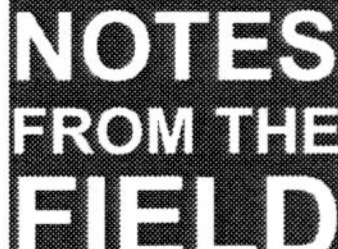

NOTES FROM THE FIELD

A Survey of Senior Leaders

Leaders of accredited organizations who were interviewed during a recent internal JCI survey advised that navigating the establishment of new processes and structures required vigilance and visibility by senior leaders who actively championed accreditation. The efforts of senior leaders to make accreditation succeed helped convince middle management leaders that quality improvement was a permanent part of operations and not just a passing fad. In addition, the board of directors at several of the hospitals made recommendations to hire new staff who had experience with accreditation. New physicians, CEOs, nurses, and quality managers were sought to complement existing staff by providing first-hand knowledge of accreditation.

---

make the biggest impact on clinical care will see the strongest benefits of clinical leadership participation. Clinical leaders are most often interested in participating if they think they can make a real and important difference in the health and safety of their patients.

Fundamentally, by explaining the benefits that accreditation offers to patients and the organization, identifying the critical role that clinical leaders play, and providing a realistic estimation of the time commitment involved, senior leaders can help gain the support of this important group.

Engaging physicians. Different types of clinicians may have varying reactions to the accreditation process. Physicians, for example, may be skeptical of accreditation and have a hard time believing the process will actually improve already existing high standards of patient care. Physicians also may worry that accreditation will result in new burdens, such as those related to documentation, credentialing, and informed consent. They may wonder if they will lose autonomy. Physicians must see accreditation standards as a framework by which organizational

NOTES FROM THE FIELD

Beijing United Family Hospital and Clinics

Beijing United Family Hospital and Clinics—a 50-bed general medical/surgical hospital with general health care clinics—pursued JCI accreditation as part of its mission to bring international health care to China. The organization sees itself as a pioneer and leader in the health care industry in China, a belief borne out by many hospitals and clinics around the country visiting every week to learn about international standards.

A large percentage of the Beijing United Family Hospital and Clinics' patients are expatriates who typically relocate to Beijing with their families for two to three years and then return to their home country. With such a diverse patient population coming from countries that do not have the same immunization regimen, the hospital felt it important to ensure that children visiting the hospital are current with their immunizations. As a result, the organization embarked on a project to increase the percentage of patients less than 6 years of age whose immunization status is up-to-date. As part of this project, the organization identified seven critical vaccinations that all children should receive. In the course of treatment, if a child is discovered to be not up-to-date, the physician recommends to the parents the necessary vaccinations. Beijing United Family Hospital and Clinics has been very successful with this approach, with 99% of the children leaving the facility current on their vaccinations.

The organization also took on a project to improve pain management in the emergency room, requiring that patients with a fracture or suspected fracture receive analgesia within 30 minutes of arrival in the emergency room.

processes will be *improved* in order to support good medical care. They also must understand that accreditation is not a peer review process or way of dictating how they will practice medicine—as physicians often suspect—but a strategic improvement process that supports the use of good clinical science and best practices.

To help gain physicians' support, both senior and medical staff leaders should take time to listen to physician concerns and provide education about how accreditation and its focus on evidence-based practices can result in improved care. Providing information at medical staff meetings and in other interactive forums will allow for questions, explanations, and discussion.

Senior and medical staff leaders should be aware that an open-ended invitation to participate in the accreditation process may not gain the physician support that is needed. Senior and medical staff leaders will need to develop a strategy to enlist the support of top physician leaders who can, in turn, make the case to their peers. To do this, organization leaders may wish to ask physicians who have expressed interest in accreditation, or who have been affiliated with accredited organizations, to act as "champions" to stimulate interest, support, and ongoing commitment.

Engaging nurses. Unlike physicians, many nurses are initially accepting of the idea of accreditation, possibly because quality improvement and standardization of patient care have been widely discussed in nursing schools for the past two decades. Members of the nursing profession also tend to be more accustomed to conforming to a disciplined routine, making the demands of accreditation easier to adopt than for physicians. Although they are more accepting, there are some challenges nurses face with accreditation. For example, nurses must learn to balance bedside patient needs and demands for quality improvement activities and formal documentation. As with physicians, identifying nursing champions to spread the word about how to successfully achieve that balance and reap the benefits of accreditation can be helpful in securing this group's support.

Establishing an Accreditation Committee

To encourage leadership's commitment to accreditation, some facilities establish a high-level accreditation committee. Such a committee could include representatives from the governing board, medical staff leaders, the chief executive officer, and leaders from the organization's quality improvement area. The committee might meet periodically to develop strategic plans to attain accreditation and to review progress toward achieving this goal. This type of leadership oversight helps drive the accreditation process and provides a mechanism for assigning responsibilities for the activities and goals related to accreditation.

Creating a high-level, written plan for the accreditation committee also might be useful to describe how the activities will be integrated and coordinated throughout the organization. This allows different staff members to see how their areas are involved in accreditation and how their activities relate to the organization's overall goals. Stating the goal of achieving accreditation in the plan, with targeted time frames for key processes, establishes a focus for all the activities and provides a measurable outcome. Sharing as much information as possible from this plan also makes accreditation a highly visible goal across the organization, promoting awareness and participation across all units and departments.

Establishing a Culture of Safety and Quality

As previously mentioned, leaders are responsible for creating an environment favorable for the implementation of accreditation principles. As a result, the next phase of the accreditation journey requires laying the groundwork for success and building a culture of safety and quality.

The word *culture* refers to the attitudes and values of a group of people. The culture of an organization mirrors the viewpoint, mind-set, and main concerns of its staff and influences the effectiveness of performance. Every organization has a culture—in many cases, more than one. A culture that reflects the beliefs, attitudes, and priorities of the majority may be dominant, but smaller, assorted subcultures that may or may not share the same values might also be present. An organization's performance can be positively or negatively affected by its dominant culture and/or its smaller subcultures, as these cultures ultimately influence how an organization accomplishes its work.

Organizations that are effective in providing safe, high-quality care work to create, support, and sustain an organizationwide culture that emphasizes safety and quality. The National Patient Safety Agency describes such a culture in health care as one in which staff and organization leaders have a constant and active awareness of the potential for things to go wrong.[8] In a safety culture, both staff and leadership are able to acknowledge mistakes, learn from them, and take action to put things right. In such a culture, all individuals focus on maintaining excellence in performance and accept that safety and quality of care, treatment, and services is a personal responsibility. Everyone in the organization knows that they cannot truly deliver the best care possible unless they are constantly striving to improve outcomes and reduce risks.

Leaders in a health care organization—including senior medical staff and nursing leaders—demonstrate their commitment to a culture of safety and quality by setting expectations related to safety and quality for themselves and for those who work in the organization. These leaders promote teamwork, open discussions of safety and quality issues, and internal and external reporting of these issues. Their attention is focused on the performance of systems and processes instead of the individual, although reckless behavior and a blatant disregard for safety are not tolerated. Leaders provide for the effective functioning of the organization, focusing on safety and quality, and they plan, support, and implement key systems critical to these efforts.

The actions and attitudes of leaders can foster an environment in which certain attitudes develop and become accepted. Leaders who are open and nonjudgmental can encourage a culture of safety and quality. For example, the governing body and organization leaders should support open communication among clinical staff about organization strengths and weaknesses, as well as adverse events. Leaders who do this demonstrate that discussions about improvements are encouraged, which in turn encourages action to make improvement. It is also important for leaders to acknowledge that improvement is always possible. If leaders act as if they do not wish to see, hear, or speak about problems, then people will not be comfortable discussing these issues or finding ways to make necessary improvements.

Staff members look to leaders for direction and priorities and closely watch the actions of leaders to see if they "walk the talk" about quality and safety or just make empty mandates and idle promises that they personally have no intention of following. For example, leadership is critical to the successful implementation of a hand-hygiene program. When leaders are involved in driving the need for such a program, support its development, and actively participate in it, the chances of successful implementation and processes improve.

Creating a culture of safety does not happen overnight. Like accreditation, it requires a continuous journey with many distinct steps. Several activities occur regularly in a culture of safety and quality. The following paragraphs take a brief look at some of the most important ones.

Ensuring the Strategic Direction Reflects the Importance of Safety and Quality

Every organization has a purpose—a reason for being. For most, if not all, health care organizations, this purpose involves the quality of care, treatment, and services provided to the population served.

To clearly identify its purpose and the way it plans to fulfill it, an organization must determine its mission, vision, and goals. These define the reasons why the organization exists, outlines what it hopes to accomplish, and identifies how it plans to achieve its desired results. The mission, vision, and goals of an organization help guide its actions, determine priorities and focus for leaders, and offer a clear-cut path to success. They also help in decisions of allocating resources and performance improvement efforts, and they influence the decision about what type of staff to hire for the organization.

Within organizations that have a culture of safety and quality, the mission, vision, and goals reflect the importance of safe, high-quality care. These strategic documents reflect the organization's emphasis on continuous improvement, proactive risk reduction, and use of evidence-based practice. Leaders should frequently review the organization's mission, vision, and goals to ensure that they properly reflect the organization's culture and encourage continuous improvement.

Fostering Teamwork

Teamwork is a cooperative, coordinated effort to achieve a common goal. It involves listening, discussing, participating, respecting, questioning, sharing, and generally communicating in a productive and interactive fashion. There has been an increased focus on teamwork in health care in recent years due to the assumption that high-performing teams produce better-quality care and fewer errors.[9] Research has supported this assumption by demonstrating better clinical outcomes and satisfaction.[10] Teamwork can also increase job satisfaction and improve organizational commitment of team members.[10]

Teamwork can thrive in an environment that supports it. Such an environment must value teamwork, provide structures that support teamwork, monitor teamwork, and refuse to tolerate behaviors that go against teamwork. Conversely, teamwork can disappear in environments that discourage teamwork and promote an individual approach to solving a problem. This type of environment seeks to blame individuals for mistakes and provides little or no support for team behaviors.

Leaders can create an environment that supports teamwork in a number of ways, including the following:

- Support the use of teams in all aspects of the organization, including in care, performance improvement, leadership, and administrative activities.
- Address hierarchies between providers and any power differences that exist.
- Provide resources for communication and teamwork training so that every member of a team is clear on his or her role and responsibilities in and to the team.
- Observe team behaviors and work to correct anti-team interactions.
- Create and enforce a policy in which anti-team behaviors are immediately addressed.

One specific way leaders can foster teamwork and the open communication that supports it is through patient safety rounds. These structured communication opportunities allow for a comprehensive exchange of safety information between senior leadership and frontline staff. During patient safety rounds, senior leadership, along with other key staff, visits units, departments, and areas of a health care organization. They engage frontline staff members in discussions over their safety concerns and help assess how ongoing or new safety efforts are being implemented. (*See* Sidebar 2-2 on page 43.)

By fostering an environment in which team behavior is the norm, leaders can ensure a collaborative, interactive approach to care. This can lead to greater acceptance and support of performance improvement projects and general readiness for change.[11]

Engaging Patients as Active Members of the Care Team

Actively involving patients in their care can improve outcomes, reduce the risk of mistakes, and improve processes. Historically, however, patients have not been involved in their care. Many organizations take the perspective that a patient is in the health care organization to receive care—not participate in it. To truly involve patients in care, leaders must set the tone for this activity and actively support the concept.

Three effective ways to involve patients in their care are to

1. encourage patients to express their concerns;

2. encourage patients to participate in the care process; and

3. educate patients so they feel more comfortable asking questions.

All patients should receive information on how to share concerns about their care. Brochures and information posted throughout the facility can help spread the word. Also, clinicians and other health care providers should actively encourage patients to speak up if they think there is a problem. Health care providers should invite patients' questions and concerns about their treatment and practitioner behaviors that are specific to safety-focused processes, such as hand washing, correct patient identification, medication teaching, and other patient-specific risk factors. Providers should allow the patient adequate time to express their concerns and ask questions. Providers should also actively listen to patients and answer their questions. (*See* Section 4, page 140, for more information on involving patients in their care.)

Using Data to Improve Performance

Data can reveal an enormous amount of information that is useful when establishing safety and quality goals and objectives. Data can be used to identify problems, prioritize issues, identify solutions, and track success. For example, data can show an organization's level of compliance with JCI standards and other requirements. Data can reveal the need for new equipment, infrastructure, and technology systems. Data can help anticipate issues in implementing new systems or programs.

When decisions are supported by data, leaders are more likely to move in directions that help them achieve organization goals. When data are analyzed and turned into information, leaders can see patterns and trends and understand the reasons for organization performance. A commitment by leadership to make data-driven decisions will permeate the organization.

Leaders should use data and information to guide decisions and understand the performance of their organization. This involves setting expectations for data use; providing the resources needed, including staff, equipment, and information systems; understanding the meanings of measures used to collect data; and understanding how data are being used throughout the organization. (*See* Section 3, pages 83–94, for more information on data use.)

Sidebar 2-2. Patient Safety Rounds

The concept of rounding is not new in health care. *Patient safety rounds* were first conceived in 2001 by Allan S. Frankel, M.D., and colleagues during an Institute for Healthcare Improvement (IHI) meeting in Boston, Massachusetts. During this meeting, patient safety rounds were designed as a means to connect senior health care organization leadership to staff in an ongoing manner.

Patient safety rounds allow management and frontline staff members to engage in a structured, two-way conversation about safety. Data from that conversation are captured, analyzed, prioritized, and addressed.

Patient safety rounds can be extremely useful in solving problems. By providing a regular, consistent presence among frontline staff and framing that presence within the context of patient safety, senior leadership can identify issues needing improvement and can also respond more effectively to those concerns. Patient safety rounds allow leaders to hear the concerns of frontline providers, gather staff opinions and perceptions of issues and risks, increase mutual understanding between senior leaders and frontline staff about safety issues, and foster a culture of teamwork and continuous learning. Rounding also helps facilitate immediate leadership responsiveness. By being visible during rounds, leaders can influence the tone of the culture.

Patient safety rounds can occur anywhere in a health care organization, including clinical care areas (nursing stations, pharmacies, ambulatory settings, outpatient offices) and nonclinical areas (billing offices, central sterilization units, transportation departments, and on floors dedicated to information technology systems). Usually lasting about an hour, they can happen as frequently as needed—weekly, quarterly, or monthly.

One specific approach to patient safety rounds is called Executive WalkRounds™. This tool not only allows for two-way communication between leaders and staff, it also serves as a method for collecting, analyzing, and responding to information gleaned during these interactions. During WalkRounds, executives ask detailed questions of staff to prompt discussion. Questions may include the following:

- What works well in the area?

- What doesn't work well?

- Are you worried about anything that could cause harm?

- Do we disclose all that we reasonably should (to patients, family, or friends), including mistakes and potential mistakes?

- How well does teamwork work in this area?

These, and questions like these, elicit different responses, and all participants are encouraged to give feedback. During the WalkRound, someone—typically a quality or safety manager—takes notes, including what was said, who said it, and what the response was. After the WalkRound concludes, participating leaders immediately discuss what went well, what went poorly, and what they learned, and begin prioritizing important issues and potential improvements. The individual taking notes adds to his or her notes any other insights generated during this discussion. To be successful at WalkRounds, organization leaders typically set up a robust system for tracking and ranking collected data, such as an interactive database that allows for sorting and prioritizing.

Sources: Frankel A., et al.: Patient safety leadership WalkRounds™. *Jt Comm J Qual Saf* 29:16–26, Jan. 2003; Frankel A., Grillo S., Pittman M.: *Patient Safety Leadership WalkRounds™ Guide.* Chicago: Health Research & Educational Trust; and Boston: Partners HealthCare, 2006. Frankel A., et al. (eds.): *The Essential Guide for Patient Safety Officers.* Oakbrook Terrace, IL: Joint Commission Resources, 2009.

Developing Systems-Based, Standardized Protocols, Processes, and Procedures

Because accreditation focuses on an organization's systems for providing safe, high-quality care, it is natural during the pursuit of accreditation to identify systems that need to be redesigned in order to maximize patient outcomes and minimize risks. This may involve redesigning, reworking, or retooling protocols, processes, and procedures. This effort may involve the use of clinical pathways and other forms of evidence-based care.

A well-designed protocol, process, or procedure is one that takes the following into consideration:

- The needs of patients, families, staff, and others
- The results of performance improvement activities
- Information about potential risks to stakeholders
- Evidence-based information
- Information about sentinel events

So how can leaders ensure that processes are well-designed? As with other aspects of performance improvement, there are many ways. For example, leaders should involve staff and those receiving care in the design of any new processes. This could include surveying staff and patients, creating a focus group or work group to help with design, or observing staff and patients to see if a new process would work effectively and meet their needs. (*See* Section 3 for more information about redesigning processes.)

Proactively Examining Risk

A culture of safety and quality relies on proactively identifying, examining, and addressing potential risk. In this context, *risks* may include incidents that result in injury, damage to property, organizational or personal risk, or other harm, loss, or danger to patients and staff.[12]

While there are many ways to proactively address risk, one effective technique is failure mode and effects analysis (FMEA). This is a team-based, systematic, proactive technique that is used to prevent process and product problems before they occur. FMEA is based on studied engineering principles and approaches to designing systems and processes. It has been successfully used in a number of industries, including the airline, automotive, and aerospace industries. Principles from this technique can be applied to the delivery of health care services. (*See* Sidebar 2-3 on page 45 for more information on FMEA.)

Identifying and Discussing Adverse Events

Mistakes happen. They are an inevitable part of any process in which human beings must work to accomplish a task. A culture based on safety and quality readily accepts mistakes and errors as learning opportunities and works to improve processes based on information gleaned from those mistakes and errors. It is important to acknowledge that mistakes and errors can happen, identify when they happen, and learn from them. So how can leaders ensure that the mistakes and errors occurring in their organization are recognized, examined, and used for improvement?

One way is by being *transparent*, meaning completely open and honest about organization performance—both good and bad—and encouraging all staff to communicate openly about mistakes, errors, and close calls.

To be transparent, leaders must regularly monitor and analyze all unfavorable events and near misses (incidents in which an error almost occurs but is caught before it happens) in a quantitative manner. Leaders should require a RCA for all adverse events that cause patient harm, perform intense analysis for undesirable trends or variations when undesired changes occur in processes (*see* page 46 for information on analyzing adverse events and RCA), search for patterns in the root causes, and communicate findings and recommendations to all stakeholders.

Senior leaders should also consider holding a series of honest, open discussions with all other leaders to develop a precise view of the safety factors facing patients, staff, and the community. Open and honest discussions should focus on improvements and not on blame or punishment.

Transparency can exist only in a "just environment" in which it is safe for everyone to talk about real and potential errors and to support each other in the effort to be error-free without fear of reprisal. As defined by James Reason, a *just environment* or *culture* is one that supports the discussion of errors so that lessons can be learned from them. It distinguishes between error that is inadvertent, unintentional, and an opportunity for learning from error that is intentional and requires immediate accountability.[13] Organization leaders must work to establish a just culture and clearly define accountability for staff, so that staff will know when they will be held accountable for an error and when the error will be used for system improvement. This knowledge can take the fear away from discussing errors.

Many organizations are fearful of transparency, as they believe it will reveal flaws, decrease market share, and

Sidebar 2-3. Failure Mode and Effects Analysis (FMEA)

FMEA is a proactive approach to identifying addressing, and ideally preventing risks. FMEA provides a look at not only what problems could occur in a process or procedure but also at how severe the effects of the problems could be. FMEA assumes that no matter how knowledgeable or careful people are, failures will occur in some situations and may even be likely to occur. The focus is on *what* could allow the failure to occur rather than *whom*.

FMEA can involve from as few as 4 to as many as 10 different steps. Following is one way to conduct an FMEA:

1. Select a high-risk process and assemble a team.

2. Describe the process.

3. Brainstorm potential failure modes (these are aspects of the process that could fail) and determine their effects.

4. Prioritize failure modes.

5. Identify root causes of failure modes.

6. Redesign the process.

7. Analyze and test the new process.

8. Implement and monitor the redesigned process.

Ideally, FMEA can be used to help prevent failures from occurring. However, if a particular failure cannot be prevented, FMEA then focuses on protections that can be put into place to prevent the failure from reaching the patient. In the worst case, FMEA helps mitigate the effects of a failure if the failure affects patient safety.

FMEA is a ready-made prospective process that has a good track record and a number of benefits. It addresses problems people have actually seen happen or errors they have almost made. It is excellent, then, for capturing incidents that can and do occur and that generally are not captured any other way. Also, the multidisciplinary process pulls several kinds of information together and allows staff to target responses in new ways.

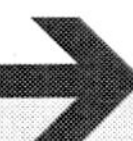

ACCREDITATION STRATEGY

Preventive Medicine

Rather than analyzing adverse events after they occur, leaders should require examinations of how such events can be prevented. Identifying and managing potential risks requires a systematic approach to determining how a process or design can fail, why it might fail, and how it can be made safer. Staff members usually have a better attitude about participating in these types of quality improvement activities because they know that they can more easily prevent bad things from happening by assessing and acting on risk.

increase lawsuits. The concerns are that if the organization exposes its weaknesses, people will, at best, seek health care elsewhere and, at worst, capitalize on published weaknesses to the detriment of the organization. However, there is research that shows that this is not what typically happens. In fact, being transparent often increases trust with patients and their families.

To further foster transparency, organization leaders should establish a reporting system through which staff can report errors, near misses, and other adverse events. These systems should not be designed to blame people but to identify system vulnerabilities that can lead to lapses in safety. Reporting systems can take many forms. but should have the following characteristics:

- Be nonpunitive. Staff must feel comfortable with reporting errors and be assured that their reports will not lead to retribution, disciplinary action, or other negative consequences. If staff believe that they will be blamed for the issues they report, then they won't report them.

- Be easy to use. If staff find it difficult or time consuming to report errors, then they will be less likely to report them. Staff must know what to report, whom to contact, how to contact them, and when to contact them.

- Have multiple venues. Leaders who allow the use of multiple venues for reporting, such as e-mail, telephone hotline, focus groups, surveys, personal meetings, or written reports, find that such a policy yields higher reporting rates.

- Examine more than just errors. By encouraging staff members to report both errors and near misses, leaders can learn about process errors as well as the errors that could occur. In addition, staff should report conditions that cause concern, because these conditions can lead to near misses or errors.

- Contain feedback mechanisms. Staff who report errors should receive feedback about their report, including an acknowledgment of the report, what was learned about the problem, what is being done to address the problem, and the results of improvement efforts. If leaders do not respond to reports, then staff may question the need for a reporting system. Staff must feel that by reporting errors they are helping to improve safety and decrease errors.

Although the data collection piece of reporting systems is important, analyzing those data is even more critical. Leaders should take information reported within a reporting system, examine that information, look for patterns and trends, and address any issues that arise. Trending error data over time can be helpful to show improvement or areas that need further work.

Responding to Adverse Events That Cause Harm

Sometimes an adverse event occurs and a patient is severely harmed. A surgeon operates on the wrong knee, a nurse inadvertently delivers a near-fatal dose of medication, a behavioral health care patient commits suicide in his room. This type of event is known as a sentinel event. A key activity that occurs in a culture based on safety and quality is consistently responding to sentinel events.

When a sentinel event occurs, an organization must conduct a thorough and credible RCA. This is a process for identifying the basic causes that underlie variation in performance, including the occurrence of a sentinel event or near miss. This process focuses primarily on systems and processes, not individual performance. RCA allows leaders to identify potential improvements in processes or systems that could decrease the likelihood that the sentinel event could occur again.

The product of an RCA is an action plan that identifies the strategies that the organization intends to implement to reduce the risk of similar events occurring in the future. The plan should address responsibility for implementation, oversight, pilot testing as appropriate, time lines, and strategies for measuring the effectiveness of the actions.

Assessing the Current Culture

When starting to establish a culture of safety, it can be helpful to determine an organization's current culture. This can be done through a cultural assessment process. Such a process allows an organization to compile a multidimensional profile of the cultural strengths and weaknesses of the organization. It can also build awareness among staff members about the importance of safety, teamwork, and quality improvement opportunities. Specifically, a cultural assessment can establish a baseline picture of the organization, make a data-driven case for change, help in selecting intervention(s) that are most appropriate for improving quality and safety, measure the success of any interventions, and track changes in safety over time. Various methods can be used for evaluation, including formal surveys, focus groups, staff interviews, and data analysis. Possible issues to consider within the assessment include the following[14]:

- Is there adequate staff?
- Do staff cooperate with each other?
- Do staff talk about the care they are providing?
- Does the organization value patient safety efforts?
- Is safety a top priority for organization leaders?
- In the staff's opinion, is making an error shameful?
- Are staff able to discuss safety concerns, issues, and errors openly and honestly?
- Are staff encouraged to report errors?
- Are staff who report issues punished by the organization?
- Does the organization proactively consider risk?
- In the respondent's opinion, who is responsible for errors—individuals or systems?

(*See* pages 49–50 for an example of how one organization assessed its culture of safety.)

Developing a Culture of Safety Statement

As work on establishing and maintaining a culture of safety begins, leaders may want to write down the characteristics they want their culture to embody. For example, a statement that says an organization is committed to

SECTION 2

systems-based processes, effective teamwork, open communication about errors, and proactive risk assessment can help build consensus around cultural improvement efforts and communicate leadership expectations. (*See* Sidebar 2-4 on page 48 for one organization's example of a culture of safety statement.)

How Can Accreditation Help Create a Culture of Safety?

Although implementing culture of safety activities—proactive risk reduction, systems improvement, data collection and analysis—may seem daunting, organization members do not have to feel that they are facing this process alone.

By participating in JCI accreditation, organizations will implement many activities, and the culture of the organization will begin to shift as a result. For example, centralizing quality improvement activities to comply with standards can help create a sense of unity in the organization around the shared goal of better patient care. A new spirit of cooperation can develop as different areas of the health care organization develop an appreciation of the roles of other departments or disciplines. The presurvey, or preparation stage, of accreditation can be helpful because it identifies specific weaknesses that offer opportunities for focused improvements.

Allocating Resources to Accreditation

As part of laying the groundwork for accreditation, leaders must allocate resources to the effort. Seeking accreditation requires a variety of different resources, including dedicated staff time, technology, education and training, equipment, and money. The following paragraphs take a further look at some of these critical resources.

Time

Achieving accreditation is a journey that takes a considerable time commitment. Leadership can contribute to the success of this journey by setting a realistic time frame for preparation. Because accreditation is a process that touches every area of an organization—for example, from the patient care areas to human resources to housekeeping—it is not practical to make the decision to seek accreditation, apply for accreditation, and undergo a survey within a matter of only a few months.

Preparing for accreditation should involve education for leaders and staff, a baseline assessment of current adherence to standards and each measurable element, collection and analysis of baseline quality data, a detailed project plan, a midpoint assessment and refinement of the project plan, and a mock survey at least 4 to 6 months in advance of the target date of the accreditation survey. In addition, JCI surveyors will be seeking data that indicate a 4-month record of standards compliance for all organizations undergoing an initial survey. (*See* Section 3 for more information on the specific aspects of accreditation preparation and the time frame for them.)

Realistically, preparing for accreditation is likely to take 12 to 24 months, with an average of 18 months (*See* Figure 2-1 on page 52.) Leaders who insist on setting an achievable time frame communicate the importance of taking a steady, comprehensive approach to accreditation. This approach seeks systems improvements that require thoughtful analysis to establish, implement, and sustain. Rushing through accreditation misses the point that quality and safety standards must become part of routine operations in order to have a meaningful, lasting impact that improves quality and safety.

Financial Resources

As discussed in Section 1, the cost of accreditation is usually surpassed by the savings realized in avoiding adverse events, improving quality, retaining staff, and enhancing patient satisfaction. With that said, organization leaders should be aware of the costs of accreditation so they can realistically compare them to the benefits realized.

Sidebar 2-4. Creating a Culture of Safety Statement

The National Guard Health Affairs (NGHA) in the Kingdom of Saudi Arabia, which has four JCI–accredited hospitals, shows how its organizations define and set expectations for its safety culture.

In any organization, a cultural concept forms its staff motivation and also governs relationships among them to distinguish its identity. Such concepts are positively or negatively reflected by the way the staff acts both inside and outside the organization. In preparing this plan, it is important to highlight the positive cultural concepts built over NGHA history as well as to recognize cultural concepts that require development in order to be a part of NGHA dynamics.

The health care organization covers the following cultural concepts:

- Patient focused—we listen to each other and treat one another with dignity and respect.

- Emphasis on the medical team concept and in a culture of involving patients and families with decision making about medical treatment

- Develop a patient's safety culture by emphasizing the role of systems rather than individuals in order to systematically develop policies to avoid future errors.

- Provision of education and skills—development opportunities to all staff

- Attracting highly qualified and skilled personnel from various countries in order to create a multicultural workforce that brings experience and achieves the NGHA organization's objectives

- Establish an NGHA culture of self-discipline, achieve decentralization, emphasize continuity and participation in decision making, encouraging teamwork and quick decision making based on scientific and objective data.

- Transparency in all health care organization activities, without breaching patient confidentiality

- Ensure fair business practices in dealing with dealers, suppliers, contractors; questioning who breaches this principle due to personal relationships, disregarding health organization interest; and avoiding personal dealing with companies.

- Justice and equality in rights and responsibilities for all staff

- Employ the principle of "Right Person in the Right Position," using a merit system in all employment and promotion decisions.

- Supporting patient's right of accessibility to the right treatment in a timely manner

- Promoting the ideal organization behavior such as punctuality, nondelay of work assignment, respecting schedules of work and assignment performance and programs, and attending meetings, committees, clinics, and scientific/training meetings

- Provision of appropriate environments for disabled persons

- Promoting smoke-free environments in all NGHA facilities

- Promoting work ethics and professional conduct in all activities such as patient care research and academic activities

- Promoting department productivity and individuals' personal growth, high performance, and loyalty

Source: National Guard Health Affairs, Saudi Arabia. Used with permission.

Case Study 2-1.   National Healthcare Group

Organization Name: National Healthcare Group (NHG)
Location: Singapore
About National Healthcare Group: NHG provides care through an integrated network of primary health care polyclinics, acute care hospitals, national specialty centers, virtual specialty centers, and business divisions. According to NHG's Web site (http://www.nhg.com.sg), the company has more than 14,000 staff in 15 different facilities.

Creating a Culture of Safety

To promote a culture of safety at NHG, different institutions in the NHG family formed a collaborative to undertake the following initiatives:

➲ Implement patient safety leadership WalkRounds. NHG senior leaders demonstrate their commitment to safety by making regular rounds to discuss safety issues with staff. During these WalkRounds (*see* Photo 1 on page 50), communication extends both ways—from leaders to staff and from staff to leaders. There is a healthy exchange of information and opinions between leaders and staff with a focused aim of improving patient safety. Across four years, NHG conducted 109 sessions and closed 81% of safety issues raised.

➲ Appoint patient safety officers (PSOs) and departmental safety champions. These leaders play pivotal roles in improving patient safety within NHG and within their own institutions. They are actively involved in the regular patient safety leadership WalkRounds, conducting patient safety workshops, promoting and implementing initiatives for safer practices, and investigating various patient safety issues. PSOs also serve as important information resources for patient safety issues within their own clinical departments. They are empowered to act and remove change barriers. PSOs also make regular presentations to the organization's governing body on safety issues and have the resources and organizational support to implement improvement work.

➲ Conduct patient safety workshops. Patient safety workshops are run by PSOs who have received local and international training. With specialized knowledge in patient safety, PSOs conduct workshops for staff from various NHG institutions. Topics covered in the workshops include the following:

⇨ Patient safety framework
⇨ Achieving safe and reliable health care
⇨ The human factor in a complex health care delivery system
⇨ Effective teamwork and communication
⇨ SBAR (situation-background-assessment-recommendation) and assertiveness (*see* Section 4, pages 142–143, for more information on SBAR)

To date, PSOs have conducted 16 patient safety workshops and trained a total of 458 physicians, 232 nurses, 55 allied health workers, and 57 administrators.

➲ Perform patient safety climate surveys. To understand patient safety perceptions of its staff, NHG has conducted a series of surveys in various NHG institutions. A survey tool adapted from one used by the Agency for Healthcare Research and Quality was used in the surveys (*see* Figure 1 on page 51). The first survey was conducted in 2005, with an overall response rate of 75%. This was followed by surveys in 2007 and 2008. The outcome of these surveys helps NHG determine the impact of its patient safety initiatives and the views of staff toward patient safety.

➲ Implement an open and fair incident reporting policy. Hospital occurrence and near-miss reporting is a key component of NHG's Quality and Patient Safety Plan. NHG employs the electronic Hospital Occurrence Reporting System (eHOR) as a platform for staff to voluntarily report medical incidents, including near misses. The organization's Open and Fair Incident Reporting Policy specifically states that incidents and near misses reported through eHOR are used solely for the purpose of improving quality and patient safety and that no information shall be used in staff performance appraisal or be documented in the staff member's personnel record. This includes counseling or reprimands. Since the implementation of

(continued on page 50)

Case Study 2-1. National Healthcare Group, *continued*

the Open and Fair Incident Reporting Policy, the eHOR reporting rates have been constantly increasing.

➲ Conduct safety briefings. Safety briefings in patient care units are a tool to increase safety awareness among frontline staff and foster a culture of safety. Based on concepts in aviation and other industries, briefings incorporate

safety consciousness into daily routines. Safety briefings help to increase staff awareness of patient safety issues, create an environment in which staff share information without fear of reprisal, and integrate the reporting of medication safety issues into daily work.

Photo 1. WalkRound at Tan Tock Seng Hospital

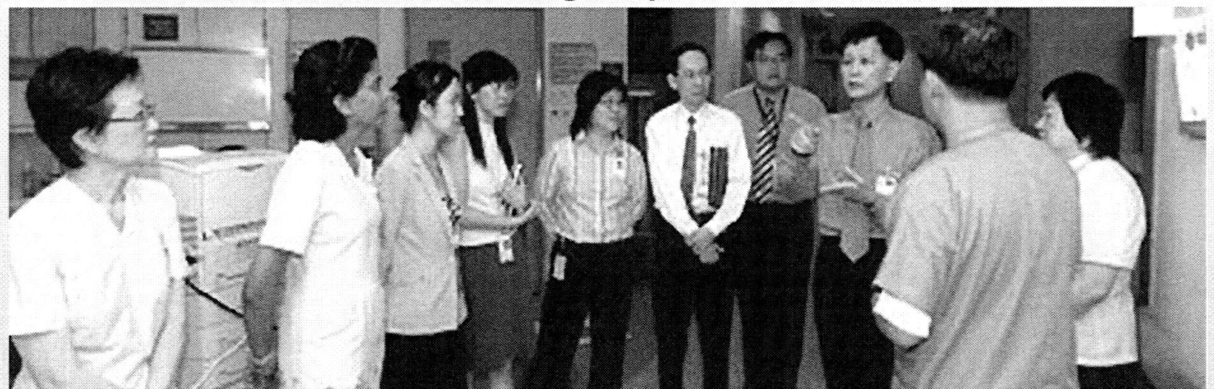

This picture shows a patient safety WalkRound under way at Tan Tock Seng Hospital in Singapore. This WalkRound—also called a "walkabout" within the hospital—is led by Dr. Lim Suet Wun, who is CEO of both National Healthcare Group and Tan Tock Seng Hospital, Singapore, as well as a member of the Joint Commission Resources Board of Directors.

Source: National Healthcare Group, Singapore. Used with permission.

The cost of accreditation can be divided into two separate parts:

1. Direct costs: These include the cost of the survey, surveyors, and other JCI fees.
2. Indirect costs: These include the cost of preparing for accreditation, including implementing new systems, purchasing new technology, hiring new staff, and so forth.

The second of the two costs is nearly impossible to estimate because different organizations enter into the accreditation process with varying levels of performance, risks, and improvement opportunities. Consequently, each organization will require a different combination of resources, and the financial price tag associated with these will vary.

The first of the two costs, however, is a little easier to predict. Although the cost of an accreditation survey depends on the unique characteristics of each health care organization seeking JCI accreditation, organizations can plan on some average costs.

JCI bases an organization's survey fees on several factors, including the volume and type of services provided, the number of surveyors, the survey's length, and the number of locations of care settings included in the survey. JCI works with the organization to determine the most efficient number of surveyors and survey days. The average cost to a hospital for an accreditation survey is US$42,000 for professional fees plus transportation and maintenance of surveyors. This is an "average" and does not correspond to any particular configuration of surveyors. (It is important to note that most hospital survey teams consist of three surveyors.) If a repeat visit is necessary, a single

Case Study 2-1. National Healthcare Group, *continued*

Figure 1. Patient Safety Climate Survey

For Office Use Only ☐☐☐☐

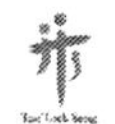

Patient Safety Climate Survey

INSTRUCTIONS

This survey asks for your opinions about patient safety issues, medical error, and event reporting in your hospital and will take about 15 minutes to complete.

- An *"event"* is defined as any type of error, mistake, incident, accident, or deviation, regardless of whether or not it results in patient harm.
- *"Patient safety"* is defined as the avoidance and prevention of patient injuries or adverse events resulting from the processes of health care delivery.

SECTION A: Your Work Area/Unit

In this survey, think of your "unit" as the work area, department, or clinical area of the hospital where you spend _most_ of your work time or provide _most_ of your clinical services.

What is your primary work area or unit in this hospital? Mark ONE answer by filling in

O 1. Many different hospital units/No specific unit

A) Medical
O 1. Division of Ambulatory & Diagnostic Medicine
O 2. Division of Medicine
O 3. Division of Surgery
O 4. NNI

B) Administration
O 1. Associate Dean's Office, Office of Clinical Governance, Clinical training, Clinical Coding
O 2. Snr Mgt Office, Exec Office, Legal Office, Corp Comms & Endowment Fund
O 3. Nursing Service-TTSH,CDC
O 4. HRM, HRD, Wellness
O 5. BO/Finance
O 6. CDC-Admin, HIV-Admin, Rehab-Admin

C) Ops/Support Ops & Services
O 1. Operations, Business Devt, Emergency planning
O 2. BME, Facilities Engineering, Comm. Sect., Estate, F&B, Security, Transport/GSS.

D) Inpatient areas
O 1. CDC-Wd 71,72,75,76/76A, 78, 82,86
O 2. Emergency,Ward 11A-EDTC
O 3. OT (includes Day Surgery, PACU)
O 4. Rehab Ward
O 5. Wards 3A, 3B
O 6. Wards 5A, 5B, 5C, 5D
O 7. Wards 6A, 6B, 6C, 6D
O 8. Wards 7A, 7B, 7C, 7D
O 9. Wards 8A, 8B, 8C, 8D
O 10. Wards 9B, 9C, 9D
O 11. Wards 10A, 10B, 10C, 10D
O 12. Wards 11B, 11C, 11D
O 13. Wards 12B, 12C, 12D
O 14. Wards 13A, 13B
O 15. Endoscopy Centre

E) Outpatient areas
O 1. Clinic 1A, 1B, 2A. 2B, B1A, B1B, Diabetic and Endocrine Clinic, Geriatric Medicine Clinic, PACE
O 2. SOC K, Preventive Services-TBC,TBCU-STEP,CDC Day Treatment Clinic, SOC J
O 3. Rehab Specialist Clinic

F) Clini Ther
O 1. D R T
O 2. Li Ti
O 3. P
O 4. C A
O 5. Ci
O 6. DI Pi O Si N Pi O
O 7. Ni
O 8. C T P

G) Othei
O Othe

1

SECTION A: Your Work Area/Unit (continued)

Please indicate your agreement or disagreement with the following statements about your work area/unit. Mark your answer by filling in the circle.

Think about your hospital work area/unit...	Strongly Disagree	Disagree	Neither	Agree	Strongly Agree	Not Applicable
1. People support one another in this unit	O	O	O	O	O	O
2. We have enough staff to handle the workload	O	O	O	O	O	O
3. When a lot of work needs to be done quickly, we work together as a team to get the work done	O	O	O	O	O	O
4. In this unit, people treat each other with respect	O	O	O	O	O	O
5. Staff in this unit work longer hours than is best for patient care	O	O	O	O	O	O
6. We are actively doing things to improve patient safety	O	O	O	O	O	O
7. We use more agency/temporary staff than is best for patient care	O	O	O	O	O	O
8. Staff feel like their mistakes are held against them	O	O	O	O	O	O
9. Mistakes have led to positive changes here	O	O	O	O	O	O
10. It is just by chance that more serious mistakes don't happen around here	O	O	O	O	O	O
11. When one area in this unit gets really busy, others help out	O	O	O	O	O	O
12. When an event is reported, it feels like the person is being written up, not the problem	O	O	O	O	O	O
13. After we make changes to improve patient safety, we evaluate their effectiveness	O	O	O	O	O	O
14. We work in "crisis mode" trying to do too much, too quickly	O	O	O	O	O	O
15. Patient safety is never sacrificed to get more work done	O	O	O	O	O	O
16. Staff worry that mistakes they make are kept in their personnel file	O	O	O	O	O	O
17. We have patient safety problems in this unit	O	O	O	O	O	O
18. Our procedures and systems are good at preventing errors from happening	O	O	O	O	O	O

SECTION B: Your Supervisor/Manager

Please indicate your agreement or disagreement with the following statements about your immediate supervisor/manager or person to whom you directly report. Mark your answer by filling in the circle.

	Strongly Disagree	Disagree	Neither	Agree	Strongly agree
1. My supervisor/manager says a good word when he/she sees a job done according to established patient safety procedures	O	O	O	O	O
2. My supervisor/manager seriously considers staff suggestions for improving patient safety	O	O	O	O	O
3. Whenever pressure builds up, my supervisor/manager wants us to work faster, even if it means taking shortcuts	O	O	O	O	O
4. My supervisor/manager overlooks patient safety problems that happen over and over	O	O	O	O	O

2

NHG used this survey tool to assess the organization's safety culture and benchmark it against a previously conducted survey. The first two of six survey pages are shown here.

Source: National Healthcare Group, Singapore. Used with permission.

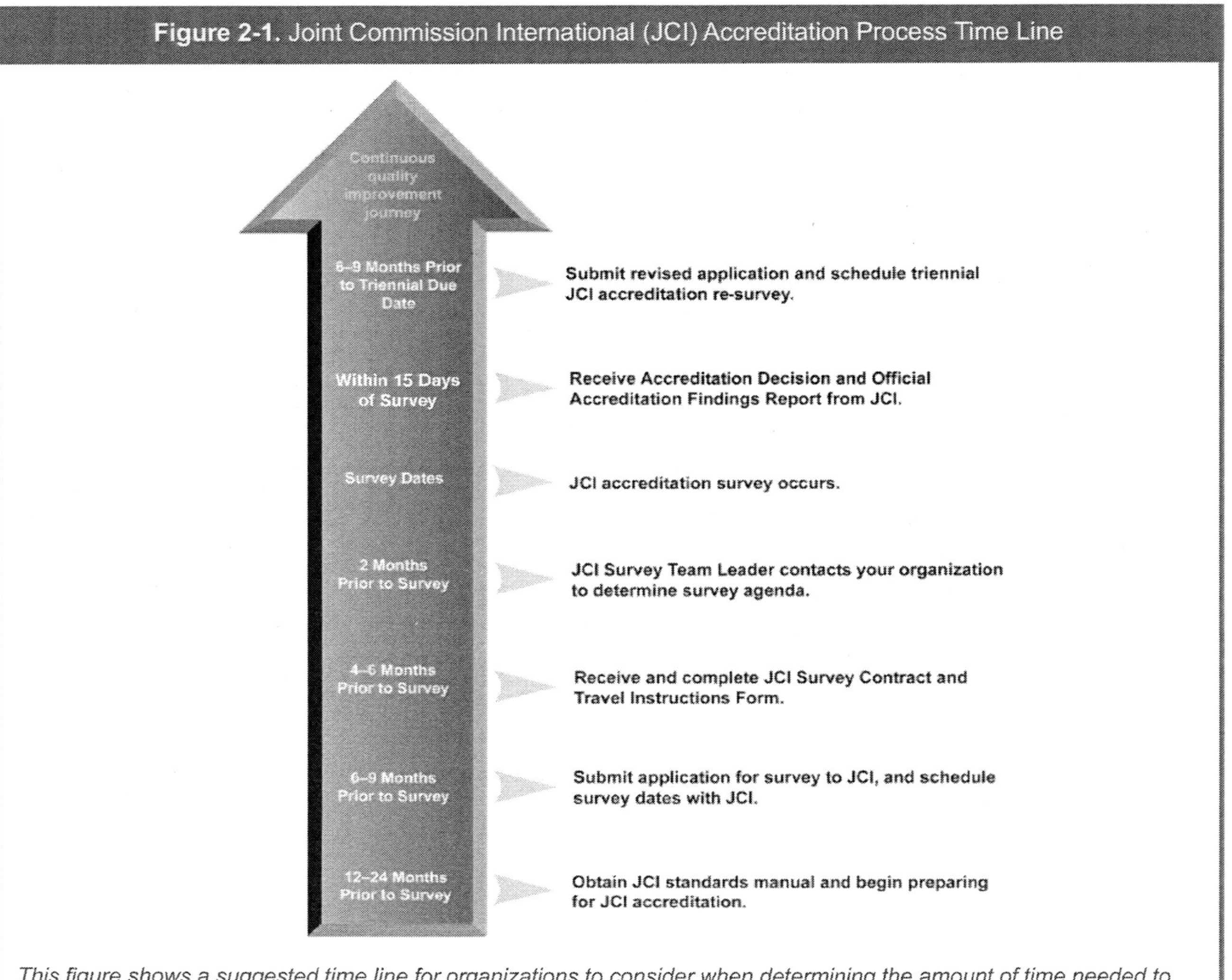

Figure 2-1. Joint Commission International (JCI) Accreditation Process Time Line

This figure shows a suggested time line for organizations to consider when determining the amount of time needed to achieve JCI accreditation.

surveyor will most likely conduct the survey, and the organization will be charged an additional fee. Surveys for other programs are priced similarly to hospitals, but in most instances only one or two surveyors are needed.

In addition to survey fees, the organization is responsible for paying all travel costs for the surveyors. This includes transportation (airfare, train, car), accommodations, meals, and incidental expenses. Maintenance expenses for lodging, transportation, meals, and incidentals will not exceed those allowed in the current JCI travel expense policy. This policy does permit business class travel for surveyors traveling from the United States to destinations in the Middle East, Turkey, India, Africa, Asia, and the Pacific Rim.

To arrive at the total cost, JCI speaks individually with each organization seeking accreditation. This one-on-one conversation provides an opportunity to explore strategies for containing costs. For example, the timing of the on-site survey may play a role in the fee. If surveys are being conducted at other organizations in the same country or region, cost efficiencies may result from travel scheduling.

Depending on the organization, other direct costs may include costs for translators (all JCI surveys are conducted in English), travel and meal costs for translators, survey training costs, outside consultant costs, and so forth.

Additional details on the cost of an accreditation survey may be found on the JCI Web site at http://www.joint commissioninternational.org/Cost-of-Accreditation/.

Capital Improvements

Health care organizations work to provide a safe, functional, and supportive facility for patients, families, staff, and visitors. To reach this goal, the physical facility must be

Allocate Enough Time

We find that when organizations rush through the accreditation preparation process they sometimes defeat the ultimate purpose, which is not only to identify and make changes that improve patient quality and safety but to sustain these changes. Building a team while preparing for accreditation leads to the capacity for self-assessment and sustaining change, which are the ultimate goals. Organizations that embrace these concepts have fewer issues during triennial reaccreditation. Organizations who just want a plaque on their wall have a very difficult time in future surveys, risk patient safety, and fail in the commitment to high-quality care that they made to their physicians and staff at the beginning of the process.

—Ann Jacobson, M.S.N., R.N., N.E.A.,
Executive Director, International
Accreditation, JCI

Old and New Facilities

Many leaders have a great deal of concern about the age of their facility. If it is a new facility, facility managers worry that something was left undone or was done incorrectly in the building process. If the building is older, the concern is that the structure and its systems are unattractive or outdated. From a standards perspective, our objective, regardless of a building's age or condition, is to assess whether an organization can safely support high-quality patient care. Has a risk assessment been done to understand where hazards exist? Is there a documented facility inspection report, and is this document actually used as an ongoing plan to meet facility needs? Having a new facility does not mean exceptional care is being provided. An older facility may not be very attractive but the care can be outstanding.

—Sherry Kaufield, M.A., F.A.C.H.E.,
Executive Director, International Services, JCI

effectively managed. Specifically, leaders must strive to reduce and control hazards and risks, prevent accidents and injuries, and maintain safe conditions. This means there must be adequate space, equipment, and resources to support the clinical services provided safely and effectively.

As part of efforts to achieve accreditation, an organization must consider issues such as facility safety and security, hazardous materials and waste disposal, emergency response, fire safety, medical equipment, and utility systems. Meeting these standards may require some capital investments, and organization leaders should be aware of these needs and plan accordingly. For example, JCI accreditation standards require that potable water and electrical power be available 24 hours a day, seven days a week to meet patient care needs. This may require the purchase of a large-capacity generator or backup system. JCI standards also require specific fire safety measures, such as a plan that includes fire prevention, early detection, suppression, and abatement, as well as methods for safe exit from the facility in response to fires and nonfire emergencies. Such a plan may require, for example, retrofitting, purchasing additional fire safety equipment, or other measures to contain smoke.

Education and Training

As an organization engages in the accreditation process, it is important for leaders to recognize and meet organization needs for immediate and ongoing education. Every member of the health care organization should be aware of what accreditation is, how it will benefit the organization, and what his or her role in the process will be. (*See* Table 2-1 on page 54.) A general knowledge of the accreditation process is essential because all staff members—from executives to frontline nurses to support personnel—play a role in efforts to deliver safe, high-quality care. This means that organizations must "live" the standards by integrating these important principles into daily operations.

When starting educational efforts, organizations should provide education for organizational leaders and managers and then progressively for all staff. The following is a list of topics to include in accreditation education:

■ Introduction to JCI accreditation as a recognized, patient-focused approach to evaluating quality and safety and reducing risk in an organization

Table 2-1. Addressing How JCI Accreditation Will Affect Staff

Activity	What It Is	Impact on You
Preaccreditation assessments	An initial, or baseline, assessment will examine our compliance with JCI standards. A mock survey will be conducted closer to our scheduled accreditation survey to evaluate progress.	You may be involved in the assessments as part of your involvement in one of the following committees *[insert committee names]*. *[Insert name]* will lead the effort to complete your assessments. *[He or She]* will communicate to you additional details about these efforts and how you will be involved.
Action planning	Use of the findings of the baseline assessment and mock survey to develop a detailed project plan with assigned responsibilities, deliverables, and time frames	You may be involved in implementing improvements. For example, *[Insert name]* will lead our efforts to carry out quality improvement actions and will be in contact with all staff members who will contribute to this effort.
On-site survey	Conducted by JCI surveyors, an evaluation of our direct care by evaluating compliance with standards and tracing the paths of patients throughout our organization	JCI surveyors will spend time speaking with staff as part of efforts to look at how care is provided on a daily basis. You may be asked to talk about how you provided care for a particular patient. There are no "trick" questions, and you should not feel like you need to be a JCI accreditation expert. You need to explain only how you did your job.

This table can help staff members understand their level of involvement in various JCI activities. It can be customized to fit each organization's needs. For example, a table could be created for each department to include only those elements that pertain to that department.

- Discussion of accreditation as a an independent audit and validation of an organization's public commitment to continuous quality improvement
- Emphasis on standards compliance as not just a goal to achieve for the on-site survey, but a continuous process that results in sound management practices in the daily delivery of high-quality and safe care
- Review of the standards and measurable elements
- Discussion of the survey process and what to expect
- Project planning and next steps

True learning takes more than one in-service training session and thus accreditation education should happen frequently. Organizations that consistently and continuously educate about accreditation through multiple venues—newsletters, staff meetings, leadership retreats, and so forth—can help ensure that everyone who works in the organization embraces this mind-set and is committed to accreditation. (*See* Sidebar 2-5 on page 55.)

By arranging specific accreditation education and training sessions for managers and staff members, leadership puts the principles and tools in place to perform accreditation preparation work, and shows that accreditation is a priority.

In addition to education about accreditation, education and training are essential to ensuring that staff members possess the knowledge and skills to perform their assigned responsibilities and provide safe, high-quality care. Training of staff has a direct impact on quality and safety of care, with knowledgeable staff making fewer mistakes, responding more quickly to issues, and providing higher-quality care. This should be the case for all organizations, regardless of accreditation, but seeking accreditation adds to expectations.

Leaders addressing resource needs should consider several factors related to training, such as the services provided by staff and the area or department in which staff work. Certain jobs require more expertise to carry out complex responsibilities. For example, staff members who are involved in meeting JCI standards related to assessing patients or managing medications may require more detailed training than an admitting clerk or individual working in laundry services.

Organizations should consider methods that can be employed to teach a specific subject and reteach it in other

Sidebar 2-5. Using a Newsletter to Educate About Accreditation

During preparation for its first JCI survey, Bangkok Hospital Medical Center (BMC) developed its *Join JCI* newsletter as a method to inform and educate staff on proper compliance with JCI requirements.

Developed by physicians, a multidisciplinary care team, and the BMC public relations department, this colorful newsletter featured a different accreditation or quality improvement topic in each issue, including the following:

- Leadership interview—Focusing on the benefits of JCI accreditation, a different member of the leadership team was interviewed. The article discussed the topic of managerial support for staff as BMC attempted to achieve JCI accreditation.

- Unit spotlight—One clinic or unit was the focal point of an article describing leadership and staff's efforts to comply with JCI requirements; this feature also included many pictures of direct care staff.

- Quality corner—Special focus on problem areas, offering solutions for continuous unit preparedness.

- Tips for tracers—Advice for successful completion of a tracer. For example, the following excerpt appeared in one *Join JCI* issue:

  ♦ A Picture Is Worth a Thousand Words—Words alone cannot come close to the added impact of a demonstration, role playing, pointing out documentation, or a storyboard. During practice tracers, the phrase "show me" is frequently repeated. If you are talking about patient education, show the surveyor the handout and point to where you documented the education in the medical record. An excellent example of this was found on the Arabic ward, where the staff have shown the initiative to meet the needs of their culturally diverse target population. A poster showed a picture of each of these unique interventions to help the patients and families feel at home.

- Physician advisor—This column discussed the areas of interest to physicians with examples of correct documentation, new policies, and educational opportunities.

- JCI Web board—An invitation to visit the online JCI Web board on the BMC intranet site, showcasing the new features that had recently been added. Staff were invited to access the JCI Web board to "join" the JCI team formally. The percentage of staff who had joined was publicized.

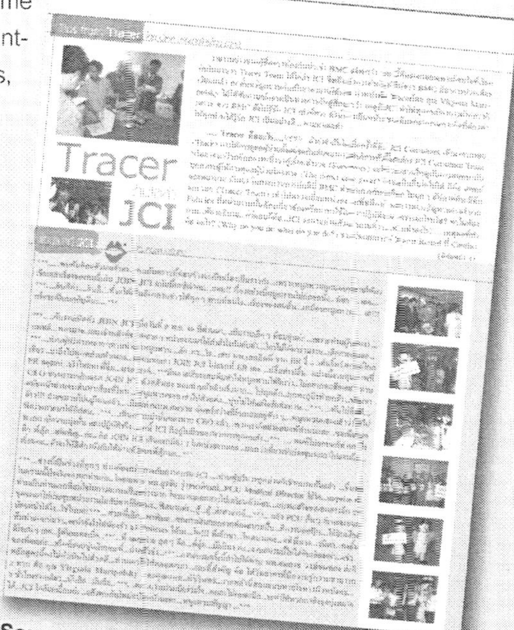

Source: Bangkok Hospital Medical Center. Used with permission

When the first issue of *Join JCI* was published, BMC staged a companywide celebration. Dr. Chatree Duangnet, CEO at BMC, along with members of his management team, personally delivered copies of the newsletter to every clinic, every inpatient unit, and even the cafeteria. (*See* Section 4, page 144, for more information on BMC.)

ways. This approach will provide staff members with opportunities to put what they have learned into action and then come back with questions. This approach also recognizes that education is a slow process that must build and deserves leadership attention. (*See* more on staff training in Section 3.

Technology

Technology has many benefits to a health care organization. It can help users avoid human error and has the potential to enhance communication, ensure complete documentation, and streamline processes. When organizations seek accreditation, technology can help the journey

NOTES FROM THE FIELD

A Survey of Senior Leaders

A recent internal survey conducted by JCI of leaders from JCI–accredited organizations revealed that one of the more common challenges associated with accreditation is overcoming resistance to change among organization leaders and staff members. Staff members who were accustomed to independent practice and decision making needed to be convinced that JCI standards should be formalized as the basis for daily operations. Documentation by all staff, using consistent parameters, also was an unfamiliar concept. Behaviorally, departments often were not accustomed to collaborating with other departments.

To overcome these challenges, leaders emphasized the importance of quality improvement and the role that standardization of care and systems plays in quality. Leaders sought opportunities to talk about the benefits of accreditation at administrative staff meetings, medical grand rounds, nursing forums, and general staff meetings. Leaders reported that this approach allowed the mission and vision of accreditation to become clearer to middle management and filter to the general staff level.

The threat to power bases and tradition was, however, unacceptable for a minority of individuals at the organizations, and leaders reported that they were still working to convince those employees that accreditation is a positive action for the greater good of the organization.

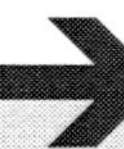

ACCREDITATION STRATEGY

Empowering Staff Understanding

To support accreditation, leaders should communicate with staff about why accreditation is important and how the organization will use accreditation on a daily basis to improve care. Leaders can help their organization obtain the greatest benefit from the accreditation process by explaining to staff why accreditation is being sought, emphasizing that the real value of accreditation is to the patients they serve, and publicly showing enthusiasm and support for quality improvement. This emphasis on building staff understanding and participation will help staff members recognize the contribution of their own work to accreditation activities, providing motivation to embrace leadership's accreditation efforts.

go a little more smoothly by ensuring better patient record management, enhancing professional communications, and allowing for quality data collection and analysis. When preparing for accreditation, organization leaders should carefully assess their organization's current technology and identify areas where adjustment or additions are necessary.

It is important to note that adding more technology will not solve performance improvement issues within a health care organization. In fact, if not used appropriately or if used in an environment that cannot support it, technology can lead to less efficiency, poor communication, decreased morale, safety risks, and, ultimately, patient error. The key to using technology well is to have it enhance safety and quality efforts and have those efforts drive the use of technology—not the other way around. In other words, technology must support an organization's safety and quality goals—not be the goal itself.[15]

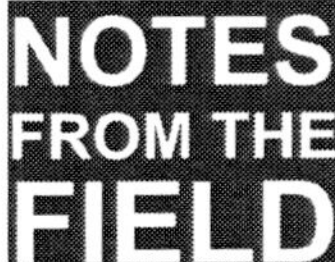

Mater Private Hospital, Dublin

Founded in 1986, Mater Private Hospital in Dublin, Ireland, has been accredited for several years. With 184 inpatient beds and a 9-bed intensive care unit, the organization provides a variety of services to patients.

Ann Higgins, infection control nurse at Mater Private Hospital, advises that feedback is essential in order to have quality improvement programs work effectively. Through feedback staff can see that certain changes produce quality improvement that benefits patient care. "It's very important, especially when you're starting out with an infection control program, that all members of staff are involved and that they realize that, regardless of what role they play in the hospital, their role has an actual impact on infection control. Whether they're a cleaner or a porter or a ward attendant or a nurse or a doctor, they can have an impact on the infection rates in the organization. Therefore, by educating those staff and letting them see that what they do has an impact, it's like having a whole team of infection control people rather than just one person involved, and everybody has ownership for what infection control actually is in the organization."

To improve infection control practices, Higgins works to ensure that staff know her well. "First of all, I meet them at the induction education sessions when they join the hospital, and that's always a good way of people getting to know the face of who infection control actually is in the organization. Then [there are] daily ward rounds throughout the hospital and constantly meeting and talking to people as you go around your work, so that they understand what infection control is and who you are. And then, of course, when you have your education sessions with staff, you can point out specific things that they can do to improve infection control." This close interaction and collaboration with staff has its rewards. "Only yesterday I had a phone call from a member of staff who works in the cleaning department, and she had been asked to clean a patient's bathroom following an MRSA [methicillin-resistant *Staphylococcus aureus*] patient, and found that before she got ready to clean it, another patient had been brought in by a nurse who was unaware that someone had used it immediately before her. She quickly phoned me and said, 'Well, should I stop this person using the bathroom?' And I was able to intervene immediately, before there was any problem."

Additional Staff

Organizations pursuing JCI accreditation may discover that additional staff are necessary to navigate the JCI accreditation process and/or meet JCI standards, which focus on ensuring an appropriate number and variety of skilled, qualified people to meet patient needs. JCI standards do not require that organizations hire a list of staff members (for example, a patient safety officer, quality manager, facility safety director, accreditation compliance officer, and so forth). But, the need for additional staff may become evident during accreditation preparation activities, such as the strategic planning process and baseline standard compliance assessment.

Although not a JCI requirement, many accredited organization have found that creating and staffing a quality manager function is beneficial in navigating the accreditation process. This leadership position is in charge of spearheading the quality improvement work of an organization. He or she continually nurtures and guides quality initiatives throughout the entire organization and enables organizations to have a centralized, consistent emphasis on quality improvement.

Outside Assistance

For organizations seeking accreditation for the first time or for those that have specific issues with which they are struggling, the use of an outside resource—such as a consultant—may be beneficial. Although such a resource is not always necessary, external assistance can be very helpful when designing new systems, processes, procedures, and

SECTION 2

EXPERT ADVICE

Overcoming Barriers

Not every staff member will embrace accreditation right away. Leaders may need to accept and work to overcome certain barriers. For example, many staff members have a fear of the unknown. Some employees think, "I'm all for change as long as *you* change, not me." Then there's the fear of failure, or being uncertain in a job they've felt certain in prior to the change: "If I learn something new, I'm not going to be efficient the first time out. I was efficient before, but now I'm not." The next step is to try to negotiate so that you change, but not that much. Then you get angry that you have to change … then that changes to depression, and then finally you arrive at resolution. Some get through these steps faster than others, some never do. When people get depressed, then leadership questions, "Should we back off?" Or leaders vacillate, and as soon as you do that, the employee goes right back to the old way of doing things. I see this with organizations that purchase new information management systems, and then don't follow through with implementation. Leadership should be quietly happy and supportive that people are going through this uncomfortable journey on the path to change.

—Helen Hoesing, R.N., M.P.H., Ph.D., *JCI Senior Consultant*

forms. Such assistance can also help with staff and leadership education, baseline standards assessments, and mock surveys. (*See* Section 3, pages 112–116, for more information on mock surveys.) Overall, they can help create a strategic approach to continuous compliance and improve organization readiness. (More information on outside resources can be found in Section 3.)

Leadership's Role in the On-Site Survey

In addition to helping organizations prepare for a successful accreditation survey, leaders play an important part in the on-site survey process. JCI surveyors will hold an opening

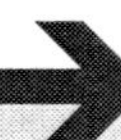

ACCREDITATION STRATEGY

The Language of Accreditation

All JCI accreditation-related communications (written and verbal) are done in English. JCI strongly recommends that the survey coordinator or primary contacts selected by the organization be able to speak and write in English fluently to facilitate and coordinate the accreditation participation process.

NOTES FROM THE FIELD

A Survey of Senior Leaders

In a recent internal survey by JCI, organization leaders from accredited organizations indicated that considerable resources, particularly in staff time, were dedicated to achieving accreditation. Information technology infrastructures also required additional resources to provide for data management and medical record capabilities that support quality improvement. Leaders interviewed assumed that their organizations had benefited from increased efficiencies by streamlining policies and procedures, but no quantitative analyses had been conducted.

conference with the chief executive officer and gather documentation needed, and then conduct a leadership interview later in the survey. An in-depth discussion of the different aspects of the on-site survey appears in Section 3, but the following paragraphs introduce the portions of the survey process in which leaders are directly involved.

Opening Conference

The purposes of the opening conference are to introduce surveyors and senior leadership of the organization to one another and to review and make any last-minute changes to the survey agenda.

Typically, the chief executive officer of an organization participates in this conference, along with the individual responsible for coordinating the organization's survey activities. Other individuals may be present at the discretion of the organization.

During the opening conference, surveyors will answer questions about the survey agenda, explain the scoring of compliance to the standards, and discuss pertinent decision rules having to do with the submission of the preliminary report to the JCI Accreditation Committee.

To facilitate the opening conference, organization leaders should have copies of the survey agenda available for all participants in the meeting. Prior to the survey, leaders should decide which member of the leadership team or staff member will accompany each surveyor throughout each survey day.

Leadership Interview

The leadership interview is an interview session conducted by the surveyors to assess communication among senior leaders of the organization and how they address organizational performance issues. Depending on the organization, different individuals will be present during this meeting. Participants typically include the following:

- Chief executive officer
- Chief financial officer
- Chief operating officer, when applicable
- Chairman of the governing body or similar representative
- Elected or appointed leader of the medical staff
- Nurse executive
- Quality improvement coordinator
- Other senior leaders, at the discretion of the organization

While the organization designates which senior leaders should be present, it is important to keep in mind that too large a group may impede an interactive process, and is thus not recommended for this interview.

During the leadership interview, collaborative involvement of the senior leaders of the organization in governing, managing, and directing the organization will be evaluated. The surveyors will all ask questions related to leadership activities and the decisions the leadership has made. They will also identify topics they wish to pursue later during the survey. Everyone present should participate in answering

the questions. Topics covered in the leadership interview may include, but will not be limited to, the following:

- Patient care, treatment, and services
- Leadership structure and decision making
- Quality improvement
- Patient rights
- Patient and family education

Participation in the Leadership Interview

The leadership interview is basically an opportunity for leaders to show they have planned for and thoroughly understand what is going on in their facility. The way leaders handle themselves will show whether they communicate well with one another and with all levels of staff in a way that gives them an understanding of the care they deliver and the environment in which they provide it. Their answers will show how leaders plan services and prioritize the resources needed. We hope to see wide participation during this interview from leaders who are clearly comfortable with one another and the work they do together.

—Marlis Daerr, R.N., Surveyor, JCI

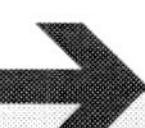

ACCREDITATION STRATEGY

Avoid Hovering During Survey

Organization leaders can help their staff feel more comfortable during an on-site survey by providing employees with a bit of space during their interactions with surveyors. A team of leadership observers standing elbow to elbow nearby can be unsettling. Leaders may want to stand off to the side, giving staff and the surveyor a chance to have a one-on-one conversation. It's important for leaders to trust their frontline staff to tell the JCI surveyor what he or she needs to know.

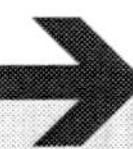

ACCREDITATION STRATEGY

Pitfalls to Avoid

Although no accreditation process goes perfectly smoothly, there are some fairly common pitfalls that leaders should try to avoid:

→ Leaders giving "lip service" to accreditation, but not providing the time and resources necessary to be successful

→ Having unrealistic expectations of how long it will take to achieve accreditation (a realistic goal being 12 to 24 months)

→ Burdening staff with "extra" accreditation work for which they are neither rewarded nor recognized

→ Making accreditation a punitive process instead of a motivating process to improve care

- Staff qualifications and education
- Information management
- Infection control

Although no documents are required to be available during the leadership interview, JCI surveyors will review documents, such as the organization chart, mission statement, budget and resource allocation, strategic planning documents, information management plan, quality management plan, and worksheet of applicable laws and regulations, as preparation for this discussion.

To help participants in the leadership interview prepare for the process, organizations may want set up mock interviews with participants. This allows leaders to feel comfortable with and think about how they will answer possible questions from surveyors. One way to frame these mock interviews is to turn the standards into questions and ask participants to answer those questions. Sample questions may include the following:

- Describe how clinical leaders in your organization collaborate to create the plans and policies needed to fulfill the organization's mission.
- Can you explain the process you, as leaders, use to approve the policies and plans used to operate your organization?
- Provide an example of how the quality and safety of clinical care provided by each staff member is evaluated.
- Describe how the organization's staffing plan is developed. How is the plan evaluated to ensure the provision of safe patient care?
- How does the organization identify the procedures and processes associated with the risk of infections?

Leadership Exit Conference

At the conclusion of the survey, the organization CEO and other senior leaders will meet with surveyors to discuss the outcome of the on-site survey, discuss any concerns with the survey, and resolve any issues of interpretation that may have been identified during the survey. At this time, surveyors will present the organization with an exit report that contains preliminary findings from the survey. Surveyors may also use this time to provide some education to organization leaders to help them in responding to negative survey outcomes.

Leaders should take this opportunity to ask surveyors any questions they may have and work collaboratively with surveyors to gather information about resolving deficiencies.

After surveyors leave the premises, organization leaders, along with quality/accreditation specialists, will want to review the exit report and examine areas for improvement. The quality/accreditation specialist at most organizations will then lead the effort in establishing Strategic Improvement Plans (SIPs) to make any required improvements. (*See* Section 3, pages 121–126, for more information on SIPs.)

Effectively leading an organization through accreditation is not a commitment to be taken lightly. All aspects of a leader's effort, including making the decision to seek accreditation, laying the groundwork for quality improvement, allocating the resources, and being involved in all aspects of the process, including the on-site survey, is a significant commitment. Management by leaders is important to keep the compliance process on track and true to its initial vision. Such oversight and participation can help smooth out problems and ensure that the process stays on course.

Case Study 2-2. OCA Hospital

Organization Name: OCA Hospital
Location: Monterrey, Mexico
Year accredited: 2008
About OCA Hospital: OCA Hospital, with 290 beds, is Monterrey, Mexico's largest private hospital. Its specialties include cardiology, surgery, emergency care, endoscopy, hemodialysis, maternity and obstetrics, oncology, and bariatric surgery.

The Decision to Pursue JCI Accreditation

Quality and safety have always been at the core of OCA Hospital's values, according to CEO Dan Levinson. "We achieved International Organization for Standardization (ISO) 9001 certification in 2003 and won the State Quality Award (a Mexican award based on the Malcolm Baldrige model) in 2007," Levinson says. "We decided that the next step in the ladder would be to seek accreditation by a health care–specific organization with health care–specific standards." OCA contacted JCI and started the planning and implementation in November of 2007.

Although the JCI accreditation process was new to OCA, the organization had a long track record of experience documenting, standardizing, and improving processes, as evidenced by its ISO 9001 certification and State Quality Award. As a result, the organization was able to easily understand the JCI requirements.

OCA's first challenge was to make the accreditation a common goal across the organization. OCA management presented its proposal to pursue JCI accreditation to its board for approval in a quarterly meeting. Following the board's consent, OCA presented the decision to pursue accreditation to the rest of the hospital through dedicated meetings in which the leadership team explained the importance of this project. "We believed that this had to be communicated in person by the hospital's leaders to create the kind of commitment and resolve we needed for this project," Levinson says.

"Fortunately, and thanks to the great management team in this hospital, this goal [accreditation] was quickly reached," Levinson said. "The way the whole staff—nurses, physicians, technicians, and so forth—aligned and worked together with the purpose of providing better care to our patients was inspiring. Considering our time frame for achieving accreditation was just one year [JCI recommends organizations budget for 13 to 24 months of preparation before an initial on-site survey], our staff did excellent work, and throughout this process our patient safety culture became even stronger."

Beginning the Pursuit of Accreditation

OCA had a quality department before starting the JCI accreditation process, but Levinson says preparation for JCI accreditation improved OCA's quality department by helping it set the following objectives and responsibilities:

- Improve the quality of patient care by identifying opportunities for improvement through assessment and evaluation of the functions, processes, and outcomes affecting patient care.
- Establish goals for organizational performance improvement, including, for example, response times.
- Establish the roles of the clinical and nonclinical staff, other personnel, team leaders, and committees.
- Define and reduce variation in clinical and business processes by developing standards of service that are clear, realistic, measurable, and responsive.
- Reduce malpractice and general liability claims by establishing operational linkages and sharing information as appropriate between departments.
- Increase organizationwide involvement in the performance improvement program by establishing multidisciplinary performance improvement teams, as appropriate, to assess and improve performance.
- Define the integration of care services by requiring each department to identify its scope of service; which services it provides, to whom,

(continued on page 62)

Case Study 2-2.　OCA Hospital, *continued*

and how; and how others interact with the department in providing the service.

- ⮑ Evaluate the expectation achievements of patients and their families, hospital personnel, and physicians through interviews, surveys, and other informal communication methods.
- ⮑ Evaluate the quality of services provided through internal indicators.

Improvement Projects

OCA made the following significant quality and safety improvements en route to their 2008 accreditation:

Decreasing Its Health Care–Associated Infection Rate

Although Levinson describes OCA's preaccreditation health care–associated infection (HAI) rate as "low compared to international standards," he and OCA leaders and staff set out to bring the rate of infection even lower. OCA developed a cross-functional project that combined the efforts of the departments involved with the care of patients in the hospital's intensive care units (ICUs). This project's conception came as a result of working with JCI and was put together with a very holistic approach, trying to incorporate teamwork and patient safety as much as possible into the project's activities with the undisclosed intention of injecting these cultural values into the group. The project started with specific goals and activities and ended up creating new ways of communicating and collaborating for the people and the departments involved.

OCA's key strategies for this project included the following:

- ⮑ Forming a multidisciplinary task force for the project, including members from all key areas involved with patient care in the ICUs
- ⮑ Revamping infection prevention and control policies via a thorough analysis of the existing policies and procedures and the creation and implementation of additional ones, as deemed necessary by the task force
- ⮑ Improvement of OCA's quality assurance program, which is based on systematic internal audits

- ⮑ Addition of more negative and positive pressure rooms to both the neonatal and adult ICUs, and the subsequent training for personnel in the correct usage of both ICUs
- ⮑ A better integration between the areas involved with patient care in the ICU, including, but not limited to, the infection control department, ICU staff, and cleaning services

"The overall hospital infection rate was already low before we started this project, and we still were able to bring it down some more, from 1.6% to 0.70%," Levinson reports. "This is considerably lower than the average of 2% that some of the best hospitals in the world have, and our ventilator-associated pneumonia rate is comparable to the U.S. top 10% hospitals using the information from the Centers for Disease Control and Prevention."

Preventing Multidrug-Resistant Microorganisms

Another important project that OCA developed concerned ensuring the correct use of antibiotics in the ICUs to prevent the creation of multidrug-resistant microorganisms. OCA developed and implemented its guidelines after gathering antibiogram data from each unit for an entire year and consulting the Pan American Health Organization guidelines on the proper prescription of antibiotics. "We have achieved tremendous results in this area, with a majority of our physicians prescribing first- or second-generation antibiotics each time when possible," Levinson says.

Clinical Pathway on Myocardial Infarction

OCA's third major performance improvement project was the implementation of a clinical pathway on myocardial infarction. The main objectives of this project were the following:

- ⮑ Reducing door-to-drug and door-to-balloon times
- ⮑ Increasing the administration of aspirin within 15 minutes of arrival in the emergency department (ED)
- ⮑ Increasing the use of beta-blockers during the hospital stay
- ⮑ Increasing the use of nonfractionated heparin in the ED (when no contraindications are given)

Case Study 2-2. OCA Hospital, *continued*

⮕ Increasing the percentage of electrocardio-
grams (EKGs) within 10 minutes of arrival

⮕ Decreasing the overall mortality rate and average length of stay

Just as with the HAI project, a multidisciplinary
task force was created. After implementation, OCA
reports successful results, including the following:

⮕ The administration of aspirin and the conducting of EKGs are each occurring with 100%
compliance.

⮕ Door-to-balloon time has also been reduced by
approximately 50%.

⮕ There have been substantial improvements with
the other indicators.

The Role of Staffing

OCA was able to complete its JCI accreditation
journey using mostly existing staff. "We had to
reinforce some departments, and therefore some
hiring was required, but nothing major was
required," Levinson says. "We mainly worked with
the current staff at the time and focused on training them in accordance with the standards and
requirements of the JCI accreditation."

Staff participation has been the leading force in
this change, says Levinson. "We have seen an
increase in staff participation throughout our different committees, as well as in medical and nursing
events," Levinson says. "We feel very proud about
the people in our organization and about how they
made this accreditation possible. We believe in
their commitment to stay on this path."

Going Forward

Levinson believes JCI accreditation, and the quality improvements OCA made on its path to accreditation, has helped the organization in a number of
ways above and beyond the paper certificate it
received when it was accredited in 2008. "OCA
Hospital owes its good reputation within our community to a constant commitment throughout the
years to deliver health care services with the
highest-quality standards," Levinson says. "JCI
accreditation has come to enrich our operation
with a more patient- and safety-focused culture
that has translated into more integrated services.
Patients, doctors, and health care providers are
working together as true teams focused on providing optimal patient care."

Case Study 2-3. National Heart Centre Singapore

Organization Name: National Heart Centre Singapore
Location: The Republic of Singapore
Years accredited: 2005, 2008
About National Heart Centre Singapore: National Heart Centre Singapore is a 185-bed national and regional referral center for cardiovascular medicine.

The Decision to Pursue Accreditation

Although the National Heart Centre Singapore (NHCS) was one of the most reputable tertiary referral centers in Southeast Asia, the senior management of the hospital decided to pursue JCI accreditation because they wanted to further strengthen the organization's position and ensure compliance with a set of established health care quality standards. Organization leaders were confident that compliance with the JCI standards would help the organization do the following:

- Improve patient care processes and outcomes
- Ensure a safe environment and continually work to reduce risks to patients and staff
- Reinforce its commitment to quality care for patients

Informing Staff and Leadership

As a first step in its accreditation journey NHCS communicated to its leadership group the senior management decision to pursue JCI accreditation, focusing on the rationale and benefits for doing so. "We have a management committee, the members of which include the senior executives of the hospital and the clinical department heads," says Tan Teing Ee, M.D., senior consultant for cardiothoracic surgery at NHCS. "After the senior management decided to pursue JCI accreditation, we discussed the decision at the management committee so that all members understood the benefits and challenges we faced."

After receiving the support of senior leadership, the organization focused on communicating with staff about the importance of accreditation. Ways in which the organization engaged in this communication include the following:

- Made use of its staff communication session—a regular communication session between the senior management and the representatives of staff from different departments—to inform the staff of the decision to pursue JCI accreditation

- Sent e-mail and memoranda to all staff
- Took actions to ensure that staff understood the benefits and challenges of pursuing JCI accreditation (department heads)
- Featured the topic of JCI accreditation in the hospital quality newsletter (*see* Figure 1 on page 65)
- Conducted slide presentations for various groups of staff
- Developed pocket-sized booklets on JCI accreditation and gave one to each member of the staff
- Created a hospital intranet Web site specifically for providing information and education on JCI accreditation.
- Printed and distributed pamphlets on the different JCI standards chapters.

Beginning Pursuit

Before embarking on their accreditation journey, members of the organization visited other accredited hospitals and invited them to share their experiences. "We also formed a JCI steering committee to take charge of our accreditation journey and working teams to take responsibility for the various areas," says Dr. Tan. "We provided the steering committee, working teams, and other key organization staff with training and education on JCI accreditation, including training sessions conducted by JCI."

Prior to embarking on its accreditation efforts, NHCS already had two different quality departments, responsible for clinical quality and service quality, respectively. "During our initial preparation for JCI accreditation in 2005, we appointed the manager of one of these departments to be the chief accreditation coordinator. He was in charge of overall survey preparation coordination," says Dr. Tan. "We also expanded the staff in these two departments so we could more effectively manage

Case Study 2-3. National Heart Centre Singapore, *continued*

Figure 1. NHCS Quality Newsletter

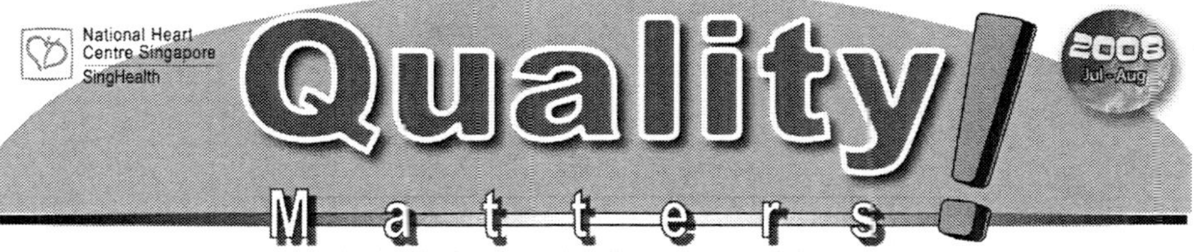

NHC JCI RE-ACCREDITATION EXPERIENCE

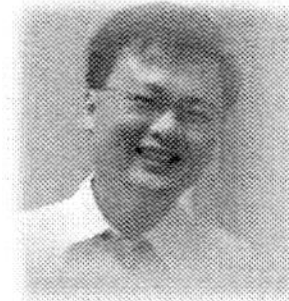

Dr Tan Teing Ee
Chairman, JCI Steering
Committee

Joint Committee International (JCI) sets uniform and high standards for patient care and safety. The JCI standards focus on the areas that most directly impact patient care, such as access to care, assessment of patient, infection control, patient and family rights and education. JCI standards also address facility management and safety, staff qualifications, quality improvement, organisational leadership, and information management.

NHC first received the JCI accreditation in 2005. From 21 to 23 July 2008, 3 JCI surveyors conducted the re-accreditation survey at NHC. Unlike the initial survey that required 4 months of track records, the re-accreditation survey required track records of 12 months. With the new standards and tracer methodology, the re-accreditation survey became more challenging. However, NHC achieved excellent results with high compliance rate.

Our success in achieving the excellent survey results would not have been possible without the concerted efforts of all NHC staff. We would like to take this opportunity to thank all staff for their hard work and commitment.

During the re-accreditation survey, the surveyors were impressed by our high standards of patient care and safe environment. However, they also pointed out some gaps in patient care, medication management, information management and facility management, such as inconsistency in care provided to patients, lack of comprehensive review of the medication management system, medication storage areas that need to be improved, insufficient documentation or illegible handwriting in medical records, fire safety plan not fully implemented in the Outram Campus, etc. We will bridge these gaps to further improve our quality of care.

On a personal note, it has been a great learning journey for me. I have seen places I have never seen and interviewed people I have never spoken to before JCI. It has been a pleasure working with many people who are supportive and also believe in quality care for our patients.

It has opened my eyes to see many things from a different perspective. When some medical staff (especially a junior one) makes a mistake, I now always question if he/she was given adequate training/briefing/orientation, if he/she was overworked/stressed, and if the system/processes/equipment under which we work can be changed to minimise these errors.

Any system that demands perfect performance from all the people involved will fail. Humans make mistakes, some more than others. We often cannot change people a lot, but we can definitely change the environment under which he/she works to minimise the errors that he/she makes. Examples of things we have done include the removal of concentrated KCl from the wards, or checking both name and NRIC just before taking blood.

Do you see something in the way we work that can be improved for the safety of our patients? Be bold - bring it up to the staff suggestion scheme, your supervisor or HOD. Make a difference.

Editors :
QM Workgroup

Layout :
Haja Mydin

Have something to share on quality improvement?
Email your articles/ comments to :
vasantha_gopal@nhc.com.sg
or
nurina.md.khamis@nhc.com.sg

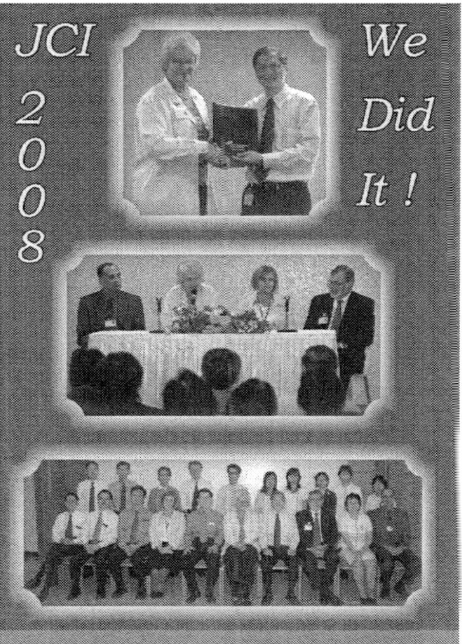

This figure shows an example of one of NHCS's quality newsletters and illustrates how it could be used to communicate about accreditation.

Source: National Heart Centre Singapore. Used with permission.

(continued on page 66)

Case Study 2-3. National Heart Centre Singapore, *continued*

the increased workload of quality improvement activities."

When seeking reaccreditation, the senior management of the organization recognized the need and benefits of long-term commitment to the accreditation process and thus formed an accreditation department in 2007. "This department is in charge of overall coordination for JCI accreditation and related matters, while the quality department focuses on quality issues and serves as the champion for the QPS ["Quality Improvement and Patient Safety"] chapter, one of the chapters of the JCI standards," says Dr. Tan.

Benefits to the Process

Since starting its accreditation journey, NHCS has seen many benefits. The following are some examples of the positive impacts on the organization:

- More emphasis is placed on the quality of care for patients.
- Patients' and families' rights are given higher priority and respect.
- Leadership and governance has been strengthened.
- A systematic approach in assessing the clinical quality/performance of individual medical specialists has been implemented.
- Storage and labeling of medications has been improved, resulting in decreased medication errors.
- A safer environment and established protocols have led to reduction in harm to patients, such as falls.
- Standardized processes of verifying patients' identities have contributed to lower risk of performing procedures on or serving medications to the wrong patients.
- Improved communications skills and enhanced patient education has increased patient satisfaction.

One specific area that has improved as a result of quality improvement work and accreditation is the organization's door-to-balloon (DTB) time for acute myocardial infarction (AMI) patients. This is the time interval between the time the patient presents to the emergency department (ED) and the time the first balloon catheter is inflated to reopen the occluded artery in the cardiac vascular laboratory (CVL). Studies have shown that the shorter the DTB time, the better the prognosis for patients with AMI, as more myocardium can be salvaged. The recommended DTB time for AMI by the American College of Cardiology and the American Heart Association is 90 minutes or less.

Through the past years, NHCS has successfully implemented several measures to reduce DTB time. The organization's latest measure expedites the transfer of AMI patients from the ED to the CVL. This is done through a new position on the primary angioplasty team—the nurse officer on night duty. Although this new position has only recently been implemented, it has shown very good results in terms of reduction in DTB time. Preliminary results show a median DTB time of 59 minutes, with 82% of the acute patients receiving the therapy within 90 minutes.

Overcoming Challenges

"One of the challenges we faced in preparing for accreditation was overcoming some staff members' resistance to the new quality standards and practices," says Dr. Tan. "Involvement of the senior management was the key to overcoming this problem. Senior leaders must support the implementation of new processes by approving the proposals and providing the material support, such as budget and manpower." With that said, the organization found that some of the departments, such as the nursing department, were particularly supportive of quality improvement initiatives. Not only did they implement many changes, they also formed teams that conducted internal audits to ensure that the changes were carried out.

NHCS also had difficulty clearly understanding some of the JCI standards/requirements. "We had many meetings at which we debated the interpretation of the requirements, attended training courses provided by JCI, consulted JCI via e-mail, and also discussed our problems with colleagues from other hospitals that had completed their JCI survey," says Dr. Tan.

Case Study 2-3. National Heart Centre Singapore, *continued*

Advice for Other Organizations

According to Dr. Tan, JCI accreditation requires some getting used to. "It seems to be very daunting at first but you will realize that once you get used to the good practice, it becomes your habit and you will do it naturally. As a result, both the patients and staff/hospital will benefit from such good practice."

Dr. Tan also recommends consulting with JCI staff on areas of confusion and keeping in touch with colleagues in other hospitals that have already been accredited by JCI. "These groups may share very useful tips and information with you, and seeking out their counsel can be quite beneficial."

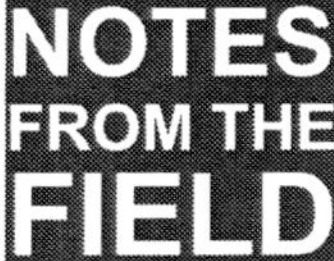

An Accreditation Journey—One Hospital Executive's Story

by John Wocher

John Wocher, executive vice president for administration at Kameda Medical Center in Kamogawa, Chiba Prefecture, Japan—the first-ever accredited hospital in Japan—is a champion of accreditation and a force for quality improvement and patient safety. In this narrative, he shares his memories of his and Kameda's journey to JCI accreditation.

Ten years ago in *The Journal of the Japan Hospital Association* (No. 18, July 1999), I authored an article titled "Hospital Accreditation in Japan—Long Overdue?" In that article, I lamented the slow progress in Japan in establishing an effective third-party, independent evaluation of hospitals. Although some activity was under way, change was slow. Fledgling efforts to promote effective evaluations had begun in 1985 when the work of the group known as the Tokyo JCAHO Research Group led to the formation of the Japan Hospital Quality Assurance Society (JHQAS) in 1990. Prior to this, hospitals completed a self-assessment using a Ministry of Health and Welfare checklist, which to me seemed very subjective. My hospital, the Kameda Medical Center, was among the approximately 60 initial JHQAS member hospitals in 1990 that desired evaluation by an external entity.

In 1995 the Ministry of Health and Welfare joined with the Japan Hospital Association and the Japan Medical Association to form the Japan Council for Quality Health Care (JCQHC). The JCQHC is the only authorized accrediting body for hospitals in Japan, and in 1999 when I wrote my article, a total of 136 hospitals had undergone accreditation, including Kameda Medical Center.

By May of 2005, just 16% of all hospitals in Japan were accredited by JCQHC. As of this writing in 2010, the JCQHC Web site reports that a total of 2,556 of 8,766 Japanese hospitals have been accredited, which, despite being an improvement, still means that fewer than 30% of Japanese hospitals are accredited.

There are many possible reasons for the increase in the percentage of accredited hospitals. For example, the introduction of Diagnosis Procedure Combinations (a Diagnosis Related Groups [DRGs] hybrid) reimbursement in 2003 for highly advanced treatment hospitals—which ties reimbursement to length of stays—

(continued on page 68)

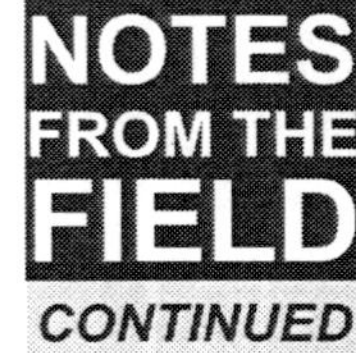

may have motivated the better hospitals to undergo accreditation. The percentage of accredited hospitals is also higher today because there are fewer hospitals in Japan now than in 2005.

Despite the lackluster percentage of accredited hospitals in Japan, much progress has been made in the areas of quality improvement over the decade since my article was published. For example, there are many evidence-based tools to evaluate quality. Some hospitals in Japan have taken additional steps to improve the quality and safety of the care delivered. Kameda Medical Center, among others, has embraced International Standards Organization (ISO) certification, specifically ISO 9001. Other certifications achieved at my hospital include United Kingdom Accreditation Services, British Standards Institute, Japan Accrediting Board, and Privacy Mark. We feel a strong moral and ethical obligation to obtain the highest standards possible, above and beyond the minimal requirements.

Kameda's JCI Journey: A 14-Year Odyssey

Kameda's accreditation journey began in 1995. Kameda Clinic, a freestanding outpatient facility, was built and opened that year, and Kameda General Hospital, a 925-bed acute care facility (which opened in 2005), was already in the planning stages. We felt we had a very sophisticated electronic medical record system established, and I felt the timing was right for us to consider attempting accreditation of our Kameda Clinic against The Joint Commission's U.S. ambulatory care standards. (At this time, JCI had not yet been formed; JCI's first accreditation survey did not occur until 1999.)

To that end, I hired a summer intern in 1996 from the University of Iowa's Graduate Program in Healthcare Administration, and that student was given the task of evaluating and predicting whether or not our clinic could successfully pass a Joint Commission survey. We arranged for the student to attend a one-week Joint Commission orientation at its headquarters near Chicago, Illinois, USA. For three months at Kameda, the student assessed our Joint Commission compliance, and when she found shortfalls she made recommendations on how to close compliance gaps. In short, the student concluded that with significant additional efforts to document the structure, processes, and outcomes at the Kameda Clinic, it could achieve Joint Commission accreditation.

Unfortunately, The Joint Commission would not accredit Kameda or any non-U.S. organization at that time, other than U.S. military health care organizations outside the United States. In 1999 Joint Commission International (JCI) was formed, and it issued its first set of international hospital standards. We reviewed those standards and concluded that we could prepare and successfully become accredited. We decided to wait for completion of the new Kameda inpatient building known as K-Tower and then have the entire Kameda complex surveyed by JCI at the same time. K-Tower was completed in 2004 and opened in 2005. In May 2007 Kameda committed to a two-year preparation plan for JCI accreditation.

The Reasons Behind the Decision

Kameda was the first hospital to pursue JCI accreditation in Japan. I had long felt that Kameda needed to grow internationally in stature and become more globally focused if it was to become a world-class medical institution. Also, my informal feedback from non-Japanese friends and colleagues living and/or working in

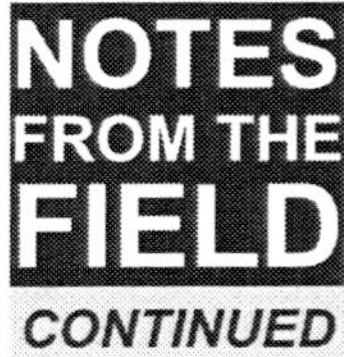

Japan was that they were generally dissatisfied with health care encounters in Japan and tended to return to their home country at any sign of what might be a serious medical condition.

Another contributing factor in our decision was the global trend, particularly in Asia, to achieve JCI accreditation. Virtually all government and private hospitals in Singapore are now JCI accredited.

Severance Hospital in Seoul was joined by Korea University Anam Hospital in July 2009. Clifford Hospital in China was first accredited by JCI in 2003 and reaccredited in 2006. A total of five Chinese hospitals are now accredited. Three hospitals in Malaysia are accredited, as well as two in the Philippines, six in Taiwan, and seven in Thailand. With the very best hospitals in Asia seeking and obtaining JCI accreditation, I felt that the great hospitals in Japan were (and still are) missing the opportunity to be recognized along with these prestigious health care institutions. While they grew in international esteem, Kameda and other Japanese hospitals were seen as remaining domestically and inwardly focused.

Kameda's decision to become JCI accredited was also motivated by a desire to improve on an existing culture of safety and quality. We wanted to instill confidence and trust in the community we serve—patients, their families, our visitors, and our staff—and convey to them in word and deed that our priority is their safety through the quality of our care. By pursuing a higher standard of JCI accreditation, we feel we demonstrate to patients and their loved ones that Kameda cares, it respects their rights and privacy, and it desires to be in partnership with them in their health care decisions. For our staff, we wanted to provide a safe working environment and, in doing so, improve employee satisfaction. And last, but not least, we wanted to improve our corporate culture by showing it is open to learning from things that don't go as planned and is fully supportive of the internal reporting of adverse events so that we can improve and prevent recurrence.

Getting Started

The first year of preparation consisted mostly of discussion between Kameda leadership and JCI regarding costs, timing, and logistical and technical questions. The cost to undergo accreditation was significant. There are both direct and indirect costs associated with major decisions, and both need careful consideration. The direct costs are precise, but indirect costs are often underestimated—they can get lost in the general overhead of doing business or get underestimated in order for them to appear more reasonable.

The direct costs of JCI accreditation had several components, including a set fee based on organization size and complexity of services, regarding which JCI based its number of surveyors and the number of days required to survey the organization. In our case, with 965 operating beds and approximately 3,000 outpatient visits per day, it was determined that we would require three surveyors and a five-day survey.

Direct costs not included in the previously mentioned set fee included

- transportation, accommodations, and tuition for two Kameda staff to attend a JCI Practicum in Bangkok;
- observation of a mock survey at Severance Hospital in Seoul four senior staff, including me;
- two mock surveys of Kameda Medical Center by experts outside of our organization; and
- translators for the on-site JCI survey (the survey is always conducted in English, regardless of the nationality). Kameda used four outside interpreters each day, and costs included interpreters' fees, transportation, accommodations, and some meals.

(continued on page 70)

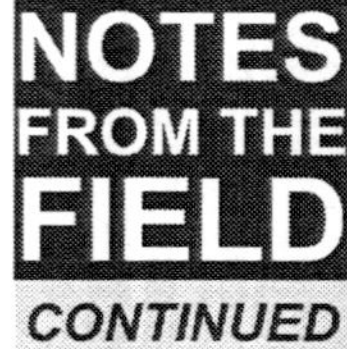

In the absence of precise methodology, there is simply no way to measure indirect costs, given no historical precedent at our medical center. Budgeted projects for cosmetic improvements initially unrelated to JCI accreditation were moved up in the scheduling process, and because the JCI survey came within a month of our JCQHC survey, it is impossible to determine the cost of each separately.

No new employees were hired to support JCI accreditation, so employee costs were fixed over the preparation period.

The Kameda JCI "team" consisted of a senior physician, a senior nurse, a project coordinator, five assistant coordinators, the University of Iowa graduate student mentioned earlier, and me. We worked mainly on the JCI survey preparation for the three months leading up to and including the actual survey. With the exception of the project coordinator, none of us worked on accreditation full time, but as the date of the survey grew closer, our time requirements grew proportionally.

Staff Buy-In

Staff awareness and education are essential components in changing corporate culture. With JCI accreditation requiring virtually all staff in the medical center to be aware of what needed to be done and the reasons for it, this became a major effort. Translation of the JCI standards—1,030 measurable elements in the 349 standards—into Japanese was done by members of the JCI team and not contracted out. After this was accomplished, every department in the medical center was provided a copy of the requirements that were specific to its areas of responsibility. Members of the team responsible for the medical staff, nursing staff, ancillary staff, and administration visited each department on numerous occasions to systematically explain and clarify the requirements.

The most important issues we dealt with pertained to how we provide documentation regarding compliance. All of Kameda's policies and procedures manuals were reviewed for accuracy. In many cases, there was ample indication of things being done properly, but documentation was poor or absent. In other cases, new policies and procedures were created to become compliant with the requirements. JCI requires at least four months of documented compliance prior to an initial survey date in order to meet the standards, another reason why early preparation was so important.

It was essential that staff understood and agreed with the spirit and intent of the standards, and with few exceptions they did. This effort by all staff to improve the documentation of the work they did was a great opportunity to improve the quality and safety of the care provided and created new opportunities to implement new policies and procedures that would further benefit patients. Were all staff enthusiastic? No. In any large organization, there are employees who, for various reasons, do not actively support organizational change. Some are unsupportive because they do not comprehend the need. This is sometimes caused by management's failure to adequately articulate the need. Some are unsupportive because the change is threatening to them or, more rarely, they fear the unknown. Everyone who works in hospitals in Japan works extremely hard and long hours without much recognition, so adding additional tasks and changes can be burdensome. However, through frequent visits by JCI team members, use of mock surveys, use of internal communication methods, and having the JCI requirements addressed at all departmental meetings, Kameda leaders and staff did a good job of staff education.

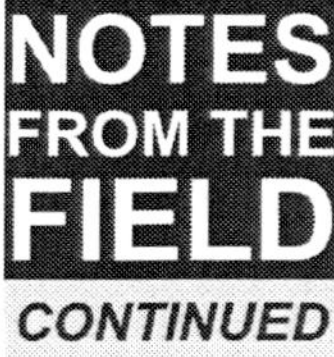

The value of mock surveys cannot be overestimated. For a health care organization facing JCI accreditation in a country where there is no precedent to rely on, mock surveys were an essential undertaking (*see* Section 3 for more information on mock surveys). To gain more experience in understanding the logistics of undergoing JCI accreditation and understanding of a mock survey process, Kameda's medical director, director of nursing, JCI team coordinator, and I visited Severance Hospital in Seoul in February of 2009 and observed a mock survey in preparation for reaccreditation in 2010. This was a valuable experience to observe not only how Severance prepared each department for interaction with surveyors but also to see how the survey process was actually carried out. When we returned to Japan, we were determined to conduct not only a mock survey but to arrange for two mock surveys using external expertise. We used external consultants to help us prepare.

Because Kameda has long been a referral site for U.S. military hospitals in Japan, combined with the fact that all of the hospitals are accredited by The Joint Commission, we asked both the U.S. Navy Hospital in Yokosuka and the U.S. Navy Hospital in Okinawa if they could provide us some assistance in preparing us for accreditation. In the true spirit of international cooperation, they agreed, and on two separate occasions we underwent a full three-day mock survey using both Joint Commission and JCI standards. Kameda then corrected all deficiencies found during the mock surveys in order to show at least a four-month compliance with JCI standards by the time of the actual JCI survey. This cooperation was of immense benefit to Kameda in our successful survey. Practice makes perfect, so to speak.

The Survey

From 3 to 7 August 2009, Kameda Medical Center underwent a very successful accreditation survey by JCI. We received a full three-year accreditation without any follow-up requirements other than creating a Strategic Implementation Plan (SIP) to improve areas identified by JCI (*see* Section 3). This SIP was accepted by JCI in a minimal time frame.

Kameda will always be able to claim being the first Japanese hospital to become JCI accredited, but it is my hope that other hospitals in Japan will consider accreditation using global standards in addition to local/domestic standards. To be clear, I am in no way advocating that JCI replace local accrediting by the JCQHC.

Is JCI Accreditation Worth It?

The answer to this question is absolutely, without reservation and resoundingly YES! Because the JCI accrediting process is educational, we learned many, many things about how to improve quality and enhance safety. Through our preparation activities we created new policies and procedures that improved many aspects of our organization.

Kameda now proudly displays the JCI Gold Seal of Approval™ as well as that of the JCQHC. In this sense, we have the best of both worlds, and both accrediting programs complement each other. Their combined value is greater than each one alone. I look forward to other hospitals in Japan considering accomplishing this, and Kameda will be pleased to provide assistance based on our experience.

REFERENCES

1. Isgar T., Ranney J., Grinnel S.: Team leaders: The key to quality. *Training & Development* 48:45–47, Apr. 1994.

2. Vaughn T., et al.: Engagement of leadership in quality improvement initiatives: Executive quality improvement survey results *J Patient Saf* 2:2–9, Mar. 2006.

3. Botwinick L., Bisognano M., Haraden C.: *Leadership Guide to Patient Safety* (IHI Innovation Series white paper). Cambridge, MA: Institute for Healthcare Improvement, 2006.

4. Institute for Healthcare Improvement: *Health Care Leaders Leading: A Dana-Farber Cancer Institute Executive Describes the Crucial Role of Leadership in Driving Patient Safety.* http://www.ihi.org/IHI/Topics/PatientSafety/MedicationSystems/ImprovementStories/HealthCareLeadersLeadingADanaFarberCancerInstituteexecutivedescribesthecrucialroleofleadershipindriv.htm (accessed 14 May 2010).

5. Reinertsen J., Bisognano M., Pugh M.: *Seven Leadership Leverage Points for Organization-Level Improvement in Health Care,* 2nd ed. (IHI Innovation Series white paper). Cambridge, MA: Institute for Healthcare Improvement, 2008.

6. Jiang H.J., et al.: Board engagement in quality: Findings of a survey of hospital and system leaders. *J Healthc Manag* 53:121–135, Mar.–Apr. 2008.

7. McAlearney A., et al.: Developing effective physician leaders: Changing cultures and transforming organizations. *Hosp Top* 83:11–18, Spring 2005.

8. National Patient Safety Agency: *Putting Patient Safety First: A Compendium of Patient Safety in Practice.* http://www.nrls.npsa.nhs.uk/EasySiteWeb/getresource.axd?AssetID=60172&type=full&servicetype=Attachment (accessed 14 May 2010).

9. Page A. (ed.): *Keeping Patients Safe: Transforming the Work Environment of Nurses.* Washington, DC: National Academies Press, 2004.

10. Rathert C., Fleming D.: Hospital ethical climate and teamwork in acute care: The moderating role of leaders. *Health Care Manage Rev* 33:323–331, Oct.–Dec. 2008.

11. Caldwell D., et al.: Implementing strategic change in a health care system: The importance of leadership and change readiness. *Health Care Manage Rev* 33:124–133, Apr.–Jun. 2008.

12. Ahlin P., Weiss R.: Risk management and compliance in pathology and laboratory medicine. *Clin Lab Med* 27:859–873, Dec. 2007.

13. Reason J.T.: *Managing the Risks of Organizational Accidents.* Aldershot, England: Ashgate, 1997.

14. Liu Y., Kalisch B., Zhang L.: Perception of safety culture by nurses in hospitals in China. *J Nurs Care Qual* 24:63-68, Jan.–Mar. 2009.

15. Frankel A., et al. (eds.): *The Essential Guide for Patient Safety Officers.* Oakbrook Terrace, IL: Joint Commission Resources, 2009.

SECTION

3

ACCREDITATION FOR THE QUALITY/ACCREDITATION SPECIALIST

This section explores the information that the quality or accreditation specialist needs in order to help ensure the success of the accreditation journey for his or her organization. It provides information on the components of accreditation and offers guidance on how to go about implementing these components.

The decision to seek accreditation represents the beginning of a journey for an organization. It requires an organizationwide commitment as well as collaborative work to assess current standards adherence, improve noncompliant areas, and maintain continuous compliance—not only with the standards but with new or improved processes that have been implemented by the organization. It requires a systematic approach to improving quality at all levels of the organization.

Section 2 discusses the significant role that leaders play in setting the stage for, supporting, and encouraging quality improvement efforts and the pursuit of accreditation, but leadership alone cannot drive the preparation process and create all of the systems necessary for continuous quality improvement. Leadership must work with quality and accreditation staff to drive the accreditation process and engage the rest of the staff in improvement efforts.

Depending on the size and scope of an organiza-

tion, there may be one or several people in charge of accreditation activities and quality improvement in an organization. Different organizations fill these roles in varying ways. For example some organizations have one individual in charge of both accreditation and quality. Others have a designated department in charge of quality improvement efforts, with the pursuit of accreditation falling within the responsibility of this group. A specific individual or individuals within this department drive and manage accreditation efforts, including conducting the baseline assessment of standards compliance, planning improvement strategies, and preparing for the on-site survey. Other organizations create an accreditation department whose sole responsibility is to manage these different aspects of accreditation and work with the quality department to achieve continuous standards compliance. Joint Commission International (JCI) recommends that an organization's survey coordinator be a full-time employee dedicated to preparation for accreditation and implementing the improvements based on survey results.

Regardless of the structure of an organization's quality improvement and accreditation preparation efforts, there are specific elements of the accreditation process that should be familiar to all involved.

Getting Started

Because accreditation affects nearly every aspect of an organization, determining how to get started can in itself present challenges. Organizations often have similar questions. How do we know where to begin? How do we know whether we comply with JCI standards? Will we need external help to achieve accreditation? How do we set priorities and determine realistic time lines? How should we coordinate accreditation activities? There are no "right" or "wrong" answers to these questions. Instead, the answers depend on the characteristics and needs of each organization. An accreditation specialist (designated from within the staff of the organization) or quality specialist is in the best position to examine each of these questions and work with leaders and staff to arrive at

the right answers for your organization. However, there are some general activities in the preparation process that all organizations must address. The following paragraphs provide some examples and suggestions on how to consider the questions associated with getting started and how to move ahead with the preparation process.

Get Familiar with the JCI Standards and Accreditation Process

Achieving JCI accreditation requires a comprehensive knowledge of JCI policies and methodologies. When an organization has committed to accreditation, quality improvement professionals and/or accreditation specialists (if the organization assigns this role), along with organization leaders, should take the time to thoroughly learn about and understand the logistics involved in the accreditation process and the time and resources that may be necessary. In addition, these individuals should familiarize themselves with the intent and implications of the JCI standards and what they mean for an organization. Specifically, the organization needs to learn how the standards are organized, their meaning and intent, and what the measurable elements require. This may involve getting a multidisciplinary group, including senior leaders, clinical leaders, quality improvement professionals, and accreditation specialists together in a room to walk through each of

---

NOTES FROM THE FIELD

Ospedale Regionale di Locarno

Achieving and maintaining JCI accreditation was a matter of rethinking all aspects of patient care and emphasizing the team aspects of performance improvement, according to Angela Greco, Quality Manager and Coordinator, JCI Project, Ospedale Regionale di Locarno, Locarno, Switzerland. "JCI accreditation was the result of a series of exacting reviews of some of our patient care and management processes established by JCI standards," says Greco. "Unlike other quality certification programs previously undertaken by our hospital, JCI accreditation has required the involvement of the hospital staff as a whole—more than 600 people. Staff members have been asked to change their professional culture significantly, as well as their day-to-day practices."

EXPERT ADVICE

Looking Outside for Help

Most organizations I know of have used some external help to prepare for accreditation. Their leaders feel that bringing in an accreditation, quality improvement, or process expert with an unbiased view of their organization is a smart long-term investment. But I do know of an organization that self-prepared for its initial survey and succeeded—this organization is accredited now. Its leaders made the decision mainly for financial reasons, but the organization had a very strong quality department with extensive hospital and physician leader involvement. It did an excellent job with its own assessment, mock survey, and all aspects of the preparation.

—Bruce Frederick, R.N., M.N.,
JCI Consultant

the standards and ask, "What does this standard mean, and how do we implement it in our organization?"

This is an excellent time, if the organization budget allows, to seek training on the standards from outside the organization. Education and training can come from a variety of sources, including JCI education and training programs and materials, other organizations preparing for accreditation, accredited organizations, outside consultants, and so forth. (*See* Sidebar 3-1 on page 76.)

It is very important for organizations to allow enough time for this familiarization process. The more an organization understands about accreditation and the intent and content of the standards, the better able it will be to successfully navigate the accreditation preparation journey.

Planning for Education

As discussed in detail in Section 2, it is important for every individual in an organization to have an introduction to the JCI accreditation philosophy and approach, as well as more detailed education about how accreditation can be used as a risk reduction strategy. This education is crucial to motivate and inspire staff commitment at all levels.

It is also important for staff members to understand how accreditation and complying with the standards fits into their current work. Because they will need to put the requirements of the standards into practice on a day-to-day

> ### ACCREDITATION STRATEGY
>
> **Resources for Accreditation**
>
> An organization does not have to be alone in its accreditation journey. Seeking information from other accredited organizations about compliance strategies, resource allocation, and evidence-based practice can help enhance an organization's efforts toward accreditation. Some further sources for accreditation strategies include patient safety literature, professional organizations, and international health care groups such as the World Health Organization.

Learn the Standards

Whether an organization does it internally or brings in outside help, learning the JCI standards and measurable elements is essential. The standards are relatively straightforward and easy to understand if an organization studies the intents and measurable elements. One question we do hear quite often is "How is this [standard or measurable element] applicable in this country?" The fact is, they have been written so they are culturally adaptable in all countries within the context of their laws and regulations. There have been standards that the field has considered to be problematic in the past, and JCI has responded to that feedback. There is an ongoing standards interpretation process, in which JCI invites feedback from organizations and reinterprets or, eventually, revises standards for clarity.

—Bruce Frederick, R.N., M.N.,
JCI Consultant

> ### ACCREDITATION STRATEGY
>
> **Translating the Standards**
>
> Several organizations that have achieved JCI accreditation have noted the benefit of having the JCI standards available to leaders and staff in the organization's native language. To see which of JCI's standards have been translated into languages other than English, go to JCI's Web page for its accreditation manuals:
> http://www.jointcommissioninternational .org/Products-and-Services/Accreditation -Manuals-Home/.

Sidebar 3-1. JCI Resources for Getting Started

The following is a list of possible resources that organizations can use to help familiarize themselves with the JCI standards and accreditation process. It is by no means a comprehensive list. Many resources are free or have a minimal cost and are readily available. More information on these tools can be found on the JCI Web site at http://www.jointcommissioninternational.org/Products-and-Services/.

- JCI Accreditation Manuals. These are the official published volumes of the international standards and are specific for each type of JCI accreditation program.

- Survey Process Guides. These are the official published guides that correspond to each of the specific JCI accreditation programs and contain important information about the survey process, including lists of required documents, definitions of terms, sample agendas, and other valuable information.

- *JCInsight*. Produced quarterly, this free, online publication provides key information for health care organizations around the world about patient safety and quality. (Note: Accredited organizations receive an additional electronic newsletter with updates on new requirements and other accreditation-related matters.)

- Books and e-Books. JCI publishes numerous references about patient care, quality improvement, medication management, infection prevention and control, patient safety, and other topics.

- Web-Based Training. JCI offers Web-based education as an effective way for organizations to participate in training without the costs and time of travel. These self-paced offerings are accessible through the Internet and can provide an introduction to the international accreditation process and JCI standards.

- JCI Practicum. This is a premium five-day education and training program that provides a comprehensive explanation of the JCI process, improvement philosophy, standards, and methodology. The Practicum is highly interactive and offers practical, hands-on sessions on key topic areas. Generally held in the Middle East, Europe, Asia Pacific, and United States (for international participants) annually, the program combines classroom education with on-site demonstrations of JCI's tracer methodology within local JCI–accredited hospitals.

- International Essentials of Healthcare Quality and Patient Safety™. Produced by JCI, this is a framework that organizations can use to assess performance in five focus areas that have the greatest impact on patient care. The International Essentials can help organizations begin the process of designing and implementing a risk reduction program that will lead to improved patient safety. Technical support and Internet tools for The International Essentials are also available. It is important to note that complying with The International Essentials is not the same as complying with JCI standards. Organizations can obtain a free copy of The International Essentials by going to http://www.jointcommissioninternational.org/International-Essentials-for-Quality-and-Patient-Safety/.

- The Center for Transforming Healthcare. Established in 2009, the Joint Commission Center for Transforming Healthcare is a division of The Joint Commission, JCI's parent organization in the United States. Through collaboration with leading U.S. hospitals and health systems, the Center is focused on solving health care's most critical safety and quality problems. Participant organizations use a proven systematic approach to analyze specific breakdowns in care and discover the underlying causes. These organizations then collaborate to develop targeted solutions that solve these complex problems. Although the Center for Transforming Health Care is based in the United States, solutions developed at the Center can be applied globally. The Web site for the Center is http://www.centerfortransforminghealthcare.org/.

ACCREDITATION STRATEGY

A Helpful Presentation

To begin an organization's journey toward accreditation, quality and accreditation professionals should consider organizing meetings for staff members to see "JCI Accreditation: Getting Started," which is an introductory slide presentation in the Online Extras section of this book. This can serve as both an introduction to JCI and the accreditation process and become the first step in ongoing education on accreditation.

basis, staff members must recognize how standards compliance makes care safer for patients. This furthers the mission not only of the organization but also the personal mission of those who choose to work in the health care field.

Although organization leaders must make and maintain a visible commitment to accreditation, most of the ongoing work involved in educating both leaders and staff typically falls to the quality or accreditation professional. Education may include providing information sessions, writing newsletter articles, posting results of quality improvement efforts, speaking at department meetings, being present and involved in leadership meetings, and so forth. Other forms of communication can be useful in providing staff with facts and dispelling any misconceptions, such as fliers and posters, an intranet section on accreditation-related activities and results, special lunchtime information sessions, in-service training, and videos.

Another approach to organizationwide education is for the quality or accreditation specialist to educate an individual from each department, who will in turn share this information with colleagues. Other organizations can also be helpful when designing education programs. Conducting joint programs with similar organizations in the accreditation preparation process can help encourage an exchange of ideas and joint learning. Topics for these sessions may include how the accreditation process works, how to handle challenging standards, and how to develop performance improvement strategies.

Developing and maintaining a schedule of programs for staff members to attend on topics related to standards,

quality improvement, and the survey process will reinforce the goal for staff to provide safer, higher-quality care to patients. Ongoing attention to education demonstrates that the organization takes the process of accreditation seriously, that everyone is important to the effort, and that the organization is open to change and improvement.

Compiling a list of frequently asked questions, with honest, direct answers, can be useful in addressing staff concerns. For example, one of the most basic questions may be, "Is accreditation really necessary?" Thinking about how to answer this question and the many other staff questions that arise during the accreditation process helps an organization to sharpen its focus on taking the actions necessary for success.

Although staff will not be expected to recite JCI standards or survey processes, successfully achieving accreditation requires that they understand how to effectively carry out their duties in a way that meets organizational goals for consistently delivering high-quality care. Staff may want to know, "Will my daily work change as the result of our organization seeking JCI accreditation?" and "Will accreditation change the way my organization operates?" The answer to both of these questions will depend on the organization. Most organizations that seek JCI accreditation do have to make some changes in operations, meaning that staff also may need to make adjustments. Staff should understand, however, that JCI accreditation is dependent upon evaluating how an organization goes about providing safe, high-quality care in its everyday care for patients. In other words, the actions undertaken to satisfy accreditation requirements should be the same actions taken to ensure that patients receive the best care possible.

Quality/accreditation specialists will find that some departments and staff will need more information about accreditation than others. For example, nurses may need more information than technicians because of their roles in overseeing care. To determine staff education needs, consider the following questions:

- How does information about accreditation fit into daily operations for both clinical and nonclinical staff?
- Do current staff receive ongoing information on the standards as necessary to successfully carry out their responsibilities?
- Do specific disciplines, departments, or units need different information about accreditation?
- How are materials or presentations tailored to specific disciplines or departments or units?

■ Have enough individuals in the organization been designated as accreditation "experts" so that staff members can easily find answers to their questions and receive information as they carry out their duties?

■ Are there measurable goals in some of the normal staff responsibilities that are carried out regularly? Examples of this might be patient education, incident reporting, fall prevention, and needlesticks. Education using outcome data can show progress in standards compliance.

■ Are new staff members assessed for their need for information on accreditation?

■ Have staff members been asked what types of information they want or need about accreditation?

Although education must be taken seriously, accredited organizations have designed many different and creative approaches to education and ongoing training of staff during the accreditation preparation process. And although it is hard work, because the process is likely to take many months or even several years, it is important to avoid creating undue stress or the feeling that the organization is in a constant state of emergency. Many organizations plan fun events to celebrate successes along the way. They highlight individuals or teams who achieve goals and spotlight best practices and great ideas. In this way, education and training can be seen as positive and helpful, rather than as disruptive or extra work.

Developing Policies and Procedures

One of the first steps in getting started down the right path is to ensure that policies and procedures are developed or revised to be consistent with the requirements in the standards and measurable elements. The policies and procedures are the foundation to ensure that all physicians and staff members are practicing in the same way in all areas for uniform patient care. Most organizations make the mistake of developing policies and procedures that are extremely long and do not follow the requirements in the standards. Policies and procedures fail when they are

■ out of date;

■ too long and wordy;

■ unclear, complicated, or difficult to understand;

■ too generic or general;

■ confusing because they use different formats;

■ poorly designed or hard to navigate; or

■ hard to find or locate.

The worth of a policy or procedure is not in its design

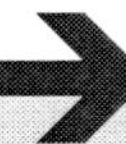

Making the Standards Available

To help staff with the familiarization process, quality and accreditation specialists may wish to make the standards manual easily available by keeping multiple copies in a resource center, break room, or other common areas where staff may congregate. JCI manuals are also available in electronic format (PDF) that can be posted on a shared internal network drive. Staff members should be encouraged to look up specific topics, read through sections that apply to or interest them, ask questions about standards or measurable elements that may seem confusing, or suggest ideas for future education events.

and level of detail but rather in its ability to be carried out regularly and consistently. Developing and approving a policy or procedure should take about 10% of an organization's time. The remaining 90% of the time will be required to implement the policy and ensure consistent adherence. If a policy or procedure is too difficult to follow or does not fit easily into daily work practices, then staff will not follow it. If staff won't follow it, then the revised policy is doing nothing to improve performance. For this reason, when designing and revising policies, organizations should ask themselves, "How are we going to implement this?" If the implementation appears to be too difficult, then revision of the policy or procedure may be indicated.

More information on developing policies and procedures can be found on page 101.

Conducting a Baseline Assessment

After an organization is familiar with the standards and a number of policies are developed and implemented, it is time to conduct a baseline assessment of the organization's level of compliance. Conducting a baseline assessment not only allows organizations to prepare for JCI accreditation, it also presents an opportunity for organizations to identify strengths and weaknesses, address possible areas of risk, and plan for improvements in the safety and quality of care provided to patients. This systematic examination process educates leaders and staff members on how the organization is performing in its daily operations. It defines a baseline from which the organization can strive for performance improvement and incorporate the quality and safety concepts in the standards into day-to-day patient care. Based on the "gap" between the standards and performance identified in the baseline assessment, the organization can plan next steps in the accreditation preparation process.

Any time an individual or organization undertakes a self-assessment, there is some question as to whether the result will be thorough and comprehensive. In the case of the baseline assessment, it is in an organization's best interests to honestly identify problem areas, create plans for improvement, and address issues. Thoroughly assessing compliance with standards during the preaccreditation period gives organizations adequate time to implement action plans, which lessens the need to handle issues with short-term "fixes" immediately before a JCI survey. Solutions that are implemented at the last minute before a survey in order to prove compliance are generally not well integrated into clinical performance, and this quickly becomes evident to the surveyors. A valid self-assessment allows organizations to plan and implement continuous standards compliance that will have a meaningful and sustainable impact on the quality and safety of patient care.

Determining Who Will Conduct the Assessment

To ensure a valid and comprehensive baseline assessment, organizations should make sure that knowledgeable and credible evaluators will critically and objectively assess each area. Depending on the organization, the approach to this assessment will vary. When internal staff are new to the accreditation process, organizations may choose to bring in external consultants to conduct this assessment. Alternatively, organizations can send new internal staff members to an outside training and education event to gain a deeper understanding of the standards and how to conduct the baseline assessment.

Some organizations use a combination of internal and external evaluation. Qualified internal evaluators may do an initial assessment, and then a team of outside evaluators may do an official baseline assessment. This gives the advantage of comparison of the results of the two assessments, offers the organization an opportunity to clarify any questions about interpretation of the standards or the accreditation process, and provides a learning opportunity for internal quality or accreditation professionals.

Other organizations use an external team for the baseline assessment as a first step, and when the results are known, an action planning session is jointly held between the external consultants and the quality or accreditation specialists and other key staff to discuss the gap analysis, plan time lines, and determine a realistic time for the accreditation survey.

Regardless of the approach for the baseline assessment, leaders should recognize the critical importance of this activity—it allows the organization to plan the time line for the accreditation survey based on a gap analysis of the current level of performance and the standards, and it forms the basis for performance improvement activities. If the assessment is not comprehensive or a realistic view of current performance, then planned activities may fall short of the standards.

There are several benefits to organizations using internal staff to conduct the baseline assessment, including the following:

- As members of the staff, internal evaluators emphasize the importance of quality and safety as organization goals. When organization leaders and staff actively lead the assessment, it underscores the importance of each staff member in improving safety and quality.
- Self-assessment enhances learning. By reviewing and assessing all standards, quality and accreditation specialists, department managers, clinical leaders, and other staff who are involved in the assessment process will become more familiar with the standards. They also will begin to recognize what is considered compliance with the standards and understand how the organization is or is not meeting those standards. This learning process can help staff understand the need for improvement activities more fully and thus can garner more support and buy-in during the improvement process.
- Self-assessment builds confidence. Internal review can build staff confidence about the standards and accreditation process, so staff feel more comfortable during the on-site survey.

elements provide performance expectations about the standard and detail specific structures, processes, or systems that must be in place for an organization to provide safe, high-quality care. The measurable elements are useful because they clearly outline the requirements of the standards. Standards compliance is based on these measurable elements, and every organization is evaluated on them. Both JCI surveyors and organizations have access to the measurable elements, so everyone knows exactly what is expected and no requirements or expectations are hidden. (*See* Sidebar 3-2 on page 84.)

Because the measurable elements clearly outline the requirements of the standards, an organization can turn them into questions to help determine the organization's level of compliance. For example, a standard in the "Prevention and Control of Infections" (PCI) chapter of the hospital accreditation manual states: "Gloves, masks, eye protection, other protective equipment, soap, and disinfectants are available and used correctly when required."

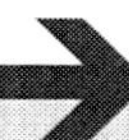

ACCREDITATION STRATEGY

Helpful Questions for Assessing Compliance

Helpful questions to ask when assessing standards compliance include the following:

→ Is evidence of the measurable element's requirement present or available?

→ Which patients or units are affected by the standard or a measurable element?

→ If a requirement is an activity that must be performed or accomplished within a particular time frame, is that time frame being met? Is there evidence of this?

→ Is the requirement in a measurable element being met completely, effectively, and appropriately?

The intent statement gives insight into the standard, explaining that

Hand hygiene, barrier techniques, and disinfecting agents are fundamental tools for proper infection prevention and control. The organization identifies those situations in which masks, eye protection, gowns, or gloves are required and provides training in their correct use. Soap, disinfectants, and towels or other means of drying are located in those areas where handwashing and disinfecting procedures are required. Hand-hygiene guidelines (use of guidelines is scored at IPSG.5, ME 2) are adopted by the organization and posted in appropriate areas, and staff are educated in proper handwashing, hand disinfection, or surface disinfection procedures.

The measurable elements for the standards are as follows:

1. The organization identifies those situations for which gloves and/or masks or eye protection are required.

2. Gloves and/or masks or eye protection are correctly used in those situations.

3. The organization identifies those areas where handwashing and hand disinfection or surface disinfecting procedures are required.

4. Handwashing and hand-disinfection procedures are used correctly in those areas.

5. The organization has adopted hand-hygiene guidelines from an authoritative source.

An organization can turn the measurable elements for this standard into the following assessment questions:

- Has the organization identified those situations for which gloves and/or masks are required?

- Are gloves and/or masks used correctly in those situations?

- Have those areas where handwashing and hand-disinfecting or surface-disinfecting procedures are required been identified?

- Are handwashing and disinfecting procedures used correctly in those areas?

- Has the organization adopted hand-hygiene guidelines from an authoritative source, such as the World Health Organization?

When assessing compliance with the various measurable elements, organizations should collect appropriate data that will help determine the level of compliance. These data should be quantifiable. It should not be acceptable for a staff member to "think" the organization complies with a standard or measurable elements; confirmation should be based on written documentation, dated checklists, written plans, policies, meeting minutes, or other data. These data should be interpreted and summarized as needed for internal use.

Data that verify compliance can take a variety of forms, including policies and procedures, outcome data, infection rates, and data about the performance of specific processes and procedures—such as hand hygiene or patient assessment. Some standards may even require a mix of data to prove compliance. The appropriate data will vary depending on the standard being evaluated and the type of organization and services available for patients. (*See* pages 85–94 for more information on using data to assess compliance.

It is also important to remember that when JCI surveyors conduct an on-site evaluation, they will be examining compliance *sustainability*. In other words, has the compliance level been maintained for a sufficient period of time to indicate that this level (or higher) will be sustained over time? To prove sustainability, organizations must understand how long the standard has been implemented in the organization. This can be accomplished by "looking back" at the compliance evidence trail over time.

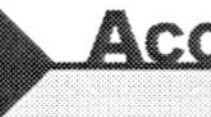

ACCREDITATION STRATEGY

Focus on Implementation

Remember that the real measure of compliance with JCI standards is implementation and outcomes. This recognizes that the goal is not complying with standards for the sake of compliance, but rather to improve the quality and safety of care. For example, JCI does not require that "an initial assessment process [be] used to identify the health care needs of all patients" because it is a good way of establishing a paper trail; JCI requires the assessment because it is in the best interest of patients that caregivers understand their health care needs when patients enter the organization.

For currently accredited organizations this look-back period covers 12 of the last 36 months of an organization's accreditation award. For an organization undergoing its initial accreditation survey, the look-back period is 4 months.

The compliance evidence trail will not be the same for all standards. A standard for which the primary evidence is gained by observation and interview will not require this trail. For example, it would be difficult to look back at evidence in the case of patient privacy (PFR) in light of the surveyor's observation that privacy is respected during examinations, procedures, and treatments. However, there may be evidence that the organization has a written document in place that informs a patient about his or her right to privacy.

For standards in which documents, documentation, or other logs or records are the primary evidence, it is possible to look back over time at compliance. Thus, the effective date of a policy or procedure can be noted by the surveyor, logs of training examined, or patient charts reviewed to evaluate the date of implementation of a new process or form.

Using Data for More Than Just Compliance Assessment

In addition to using data to determine standards compliance in the baseline assessment, organizations should use data to look for trends and patterns and identify possible areas of improvement. This process may include watching data over time. Analysis could reveal strengths or weaknesses in a particular location, shift, or procedure or at a particular time of day. For example, analysis of data collected on placing central lines may identify an increased number of infections during a particular shift, just after new nurses are hired, among certain types of patients (such as those who have central lines in place for more than seven days), or because of certain types of procedures, such as inserting femoral lines. This type of data collection and analysis is the foundation of quality improvement.

In addition, data analysis can be used to compare data between programs or departments in order to highlight problem-prone areas. For example, an organization may use restraints to prevent patients from pulling out tubes, falling from a bed, or interfering with care. Alternatives to restraints may be sought by the organization because of the great risk of injury or death. By comparing restraint use against other programs or departments, the organization can compare the number of times that restraints are used

Sidebar 3-2. Most Challenging Standards in 2009

From January through December 2009, the following hospital chapters and standards were most challenging to organizations undergoing JCI on-site surveys, grouped by the standards chapter; the ranking of chapters by number of noncompliant standards found; the most frequently noncompliant standards in that chapter; and the issue covered in the named noncompliant standard.

Standards Chapter	Ranking by Most Noncompliant Standards Found	Most Frequently Noncompliant Standard in Chapter	Subject Matter of Most Frequently Noncompliant Standard
Facility Management and Safety (FMS)	1	FMS.7.1	Fire safety—safe exit from the facility
Medication Management and Use (MMU)	2	MMU.3	Labeling medications
Assessment of Patients (AOP)	3	AOP.1.2	Medical assessment contains health history and physical exam.
Staff Qualifications and Education (SQE)	4	SQE.11	Ongoing professional practice evaluation
Prevention and Control of Infections (PCI)	5	PCI.7.1	Equipment cleaning, disinfection, and sterilization
Management of Communication and Information (MCI)	6	MCI.19.3	Clinical record entries identify the author, when entered, and, if required, time of entry.
International Patient Safety Goals (IPSG)	7	IPSG.4	Correct-patient, correct-procedure, and correct-site surgery—use of a checklist and time-out
Care of Patients (COP)	8	COP.2.1	Care plan
Patient and Family Rights (PFR)	9	PFR.6.4	Informed consent
Anesthesia and Surgical Care (ASC)	10	ASC.3	Presedation assessment
Access to Care and Continuity of Care (ACC)	11	ACC.3.2	Discharge summary
Quality Improvement and Patient Safety (QPS)	12	QPS.6	Data analyzed when undesirable trends or patterns are found
Governance, Leadership, and Direction (GLD)	13	GLD.1	Governance performance evaluation
Patient and Family Education (PFE)	14	PFE.2	Educational needs assessment and documentation of education

Source: Joint Commission International.

instead of alternative means. This type of data analysis gives the organization insight into how its quality improvement efforts are progressing and can highlight issues that need immediate attention.

An organization may also be able to compare data about issues, such as particular types of medication errors, infections, patient falls, and so forth, with outside organizations. External comparisons can provide meaningful assessments of organization performance and highlight areas for improvement, as well as generate ideas for quality initiatives.

Types of Data

Data are critical elements in the baseline assessment process. They can clearly show compliance or noncompliance and help indicate the sustainability of the compliance effort. Many different types of data can be used when determining compliance, including outcome, patient satisfaction, quality, process variation, and staff perception.

Overall, there are two main types of data:

1. Primary data

2. Secondary data

Primary data are more clinically oriented than secondary data. Primary data are typically recorded by clinicians as opposed to administrative staff. Examples of primary data include disease-specific data, blood use data, operative and invasive procedure data, and behavior management and treatment data. Primary data can be used to understand the care delivered in an organization.

Secondary data are more administrative in nature and include such information as demographics, diagnoses, treatments, medications, laboratory data, and morbidity and mortality data. Secondary data are typically, but not always, collected for financial reimbursement and can also highlight issues or problems in an organization that need attention. This type of data does not show the reasons behind any issues or how those issues may be addressed. Primary data are more suitable for that task.

Both primary and secondary data can be helpful when assessing standards compliance. Sources for data will vary depending on the organization. For example, primary and secondary data that are helpful for assessing compliance can be found in shift reports, documented incidents in an adverse event reporting system, satisfaction data in surveys, and quality data from measures collected to satisfy regulatory requirements.[1] Some of the more common data sources are the following:

- **Clinical records.** Because of all the personal health information this record contains, such as assessment findings, treatment details, and progress notes, the clinical record is a valuable source of primary data, including interventions, screenings, and outcomes. When using these data to verify compliance, organizations should select an appropriate sample and establish reasonable thresholds for compliance.

- **Admission and billing records.** These sources can provide information on demographics, scheduled procedures, treatments received, and outcomes.

- **Policies and procedures.** Verifying the existence of a policy or procedure is not enough to determine compliance; the content of a policy and whether performance is consistent with the policy are the determining factors.

- **Human resources data.** These data may include personnel files, performance reviews, and orientation surveys.

- **Shift reports.** Because these reports offer a comprehensive picture of what occurred during a particular shift, including the status of each individual served, medications administered, a description of any incidents, and other information, these reports can be analyzed for a variety of information, such as data on falls, patient education, and reactions to medications.

- **Surveillance data.** The process of clinical care involves recording specific outcomes of care in a particular population. Surveillance data can highlight a safety issue and help an organization track its performance over time. Surveillance is relatively easy to do and can be low cost; however, it focuses on particular data points and may not highlight more global issues.

- **Infection control data.** These data can illustrate compliance with infection-reducing practices, such as hand hygiene, surgical-site preparation, environmental cleaning, and so forth.

- **Observations.** In some cases, merely observing staff can yield a source of primary data. For example, if measuring compliance with recently instituted hand-hygiene initiatives, organizations can observe staff over time to determine compliance. One caution with direct observation is the presence of the Hawthorne effect. This occurs when individuals change their behavior because they are being watched. In the case of hand-hygiene initiatives, for example, staff members may be more or less likely to comply with hand-washing guidelines when they are being observed.

- **Meeting minutes.** These can provide valuable insight

into whether a meeting took place, what was discussed, and the action items that resulted from the meeting.

- **Building tours.** Environmental safety tours, fire safety tours, and any other tours that involve an assessment of the building and its features can be helpful in identifying areas of compliance and noncompliance.
- **Planning documents.** These may include the organization's strategic plan, safety plan, quality improvement plan and others.
- **Performance improvement data.** Data from performance improvement projects that are under way can help illustrate compliance.
- **Adverse event reporting system.** As discussed in Section 2, organizations should have a method for collecting information on sentinel events, near misses, and other adverse events that occur in the organization. This system may involve staff filling out written reports, sending in e-mail forms, or using a telephone hotline. Information from this reporting system should be transferred to a database or spreadsheet for analysis and response. These adverse events can be analyzed to show patterns of risk or areas needing improvement.
- **Complaint data.** These data are usually collected from satisfaction surveys, written complaints, or complaints made by telephone. This type of data can be a good source of information on areas that need improvement.

Electronic data sources. Computers play an increasingly important role in the data management process. Many health care organizations access data electronically through a variety of sources, including, but not limited to, the following:

- Electronic admission and billing data
- Electronic clinical records
- Electronic medication administration records
- Computerized prescriber order entry systems
- Bar-coding systems for medication management
- Internal databases or spreadsheets
- Laboratory software

The advantages of electronic data are that they are easily accessible and reliable. A computer can retrieve data efficiently, accurately, and consistently. Electronic data can be shared more easily and efficiently than manual data and are easier to manipulate for data analysis, if needed.

However, electronic data do have some disadvantages. For example, even if an organization has access to many electronic data sources, data systems are often incompatible, and combining or transferring between sources can be challenging. Also, when departments of a large organization work very independently, and data systems and the types of data collected are not known to one another, there is the potential for misunderstanding the organization's overall performance.

Despite potential limitations, recent advances in Internet software and architecture have made it easier to share data. The advent of decision-support software is helping organizations overcome the issues associated with sharing data electronically.

Tools for Data Collection

There are a variety of tools organizations can use to collect data for compliance assessment. Some of the more common are the following:

- **Checklists.** A checklist is a common form for gathering data. An example of a checklist might be a discharge summary sheet of instructions to be given to a patient upon discharge from the emergency department. Sometimes a checklist will have blank lines for physicians or nurses to document specific instructions given to a particular patient and to check off when the instructions have been delivered. For example, in community-based care settings, a checklist is often used to record a resident's skin integrity on a weekly basis.

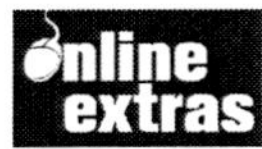

A sample data collection checklist is available in the Online Extras at www.jcrinc.com/JCIGS10/Extras.

- **Logbooks.** Many departments or units keep logbooks to record such things as patient falls, including the time of the fall, the environmental conditions, and the outcome of the fall. A long term care organization may keep a logbook of residents' weekly weights or the activities residents have participated in, with additional notations that are pertinent to each. A hospital may keep logbooks to record functioning of generators and water treatment systems. If additional data are required for a performance improvement project, a column(s) may be added to these logbooks to facilitate ease of data collection. Logbooks can be efficiently transformed into electronic files by using spreadsheet or database software packages that are readily available and easily customized to an organization's special needs. After the hard copy data are computerized, sharing data with appropriate health care team members is easily facilitated (as long as the same software for data collection is available to all those needing the information), particularly through an intranet system.

- **Records of events.** Often, forms are used to gather information and can be modified to collect needed data in a routine and reliable way. For example, patient assessment forms can be used to calculate composite scores or values for the overall health status of patients. Some performance measures can be derived based on a patient's assessment score change from admission to discharge. Forms such as operating room records and birth records also fall into this category. (*See* page 89 for more information about performance measures.) Forms must be made useful to the organization's specific services and populations.

- **Specially designed data collection tools.** At times, data collection may be facilitated by using a specially created tool or form containing closed-ended questions and a predefined choice of responses. For example, a specially designed data collection tool related to pain management is the pain scale. Patients are asked to rate their level of pain on a scale of 0 to 10, with 0 equal to no pain, and 10 equal to excruciating pain. This information is documented on the tool. After information is

collected, data can be entered into an electronic file (spreadsheet or database) or other information system for efficient and effective data analysis and information sharing.

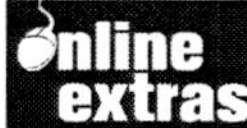

A sample data collection tool can be found in the Online Extras at www.jcrinc.com/JCIGS10/Extras.

- **Surveys.** Surveys can be used to capture people's opinions, feelings, and level of satisfaction with a particular process, event, episode, and so forth. Survey data can be obtained many different ways, including via e-mail, the Internet, personal interviews, telephone conversations, focus groups, or mailing a survey instrument to the individual's home. One important aspect of a survey is the response rate. Ideally, a response rate of more than 50% is desired for a valid survey. If the response rate to a survey is significantly less than 50% (such as 20% to 30%) the organization may need to brainstorm ways to increase response rates. This may mean shortening the survey tool so it can be filled out more quickly or offering some incentive to those who respond. In addition, those who do not respond can be contacted to understand the reason for nonresponse. If constructed, implemented, and analyzed effectively, a survey can yield data that can be a valuable resource for organizations. However, survey data that lack credibility and objectivity may very well be useless information. If decisions are being made based on survey data, a basic understanding of sampling methodologies, response rates, and survey errors is necessary to make correct decisions.

Ensuring Effective Data Collection

To ensure that data used for assessment are valid, appropriate, and accurate, organizations should take time to examine their data collection processes. Without consistent and well-defined ways of collecting data, the resulting data can be flawed. Without specific and straightforward methods of data collection, the process can be a burden and a waste of precious health care resources. Without a well-considered use for data, data can be collected unnecessarily just for the sake of collecting data. Organizations must be careful to refrain from collecting data that are not useful and prevent or minimize duplicative data collection.

Data collection efforts are more effective if there is a plan that controls the efforts. Having a well-considered, well-conceived plan can help ensure that the data collection process is efficient, is effective, and yields useful, accurate, and reliable data. When considering a data collection plan, organizations should answer the following questions:

What data are needed? The answers to this question should be specific and precise to ensure that the appropriate information is gathered. For example, organizations that want to collect data on infection control rates need to identify what infections they want to monitor and among what groups of patients. Figuring out what to measure can sometimes seem like the most difficult part of the data management process. Some organizations might set their sights too low, measuring what they have always measured because it is easy and familiar, even if those data will not verify standards compliance or show improvement in quality and safety. Other organizations might go to the opposite extreme and try to measure everything, spreading resources too thin to allow anything useful to be collected. Another problem arises when organization leaders decide what to measure without getting input from frontline staff who actually know and work with the processes.

Are the data already being collected? In some cases, an organization may already be collecting data that can be useful in assessing compliance, and there is no need to duplicate efforts. In other cases, small modifications to existing data collection strategies may yield the necessary information. Organizations may be collecting more data than they realize. By taking a close look a the activities of risk management, quality management, facility safety, and so forth, organizations may be able to combine data collection efforts and use the resulting information to assess standards compliance and improve quality in multiple areas.

If not already collected, how will data be collected? This includes defining the way to collect the data and the processes involved in collecting them. Data definitions should be easy to understand, and the process of data collection should easily fit within daily workflow. It is important to involve the staff responsible for collecting the data in determining the definition. In addition, organizations should consult representatives from the information technology (IT) department, quality department, and health information (medical record) department because these individuals can provide insight about which data collection strategies are appropriate for the organization. IT professionals can help make changes to the electronic medical record, while health information

department personnel can identify better ways to collect data.

Who will collect the data? This could be an individual, a group, a committee, or a specific job title or function within an organization. Data should be collected by whoever has the easiest and most reliable access to the data within the organization.

How often will data be collected? Deciding how often to collect data will depend on what is being examined. Organizations may collect some information on a daily basis, while other data might be abstracted on a monthly basis. For example, an organization might engage in frequent data collection related to safety efforts (medication errors, patient identification) or assessment of patients, while data might be collected at longer intervals for issues related to patient and family rights, pain management, and patient education.

How will data collectors be trained? Training data collectors is a critical step to gathering complete and accurate data while minimizing variation. Everyone responsible for collecting data should know how and why they are collecting data. Staff must clearly understand the required data elements and their definitions in order to collect accurate data consistently. In addition, staff need to know when to collect the data (such as concurrently at admission, prior to a procedure, after a procedure, or retrospectively after the patient is discharged) and how frequently (daily, weekly, monthly, quarterly, and so forth).

Is there enough time for data collection? Individuals working in a health care organization are busy, and adding one more responsibility can cause anxiety and frustration, lead to poor data collection, and, in the worst case, compromise patient safety. Leaders and quality professionals should review staff responsibilities and ensure that the appropriate level of human and other resources are available for data collection activities. In addition, data collection should be easy and not require too much extra work. For example, organizations that have an electronic medical record might want to use it to help capture data. Staff can enter data into a field on the record so that information can be tracked and compared. When designing electronic medical records, organizations should consider leaving some fields blank so they can be used for future data collection. Doing so allows organizations to collect data for a short period in one of the empty fields. When data collection on that topic is

SECTION 3

no longer necessary, the field can be used to store other data.

- **How will the organization be sure that data are collected consistently?** Scheduled and random audits are effective methods of determining whether the process is being carried out consistently. If the audits reveal inconsistency in data collection, further training may be necessary.

- **Who will oversee data collection efforts?** Organization leaders should assign an individual to oversee the data collection process. This person may be a quality or accreditation specialist, member of the quality department, manager in the department where data are to be collected, or other appropriate staff member. As the primary resource person, this individual should be able to answer questions regarding the data collection, aggregation, and analysis processes, and be able to examine trends indicated by the data. He or she must also be able to interpret the data and transform results into information that is useful for quality improvement activities.

- **How will data validity be ensured?** Organizations should periodically evaluate data quality to ensure that the collected data are accurate and complete. Any inconsistencies should be identified and removed. A common reaction is to "blame the collector" for invalid data, when what is needed for improvement are management processes for retraining or educating the workers involved, allowing more time for data collection, redesigning data collection tools, and so on. Beginning 1 January 2011, JCI hospital requirements state that an internal process for data validation must be in place and that the process must be performed by a minimum of two people—a person to collect and one to reabstract the same data. JCI also requires that data validation accuracy totals of less than 90% must be reviewed for causes and then corrected. (Other programs should check the appropriate comprehensive accreditation manual for JCI's current requirements.)

- **How is data security ensured?** Data should be readily available yet protected from unauthorized disclosure or misuse. Security policies and procedures should address every point at which data can be accessed. User responsibilities include password protection, physical security of computers, and protection of hard copy reports containing sensitive information. Staff members who are responsible for information systems must protect access to computer files and database management systems. An

organization's leaders must strike a balance between security and utility.

- **How will the data be analyzed?** Collecting data does not ensure proper use of the data for compliance assessment. Quality or accreditation specialists must analyze the data and turn them in to useful information. There are many ways to analyze data, including statistical methods. While the scope of this publication does not allow for an in-depth discussion of data analysis, some strategies can be found in Sidebar 3-3 on pages 90–93.

- **Are any external benchmarks available?** Organizations should determine whether there are any benchmark data available to compare performance. Such data may be available from government sources, safety-focused organizations, sister organizations, parent organizations, and others.

Defining Performance Measures to Collect Data

A measure, also known as an indicator, is one way to collect data. It is a precisely defined, often standardized way to determine, over time, an organization's performance of functions, processes, and outcomes. Measures can reflect performance in care appropriateness, availability, continuity, effectiveness, efficacy, efficiency, safety, or timeliness. No matter its purpose, a measure can also be used to verify compliance with JCI standards.

Many organizations use a few key measures to assess performance and quality, such as the following:

- Key internal process measures
- Key financial measures
- Innovation and improvement measures
- Customer satisfaction and operational measures

An effective measure is reliable, is valid, can be interpreted easily, and is reasonable to collect. It is well defined and includes a description of its rationale or intent, a defined sampling procedure, and a specific calculation method.

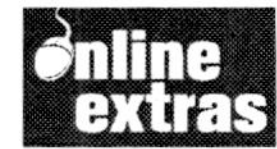

A sample measure profile form is included in the Online Extras at www.jcrinc.com/JCIGS10/Extras.

Sidebar 3-3. Tools for Analyzing Data

Although there are many tools for analyzing data, following is a brief description of some of the more common.

Boxplots

Boxplots provide a way of displaying comparison data for quick analysis. Data are broken down into groups based on where they fit into the overall standard distribution (sometimes known as a bell curve). Data are considered significant if they fall between the 25th percentile and 75th percentile of the distribution. Anything above the 75th percentile or below the 25th percentile is regarded as atypical, or "outlier" data. Boxplots are useful for looking at the overall pattern of data rather than scrutinizing data in great detail. In other words, they show the "big picture."

Figure 1 shows a sample boxplot.

This boxplot shows the 25th, 50th, and 75th percentile of surgical patients at Joint Commission (U.S.)–accredited hospitals whose antibiotic was stopped within 24 hours after surgery (or 48 hours after having coronary artery bypass graft surgery or other cardiac surgery).

Comparison Chart

A comparison chart is a graph that is set up to compare two or more separate groups of data. While a boxplot can serve as a rough comparison chart, more sophisticated analyses may require risk adjustment so that the data from different groups are truly comparable. Not all data lend themselves to risk adjustment. Risk adjustment should be performed wherever it can be.

Figure 2 shows a sample comparison chart.

Control Chart

The control chart was first developed in the 1920s by Walter Shewhart. Like many other performance

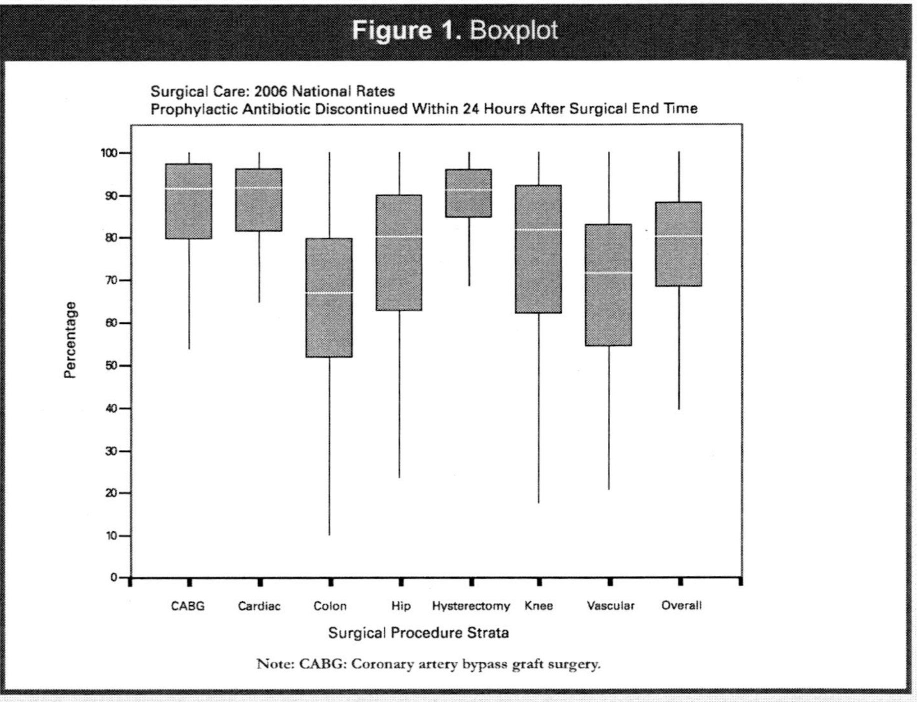

Figure 1. Boxplot

Note: CABG: Coronary artery bypass graft surgery.

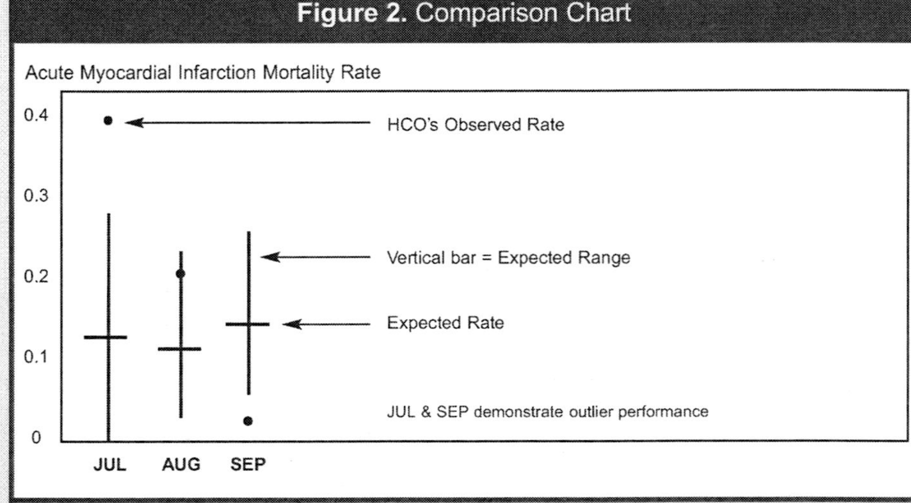

Figure 2. Comparison Chart

Sidebar 3-3. Tools for Analyzing Data, *continued*

measurement tools, control charts are borrowed from manufacturing. The control chart has been applied to health care as the field has tried to standardize the delivery of patient care. The advantage of a control chart is that it can help determine scientifically whether a process is in control or out of control. Control charts show what processes have problems that need to be solved and can indicate whether improvement efforts have been successful. Control charts are most valuable when data collection has taken place over a significant period of time; they are not the best choice for short-term studies.

Figure 3 shows a sample control chart.

Histogram

The histogram, also called a bar chart or a frequency distribution, is one of the oldest tools for statistical analysis.

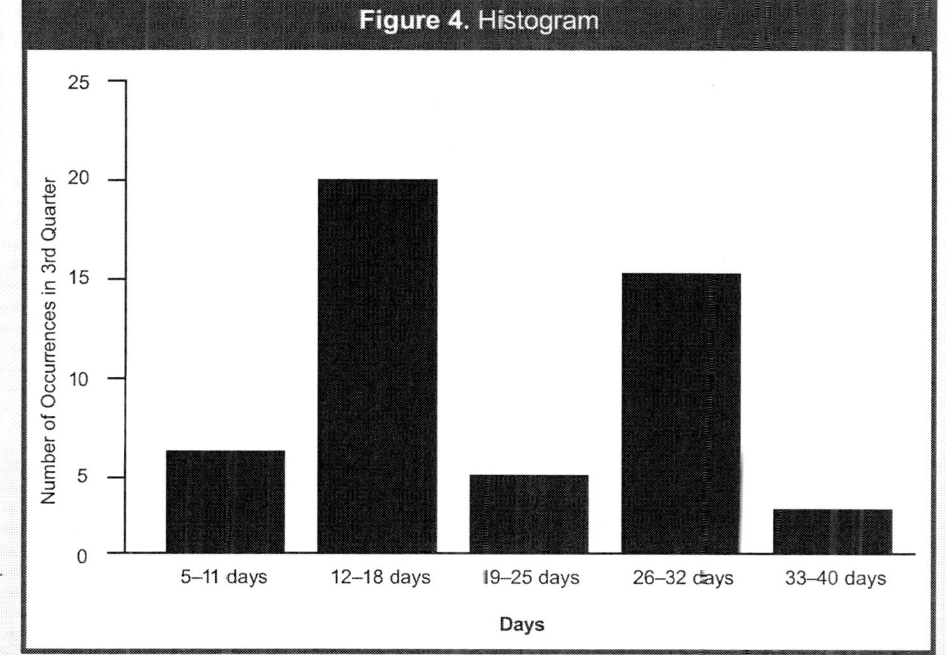

Figure 3. Control Chart

Figure 4. Histogram

Histograms do not show changes over time but, like a photograph, they portray what is happening within a process at a single moment. Histograms are useful for analyzing variable data and evaluating results. Histograms are helpful when an organization's processes have a wide variety of possible values rather than a simple yes-or-no result.

Figure 4 shows a sample histogram.

Line Graph

One of the simplest performance tools to create and interpret, the line graph is used to show measurements made over specific periods of time. This tool functions basically as a running tally and is used to identify trends and other patterns in a process or to help decide whether a target level has been reached. It can indicate how a process is working and reveal which areas need improvement. It can also reveal which areas are already improving. It also allows users to spot trends even in the early stages of data collection, long before there is

(continued on page 92)

Sidebar 3-3. Tools for Analyzing Data, *continued*

enough information to draw a control chart.

Figure 5 shows a sample line graph.

Run Chart

A run chart is a more sophisticated version of a line graph. It plots data points in a time sequence as does a line graph, but it does so in a way that reveals whether patterns or trends can be attributed to common or special causes of variation. It is less sensitive than a control chart for identifying special-cause variation, but it is quicker and easier to use, and it provides a good starting place for data analysis.

Figure 6 shows a sample run chart.

Pareto Chart

The Pareto chart (or Pareto diagram) combines analysis of frequency (or some other quantity) of a problem with analysis of its causes. It is named after Vilfredo Pareto (1848–1923), an Italian economist. Pareto analysis breaks down into two basic steps: (1) collecting data and (2) displaying the data in a user-friendly way. The most common type of display is a bar graph in which the percentages of various factors are plotted on the chart in order of size.

Figure 7 shows a sample Pareto chart.

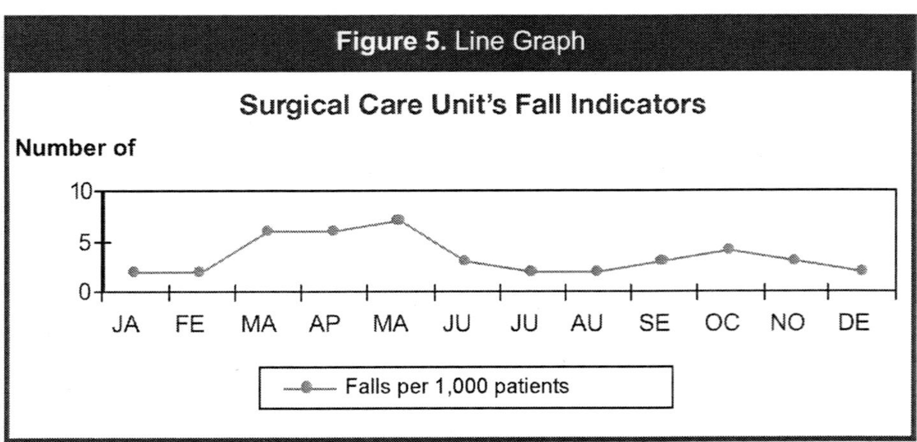

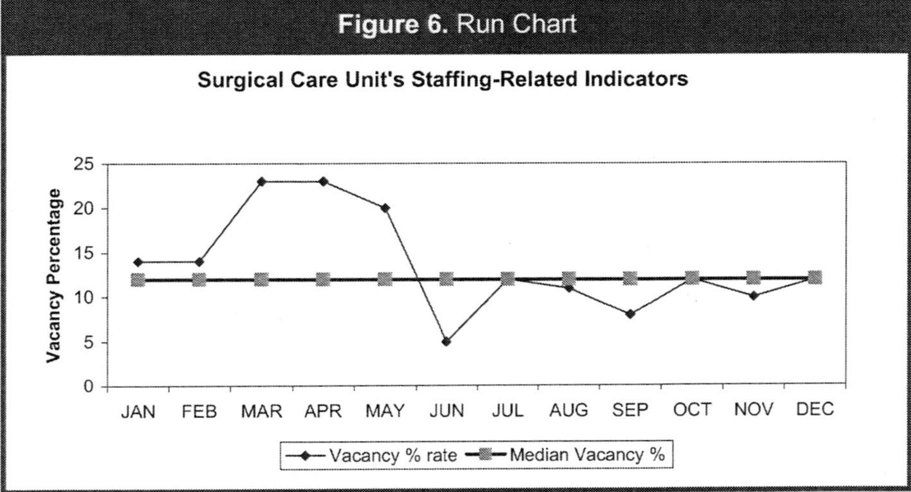

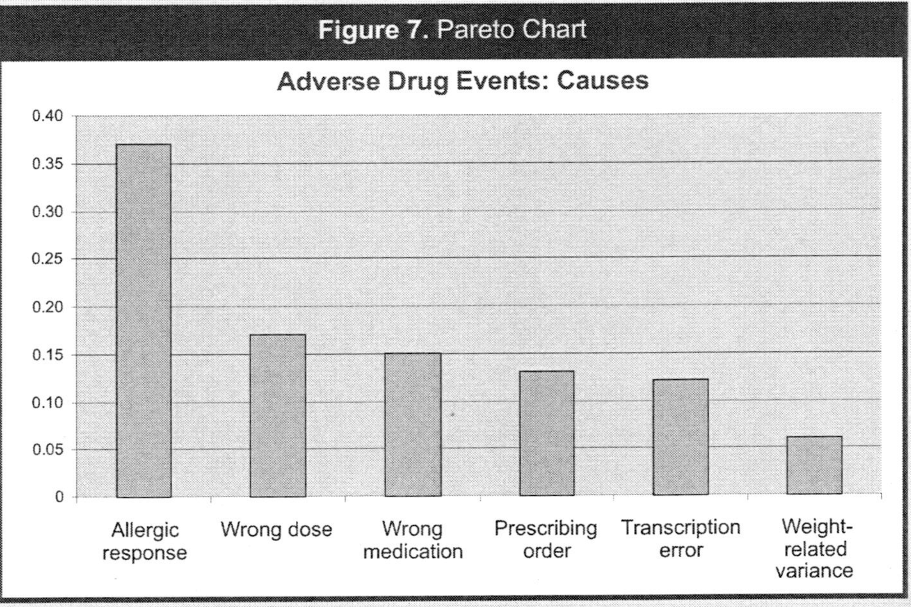

Sidebar 3-3. Tools for Analyzing Data, *continued*

Stratification Chart

Stratification is the process of breaking down a population or process into its component parts. It is useful for discovering root causes of problems in situations in which data of different types have been placed in the same general category. Stratification divides the data into subcategories so users can see underlying distinctions and interpret the data accurately. Stratification is used in conjunction with other tools, such as Pareto charts, scatter diagrams, and histograms, when data on those graphs come from different sources.

Figure 8 shows a sample stratification chart.

Balanced Scorecard or Dashboard

The balanced scorecard was developed in the mid-1990s at Harvard Business School. It is a strategic management approach that helps align and sustain four broad performance areas: financial performance, customer knowledge, internal business processes, and learning and growth. In recent years, it has been adapted for health care.

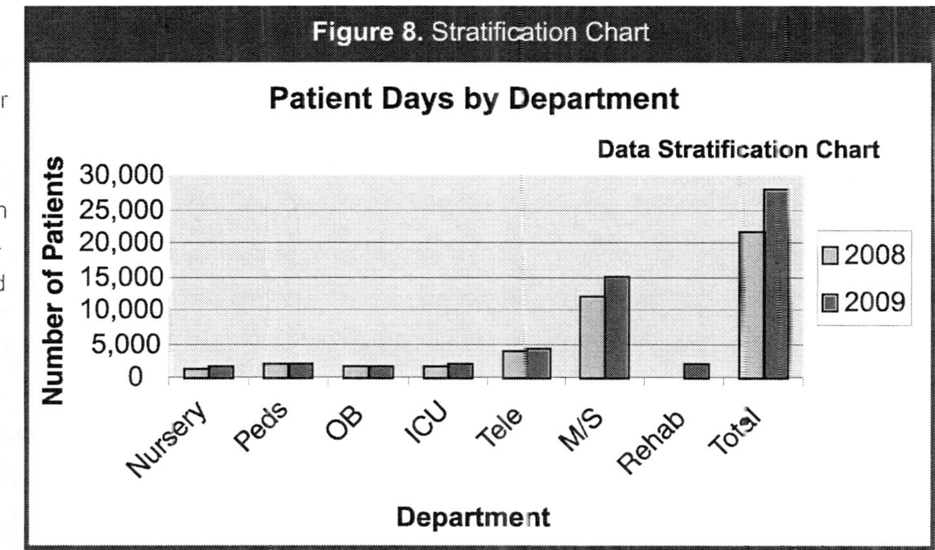

Figure 8. Stratification Chart

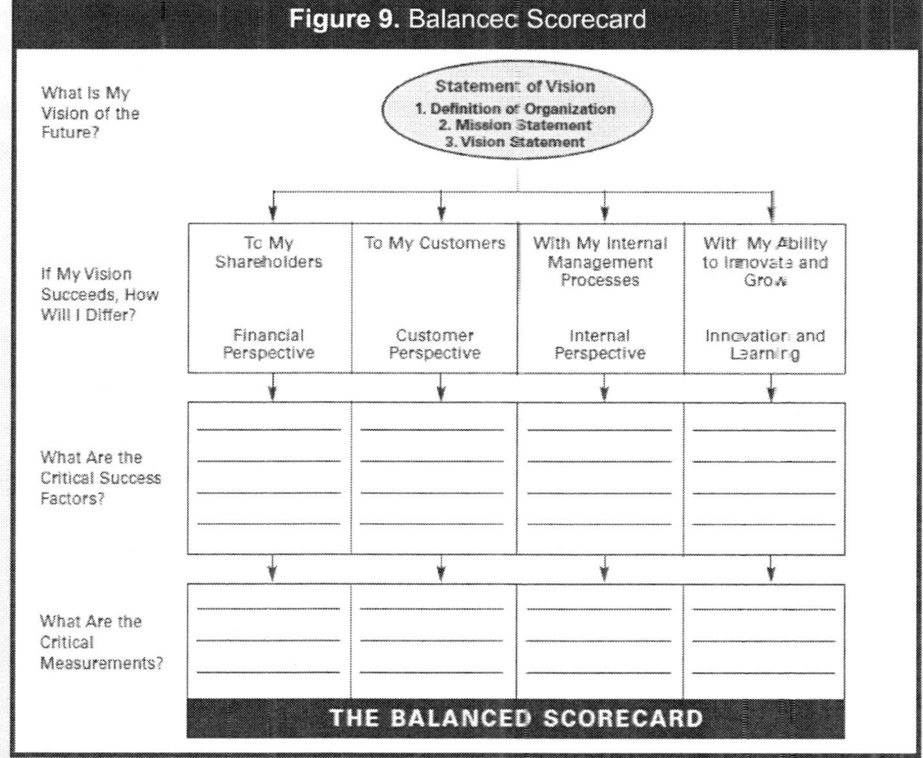

Figure 9. Balanced Scorecard

The underlying concept of a balanced scorecard or dashboard is that the four performance areas should be balanced—that is, all four are equally important and equally excellent. The terms *dashboard* and *balanced scorecard* are sometimes used interchangeably to indicate the presentation tool used to show organizations' performance and goals. The dashboard display is the end product of the balanced scorecard planning tool; in other words, it presents the outcome of that strategic plan.

Figure 9 shows a sample balanced scorecard.

There are two main types of measures:

1. Process measures

2. Outcome measures

A *process measure* focuses on one or more steps that lead to a certain outcome, such as whether preventive skin care was given to patients at risk for developing pressure ulcers. An *outcome measure* focuses on the result of the performance or nonperformance of the process, such as which patients who did or did not receive care developed pressure ulcers.

Health care measures can be taken from any point along the patient care time line: at admission or during treatment, after instructions/education, at discharge, or after the patient is billed. Data collection may occur while the patient is receiving treatment or services (concurrent method) or after the patient is discharged (retrospective method).

Starting 1 January 2011, organizations must choose one measure per JCI–approved category and collect, analyze, and use those date in 2011. The organization must submit the data to JCI on a quarterly basis starting in 2012.

The JCI standards require organizations to define and collect key measures to monitor the organization's clinical and managerial structures, processes, and outcomes and the International Patient Safety Goals. These measures vary depending on the program, but general topics include the following:

- Completeness and appropriateness of patient assessments
- Laboratory safety and quality
- Radiology safety and quality
- Use of evidence-based care
- Use of antibiotics
- Use of medications and medication compliance by patients
- Infection control, surveillance, and reporting
- Clinical research activities, as applicable
- Effectiveness of patient and family education
- Adequate supplies and medications
- Patient and family expectations and perceptions of care
- Staff expectations and satisfaction
- Patient demographics and diagnoses
- Financial management
- Adverse events

While organizations must define these measures and collect them according to their definition in order to be in compliance with the Quality Improvement and Patient Safety (QPS) standards, data collected as part of these measures can also help validate compliance with other standards as well. For example, measures related to the completeness and appropriateness of assessment can show compliance with both the quality standards and those relating to patient assessment.

Defining, collecting, and responding to measures supports quality improvement efforts and provides a valid base for local, national, and international comparisons. (*See* Sidebar 3-4 on page 95). A well-rounded measurement program requires the combination of different types of measures to address the different aspects of care in health care organizations. Process measures and outcome measures are both necessary to identify the need for improvement, establish baseline performance, compare performance to other organizations, and verify the effectiveness of improvement activities.

Defining performance measures should be done systematically. Many aspects of measurement should be considered in determining an effective set of measures. The purpose of the measure, the dimensions of performance being measured, and the ultimate strategic goals of the organization must all be considered when choosing and defining effective measures. In addition, literature reviews show that implementation of quality and performance measures is most effective when education and feedback are part of the implementation, and measures are used to help develop a quality improvement plan.[2] As mentioned earlier, JCI hospital requirements starting 1 January 2011 require organizations to select some measures from a JCI "library" of measures to enhance consistency in data collection and reporting, which will then enhance benchmarking capabilities. Measures will be expected to be validated internally and externally; measures reported on an organization's Web site or elsewhere must be validated by a neutral, qualified third party.

Planning Improvement Actions

As an organization proceeds through its baseline assessment, it will identify areas that require improvement. Using these findings, organizations must develop a detailed action plan that assigns responsibilities, deliverables, and time frames for improvement. (*See* Sidebar 3-5 on page 99.)

Organizations should create an action plan for each JCI standard that is determined to be noncompliant and address each related measurable element found to be in partial or insufficient compliance.

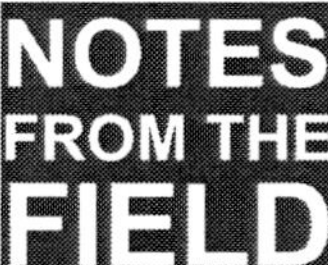

Santa Chiara Hospital

Located in Trento, Italy, Santa Chiara Hospital is a 682-bed acute care facility that services a thriving community in Northern Italy. The organization first achieved accreditation five years ago and continues to work at continuous compliance with JCI standards.

Santa Chiara chose to pursue JCI accreditation because of its deep-rooted interest in effective quality improvement and patient safety. Being part of the JCI network of accredited hospitals provides the organization with clear affirmation of its work and distinct goals toward which to strive.

According to Enrico Baldantoni, the organization's former chief medical officer, "JCI accreditation provides a conceptual model to 'read' the hospital as a living body with interconnected functions, and this alone is a very powerful tool to understand where we are and where we want to go."

Data collection and analysis are key elements in the hospital's accreditation journey. The organization gathers performance data from clinical units and has built more than 50 clinical indicators that are analyzed for corrective actions by the hospital's quality committee. Santa Chiara also closely evaluates medication errors and heath care–associated infections and uses a checklist to monitor samples of medical records to assess their quality and consistency. "JCI acted as a booster to give more power to our actions, giving us also a sense of direction for improvement and teaching us to use the best approaches," says Baldantoni.

To further measure its performance, Santa Chiara Hospital joined the International Quality Indicators Project® and collected data on such performance indicators as acute care inpatient mortality, neonatal mortality, unscheduled returns to the emergency department (ED), and length of stay in the ED. The data are analyzed for plausibility by the Center for Performance Sciences (a subsidiary of the Maryland Hospital Association) and benchmarked internally and with other similar hospitals in Europe and the United States.

In recommending the accreditation process to other organizations, accreditation project manager Maria Grazia Allegretti offers the following comment: "Our experience has been that of a learning quest toward an unforeseen destination, meaning that we have had more insights about ourselves and have received more than a 'simple award.' The most valuable part of this quest was, and still is, the journey itself."

Sidebar 3-4. The International Cardiac Surgery Benchmarking (ICSB) Project

High-risk clinical areas are ideal candidates for quality and safety improvement efforts. Recently, JCI began a benchmarking project that will enable hospitals to evaluate the current status of their coronary artery bypass graft (CABG) and valve surgery risk-adjusted mortality rates. The purpose of the project is to provide a quality improvement and benchmarking opportunity for JCI–accredited organizations performing CABG and cardiac valve procedures and encourage participating hospitals to implement quality programs and measure rates of improvement.

The project provides participating hospitals with information to assist them in assessing patients' risk factors and improving their quality of care. The long-term goal of the project is to support the improvement of outcomes of cardiac surgical procedures in accredited organizations.

As of this writing, the ICSB project is in the pilot phase, with the initial group of JCI–accredited hospitals located in Asia, Europe, Latin America, and the Middle East. The pilot phase of this project is anticipated to last 18 to 24 months from implementation.

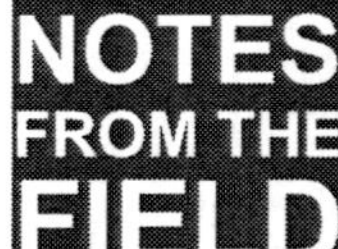

Changi General Hospital

As mentioned in Section 1 (*see* page 23), Changi General Hospital is a 788-bed 26-ward hospital located in Singapore. For more than 10 years, the organization has benchmarked itself against world-class standards of business excellence and quality, including those of the International Organization for Standardization (ISO). Seeking to benchmark itself against quality health care standards, Changi embarked on a journey toward JCI accreditation several years ago. JCI's focus on quality management, teamwork, staff and patient safety, patient satisfaction, continuity of care, and respecting the rights of patients and their families was aligned with the organization's quality vision.

A key aspect of Changi's accreditation journey is the organization's focus on performance measurement and improvement. One of the ways Changi tracks its performance is through the International Quality Indicator Project®, as well as through Specialty Specific Quality Indicators. Through these indicators, Changi measures how it is performing in key patient safety and quality care areas, such as ventilator-associated pneumonia, thrombolysis initiation within 1 hour of a patient presenting with acute myocardial infarction, CT/MRI for stroke within 24 hours of admission, unplanned readmissions, total inpatient mortality, perioperative mortality, and so forth.

As a result of its data collection and analysis process, the organization embarked on projects to improve patient and staff safety and deliver better care. Among the many projects are those involving medication safety, fire safety, and reduction of needlestick injuries among health care workers.

Reducing Needlestick Injuries

After Changi experienced an increase in needlestick injuries, from 45 cases to 78 cases in one year, a team was appointed to address the issue. The team determined that most needlestick injuries occurred during disposal and when a syringe and needle was used for venipuncture instead of using a blood collection needle system. As a result, Changi implemented the following changes:

- Reinforced the use and benefits of the blood collection needle system to minimize needle exposure and eliminate the transfer of blood specimens to a specimen container.
- Implemented use of a blood-taking tray with a customized sharps container for immediate disposal of sharps.
- Conducted road shows to improve needlestick awareness.
- Presented awards to departments that had no needlestick injuries for three months.
- Incorporated needlestick injury reduction as a departmental key performance indicator.
- Followed up on every needlestick injury to ensure that corrective actions were taken.

The team also benchmarked needlestick data against a local hospital that had a low needlestick rate.

After implementing these changes, Changi General Hospital experienced a reduction in needlestick injuries from 6.5 cases per month to 2.9 cases per month. This saved the organization almost US$15,000 per year.

SECTION 3

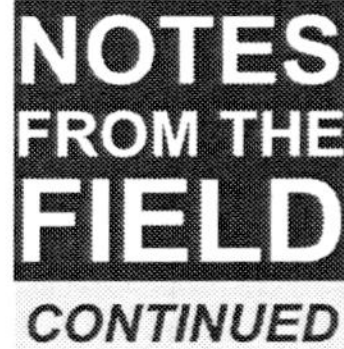

Culture of Safety Survey

Another way Changi measured its performance was through a culture of safety survey. The organization selected 287 Changi staff, ranging from medical consultants to health care attendants to engineers, to participate in the survey. Participants were selected through stratified, systematic, random sampling. The survey covered five dimensions of patient safety climate and used an anonymous, self-administered, 5-point Likert scale survey questionnaire that had been revised since an earlier survey process. Final data results were compared to the earlier results and served as a benchmark. The organization garnered a 92% response rate to the survey, with the rate varying by type of staff. For example, 100% of radiographers and house officers responded to the survey, while only 65% of medical officers did.

Within the survey, most staff acknowledged hospital senior management's commitment toward patient safety as a priority and confirmed that there is a link between patient safety and high-quality care. Staff indicated that there had been significant improvement in the medical error reporting system and improvement in resources and training to facilitate patient safety practices. Staff also communicated that greater progress can still be made to increase staff understanding that medical errors are due to systems failures rather than mistakes by individuals.

Findings from this study were used to review current staff workload as well as the availability of training to include all groups of staff.

As with the baseline assessment, how action plans are developed will vary from organization to organization. Some organizations may choose to create action plans as they progress through the baseline assessment, but others may go through the action-planning process after they are finished assessing all the standards. Creating action plans when compliance issues are identified helps ensure timely attention to areas that require improvement and results in more manageable projects. It also allows organizations to give immediate feedback to those involved in the processes or behaviors that are a cause for concern.

However, creating action plans after all of the standards have been assessed allows organizations to set improvement priorities and explore systems throughout the organization that relate to a particular standard or series of standards. This may lead to more comprehensive projects that address multiple standards at one time, thus making efficient use of different resources, such as staff time.

Developing a Detailed Plan

An appropriate and effective action plan includes the facts about the project and considers the "who," "when," and "how" of the plan (*see* Figure 3-1 on page 100). For example, the elements of the plan may include the following:

■ The name of the person or persons responsible for implementing the plan. Any action plan should have a champion who is in charge of recruiting others to help with implementation and driving the implementation process. Ideally, this individual should be committed to the project and have good people, time management, communication, and consensus-building skills. Who an organization chooses to champion a plan will depend on the organization, the standard, and the action plan. It is important, however, to consider involving physicians, staff members who provide care, and organization leaders. Regardless of who is chosen to oversee an action plan, organizations should be prepared for changes in the team as new champions emerge, and some leaders or participants depart.

■ The date by which the plan will be implemented. This date should take into consideration the scope of the compliance issue and the four-month record of compliance that JCI surveyors will be seeking when conducting the on-site accreditation survey.

■ The nature and scope of the compliance issue. Each measurable element that is identified as partially compliant or not compliant should be addressed. The problem should be outlined in a few sentences or even a paragraph, with attention focusing on how to correct the issue and validate the correction.

SECTION 3

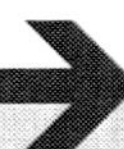 **ACCREDITATION STRATEGY**

Quality Monitors

Although data are important for the JCI survey process, organizations preparing for accreditation should not delay progress or improvement in order to meet the four-month record of compliance. Surveyors understand that new policies and procedures, better documentation methods, new types of training, and so on are continually introduced. In such instances, the look-back period would apply only to the introduction of the improvement at the time this improvement began.

This is particularly true for the quality monitors listed in the Quality Improvement and Patient Safety standards. For example, it is expected that the specific measure chosen that relates to anesthesia monitoring will change over time. JCI surveyors will want to know that anesthesia monitoring has been continuous over previous months, not that a particular monitor has been in use over a specific period. The surveyor would expect to see that the quality monitoring cycle—data collection, data analysis, improvement when indicated, and new data collection—has been ongoing even if the specific measure has changed.

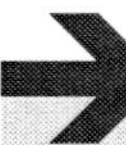 **ACCREDITATION STRATEGY**

Prioritizing High-Risk Issues

Depending on how many compliance issues need to be addressed and the resources of the organization, an organization may need to prioritize which issues are addressed first. When prioritizing, organizations should consider high-risk, problem-prone compliance issues first, as well as those that will take the longest time to address, such as the quality monitoring system for quality and patient safety measures.

■ How the organization will resolve the issue. Organizations can determine how to resolve the issue by asking the following questions:
  - What actions can bring the measurable element into compliance?
  - How will these actions bring the measurable element into compliance?

  These actions do not necessarily need to be complex or research supported, but they should fit the problem identified and be appropriate for the organization.
■ How the proposed actions will be implemented. (*See* page 102 for more information on implementation.)
■ How leaders and staff will be held accountable for accomplishing the plan
■ How the success of the plan will be measured. The action plan should contain measurable, objective criteria that will be used to show that the measurable elements are in compliance. For example, medical records, staff interviews, facility inspections, or performance improvement data—any data that can show a track record of compliance.

SECTION 3

Sidebar 3-5. Defining the Term *Action Plan*

An action plan is a detailed plan that outlines an organization's intentions and the activities that support those intentions to improve performance. Organizations have several different opportunities to use action plans. For example, action plans can be used to respond to a shortfall in standards compliance after the baseline assessment. They can also be used as a part of a root cause analysis (*see* Section 2). Within a root cause analysis action plan, an organization must identify the strategies the organization intends to implement to reduce the risk of the event under study from occurring in the future. A sample action plan is shown in Figure 3-1 on page 100.

Another type of action plan, called a Strategic Improvement Plan (SIP), is required in response to "Not Met" findings identified in the Official Survey Findings Report. (*See* more information on page 121.) This, too, requires detailed information on actions, oversight, and measures of success.

Regardless of when an organization uses an action plan, the basic structure is the same. Such a plan should address responsibility for implementation, oversight, pilot testing as appropriate, time lines, and strategies for measuring the effectiveness of the actions.

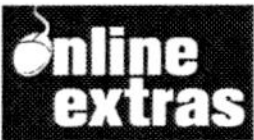 A useful template—the JCI Action Plan—is included in the Online Extras at www.jcrinc.com/JCIGS10/Extras.

In addition to these components, it may be helpful to identify how a measurable element was determined to be not compliant or partially compliant. Examining what data or criteria were used allows an organization to use this information when implementing the action plan. It also may be helpful to identify possible causes of the compliance problem. The focus should be on organization systems, rather than on individuals. For example, causes might relate to allocation of resources, lack of policies, or lack of leadership support. By examining possible causes, organizations may be able to identify a larger problem that should be addressed. Several areas of noncompliance around a particular issue may point to a system or organization problem.

Using a Team Approach to Creating an Action Plan

Action plans that result from the baseline assessment can be thought of as strategic priorities for the organization. These plans are more than just a means to achieve accreditation; the plans represent real opportunities for improved patient care and patient safety.

To successfully implement these plans, organizations must create an atmosphere that makes them an organizationwide priority. Using a team approach allows various staff members throughout the organization to unite to create achievable solutions, rather than simply carry out

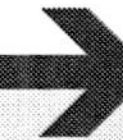

ACCREDITATION STRATEGY

Is the Issue Systemwide?

When creating an action plan, organizations may want to consider whether a deficiency identified during the baseline assessment is specific to the area in which it was identified or whether it is a system problem appropriate for organizationwide improvement. Give staff involved in creating and carrying out the action plan approximately one to two weeks to accomplish this task.

ACCREDITATION STRATEGY

Leveraging Technology

If available, organizations should consider using a software program, such as MS Project or Excel, to create, modify, and distribute the plan. This technology allows for easy updates to the plan and facilitates sharing between multiple parties. It also allows the plan to be confirmed in writing.

Figure 3-1. Sample Action Plan

Standard AOP.1.4

☐ Assessments are completed in the time frame prescribed by the organization.

Measurable Elements of AOP.1.4

☐ 1. Appropriate time frames for performing assessments are established for all settings and services.
☐ 2. Assessments are completed within the time frames established by the organization.
☐ 3. The findings of all assessments performed outside the organization are reviewed and/or verified at the time of admission to inpatient status.

Areas of Noncompliance

The organization does not consistently complete medical assessments within the 24-hour time frame prescribed by the organization. This issue was identified through interviews with staff members during the baseline assessment and chart reviews.

Action Plan

☐ 1. Meet with nursing and medical staff to discuss the approach to assessment in light of patient safety and quality of care.
☐ 2. Develop and/or revise in writing the time frame and criteria for a complete assessment.
☐ 3. Revise the medical assessment form to more clearly emphasize the time frame and criteria for performing a complete assessment.
☐ 4. Conduct an in-service for medical staff.

Due Date

4 January 2011

Responsible Individual

Medical Director

Data to Determine Compliance

Monthly audit of patient records indicating that 90% or more of all patients receive a complete medical assessment within 24 hours of inpatient admission

---

This example shows how a hospital might go about creating an action plan for an Assessment of Patients (AOP) standard found to be not compliant during the baseline assessment. Please note: This standard was effective for accredited hospitals as of the publication date of this product; see the appropriate updated JCI accreditation manual for the standard that is effective now.

orders from leadership. Staff can be creative in examining the problem and take pride in creating strategies for improving their jobs and, therefore, the care provided by the organization as a whole.

A team approach to action planning also brings specific problems to the attention of staff throughout the organization by taking these problems out of the realm of "JCI issues" or "that is the way it has always been" into the realm of problems that they can help solve. Team members can clearly understand how their daily work contributes to better care.

Choosing a team approach to the action planning process also allows the effort to include and leverage multiple perspectives. As previously mentioned, an organization should appoint a "champion" or someone who will be accountable for creating, implementing, and monitoring specific action plans. For a chapter relating to patient care, for example (such as the "Patient Care and Continuity of Care" [PCC] chapter for ambulatory programs; the "Care, Services, and Support" [CAS] chapter for care continuum programs; or the "Care of Patients" [COP] chapter for hospital programs), a nursing or physician leader might serve as the champion. This individual can then identify team members from throughout the organization who should be part of the action planning team.

When choosing members of an action planning team, champions should consider staff who see the organization's strengths and weaknesses related to the project on a daily basis as part of their jobs. These individuals are most qualified to develop and implement action plans that are meaningful to the organization. Such staff should not be limited to clinical areas. For example, staff from such areas as information technology, human resources, or environmental services, who may not consider themselves part of the standards evaluation and compliance process, may provide critical insight to improving performance. Staff in some areas within an organization might not immediately recognize how their work contributes to accreditation and improved care, but involvement in action planning can provide this understanding.

It can also be helpful to involve individuals who are skeptical of the issues in the improvement project on the action planning team. This will allow them to directly see the nature of the problem and how it can be addressed.

Action planning also helps leadership and managers by focusing their efforts. Supervisors, for example, can make a compelling case to leaders for investing time and resources to improve noncompliant areas. Or leaders can use the process as a tool to guide improvement and education efforts more effectively. By focusing on specific objectives, organizations can reinforce the idea of a systems approach to providing safe, high-quality care for patients that involves working across disciplines and departments in order to achieve stated goals.

Policies and Procedures

During the action planning process, it is often helpful for the quality improvement or accreditation specialist to compile a list of required policies and procedures that need to be either developed or revised. While JCI surveyors are most interested in how policies and procedures are carried out to benefit patients, these policies and procedures are a crucial starting point for accreditation preparation. This is

because they make clear how an organization operates, and they provide direction for leaders and staff.

As previously mentioned, organizations should be prepared to spend adequate time on the process of developing or revising policies and procedures, submitting the proposed policies and procedures for organizational review, testing as necessary, obtaining final approval for implementation, and educating staff on new policies to ensure understanding and compliance.

Consider the example of one organization that found it needed new policies and procedures for ensuring the qualifications of its 5,000 nurses. Establishing policies and procedures to address this accreditation requirement required significant time and planning. Not only were there large numbers of nursing qualifications to verify, but more than 85% of the organization's nurses are recruited from abroad—representing 35 countries. It was a major challenge for the organization and it took a lot of time to address the issue because there is no board of nursing in many countries. Instead, the organization had to establish its own system to ensure that licenses of all professional nurses were verified from their original source before nurses were allowed to practice within the organization

Being Transparent About Progress

Preparing action plans should be an open process in which staff and leadership are kept informed every step of the way. Quality and accreditation specialists should ensure that all members of an organization are aware of how preparation efforts are going and what work is necessary to

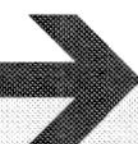

➤ ACCREDITATION STRATEGY

Make Sure Policy Reflects Practice

Often when organizations begin revising a policy, they turn to outside resources. This is a great starting place; however, it is important to remember that policies should reflect actual practices in the organization, as this is what JCI surveyors will evaluate an organization against during the accreditation survey. To ensure that policies reflect practice, organizations should test and revise them as necessary.

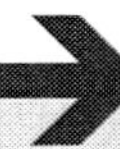

ACCREDITATION STRATEGY

Creating a Quality Council

To help prepare for accreditation, organizations may want to create a quality council. Although not required by the JCI standards, this interdisciplinary group can serve as a catalyst for quality improvement activities, taking responsibility for making final decisions. From the quality council, organizations can form task forces and committees related to each of the chapters in the accreditation manual. Made up of representatives from departments across the organization as well as organization leaders, these committees and task forces can then develop policies, procedures, and guidelines based on the requirements in each chapter. As a result of these committees, quality improvement discussions can become a regular part of the agenda at department meetings. Departments can take responsibility for developing specific continuous quality improvement projects, including developing methods for collecting measurable data to gauge progress.

achieve compliance and improve care. For example, information about what issues arose during the baseline assessment, how the organization plans to make improvements, and the results of those improvements should be shared with staff and leaders at regular intervals. Staff should be aware of how processes might be changing and why, so they can understand how improvement will influence the way they practice. Awareness increases when information is shared through multiple venues, such as newsletters, e-mails, posters, and so forth.

Action Planning Should Not Be a One-Time Exercise

Completing the baseline assessment and planning necessary improvement actions is just the beginning of preparation efforts for accreditation. Organizations should also consider strategies to sustain progress and identify areas requiring further attention. While each organization must create its own detailed plan to meet its own unique needs, consider the following ideas:

- Continue monitoring progress toward meeting JCI standards. For example, conduct a minievaluation of each chapter of the accreditation manual at regular intervals. This could be on a quarterly basis or, as the target date for accreditation approaches, on a monthly basis.

- Adjust the accreditation project plan. After getting started, it may become clear that changes in policies and procedures will take longer than expected. Or perhaps data collection efforts have revealed unexpected areas for improvement. Being realistic about the actions necessary and time needed to complete those actions will help keep accreditation efforts on track.

- Continue to involve as many staff as possible in the process. Making organizational quality a goal that can be achieved only by working together will ensure the success of projects.

Implementing Planned Actions

Although identifying areas of improvement and outlining action plans to achieve compliance are critical steps in preparing for JCI accreditation, implementing planned actions and measuring their success are even more important elements of the process. The implementation piece of the preparation efforts allows organizations to truly realize improvement and enhance safety and quality.

How an action plan is implemented will depend a lot on the nature of the issue being addressed, how much of the organization the issue affects, and whether the improvement project can be incorporated into an organizationwide improvement process. For example, improving an organization's informed consent policy may involve one or two individuals developing a draft and a small group reviewing, refining, testing, and finalizing it. Conversely, compliance issues associated with the medication management process may be addressed through an organizationwide improvement project designed to improve the safety of the medication management process.

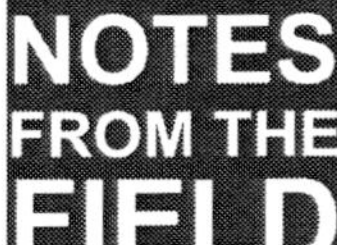

The Institute of Mental Health

Based in Woodbridge Hospital, the Institute of Mental Health (IMH) is the main psychiatric hospital in Singapore. It provides multidisciplinary, tertiary psychiatric services. More than five years ago, as IMH began its journey to prepare for JCI accreditation, IMH's nursing department decided to critically appraise its existing nursing competencies against JCI's Staff Qualifications and Education standards. Nursing leaders from the education, clinical, and management areas formed a work group to plan and design an organized, systematic, and comprehensive framework to ensure the delivery of competent to superior nursing care to the patients within the nurses' various psychiatric disciplines.

The work group's ultimate challenge was to develop competencies that support IMH nurses in achieving safe, high-quality, patient-centered care. Various resources were used, including JCI's standards, existing IMH practices, and an extensive literature review. The result of the task force's work was the Nursing Competency Assessment Checklists for two grades of staff—registered nurses and enrolled nurses. These checklists addressed competencies for newly recruited nurses as well as specialty areas, including child and adolescent psychiatric, psychiatric rehabilitation, and forensic psychiatric care, to name a few. (*See* Figure 1, below, and Figure 2 on page 104 for samples of some of the different competency checklists.)

Figure 1. A Sample Generic Competency Checklist for Registered Nurses

Section II: Generic Nursing Competency Assessment Checklist

* Competencies to be achieved within two months.

Designation and Name: ___________________ **Ward/Department:** ___________________
Date Commenced Work: ___________________

Evaluation Methods:
O – Observation
P – Paper-Pencil Test
R – Review Documentation in Chart
V – Verbal Discussion
RD – Return Demonstration

Items	Preceptor's Signature and Date	Evaluation Methods					Competent		Remarks
		O	P	R	V	RD	Yes	No	
1. Patient Management									
Perform patient assessment on admission to ward (refer to DNA P01 Admission)									
Perform history taking on admission (refer to DNA P01 Admission)									
Practice safekeeping of patients' properties (refer to DNA I07 Management of Patient's Property)									

Source: Institute of Mental Health, Singapore. Used with permission.

The development process of the competency checklists took about 14 weeks. During this time, there were numerous collaborative discussions, modifications, and validations of the competencies with clinical experts and frontline staff. These efforts facilitated the development of a tool that is comprehensive, is user friendly, and can best support the nurses' chances of achieving higher standards of performance.

(continued on page 104)

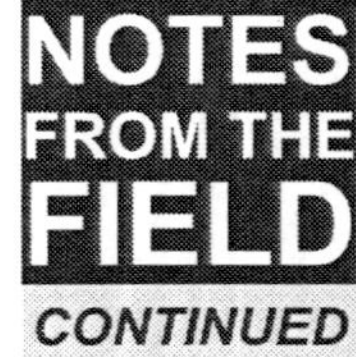

After the checklists were developed, the organization had the large task of identifying and providing training to bridge practice gaps for all the clinical staff. To ensure buy-in from the nurses, several workshops were conducted to introduce and familiarize nurses with the new checklists. Continuous training and "road shows" were conducted to disseminate to the nurses this new assessment paradigm. This quickly led to mass acceptance and mind-set change and corresponding boosts in the nurses' confidence level.

IMH Nursing Competency Assessment Checklists developed professionalism and advanced training opportunities for the nurses to achieve evidence-based, standardized, patient-centered care. However, the development of appropriate evaluation tools to measure competence remains the challenge now. It therefore behooves the nursing leadership to continue to challenge paradigms, review existing processes, and devise innovative approaches to foster a climate of continual growth and learning. This in turn will help develop competent nurses who are always prepared with the most current information and training.

Figure 2. A Sample Psychiatric-Specific Competency Checklist of Registered Nurses

Section III: Psychiatric-Specific Nursing Competency Assessment Checklist

* Competencies to be achieved within three months.

Designation and Name: ____________________ **Ward/Department:** ____________________
Date Commenced Work: ____________________

Evaluation Methods:
O – Observation
P – Paper-Pencil Test
R – Review Documentation in Chart
V – Verbal Discussion
RD – Return Demonstration

Items	Preceptor's Signature and Date	Evaluation Methods					Competent		Remarks
		O	P	R	V	RD	Yes	No	
1. Therapeutic Use of Self									
Verbalize knowledge and application of therapeutic nurse patient relationship									
Verbalize the dynamics of human behavior									
Recognize and identify own feelings									
Recognize and identify feelings of others									
Recognize the effect of one's behavior on others e.g. client/family, staff									
Demonstrate empathy, warmth and respect during patient interactions									
Utilize, as appropriate, problem-solving techniques during interactions									
Identify individuals' communication limitations and utilizes alternative forms of communication as appropriate									

Source: Institute of Mental Health, Singapore. Used with permission.

There are several tools available that can help organizations with their implementation efforts. While the scope of this publication does not allow an in-depth discussion of these tools, following is a brief overview of five tools with which quality/accreditation specialists should be familiar.

Plan-Do-Study-Act

Perhaps the most famous implementation tool is known as the plan-do-study-act (PDSA) cycle. Based on the scientific method, this well-established process for improvement can help guide the implementation process and ensure that any changes are effective. Development of the PDSA cycle (also called the PDCA cycle, with the word *check* replacing the word *study*) is attributed to Walter Shewhart, a quality improvement pioneer with the U.S.-based company Bell Laboratories in the 1920s and 1930s. The cycle is also widely associated with W. Edwards Deming, student and colleague of Shewhart.

The PDSA cycle includes the following aspects:

- "Plan" refers to first understanding the process, then proposing an improvement, and finally deciding how an improvement action will be tested and how data will be collected to determine what effect the action has on the process.
- "Do" means to perform the test by implementing the action on a small scale.
- "Study" involves analyzing the effect of the action being tested.
- "Act" means to fully implement the action or reassess the improvement action taken and perhaps then choose another action.

The cycle is continuous and can be entered at any point. PDSA cycles are meant to test changes on a small scale to see if they result in improvement. Small-scale tests may involve 1 individual or 10 individuals and should never be considered successes or failures but merely opportunities for learning.

When implementing a complicated process, organizations should plan for multiple PDSA cycles, with each cycle focusing on one aspect of the process. Testing changes in this way can help verify that a change will result in improvement, predict how much improvement can be expected from a change, and minimize resistance upon full implementation.

After testing a change on a small scale, learning from each test, and refining the change through several PDSA cycles, organizations can implement the change on a broader scale—for example, for an entire pilot population or on an entire unit.[3]

Lean Thinking

Lean thinking, sometimes known as Lean methodology or simply Lean, was developed initially in the 1930s as a response to the need to eliminate waste and improve quality in manufacturing. Since the 1980s, it has been expanded and adapted to meet the needs of the health care profession. Lean thinking embraces the concept of "doing more with less"—less human effort, less time, less space, less equipment—while providing customers with exactly what they want when they want it. Translated to health care, Lean thinking emphasizes patient service, safety standards, improved quality, staff satisfaction, and economic vitality.

A primary concept underlying Lean thinking is the elimination of waste. In fact, proponents of Lean thinking, not only in Japan but everywhere, use the Japanese word for waste—*muda*—when discussing any activity that uses resources but creates no value. In other words, *muda* is anything that creates mistakes, stockpiles unnecessary inventory, requires unnecessary process steps, moves employees from one place to another for no logical reason, forces workers to wait for an earlier snag to be fixed, or produces products/services that do not meet the demands of the customer. The rationale behind eliminating waste is that, by so doing, an organization can carry out the task of providing the customers/patients with what they want when they want it with the minimum of resources.

Lean methodology departs from the usual practice of convincing the customers to accept products or services that an organization already provides or wants to provide. Instead, Lean thinking turns the concept around and begins with the customers, asking them what they want and how and when they want it. In other words, the customers become the focus, and they specify value in the end "product."

Lean thinking in health care is one effective way to enhance patient safety. Because multiple steps in a process can lead to multiple opportunities for errors, and Lean thinking reduces steps, Lean thinking therefore reduces opportunities for errors. In addition, Lean thinking exposes waste, flaws, and barriers. As staff members tackle these impediments, they begin to perfect processes and make them more patient focused.[4]

The Lean thinking system also delivers fast and dramatic results. Careful preplanning, and critical examination of the value-added and non–value-added aspects of a process, can provide improvement in a matter of days—rather than weeks or months—without closing down a function or department.

Lean thinking also engages and empowers staff members at all levels—from senior managers to frontline staff. Consequently, organizations adopting Lean thinking have often developed improvement *cultures*, not just improvement training or programs. (*See* page 106 for an example of one organization that used Lean methodology to realize organizationwide improvement.)

Six Sigma

Developed by Motorola and adopted by General Electric, Six Sigma is a quality measurement and improvement program that aims to improve the capability of business processes. Fundamentally, Six Sigma focuses on making every step in a process as reliable as it can be. There is often

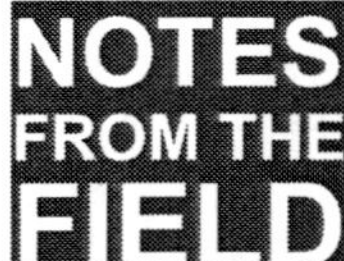

Singapore General Hospital

Singapore General Hospital is a 1,400-bed acute tertiary care public hospital. Besides being the largest hospital in Singapore, it is also the oldest, at more than 180 years. It has long been a health care institution that the public has looked up to and trusted for quality care.

Although it is a public hospital, it also attracts patients from outside Singapore because of its reputation for its standard of care in various medical and surgical specialties. The hospital started its quality journey as early as 1996 by attaining International Organization for Standardization (ISO) 9001 certification, and then in subsequent years it obtained other certifications, including Singapore Quality Class, ISO 14001, College of American Pathologists, and Hazard Analysis and Critical Control Points.

Singapore General Hospital chose to pursue JCI accreditation to affirm its belief, as well as the public's, that it is an excellent organization that delivers care with a patient-centered focus. This is in line with the mission statement: "We deliver quality care to every patient through comprehensive integrated clinical practice, medical innovation, and lifelong learning," as well as the vision statement: "To be a renowned organization at the leading edge of medicine, providing quality health care to meet our nation's needs."

Within Singapore General Hospital, incremental improvement is achieved through numerous quality improvement projects conducted by cross-functional teams using the rapid plan-do-check-act cycle (*see* pages 104–105 for more information on PDCA). These projects are initiated primarily by staff and arise from the identification of improvement opportunities through suggestions or analysis of performance indicators. Successful projects are shared at monthly Quality Showcase meetings or during the organization's annual Quality Week. Projects are also featured in presentations at selected quality conferences. Examples include such innovative initiatives as early ambulation of postoperative orthopedic patients, which won the 2005 Hospital Management Asia Award for Customer Service Project; improving cholectomy clinical pathway utilization; improving hand-hygiene compliance; and reducing health care–associated, methicillin-resistant *Staphylococcus aureus* infections.

The organization also uses Lean thinking (*see* page 105) to improve performance throughout the organization. Examples of successful projects using Lean thinking include early discharge of inpatients by 11 A.M. instead of the previous 1 P.M. discharge time, and timely arrival of first case patients at the operating theaters. These projects are large scale and driven mainly by management, with the participation of key staff from selected areas. This model of quality improvement has worked well for the hospital in ensuring a healthy growth gradient of improvement across the facility.

confusion between Lean thinking and Six Sigma. One easy way to remember remember which is which is that Lean helps reduce waste, while Six Sigma increases reliability by reducing variation.

Six Sigma focuses on high-quality production and depends heavily on statistical data to measure success. Six Sigma accomplishes its goals by means of improvement projects, which apply two Six Sigma improvement methods: define, measure, analyze, improve, control (DMAIC)

and define, measure, analyze, design, verify (DMADV). The DMAIC process is an improvement system for existing processes that do not meet specifications and therefore need improvement. DMADV is a system to develop new products or processes to Six Sigma specifications.

Case histories show that implementing Six Sigma methods have saved companies more than US$200,000 per project and have permitted trained employees to complete four to six performance improvement projects per year. Furthermore, the focus on statistical data and verification is particularly relevant to performance improvement programs in health care settings because it provides a balance to more intuitive improvement methods.[5]

Beginning on page 108 is a case study demonstrating how Apollo Hospitals, which at the time of this publication had seven JCI–accredited hospitals in India and Bangladesh, used Six Sigma as part of a larger performance improvement project to reduce ventilator-associated pneumonia (VAP) in its organizations.

Lean/Six Sigma

Sometimes it is difficult for an organization to select the most appropriate quality improvement and implementation method for its needs. Many companies, deciding that a combination of methods may be the most suitable, recognize that Lean thinking and Six Sigma work well together. As a team, these strategies can help organizations achieve rapid product/service improvement and better product/service consistencies. Lean aims for zero waste; Six Sigma aims for zero defects. Lean encourages improvement as the outcome of a broad horizontal process directed by an empowered staff at all levels, from management to front-line team members. Six Sigma employs statistical analysis and analytical discipline to identify root causes of problems and incorporate improvement strategies. Together, the tools of each system maximize the improvement outcomes.

An additional benefit is that the methods overlap. Lean's ongoing efforts to eliminate waste contribute to Six Sigma's effort to reduce variations. In addition, just as Six Sigma strives for zero defects, Lean, too, tries to prevent errors. In many cases, combining the two methods results in a process improvement methodology that, under the right circumstances, can be more effective than either method alone.[6]

Robust Process Improvement

Robust Process Improvement™ (RPI) is The Joint Commission's—JCI's United States–based parent—systematic methodology for improving business processes and seeks to continuously increase the quality and efficiency of products and services. The successful adoption of RPI techniques can produce substantial improvements in the quality of processes and products as well as increase consistent effectiveness of customer service.

RPI consist of a set of strategies, tools, methods, and training programs aimed at achieving the following:

- Recognizing and seeking the voice of the customer
- Defining factors critical to quality
- Using data and data analysis to design improvement
- Enlisting stakeholders and process owners in creating and sustaining solutions
- Eliminating defects and waste
- Drastically decreasing failure rates
- Simplifying and increasing the speed of processes
- Partnering with staff and leaders to seek, commit to, and accept change

For more information on this process, go to http://www.centerfortransforminghealthcare.org/about/qualitysolutions.aspx.

Although using a formalized implementation strategy, such as the ones discussed earlier in this chapter, is not a JCI requirement, these tools can help organizations focus their implementation efforts and ensure an efficient, effective, and appropriate process that results in improved safety and quality. Using these processes can also help reinforce a culture of safety in which organizations are transparent about issues and actively work to proactively reduce risk.

Training Is Critical Within Implementation Efforts

Humans resist change. To do so is a natural response that everyone experiences to some degree. For this reason, it is important for health care organizations to empower staff to embrace change during implementation processes. That empowerment comes from education and familiarity with change concepts. Whether an organization uses a formalized implementation method or not, staff throughout the organization should be familiar with whatever implementation strategies the organization uses and understand how to use those strategies effectively. In addition, staff should be educated on the details of new processes, procedures, or policies and how they affect their day-to-day work.

Staff need to be reassured that it is natural to feel uncertain about change and that others across the organization are likely feeling the same way. By following a specific strategy for change, processes can be implemented incrementally, resulting in a smoother transition to a higher level of care.

To help with implementation efforts, one organization—Changi General Hospital in Singapore—produced a publication, the *CGH Pocket Guide*. This is a 20-page,

Case Study 3-1. A Project to Reduce Ventilator-Associated Pneumonia (VAP) at Apollo Hospitals

by Gaurav Loria, Quality Coordinator, Apollo Hospitals Group

Organization Name: Apollo Hospitals Group
Location: Chennai, India
About Apollo Hospitals Group: The Apollo Hospitals Group includes 46 hospitals with more than 8,000 beds in India and elsewhere, including Bangladesh. At the time of this publication, 7 hospitals in the Apollo Hospitals Group—including Apollo Hospitals, Hyderabad (where this project was implemented)—were accredited by JCI.

Project Description

The standard treatment for patients who are unable to breathe on their own is to sedate them and put them on a ventilator. The longer a patient is on a ventilator, the less his or her lungs will work naturally. There is a "honeymoon" period during which it is advisable to be on a ventilator; after that, however, patients who are not weaned off ventilation soon enough are in danger of developing many complications, including VAP, internal infections, oral ulcers, pressure ulcers (bed sores), and more.

VAP has been shown to increase intensive care unit length of stay (ICU LOS), the cost of treatment, and patient mortality. As patient days increase in number, the cost to treat the patient goes up due to the increasing number of bed turns (the number of days a patient occupies a bed). The number of ventilator days is directly proportional to ICU LOS, and as the ventilator days increase VAP rates also increase.

In February 2009, Apollo Hospitals began a project to reduce the number of ventilator days in ICUs in order to decrease the chances of VAP by 50%. A secondary goal of the project was to reduce the overall ICU LOS and mortality rate. When the project began, ICU LOS at Apollo Hospitals was on average 3.9 days, the total number of ventilator days was 357, and the mortality rate was 12% for ventilated patients. Apollo Hospitals hoped its improvement project would translate to fewer complications and improved quality of patient care. Leadership also hoped to improve the hospital's bottom line by decreasing the cost per case and lowering the cost of care to the end user—the patient—through shorter stays, fewer procedures, and less follow-up care.

Project Method

Apollo Hospitals adopted a Six Sigma strategy for defect reduction in its VAP procedure, using the DMAIC project methodology as follows:

Define

During the *define* stage, the organization identified the problem and contributing factors using the following processes:

- **Completing the project charter**—Laying out the team's mission and goals (as identified earlier)
- **Conducting an infection control risk assessment**—The organization performed a thorough infection control risk assessment in the ICU, examining the following areas of risk:
  - Surveillance indices
  - Communicable diseases
  - Hand hygiene
  - Compliance with International Patient Safety Goal 5 (IPSG.5), Reduce the Risk of Health Care–Associated Infections (*see* Section 1)

  Scoring was done on the basis of the following:
  - Probability of occurrence
  - Potential severity
  - Required organizational care response
  - Preparedness
- **Developing a "Suppliers, Inputs, Processes, Outputs, Customers" (SIPOC) map**—Identifying all suppliers, inputs, processes, outputs, and customers involved (*see* Figure 1 on page 109).
- **Creating a macro-level process map**—A visual representation of the task sequence, including people, duties, and transactions, involved in delivering the ventilator assistance.
- **Creating a fishbone diagram**—Another visual representation of causes to discover the

Case Study 3-1. A Project to Reduce Ventilator-Associated Pneumonia (VAP) at Apollo Hospitals, *continued*

ultimate root causes of the defect (*see* Figure 2 on page 110)

Measure

The organization developed a process map using a visual dashboard and infection control surveillance tool (*see* Figure 3 on page 111).

Analyze

The organization analyzed data on ICU LOS and mortality and also performed a cost analysis, using failure mode and effects analysis (FMEA) for patients on ventilators for more than 48 hours, as shown in Table 1 on page 111.

Because the risk priority numbers were highest for the categories "No proper follow-up as per protocol" and "Lack of hand hygiene," Apollo Hospitals focused most of its attention on these two factors.

The organization also included the other risk points in one way or another in all other programs.

Improve

As a result of the project, Apollo Hospitals implemented the following improvements:

- ⮑ Instituted the VAP green star project in all three ICUs, which consisted of the complete implementation of protocols, training, strict monitoring, and using the green star dashboards. The infection control team, the intern in charge, and a quality department representative conducted three inspections per day, the results of which were communicated directly to the chief executive officer.

- ⮑ Enforced strict compliance with the VAP bundle by the Institute for Healthcare Improvement.[1]

- ⮑ Devised and executed a hand-hygiene study in the ICUs consisting of daily surveillance by a "mystery shopper"—an observer whose role was unknown to staff—who reported findings to management. As a result, hand-hygiene compliance increased from 68% to 82% in 30 days.

- ⮑ Initiated interdisciplinary rounds (IDR). These consisted of daily rounds by an infection control nurse, an intensivist, and a pharmacologist (to check on all ventilated cases and antibiotics).

- ⮑ Instituted an Infection Control Week. During this week, VAP training was given to applicable staff. Other educational events and tools were also employed, such as hanging educational/reminder posters throughout the organization, distributing VAP–themed crossword puzzles and quizzes to staff, and inviting staff to share their VAP thoughts and concerns with leaders.

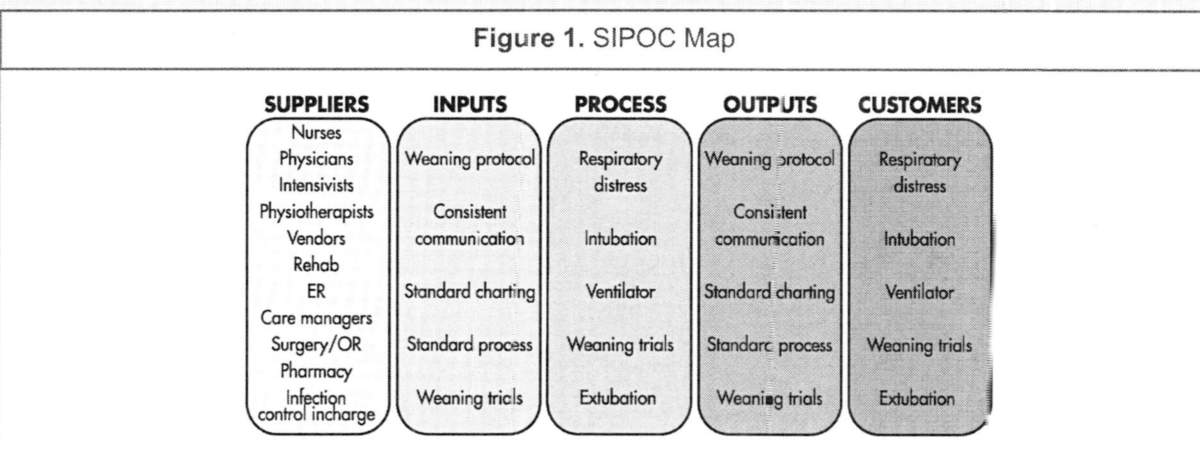

Figure 1. SIPOC Map

Source: Apollo Hospitals Group, Chennai, India. Used with permission.

(continued on page 110)

Case Study 3-1. **A Project to Reduce Ventilator-Associated Pneumonia (VAP) at Apollo Hospitals, *continued***

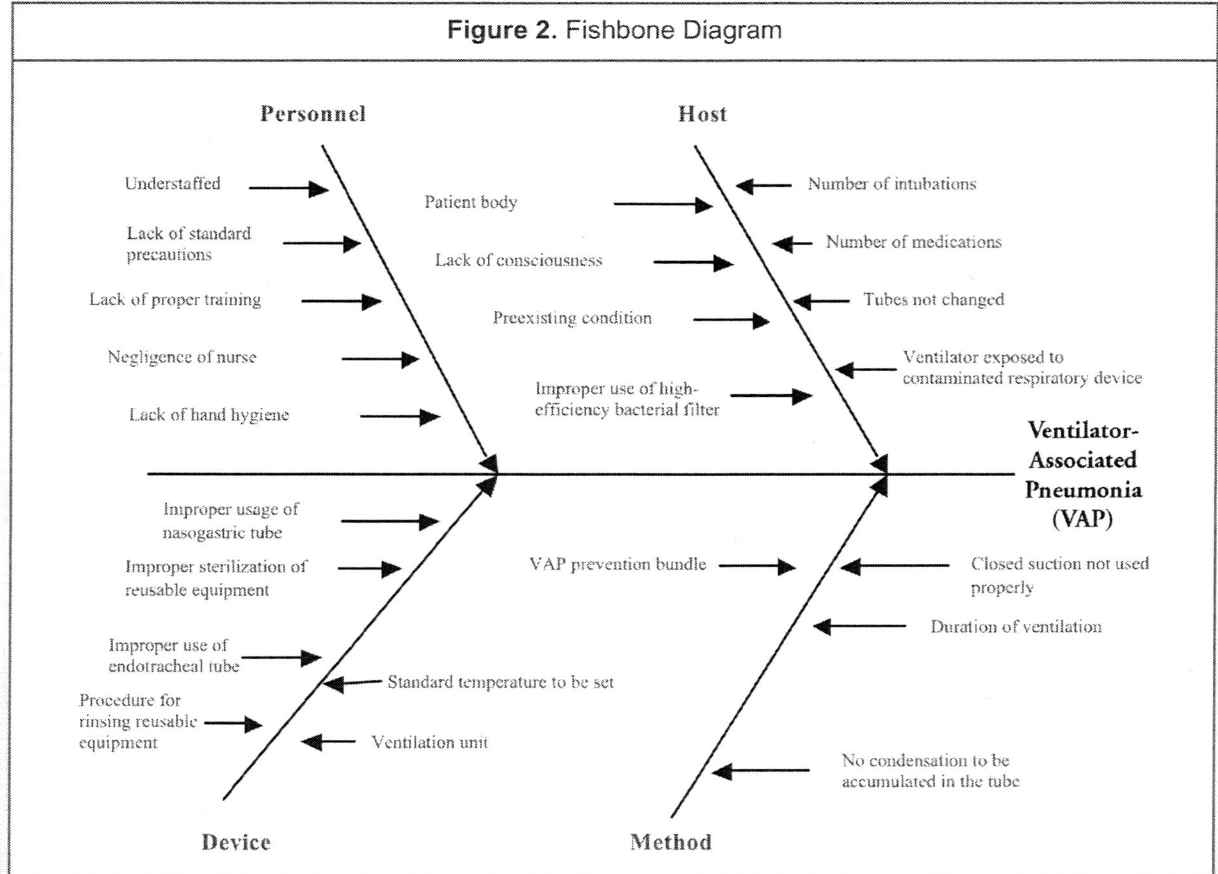

Figure 2. Fishbone Diagram

Source: Apollo Hospitals Group, Chennai, India. Used with permission.

- ➲ Conducted a certificate course in hospital epidemiology and infection control for applicable staff.
- ➲ Created and distributed a monthly VAP dashboard to make the entire organization aware of results and to reward the best-performing staff.

Control

In the *control* phase, Apollo Hospitals continued the following initiatives:
- ➲ Strict monitoring
- ➲ Including infection control on monthly performance dashboards of each unit
- ➲ Continuous training

- ➲ Separate module of training included in new staff orientation
- ➲ Daily rounds
- ➲ Letters from CEO to specific leaders or staff if they are not doing their work as they are supposed to do
- ➲ Daily data analysis
- ➲ Dedicated team to perform these functions

Apollo also extended its efforts to other areas of the organization, which were very successful.

Results of the Project

The results of the project are as follows:

Case Study 3-1. A Project to Reduce Ventilator-Associated Pneumonia (VAP) at Apollo Hospitals, *continued*

Figure 3. Daily Infection Control Surveillance for Ventilator-Associated Pneumonia Patients

Patient Number	Patient Name/Age	Diagnosis	Comorbid Condition	VAP Yes No	Date/Time of Intervention with VAP Bundle	Outcome	Remarks

Source: Apollo Hospitals Group, Chennai, India. Used with permission.

Table 1. FMEA for Patients on Ventilators for More Than 48 Hours

Failure Mode	Effect	Severity Rating*	Classification	Cause(s)	Occurrence Rating*	Detection Rating*	Risk Priority Number†	Recommended Actions
No proper follow-up as per protocol	VAP	8	Critical	Ignorance	7	6	336	Constant monitoring; should comply with the VAP bundle
Patient body posture	Increase in bacterial passage	6	Critical	Increased workload, ignorance	4	4	96	Maintain 30° head-of-bed elevation
Lack of hand hygiene	Improper treatment, discomfort to patient	7	Critical	Unaware of procedure, increased workload	7	6	294	Retraining to be given to nurses and newly appointed nurses
Lack of standard precaution	Improper treatment, death	6	Critical	Unaware of procedure	4	6	144	Display of charts in ICU, training, monitoring
Condensation accumulated in tube to be removed	Allows free passage of bacteria	4	Critical	Ignorance, lack of proper training	5	4	80	Tube to be changed within 48 hours, filter to be changed within 24 hours
Rinsing reusable equipment	Increased rate of infection	5	Critical	Unavailability of sterile equipment, ignorance of caregiver	5	5	125	Rechecking to be done before use
Improper antiseptic mouthwash	Improper treatment, VAP	6	Critical	Lack of knowledge about the procedure, increased workload, ignorance	3	8	144	To be done every 3–4 hours, conducting oral hygiene program, constant monitoring
No proper selective decontamination of digestive tract	VAP	4	Critical	Improper training provided to new caregivers, ignorance	5	6	120	Selective digestive tract disinfection (SDD) to be done regularly following proper procedure
Insertion of nonsterile catheter	VAP	4	Critical	Improper checking done	6	7	168	2 nurses required for suctioning

*Ratings are on a 1–10 scale, with 10 = most severe ("very high severity ranking when a potential failure mode affects safe system operation without warning"), 5 = low severity ("system inoperable without damage"), and 1 = no severity ("no effect").

†Risk Priority Number = Severity x Occurrence x Detection.

Source: Apollo Hospitals Group, Chennai, India. Used with permission.

(continued on page 112)

<table>
<tr><td>Case Study 3-1.</td><td>A Project to Reduce Ventilator-Associated Pneumonia (VAP) at Apollo Hospitals, continued</td></tr>
</table>

- ➲ The organization reached and has sustained a VAP rate as low as 2.1 device days (reaching zero at times in some ICUs) and an ICU LOS of 2.3 days for these patients.
- ➲ Bed turns increased an average of 1.5 times in all three ICUs.
- ➲ ICU infection rates decreased by 50%, and overall billing to ICU patients decreased by 57%.

- ➲ On the whole, the average number of ventilator days was reduced by 50% to 7 days.
- ➲ Six Sigma level was achieved.

Reference

1. Institute for Healthcare Improvement: *Implement the Ventilator Bundle.* http://www.ihi.org/IHI/Topics/CriticalCare/ IntensiveCare/Changes/ImplementtheVentilator Bundle.htm (accessed 21 May 2010).

Author's note: The author extends gratitude to K. Hari Prasad, M.D., Chief Executive Officer, Apollo Health City, for permitting the study and is grateful for the hard work put in by the complete hospital team, including infection control in-charges, Dr. Ratna Rao, Dr. Ratnamani, Dr. Saritha, Dr. Sanjiv, Ms. Remya, all infection control nurses, intensive care unit in-charges, and the intensive care unit teams.

pocket-sized manual containing materials essential to working in what hospital management feels is an environment "good enough for our own mothers." (Samples from that booklet are featured in the case study on Changi General Hospital on pages 23–30.)

Conducting a Mock Survey

Overall, the best way to prepare for a JCI survey is to consistently assess, monitor, and improve the systems and processes already in place to provide safe, high-quality care. In other words, using JCI standards as a basis for routine operations "prepares" an organization for survey.

With that said, however, some organization find it beneficial to conduct a mock survey—a trial run of the on-site survey which helps the organization see if the standards are being met in practice. Although this is not a JCI requirement, this approach does provide a method for identifying areas of noncompliance, assessing improvement efforts, preparing staff for the survey process, getting familiar with the standards scoring process, and increasing staff comfort in speaking with surveyors.

The process for conducting a mock survey should follow the model for the baseline assessment described earlier—that is, addressing organization adherence to JCI standards in day-to-day operations.

To help the mock survey mirror an actual accreditation survey, organizations can use the JCI accreditation manual and the JCI survey process guide that all organizations receive when applying for accreditation. The survey process guide provides a sample survey agenda and explains each portion of the survey, from the opening conference to the facility tour, from the leadership interview to the closing conference. (More information on these guides can be found on page 76.) The guide also contains survey planning reference lists that detail required quality monitors; organization plans; policies, procedures, written documents, or bylaws; and a law and regulation worksheet.

Within the mock survey, organizations may want to score the standards as a surveyor would score them during the actual on-site survey. (*See* Sidebar 3-6 on pages 115–116 for information about the scoring process.) This can help staff and leadership become familiar with the scoring process and what it means for compliance.

A mock survey should result in a detailed document of mock survey results. From these results, organizations most likely will need to do further action planning to determine how to resolve the issues that were revealed during the mock survey process and set aside time and resources for implementation. It's very important that someone in an oversight position in leadership makes sure that the resulting action plans are implemented.

ACCREDITATION STRATEGY

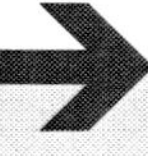

Sharing Best Practices

To help staff educate each other about change management, quality/accreditation specialists should encourage staff to share their best practices with others in the organization. These strategies could be posted on the intranet, distributed at staff meetings, or included as part of in-service training sessions.

Some organizations have a second mock survey after they believe that most of their issues in the first mock survey are resolved to see if performance is truly consistent throughout the organization.

Approximately four to six months before the actual survey, an organization may want to do a "dress rehearsal"—the final mock survey, evaluating everything, including what was proposed in the action plans. The organization will thus have time to fix anything that isn't compliant prior to its actual survey.

It may be useful for the final mock survey to use evaluators who were not involved in the baseline assessment and accreditation preparations that have taken place to date. These evaluators could be internal staff or external consultants. The idea in turning to other individuals to conduct the mock survey is to find evaluators who will look at the organization objectively, without the unintended biases or attachments that may come from having participated in the baseline assessment and other accreditation preparation efforts.

After completing the final mock survey, organizations should plan for any final revisions to systems, policies, procedures, and so forth. The process for any improvements after the final mock survey should follow the model for the action planning described earlier.

The weeks and months following the final mock survey and leading up to the JCI survey offer new opportunities to bring specific problems to the attention of staff, consider new methods for achieving organization goals, and make improvements.

Encourage Staff to Participate in Mock Surveys

Involving staff in mock surveys makes them part of the accreditation preparation process. This enhances individual learning and can serve as a powerful vehicle for knowledge retention and staff acceptance of accreditation. Sharing information during and after mock surveys helps foster understanding about the standards and the role they play in daily operations. By sharing this information, organizations can help staff better understand how JCI accreditation works and how their daily duties contribute to delivering care that improves patient outcomes and reduces risks. Staff on the front lines of care can be valuable in conducting mock surveys, or staff who might not ordinarily be involved in the accreditation process can be asked to serve on the mock survey planning team.

Using Tracer Methodology During the Mock Survey

As discussed in Section 1, tracer methodology is a focused survey tool that provides a framework for JCI surveyors to assess standards compliance and patient safety during on-site surveys. The tracer process allows surveyors to select a patient and use that individual's record as a road map. This guides the surveyor through an organization to assess and evaluate the organization's compliance with selected standards and the organization's systems of providing care and services.

Tracer methodology is not just for surveyors. Organizations can benefit from applying this methodology to self-assessment activities, including mock surveys. There are many benefits to conducting mock tracers, including the following:

- Connects actual patient care to specific JCI standards, strengthening the connection between standards and patient care in the minds of staff. This also helps staff better understand how their actions have an impact on safety and quality, even after they leave a patient's bedside.

- Helps determine how well performance matches process design in delivering safe, high-quality care.

- Encourages a continuous standards compliance approach rather than simply preparing for the survey "exam" on a periodic basis. This improves the ability of organizations to deliver safe, effective care every day.

- Offers insight into how surveyors conduct their evaluation.

- Spurs new ideas for process improvements.

Managing Change

Have your staff know how to manage change. First-line managers tend to have the biggest job, and we rarely give them the training they deserve. They are among the least experienced—they are told to change, and staff members tell them they don't want to change, so they're in the middle. The manager of a unit, supervisor of the night shift, the person to whom staff report directly: They are the first step.

—Helen Hoesing, R.N., M.P.H., Ph.D.,
JCI Senior Consultant

How to conduct a tracer. The following five tracer steps can be used for self-assessment purposes to evaluate performance and make necessary improvements:

1. Select current patients within the organization who have received care across a number of departments and consider which organizational systems or processes are used to deliver the necessary services for those patients.

2. Plan the tracers. This process involves listing all of the disciplines and areas involved in the patient's care, applicable JCI standards and International Patient Safety Goals, and relevant staff.

3. Conduct the tracers. A designated person familiar with JCI standards should visit the areas involved in the mock tracers, interview staff, and conduct any follow-up.

4. Analyze results to identify areas for improvement. Information gleaned from the mock tracers can be used to identify trends and prioritize improvement efforts.

5. Document next steps. After determining areas of improvement, organizations should outline how they plan to pursue those areas. This may involve creating action plans.

> **Online extras** Figure 3-2 on page 118 offers a tool to help plan for the tracer activity. More tools can be found in the Online Extras at www.jcrinc.com/JCIGS10/Extras.

Tips for conducting an effective mock tracer.

Although every tracer will be slightly different depending on the patient or system being traced, organizations can

Mock Surveys

Mock surveys are extremely important, but only after a considerable amount of foundation work is done. First, there's the need to educate staff, leaders, and physicians to the JCI standards. Then, your lead person or team does an initial assessment to determine the level of compliance with the standards and measurable elements, which results in identification of the priority areas for improvement. When those steps have been taken, when priority areas are completely addressed, and when processes are changed and implemented, you are ready for a mock survey.

—Bruce Frederick, R.N., M.N.,
JCI Consultant

make the most of the tracer methodology by consider the following strategies:

- Trace the patient, not departments.
- Ask open-ended questions.
- Use different ways of asking for information and encourage staff to provide different evidence of standards compliance.
- Listen to staff answers—the answers may be unexpected.
- Ask staff to provide documents and policies and demonstrate a process.
- Involve staff in conducting the tracers. As in the mock surveys, staff conducting mock tracers can work together to come up with the types of questions surveyors might ask. For example, if a hospital performing a mock tracer selects the record of a 60-year-old male admitted through the emergency department with cardiac disease, who went to the cardiac catheter lab, the operating room, and the intensive care unit before developing VAP, how does this patient's care relate to standards found in the "Assessment of Patients," "Care of Patients," "Prevention and Control of Infections," and "Staff Qualifications and Education" chapters of the hospital accreditation manual? The mock tracer team can go through each of the standards in these areas to determine compliance and develop questions.
- Validate discrepancies from policy, best practices, or systems failures.

Sidebar 3-6. The Scoring Process

During the on-site survey, each standard and International Patient Safety Goal is scored based on whether or not the measurable elements of the standard are met, partially met, or not met, and the organization demonstrates acceptable compliance with each standard. A score of at least "5" on each standard is considered acceptable compliance.

As previously mentioned, measurable elements (MEs) are the components of the standard that are scored by the surveyors on site. Each standard *and* each ME of a standard is scored "Fully Met," "Partially Met," "Not Met," or "Not Applicable" as follows:

- 0 = Noncompliance or "Not Met"
- 5 = Partial Compliance or "Partially Met"
- 10 = Satisfactory Compliance or "Fully Met"

The following are some further guidelines for the scoring for both standards and the International Patient Safety Goals:

- The use of percentages or numbers is not absolute. For example, 12 incomplete orders by one physician (could be "Partially Met") should be considered differently than 12 incomplete orders by 12 physicians (could be "Not Met" if 12 out of 14 physician records were reviewed).
- Sometimes it is the criticality of the finding rather than the number that is weighted. For example, 2 exits blocked out of 12 total exits could become a "Not Met" finding if the exits are considered critical points of egress by the on-site surveyor.

"Fully Met" Score

An ME is scored "Fully Met" if the answer is "Yes" or "Always" to the specific requirements of the ME. Also considered are the following:

- A single negative observation may not prevent a score of "Fully Met" (*also see* Consideration of Impact and Criticality below).
- If 90% or more (for example, 9 out of 10) of observations or records are met

The track record related to a score of "Fully Met" is as follows:

- A 12-month look-back period of compliance for triennial surveys
- A 4-month look-back period of compliance for initial surveys

"Partially Met" Score

An ME is scored "Partially Met" if the answer is "Usually" or "Sometimes" to the specific requirements of the ME. Also considered are the following:

- If 50% to 89% (for example, 5 through 8 out of 10) of records or observations demonstrate compliance
- Evidence of compliance cannot be found in all areas/departments in which the requirement is applicable (such as inpatients but not outpatients; surgery but not day surgery; sedating areas except dental)
- When there are multiple requirements in one ME, at least half (50%) are present
- A policy/process is developed, implemented, and sustainable, but does not have the track-record required for "Fully Met"
- A policy/process is developed and implemented but does not seem to be sustainable

The track record related to a score of "Partially Met" is as follows:

- The requirements of the ME are "Fully Met"; however, there is
  ◆ a 5–11 month look-back period of compliance for triennial surveys; or
  ◆ a 1–3 month look-back period of compliance for initial surveys.

"Not Met" Score

An ME is scored "Not Met" if the answer is "Rarely" or "Never" to the specific requirements of the ME. Also considered are the following:

- If 49% or fewer (for example, 4 or less out of 10) records or observations demonstrate compliance

(continued on page 116)

Sidebar 3-6. The Scoring Process, *continued*

- A finding of "Not Met" for the ME during the last full survey and now the finding is 67% or fewer observations of compliance
- When there are multiple requirements in one ME, 49% or fewer are present
- A policy/process is developed but is not implemented

The track record related to a score of "Not Met" is as follows:

- The requirements of the ME are "Fully Met" however, there is only
  - ♦ a less than 5-month look-back period of compliance for triennial surveys; or
  - ♦ a less than 1-month look-back period of compliance for initial surveys

If an ME was scored "Not Met" and some or all of the other MEs are dependent on the one scored "Not Met," then the remaining ME(s) tied to the prior ME is scored as "Not Met". For example, AOP.1.4, ME 1 states "Appropriate time frames for performing assessments are established for all settings and services." ME 2 states "Assessments are completed within the time frames established by the organization." If ME 1 is not met, ME 2 cannot be met, so both MEs are scored "Not Met."

"Not Applicable" Score:

If the requirements of the MEs do not apply based on the organization's services, patient population, etc. (for example, the organization does not conduct research), the ME is scored "Not Applicable."

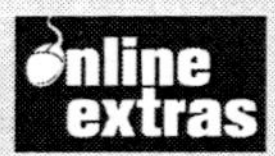

For additional information on the scoring of JCI standards, including information on look-back periods, impact and criticality, and MEs will multiple expectations, see the online extras at www.jcrinc.com/JCIGS10/Extras.

- Go beyond interviews with the nurse by seeking out dietitians, physicians, therapists, clerks, and so forth.
- Include the department or area supervisor as an observer, which allows leaders to provide private coaching or clarification as necessary.
- Trace often. Some organizations see value in conducting tracers of different areas monthly. This allows interviewers and responders to get comfortable with the process and the standards themselves.
- Thank staff members for their participation.
- Share results. The tracer findings should be part of discussions at department meetings, performance improvement meetings, and leadership meetings.

Submitting an Accreditation Application

At around the same time an organization begins conducting its final mock survey, it is also time to submit an application for survey. Submitting an application to JCI at least six months in advance of the desired date for an on-site survey will give both the organization and JCI time to make all the necessary arrangements.

To submit the application, first download the official application for your program from the JCI Web site (www.jointcommissioninternational.org). Complete the application—a process usually done by organization leaders and quality improvement/accreditation specialists—and submit it electronically to the JCI accreditation department via e-mail (JCIAccreditation@jcrinc.com). Call the JCI accreditation department if you encounter questions during the process.

If there are any changes within the organization after the application is completed but before the survey is conducted that would alter the information contained in the application, the organization must inform JCI.

After the application is submitted, JCI will determine mutually agreeable survey dates with the organization and assemble a surveyor team. The appropriate-size survey team is based on the size, services, and complexity of the organization. JCI will then send a contract agreement for the accreditation survey to the organization.

As mentioned in Section 1, upon receipt of the signed contract agreement, JCI will commence development of

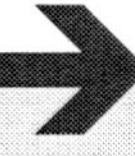 ## ACCREDITATION STRATEGY

Involving Staff in Mock Surveys

To involve staff in the mock survey process, each department or unit might work with the quality or accreditation specialist to create a list of sample survey questions that deal with how it delivers safe, high-quality care. For example, staff on the medical/surgical ward of a hospital might develop questions about infection control, such as, "What are the most common infections?" and "How do you and the organization work to prevent these infections?" In addition to helping staff become more comfortable in thinking about the role that their daily work plays in meeting standards, the thought that goes into creating and answering these questions may spur new quality improvement initiatives in the organization. Also, remember to include staff on all shifts, all days of the week, and in all units to ensure that implementation of policies and procedures is consistent organizationwide and systemwide.

the survey agenda. A JCI survey team leader will seek input from organization staff in the development of the agenda. The survey team leader will contact the organization's primary survey contact to work out the details of the survey agenda to ensure that staff are available and the schedule is comfortable. Assistance should be provided during agenda development to ensure that unit visits in the same building or in close proximity are scheduled at similar times, when possible, to prevent frequent moving from one building to another during the day. This will save time during the survey. It is also important for the team leader to be aware of the distance from the main campus for all sites where services are provided, so he or she can calculate travel time when planning the agenda.

The On-Site Survey

When JCI surveyors arrive at an organization, all of the components of an organization's quality improvement initiatives and accreditation preparation activities will be put into action. This is likely to be a time of great anticipation for leaders and staff, but the months of education that have already taken place can help staff and leaders feel confident that they are ready individually and that the organization is ready as a whole to achieve accreditation. Every individual in the organization should also find satisfaction in knowing that the organization's focus on standards compliance means that it is doing its best to provide safe, high-quality care and is using the JCI standards as an operational guide.

In the days leading up to the on-site survey, the quality/accreditation specialist should review the final survey agenda with involved staff and may wish to once again go over the events that are likely to occur during the survey process.

As mentioned in Section 1, the bulk of the on-site survey for all programs will be made up of individual and system tracers. These will help surveyors assess compliance and directly see how an organization follows its own policies and procedures.

In addition to tracers, the survey has several critical interviews that further help surveyors assess compliance. Although each survey is unique, the following provides a brief summary of some of the key activities

Opening Conference, Orientation to Organization, and Document Review

As discussed in Section 2, this opening conference allows for introductions among key organization staff and the surveyors. The organization provides information about its purpose and structure to help guide the survey process. The chief executive officer, other leaders, and the individual(s) responsible for coordinating the survey agenda should attend this session to discuss their responsibilities and the survey agenda.

The purpose of the document review is to survey standards that require some written evidence of compliance, such as an emergency preparedness plan or a patient rights document. Almost all standards chapters make reference to plans, policies, procedures, and so forth that are to be written. In addition, the document review session orients the survey team to the organizational structure and management structure. Participants should include organization staff members who are familiar with the documents, can

Figure 3-2. Planning Tool for Tracer Activity

Steps:	Specific Information		
Type of Tracer	❏ Individual ❏ Facilities	❏ Medication ❏ Unit/Department	❏ Infection
Selection of Team Members	Members:		
Determine Structure	Scribe: Interviewer(s): Observers:		
Identify Standards of Focus			
Identify Patient Safety Goals of Focus			
Determine Areas to Visit			
Identify Types of Staff Members to Participate			

This tool helps begin discussions on and frame thought processes around where the tracer should focus.

Source: © 2010 Joint Commission International. Provided by Helen Hoesing, R.N., M.P.H., Ph.D., Senior Consultant, Joint Commission International.

translate them, and can respond to any surveyor questions. The surveyors will refer to or read additional documents during the survey, so those documents should be available throughout the survey. Translators will be used, if needed, to assist the surveyors in understanding the documents.

Leadership Interview

As discussed in Section 2, surveyors assess communication among senior leaders of the organization and how leaders address organizational performance issues in this interview. This session gives surveyors an opportunity to talk with leaders about their roles in governing, managing, and directing the organization, as well as improvement activities for systemwide issues.

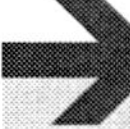

ACCREDITATION STRATEGY

Create an Award for Tracer Participation

Using the tracer methodology helps maintain motivation to achieve organization goals related to quality and safety. To involve the entire organization in tracers, organizations can create reward systems for participants and establish rewards for desired performance in tracers.

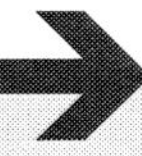

➜ ACCREDITATION STRATEGY

Tracer Feedback

Create a system for feedback of tracer findings to leadership, the appropriate performance improvement or accreditation teams, physicians, and staff. Communicating the results of the tracer process increases the involvement of staff in the process and allows them to take action to improve the way they carry out their daily work to benefit patients.

Staff Qualifications and Education

During this session, staff and surveyors will discuss orientation, training, and education for staff. In addition, the interview addresses the organization's process for evaluating the credentials of the medical staff, nursing staff, and other health care professional staff. The interview also addresses staff's ability to provide clinical services consistent with their qualifications. Staff who will participate in the session should include the individuals responsible for human resources, education, and assessment of staff competency. The chief nurse and medical director or leader of the medical staff also should be present.

Facility Tour

The purpose of the facility tour is to address issues related to the physical facility, medical and other equipment, patient and visitor safety, and infection control. The surveyors will also identify high-risk areas that must be visited after reviewing the organization's application and reading the organization's documents required in the Facility Management and Safety (FMS) standards. This "top-to-bottom" review is just that; the tour usually begins at the roof, working downward in the building. The surveyors will be looking to see that the corridors and exit paths of travel are free for safe exit of the facility in an emergency. In all areas, the surveyors will observe the facility and interview staff to learn how the organization

- reduces and controls hazards, infections, and security risks;
- reduces fire safety risks;
- prevents accident and injuries; and
- maintains safe conditions.

During the course of the tour, surveyors will visit selected patient care settings, inpatient and ambulatory units, treatment and diagnostic areas, and other areas, including registration, admitting, kitchen, pharmacy, central storage, laundry, and power plant, as applicable. Depending on the organization, the tour may also extend to other types of settings, such as individuals' homes, assisted living environments, and hospice settings. Tours of these settings will be conducted as appropriate.

Prior to the facility tour, the surveyors will have reviewed the facility management and safety plans. They will then visit different areas of the facility to check on the implementation of these plans. The surveyors will also review selected portions of the facility inspection report prepared by the organization.

Participants in the facility tour include the chief engineer, safety officer, and staff who coordinate facility management activities. In addition, individuals in charge of specific areas under review—such as admitting or pharmacy—may need to be present.

The Leadership Conference

As discussed in Section 2, this occurs at the close of survey before JCI surveyors leave the premises. During this meeting, surveyors share a Preliminary Survey Findings Report with organization leadership, clarify any issues and concerns of leadership, and provide education as necessary. For example, the surveyors will also offer the leaders a session to review the scoring guidelines and decision rules toward the end of the survey. Surveyors will also provide instructions in completing the postsurvey follow-up activities, including completion of the Strategic Improvement Plan (SIP), using an example of a finding from the preliminary/exit report.

Other Key Interactions

There are several other key meetings and interactions with surveyors that are dependent on the organization's program, size, and scope of services. A detailed explanation of each of these applicable surveyor visits and interviews can be found in the JCI survey process guide, which is provided to all organizations that have applied for accreditation.

The Accreditation Decision

As previously mentioned, while JCI surveyors are still on site they issue an exit report—containing preliminary survey findings—to an organization's leadership. This report is subject to approval from JCI's accreditation leadership and JCI's Accreditation Committee, but it offers the organization a clear view of its performance. Surveyors leave this report with the organization to allow leaders and staff to begin focusing attention on addressing the recommendations cited in the report.

The surveyors' report is submitted to JCI's accreditation leadership, which analyzes findings and data collected during the on-site survey; the report is compared to the current JCI decision rules to render an accreditation decision; and then JCI issues a report with one of the following decisions:

1. Accredited. This means the organization demonstrates acceptable compliance with all measurable elements and International Patient Safety Goals. Should this be the

Seek JCI's Help Throughout the Process

Joint Commission International Accreditation and Standards Development and Interpretation staff are available to assist organizations at all stages of the three-year accreditation cycle. Our staff work with the key leaders from the organization—including the CEO, survey coordinator, and clinical care program director—in facilitating communication of vital information through e-mail, telephone conference calls, and webinars. JCI staff provide guidance and support, answer questions, and clarify expectations related to a variety of activities, such as completing the survey application, developing the contract, understanding the intent of the standards, and scheduling the survey and surveyors, as well as providing help understanding and completing the SIP after the survey is over.

—Ann Jacobson, M.S.N., R.N., N.E.A., Executive Director, International Accreditation, JCI

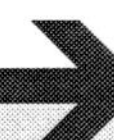

ACCREDITATION STRATEGY

Prepare Early and Often

Help staff members prepare for interaction with surveyors and feel more comfortable with their knowledge by randomly posing questions during the months leading up to the on-site survey. For example, the quality/accreditation specialist may want to ask a member of the medical records staff how he or she ensures that summary lists for a particular patient are up-to-date. Or a variety of staff could be asked about the process used for the read-back of verbal orders (International Patient Safety Goal). Physicians might be asked how they are involved in improving patient safety.

Supervisors or department managers could also conduct these activities as a means of involving more individuals in the process.

decision, the organization would receive an Official Survey Findings Report and a Gold Seal of Quality Approval™.

2. At Risk for Denial of Accreditation. This means the organization does not demonstrate acceptable compliance with all measurable elements and International Patient Safety Goals. Should this be the decision, the organization will receive a Preliminary Survey Findings Report that includes the follow-up activities, such as a focused survey conducted on site within 90 days to review the organization's current compliance with all the not-met and partially met findings from the preliminary report.

At Risk for Denial of Accreditation is the more likely of the two initial decisions, as perfect compliance during the first on-site survey is almost never achieved. Most organizations have areas in which they must improve, and these are indicated in the Official Survey Findings Report as requirements "Not Met."

When an organization receives a decision of Accredited, the organization is still required to address any noncompliant areas using an SIP. As previously mentioned, the SIP describes the specific actions the organization will use to achieve compliance with the "Not Met" standards/measurable elements cited. The SIP must also outline the organization's methodology to prevent recurrence and sustain improvement over time. It should also include measures that will be used to evaluate the effectiveness of the improvement plan (including the submission of data that will occur over the subsequent three years). Fundamentally, SIPs must demonstrate that an organization's actions lead to full compliance with the standards and measurable elements. Figure 3-3 on page 123 shows a sample page for JCI's SIP electronic tool.

Typically, the quality improvement/accreditation specialist will take the lead on developing appropriate SIPs for the organization. As with other action plans discussed in this section, a collaborative effort with leadership, department managers, and frontline staff will be necessary. (*See* Sidebar 3-7 on pages 124–126 for a list of suggested content for an SIP and a sample.)

If an accredited organization is unable to achieve an acceptable SIP after two submissions, the organization will be placed in the category of At Risk for Denial of Accreditation and scheduled for a Follow-Up Focused Survey to determine current compliance. If the organization does not demonstrate acceptable compliance at that time, the organization's status is changed to Accreditation Denied. If the organization demonstrates compliance, the organization is classified as Accredited and proceeds to the SIP process.

Intracycle Performance Review

After an organization's SIP is accepted, the next JCI evaluation for all accredited organizations is its Intracycle Performance Review, which occurs approximately halfway between an organization's triennial on-site surveys. The organization submits written reports of compliance data, particularly in those areas identified as noncompliant dur-

---

Changes in the Agenda

During a survey it is very common for a surveyor to change the sequence of tracer activities from plans initially outlined in the morning briefing. For example, a maternity tracer was going to start in the prenatal clinic and continue to the labor and delivery suites. But while in the clinic, a surveyor decides to make a change and stop in the emergency department and follow the path of an emergency delivery. Other changes in an agenda that may happen are that surveyors may trade activities assigned to them. The nurse may do the medication tracer, or one of the surveyors may not participate in the data sessions but instead follows up on issues that need clarification or gathers additional information that was not captured as part of the individual patient or systems tracer activities. The intention is not to put organizations off guard but to get the most accurate information possible. Do not let this create undue concern. Be prepared to rewrite the agenda, alert the necessary staff, and just carry on.

—*Ann Jacobson, M.S.N., R.N., N.E.A.,*
Executive Director, International
Accreditation, JCI

The Daily Briefing

Note that the agenda has time for a "Daily Briefing" each morning. This can be a critical 30-to-60 minutes for your organization. You should have persons from the areas visited the previous day attending the briefing, and they can discuss the topics the surveyors have already covered with them. You have an opportunity during this time to respond to the findings that your surveyors noted from the day before. You can correct information, provide additional data, explain a process, or direct the surveyors to other resources. You should never let the surveyors leave a debriefing with a misconception that a finding stated during the daily briefing session reflects your organization.

—*Marlis Daerr, R.N., Surveyor, JCI*

ing the previous on-site survey (and therefore targeted for improvement in the SIP). The representations made during the Intracycle Performance Review are then verified during the organization's next on-site survey.

Communicating About Survey Results

When the survey ends, organization leaders and quality/accreditation specialists should work together to communicate survey findings to other leaders and organization staff. The results of accreditation should not be secret but should be shared and discussed throughout the organization.

Although an organization will not have its official accreditation decision for 10 to 15 days following the survey, this should not cause a delay in communicating with staff and leaders about how the survey went and how the organization proceeds. Silence on this issue can breed speculation, and it's better to be up-front and open with everyone about how the organization did. However, the leaders are not to communicate the accreditation decision to the public until they receive the official accreditation report from JCI.

Explaining the meaning of the survey report will help staff members see how their work contributed to the process. In addition, this offers an opportunity to emphasize that continuous quality improvement is an institutional goal and that the survey report supports that goal by highlighting areas in which improvement is of the highest priority.

There are many ways to foster open communication in the immediate aftermath of a JCI survey, including the following:

- Send an e-mail or memo to all organization staff, giving them an update and outlining next steps.
- Make a booklet that includes the findings and suggestions by the surveyors and distribute it to all quality, accreditation, and performance improvement committees.
- Emphasize and explain the issues addressed in the findings, and review the related standards item with the departments and committees.
- Solicit staff opinions on how to achieve compliance. Seeking the advice of staff in relevant areas can help solicit ideas for complying with the identified standards and ensuring that compliance is part of daily staff routines.
- Encourage teamwork in efforts to come into compliance and avoid placing blame. Listing the relevant standards and measurable elements for staff will help to make everyone in

the organization aware of improvement priorities.

Consistent and open communication in the weeks following the survey can keep up organizationwide morale, momentum, and commitment.

After Achieving Accreditation

When an organization achieves "Accredited" status, it is time to celebrate success! An organizationwide celebration may be in order, or an all-staff memo or voice mail may be used to share information about the accreditation decision. Use the JCI Gold Seal as appropriate to show internal and external customers your compliance with JCI requirements. (Note: The organization's CEO will be given a password by JCI Accreditation for a one-time download of the Gold Seal from the JCI Web site and will also receive a publicity kit that provides the guidelines for use of the Gold Seal in marketing materials and promotions.) Other ideas to celebrate this accomplishment include the following:

- Hang banners both inside and outside the facility to announce that the organization is JCI accredited. (Note: organizations should ensure that these banners do not present a fire hazard or violate standards relating to fire hazards.)
- Send a news release to local media.
- Conduct a news conference. Invite local reporters to meet with the CEO, medical director, quality assurance/improvement director, and other key staff members. Discuss how staff involvement was vital to the on-site survey because of the focus on patient care. Emphasize the thoroughness of the on-site survey and stress the organization's ongoing continuous compliance with standards 24/7/365.
- Place news of JCI accreditation in a prominent position on the organization's Web site.
- Notify any regional or metropolitan provider association in which the organization is a member. Many of these associations publicize accreditation information in their newsletters.
- Notify the benefit manager at insurance carriers and/or health plans whose clients use or might use organization services.
- Include information on the benefits of accreditation in organization newsletters and in presentations to staff, board members, and community groups.
- Celebrate the accreditation award by sponsoring a "Quality Day" at the organization. Honor special staff,

SECTION 3

Figure 3-3. Sample Page of Joint Commission International Strategic Improvement Plan (SIP) Electronic Tool

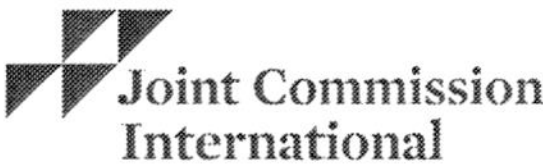

Joint Commission International (JCI) Accreditation Strategic Improvement Plan (SIP) Form (Effective 10 Feb 2010)

SECTION I – Survey Findings

INSTRUCTIONS:
Please copy the cited survey findings from the survey finding reports to the table below.

Chapter:
Standard:
Measurable Element(s) with surveyor's scoring and findings:

SECTION II - Strategic Improvement Plan (SIP) and/or Corrective Action(s)

INSTRUCTIONS:
Please provide a detailed description of the sustainable Strategic Improvement Plan (SIP) and/or corrective action(s) that will be implemented to achieve full compliance with the standard's requirement. If the plan involves change to the policy and procedure, please provide the high-level details for the key elements of the intended changes.

Strategic Improvement Plan (SIP) and/or Corrective Action(s)		
What and Where (Action Plan[s]) and Areas for Implementation)	Who (Owner—Staff Name/Title)	When (Completion Date)

Source: © 2010 Joint Commission International.

volunteers, or donors and offer tours of the facility.

■ Demonstrate ongoing efforts to comply with JCI standards which can provide additional positive publicity. For example, invite the news media to cover emergency drills. This is a highly visible, graphic story and generates positive media exposure.

Maintaining Accreditation

Achieving accreditation, while an accomplishment to be celebrated, should not end an organization's pursuit of high-quality care. JCI accreditation is a continuous process. Every time a nurse double-checks a patient's identification before administering a medication, and every time a surgical team calls a "time-out" to verify that they agree they're about to perform the correct procedure, at the correct site, on the correct patient, these individuals are living and breathing the accreditation process. JCI accreditation is woven into the fabric of a health care organization's operations.

To maintain the momentum of safety and quality improvement activities during the postsurvey period, organizations should establish structures and systems that encourage and support ongoing standards compliance and survey readiness. This may include hosting regular in-services about standards and compliance strategies, researching and implementing improvement methods such as Lean and Six Sigma to help guide improvement efforts, conducting monthly mock tracers to assess how patient care is being provided in the organization, writing newsletter articles about performance improvement and standards compliance activities, and so forth. Organizations may even want to establish an accreditation department whose sole focus is to encourage, support, and maintain an organization's continuous compliance with standards.

Many of the structures, activities, and approaches an organization uses in preparing for accreditation will be beneficial in maintaining accreditation. The key is to

Sidebar 3-7. Content of a Strategic Improvement Plan (SIP)

To be effective, an SIP must include specific content that shows how the organization will achieve sufficient and sustainable compliance with "Not Met" measurable elements. Following is a list of the recommended content:

- Standard number
- Measurable Element number
- Description of the finding. This should be stated as it was in the survey report.
- Activity plan. This should include a brief description of the planned activities for improvement.
- Specific actions. This is similar to a "to do" list and should include a detailed list of each activity to achieve the sustainable improvement.
- Responsible department/people. This should indicate which department, committee, or improvement team is in charge of implementing the SIP as well as who is assigned to do the work associated with the SIP.
- Planned completion date. This is the date that the organization anticipates the system will be in place and the date on which measurement begins
- Measurement criteria. This may include pictures, measures, and/or documents that will show how JCI will understand if an organizaiton has improved the "Not Met" issue.
- Needed documents/evidence. This may include policies, procedures, forms, education materials, meeting minutes, memos, measure definition forms, and performance improvement graphs as evidence of the corrective actions done and performance level achieved.

Following is a brief example of a possible SIP related to infection prevention and control.

Standard number

IPSG.5

Measurable element number

ME 3

Description of the finding

An insufficient number of sinks and hand sanitizer dispensers were noted in the ambulatory clinics and in the Family Medicine Center. For example, in the polyclinic, the blood draw room and the medication room had neither sinks nor hand sanitizer dispensers mounted.

Activity plan

Increase the number of hand sanitizer dispensers

Specific actions

- Establish an improvement project team to work on this finding.
- Choose the appropriate hand sanitizer.
- Specify the needed areas in which to place the dispensers.
- Purchase additional required dispensers.
- Distribute the dispensers to the needed areas (these areas include the blood draw room and the medication room at the Family Medicine Center, each inpatient room, polyclinic areas).

| **Sidebar 3-7.** | **Content of a Strategic Improvement Plan (SIP),** *continued* |

- Review the material safety data sheets (MSDSs) and manufacturer's guidelines of the hand sanitizer.
- Prepare appropriate labels for "irritation sign," "flammable sign," and "date of opening and due date" to be put on the dispensers (the hand sanitizer was suggested to be used within three months after it has been opened and it was flammable and possible irritant).
- Label the dispensers.
- Prepare an instruction leaflet on how to use the dispensers and hand sanitizers and hang a copy on each dispenser.
- Place the dispensers in the identified areas.
- Revise the hospital policy on "General and Surgical Handwashing Techniques/Wearing Gloves" to reflect the guidelines on how to use the new hand sanitizer.
- Address the issue in the June issue of the internal Continuous Quality Improvement (CQI) bulletin.
- Prepare a checklist for on-site control of the revised system and train the staff.
- Prepare information leaflets and distribute them to the units as a training tool.
- Measure performance.

Responsible department/people

- Infection Control Committee
- Risk Management Committee
- Family Medicine Center Manager
- Purchasing and Logistics Manager
- Maintenance Manager
- Nursing Services Managers
- Patient Safety Supervisor
- CQI Manager
- CQI Staff

Planned completion date

1 January 2011

Measurement criteria

In addition to the current measure followed on hand-wash rate, we will define "alcohol-based hand-rub usage rate" as a performance indicator. We will collect data, aggregate data to measure the performance, calculate performance improvement, and prepare graphs to see the trend of the performance improvement. We will analyze the trend of "alcohol-based hand-rub usage rate" and evaluate the correlation with the "handwash rate." Quality improvement personnel will review the results with the Infection Control Committee and write the summary report related to the finding.

Needed documents/evidence

Following is the evidence we will submit to show sustained improvement:

- Relevant Infection Control Committee meeting minutes

(continued on page 126)

<table>
<tr><td>Sidebar 3-7.</td><td>Content of a Strategic Improvement Plan (SIP), continued</td></tr>
</table>

- Relevant Head Nurse meeting minutes
- Relevant Risk Management Committee meeting minutes
- List of hand sanitizer dispenser locations
- Pictures of the hand sanitizer dispensers at the Family Medicine Center
- General and surgical handwashing techniques/wearing gloves policy
- Indicator definition form for alcohol-based hand-rub usage rate
- PI graphs for alcohol-based hand-rub usage rate (%)
- Handwash rate (%)

Source: Özlem Yildirim, Ph.D., Continuous Quality Improvement Manager, Amerikan Hastanesi Saglik Hizmetleri A.S, Istanbul, Turkey. Used with permission. Ms. Yildirim credits the members of the team responsible for this SIP, including Infection Control Committee Chairperson Birsen Cetin, Infection Control Committee member and nurse Nilufer Dogan Kazanci, Risk Management Committee Chairperson Omur Ercelen, Family Medicine Center Manager Hakan Sezer, Purchasing and Logistics Manager Vedat Peker, Maintenance Manager Ali Süngü, Nursing Services Managers Secil Aksayan and Nuray Erdemir, Patient Safety Supervisor Fatma Küçükerenköy, and CQI staff member Demet Yigit.

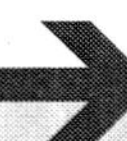

ACCREDITATION STRATEGY

Helping Organizations Celebrate

To help organizations celebrate the accreditation award, they will receive the following from JCI:

→ A certificate of accreditation for display

→ A publicity kit, including a sample press release announcing the organization's accreditation

→ Publication of the accreditation decision on JCI's Web site, http://www.jointcommissioninternational.org.

Organizations should consider using these tools to help promote their accreditation status to the staff, patients, and community at large.

Maintaining Focus

It is a natural organizational tendency to let up a bit after becoming accredited. But the message has to be, "Just keep doing what you've been doing," which is continuously improving. Another time when an organization needs to stay focused is when there are key leadership or personnel changes in the organization that may influence the accreditation process. Those are times when it's easy for an organization to become lax or lose focus.

—Bruce Frederick, R.N., M.N.,
JCI Consultant

Embracing the Journey

To maintain accreditation, organizations must accept the concept that accreditation is a journey. This is not a licensure, where you do everything the same way at that same time every year. The journey is a step-by-step process. The first survey is the foundation, and then with the next survey, you move to the next level, and so on. For example, staff at one organization I work with were shocked at how much easier their second survey was than their first. It all goes back to the principle of quality improvement—constant improvement. Surveys are more rigorous the second time around, but the organizations that make constant improvement their goal find that they are equal to the challenge.

—Helen Hoesing, R.N., M.P.H., Ph.D.,
JCI Senior Consultant

continue those activities to sustain compliance and continuously strive for high-quality care. Regardless of the structures an organization puts in place, organization leaders and quality/accreditation specialists must work together to keep the pursuit of quality and safety in the forefront of organization priorities and activities.

Case Study 3-2. Tawam Hospital

Organization Name: Tawam Hospital
Location: Al Ain, Abu Dhabi, United Arab Emirates
Years Accredited: 2006, 2009
About Tawam Hospital: Tawam Hospital is a 477-bed tertiary care facility that serves as a regional referral center for specialized medical care and a national referral center for oncology services. The hospital is best known for its neonatal care, emergency medicine, intensive care, cardiac care, and oncology services.

Making a Commitment to Quality Through Accreditation

Almost five years ago, Tawam Hospital, entered into a management agreement with Johns Hopkins Medicine. As part of this agreement, Tawam began a patient safety program to promote patient safety within the hospital and local community. This program includes a safety awareness campaign that helps educate staff members on how to use the International Patient Safety Goals and provide safe, high-quality patient care in accordance with JCI standards.

To promote the campaign, the hospital posted campaign slogans titled "Patient Safety Top Priority" in numerous places around the hospital. Employees were sent text messages with safety awareness tips, and even employee pay slips had reminders about the campaign.

During the campaign itself, the hospital hosted a continuing medical education session about patient safety and played a video—translated into Arabic—about safety in patient waiting areas. Other topics covered within the campaign included medication safety and infection control.

Medication Safety

One of the ways Tawam addressed medication safety in the organization was through a project to assess the current medication cabinet in the intensive care unit and implement changes to improve the cabinet's organization. Tawam used a Lean/Six Sigma approach (*see* page 107) to identify waste within the cabinet; remove clutter; ensure logical organization; review policies, procedures, and guidelines; and maintain improvement processes.

Within the project, a performance improvement team assessed the medication cabinet, conducted a nursing survey, identified and implemented improvement processes, and provided education on the new organization of the cabinet. Improvement processes implemented included the following:

- Alphabetizing drugs
- Properly labeling drugs with an appropriate font size and color
- Segregating drugs, including oral medications from parenteral medications, inhalers from nebulizers, and adult doses from pediatric doses
- Reviewing all look-alike, sound-alike medications and developing a policy to ensure their proper storage
- Identifying high-alert medications and developing a policy for an independent double check

By engaging in this effort, the organization was able to improve efficiency and safety associated with the medication cabinet.

Infection Control

Part of the hospital's efforts to improve infection control centered around hand hygiene. Each month, members of the hospital's infection control committee observe most of the departments in the hospital to monitor the practice and adequacy of hand hygiene efforts. All disciplines are observed, including nurses, physicians, ancillary staff, and support staff. Periodically, a report is generated and given to department managers and administrators so they can track and trend compliance results. The infection control department collates these reports and, based on its findings, selects a department to receive a hand hygiene award. This award helps promote awareness of the importance of hand hygiene and celebrates staff work toward improvement in this area.

Case Study 3-3. Severance Hospital, Yonsei University College of Medicine

Organization Name: Severance Hospital, Yonsei University College of Medicine
Location: Seoul, Republic of Korea
Years accredited: 2007, 2010
About Severance Hospital, Yonsei University College of Medicine. Established in 1885, Severance Hospital, Yonsei University College of Medicine has grown to include more than 6,000 staff, facilitating more than 7,000 outpatient visits per day, with specialty organizations such as a Cancer Center, Rehabilitation Hospital, Cardiovascular Hospital, Eye and ENT Hospital, Children's Hospital, Emergency Care Center, Diabetes Center, Allergy and Asthma Clinic, Neuroscience Center, and intensive care unit. Severance introduced its first "Patient's Bill of Rights" in 1993.

Starting the JCI Accreditation Journey

Severance, under the leadership of former general director Dr. Chang-Il Park, committed to seeking JCI accreditation in 2005, when construction on its new facility was complete. A team of Severance's Office of Quality Improvement (OQI) leaders attended a JCI Practicum in Chicago, Illinois, USA, and returned to the hospital to endorse the prospect of accreditation to executive leadership.

After leadership approved the plan to apply for JCI accreditation, Severance formed its JCI Basecamp, a team including physicians, nurses, pharmacists, a radiology technician, a safety manager, and representatives from the following departments:

➲ Nursing
➲ OQI
➲ Pharmacy
➲ Medical records
➲ Information systems
➲ Infection control
➲ Safety management
➲ Education and training

The JCI Basecamp was responsible for communicating information about the JCI accreditation to the staff. The Basecamp team met weekly to study the standards and prepare the hospital for the accreditation survey.

Although the OQI existed before Severance began its path to JCI accreditation, the department's responsibilities multiplied during accreditation preparation. Among the many new responsibilities of the OQI were coordinating the JCI Basecamp meetings, developing educational materials on JCI standards and initiatives (*see* Figure 1 on page 130), educating the staff using those materials, and coordinating logistics of the on-site survey with JCI.

Overcoming Obstacles

Tailoring hospital processes and procedures to fit JCI requirements was an achievable challenge for Severance leaders and staff, but not one without significant challenges.

"One of the difficulties was to convince the entire hospital to accept JCI, especially on the standards," says Dongsik Bang, M.D., Ph D., vice director for clinical affairs. "Some staff had disagreement with the standards due to the cultural differences. Another difficulty was to convey the message of JCI requirements and to educate over 6,000 staff members. Since this is a very busy hospital with over 7,000 outpatient visits per day, it was difficult to implement some of the standards."

Ja-Young Kwon, M.D., Ph.D., says standardization of processes and implementing new practices challenged management and staff. "There were an infinite number of meetings held to share processes and understand each other's practices," says Kwon. "We had to reach a unified and standardized process to fit us all in a practical way. Then, making physicians, professors, residents, and interns implement something that was new and that they were not used to—for example, setting the care plan, conducting time-outs, engaging in read-backs, etc.—was difficult for us."

(continued on page 130)

Case Study 3-3. Severance Hospital, Yonsei University College of Medicine, *continued*

Figure 1. Severance Hospital Newsletter on Sound-Alike, Look-Alike Drugs

QI Newsletter

2009.3.

- 유사이름, 유사모양 약물 주의-
(Sound Alike, Look Alike Drug)

◈ 유사이름 약물 (약 이름으로 혼동될 수 있는 약)

Carmazepine(흰색)	↔	CARMAZEPINE CR(주황색)
Citopcin	↔	Cytotec
Clidol	↔	Clid
★Depakine chrono	↔	DepakOTE ER(회색)
Diamox	↔	Doxium
Dilatrend(흰색)	↔	Dichlozide
Dinol	↔	Denol
Ebastel	↔	Etravil(파랑색)
Endapen	↔	Enaprin
Foipan	↔	Folin(엽산)
Ganaton	↔	Gasmotin
Lopid	↔	Lipidil supra
MyAlone(파랑)	↔	Malarone(분홍)
Neomazin	↔	Neurontin(흰색)
Olbetam	↔	Ostemin
Phenobarbital	↔	Phenytoin
Suprax	↔	Sporanox
★Tenormin	↔	Tenoretic

◈ 유사모양 약물

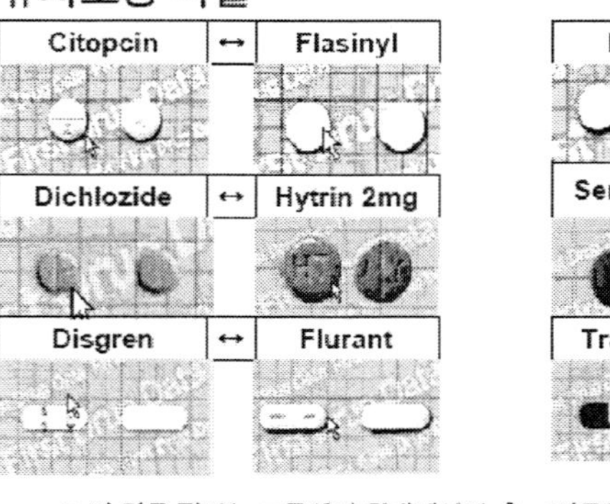

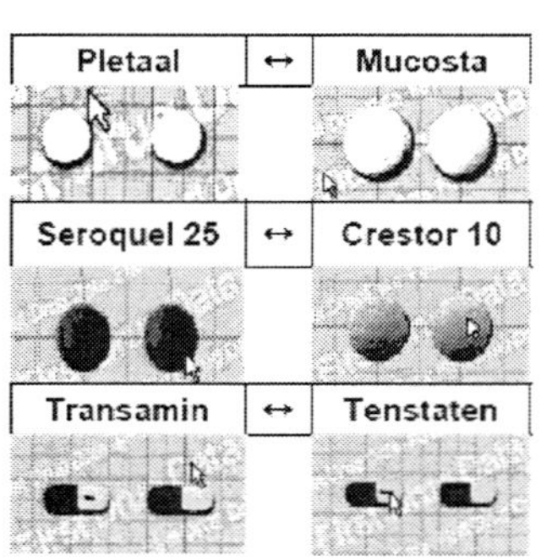

※ 더 많은 정보는 그룹웨어 원내게시판 → '약무국' 에서 찾아볼 수 있습니다.

세 브 란 스 병 원 장

This one-page pamphlet is an example of educational materials used by Severance Hospital during its preparation for its initial JCI on-site survey.

Source: Severance Hospital, Seoul, Republic of Korea. Used with permission.

Case Study 3-3. Severance Hospital, Yonsei University College of Medicine, *continued*

After Severance had instituted new policies and procedures and had implemented them long enough for leaders and staff to feel more comfortable with them, the JCI Basecamp initiated a mock survey to measure compliance. As previously mentioned, the mock survey is a thorough duplication of the JCI on-site survey, and it produces evidence of compliance and noncompliance with JCI requirements that inform the organization of the steps it needs to be ready for an actual JCI survey (*see* page 112 for more information on the mock survey).

Additional Resources
In addition to modifying existing processes and creating new ones, Severance did increase resources in order to meet JCI requirements. Among its new initiatives were the following:

- Increasing the number of infection control nurses from two to seven
- Adding a triage system with a triage nurse in the emergency department
- Adding a pediatric sedation room
- Increasing the number of pharmacists
- Establishing an interface system between the patient monitor and the electronic medical records

Just as important was a significant increase in staff education and training sessions. "There were infinite numbers of education sessions, meetings with each and every department, and interdisciplinary, small-group talks to convey the importance of compliance and to inspire them to act,' says Kwon.

Advice to Organizations Considering JCI Accreditation
Dr. Kwon says organizations contemplating JCI accreditation should make certain to involve physicians and leaders in as many parts of the preparation as possible. 'Recruit as many doctors as possible to participate in the accreditation preparation," Kwon says. "Doctors should take an active part in educating medical staff. Leaders of the organization should understand that JCI accreditation is about upgrading the hospital process and employee quality to make the organization a safe and better place for patient care."

To Dr. Kwon's point, patients' satisfaction with their care at Severance Hospital has increased significantly since the hospital initiated its path to accreditation. In 2005, when Severance made the decision to pursue JCI accreditation, inpatient and outpatient customer satisfaction numbers were measured at 64% and 64.1%, respectively. By 2007, when JCI first accredited Severance, customer satisfaction had risen to 89.3% for inpatient satisfaction and 81.6% for outpatient satisfaction. Inpatient and outpatient satisfaction increased again in 2008 (92.3% and 83.5%, respectively).

SECTION 3

Case Study 3-4. Na Homolce Hospital

Organization Name: Na Homolce Hospital
Location: Prague, Czech Republic
Years Accredited: 2005, 2008
About Na Homolce Hospital: Na Homolce Hospital is a 357-bed hospital offering comprehensive medical services in the field of cardiovascular medicine, as well as in neurology and neurosurgery, with an emphasis on minimally invasive methods of treatment.

Making the Decision to Pursue JCI Accreditation

Na Homolce Hospital management made the decision to pursue JCI accreditation mainly as a testament to JCI's standards. "The standards are concise, coherent, and well-defined," says Barbora Vaculíková, R.N., manager of Na Homolce's quality control department. "Our hospital wants to provide safe and quality care, and the implementation of international accreditation standards serves as a guide towards this goal."

Na Homolce leaders made their first commitment to seek JCI accreditation in 2003. Initial steps taken included the following:

1. Initiation to JCI's accreditation process and standards by top and midlevel management

2. Allocation of responsibilities, setting up the following teams and working groups:
   - An **accreditation preparatory team,** consisting of physicians, nurses and non–health employees, all working at middle management level. This team was later renamed the Commission on Quality and Safety.
   - **Internal auditors,** a team of physicians and nurses from all disciplines, responsible for quality management at individual work centers
   - **A hospital-acquired infections team,** composed of physicians and nurses

3. Review and preparation of internal policies and procedures

4. Training of hospital staff at all levels on JCI requirements

Establishing a Quality Control Department

The decision to establish an independent quality control department at Na Homolce followed the decision to seek accreditation. The main duties of the staff of the quality control department are as follows:
- Coordinating activities relating to quality and safety assurance
- Identifying and analyzing risk areas of both the medical and technical operations
- Implementing the requirements of international standards into internal regulations and practice
- Monitoring and evaluating quality indicator data
- Organizing seminars and training in quality and safety enhancement, among other related topics

The head of the quality control department—a position now held by Barbora Vaculíková—is a member of the hospital management, which ensures that other members of the management receive feedback on quality and safety enhancement processes and which gives the entire management team a chance to take an active part in quality control decision making. The quality control department also employs three specialists, as well as technicians focusing on safety and health protection for workers, fire protection, and crisis management.

Encountering and Overcoming Obstacles

One obstacle Na Homolce management encountered en route to JCI accreditation was a somewhat hostile perception of the accreditation process by staff because of an increase in the amount of documentation of patient care linked to

Case Study 3-4.   Na Homolce Hospital, *continued*

accreditation. Management responded by reinforcing that every step taken in patient care must be properly documented, and not only "because of accreditation." "Patient care is a multidisciplinary activity, and every specialist needs to get relevant and accurate information from the patient's documents," says Vaculíková. "Properly kept and legible documentation definitely does reduce the risk of error in various parts of the diagnostic and therapeutic process. Patients are better informed about their treatment and medical options than they had been until recent times, and they have the right to look into and make copies of their medical files."

One of the more demanding aspects of documentation was the development of unified documents for all the hospital departments. Na Homolce Hospital is focused on patient care provided under three basic programs—cardiovascular, neurological and neurosurgical, and general care. Leaders and staff found difficulty with defining common starting points for the unification of the content, but they have since succeeded in developing the following unified documents:

- Medication and infusion lists
- General nursing records (*see* Figure 1 on page 134)
- Pain treatment
- Daily record of intensive care for all surgical disciplines

The unification of documentation procedures resulted in improved communication among staff and in better interdisciplinary cooperation within the entire hospital. Presently, quality leaders are recruiting additional specialists for the clinical pharmacy department with a view toward enhancing safety during the administration of medication.

An Increase in Patient Satisfaction

One of the results of the processes associated with the implementation of accreditation standards was a better quality of cooperation from patients and their families during treatment. Na Homolce Hospital placed second among all Czech Republic hospitals in a national patient satisfaction survey in 2009. "This gives us reason to believe that this excellent result is connected with the process of continuous quality and safety enhancement," says Vaculíková

Quality Improvement Program— Prevention and Control of Hospital-Acquired Infections

Na Homolce Hospital has been accredited twice by JCI—in 2005 and in 2008. The hospital has maintained its commitment to continuous quality improvement beyond the requirements of the on-site survey. Examples of specific, data-supported improvements made by Na Homolce in conjunction with its JCI accreditation efforts include its Prevention and Control of Hospital-Acquired Infections initiative. The program required intensive training of all health care professionals, which contributed to a reduction of hospital-acquired bloodstream infections from 2.47 incidents per 1,000 patient days in 2007 to 2.04 per 1,000 patient days in 2009.

The program has also contributed to a significant reduction in the number of hospital-acquired methicillin-resistant *Staphylococcus aureus* (MRSA) cases although rates of MRSA imported from other health care facilities increased. The incidence of hospital-acquired MRSA bloodstream infections has also dropped significantly, with 10 cases in 2007, 6 in 2008, and only 1 registered case in 2009.

Advice to Organizations Seeking JCI Accreditation

Vaculíková says organizations making the decision of whether or not to seek JCI accreditation should not run from a challenge. "A risk that is always present in an organizational culture of continuous quality and safety enhancement is that staff will be resistant to such processes," Vaculíková says. "This is caused, *inter alia*, by human nature with its encoded aversion to novelties and change—'We have always done it this way and it worked, so why change it now?' This attitude can be changed only by communicating,

(continued on page 134)

Case Study 3-4. Na Homolce Hospital, *continued*

Figure 1. Nursing Admission Report

NA HOMOLCE NEMOCNICE

Nursing Admission Report

☐ Admission ☐ During hospitalisation

DEPARTMENT **PID**

Admission

Date: Time:

Admitted from: ☐ From home ☐ NNH Department .... ☐ EMS (emergency medical services) ☐ Other healthcare facility ....

Repeated admission: ☐ Yes ☐ No

Dg.: ....

Patient handed in medication: ☐ No ☐ Yes

Relatives informed: ☐ Yes ☐ No

Physiological functions: TK: PHK .... LHK .... P .... TT .... D ....

Risks: ☐ Fall risk, score .... ☐ Risk of decubitus ulcers development .... ☐ Infection (please specify) ....

Allergy: ☐ No ☐ Yes Allergen: ....

Consciousness: ☐ Conscious ☐ Disturbance of consciousness ☐ Unconscious ☐ Worsened

Contact: ☐ Without limitations ☐ No contact possible

Mental condition: ☐ Cooperative ☐ Calm ☐ Well-oriented ☐ Non-cooperative ☐ Agitated ☐ Confused ☐ Fear

Disturbed sleep: ☐ No ☐ Yes Medication: ....

Ability to receive education:

PATIENT ☐ Yes ☐ No

FAMILY ☐ Yes ☐ No

Requested spiritual services: ☐ No ☐ Yes

Breathing: ☐ Undisturbed ☐ Cough ☐ Dyspnoea ☐ Effort dyspnoea ☐ Rest dyspnoea ☐ Night ☐ Smoker

Nutrition: ☐ Self-attending ☐ Not self-attending ☐ Parenteral ☐ Probe ☐ Diet ☐ Diabetic ☐ OAD ☐ INS

Pain: ☐ No ☐ Yes ☐ Acute ☐ Chronic

Localisation:

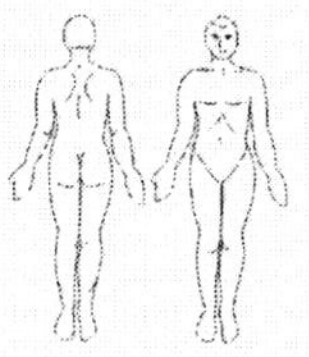

Intensity: 1 2 3 4 5

Skin: ☐ Without change ☐ Intertrigo ☐ Oedema ☐ Decubitus ulcers ☐ Other lesions ☐ Surgical wound ☐ Burn ☐ Atony ☐ Chronic wound ☐ Other skin integrity impairment ....

Localisation:

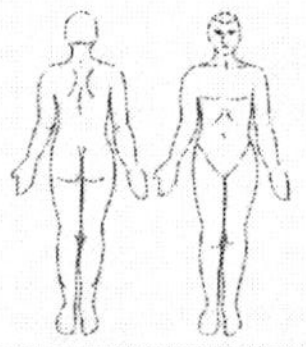

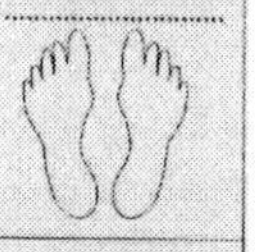

Self-attendance and mobility: ☐ Self-attending ☐ Partially self-attending, limitations........ ☐ Not self-attending ☐ When walking ☐ At meals ☐ During hygiene procedures ☐ When dressing ☐ When voiding

Significant limitation: ☐ None ☐ Eyesight problems ☐ Hearing problems ☐ Speech problems ☐ Physical handicap (please specify) .... ☐ Foreigner, spoken language: .... ☐ Other: ....

Compensatory aids: ☐ No ☐ Spectacles ☐ Contact lenses ☐ Hearing aid ☐ Denture ☐ Upper denture ☐ Lower denture ☐ Wheelchair ☐ Crutches / walking stick ☐ Others ....

Voiding:

Urine: ☐ No problems ☐ Burning sensation, strangury ☐ Retention ☐ Incontinence ☐ Other ....

Defecation: ☐ Without problems, regular ☐ Diarrhoea ☐ Constipation ☐ Ostomy ☐ Incontinence

Date of last defecation: ....

Assessment of nutritional condition:

Usual weight .... kg

Actual weight .... kg

Stature .... Cm

Significantly emaciated ☐ No ☐ Yes (BMI below 18,5)

Eats considerably less ☐ No ☐ Yes (1 week 1/2 a portion and less)

Considerable weight loss ☐ No ☐ Yes (10% and more in ½ a year)

In case of at least one positive answer, please inform the nutritional therapist.

Nutritional therapist was contacted. ☐ No ☐ Yes

Social history
Discharge plan

The patient is capable of performing everyday life activities and is self-attending. ☐ Yes ☐ No

The patient is well-oriented (as regards time, place, persons) and is able to take decisions himself/herself. ☐ Yes ☐ No

The patient has problems with the administration of medication, or ostomy or invasive device site care. ☐ No ☐ Yes ....

Requires follow-up rehabilitation. ☐ No ☐ Yes

The patient has problems whit accommodation. ☐ No ☐ Yes

The patient has a contact person who will help him/her after discharge from hospital. ☐ Yes ☐ No

The post-hospitalisation care co-ordinator has been contacted. ☐ Yes ☐ No

A nursing admission report is one of the unified documents used across all departments at Na Homolce Hospital.

Source: Na Homolce Hospital Prague, Czech Republic. Used with permission.

Case Study 3-4.　**Na Homolce Hospital,** *continued*

explaining, and presenting data to make personnel understand the essence and importance of the measures that are being introduced. A key factor is the inclusion of employees into the development of internal procedures and regulations that have an immediate impact on their everyday work."

REFERENCES

1. Dlugacz Y., Restifo A., Greenwood A.: *The Quality Handbook for Health Care Organizations: A Manager's Guide to Tools and Programs.* San Francisco: Jossey-Bass, 2004.

2. De Vos M., et al.: Using quality indicators to improve hospital care: A review of the literature. *Int J Qual Health Care* 21:119–129, Apr. 2009.

3. Frankel A., et al. (eds.): *The Essential Guide for Patient Safety Officers.* Oakbrook Terrace, IL: Joint Commission Resources, 2009.

4. Womack J.P., Jones D.T.: *Lean Thinking: Banish Waste and Create Wealth in Your Corporation.* 1st Free Press (ed., rev., and updated). New York: Free Press, 2003 (original edition: New York: Simon & Schuster, 1996).

5. iSixSigma LLC: *Six Sigma—What Is Six Sigma?* http://www.isixsigma.com/sixsigma/six_sigma.asp (accessed 15 Jan., 2010).

6. Sunyog M.: Lean Management and Six-Sigma yield big gains in hospital's immediate response laboratory. *Clin Leadersh Manag Rev* 18:255–258, Sep.–Oct. 2004.

SECTION 3

Joint Commission International Accreditation: Getting Started, Second Edition

SECTION

4

ACCREDITATION FOR HEALTH CARE STAFF

Section 4 discusses the role of the frontline staff person in an organization's accreditation journey and offers specific actions staff should take to support the process. Many of the topics covered in this section are addressed in other sections as well. For that reason, this section offers brief synopses of different topics and shows the reader where to refer back for further information.

Although the focus of Joint Commission International (JCI) accreditation is on the entire health care organization rather than on individual staff members or departments and services, planning and preparation by every single person in the organization are necessary in order to have a successful survey and continued operational improvement. It is not enough for the leaders of the organization to prepare for accreditation, nor is it appropriate for the entire accreditation effort to rest on the shoulders of quality/accreditation specialists. Individual staff members must be committed to the process of accreditation and be active participants in the organization's efforts to improve quality and safety.

Learn About the Accreditation Process

As discussed in Section 1, JCI accreditation is a process of continuously complying with international standards, which focus on key systems, patients, and performance improvement. This compliance effort creates a cultural shift toward quality and safety. Achieving JCI accreditation requires everyone in an organization, including—and particularly—the staff providing care and treatment every day, to be committed to providing the best, safest, most appropriate care they can.

A first step in supporting an organization's accreditation journey requires staff to learn about the accreditation process and what's involved. Staff should familiarize themselves with the concepts contained in JCI accreditation standards, understand how these standards affect their work duties, and be aware of the process used to evaluate standards compliance. They should also learn about the International Patient Safety Goals and how they relate to their daily work life.

There are many ways staff members can familiarize themselves with the ins and outs of accreditation. One way is to review Section 1 of this publication, which outlines what accreditation is and specifically what is involved in JCI accreditation. It also discusses the standards, the International Patient Safety Goals, and other key information.

The leaders of an organization as well as quality/accreditation specialists will also provide additional opportunities for staff to learn about accreditation and the role they play in it. Staff must take advantage of these opportunities. They should attend education sessions about accreditation and the standards, read newsletter articles on the topic, review any Web-based opportunities for learning, and interact with other organizations that have achieved accreditation. In general, they must be available and willing to learn about, understand, and embrace the accreditation process.

When learning about the accreditation process, staff may come across terms with which they are not familiar. Sidebar 4-1 on page 139 offers a brief list of some of these accreditation terms. Further definitions can be found in an organization's accreditation manual and survey process guide.

After a basic introduction, staff should begin to further educate themselves on the standards and how they relate to their daily work. Staff members should read and understand portions of the accreditation manual that are applicable to their duties. Nurses, for example, should be generally familiar with JCI's patient-centered standards that address access to care and continuity of care, patient and family rights, assessment of patients, care of patients, and patient and family education; but they will also need to understand their responsibilities regarding the infection prevention and control and quality improvement requirements.

Infection control staff will need to understand how standards related to prevention and control of infections as well as emergency management, affect their job responsibilities. Those staff involved in maintaining the facility will need to understand the facility management and safety standards, while information technology staff should learn about the management of information standards.

Staff at health care organizations have many demands on their work hours. At times, it can seem as though there are not enough hours in the day to provide the best care possible and complete administrative duties. Accreditation preparation and its related activities may initially provoke worries that staff are being asked to do even more. Although achieving accreditation is demanding, the ideas behind this process are not to perform certain tasks just for the sake of putting a check mark beside an accreditation to-do list and moving on to the "real" work of the organization. Accreditation provides a detailed framework that gives staff members efficient, effective methods for carrying out their jobs.

Play a Role in Quality and Safety Efforts

To achieve accreditation, organizations must lay the foundation to support it. This foundation is a culture that supports safety and quality and ensures open and proactive communication about risks, errors, and opportunities for improvement. As discussed in Section 2, organization leadership is critical to establishing, supporting, and fostering a culture of safety. However, leadership cannot achieve such a culture alone. Each staff member must personally commit to a proactive approach to error prevention, embrace open communication practices, and actively work to ensure a safe environment. Following are some specific ways to do this:

■ **Look for potential safety problems and quality improvement opportunities.** This can involve large-scale issues, such as staffing concerns, or seemingly small issues, such as a loose handrail. Staff members who view their work environment from a quality and safety perspective can help identify and address all types of concerns. These concerns could include hazards that could cause patient falls, written policies or assessment forms that are unclear, or written patient education materials that may be confusing.

■ **Report concerns or ideas to the appropriate supervisor or through the organization's reporting system.** Leaders may not be aware of a particular potential problem or opportunity for improvement. Sharing concerns and ideas also can lead to the realization that there is a larger issue throughout the organization.

In addition to concerns, staff members should report any adverse events that occur within the organization. Such events present opportunities for improvement. By using risk reduction methodologies such as root cause

Sidebar 4-1. Terms Associated with Accreditation

Following is a basic list of accreditation terms with which staff should be familiar:

- **Accreditation.** A process in which an organization outside the health care organization, usually nongovernmental, assesses the organization to determine if it meets a set of standards designed to improve quality of care; the outcome of the review by an accrediting organization. Also, the decision that an eligible organization meets an applicable set of standards.

- **Accreditation process.** A continuous process whereby health care organizations are required to demonstrate to JCI that they are providing safe, high-quality care, treatment, and services as determined by compliance with JCI standards. A key component of this process is an on-site evaluation of an organization by JCI surveyors.

- **Accreditation survey.** An evaluation of an organization to assess its compliance with applicable standards and to determine its accreditation status. The JCI survey includes evaluation of documents provided by organization staff that show compliance; verbal information about the implementation of standards, or examples of their implementation, that enables compliance to be determined; on-site observations by surveyors; and education about standards compliance and performance improvement.

- **Joint Commission International (JCI).** A not-for-profit organization dedicated to continuously improving the safety and quality of care in the international community through the provision of education and consultation services and international accreditation.

- **Standards.** For the purposes of accreditation, a set of expectations predetermined by a competent authority. A standard describes the acceptable level of performance of an organization or individual. It relates to structures in place, conduct of a process, or measurable outcome achieved.

- **Measurable elements**. These are the requirements of JCI standards that will be reviewed and assigned a score during the accreditation survey process.

- **Tracer.** Tracer methodology is an evaluation method in which surveyors select a patient and use that individual's record as a road map to move through an organization to assess and evaluate the organization's compliance with selected standards and the organization's systems of providing care and services. Surveyors retrace the specific care processes that an individual experienced by observing and talking to staff in areas where the individual received care. As surveyors follow the course of a patient's treatment, they assess the health care organization's compliance with JCI standards. They conduct this compliance assessment as they review the organization's systems for delivering safe, high-quality health care.

---

analysis (RCA) and failure mode and effects analysis (FMEA), staff can work with organization leaders to identify issues and effectively respond to adverse events. (*See* Section 2, pages 44–46, for more information on the topics of reporting systems, adverse events, FMEA, and RCA.)

- **Participate in quality improvement and safety activities.** This could take the form of volunteering to serve on a committee charged with addressing a particular topic, offering to participate in revising a policy or procedure, taking part in a mock survey (*see* Section 3, beginning on page 112), participating in the review of medical record documentation, or encouraging colleagues to embrace

quality improvement initiatives. Quality improvement initiatives are successful only if they receive the full support of staff.

- **Embrace teamwork strategies that promote safe care.** The provision of care, treatment, and services is most productive when a team of providers works collaboratively toward a common goal. Health care teams that function in this fashion can provide timely, efficient, and safe patient care and also improve staff satisfaction and morale. Such teams can contribute toward reduced patient lengths of stay, higher perceived care quality, and improved patient outcomes.[1] Interactive, effective, interdisciplinary care can be particularly important for patients with multiple comorbidities, as these patients need coordinated resources across time, within multiple settings of care, and from diverse disciplines. To be effective, teamwork requires listening, discussing, participating, respecting, questioning, sharing, and generally communicating in a productive and interactive fashion. Staff members should try to model team behaviors and participate in any organizationwide efforts to improve teamwork. (*See* Section 2, pages 41–48 for more discussion on teamwork and a culture of safety.)

- **Use effective communication techniques when communicating with colleagues.** Communication between staff in a health care setting is often informal, disorganized, and variable. In situations where specific and complex information must be communicated and responded to in a timely manner, and where the consequences of omitting critical information can be dire, it is essential to add structure to the exchange.[2] One way to do this is through structured communication techniques. These techniques provide prescriptive steps, which ensure that the proper information is conveyed at the correct time to the correct people. Just as clinical practice guidelines can assist practitioners in making decisions and taking actions for specific clinical circumstances, structured communication techniques can assist practitioners in communicating specific, critical information. (*See* Sidebar 4-2 on page 142 for some specific techniques staff should consider using.)

- **Actively involve patients in their care.** The patient represents a key voice in the patient care team. Involving patients in their care can yield many benefits, including improved patient outcomes, patient satisfaction, and staff satisfaction, just to name a few. Such involvement is also important from an ethical perspective. Patients have the right to be treated respectfully, to be included in their care decisions, and to be fully informed about all aspects of their care. Organizations that achieve accreditation emphasize involving patients in their care.

There are several ways that staff can involve patients in their care. For example, when communicating with patients, staff should remain open and respectful. Patients should feel comfortable asking questions and sharing concerns. They should feel that health care providers are concerned about their well-being and are willing to work together to provide the best possible care. Providers should speak slowly and clearly and avoid using medical terminology and other difficult-to-

understand words. Providers should also respect a patient's specific cultural, religious, or emotional needs or expectations. Providers should also be aware of how the patient is responding to information provided.

- **Seek out ways to improve quality and safety.** This may involve attending seminars and training programs, reading literature, talking with colleagues, learning about structured improvement methodologies—such as Lean and Six Sigma—or simply being receptive to the idea of change. (*See* Section 3 pages 105–107, for more information about Lean, Six Sigma, and other improvement methodologies.)

Participate in a Baseline Assessment

When an organization has committed to seeking accreditation, it must conduct a baseline assessment of its current standards compliance. This involves going through all the standards and measurable elements and determining, through data analysis and policy review, whether the organization is meeting JCI requirements. Staff should be involved in this process. This may involve participating on teams that conduct an entire assessment or taking on assessment responsibilities for the standards that relate to specific departments. Section 3 provides a detailed description of the baseline assessment process. Staff members should con-

ACCREDITATION STRATEGY

Trouble Spots

Staff can contribute to a successful accreditation experience by identifying trouble spots in the organization. Staff can determine how each trouble spot affects the quality and safety of care, suggest possible solutions, and identify methods to measure the effectiveness of proposed actions. Using a simple compliance-issue logbook, staff can document a deficiency, the standards to which the deficiency relates, and whether the issue is specific to an area or is organizationwide.

<table>
<tr><td>

Ospedale Regionale di Locarno

Management and staff at Ospedale Regionale di Locarno in Locarno, Switzerland, discovered that working as a team was crucial to the organization's successful accreditation and overall performance improvement efforts. Following are some thoughts from different members of the organization:

- *The standards that pertain to my area of business have allowed me to implement changes that have turned out to be positive and useful. Undoubtedly, today, some of our processes are smoother and there is greater awareness among the staff not only in terms of everyone's job but also with respect to the organization as a whole.* —Michele Gustarini, Hotel Service Manager

- *The process of becoming accredited required a different mental process. It required thinking differently about uniformity, so we had to work in clusters rather than only focus on our own areas.* —Rita Monotti, M.D., Deputy Chief Physician of Medicine

- *Becoming accredited caused us to have a well-rounded vision of a problem. We had to collaborate. Physicians, nurses, and others had to work together to solve the problem. We could not do it alone, to the benefit of the patient.* —Chiare Canonica, R.N., Chief of Nursing

</td><td>

sider reviewing this section to become better acquainted with the process and how they may become involved.

Participate in Mock Surveys

Before an organization goes through an actual on-site survey, it may choose to hold one or more mock surveys—a trial run of the on-site survey that helps the organization see if standards are being met in practice. As with the baseline assessment, staff participation in mock surveys is critical to identifying and responding to quality and safety issues. During mock surveys, health care staff can see how accreditation will ultimately affect and improve the care they personally provide or that the organization as a whole provides. By participating in mock surveys, staff can see how accreditation relates to their jobs and to the patients that depend on these jobs being done well.

Taking part in mock surveys can also minimize concerns or apprehension about the on-site survey process by giving staff a better idea of how the process works and what type of interaction with surveyors will take place during the actual on-site survey.

Staff should familiarize themselves with the mock survey process. The more staff is aware of how the process works and what its goals are, the more effective they will be in participating in the process. With that said, Section 3, pages 112–116, provides an in-depth discussion of the mock survey process, and staff members should consider reviewing this section to understand the many benefits of mock surveys.

When they are familiar with the mock survey process, staff can get involved in a variety of ways. For example, they can help develop questions to be used during the survey. Such questions should relate to the care provided to patients and reflect areas of compliance for the organization. Staff can also participate on mock survey teams that travel through the organization assessing standards compliance and promoting quality of care.

Understand Tracer Methodology

As discussed in Section 1, tracer methodology is an evaluation method in which surveyors select a patient and use that individual's record as a road map to move through an organization. During this process, surveyors assess and evaluate the organization's compliance with standards and

</td></tr>
</table>

Sidebar 4-2. Structured Communication Techniques

Although there are many different techniques to improve communication between staff members, following is a brief discussion of some important methods of which staff should be aware:

- **Closed Communication Loops.** These help improve the reliability of communication by having the person receiving the communication restate what the sender has said to confirm understanding. One specific type of closed-loop communication is the repeat-back. This tool involves the following four distinct actions:

  1. The "sender" concisely states information to the "receiver."
  2. The receiver then repeats back what he or she heard.
  3. The sender then acknowledges that the repeat-back was correct or makes a correction.
  4. The process continues until a shared understanding is verified.

  Within this model, responding to a message with an "OK" or a nod of the head is not sufficient to close the communication loop. The message must be explicitly restated and acknowledged. Organizations requiring this type of closed-loop communication during times when communication must be reliable and effective can help smooth the communication process and ensure that no critical information is lost.

  The International Patient Safety Goals require staff to use a repeat-back when confirming verbal and telephone orders. Closed-loop communication can also be helpful in such situations as during surgery to confirm sponge count, during high-risk patient handoffs to ensure comprehensive information exchange, and during medication ordering to ensure that the right medication, right dose, and right route are communicated.

  If staff practice this type of communication during routine circumstances, they will be well prepared to use it during acute situations when time pressure and urgency play a role.[1]

- **Briefings.** Briefings are a critical element in team effectiveness and can determine whether people work together as a cohesive team or as a group of individuals with different ideas and goals sharing the same space. Briefings are short discussions between team members that aim to get all clinicians at the same starting point. They can help identify risk points in a procedure, plan for contingencies, avoid surprises, promote a sense of collaboration between team members, and set the tone for open communication. Briefings can be used at any point in any clinical care situation. They can, for example, help prepare for a particular process (such as surgery), be useful at the beginning of a shift, and help a team refocus during times of change (such as a sharp decline in a patient's status). Effective briefings can establish predictability, reduce interruptions, prevent delays, and build social relationships and capital for future interactions.[2]

- **Situation-Background-Assessment-Recommendation (SBAR).** Whenever critical information must be shared between two parties, staff may want to use the Situation-Background-Assessment-Recommendation (SBAR) structured communication technique. This technique can be used to standardize communication between two or more people.[3] Within this technique, individuals offer a brief description of the situation at hand, any relevant

(continued on page 143)

the organization's systems of providing care and services. Tracers can be customized to an organization's settings, services, patient population, and demographics, so the organization is surveyed only on the care it provides. Tracers require fewer formal interviews and less paperwork, which allows caregivers to focus on telling surveyors how they do their job rather than filling out forms or documents.

Just as conducting mock surveys helps an organization prepare for JCI accreditation, conducting mock tracers can be useful in assessing standards compliance and patient safety. Staff members can learn from this process by seeing how their individual responsibilities affect the organization as a whole. Staff also can identify performance issues and examine how processes in the organization are linked. This in turn supports organization efforts for integrating ongoing standards assessment and compliance into the everyday practices of staff.

Sidebar 4-2. Structured Communication Techniques, *continued*

information to help understand the situation, an assessment of any issues present, and a recommendation for further action. SBAR is an easy-to-remember, specific mechanism useful for framing any conversation, particularly critical ones requiring a clinician's immediate attention and action.[4] SBAR helps set the expectation within a conversation that specific, relevant, and critical informational elements are going to be communicated every time a patient is discussed.

References

1. Brow J.P.: Closing the communication loop: Using readback/hearback to support patient safety. *Jt Comm J Qual Patient Saf* 30:460–464, Aug. 2004.

2. Makary M.A., et al.: Operating room briefings: Working on the same page. *Jt Comm J Qual Patient Saf* 32:351–355, Jun. 2006.

3. Haig K.M., Sutton S., Whittington J.: SBAR: A shared mental model for improving communication between clinicians. *Jt Comm J Qual Patient Saf* 32:167–175, Mar. 2006.

4. Kaiser Permanente of Colorado: *SBAR Technique for Communication: A Situational Briefing Model.* Institute for Healthcare Immprovement. http://www.ihi.org/IHI/Topics/PatientSafety/SafetyGeneral/Tools/SBARTechniquefor CommunicationASituationalBriefingModel.htm (accessed 21 May, 2010).

EXPERT ADVICE

Communication During Mock Surveys

Staff should practice effective communication techniques during mock surveys. This will help them feel more comfortable and respond more effectively during the actual accreditation survey. Staff should listen carefully, and if they do not understand a question, they should ask for clarification before answering. They should never make up an answer if they are unsure of what to say. It is much better to say they do not know the answer but they know where to find the information being asked for. Staff should answer each question thoroughly but succinctly, and then wait for any follow-up questions. If the surveyor asks for additional information, such as copies of policies or protocols, it should be provided when promised. And finally, staff should not hesitate to let the pride in the work they do show in their answers.

—Sherry Kaufield, M.A., F.A.C.H.E.,
Executive Director, International Services, JCI

Participate in the On-Site Survey

A significant benchmark along an organization's journey to improve quality and safety is the accreditation survey. This on-site survey occurs every three years in an organization and includes several interviews with leadership, individual and system tracers (depending on the program), and other important meetings. Section 3, beginning on page 117, provides an introduction to the on-site survey and its various components. Staff members should consider reviewing this section to learn more about each element of the process and how to participate effectively in the process.

Overcoming Any Anxiety Associated with Accreditation

Health care is pressure-packed work. But even frontline caregivers, such as nurses, therapists, physicians, and others who are accustomed to dealing with stressful situations every day, are sometimes nervous about talking with a JCI surveyor. Accreditation is important to health care organizations and staff, so a bit of anxiety is natural. With that said, keeping the following ideas in mind will help staff feel more comfortable during the on-site survey process:

SECTION 4

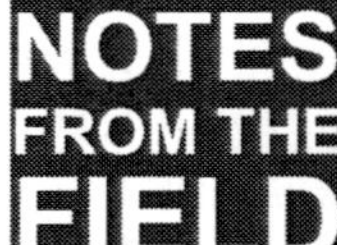

Bangkok Hospital Medical Center

Bangkok Hospital Medical Center (BMC), a large multihospital medical center located in Bangkok, Thailand, offers the following recommendations to staff on how they can best perform during a tracer:

First, make arrangement to have a conference room ready to meet with the surveyors when they arrive at your unit. In the conference room, you will need to share several resources with the surveyor. Some we recommend are the following:

- Manuals or work instructions for equipment unique to your unit
- Evidence of daily crash cart checks and daily refrigerator checks
- Written evidence of a system for checking for expired supplies, and evidence that such checks are done regularly
- Binder of unit orientation practices, on-the-job training, and attendance records for ongoing staff education
- Employee portfolios with certificates from staff members who have attended outside education (the originals are kept in the human resources department)
- Binders with clinical pathways, scientific articles related to the unit's work, and agreed-upon standards and benchmarks
- Copies of staff schedules
- The unit's scope of services, including the top five diagnoses
- The most recently approved unit policies and procedures
- Written evidence of quality monitoring that takes place on your unit
- Evidence of any quality improvement projects on your unit and the outcome(s)

    You can organize your materials on a rolling cart to enable you to follow the surveyor as he or she travels the unit, bringing your reference materials with you.

    Other good practices for a successful tracer in your unit include the following:

- Prepare a short slide presentation to show in an animated way the main components of your unit. Even if you do not show the presentation to the surveyor, preparing it helps you and other staff organize your thoughts about your unit (and can be a good teaching tool for new staff).
- Prepare a poster or storyboard that enhances the meaning and outcomes of a recent project by utilizing pictures, graphs, and statistics to focus on the successes of your unit. "A picture is worth a thousand words."
- Display patient education brochures specific to your specialty.
- Decorate and display a unit bulletin board with staff education, relevant meeting minutes, and other announcements important for your staff to know.
- Have a continuous quality improvement bulletin board on display for easy reference.

- This is not a test. Staff don't need to memorize and recite JCI standards or measurable elements. Surveyors want to know how staff provide treatment. It's the surveyor's job to evaluate how that care relates to JCI requirements. The surveyor is interested only in what staff do on a daily basis and what their role is on the health care team. The surveyor is not there to quiz staff or test their knowledge of JCI standards.

- There are no "wrong" answers. Staff members can expect to be asked basic questions about their training and role in care. None of the questions are trick questions. Staff should know all of this information—they use it in their jobs every day. When asked a question by a surveyor, the best approach for staff is to listen carefully and answer honestly. If they don't know the answer, they should just tell the surveyor, "Sorry, I don't know the answer, but I do know how to find it." Then, the staff member can go to the policy book or access the information in some way, or even ask another staff member. Staff should not worry if another staff member is asked the exact same question. Surveyors are going to ask the same questions over and over. It's because they want to see if they get the same answer. It's called "convergent validity," and it helps the surveyor understand what staff are supposed to be doing and how management has trained staff to carry out their duties.

■ Try to relax. The purpose of accreditation is not to make staff nervous. Staff should try not to worry about the standards when talking with surveyors and just speak from the heart. For example, it is not necessary to cite standards and measurable elements when talking to surveyors; staff can merely say, "This is how I would register Mrs. Jones" or "If I need to do an order, this is how I contact the doctor." It comes very naturally if staff do it that way and it's a more free-flowing conversation for everyone.

Fundamentally, surveys shouldn't bring anxiety to staff if they know what their jobs require and how to do those jobs effectively. By demonstrating how care is provided every day, staff can show surveyors the level of quality and safety within the organization.

Keep Striving for Continuous Compliance

Achieving JCI accreditation is not meant to be a one-time accomplishment, but an ongoing journey in which the organization continuously monitors its performance, searches for areas of improvement, and implements initiatives to respond to safety issues and areas of risk. Staff members must be committed to this process. They must understand the key role they play in continuously providing care of the highest quality to patients in a way that ensures patients' safety and satisfaction.

Committing to a continuous compliance approach requires staff to consistently engage in improvement efforts, consciously look for ways to be better, and support change and improvement across the organization.

Survey Anxiety

In every organization I went into (when I was a surveyor), there was a high level of anxiety. That's natural. At the point of the survey, the organization has done a lot of preparation and there is a lot on the line. But once the process of the survey begins, many organizations find that it's not as bad as they expected. The most important thing to know in advance is that there are no trick questions, and by the time the surveyor or surveyors leave, nothing is a surprise. The organization knows in what areas they're deficient and is given direction as to how to become compliant.

—Bruce Frederick, R.N., M.N.,
JCI Consultant

You Only Know What You Know

Tests tend to bring on anxiety, particularly if you need to memorize answers. However, in surveys, you do not need to memorize any answers—only be able to discuss your job and how you perform it. Survey questions are not tricks. Surveyors ask questions about the policies and procedures—it's what you should be doing, per your job description. If you are asked a question that's outside of your area … you don't answer it. You tell the surveyor that it is not something you do in your job. There's no memorizing . . . just talking about what you do when you are doing your job.

—Helen Hoesing, R.N., M.P.H., Ph.D.,
JCI Senior Consultant

Conclusion

After reading this publication, organizations may be a little overwhelmed by the depth and breadth of effort required to achieve JCI accreditation. However, organizations should know that they control the process and the pace of the accreditation journey, and there are many resources available to help along the way. Although this book has introduced the accreditation process and what it can mean for an organization, reading this publication should not be an organization's only step along the journey. Seeking out other resources, communicating with other organizations, asking questions, and working with all members of the organization to learn, change, and improve will help make this process a smooth one.

Although an organization may be concerned it is not ready for the accreditation process, if it has the desire to provide safe, quality-driven patient care and the commitment to make it happen, then it has what it takes to be successful. Not one organization that has achieved accreditation has ever expressed regret over the decision. When the time is right, make the decision, take the first step, and don't look back.

REFERENCES

1. Temkin-Greener H., et al.: Measuring interdisciplinary team performance in a long-term care setting. *Med Care* 42:472–481, May 2004.

2. Frankel A., et al.: *The Essential Guide for Patient Safety Officers.* Oakbrook Terrace, IL: Joint Commission Resources, 2009.

ONLINE EXTRAS

Available at www.jcrinc.com/JCIGS10/Extras

Tools
- Data Collection Tool
- Measure Profile
- JCI Action Plan
- Tracer Activity Data Collection Tool
- Tracer Methodology Tool
- Summary Results/Actions of Tracer
- Tracer Case Studies

Slide Presentations
- Use of Tracers as a Leadership Tool
- JCI Accreditation: Getting Started

Videos (Windows Media)
- Leonardo la Pietra, M.D., Chief Medical Officer, European Institute of Oncology, talks about the leader's role in patient safety and how patient-safe care has a variety of benefits for health care organizations.
- Helen Oh, M.D., Changi General Hospital, discusses staff infection control education in her organization.
- Paul Tighe, Deputy Pharmacy Manager, Mater Private Hospital, discusses his organization's policy for reporting adverse incidents.
- Muayad Kasim Khalid, M.D., Consultant Physician, Emergency Department, Hamad General Hospital, talks about patients' involvement in their own care.
- Annie Chia, Pharmacy Manager, Tank Tock Seng Hospital, discusses medication error reporting and following up to make sure incidents are not repeated.
- Jonathan Seah, Pharmacist, Changi General Hospital, talks about his organization's multi-pronged approach to medication safety.

Links to JCI Web Site

JCI Accreditation
http://www.jointcommissioninternational.org/Accreditation-andCertification-Process

JCI Accreditation and Certification Programs
http://www.jointcommissioninternational.org/Why-Become-Accredited

Find an Accredited Organization
http://www.jointcommissioninternational.org/JCI-Accredited-Organizations

Submit a Standards Interpretation Question
http://www.jointcommissioninternational.org/interpretation-question

JCInsight (the quarterly JCI newsletter)
http://www.jointcommissioninternational.org/Joint-Commission-Internationa-eZine

Meet the JCI Teams
http://www.jointcommissioninternational.org/Meet-the-JCI-Teams

JCI Regional Offices
http://www.jointcommissioninternational.org/Regional-Offices

Report a Complaint About a Health Care Organization
http://www.jointcommissioninternational.org/reporting-quality-and-safetyissues

JCI Advisory Services
http://www.jointcommissioninternational.org/JCI-Advisory-Services

Products and Services
http://www.jointcommissioninternational.org/Products-and-Services

Quality and Safety Risk Areas
http://www.jointcommissioninternational.org/Quality-andSafety-Risk-Areas

About JCI
http://www.jointcommissioninternational.org/about-jci

INDEX

A

staff participation in, 140–141
Assessment of Patients (AOP) standard, 17–18
At Risk for Denial of Accreditation, 120–121

B

Balanced scorecard, 93
Baldantoni, Enrico, 95
Bangkok Hospital Medical Center (BMC), 55, 144
Bar chart. *See* Histogram
Baseline assessment. *See* Assessment
Beijing United Family Hospital and Clinics, 39
Best practices, sharing, 81, 113
Billing records, 85
Boxplots, 90
Briefings, 142
British Standards Institute (BSI), 68
Building tours, 86

C

Capital improvements, 52–53
Cardiac vascular laboratory (CVL), 66
Care continuum standards, 13–14
Care decisions/processes, 10
Caregivers, improving communication among, 20
Care team
 multidisciplinary, 55
 patients as member of, 42, 140
Case study
 Apollo Hospitals, 108–112
 Changi General Hospital, 23–25, 29–30
 Na Homolce Hospital, 132–135
 National Healthcare Group, 49–51
 National Heart Centre Singapore, 64–67
 OCA Hospital, 61–63
 Severance Hospital, 129–131
 Tawam Hospital, 128
Center for Transforming Healthcare, 76
Certification
 vs. accreditation, 3
 case study, 23–25
 programs, 15
CGH Pocket Guide, 28, 107
Changi General Hospital
 case study, 23–25, 29–30
 performance measurement at, 96
 publication by, 107
Checklists, obtaining data through, 86–87
Clifford Hospital, 69
Clinical Care Program Certification (CCPC), 15
Clinical laboratories standards, 14
Clinical records, 85
Clinicians
 gaining support of, 37–39
 JCI accreditation case study and, 23
Closed communication loops, 142
College of American Pathologists, 106
Communication
 about accreditation process, 37, 56
 about survey results, 122
 improving effectiveness of, 20
 during mock surveys, 143
 with patients, 140

between staff members, 140
 techniques for, 142–143
Comparison chart, 90
Complaint data, 86
Control chart, 90–91
Convergent validity, 145
Coronary artery bypass graft (CABG), 95
Correct-site, correct procedure, and correct-patient surgery, 21
Cost issues
 case study, 108–109
 JCI accreditation and, 10–11, 47, 50, 52, 69–70
 quality improvement and, 34
 self-assessment and, 80
Cultural and religious issues, 18

D

Dashboard, 93
Data
 analysis, 83, 85, 89–93
 complaint, 86
 electronic, 86
 evaluation methodology, 86
 performance improvement, 86
 purpose of, 86
 security, 89
 sources, 85–86
 tracer, 5
 types of, 85
 validity, 89
Data collection
 ensuring effective, 87–89
 frequency of, 88
 IPSG related, 19
 performance measures and, 89, 94
 Santa Chiara Hospital case study and, 95
 standards compliance assessment and, 82–83
 tools for, 86–87
Data-driven decisions, 42
Define, measure, analyze, design, verify (DMADV) process, 106
Define, measure, analyze, improve, control (DMAIC) process, 106
Deming, W. Edwards, 104
Diagnosis Procedure Combinations, 67
DMADV process, 106
DMAIC process, 106
Documentation
 case study, 29
 for compliance, 19, 70
 increase in amount of, 132, 133
 for policies and procedures, 71
 unification of, 133
Document review, purpose of, 117
Door-to-balloon (DTB) time, 66

E

Education and training
 about accreditation, 53–55, 70–71, 75, 77–78, 137–138
 about JCI standards, 75–76
 for assessment benefits, 81
 for data collection, 88
 determining need for, 77–78
 for managing changes in organizations, 114
 for planned actions, 107, 112

P

Q

R

S